CONVERSION TO SYSTEME INTERNATIONAL (
FOR COMMON SERUM CHEMISTRY DA

MW00844858

Measurement	SI Unit	Common Unit		
Albumin	g/L	g/dL	10.0	0.100
Bile acids	μmol/L	mg/L	2.55	0.392
Bilirubin	μmol/L	mg/dL	17.10	0.058
Calcium	mmol/L	mg/dL	0.250	4.00
Carbon dioxide content	mmol/L	mEq/L	1.00	1.00
Cholesterol	mmol/L	mg/dL	0.026	38.7
Chloride	mmol/L	mEq/L	1.00	1.00
Creatinine	μmol/L	mg/dL	88.40	0.011
Creatinine clearance	mL/s	mL/min	0.017	60.0
Glucose	mmol/L	mg/dL	0.056	18.0
Inorganic phosphorus	nmol/L	mg/dL	0.323	3.10
Magnesium	mmol/L	mg/dL	0.41	2.44
Osmolality	nmol/kg	mOsm/kg	1.00	1.00
Potassium	mmol/L	mEq/L	1.00	1.00
Protein, total	g/L	g/dL	10.0	0.100
Sodium	mmol/L	mEq/L	1.00	1.00
Triglycerides	mmol/L	mg/dL	0.01	10.0
Urea nitrogen	mmol/L	mg/dL	0.357	2.8

*Factor to multiply to convert from one unit to other.

Canine & Feline
ENDOCRINOLOGY

Fourth Edition

Canine & Feline ENDOCRINOLOGY

Edward C. Feldman, DVM, DACVIM (Internal Medicine)
Professor, Department of Medicine and Epidemiology
School of Veterinary Medicine
University of California, Davis
Davis, California

Richard W. Nelson, DVM, DACVIM (Internal Medicine)
Professor, Department of Medicine and Epidemiology
School of Veterinary Medicine
University of California, Davis
Davis, California

Claudia E. Reusch, DVM, DECVIM-CA
Professor
Clinic for Small Animal Internal Medicine
Vetsuisse Faculty
University of Zurich
Zurich, Switzerland

J. Catharine R. Scott-Moncrieff, MA, Vet MB, MS, DACVIM (Small Animal Internal Medicine), DSAM, DECVIM-CA
Professor, Department of Veterinary Clinical Sciences
College of Veterinary Medicine
Purdue University
West Lafayette, Indiana

CONTRIBUTING AUTHOR

Ellen N. Behrend, VMD, PhD, DACVIM (Small Animal Internal Medicine)
Joezy Griffin Professor, Department of Clinical Sciences
Auburn University
Auburn, Alabama

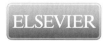

ELSEVIER
SAUNDERS

3251 Riverport Lane
St. Louis, Missouri 63043

CANINE AND FELINE ENDOCRINOLOGY, EDITION 4   ISBN: 978-1-4557-4456-5

Copyright © 2015 by Saunders, an imprint of Elsevier Inc.
Previous editions copyrighted 2004, 1996, 1987

All rights reserved. No part of this publication may be reproduced or transmitted in any form or by any means, electronic or mechanical, including photocopying, recording, or any information storage and retrieval system, without permission in writing from the publisher. Details on how to seek permission, further information about the Publisher's permissions policies and our arrangements with organizations such as the Copyright Clearance Center and the Copyright Licensing Agency, can be found at our website: www.elsevier.com/permissions.

This book and the individual contributions contained in it are protected under copyright by the Publisher (other than as may be noted herein).

Notices

Knowledge and best practice in this field are constantly changing. As new research and experience broaden our understanding, changes in research methods, professional practices, or medical treatment may become necessary.

Practitioners and researchers must always rely on their own experience and knowledge in evaluating and using any information, methods, compounds, or experiments described herein. In using such information or methods they should be mindful of their own safety and the safety of others, including parties for whom they have a professional responsibility.

With respect to any drug or pharmaceutical products identified, readers are advised to check the most current information provided (i) on procedures featured or (ii) by the manufacturer of each product to be administered, to verify the recommended dose or formula, the method and duration of administration, and contraindications. It is the responsibility of practitioners, relying on their own experience and knowledge of their patients, to make diagnoses, to determine dosages and the best treatment for each individual patient, and to take all appropriate safety precautions.

To the fullest extent of the law, neither the Publisher nor the authors, contributors, or editors, assume any liability for any injury and/or damage to persons or property as a matter of products liability, negligence or otherwise, or from any use or operation of any methods, products, instructions, or ideas contained in the material herein.

Library of Congress Cataloging-in-Publication Data
Feldman, Edward C., author.
 [Canine and feline endocrinology and reproduction]
 Canine and feline endocrinology / Edward C. Feldman, Richard W. Nelson, Claudia E. Reusch, J. Catharine R. Scott-Moncrieff. -- Fourth edition.
    pages ; cm
 Preceded by Canine and feline endocrinology and reproduction / Edward C. Feldman, Richard W. Nelson. 3rd ed. c2004.
 Includes bibliographical references and index.
 ISBN 978-1-4557-4456-5 (hardcover : alk. paper) 1. Dogs--Diseases. 2. Cats--Diseases. 3. Dogs--Endocrinology. 4. Cats--Endocrinology. 5. Dogs--Reproduction. 6. Cats--Reproduction. I. Nelson, Richard W. (Richard William), author. II. Reusch, Claudia, author. III. Scott-Moncrieff, J. Catharine R., author. IV. Title.
 [DNLM: 1. Dog Diseases. 2. Endocrine System Diseases--veterinary. 3. Cat Diseases. 4. Genital Diseases, Female--veterinary. 5. Genital Diseases, Male--veterinary. SF 992.E53]
 SF992.E53F45 2015
 636.7'08964--dc23
          2014034827

Vice President and Publisher: Loren Wilson
Content Strategy Director: Penny Rudolph
Content Development Specialist: Brandi Graham
Publishing Services Manager: Deborah Vogel
Senior Project Manager: Brandilyn Flagg
Designer: Ashley Miner

Printed in the United States of America

Last digit is the print number: 9 8 7 6 5 4 3 2 1

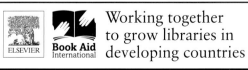

Editors

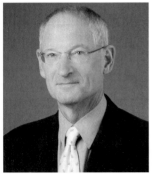

Edward C. Feldman, DVM, DACVIM (Internal Medicine), is a Professor of Small Animal Internal Medicine in the Department of Medicine & Epidemiology, School of Veterinary Medicine, University of California, Davis. Dr. Feldman earned his DVM from the University of California in 1973. He joined the Davis faculty in 1979 after an internship at the Animal Medical Center in New York City, a residency with Dr. Stephen Ettinger in the world's first referral-only private-veterinary-practice in Berkeley California, a year in general practice, and another 2 years on faculty at the University of Saskatchewan in Canada. Dr. Feldman has authored more than 160 peer-reviewed scientific publications, 110 scientific abstracts, and 75 book chapters. He is co-editor with Dr. Ettinger of the *Textbook of Veterinary Internal Medicine,* now in its 7th edition and translated into six foreign languages. He has also served as co-author with Dr. Nelson on the first three editions of this book, which have been translated into five foreign languages. Dr. Feldman has lectured in more than 40 of the 50 United States and 25 countries. He has served on the Board of Directors for Guide Dogs for the Blind and on the Board of Directors for the Western Veterinary Conference (one of the two largest veterinary conferences in the United States), and he is a member of the Scientific Advisory Board of the Annette Funicello Foundation for Multiple Sclerosis. He is a co-founder and two-term past-president of the Society for Comparative Endocrinology. Dr. Feldman's teaching awards include the Faculty Teacher of the Year Award from the University of Saskatchewan Western College of Veterinary Medicine, the UC Davis Norden Distinguished Teaching Award, the North American Veterinary Conference Speaker of the Year Award, and the California Academy of Veterinary Medicine's Award for Excellence in Continuing Education. Dr. Feldman has been honored with several research awards, including the Ralston Purina Small Animal Research Award, the American Association of Feline Practitioners Research Award, the SmithKline Beecham Award for Research Excellence, eight Daniels / Oxford Laboratory Awards for authoring one of the two or three best clinical veterinary endocrine research publications for a given year, and the American Veterinary Medical Foundation / AKC Career Achievement Award in Canine Research. Additional recognitions received by Dr. Feldman include the FIDO Award from the American Veterinary Medical Association, the Distinguished Alumnus Award from the Animal Medical Center in New York City, and the UC Davis Alumni Achievement Award.

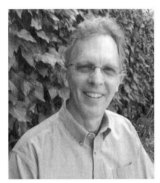

Richard W. Nelson, DVM, DACVIM (Internal Medicine), is a Professor in the Department of Medicine & Epidemiology, School of Veterinary Medicine, University of California, Davis. Dr. Nelson received his DVM degree from the University of Minnesota in 1979. After graduation he completed an internship at Washington State University and a medicine residency at the University of California, Davis. In 1982 he joined the small animal medicine faculty at Purdue University. In 1989 he moved to the University of California, Davis, where he is currently a professor in small animal internal medicine. Dr. Nelson's interest lies in clinical endocrinology, with an emphasis on disorders of the endocrine pancreas, thyroid gland, and adrenal gland. Dr. Nelson has authored numerous scientific publications and book chapters; has co-authored two textbooks, *Canine and Feline Endocrinology and Reproduction* with Dr. Feldman and *Small Animal Internal Medicine* with Dr. Guillermo Couto; and has lectured extensively nationally and internationally. He was an associate editor for the *Journal of Veterinary Internal Medicine* and serves as a reviewer for several veterinary journals. Dr. Nelson is a co-founder and member of the Society for Comparative Endocrinology and a member of the European Society of Veterinary Endocrinology. Dr. Nelson has served as Chair of the Department of Medicine and Epidemiology and as Director of the Small Animal Clinic at UC Davis. Dr. Nelson has received the Norden Distinguished Teaching Award, the BSAVA Bourgelat Award, and the ACVIM Robert W. Kirk Award for Professional Excellence.

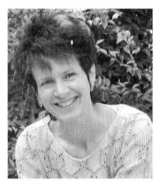

Claudia E. Reusch, DVM, DECVIM-CA, Professor, Clinic for Small Animal Internal Medicine, Vetsuisse Faculty, University of Zurich, Switzerland. After graduation Claudia Reusch worked in private small animal clinics for several years before moving to the University of Munich, where she became Professor for Small Animal Internal Medicine in 1992. Since 1996 she has been the director of the Clinic for Small Animal Internal Medicine at the University of Zurich in Switzerland. She is founding member of the European Society of Veterinary Endocrinology (ESVE) and was its president from 2001 to 2003. From 2003 to 2006 she was president of the European College of Veterinary Internal Medicine-Companion Animals (ECVIM-CA). Since 2011 she has been a member of the University Council of the University of Veterinary Medicine in Vienna, Austria, and since 2013 she has been a member of the Scientific Advisory Board of the same university. In 2014 she was given the Bourgelat Award by the British Small Animal Veterinary Association (BSAVA) for outstanding international contributions to the field of small animal practice. Her research focus is on clinical endocrinology in dogs and cats.

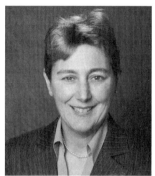

J. Catharine R. Scott-Moncrieff, MA, Vet MB, MS, DACVIM (Small Animal Internal Medicine), DSAM, DECVIM (Companion Animal), Professor, Department of Veterinary Clinical Sciences, College of Veterinary Medicine, Purdue University, West Lafayette, Indiana. Catharine Scott-Moncrieff received her veterinary degree from the University of Cambridge in 1985. She completed an internship in small animal medicine and surgery at the University of Saskatchewan, Canada, and a residency and Master of Science degree in internal medicine at Purdue University. In 1989 she joined the faculty of Purdue University, where she is currently Professor of small animal internal medicine and Head of the Department of Veterinary Clinical Sciences. She is a Diplomate of the American College of Veterinary Internal Medicine (small animal) and the European College of Veterinary Internal Medicine (companion animal), and has a diploma in Small Animal Medicine from the Royal College of Veterinary Surgeons. She is a past president of the Socety for Comparative Endocrinology and has lectured extensively nationally and internationally. Her research focus is clinical endocrinology of the dog and cat with an emphasis on disorders of the thyroid and adrenal glands. She has authored numerous scientific publications and lectured extensively both nationally and internationally. She served as Associate Editor of the *Journal of Veterinary Internal* from 2002 to 2010 and is a member and past president of the Society of Comparative Endocrinology. She has received the Daniels Award for Excellence in Small Animal Endocrinology on three occasions.

CONTRIBUTING AUTHOR

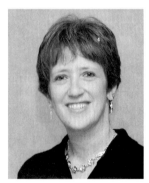

Ellen N. Behrend, VMD, PhD, DACVIM (Small Animal Internal Medicine), Joezy Griffin Professor, Department of Clinical Sciences, Auburn University, Auburn, Alabama. Dr. Behrend received her VMD degree from the University of Pennsylvania in 1988 and her PhD from Auburn University in 2001. Dr. Behrend's research interest lies in clinical endocrinology with an emphasis on diagnostic testing and diseases of the canine adrenal glands. She has authored numerous scientific publications and book chapters, served as Endocrine section editor for editions of *Consultations in Feline Internal Medicine* and *Kirk's Current Veterinary Therapy*, and was the editor for the canine chapters of *Clinical Endocrinology of Companion Animals*. Dr. Behrend has been on the review board for two journals and is currently serving on the Small Animal Advisory Panel for Morris Animal Foundation and holds a position on the ACVIM Board of Regents. She has provided numerous continuing education lectures at national and international conferences. Dr. Behrend has received the Daniels Award for Excellence in Small Animal Endocrinology and has twice won the Norden Distinguished Teaching Award.

Preface

The goal of the fourth edition of our textbook on canine and feline endocrinology is similar to that of the first three editions: to provide veterinarians and readers of this textbook with a concise but complete source of information on pathophysiology, clinical signs, diagnosis, and treatment of endocrine disorders in dogs and cats. Because of the tremendous expansion of information on these disorders since publication of the last edition more than a decade ago, the fourth edition required a complete overhaul of the previous edition. To help accomplish this, we brought three additional world-renowned clinical endocrinologists on board, Claudia Reusch, Catharine Scott-Moncrieff, and Ellen Behrend, whom are superb clinician scientists; all are actively involved in patient care, clinical investigative studies, and publications in the field of small animal endocrinology.

The fourth edition has significant changes starting with the removal of the reproduction section, thereby allowing us to focus entirely on our primary passion: endocrine disorders of dogs and cats. There are many additions to this book we believe will enhance the clinical usefulness of this resource. All chapters have undergone extensive rewriting and updating of material, provision of new or updated tables, and addition of new or updated figures and algorithms. Diagnostic strategies are presented with the intent of making them practical, cost-effective, and expedient while ensuring they represent standard of care backed by research and experience. Treatment recommendations were also consistently developed with practicality, cost-effectiveness, and compassionate care in mind, backed by research and experience.

The development of this textbook provided us with a challenging, informative, and laborious but rewarding task. We are confident this textbook provides the reader with complete, current, and applicable information on endocrine disorders of dogs and cats and will help veterinary students, practitioners, interns, residents, and owners. We do not claim that the information is presented completely without bias. Indeed, our extensive clinical experience creates bias, which we are convinced provides a positive and well-established foundation to our recommendations on diagnostic and treatment strategies. We hope you will find our textbook a valuable resource for information on endocrine disorders of dogs and cats.

Edward C. Feldman
Richard W. Nelson

To our colleagues and clients who have provided us with cases
and supported our work through the years.
To Claudia, Catharine, and Ellen for their willingness to become involved
in this project and for their hard work and dedication.
To Penny Rudolph, Brandi Graham, Brandi Flagg, Katie Stark,
and many others at Elsevier for their commitment, patience, and latitude
in the development of this textbook.
Also, with special thanks to our residents, technicians, and students who have
helped perform much of our clinical research and who refuse to allow
us to stop searching for answers.
ECF & RWN

To our students, interns, residents, staff members, referring veterinarians,
pet owners, and colleagues: thank you for asking the questions whose answers
would improve the quality of life for our patients. To the late Ruth Johnston, whose contributions
allowed us to complete so many clinical research studies. Regarding both veterinary
medicine and ourselves: we have learned much, we have much to learn.
ECF

To my soul mate Kay who has been with me for 40 years and has had
to endure all of the trials and tribulations affiliated with all of my publication
endeavors; it would not have been possible without you.
RWN

To my family for their love and continuous support.
CER

To my husband Wallace who has supported all my endeavors. To the students,
interns, residents, and colleagues who have asked thought provoking questions
about endocrinology and the pets and pet owners who have helped answer
some of those questions.
CSM

To my parents, Erika and Stephen, who gave me immeasurable support and
the drive to ask questions, to learn, and to succeed. To Charles, for continuing
their tradition.
ENB

Contents

CHAPTER 1

Water Metabolism and Diabetes Insipidus

Richard W. Nelson

CHAPTER CONTENTS

Water consumption and urine production are controlled by complex interactions between plasma osmolality, fluid volume in the vascular compartment, the thirst center, the kidney, the pituitary gland, and the hypothalamus. Dysfunction in any of these areas results in the clinical signs of polyuria and polydipsia. Arginine vasopressin (AVP) plays a key role in the control of renal water resorption, urine production and concentration, and water balance. In the presence of vasopressin and dehydration, the average dog and cat can produce urine concentrated to or above 2300 mOsm/kg of H_2O. In the absence of vasopressin or vasopressin action on the kidneys, the urine may be as dilute as 20 mOsm/kg of H_2O.

Diabetes insipidus results from deficiencies in secretion of vasopressin or in its ability to interact normally with receptors located in the distal and collecting tubular cells of the kidney. The result of either disorder is impaired ability to conserve water and concentrate urine, with production of large volumes of hypotonic dilute urine and compensatory often severe polydipsia to minimize dehydration. Because of the dramatic polyuria and polydipsia associated with diabetes mellitus and diabetes insipidus, the term *diabetes* (secretion of a large volume of urine) was historically used for both conditions. However, the urine is tasteless (insipid) with diabetes insipidus because, unlike in diabetes mellitus (in which the urine is sweet from sugar), polyuria in

1

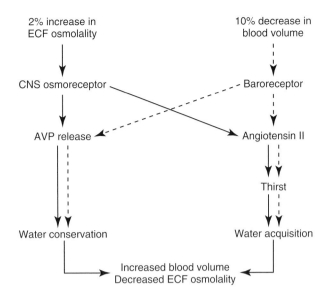

FIGURE 1-1 Schematic illustration of the primary mechanisms involved in maintenance of water balance. *Solid lines* indicate osmotically stimulated pathways, and *dashed lines* indicate volume stimulated pathways. (Adapted from Reeves WB, Andreoli TE: The posterior pituitary and water metabolism. In Wilson JD, Foster DW, editors: *Williams textbook of endocrinology*, ed 8, Philadelphia, 1992, WB Saunders, p. 311.) *AVP,* Arginine vasopressin; *CNS,* central nervous system; *ECF,* extracellular fluid.

diabetes insipidus is not the result of a glucose-induced osmotic diuresis.

 ## PHYSIOLOGY OF WATER METABOLISM

Plasma osmolality and its principal determinant, the plasma sodium concentration, are normally maintained within remarkably narrow ranges. This stability is achieved largely by adjusting total body water to keep it in balance with the serum sodium concentration. Water balance is controlled by an integrated system that involves regulation of water intake by the thirst center and control of urine volume by plasma vasopressin (Fig. 1-1). The physiologic regulation of vasopressin synthesis and secretion involves two systems: extracellular fluid (ECF) osmolality and blood pressure and volume. Vasopressin is the main hormone involved in the regulation of water homeostasis and osmolality and the renin-angiotensin-aldosterone system (RASS) is mainly responsible for regulation of blood pressure and volume (Robinson and Verbalis, 2011). Regarding osmoregulation, vasopressin secretion is relatively uncomplicated, with small increases in osmolality producing a parallel increase in vasopressin secretion and small decreases in osmolality causing a parallel decrease in vasopressin secretion.

The Neurohypophysis

The neurohypophysis consists of a set of hypothalamic nuclei (supraoptic and paraventricular) containing magnocellular neurons responsible for the synthesis of oxytocin and vasopressin; the axonal processes of these cells, which form the supraopticohypophysial tract; and the termini of these cells within the posterior lobe of the pituitary (Fig. 1-2; Reeves et al, 1998). The magnocellular neurons in the paraventricular and supraoptic nuclei secrete vasopressin or oxytocin in response to appropriate stimuli. The magnocellular neurons producing vasopressin receive neurogenic input from various sensor elements, including high-pressure arterial baroreceptors

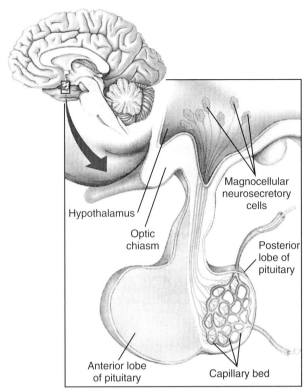

FIGURE 1-2 Midsagittal view of the hypothalamus and pituitary gland illustrating the cell bodies of the magnocellular neurons in the hypothalamus and extension of their axons into the pituitary gland where vasopressin and oxytocin are secreted directly into capillaries in the posterior lobe of the pituitary gland. (From Bear MF, et al.: *Neuroscience: exploring the brain,* ed 3, Baltimore, 2007, Lippincott Williams & Wilkins, p. 486.)

located in the carotid sinus and aortic arch and low-pressure volume receptors located in the atria and pulmonary venous system (Thrasher, 1994). Baroreceptors and volume receptors normally inhibit the magnocellular neurons, and decreases in this tonic inhibition result in the release of vasopressin. Arterial and venous constriction induced by vasopressin action on V_{1a} receptors on blood vessels contracts the vessels around the existing plasma volume to effectively "increase" plasma volume and reestablish the inhibition of secretion of vasopressin (Robinson and Verbalis, 2011). Vasopressin's action at the kidney to retain water does help replace volume, but the major hormonal regulation to control blood volume is the RAAS, which stimulates sodium reabsorption in the kidney.

Vasopressin: Biosynthesis, Transport, and Metabolism

Vasopressin and oxytocin are nonapeptides composed of a six-membered disulfide ring and a three-membered tail on which the terminal carboxyl group is amidated (Fig. 1-3). AVP is the antidiuretic hormone in all mammals except swine and other members of the suborder Suina, in which lysine vasopressin is synthesized (Reeves et al, 1998). Vasopressin differs from oxytocin in most mammals only in the substitution of phenylalanine for isoleucine in the ring and arginine for leucine in the tail. The ratio of antidiuretic to pressor effects of vasopressin is increased markedly by substituting d-arginine for l-arginine at position 8. This modification, as well as removal of the terminal amino group from cysteine, yields desmopressin acetate (DDAVP), a synthetic commercially available product (see Fig. 1-3). DDAVP is a clinically useful analogue with prolonged and enhanced antidiuretic activity that does

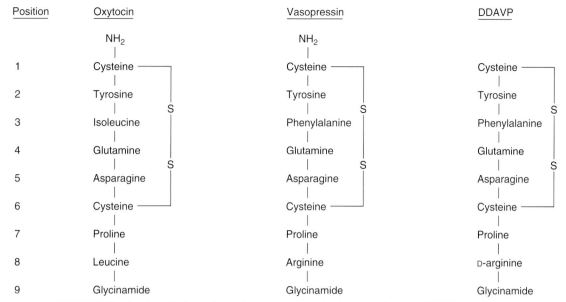

FIGURE 1-3 The chemical structures of oxytocin, vasopressin, and 1 desmopressin acetate (DDAVP).

not require injection to be effective and is commonly used to treat central diabetes insipidus (CDI) in dogs and cats.

The production of vasopressin and oxytocin is associated with synthesis of specific binding proteins called *neurophysins.* One molecule of neurophysin I binds one molecule of oxytocin and one molecule of neurophysin II binds one molecule of vasopressin (Reeves et al, 1998). The neurophysin peptide combination, often referred to as *neurosecretory material,* is transported along the axons of the hypothalamo-neurohypophyseal nerve tract and stored in granules in the nerve terminals located in the posterior pituitary gland (see Fig. 1-2). Release of vasopressin into the bloodstream occurs following electrical activation of the magnocellular neurons containing AVP. Secretion proceeds by a process of exocytosis, with release of vasopressin and neurophysin II into the bloodstream. In plasma, the neurophysin-vasopressin combination dissociates to release free vasopressin. Nearly all of the hormone in plasma exists in an unbound form, which because of its relatively low molecular weight, readily permeates peripheral and glomerular capillaries. Metabolic degradation of AVP appears to be mediated through binding of AVP to specific receptors, with subsequent proteolytic cleavage of the peptide (Reeves et al, 1998). Renal excretion is the second method for elimination of circulating AVP and accounts for about one-fourth of total metabolic clearance.

Actions of Vasopressin

AVP binds to cellular receptors at the end organs of response. The antidiuretic action of AVP is mediated through V_2 cyclic adenosine monophosphate (AMP)-dependent receptors on renal collecting duct epithelia, whereas its vasoconstrictive action is mediated through V_{1a} phosphatidylinositol dependent receptors on blood vessels. A third receptor (V_3 or V_{1b}) is responsible for the nontraditional biologic action of vasopressin to stimulate adrenocorticotropic hormone (ACTH) secretion from the anterior pituitary. V_2 receptors also regulate the nontraditional action of vasopressin to stimulate production of factor VIII and von Willebrand factor (Robinson and Verbalis, 2011). The vasopressin analogue, DDAVP, which is commonly used for the treatment of CDI, has a strong affinity for V_2 receptors with minimal pressor (V_1) activity.

The primary receptors for sensing changes in osmolality are located in the brain and, specifically cells in the organum vasculosum of the lamina terminalis and in areas of the adjacent anterior hypothalamus near the anterior wall of the third cerebral ventricle (Robinson and Verbalis, 2011). Because cells in these areas are perfused by fenestrated capillaries, the blood brain barrier is deficient, the cells are influenced by the composition of plasma rather than cerebrospinal fluid (CSF) and are able to invoke a rapid change in vasopressin secretion in response to changes in plasma osmolality. As little as a 1% increase or decrease in plasma osmolality causes a rapid increase or decrease of vasopressin from the store of hormone in the posterior pituitary. Rapid metabolism of vasopressin (half-life of approximately 15 minutes) also allows rapid changes in the concentration of vasopressin in plasma.

In the kidney, water is conserved by the combined functions of the loop of Henle and the collecting duct. The loop of Henle generates a high osmolality in the renal medulla by means of the countercurrent multiplier system. Vasopressin acts to increase the water permeability of the collecting duct, thereby allowing osmotic equilibration between the urine and the hypertonic medullary interstitium. The effects of AVP are mediated primarily by the intracellular second messenger cyclic adenosine monophosphate (cAMP) (Fig. 1-4). AVP binds to the V_2 receptors of hormone-responsive epithelial cells and activates membrane-associated adenylate cyclase to catalyze cAMP generation from adenosine triphosphate (ATP). cAMP-dependent activation of protein kinase A leads to an increase in water permeability of the luminal membrane of the cell as a result of insertion of aquaporin-2 water channels into the apical membrane of the epithelial cell. Transmembrane water movement occurs through these water channels, rather than by diffusion across the lipid bilayer or through junctional complexes (Fig. 1-5; Robben et al, 2006). In essence, AVP, working via cAMP and protein kinase A, alters water transport in hormone-responsive epithelia by causing the microtubule-dependent insertion of specialized membrane units (aquaporin-2 water channels) into the apical plasma membranes of these cells. The increase in water permeability in these segments augments osmotic water flow from the tubular lumen into a hypertonic medullary interstitium. Blood vessels in the interstitium (i.e., vasa recta) distribute absorbed water into the systemic circulation, maintaining the hypertonicity of the medullary interstitium. The net effect of this process is to extract water from the

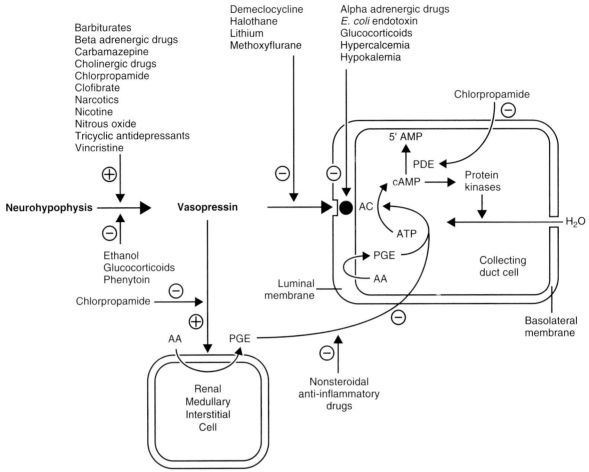

FIGURE 1-4 Effects of selected drugs and electrolytes on vasopressin release and action. (From DeBartola SP: Disorders of sodium and water: hypernatremia and hyponatremia. In DiBartola SP, editor: *Fluid therapy in small animal practice*, ed 2, Philadelphia, 2000, WB Saunders, p. 52.) *5'AMP*, 5'-adenosine monophosphate, *AA*, arachidonic acid; *AC*, adenyl cyclase; *ATP*, adenosine triphosphate; *cAMP*, cyclic adenosine monophosphate; *PDE*, phosphodiesterase; *PGE*, prostaglandin E.

urine, resulting in increased urine concentration and decreased urine volume. Dissociation of AVP from the V_2 receptor allows intracellular cAMP levels to decrease and the water channels are then reinternalized, terminating the increased water permeability.

The primary effect of AVP is to conserve body fluid by reducing the volume of urine production (Table 1-1). This antidiuretic action is achieved by promoting the reabsorption of solute free water in the distal and/or collecting tubules of the kidney. In the absence of AVP, the membranes lining this portion of the nephron are uniquely resistant to the diffusion of both water and solutes. Hence the hypotonic filtrate formed in the more proximal portion of the nephron passes unmodified through the distal tubule and collecting duct. In this condition, referred to as *water diuresis,* urine osmolality is low and urine volume is great (see Fig. 1-5).

The amount of water reabsorbed in the distal nephron depends on the plasma AVP concentration and the existence of a significant osmotic gradient in the renal interstitium. Vasopressin does not cause an active (i.e., energy-requiring) reabsorption of solute free water. It merely "opens the water channels" in the luminal membrane to allow water to flow in the direction of the higher osmolality (along the osmotic gradient). In the normal animal, the osmolality of the filtrate entering the distal tubule is low, whereas that of the renal interstitium is high, promoting reabsorption of water when the pores are open. Increasing the renal medullary interstitial osmolality increases the ability to reabsorb water and

concentrate urine; thus desert rodents with extremely concentrated medullary interstitium can produce urine more concentrated than that of dogs and are remarkably capable of conserving fluid. Conversely, loss of the renal medullary hypertonicity may inhibit vasopressin's antidiuretic activity (see Fig. 1-5). Decreased medullary hypertonicity (or lack thereof) can result from various causes, such as chronic water diuresis or reduced medullary blood flow. However, because a majority of fluid flowing from the loop of Henle can still be reabsorbed isotonically in the distal convoluted tubule and proximal collecting duct, loss of the hypertonic medullary concentration gradient alone rarely results in marked polyuria (Robertson, 1981).

It should be noted that 85% to 90% of the fluid filtered by the glomerulus is reabsorbed isosmotically with sodium and glucose in the proximal portion of the nephron. Sodium is then selectively reabsorbed from the remaining fluid, making the fluid hypotonic as it reaches the distal nephron. An additional 90% of this remaining fluid can be reabsorbed under the influence of AVP (Robertson, 1981). However, if the oral intake of salt is high or if a poorly reabsorbed solute such as mannitol, urea, or glucose is present in the glomerular filtrate, fluid resorption from the proximal tubule is impaired. The resultant increase in fluid volume presented to the distal nephron may overwhelm its limited capacity to reabsorb water. As a consequence, urine osmolality decreases and volume increases, even in the presence of large amounts of vasopressin.

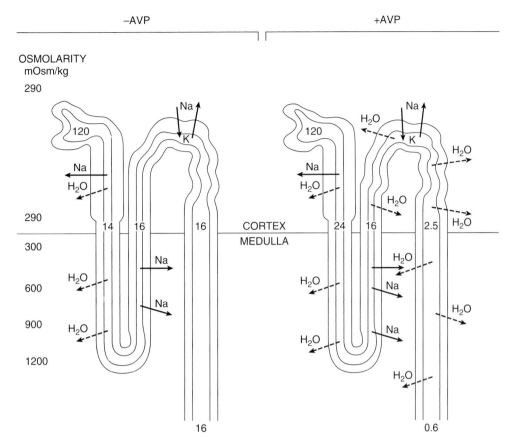

FIGURE 1-5 Schematic representation of the effect of vasopressin on the formation of urine by the human nephron. The osmotic pressure of tissue and tubular fluid is indicated by the density of the shading. The numbers within the lumen of the nephron indicate typical rates of flow in milliliters per minute. *Arrows* indicate reabsorption of sodium (Na) or water (H_2O) by active *(solid arrows)* or passive *(broken arrows)* processes. Note that vasopressin acts only on the distal nephron, where it increases the hydro-osmotic permeability of tubular membranes. The fluid that reaches this part of the nephron normally amounts to between 10% and 15% of the total filtrate and is hypotonic owing to selective reabsorption of sodium in the ascending limb of the loop of Henle. In the absence of vasopressin, the membranes of the distal nephron remain relatively impermeable to water, as well as to solute, and the fluid issuing from the loop of Henle is excreted essentially unmodified as urine. With maximum vasopressin action, all but 5% to 10% of the water in this fluid is reabsorbed passively down the osmotic gradient that normally exists with the surrounding tissue. Remember that the concentration of the canine renal medullary interstitial fluid can be greater than 2500 mOsm/kg. (Reprinted with permission from Robertson GL: Posterior pituitary. In Felig P, et al. (eds): *Endocrinology and metabolism*, ed 2, New York, 1987, McGraw Hill Book Co, p. 351.)

TABLE 1-1	**ACTIONS OF VASOPRESSIN**	
TARGET ORGAN	**TYPE OF RECEPTOR**	**ACTION**
Kidney		
Cortical and medullary collecting ducts	V_2	Enhances water permeability
Thick ascending limb of the loop of Henle	V_2	Enhances Na^{2+}, Cl^-, K^+ reabsorption
Juxtaglomerular cells	V_1	Suppresses renin release
Cardiovascular system		
Arterioles	V_1	Vasoconstriction
Coagulation system	V_2	Stimulate von Willebrand factor Stimulate antihemophiliac factors
Pituitary gland	V_3	Stimulate ACTH secretion

ACTH, Adrenocorticotropic hormone.

This type of polyuria is referred to as solute diuresis to distinguish it from that due to a deficiency of vasopressin action.

Thirst

Consumption of water to preserve body fluid tonicity is governed by the sense of thirst, which in turn is regulated by many of the same factors that determine AVP release (Fig. 1-6). Thirst can be stimulated by increases in ECF osmolality and by decreases in intravascular volume. Osmoreceptors in the anterior hypothalamus and low- and high-pressure baroreceptors in the thorax mediate the thirst stimulus. Circulating angiotensin II may also stimulate thirst when hypovolemia and hypotension are severe (Stocker et al, 2000). Studies in humans using quantitative estimates of subjective symptoms of thirst have confirmed that increases in plasma osmolality of 2% to 3% are necessary to produce an unequivocal sensation of thirst (Baylis and Thompson, 1988).

Satiation of Thirst

Dehydrated animals have a remarkable capacity to consume the appropriate volume of water to repair a deficit. It has been

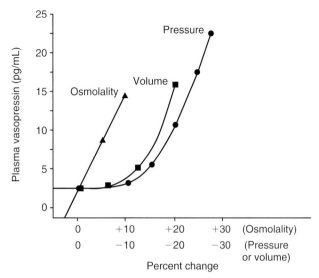

FIGURE 1-6 The relationship between plasma osmolality and plasma vasopressin level. (Adapted from Robertson GL, Berl T: Water metabolism. In Brenner BM, Rector FC Jr, editors: *The kidney*, ed 3, Philadelphia,1986, WB Saunders, p. 385.)

demonstrated that dogs deprived of water for various periods of time drink just the volume of water needed to meet the deficit within 5 minutes. All animals have this capacity, although some species take longer to ingest the required amount of fluid. Satiation of thirst in dogs and cats requires restoration of normal plasma osmolality and blood volume, with correction of plasma osmolality playing the major role. In dogs with hypertonic volume depletion, restoration of osmolality in the carotid circulation without correcting osmolality outside the central nervous system (CNS) caused a 70% decrease in drinking (Reeves et al, 1998). Restoration of blood volume in these dogs without ameliorating plasma hypertonicity reduced drinking by about 30%. Additional mechanisms may also play a minor role, including gastric distention and perhaps the participation of receptors in the liver. Similar inhibitory influences affect vasopressin secretion. Following voluntary rehydration in dehydrated animals, plasma vasopressin secretion returns to normal before redilution of the body fluids has been completed.

DIFFERENTIAL DIAGNOSES FOR POLYDIPSIA AND POLYURIA

Increased thirst (polydipsia) and urine production (polyuria) are common owner concerns in small animal veterinary practice. In dogs, normal water intake is usually less than 80 mL/kg of body weight/24 h. Water intake between 80 and 100 mL/kg/24 h is suggestive of polydipsia but may be normal in some dogs. Water intake greater than 100 mL/kg/24 h confirms polydipsia. Similar values are used for cats, although most cats drink considerably less than these amounts. Normal urine output varies between 20 and 45 mL/kg/24 h (1 to 2 mL/kg/h; Barsanti et al, 2000). Polyuria in the dog and cat has been defined as urine production greater than 50 mL/kg/24 h, respectively, although it is possible for urine production to be abnormal within the limits of these normal values in individual dogs and cats. Polyuria and polydipsia usually exist concurrently, and determining the primary component of the syndrome is one of the initial diagnostic considerations when approaching the problem of polydipsia and polyuria (see Diagnostic Approach to Polyuria and Polydipsia later in this chapter).

A variety of metabolic disturbances can cause polydipsia and polyuria (Table 1-2). Primary polyuric disorders can be classified on the basis of the underlying pathophysiology into primary pituitary and nephrogenic diabetes insipidus (NDI), secondary NDI, osmotic diuresis-induced polyuria, and interference with the hypothalamic-pituitary secretion of AVP. The most common form of diabetes insipidus is acquired secondary NDI. This form includes a variety of renal and metabolic disorders in which the renal tubules lose the ability to respond adequately to AVP. Most of these acquired forms are potentially reversible after elimination of the underlying illness.

Secondary NDI results from interference with the normal interaction of AVP and renal tubular AVP receptors, problems with the generation of intracellular cAMP, problems with renal tubular cell function, or loss of the renal medullary interstitial concentration gradient. Primary polydipsic disorders occur in dogs and usually have a psychogenic or behavioral basis for the compulsive water consumption.

Osmotic Diuresis

Diabetes Mellitus

Diabetes mellitus is one of the most common endocrinopathies in the dog and cat. As glucose utilization diminishes as a result of relative or absolute insulin deficiencies, glucose accumulates in the blood. When the rising blood glucose concentration exceeds the renal tubular capacity for glucose reabsorption, glucose appears in the urine and acts as an osmotic diuretic, causing increased water loss into the urine. The water loss results in hypovolemia, which in turn stimulates increased water intake. Urinalysis and fasting blood glucose measurement are usually sufficient screening tests for diagnosing diabetes mellitus.

Primary Renal Glycosuria

This uncommon disorder is seen primarily in the Basenji and Norwegian Elkhound. Primary renal glycosuria is a congenital renal tubular disorder resulting in an inability to reabsorb glucose from the ultrafiltrate in the nephron. In some dogs and cats, renal glycosuria may also be a component of a Fanconi-like syndrome, in which phosphate, potassium, uric acid, amino acids, sodium, and/or bicarbonate may also be inadequately reabsorbed from the ultrafiltrate. As in diabetes mellitus, glucose appears in the urine and acts as an osmotic diuretic, causing polyuria and, in turn, polydipsia. Primary renal glycosuria should be suspected in a dog with polyuria and polydipsia, persistent glycosuria, and normal blood glucose and serum fructosamine concentrations. Urinalysis and fasting blood glucose measurement are sufficient initial screening tests for this disorder.

Chronic Renal Failure

Chronic renal failure is a syndrome in which the number of functioning nephrons progressively decreases as a result of structural damage to the kidney, as occurs with chronic interstitial nephritis, medullary interstitial amyloidosis, and chronic pyelonephritis. A compensatory increase is seen in glomerular filtration rate (GFR) per surviving nephron, but the amount of fluid presented to the distal renal tubules is increased. Increased tubular flow rate causes less urea, sodium, and other substances to be reabsorbed. The result is an osmotic diuresis that is further complicated by a reduced renal medullary concentration gradient. These factors contribute to polyuria. The water loss results in hypovolemia, which causes compensatory polydipsia. Findings on routine blood and urine tests include increased blood urea nitrogen (BUN), creatinine, and inorganic phosphorus concentrations, nonregenerative anemia and isosthenuric urine (urine specific gravity of 1.008 to 1.015).

TABLE 1-2 DIFFERENTIAL DIAGNOSIS FOR POLYDIPSIA AND POLYURIA AND USEFUL DIAGNOSTIC TESTS

DISORDER	DIAGNOSTIC AIDS
Diabetes mellitus	Fasting blood glucose, urinalysis
Renal glycosuria	Fasting blood glucose, urinalysis
Chronic renal failure	History, physical exam, BUN, creatinine, Ca:P, urinalysis
Polyuric acute renal failure	History, physical exam, BUN, creatinine, Ca:P, urinalysis
Postobstructive diuresis	History, monitoring urine output
Pyometra	History of recent estrus, CBC, abdominal radiography, abdominal ultrasonography
Escherichia coli and septicemia	Blood cultures
Hypercalcemia	Serum calcium
Hepatic insufficiency	Biochemistry panel, bile acids, ammonia tolerance test, abdominal radiography and ultrasonography
Hyperadrenocorticism	Physical exam, chemistry panel, abdominal ultrasonography, urine cortisol/creatinine ratio, low-dose dexamethasone suppression test
Primary hyperaldosteronism	Serum sodium and potassium, blood pressure, abdominal ultrasonography, baseline plasma aldosterone
Bacterial pyelonephritis	Urine culture, abdominal ultrasonography, excretory urography
Hypokalemia	Serum potassium
Hyponatremia	Serum sodium
Hypoadrenocorticism	Na:K, baseline serum cortisol, ACTH stimulation test
Hyperthyroidism	Serum T_4 and TSH
Diabetes insipidus	Modified water deprivation test, response to DDAVP
Psychogenic polydipsia	Modified water deprivation test, response to gradual water restriction
Renal medullary solute washout	Response to gradual water restriction
Polycythemia	CBC
Acromegaly	Physical exam, serum GH and IGF-I, CT scan
Paraneoplastic Disorders	
Intestinal leiomyosarcoma	Abdominal ultrasonography, biopsy
Iatrogenic; medications	History
Very low protein diet	History

ACTH, Adrenocorticotropic hormone; *BUN,* blood urea nitrogen; *Ca:P,* calcium:phosphorus; *CBC,* complete blood count; *CT,* computed tomography; *DDAVP,* desmopressin acetate; *GH,* growth hormone; *IGF-I,* insulin-like growth factor-I; T_4, thyroxine; *TSH,* thyroid stimulating hormone.

Postobstructive Diuresis

Postobstructive diuresis may occur in any animal but is most common after urethral obstruction by a urolith or urethral plug is relieved in male cats with feline lower urinary tract disease (e.g., feline interstitial cystitis). Obstructed male cats often develop postrenal azotemia and electrolyte and acid-base disturbances that can be severe. A marked osmotic diuresis usually occurs once the obstruction is relieved. The veterinarian must be aware of this problem and maintain the animal's hydration through frequent adjustments in intravenous (IV) fluid administration aimed at matching urine production. Postobstructive diuresis is self-limiting and the rate of fluid administration should be slowly decreased over several days as the uremia resolves and the osmotic diuresis declines.

Primary Pituitary (Central) Diabetes Insipidus

Partial or complete lack of vasopressin production by the magnocellular neurons located in the supraoptic and paraventricular nuclei in the hypothalamus is called *primary CDI.* This syndrome is discussed in subsequent sections.

Primary Nephrogenic Diabetes Insipidus

A partial or complete lack of response of the renal tubule to the actions of AVP is called *nephrogenic diabetes insipidus (NDI).*

Primary NDI results from a congenital defect involving the cellular mechanisms responsible for "opening the water channels" that allow water to be absorbed from the renal tubular ultrafiltrate. This syndrome is discussed in subsequent sections (see Primary Nephrogenic Diabetes Insipidus).

Acquired (Secondary) Nephrogenic Diabetes Insipidus

Several disorders may interfere with the normal interaction between AVP and its renal tubular AVP receptors, affect the generation of intracellular cAMP, create problems with renal tubular cell function, or result in loss of the hypertonic renal medullary interstitial gradient. Polyuria with a compensatory polydipsia results and can be quite severe. These disorders resemble primary NDI but are referred to as acquired or secondary because AVP, AVP receptor sites, and postreceptor mechanisms responsible for water absorption are present.

Bacterial Endotoxins (Pyometra)

Bacterial endotoxins, especially those associated with *Escherichia coli,* may compete with AVP for its binding sites on the renal tubular membrane, causing a potentially reversible renal tubular insensitivity to AVP, interference with the insertion of aquaporin-2 water channels in renal tubular cells or reversible renal tubular cell lesions (Heiene et al, 2004). The kidneys have an impaired ability to concentrate urine and conserve water, and polyuria with compensatory polydipsia develops. Pyometra is the most common infectious disorder associated with the development of polyuria and polydipsia, although it has also been reported with prostatic abscessation, pyelonephritis, and septicemia (Barsanti et al, 2000). Affected bitches and queens may produce extremely dilute urine, causing fluid depletion and compensatory polydipsia. Normal urine-concentrating ability usually returns within days of successfully eliminating the source of the infection.

Hypercalcemia

Increases in serum calcium concentration are associated with downregulation of aquaporin-2 water channels and decreased function of AVP by inhibiting binding of AVP to its receptor site, damage to AVP receptors in the renal tubules, inactivation of adenylate cyclase, or decreased transport of sodium and chloride into the renal medullary interstitium (Sands and Bichet, 2006; Robben et al, 2006). Polydipsia and polyuria are common early signs of hypercalcemia, which is easily diagnosed with a serum biochemistry panel. Once hypercalcemia is identified, the clinician must undertake an often extensive diagnostic evaluation to determine its cause (see Chapter 15).

Hepatic Insufficiency and Portosystemic Shunts

Liver insufficiency and portosystemic shunts are recognized causes of polyuria and polydipsia. Many of the metabolic causes of polyuria and polydipsia (e.g., diabetes mellitus, hyperadrenocorticism, hypercalcemia) secondarily affect the liver, making it difficult to determine the role of the liver in causing polyuria and polydipsia. The exact cause of the polyuria is not known but may involve loss of medullary hypertonicity secondary to impaired urea nitrogen production or altered renal blood flow, increased GFR and ultrafiltrate volume, hypokalemia, impaired metabolism of cortisol, and primary polydipsia (Deppe et al, 1999). Urea nitrogen is a major constituent in the establishment and maintenance of the renal medullary concentration gradient. Without urea nitrogen, the kidney loses the ability to concentrate urine, causing polyuria and compensatory polydipsia. Hepatic insufficiency and portosystemic shunts are usually suspected after evaluation of a complete blood count (CBC), serum biochemistry panel, urinalysis, and abdominal ultrasonography; these causes are confirmed with a liver function test (e.g., pre- and postprandial bile acids), specialized diagnostic imaging (e.g., positive contrast portogram, technetium scan) and histologic evaluation of a hepatic biopsy.

Hyperadrenocorticism (Cushing's Syndrome)

Polyuria and polydipsia are common clinical signs of hyperadrenocorticism. Glucocorticoids inhibit AVP release by a direct effect within the hypothalamus and/or neurohypophysis (Papanek and Raff, 1994; Papanek et al, 1997). This inhibition of AVP release is characterized by both an increase in osmotic threshold and a decrease in the sensitivity of the AVP response to increasing osmolality (Biewenga et al, 1991). Glucocorticoids also increase glomerular filtration rate, proximal tubular epithelial sodium transport, and free water clearance and cause resistance to the effect of AVP in the kidney, possibly through interference with the action of AVP at the level of the renal collecting tubules or direct depression of renal tubular permeability to water (Marver, 1984; Quinkler and Stewart, 2003). In a few patients, a deficiency in AVP may result from direct compression of magnocellular neurons by a pituitary macrotumor that has extended beyond the sella. Suspicion of hyperadrenocorticism is usually aroused after careful review of the history, physical examination, and results of CBC, serum biochemistry panel, and urinalysis. Confirmation requires appropriate pituitary adrenocortical function tests (see Chapter 10).

Primary Hyperaldosteronism

Polyuria and polydipsia have been reported in cats and dogs with primary hyperaldosteronism. The mechanism for polyuria and polydipsia is not clear, although mineralocorticoid-induced renal resistance to the actions of AVP and disturbed osmoregulation of AVP release have been documented in a dog with primary hyperaldosteronism (Rijnberk et al, 2001). Similar abnormalities have been identified in dogs with glucocorticoid excess, suggesting similar mechanisms of action for the polyuria and polydipsia in hyperaldosteronism and hyperadrenocorticism. Hyperaldosteronism-induced hypokalemia may also result in downregulation of aquaporin-2 water channels and urea transporters, thereby interfering with the ability to concentrate urine (Robben et al, 2006; Sands and Bichet, 2006). Baseline plasma aldosterone concentrations are markedly increased, and plasma renin activity is suppressed (see Chapters 10 and 11).

Pyelonephritis

Infection and inflammation of the renal pelvis can destroy the countercurrent mechanism in the renal medulla and the collecting ducts, resulting in isosthenuria, polyuria, polydipsia, and eventually renal failure. Bacterial endotoxins, especially those associated with *E. coli,* can also compete with AVP for its binding sites on the renal tubular membrane, causing a potentially reversible renal tubular insensitivity to AVP. A dog or cat with acute bacterial pyelonephritis may develop nonspecific systemic signs of lethargy, anorexia, and fever, and a neutrophilic leukocytosis may be identified on a CBC. Systemic signs are usually not present with chronic pyelonephritis. Pyelonephritis should also be suspected in a patient with recurring urinary tract infection. Urinalysis may reveal white blood cells and white blood cell casts, bacteria, and occasionally red blood cells. Culture of urine obtained by antepubic cystocentesis should be positive for bacterial growth. Abdominal ultrasonography and excretory urography may reveal abnormalities consistent with pyelonephritis (e.g., renal pelvis dilatation).

Hypokalemia

Hypokalemia is believed to render the terminal portion of the nephron less responsive to AVP by causing downregulation of aquaporin-2 water channels, thereby interfering with the ability to concentrate urine (Robben et al, 2006; Sands and Bichet, 2006). Hypokalemia may also alter the hypertonic medullary interstitial gradient by causing downregulation of urea transporters and interfering with solute accumulation and may interfere with release of AVP from the pituitary. Polyuria and polydipsia are not common clinical signs of hypokalemia. The most common clinical signs are related to neuromuscular dysfunction of skeletal, cardiac, and smooth muscle (e.g., weakness, cervical ventriflexion). Hypokalemia usually develops secondary to another disorder, many of which also cause polyuria and polydipsia.

Hypoadrenocorticism (Addison's Disease)

Adrenocortical insufficiency results in impaired ability to concentrate urine (see Chapter 12). Despite normal kidney function and severe hypovolemia, many dogs with hypoadrenocorticism have a urine specific gravity of less than 1.030 and in some dogs urine specific gravity is in the isosthenuric range. Mineralocorticoid deficiency results in chronic sodium wasting, renal medullary solute washout, and loss of the medullary hypertonic gradient. Adrenalectomy in rats also decreases AVP-stimulated activation of renal medullary adenylate cyclase, primarily because of impairment in the coupling between the AVP receptor complex and adenylate cyclase. Treatment with dexamethasone corrects the defect. Hypercalcemia occurs in some patients with hypoadrenocorticism and may also play a role in the generation of polyuria and polydipsia.

Polyuria and polydipsia typically develop early in the course of the disease and are quickly overshadowed by the more worrisome and obvious vomiting, diarrhea, anorexia, weakness, and lethargy seen in these patients, although occasionally polyuria and polydipsia are the primary owner complaints. The polyuria of hypoadrenocorticism can be difficult to differentiate from primary renal failure unless specific tests of the pituitary adrenocortical axis (e.g., ACTH stimulation test) are performed. Initial suspicion for hypoadrenocorticism usually follows evaluation of serum electrolytes, although hyperkalemia and hyponatremia can also occur with renal insufficiency.

Hyperthyroidism. Polyuria and polydipsia are common findings in cats and dogs with hyperthyroidism. The exact mechanism for the polyuria and polydipsia is not clear. Increased renal medullary blood flow may decrease medullary hypertonicity and impair water resorption from the distal portion of the nephron. Psychogenic polydipsia secondary to thyrotoxicosis and, in some patients, concurrent renal insufficiency may also contribute to the polyuria and polydipsia. The tentative diagnosis of hyperthyroidism is usually based on clinical signs, palpation of an enlarged thyroid lobe or lobes (i.e., goiter), and measurement of serum thyroxine (T_4) concentration.

Acromegaly

Excessive secretion of growth hormone (GH) in the adult dog or cat results in acromegaly (see Chapter 2). Acromegaly causes carbohydrate intolerance and the eventual development of overt diabetes mellitus. In most cats and dogs with acromegaly, the polyuria is assumed to be caused by an osmotic diuresis induced by glycosuria. Renal insufficiency from a diabetic or GH-induced glomerulonephropathy may also play a role (Peterson et al, 1990).

Polycythemia

Polyuria and polydipsia may occur with polycythemia. Studies in two dogs with secondary polycythemia identified an increased osmotic threshold for AVP release, resulting in a delayed AVP response to increasing plasma osmolality (van Vonderen et al, 1997a). The authors attributed the abnormal AVP response to increased blood volume and hyperviscosity, which stimulate atrial natriuretic peptide (ANP) secretion and atrial and carotid bifurcation baroreceptors. ANP inhibits AVP release from the pituitary gland and the renal collecting duct's responsiveness to AVP (Dillingham and Anderson, 1986; Lee et al, 1987).

Primary and Psychogenic Polydipsia

Primary polydipsia is defined as a marked increase in water intake that cannot be explained as a compensatory mechanism for excessive fluid loss. In humans, primary polydipsia results from a defect in the thirst center or may be associated with mental illness (Reeves et al, 1998). Primary dysfunction of the thirst center resulting in compulsive water consumption has not been reported in the dog or cat, although an abnormal vasopressin response to hypertonic saline infusion has been reported in dogs with suspected primary polydipsia (van Vonderen et al, 1999). A psychogenic or behavioral basis for compulsive water consumption does occur in the dog but has not been reported in the cat. Psychogenic polydipsia may be induced by concurrent disease (e.g., hepatic insufficiency, hyperthyroidism) or may represent a learned behavior following a change in the pet's environment. Polyuria is compensatory to prevent overhydration. Psychogenic polydipsia is diagnosed by exclusion of other causes of polyuria and polydipsia and by demonstrating that the dog or cat can concentrate urine to a specific gravity in excess of 1.030 after water deprivation. This syndrome

---

BOX 1-1 Drugs and Hormones Causing Polyuria and Polydipsia in Dogs and Cats

Anticonvulsants*
  Phenobarbital
  Primidone
  Dilantin
Glucocorticoids*
Desoxycorticosterone pivalate (DOCP)*
Diuretics*
Mannitol
Synthetic thyroid hormone supplements
Amphotericin B
Lithium
Methoxyflurane
Sodium bicarbonate
Salt Supplementation*
Vitamin D (toxicity)

*Common cause

---

is discussed in more detail in subsequent sections (see Primary or Psychogenic Polydipsia later in this chapter).

Iatrogenic (Drug-Induced) Causes of Polydipsia and Polyuria

Several drugs have the potential to cause polyuria and polydipsia (Box 1-1). The most commonly encountered in small animal veterinary practice are glucocorticoids, diuretics, anticonvulsants (e.g., phenobarbital), synthetic levothyroxine, and salt supplementation. Drug-induced polyuria and polydipsia do not usually pose a diagnostic challenge. The polyuria and polydipsia should resolve following discontinuation of the drug; the time to resolution being dependent on the duration of action of the drug (e.g., prednisone versus long-acting depot glucocorticoid preparation). If polyuria and polydipsia persist, a concurrent disorder causing polyuria and polydipsia or renal medullary solute washout should be considered.

Renal Medullary Solute Washout

Loss of renal medullary solutes, most notably sodium and urea, results in loss of medullary hypertonicity and impaired ability of the nephron to concentrate the ultrafiltrate. Renal medullary solute washout is usually caused by one of the disorders previously described. It has also been associated with chronic diuretic therapy and abnormalities in circulation, such as hyperviscosity syndromes (polycythemia, hyperproteinemia), renal lymphatic obstruction (lymphosarcoma, lymphangiectasia), and systemic vasculitis (septicemia, systemic lupus erythematosus). Perhaps the most important clinical ramification of renal medullary solute washout is its potential to interfere with results of the modified water deprivation test (see Misdiagnosis [Inaccuracies] Using the Modified Water Deprivation Test). Hypertonicity of the renal medulla is usually restored once the underlying cause of the polyuria and polydipsia is corrected.

DIAGNOSTIC APPROACH TO POLYURIA AND POLYDIPSIA

Depending on the cause, the cost and time expenditure for evaluating a dog or cat with polyuria and polydipsia may be brief and inexpensive (e.g., diabetes mellitus) or time-consuming and costly

		Urine Specific Gravity			
DISORDER	**NUMBER OF DOGS**	**MEAN**	**RANGE**	**PROTEINURIA**	**WBC (> 5/HPF)**
CDI	20	1.005	1.001-1.012	5%	0%
Psychogenic polydipsia	18	1.011	1.003-1.023	0%	0%
Hyperadrenocorticism	20	1.012	1.001-1.027	48%	0%
Renal insufficiency	20	1.011	1.008-1.016	90%	25%
Pyelonephritis	20	1.019	1.007-1.045	70%	75%

TABLE 1-3   URINALYSIS RESULTS IN DOGS WITH SELECTED DISORDERS CAUSING POLYURIA AND POLYDIPSIA

CDI, Central diabetes insipidus; *HPF,* high power field; *WBC,* white blood count.

(e.g., partial CDI). Therefore, the clinician should be reasonably sure that polyuria and polydipsia exist, preferably based on a combination of history, multiple random urine specific gravity determinations, and if necessary, quantitation of water consumption over several days with the dog or cat in the home environment. In dogs, normal water intake is usually less than 80 mL/kg of body weight/24 h. Water intake between 80 and 100 mL/kg/24 h is suggestive of polydipsia but may be normal in some dogs. Water intake greater than 100 mL/kg/24 h confirms polydipsia. Similar values are used for cats, although most cats drink considerably less than these amounts. If an owner knows the volume of water the pet is consuming in an average 24-hour period and if that amount exceeds the upper limit of normal, a diagnostic evaluation to determine the cause is warranted. If 24-hour water intake is normal, pathologic polyuria and polydipsia are unlikely and another inciting factor (e.g., hot weather) should be sought, or misinterpretation of polyuria (e.g., pollakiuria instead of polyuria) should be considered. If the owner is certain that a change in the volume of water consumption or urination exists, even though water consumption is still in the normal range, a diagnostic evaluation may still be warranted.

Assessment of urine specific gravity may be helpful in identifying polyuria and polydipsia and may provide clues to the underlying diagnosis, especially if multiple urine specific gravities are evaluated (Table 1-3). Urine specific gravity varies widely among healthy dogs and, in some dogs, can range from 1.006 to greater than 1.040 within a 24-hour period (van Vonderen et al, 1997b). Wide fluctuations in urine specific gravity have not been reported in healthy cats.

We prefer to have the owner collect several urine samples at different times of the day for 2 to 3 days, storing the urine samples in the refrigerator until they can be brought to the veterinary hospital for determination of urine specific gravity. Urine specific gravities measured from multiple urine samples that are consistently less than 1.020 support the presence of polyuria and polydipsia and the need for a diagnostic evaluation to determine the cause; the lower the urine specific gravities, the stronger the support for the existence of a polyuria/polydipsia disorder. Identification of one or more urine specific gravities greater than 1.030 supports normal urine concentrating ability and an intact, functioning pituitary vasopressin-renal tubular cell axis. Dogs and cats may still have polyuria and polydipsia despite identification of concentrated urine; possible differential diagnoses include disorders causing an osmotic diuresis (e.g., diabetes mellitus), psychogenic polydipsia, and disorders in the regulation of AVP secretion (van Vonderen et al, 1999).

Many potential causes exist for the development of polyuria and polydipsia in dogs and cats (see Table 1-2), one of the least

common being diabetes insipidus. An animal with a history of severe polyuria and polydipsia should be thoroughly evaluated for other causes of polyuria and polydipsia prior to performing specific diagnostic procedures for diabetes insipidus or psychogenic polydipsia (Fig. 1-7). Our diagnostic approach to the animal with polyuria and polydipsia is initially to rule out the more common causes. In the dog, these include chronic renal failure, diabetes mellitus, hyperadrenocorticism, liver insufficiency, and hypercalcemia. In the cat, these include chronic renal failure, diabetes mellitus, and hyperthyroidism. Recommended initial diagnostic studies include a CBC, serum biochemistry panel, and urinalysis with bacterial culture of urine obtained by antepubic cystocentesis. A serum T_4 concentration should be measured in older cats. Depending on the history and physical examination findings, abdominal ultrasonography may be warranted to evaluate the liver, kidneys, adrenal glands, and uterus or uterine stump in the female dog. Careful evaluation of the history, physical examination findings, and results of initial blood, urine, and diagnostic imaging results usually provides the diagnosis outright (e.g., diabetes mellitus, pyometra) or offers clues that allow the clinician to focus on the underlying cause (e.g., increased serum alkaline phosphatase and cholesterol in hyperadrenocorticism, hypercalcemia of malignancy).

Occasionally, the physical examination and initial data base are normal in the dog and, less commonly, the cat with polyuria and polydipsia. Viable possibilities in these dogs include diabetes insipidus, psychogenic water consumption, hyperadrenocorticism, renal insufficiency without azotemia, and possibly mild hepatic insufficiency and the early stages of hypoadrenocorticism. Viable possibilities in cats include renal insufficiency without azotemia, mild hepatic insufficiency, and diabetes insipidus. Hyperadrenocorticism, renal insufficiency, and hepatic insufficiency should be ruled out before performing tests to establish a diagnosis of diabetes insipidus or psychogenic polydipsia. Diagnostic tests to consider include tests of the pituitary adrenocortical axis, liver function tests (e.g., pre- and postprandial bile acids), urine protein-to-creatinine ratio, endogenous or exogenous creatinine clearance studies, contrast imaging of the kidney, and, if indicated, renal biopsy.

Careful evaluation of urine specific gravity and urine protein loss may provide clues to the underlying diagnosis (see Table 1-3). For example, if the urine specific gravity measured on multiple urine samples is consistently in the isosthenuric range (1.008 to 1.015), renal insufficiency should be considered the primary differential diagnosis, especially if the BUN and serum creatinine concentration are high normal or increased (i.e., ≥ 25 mg/dL and ≥ 1.6 mg/dL, respectively) and proteinuria is present. Although isosthenuria is relatively common in dogs with hyperadrenocorticism,

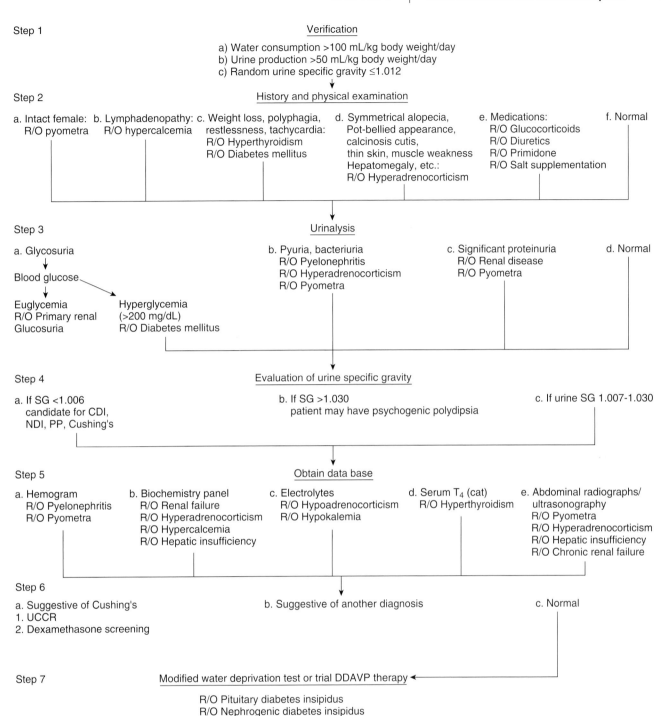

FIGURE 1-7 The diagnostic plan in a dog or cat with severe polydipsia and polyuria. *CDI,* Central diabetes insipidus; *DDAVP,* desmopressin acetate; *NDI,* nephrogenic diabetes insipidus; *PP,* primary (psychogenic) polydipsia; *R/O,* rule out (a diagnosis); *SG,* specific gravity; $T_4,$ thyroxine; *UCCR,* urinary cortisol creatinine ratio.

psychogenic water consumption, hepatic insufficiency, pyelonephritis, and partial CDI with concurrent water restriction, urine specific gravities tend to fluctuate above (hyperadrenocorticism, hypoadrenocorticism, psychogenic water consumption, hepatic insufficiency, pyelonephritis) and below (hyperadrenocorticism, hepatic insufficiency, psychogenic water consumption, partial CDI) the isosthenuric range in these disorders. In contrast, if the urine specific gravity is consistently less than 1.006, renal insufficiency is ruled out and central and primary NDI, psychogenic water consumption, hyperadrenocorticism and hepatic insufficiency should

be considered the primary differential diagnoses. CDI and primary NDI are ruled out if the urine specific gravity exceeds 1.025. Urine specific gravities that range from less than 1.005 to greater than 1.030 are suggestive of psychogenic polydipsia.

All realistic causes of secondary acquired NDI should be ruled out before performing tests (especially the modified water deprivation test) to diagnose CDI, primary NDI and psychogenic polydipsia. An index of suspicion for CDI and primary NDI versus psychogenic polydipsia can often be gained after reviewing the history and findings on physical examination and routine blood

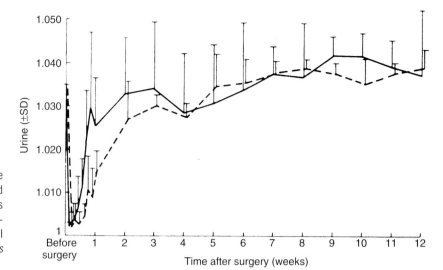

FIGURE 1-8 Mean urine specific gravity obtained before and for 3 months after hypophysectomy in four dogs treated with intraoperative polyionic fluids *(solid line)* and four dogs treated with intraoperative polyionic fluids and dexamethasone *(dashed line)*. (From Lantz GC, et al: Transsphenoidal hypophysectomy in the clinically normal dog, *Am J Vet Res* 49[7]:1134-1142, 1988.)

and urine tests. CDI and primary NDI are polyuric disorders with compensatory polydipsia to minimize dehydration. The presence of neurologic signs, serum sodium concentrations at the upper limit of the reference range, urine specific gravities consistently in the hyposthenuric range, and rapid onset of dehydration with water restriction support the presence of CDI or primary NDI. In contrast, psychogenic polydipsia is a polydipsic disorder with compensatory polyuria to prevent water intoxication. The identification of behavioral issues in the dog, serum sodium concentrations at the lower limit of the reference range, urine specific gravities that fluctuate below and above the isosthenuric range, and a relatively prolonged time interval to develop dehydration after water restriction support the presence of psychogenic polydipsia. The definitive diagnosis of CDI, primary NDI and psychogenic water consumption should be based on results of the modified water deprivation test, measurement of plasma osmolality, and response to synthetic vasopressin therapy (see Confirming the Diagnosis of Diabetes Insipidus).

ETIOLOGY OF DIABETES INSIPIDUS AND PRIMARY POLYDIPSIA

Vasopressin Deficiency—Central Diabetes Insipidus

Definition

CDI is a polyuric syndrome that results from a lack of sufficient AVP to concentrate the urine for water conservation. This deficiency may be absolute or partial. An absolute deficiency of AVP causes persistent hyposthenuria and severe diuresis. Urine specific gravity in dogs and cats with complete lack of AVP remains hyposthenuric (≤ 1.006), even with severe dehydration. A partial deficiency of AVP, referred to as a *partial CDI,* also causes persistent hyposthenuria and a marked diuresis as long as the dog or cat has unlimited access to water. During periods of water restriction, however, dogs and cats with partial CDI can increase their urine specific gravity into the isosthenuric range (1.008 to 1.015) but cannot typically concentrate their urine above 1.015 to 1.020, even with severe dehydration. For any dog or cat with partial CDI, maximum urine-concentrating ability during dehydration is inversely related to the severity of the deficiency in AVP secretion; that is, the more severe the AVP deficiency, the less concentrated the urine specific gravity during dehydration.

Pathophysiology

Destruction of the production sites for vasopressin—the supraoptic and paraventricular nuclei of the hypothalamus—and/or loss of the major ducts (axons) that carry AVP to the storage and release depots in the posterior pituitary (see Fig. 1-2) result in CDI. Permanent CDI requires an injury that is sufficiently high in the neurohypophyseal tract to cause bilateral neuronal degeneration in the supraoptic and paraventricular nuclei. Transection of the hypothalamic hypophyseal tract below the median eminence or removal of the posterior lobe of the pituitary usually causes transient (albeit severe) CDI and polyuria because sufficient hormone can be released from fibers ending in the median eminence and pituitary stalk to prevent occurrence of permanent diabetes insipidus (Fig. 1-8; Ramsay, 1983).

Etiology

CDI may result from any condition that damages the neurohypophyseal system. Recognized causes for CDI in the dog and cat are listed in Box 1-2. Idiopathic cases of CDI are the most common, appearing at any age in any breed in either gender. Necropsies performed in dogs and cats with idiopathic CDI fail to identify an underlying reason for the AVP deficiency.

Autoimmune hypothalamitis has been suggested as a possible cause of idiopathic CDI in humans (Salvi et al, 1988). Circulating AVP cell antibodies, which bind to cell membranes of hypothalamic preparations, have been identified in some humans with CDI (Scherbaum, 1987). AVP cell antibodies have been identified prior to the development of CDI, and titers of AVP cell antibodies decline eventually to negative values with increasing duration of the disease (Bhan and O'Brien, 1982; Scherbaum et al, 1986). These patients also show a significant association with other endocrine disorders (e.g., immune thyroiditis, Addison's disease), suggesting that, at least in some cases, polyendocrine autoimmunity may also involve the hypothalamus (see Chapter 3). A similar association between CDI and other endocrinopathies has not been identified in dogs and cats. However, lymphocytic hypophysitis has been documented in a dog with CDI, an inflammatory mass compressing the hypothalamus, and marked lymphocytic infiltration of the adenohypophysis (Meij et al, 2012). In humans, lymphocytic inflammation involving the posterior pituitary lobe and infundibulum is called *lymphocytic infundibuloneurohypophysitis* and humans typically develop acute onset of diabetes insipidus with intracranial mass-effect symptoms (Abe, 2008).

BOX 1-2 **Recognized Causes of Central Diabetes Insipidus in Humans, Dogs, and Cats**

Humans	Dogs/Cats
Acquired	**Acquired**
Idiopathic	Idiopathic
Head trauma	Head trauma
Neoplasia	Neoplasia
Craniopharyngioma	Craniopharyngioma
Germinoma	Chromophobe adenoma and
Meningioma	adenocarcinoma
Lymphoma	Meningioma
Leukemia	Metastases
Adenoma	Hypothalamic/pituitary malforma-
Metastases	tion
Granulomatous disease	Cysts
Infectious	Inflammation (lymphocytic hypophy-
Viral	sitis)
Bacterial (abscess)	Parasite migration
Vascular	Transsphenoidal hypophysectomy
Sheehan syndrome	
Aneurysms	**Familial (?)**
Immune-mediated	
Lymphocytic infundibulohy-	
pophysitis	
Hypophysectomy	
Familial	

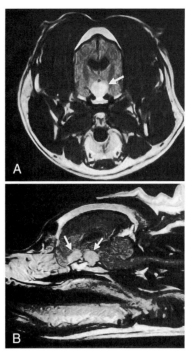

FIGURE 1-9 Transverse **(A)** and sagittal **(B)** magnetic resonance images of the pituitary region in a 12-year-old male Boxer with central diabetes insipidus (CDI), hypothyroidism, and neurologic signs. A mass is evident in the region of the pituitary gland, hypothalamus, and rostral floor of the calvarium *(arrows)*.

The most common identifiable causes for CDI in dogs and cats are head trauma (accidental or neurosurgical), neoplasia, and hypothalamic/pituitary malformations (e.g., cystic structures). Head trauma may cause transient or permanent CDI, depending on the viability of the cells in the supraoptic and paraventricular nuclei. Trauma-induced transection of the pituitary stalk often results in transient CDI, usually lasting 1 to 3 weeks (see Fig. 1-8; Lantz et al, 1988; Authement et al, 1989). The duration of diabetes insipidus depends on the location of the transection of the hypophyseal stalk relative to the hypothalamus. Transection at more proximal levels, close to the median eminence, is associated with a longer time for hypothalamic axons to undergo regeneration and secretion of AVP. Trauma-induced CDI should be suspected when severe polydipsia and polyuria develop within 48 hours of head trauma or when hypernatremia, hyposthenuria, and hypertonic dehydration develop in a traumatized dog or cat that is being treated with IV fluids rather than water ad libitum (see Complications of the Modified Water Deprivation Test: Hypertonic Dehydration and Hypernatremia later in this chapter).

Transient or permanent diabetes insipidus commonly occurs following transsphenoidal hypophysectomy for the treatment of pituitary-dependent hyperadrenocorticism in dogs. In one study evaluating hypophysectomy in 127 dogs with pituitary-dependent hyperadrenocorticism, postoperative CDI was transient in 78% of the dogs with DDAVP discontinued 2 weeks after surgery in 47% and eventually discontinued in 31% a median of 133 days (range, 28 to 1329 days) postsurgery (Hanson et al, 2005). CDI was present until death or until latest available follow-up in 22% of the dogs. In another study, the incidence of postoperative permanent CDI in dogs undergoing transsphenoidal surgery for Cushing's disease was strongly influenced by the size of the pituitary tumor; the larger the tumor, the more likely CDI was permanent after surgery (Teshima et al, 2011).

Neoplastic destruction of magnocellular neurons may also cause CDI. However, 90% of the magnocellular neurons must be destroyed to produce symptomatic diabetes insipidus. To produce CDI, a mass lesion would have to destroy a large area of the hypothalamus or be located where the tracks of the nuclei converge at the base of the hypothalamus and the top of the pituitary stalk (Robinson and Verbalis, 2011). Tumors confined to the sella do not cause CDI. Primary intracranial tumors associated with diabetes insipidus in dogs and cats include craniopharyngioma, pituitary chromophobe adenoma, and pituitary chromophobe adenocarcinoma (Fig. 1-9; Neer and Reavis, 1983; Goossens et al, 1995; Harb et al, 1996). Tumor metastases to the hypothalamus and pituitary gland can also cause CDI. In humans, metastatic tumors most often spread from the lung or breast (Reeves et al, 1998). Metastatic mammary carcinoma, lymphoma, malignant melanoma, and pancreatic carcinoma have been reported to cause CDI by their presence in the pituitary gland and hypothalamus in dogs (Capen and Martin, 1983; Davenport et al, 1986). Metastatic neoplasia as a cause for CDI has not yet been reported in the cat.

A rare, hereditary form of CDI occurs in humans, is transmitted as an autosomal dominant trait, has equal occurrence in males and females, displays father-to-son transmission, and shows variable expression among affected individuals (Baylis and Robertson, 1981). This condition is believed to result from a degenerative disorder affecting the magnocellular neurons (Kaplowitz et al, 1982). Although CDI is well documented in kittens and puppies, hereditary CDI has not yet been documented. In one report, hereditary CDI was suggested in two sibling Afghan Hound pups that developed CDI at younger than 4 months of age and were from a bitch suffering from polyuria and polydipsia "all her life" (Post et al, 1989). Necropsy of these puppies revealed vacuolated areas in the neurohypophysis and hypothalamohypophysial tracts of the median eminence of the tuber cinereum, findings that suggested hypomyelination or demyelination. We have also diagnosed CDI in a litter of five 8-week-old German Short-Haired Pointers and three of five 7-week-old Schnauzers, suggesting possible familial CDI in these dogs.

Primary Nephrogenic Diabetes Insipidus

Definition

NDI is a polyuric disorder that results from impaired responsiveness of the nephron to the actions of AVP. Plasma AVP concentrations are normal or increased in animals with this disorder. NDI is classified as primary or secondary (acquired). Secondary or acquired NDI is common in dogs and cats and is discussed in an earlier section (see Acquired [Secondary] Nephrogenic Diabetes Insipidus). Primary NDI is a rare disorder in dogs and cats; polydipsia and polyuria typically become apparent by the time the dog or cat is 8 to 12 weeks of age suggesting that primary NDI may be a congenital disorder.

Etiology

Two types of congenital NDI have been identified in humans: mutations of the V_2 receptor and mutations of the aquaporin-2 water channels (van Lieburg et al, 1999; Bichet, 2006). More than 90% of cases of congenital NDI in humans are X-linked recessive disorders in males who have one of more than 200 different mutations of the V_2 receptor (Spanakis et al, 2008). When congenital NDI is identified in a girl, it is likely that the defect is a mutation of the aquaporin-2 water channel gene producing an autosomal recessive disease (Sands and Bichet, 2006). For both disorders, clinical signs are apparent shortly after birth. The diagnosis of congenital NDI is established by high concentrations of AVP in the presence of hypotonic polyuria and the lack of response to DDAVP administration.

Only a few reports of primary NDI in dogs have appeared in the veterinary literature (Breitschwerdt et al, 1981; Grunbaum et al, 1990; Grunbaum and Moritz, 1991). Primary NDI has not yet been reported in the cat. The cause of primary NDI in dogs and cats is unknown. Electron microscopic examination of the renal medulla in a Miniature Poodle with primary NDI revealed vacuoles in the cells of the Henle loops, blood vessels, and interstitium, but the significance of these lesions is not known. Necropsy failed to identify any lesions in the kidney of a German Shepherd dog with primary NDI.

Familial NDI has been reported in a family of Huskies, in which the female parent was diagnosed as a carrier of the NDI gene, and three of four male puppies in her litter had NDI (Grunbaum et al, 1990). Affected puppies possessed normal V_2 receptor numbers in the kidney inner medulla, but the receptors had a ten-fold lower binding affinity for AVP than in normal dogs (Luzius et al, 1992). Adenylate cyclase stimulation by AVP was similarly reduced in a dose-response manner; however, stimulation of adenylate cyclase by non–AVP-mediated chemicals was comparable for normal and NDI-affected dogs, implying normal adenylate cyclase in the affected Huskies. The NDI-affected dogs also had antidiuretic responses to high doses of DDAVP, consistent with their possessing V_2 receptors of lower binding affinity.

In an older dog and cat, primary NDI should only be considered if polyuria and polydipsia has been present the animal's entire life. The onset of polyuria and polydipsia later in life in a dog or cat suspected to have NDI is suggestive of acquired NDI. A complete evaluation of the kidney, including creatinine clearance studies, IV pyelogram, computed tomographic (CT) or magnetic resonance imaging (MRI) scan, and kidney biopsy should be considered in these dogs and cats if another cause of for acquired NDI is not identified.

Primary and Psychogenic Polydipsia

Primary polydipsia (compulsive water consumption) is a syndrome characterized by ingestion of excess water resulting in compensatory polyuria to prevent water intoxication. In humans, primary polydipsia is most commonly found in individuals with underlying psychiatric illness (Cronin, 1987; Victor et al, 1989) and rarely, in individuals with lesions involving the thirst center. The cause of the polydipsia in individuals with psychiatric illness is uncertain, and most patients have, in addition to polydipsia, some abnormality in water excretion, such as excessive AVP secretion (Goldman et al, 1988).

Primary polydipsia caused by a hypothalamic lesion affecting the thirst center has not been reported in the dog or cat. A psychogenic basis for compulsive water consumption occurs uncommonly in the dog and has not been reported in the cat. Affected animals are usually hyperactive dogs that are placed in exercise-restrictive environments. Some of these dogs have had significant changes to their environment, resulting in unusual stress. In some dogs, compulsive water consumption is a learned behavior to gain attention from the owner. Dogs with psychogenic water consumption can concentrate urine to greater than 1.030 during water deprivation, although the latter may take hours because of concurrent renal medullary solute washout. Urine specific gravity may vary widely over time, and concentrated urine may be identified on random urine evaluation. Identification of concentrated urine implies hypothalamic AVP production, pituitary AVP secretion, and renal tubular responsiveness to AVP.

Abnormal AVP release in response to hypertonic saline stimulation was described in four dogs with suspected primary polydipsia (van Vonderen et al, 1999). All dogs presented for polyuria and polydipsia and had normal routine laboratory examinations except for hyposthenuria and concentrated urine during the water deprivation test. During serial measurements, urine osmolality spontaneously reached high concentrations (i.e., greater than 1000 mOsm/kg of H_2O) in two dogs. During water deprivation, plasma AVP concentrations remained relatively low in all dogs. The AVP response to hypertonic saline infusion was abnormal in all dogs, with an increased threshold value in three dogs, an increased sensitivity in two dogs, and an exaggerated response in one dog. These findings suggested a primary disturbance in the regulation of AVP secretion, although chronic overhydration may have caused downregulation of AVP release in response to hypertonicity (Moses and Clayton, 1993). Subnormal AVP release during water deprivation and hypertonic stimulation has been documented in humans with primary polydipsia (Zerbe and Robertson, 1981); these individuals were subsequently classified as having partial diabetes insipidus. It is not clear whether the dogs described by van Vonderen, et al., (1999) represent a variant or early stage of partial diabetes insipidus. They were classified as having primary polydipsia based on their ability to concentrate urine to a specific gravity greater than 1.030, but the identified abnormalities suggest a problem with AVP release rather than the thirst center, per se.

 CLINICAL FEATURES OF DIABETES INSIPIDUS AND PSYCHOGENIC POLYDIPSIA

Signalment

Central Diabetes Insipidus

There is no apparent breed, gender, or age predilection for CDI (Fig. 1-10). Of 60 dogs diagnosed with CDI at University of

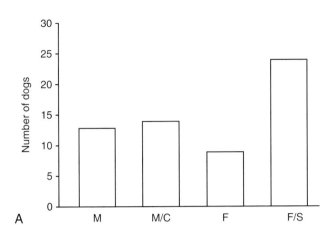

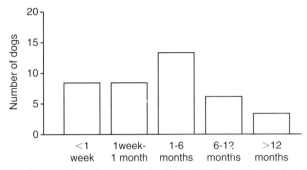

FIGURE 1-11 Duration of polyuria and polydipsia in 38 dogs with central diabetes insipidus (CDI) before owners presented their pet to the veterinarian for examination.

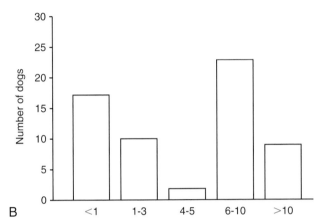

FIGURE 1-10 Gender (A) and age (B) distribution of 60 dogs diagnosed with central diabetes insipidus (CDI). *F*, Female; *F/S*, female/spayed; *M*, male; *M/C*, male/castrated.

California, Davis, 25 different breeds were represented. The Labrador Retriever (eight dogs), Boxer (five dogs), and German Shepherd (five dogs) were the breeds most commonly affected. The age at time of diagnosis in these 60 dogs ranged from 7 weeks to 14 years, with a median age of 6 years. Most dogs diagnosed with CDI were younger than 2 years or older than 5 years of age.

Twelve cats with CDI have been reported in the literature (Burnie and Dunn, 1982; Winterbotham and Mason, 1983; Kraus, 1987; Brown et al, 1993; Pittari, 1996; Aroch et al, 2005), and we have diagnosed an additional four cats at UC Davis. Thirteen of these sixteen cats were Domestic Short- or Long-Haired, two were Persian, and one was an Abyssinian. Eight of the cats were female or female/spayed, and eight were male or male/castrated. The age at the time of diagnosis of CDI ranged from 8 weeks to 6 years, with a mean of 1½ years.

Primary Nephrogenic Diabetes Insipidus

Primary NDI is rare in dogs and cats. To date, primary NDI has been reported in a 13-week-old male German Shepherd dog, an 18-month-old male Miniature Poodle, an 18-month-old female Boston Terrier, and a family of Huskies (Breitschwerdt et al, 1981; Grunbaum et al, 1990). We have also diagnosed NDI in a 5-month-old Norwegian Elkhound and a 1-year-old Boston Terrier. Both dogs had polyuria and polydipsia since being acquired by their owners at 6 to 8 weeks of age. Primary NDI has not yet been reported in the cat.

Psychogenic Polydipsia

Psychogenic polydipsia can be diagnosed in dogs of any age, either gender, and numerous breeds. Fifteen different breeds were represented in 18 dogs diagnosed with psychogenic polydipsia at UC Davis. Eleven dogs were female or female/spayed, and the age at time of diagnosis ranged from 6 months to 11 years, with a mean and median age of 4½ and 4 years, respectively. Psychogenic polydipsia has not yet been reported in the cat.

Clinical Signs

Polyuria and polydipsia are the hallmark clinical signs for diabetes insipidus and psychogenic polydipsia. Polyuria and polydipsia can be quite severe, with 24-hour water intake exceeding 200 mL/kg. Polyuria and polydipsia have usually been present for 1 to 6 months before veterinary care is sought (Fig. 1-11). Many owners also report urinary incontinence, in part because of the frequency of urination and loss of normal "house broken" behavior and in part because of the inability to maintain continence because of the large volume of urine being produced, especially when the dog or cat is sleeping. Owners of cats with diabetes insipidus also complain about the increased frequency of changing the litter, which often needs to be done two or three times a day. An insatiable desire for water may result in the consumption of any liquid, including ice, snow, and urine. Occasionally, the afflicted pet's strong desire for water overrides its normal appetite (i.e., they would rather drink than eat), resulting in weight loss.

Additional clinical signs depend, in part, on the underlying cause. Other historical abnormalities (e.g., vomiting, diarrhea, coughing) are usually not present in dogs or cats with congenital, idiopathic, or trauma-induced forms of diabetes insipidus. These pets are typically alert and playful and have normal exercise tolerance. However, dogs with acquired CDI secondary to a growing pituitary or hypothalamic neoplasm may develop additional signs related to the nervous system, including inappetence, stupor, disorientation, pacing, ataxia, seizures, and tremors (Harb et al, 1996). Neurologic signs may be present at the time CDI is diagnosed or, more typically, develop weeks to months after CDI is identified. In one study, 6 of 20 dogs with CDI developed neurologic signs from 2 weeks to 5 months (median, 1 month) after CDI was diagnosed (Harb et al, 1996). A tumor in the region of the hypothalamus and pituitary was identified by CT scan or necropsy in all six dogs. Neurologic signs may also develop secondary to hypertonic dehydration and severe hypernatremia.

Physical Examination

As with the history, the abnormalities found during the physical examination depend on the underlying cause. For most animals, the physical examination is unremarkable, although some dogs tend to be thin. Abnormalities of the cardiovascular, respiratory, gastrointestinal, and urogenital systems are usually absent. Animals with idiopathic or congenital diabetes insipidus are alert and active. Typically, as long as access to water is not restricted, hydration, mucous membrane color, and capillary refill time remain normal. The presence of neurologic abnormalities is variable in dogs and cats with trauma-induced CDI or neoplastic destruction of the hypothalamus and/or pituitary gland. Many of these animals have no perceptible neurologic alterations on physical examination. A few show mild to severe neurologic signs, including stupor, disorientation, ataxia, circling, and pacing.

Clinical Pathology Abnormalities

Complete Blood Count

The CBC in dogs and cats with CDI or NDI is usually unremarkable. The white blood cell count and differential are normal. The red blood cell count is normal or mildly increased. Polycythemia is not common and is the result of a mild, clinically imperceptible state of dehydration. Diabetes insipidus is a primary polyuric disorder with compensatory polydipsia, and affected dogs and cats are chronically, albeit mildly, fluid-depleted to stimulate the compensatory thirst response. Owners commonly tire of their pets' polyuria and polydipsia and begin restricting access to water, further exacerbating dehydration. Fluid depletion results in hemoconcentration with a mild increase in hematocrit, red blood cell count, and serum total protein concentration. The CBC in dogs with psychogenic polydipsia is rarely abnormal.

Urinalysis

Random urinalysis in dogs and cats with CDI, NDI, or psychogenic polydipsia typically reveals a urine specific gravity less than 1.006, with values of 1.001 and 1.002 occurring commonly (Fig. 1-12). The corresponding urine osmolality is usually less than 300 mOsm/kg. A urine specific gravity in the isosthenuric range (1.008 to 1.015) does not rule out diabetes insipidus (see Fig. 1-12) or psychogenic polydipsia (see Table 1-3), especially when the urine has been obtained after water is knowingly or inadvertently withheld (e.g., a long car ride and wait in the veterinary office). Dogs and cats with partial diabetes insipidus can concentrate their urine into the isosthenuric range if dehydrated. The remaining components of the urinalysis in these animals are usually normal.

Extremely dilute urine is not commonly seen in veterinary practice, being limited usually to animals with postobstructive diuresis, excessive IV fluid administration, diuretic use, and hyperadrenocorticism, as well as CDI, NDI, and psychogenic polydipsia. Although numerous disorders can result in polydipsia and polyuria (see Table 1-2), most of these disorders do not cause the severe polyuria suggested by remarkable depression in the specific gravity (< 1.005). Although we have seen animals that were polyuric owing to hypercalcemia, hypokalemia, pyometra, pyelonephritis, and other disorders, the degree of urine dilution is less dramatic and typically in the 1.006 to 1.020 range. However, even mild disturbances in the ability to concentrate urine, resulting in urine specific gravities of 1.008 to 1.015, often alter behavior sufficiently to allow an owner to realize the change.

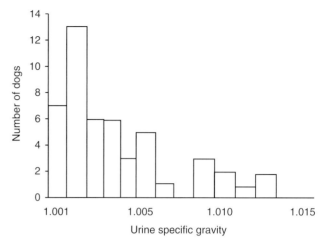

FIGURE 1-12 Urine specific gravity measured in 49 dogs with central diabetes insipidus (CDI) at the time of initial presentation to the veterinarian.

Serum Chemistries

The serum biochemistry panel is normal in most dogs and cats with diabetes insipidus and psychogenic polydipsia. The chronic and severe diuresis associated with CDI, NDI, and psychogenic polydipsia causes excessive loss of urea via the kidneys and may cause a subsequent reduction of BUN to concentrations of 5 to 10 mg/dL. Ten of 40 dogs with CDI had a BUN less than 10 mg/dL at the time of initial presentation to UC Davis. Inadequate access to water can cause severe dehydration and prerenal azotemia with hyposthenuria. The combination of prerenal azotemia, hypernatremia, and hyposthenuria was identified in 3 of our 40 dogs with CDI at the time of initial presentation to our hospital. These clinicopathologic abnormalities resolved after allowing the dogs to have access to water and initiating DDAVP therapy. Owners had restricted access to water in all three dogs.

Serum Electrolytes

Serum electrolytes are usually normal in dogs and cats with diabetes insipidus and psychogenic polydipsia. Mild hyponatremia and hypokalemia have been identified in 20% of our dogs with CDI and psychogenic polydipsia. More important, severe hypernatremia (serum sodium, 159 to 165 mEq/L) and hyperkalemia (5.4 to 5.9 mEq/L) have been identified in 15% of our dogs with CDI, abnormalities presumably developing secondary to water restriction and dehydration. An intact renin-angiotensin-aldosterone axis succeeds in maintaining electrolyte homeostasis in most dogs and cats despite the remarkable urine output associated with CDI, NDI, and psychogenic polydipsia. Maintenance of fluid and electrolyte balance depends on functioning thirst and hunger centers in the hypothalamus. Water restriction can cause severe dehydration in a matter of hours. Because free water diuresis continues despite water restriction, vascular and systemic hyperosmolarity develops. Increases in serum sodium contribute significantly to this hyperosmolarity. Hypertonic dehydration, severe hypernatremia, and neurologic signs may develop in a dog or cat with diabetes insipidus that is unable to drink (e.g., posttraumatic episode) or has restricted access to water (Reidarson et al, 1990). Severe hypernatremia is associated with significant metabolic consequences and is a difficult therapeutic challenge. Water deprivation studies to confirm the diagnosis of diabetes insipidus are not without complications and require careful patient monitoring to avoid dangerous consequences (see Complications of the Modified Water Deprivation Test: Hypertonic Dehydration and Hypernatremia).

CONFIRMING THE DIAGNOSIS OF DIABETES INSIPIDUS

Diagnostic tests to confirm and differentiate among CDI, primary NDI, and psychogenic water consumption include the modified water deprivation test, random plasma osmolality determination, and the clinical response of the dog or cat to DDAVP treatment. The results of these tests can be interpreted only after the causes for acquired NDI have been ruled out. Recommended initial diagnostic studies to rule out acquired NDI include a CBC; serum biochemistry panel; serum T_4 concentration (older cat); urinalysis with bacterial culture; abdominal ultrasonography; a urine cortisol-to-creatinine ratio, low-dose dexamethasone suppression test, or both in dogs; baseline serum cortisol concentration if hypoadrenocorticism is suspected (dogs); and pre- and postprandial bile acids if hepatic insufficiency is suspected. Results of these screening tests are normal in dogs and cats with CDI, primary NDI, and psychogenic water consumption, although a low-normal serum urea nitrogen concentration may be identified in animals with unrestricted access to water and erythrocytosis, hyperproteinemia, hypernatremia, and azotemia may be found if access to water has been restricted.

Pituitary-dependent hyperadrenocorticism can mimic CDI in the adult dog. Pituitary-dependent hyperadrenocorticism commonly causes severe polyuria and polydipsia and occasionally dogs have no other clinical signs, do not have the typical abnormalities (e.g., increased serum alkaline phosphatase activity, hypercholesterolemia) associated with the disease, and adrenal gland size is at the upper end of the reference interval with ultrasonography. Results of the modified water deprivation test in dogs with hyperadrenocorticism are similar to results in dogs with partial CDI (see Fig. 1-18) and, sometimes, dogs with psychogenic polydipsia. Severity of polyuria and polydipsia may improve noticeably to the owner after initiating treatment with DDAVP in these dogs but improvement tends to be transient, lasting only a few months, and the dog typically re-presents to the hospital with owner concerns that the DDAVP is no longer working. For these reasons, we always perform screening tests for hyperadrenocorticism (i.e., urine cortisol-to-creatinine ratio on urine collected at home; low dose dexamethasone suppression test) in an adult dog in which CDI and psychogenic polydipsia have risen to the top of the differential diagnoses and always before initiating DDAVP treatment.

An index of suspicion for CDI and primary NDI versus psychogenic polydipsia can often be gained after reviewing the history and findings on physical examination and routine blood and urine tests. The presence of neurologic signs or behavioral issues, the serum sodium concentration (i.e., upper versus lower limit of the reference range), the consistency of hyposthenuric urine, and the dog's susceptibility to dehydration after water restriction provide clues to the underlying diagnosis. The definitive diagnosis is based on results of the modified water deprivation test, measurement of plasma osmolality, measurement of plasma AVP concentration and response to synthetic vasopressin therapy.

Historically, the modified water deprivation test has been considered the best diagnostic test to differentiate between CDI, primary NDI and psychogenic polydipsia. However, the test can be labor-intensive, time-consuming, and expensive, especially if urine and plasma osmolalities and plasma AVP concentrations are measured. Results of the test can also be confusing, especially with partial deficiency syndromes. Currently, we consider performing a water deprivation test only in dogs (and rarely cats) that have a poor response to trial DDAVP treatment and when we suspect either partial CDI or psychogenic polydipsia. In these cases,

response to water deprivation provides insight into the animal's ability to concentrate urine (i.e., can the patient concentrate urine to a specific gravity above 1.030).

A simpler approach that is especially appealing in a busy practice is the evaluation of response to trial therapy with DDAVP and, if available, measurement of plasma osmolality obtained while the dog or cat has free access to water (see Random Plasma Osmolality as a Diagnostic Tool).

RESPONSE TO TRIAL THERAPY WITH DESMOPRESSIN ACETATE

CDI, primary NDI, and psychogenic polydipsia are uncommon to rare causes of polyuria and polydipsia in dogs and cats; and of these three differential diagnoses, partial CDI and psychogenic polydipsia are the most common. Because CDI is treated with DDAVP, a viable approach to establishing the diagnosis is to evaluate the animal's response to trial therapy with DDAVP (Aventis Pharmaceuticals). Oral DDAVP tablets or conjunctival drops of DDAVP nasal spray (see Treatment) should be administered every 12 hours for 7 days. The effect of DDAVP should not be critically evaluated until after 5 to 7 days of therapy because renal medullary solute washout may prevent a dog or cat with CDI from concentrating its urine and decreasing water intake after only 1 or 2 days of DDAVP treatment. Clients should notice a definite improvement in the severity of polyuria and polydipsia by the end of the treatment period if the polyuria and polydipsia are caused by CDI. Urine specific gravity should be measured on several urine samples collected by the client on the last couple of days of trial therapy. An increase in urine specific gravity by 50% or more, compared with pretreatment specific gravities, supports the diagnosis of CDI, especially if the urine specific gravity exceeds 1.030. There should be only minimal improvement in dogs and cats with primary NDI, although a response may be observed with very high doses of DDAVP (Luzius et al, 1992). Dogs and cats with psychogenic water consumption may exhibit a mild decline in urine output and water intake because the chronically low serum osmolality tends to depress AVP production. Theoretically, dogs with psychogenic polydipsia could develop clinical signs of hyponatremia during DDAVP therapy but we have not yet identified this complication (see Syndrome of Inappropriate Vasopressin Secretion: Excess Vasopressin). A thorough review of the diagnostic evaluation of the patient, owner compliance in treating the pet, and adjustments in the DDAVP treatment protocol should be undertaken in dogs and cats that fail to respond to DDAVP before considering the modified water deprivation test.

MODIFIED WATER DEPRIVATION TEST

Principle of the Test

The modified water deprivation test is designed to determine whether endogenous AVP is released in response to dehydration and whether the kidneys respond to this stimulus. The modified water deprivation test consists of two phases. In phase I the AVP secretory capabilities and renal distal and collecting tubule responsiveness to AVP are evaluated by assessing the effects of dehydration (i.e., water restriction until the animal loses 3% of its body weight) on urine specific gravity. The normal dog and cat, as well as those with psychogenic water consumption, should be able to concentrate urine to greater than 1.030 (1.035 in the cat) if dehydrated. Dogs and cats with partial and complete CDI and primary NDI have an impaired ability to concentrate urine in the face of dehydration (Table 1-4 and see Figure 1-17). Phase II of the water deprivation test is indicated for dogs and cats that do not concentrate urine to greater than 1.030 during phase I of the test. Phase II determines the effect, if any, that exogenous AVP has on the renal tubular ability to concentrate urine in the face of dehydration (see Fig. 1-19). This phase differentiates impaired AVP secretion from impaired renal tubular responsiveness to AVP (see Table 1-4). The modified water deprivation test is not indicated to study the function of any organ system other than renal tubular response to AVP. This protocol is specifically contraindicated in patients suspected or known to have renal disease, those that are uremic owing to prerenal or primary renal disorders, and animals with suspected or obvious dehydration (see Approach if the Dog or Cat Is Brought into the Hospital Dehydrated).

Protocol

See Box 1-3.

Preparation for the Test

The severity of renal medullary solute washout is a difficult variable to evaluate in an animal with severe polydipsia and polyuria; yet it may have an effect on test results. Theoretically, correction of renal medullary solute washout improves renal tubular concentrating ability and the accuracy of the modified water deprivation test in differentiating among CDI, primary NDI, and psychogenic polydipsia. However, in animals with CDI, water restriction alone may not improve renal medullary solute washout; only after correction of polyuria and polydipsia with vasopressin therapy can the capacity of the renal tubule to concentrate urine be fully appreciated (Fig. 1-13). Nevertheless, we attempt to minimize the effects of severe medullary washout on the results of the modified water deprivation test, using progressive water restriction before initiating total water deprivation. The goal is to decrease 24-hour water intake to approximately 100 mL/kg the day prior to performing the water deprivation test. This goal can be hard to attain, especially in dogs or cats with severe polyuria and polydipsia. Total water intake per 24 hours should be determined by the owner and based on unrestricted access to water. Water restriction is begun once total 24-hour water intake has been quantified. We arbitrarily decrease daily water intake by 10% every 1 to 2 days and continue until the goal of 100 mL/kg/24 h is attained, the animal becomes aggressive for water, or begins to develop clinical signs suggestive of hypertonic dehydration (e.g., change in mentation; see Complications of the Modified Water Deprivation Test: Hypertonic Dehydration and Hypernatremia). Each day's 24-hour allotment of water should be divided into six to eight aliquots with the last aliquot given at bedtime. No food is given within 12 hours of beginning the test or during the procedure.

Phase I of the Test

The water deprivation test should always be started at the beginning of the workday, because animals undergoing this test must be observed and evaluated frequently. Most dogs and cats with CDI or primary NDI dehydrate and lose 3% of their body weight (end point for this phase of the test) within 3 to 10 hours (see Table 1-4). Withholding water and leaving the dog or cat with diabetes insipidus unattended for several hours or throughout the night may result in the development of severe complications and possibly death (see Complications of the Modified Water Deprivation Test: Hypertonic Dehydration and Hypernatremia). Frequent observation of the animal helps avoid complications or severe dehydration.

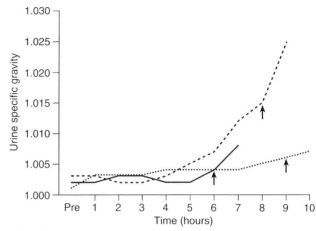

FIGURE 1-13 Results of the modified water deprivation test in a 1-year-old Persian cat with congenital central diabetes insipidus (CDI). *Solid line,* Initial water deprivation test results. *Dotted line,* Water deprivation test results after gradually restricting water consumption for 7 days prior to performing the test. *Dashed line,* Water deprivation test results after gradual water restriction and twice-daily injections of arginine vasopressin (AVP) for 7 days prior to performing the test. AVP injections were discontinued 24 hours prior to performing the test. ↑, 5% loss of body weight and aqueous AVP injection.

At the start of the test, the dog's or cat's bladder is emptied by micturition (walking outside) or catheterization; then an exact body weight is obtained and water is completely withheld from the patient. Urine specific gravity and, if possible, osmolality should be determined on a pretest urine sample. Periodic evaluation of BUN and serum sodium concentration, beginning at the start of the test, is helpful in identifying the development of azotemia or hypernatremia. The onset of azotemia or hypernatremia is a criterion for ending the test.

Although urine osmolality is more consistent and accurate than urine specific gravity, determination of urine specific gravity allows differentiation between CDI, primary NDI and psychogenic polydipsia in most situations, is readily available, inexpensive, and provides immediate information on urine concentration. Prior to starting the modified water deprivation test, the clinician should check the accuracy of the refractometer by ensuring that a reading of 1.000 is obtained with distilled water (Barsanti et al, 2000).

During Phase I of the Test

The urinary bladder should be emptied by micturition or catheterization every 1 to 2 hours. For cats, an indwelling urinary catheter is usually required. The specific gravity should be determined on each urine sample and an aliquot stored for osmolality determination, should it be desired at the end of the test. Most important, the dog or cat must be carefully weighed at least once an hour. Phase I ends when 3% of body weight has been lost or urine specific gravity exceeds 1.030. Additionally, the dog or cat should be assessed for clinical evidence of dehydration and changes in mentation or behavior. Periodic evaluation of BUN and serum sodium concentration should also be done. The test should be halted if the dog or cat becomes azotemic, hypernatremic, or severely dehydrated or develops changes in mentation or behavior.

End of Phase I

Maximal secretion of AVP and concentration of urine are achieved when an animal loses 3% of its body weight owing to loss of fluid in the urine with simultaneous water deprivation. At that point the urinary bladder should be completely emptied, the urine checked for specific gravity and osmolality, and phase II of the water deprivation test initiated (see Box 1-3). If available, a plasma vasopressin concentration obtained at this time is helpful in interpreting the test (see Plasma Vasopressin Determinations).

Normal dogs typically require more than 24 hours to lose 3% of body weight following water deprivation. In contrast, water deprivation usually causes 3% or greater loss of body weight within 3 to 10 hours if the animal has CDI or primary NDI (see Table 1-4). Dogs or cats with partial CDI or psychogenic polydipsia may require considerably longer than 10 hours to achieve 3% loss of body weight. The clinician should always be prepared to continue the water deprivation test into the late evening hours. If this is not possible and the dog or cat has not yet lost 3% body weight or attained a urine specific gravity greater than 1.030 by the end of the working hours, the dog or cat can be transferred to a veterinary hospital with overnight care so the test can be continued.

Alternatively, the study can be stopped and water offered, initially in small amounts to prevent overzealous intake. The modified water deprivation test can then be repeated in a few days with the following adjustments in protocol: body weight is measured and water withheld beginning at midnight; the dog or cat is kept in a cage (or at home) for the remainder of the night, ideally with periodic visual assessment by individuals working at night (or by the owner if the patient is at home); the urinary bladder is completely emptied first thing in the morning and urine specific gravity and/or osmolality are measured; body weight is recorded; and phase I is continued as previously discussed. With this modification, the clinician is already 6 to 8 hours into phase I of the test at the beginning of the workday. Complete CDI and primary NDI must be ruled out before this modification to the modified water deprivation test is used; that is, the clinician must prove that the dog or cat requires at least 10 hours of water deprivation before 3% loss of body weight occurs. The modification described here should never be incorporated into the initial modified water deprivation test performed on the dog or cat.

Serial evaluation of body weight is a simple, inexpensive, reliable, and readily available method to determine the end point of phase I of the test. The goal is to lose 3% body weight during water deprivation. A 1% to 2% loss of weight due to dehydration may fail to maximally stimulate AVP secretion. False plateaus in urine osmolality and urine specific gravity have been observed with weight loss in the range of 2%, which can be misleading.

Other criteria have been used to determine whether and when maximal urinary concentration has been achieved through water deprivation. One method is recognition of a "plateau," or lack of increase, in urine osmolalities. This criterion is based on the knowledge that after the maximal renal response to water deprivation is achieved, the urine osmolality becomes relatively constant. This plateau in urine concentration is defined as a change in osmolality between three consecutive urine collection periods, 1 hour apart, of less than 5% or 30 mOsm/kg of H_2O. Monitoring urine specific gravity in lieu of osmolality or body weight is less reliable because false plateaus in urine specific gravity are common, even before 3% loss of body weight has occurred. Although the ability to ascertain a specific gravity is readily available, it is not sufficiently accurate to use as a criterion for ending phase I of the study, unless the urine specific gravity exceeds 1.030.

Monitoring skin turgidity and measuring the packed cell volume of blood have not proved to be reliable or consistent tools for recognizing dehydration. Measurement of total plasma protein concentration may be more reliable than the former two

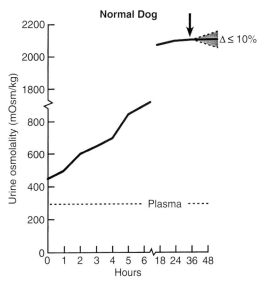

FIGURE 1-14 The effect of water deprivation on the urine osmolality of a normal dog. ↓ represents an injection of aqueous vasopressin, which alters urine osmolality 10% or less.

parameters, but monitoring cannot be considered as consistent or informative as body weight and patient observation. One important aid during phase I of the modified water deprivation test is the periodic check of the BUN and serum sodium concentration. Whenever the BUN rises above 30 mg/dL, the patient is azotemic and phase I should be ended; development of azotemia suggests occult renal disease. Azotemia developing during the modified water deprivation test has not resulted in problems in dogs and cats monitored as suggested earlier. Similarly, hypernatremia and increased plasma osmolality are potent stimulants of AVP secretion; when identified, these findings suggest that phase I of the water deprivation test be ended.

Response to Exogenous Arginine Vasopressin (Phase II)

Phase I determines the effects of dehydration on endogenous AVP secretion and AVP action on the renal tubules. Phase II determines what effect, if any, exogenous AVP has on renal tubular ability to concentrate urine in the face of dehydration. This phase differentiates impaired AVP secretion from impaired renal tubular responsiveness to AVP. Synthetic aqueous vasopressin (Pitressin) at a dosage of 0.2 to 0.4 U/kg up to a maximum of 5U, is administered with a intramuscular (IM) injection, urine samples are obtained, and the bladder is emptied 30, 60 and 120 minutes following the injection. Alternatively, DDAVP injection may be administered at a dose of 5 μg subcutaneously (SC) and urine samples obtained and the bladder emptied 2 and 4 hours following injection. Specific gravity and/or urine osmolality are determined on these urine samples and the dog or cat is offered small amounts of water over the next 2 hours. Ultimately, the animal is returned to free-choice water. The water is initially offered in small amounts to prevent overzealous intake, which could result in vomiting or water intoxication.

Responses to the Modified Water Deprivation Test

Normal Dogs

Normal dogs dehydrate quite slowly (Fig. 1-14). The secretion of AVP in the normal dog results in exquisite conservation of fluid over long time periods. Random urine samples from normal dogs with free access to water reveal a specific gravity of 1.006 to greater than 1.040 and an osmolality of 160 to greater than 2500 mOsm/kg of H_2O (uOsm; van Vonderen et al, 1997b). In a report on laboratory dogs, the range of values was narrower and maximal urine concentration was achieved in 20 dogs after an average of approximately 40 hours of water deprivation (Hardy and Osborne, 1979). Maximal urine osmolality ranged from 1700 to 2700 uOsm and specific gravity from 1.050 to 1.075. Urine concentration indices (specific gravity and osmolality) did not plateau after reaching maximal values. Most dogs reached a peak in urine concentration, followed by slight fluctuations below that value for the remaining period of water deprivation. No difference in testing parameters occurred between males and females. Although not specifically evaluated, similar findings are expected in the cat.

In a clinical setting, normal for the modified water deprivation test is defined as a urine osmolality significantly greater than plasma osmolality. Normal dogs and cats have urine that is typically greater than 1100 uOsm and a urine specific gravity greater than 1.030 after dehydration. If urine osmolality and specific gravity exceed these values, pituitary AVP secretion and renal responsiveness to AVP are considered intact, and there is no need to evaluate renal responsiveness to exogenous AVP.

What happens if AVP is injected after maximal urine concentration is reached via water deprivation in normal dogs and cats? As expected, such animals are experiencing maximal endogenous AVP secretion, and no further urine concentration can occur. Therefore, exogenous AVP should have little effect on urine concentration in these animals. After dehydration, changes in urine concentration of 10% or less of preinjection levels are not considered significant. Such lack of change is typical in dogs and cats with normal AVP secretion rates and renal responsiveness to AVP (see Fig. 1-14).

Central Diabetes Insipidus

Dogs and cats with severe (complete) CDI cannot concentrate urine to levels greater than plasma osmolality (280 to 310 mOsm/kg [pOms]), even with severe dehydration. In fact, the parameters of urine concentration change little, if any, with continuing water deprivation (Fig. 1-15). CDI may be subdivided into severe or partial deficiencies of AVP. The modified water deprivation test has been used to help differentiate between mild and severe forms of CDI. As previously described, mild states of dehydration, resulting in a 1% to 2% loss in body weight, cause sustained release of AVP in the normal subject. After maximal urine concentration occurs in the normal animal, it does not increase more than an additional 10% with the injection of aqueous vasopressin. If the administration of AVP to a dehydrated dog or cat causes a significant increase in the concentration of the urine, endogenous AVP production and/or secretion must be insufficient. In dogs and cats with severe AVP deficiency, the urine osmolalities do not reach 300 mOsm/kg with dehydration; however, the increase in osmolality after administration of vasopressin ranges from 50% to 600% greater than the preinjection level (Figs. 1-16 and 1-17).

Dogs and cats with partial AVP deficiencies can increase their urine osmolality above 300 mOsm/kg after dehydration, but they also experience a further 10% to 50% or greater increase in urine osmolality following administration of vasopressin

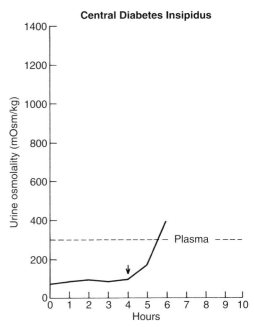

FIGURE 1-15 The effect of water deprivation on the urine osmolality of a dog with severe central diabetes insipidus (CDI). ↓ represents an injection of aqueous vasopressin administered after 5% or more body weight is lost, causing greater than 50% increase in urine osmolality. Note how quickly these dogs lose 5% of their body weight.

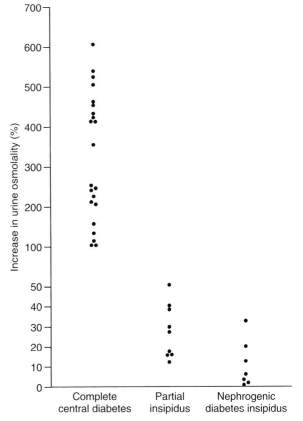

FIGURE 1-16 Increase in urine osmolality during phase III of the modified water deprivation test, that is, after intramuscular (IM) administration of aqueous vasopressin, in 22 dogs with complete central diabetes insipidus (CDI), 9 dogs with partial CDI, and 7 dogs with primary nephrogenic diabetes insipidus (NDI). Note the marked increase in urine osmolality after vasopressin administration with complete CDI versus partial CDI or primary NDI.

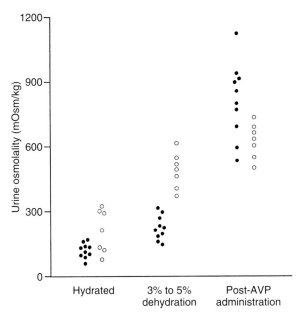

FIGURE 1-17 Urine osmolality in 10 dogs with complete central diabetes insipidus (CDI; *solid circle*) and 7 dogs with partial CDI *(open circle)* at the beginning (hydrated), end of phase II (3% to 5% dehydration), and end of phase III (post-arginine vasopressin [AVP] administration) of the modified water deprivation test. Note the relative failure of dogs with complete CDI to increase urine osmolality with dehydration and the marked increase in urine osmolality after aqueous vasopressin administration. The opposite occurred in the dogs with partial CDI.

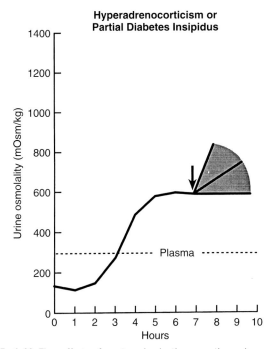

FIGURE 1-18 The effect of water deprivation on the urine osmolality of a dog afflicted with partial central diabetes insipidus (CDI) or canine hyperadrenocorticism. ↓ represents an injection of aqueous vasopressin administered after 5% or more body weight is lost owing to fluid loss via the urine. The urine osmolality did increase, but subnormally, in response to dehydration. Vasopressin results in a further 10% to 50% increase in urine osmolality. Note that the dog with partial CDI takes longer to dehydrate than one with severe CDI (see Fig. 1-15).

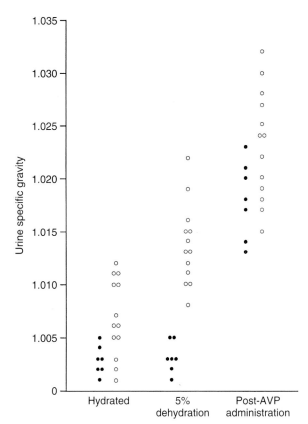

FIGURE 1-19 Urine specific gravity in 7 dogs with complete central diabetes insipidus (CDI; *solid circle*) and 13 dogs with partial CDI *(open circle)* at the beginning (hydrated), end of phase II (5% dehydration), and end of phase III (post-arginine vasopressin [AVP] administration) of the modified water deprivation test. Note the similarity of response between urine specific gravity and urine osmolality (see Fig. 1-17).

(Fig. 1-18; see Fig. 1-17). Changes in urine specific gravity often behave in a manner similar to changes in urine osmolality (Fig. 1-19; see Table 1-4). However, in some dogs and cats, urine specific gravity is not as easy to interpret as is urine osmolality (Fig. 1-20).

Primary Nephrogenic Diabetes Insipidus

Dogs, and presumably cats, afflicted with primary NDI cannot concentrate urine to levels greater than plasma osmolality (280 to 300 pOsm), even after severe dehydration. As with CDI, the parameters of urine concentration change little, if any, with continuing water deprivation (Fig. 1-21; see Table 1-4). Unlike CDI, however, minimal to no increase in urine osmolality and urine specific gravity occurs after administration of AVP (see Fig. 1-16).

Similar to dogs with severe CDI, dogs with primary NDI dehydrate quickly without water (see Table 1-4). The only difference between primary NDI and severe CDI is the lack of response to DDAVP seen in primary NDI versus the dramatic increase in urine concentration seen in CDI after DDAVP administration. Dogs with primary NDI are young and have a history of polyuria and polydipsia their entire life. In contrast, dogs and cats with acquired NDI are usually adults with a concurrent illness that interferes with AVP action at the renal tubular level and have a history of normal water intake and urination habits prior to the onset of polyuria and polydipsia. Acquired NDI patients are usually differentiated from those with CDI or primary NDI after review of the history, physical examination, and results of routine blood and urine tests and diagnostic imaging, eliminating the need for the modified water deprivation test.

Psychogenic Polydipsia

Dogs, and presumably cats, with psychogenic polydipsia have an intact hypothalamic pituitary renal tubular axis for controlling fluid balance and variable severity of renal medullary solute washout. These dogs can concentrate urine to an osmolality above that of plasma with complete water deprivation and, given enough time, can attain urine specific gravities in excess of 1.030. Depending on the severity of renal medullary solute washout, it may take 24 hours or longer of water deprivation to attain concentrated urine. The previously described progressive water restriction procedure preceding the water deprivation test aids in reestablishing the renal medullary concentration gradient in these dogs and shortens the time to attain concentrated urine. Phase II (response to DDAVP administration) is rarely needed in dogs with psychogenic polydipsia. If phase II is performed, administration of DDAVP to a dehydrated dog with psychogenic polydipsia causes little change (< 10%) in urine osmolality (Fig. 1-22). This lack of change reflects the competent AVP secretory response of the posterior pituitary to dehydration and a response to AVP by the renal tubules.

Misdiagnosis (Inaccuracies) Using the Modified Water Deprivation Test

The modified water deprivation test is an excellent study to differentiate primary NDI from CDI, but it may not differentiate partial CDI from psychogenic polydipsia with complete certainty (Fig. 1-23). Difficulties in differentiating partial CDI from psychogenic polydipsia may be explained by two associated changes in the renal response to AVP. First is the reduction in maximal concentrating capacity resulting from chronic polyuria itself (i.e., renal medullary solute washout), which is manifested as subnormal urine concentrations in the presence of excess levels of plasma vasopressin. Second, there appears to be an enhanced antidiuretic response to low levels of plasma AVP in patients with CDI; that is, these patients have a supersensitive response to the small amount of AVP they secrete endogenously (Block et al, 1981).

| | **TABLE 1-4   GUIDELINES FOR INTERPRETATION OF THE WATER DEPRIVATION TEST*** | | | | |

	Urine Specific Gravity			**Time to 5% Dehydration (Hours)**	
DISORDER	**INITIALLY**	**5% DEHYDRATION**	**POST-ADH**	**MEAN**	**RANGE**
CDI					
Complete	< 1.006	< 1.006	> 1.010	4	3-7
Partial	< 1.006	1.008–1.020	> 1.015	8	6-11
Primary NDI	< 1.006	< 1.006	< 1.006	5	3-9
Primary polydipsia	1.002-1.020	> 1.030	NA	13	8-20

ADH, Antidiuretic hormone; *CDI*, central diabetes insipidus; *NA*, not applicable; *NDI*, nephrogenic diabetes insipidus.
*Based on results from 20 dogs with CDI, 5 dogs with primary NDI, and 18 dogs with primary (psychogenic) polydipsia.

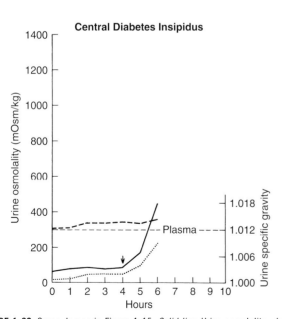

FIGURE 1-20 Same dog as in Figure 1-15. *Solid line*, Urine osmolality; *dashed line*, increasing plasma osmolality caused by dehydrating a dog with central diabetes insipidus (CDI); *dotted line*, urine specific gravity, illustrating why it is a less precise and less obvious diagnostic marker with severe CDI (see Fig. 1-15).

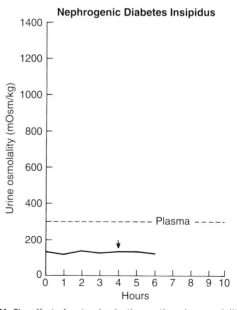

FIGURE 1-21 The effect of water deprivation on the urine osmolality of a dog afflicted with primary nephrogenic diabetes insipidus (NDI). Vasopressin is administered (↓) after 5% or more of body weight is lost (in this dog, after only 4 hours). Note the rapid loss of weight and the absence of any increase in urine concentration following 5% or more loss in body weight. The urine osmolality is not increased by vasopressin administration (< 10% change).

The consequence of the enhanced antidiuretic effect is the amelioration of the urinary manifestations of partial AVP deficiency. Therefore, patients with partial CDI and those with psychogenic polydipsia (that have not attained 3% loss of body weight) may respond to fluid deprivation with similar levels of urine concentration that cannot be increased further by injections of AVP (see Figs. 1-17 and 1-21). Thus neither the absolute level of urine osmolality achieved during fluid deprivation nor the percentage of increase evoked by exogenous AVP consistently permits a clear distinction between the two disorders (Zerbe and Robertson, 1981).

The modified water deprivation test may also occasionally misdiagnose human patients with congenital NDI. This inconsistency arises because a small percentage of these patients are only

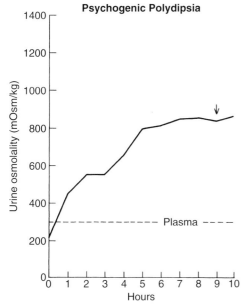

FIGURE 1-22 The effect of water deprivation on the urine osmolality of a dog afflicted with psychogenic polydipsia. Although these dogs are hormonally normal, the chronic diuresis may inhibit normal concentrating ability. ↓ represents an injection of aqueous vasopressin administered after 5% or more body weight is lost as a result of the unabated diuresis. The urine does show mild concentrating ability with dehydration, but less than 10% change in concentration following vasopressin administration.

partially resistant to the antidiuretic effect of vasopressin and can concentrate their urine to some degree if the plasma levels of the hormone are quite high (Robertson and Scheidler, 1981). Because the standard diagnostic dose of aqueous AVP customarily produces marked hypervasopressinemia, patients with partial resistance may respond in this phase of the modified water deprivation test as though they had CDI (Zerbe and Robertson, 1981). Partial resistance to the antidiuretic actions of vasopressin has been documented in Huskies with primary NDI (Luzius et al, 1992), raising the possibility, albeit an uncommon one, that the modified water deprivation test could misdiagnose primary NDI in dogs too.

A number of humans have been incorrectly diagnosed as having primary (psychogenic) polydipsia. The diagnosis was initially based on results of a modified water deprivation test similar to that illustrated in Fig. 1-22. However, sophisticated studies have revealed that some individuals have a metabolic explanation for such a test result. These patients have an abnormal "osmostat" (i.e., an abnormally elevated set point in their osmoreceptors for stimulating release of AVP). Therefore, at a relatively high plasma osmolality, which should cause release of AVP, these individuals remain "AVP free," polyuric, and thus polydipsic. Similarly, such patients may have a lower than normal set point for thirst (i.e., thirst may be stimulated at a plasma osmolality of 290 pOsm when it should not be stimulated until the osmolality reaches 295 or 300 pOsm). A similar phenomenon has been described in four dogs with suspected primary polydipsia, in which the AVP response to hypertonic saline infusion was abnormal and suggested a primary disturbance in the regulation of AVP secretion (van Vonderen et al, 1999).

Approach If the Dog or Cat Is Brought into the Hospital Dehydrated

Occasionally, pets with severe polydipsia and polyuria appear clinically dehydrated or have developed hypernatremia before the modified water deprivation test can be undertaken. The most common cause for this dehydration is the owner's withholding of water in an attempt to reduce the likelihood of urination in the home. If the dehydrated dog or cat exhibits CNS signs, immediate fluid therapy should be initiated. However, if the pet is in no apparent distress, the bladder can be drained and the urine checked for specific gravity and osmolality. A serum sample can be obtained to assess BUN, sodium, osmolality, and vasopressin concentrations.

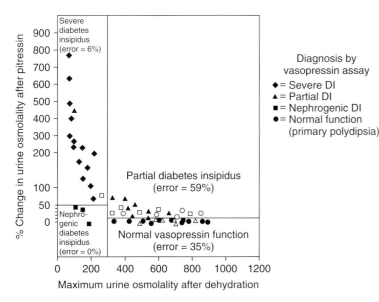

FIGURE 1-23 Relationship between maximum urine osmolality after dehydration and percentage of increase in urine osmolality after vasopressin administration in humans with central diabetes insipidus (CDI) and nephrogenic diabetes insipidus (NDI) and primary polydipsia. Note the overlap in results between patients with partial CDI and patients with normal vasopressin function (i.e., primary polydipsia). (From Robertson GL: *The Endocrine Society 41st postgraduate annual assembly syllabus*, New Orleans, October, 1989, p. 25.)

BOX 1-3   Protocol for the Modified Water Deprivation Test

Preparation for the Test
A. Determine total water intake per 24 hours based on unrestricted access to water
B. Several days prior to the test, gradually decrease total 24 hour water intake by approximately 10% every 1 to 2 days; continue until the goal of 100 mL/kg/24 h is attained or the animal becomes aggressive for water
C. Withhold food beginning 12 hours before the test

Phase I: Water Deprivation
A. Prior to initiation
   1. Withdraw food and all water
   2. Empty bladder completely
   3. Obtain exact body weight
   4. Check urine specific gravity and, if available, osmolality
   5. Obtain serum osmolality
   6. Obtain BUN and serum electrolytes
   7. Check hydration and CNS status
B. During the test
   1. Empty bladder every 60 to 120 min
   2. Check exact body weight every 60 min
   3. Check urine specific gravity/osmolality at each interval
   4. Check hydration and CNS status at each interval
   5. Periodically recheck BUN and serum electrolytes

C. End of phase I
   1. If urine specific gravity exceeds 1.030
   2. When dog is clinically dehydrated or appears ill
   3. When dog has lost 3% body weight
      a. Obtain plasma for vasopressin concentration if available
      b. Empty bladder
      c. Check urine specific gravity/osmolality
      d. Check BUN and serum electrolytes
      e. Check serum osmolality

Phase II: Response to Exogenous AVP
A. Administer aqueous vasopressin 0.2 to 0.4 U/kg (max, 5U) IM or desmopressin acetate injection 5 μg SC
B. Continue withholding food and water
C. Monitor patient
   1. Empty bladder every 30 minutes for 2 hours maximum (aqueous vasopressin) or at 2 and 4 hours (desmopressin)
   2. Check urine specific gravity/osmolality
   3. Monitor hydration and CNS status

At End of Test
A. Introduce small amounts of water (10 to 20 mL/kg) every 30 minutes for 2 hours and monitor patient
B. If patient is well 2 hours after ending test, return to ad libitum water

AVP, Arginine vasopressin; *BUN,* blood urea nitrogen; *CNS,* central nervous system; *IM,* intramuscular; *SC,* subcutaneous.

The clinician can then proceed with the next phase of the modified water deprivation test (phase II; see Box 1-3) if the urine present in the bladder has a specific gravity of less than 1.030 (osmolality < 1100 uOsm) and the dog or cat is not uremic or hypernatremic. If the urine is more concentrated than 1.030 (1100 uOsm), a normal pituitary-renal tubular concentrating axis probably exists. If the animal is truly polyuric/polydipsic, psychogenic polydipsia and hyperadrenocorticism remain possible diagnoses. If the urine is dilute, response to exogenous vasopressin administration should help to establish the diagnosis.

Complications of the Modified Water Deprivation Test: Hypertonic Dehydration and Hypernatremia

An adult dog or cat is composed of 60% water. This water is subdivided into an intracellular compartment, which accounts for two-thirds of the total, and an extracellular compartment, which is one-third (Fig. 1-24). Movement of solutes that readily diffuse across all membranes (e.g., urea) is not accompanied by appreciable fluid shifts, because these solutes generate equal osmotic forces on either side of the cell membrane. Increased concentration of these solutes creates hyperosmolality in all fluid compartments because of a lack of water redistribution.

Solutes that are less permeable across cell membranes by virtue of molecular size, electrical charge, or active membrane pumps create an effective osmotic force. Intracellular solutes of this kind include potassium, phosphate, glucose and protein. Sodium and its anions serve the same purpose in the extracellular fluid (ECF). Increased concentrations of such solutes in the ECF produce hyperosmolality and hypertonicity. The osmotic gradient that is formed results in movement of intracellular fluid (ICF) into the extracellular space. Therefore, extracellular volume increases at the expense of cellular hydration. Alternatively, decreased concentrations of extracellular solutes produce a hyposmotic, hypotonic ECF that necessitates intracellular

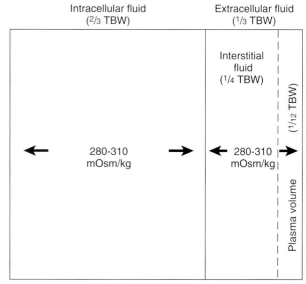

FIGURE 1-24 In the hydrated state, uniform total body water (TBW) distribution is maintained between the intracellular fluid (ICF) and extracellular fluid (ECF) compartments by osmotic forces (normal range, 280 to 310 mOsm/kg; average, 295 mOsm/kg) generated by solutes. (From Edwards DF, et al.: Hypernatremic, hypertonic dehydration in the dog with diabetes insipidus and gastric dilatation volvulus, *J Am Vet Med Assoc* 182[9]:973-977, 1983.)

movement of water, causing both hypovolemia and cellular overhydration (Edwards et al, 1983).

Three chemically distinct forms of dehydration (isotonic, hypotonic, and hypertonic) occur in veterinary practice. Isotonic dehydration is produced by proportional loss of water and electrolytes (solutes) (Fig. 1-25, *A*). Protracted vomiting and diarrhea are one cause of isotonic dehydration, in which water and electrolyte losses occur predominantly from the ECF compartment to the external

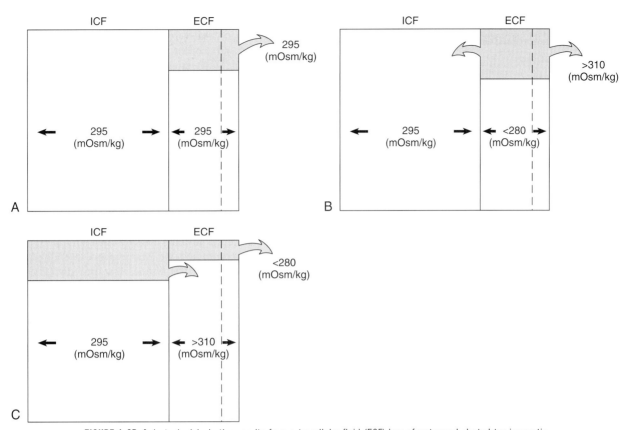

FIGURE 1-25 A, Isotonic dehydration results from extracellular fluid (ECF) loss of water and electrolytes isosmotic (295 mOsm/kg) to total body water (TBW). Because compartmental osmolality and tonicity remain unchanged (295 mOsm/kg), no major shift of intracellular fluid (ICF) occurs. **B,** Hypotonic dehydration results from ECF loss of water and electrolytes hyperosmotic (> 310 mOsm/kg) to TBW. The ECF becomes hypo-osmolar and hypotonic (< 280 mOsm/kg) to ICF. The intracellular movement of ECF reestablishes compartmental equilibrium at a lower osmotic pressure (<295 mOsm/kg) and minimizes fluid loss from the ICF space. **C,** Hypertonic dehydration results from ECF loss of water and electrolytes hyposmotic (< 280 mOsm/kg) to TBW. The ECF becomes hyperosmolar and hypertonic (> 310 mOsm/kg) and minimizes fluid loss from the ECF space. (From Edwards DF, et al.: Hypernatremic, hypertonic dehydration in the dog with diabetes insipidus and gastric dilatation volvulus, *J Am Vet Med Assoc* 182[9]:973-977, 1983.)

environment. Serum sodium concentrations are generally normal, and clinical signs (e.g., skin turgidity/elasticity) are proportional to the degree of hypovolemia.

Hypotonic dehydration is produced by loss of electrolytes in excess of water, as is seen in hypoadrenocorticism. In this example, excessive sodium is lost in the urine and gastrointestinal tract, creating a hypotonic extracellular compartment that loses water to both the external environment and the intracellular space. Serum sodium values are generally low in this condition, prerenal azotemia is common, and these animals exhibit more obvious signs of hypovolemia than those with isotonic dehydration (Fig. 1-25, *B*).

Hypertonic dehydration is produced by loss of water in excess of electrolytes and is the major concern after water deprivation in a dog or cat with CDI, primary NDI, or psychogenic polydipsia and in dogs and cats with inadequate fluid intake following the onset of trauma-induced CDI (Fig. 1-25, *C*). The hypertonic extracellular compartment preserves volume by dehydrating the intracellular compartment. The total water deficit is shared by fluid compartments in proportion to their normal content of water (Edwards et al, 1983). The cells, which contain two-thirds of the total body water, lose substantially more fluid than does the extracellular compartment. Plasma volume, constituting only one-twelfth of the total body water, is relatively well preserved under these circumstances. Thus hypertonic dehydration results in few of the expected signs of severe fluid depletion. Tachycardia,

lack of skin turgidity/elasticity, decreased pulse pressure, and decreased vascular volume are not detected until severe dehydration is present. Weight loss is consistently seen much sooner and further emphasizes the importance of monitoring body weight during a water deprivation test.

Severe hypernatremia with hyposthenuria are classic markers for hypertonic dehydration in the dog or cat with CDI or primary NDI. Other causes of hypernatremia are not typically associated with hyposthenuria (Box 1-4). The predominant clinical signs associated with hypertonic dehydration result from CNS dysfunction. The initial critical signs include irritability, weakness, and ataxia; as the hypernatremia worsens, stupor progresses to coma and seizures. The progression and severity of these signs depend on the rate of onset, degree, and duration of hypernatremia. Sodium has limited access to brain cells and is slow to equilibrate with the CSF. Rapidly developing severe hypernatremia results in a shift of water from the intracellular to the extracellular space and forces reduction in CSF volume as water crosses into the hyperosmotic fluid outside the CSF, causing shrinkage of the brain. Reduction in brain size leads to tearing of veins, subdural hemorrhage, and venous thrombosis. The brain synthesizes intracellular cerebral osmolar active substances (i.e., polyols) to compensate for the hyperosmolar ECF and to minimize the shift of fluid into the extracellular space. Osmolytes are produced in the brain beginning within 1 hour after induction of persistent hyperosmolality of ECF (Pollock and Arieff, 1980).

BOX 1-4   **Causes of Hypernatremia in Dogs and Cats**

Caused by Pure Water Loss
Central diabetes insipidus (CDI)*
Nephrogenic diabetes insipidus (NDI)*
Hypodipsia-adipsia
    Neurologic disease
    Abnormal thirst mechanism
    Defective osmoregulation of vasopressin release
Inadequate access to water
High environmental temperature (heat stroke)
Fever

Hypotonic Fluid Loss
Gastrointestinal fluid loss*
    Vomiting
    Diarrhea
Chronic renal failure*
Polyuric acute renal failure*
Osmotic diuresis
    Diabetes mellitus
    Mannitol infusion
Diuretic administration
Postobstructive diuresis
Cutaneous burns
Third-space loss
    Pancreatitis
    Peritonitis

Excess Sodium Retention
Primary hyperaldosteronism
Iatrogenic
    Salt poisoning
    Hypertonic saline infusion
    Sodium bicarbonate therapy
    Sodium phosphate enemas
    Parenteral nutrition*

Modified from DiBartola SP: Disorders of sodium and water: hypernatremia and hyponatremia. In DiBartola SP, editor: *Fluid, electrolyte and acid-base disorders in small animal practice,* ed 3, St Louis, 2006, Saunders/Elsevier.
*Common causes.

The goal in treating hypernatremic, hypertonic dehydration is to restore the ECF volume to normal and correct water deficits at a fluid rate that avoids significant complications. Because the brain adjusts to hypertonicity by increasing the intracellular solute content via the accumulation of idiogenic osmoles, the rapid repletion of body water with ECF dilution causes translocation of water into cells and can cause cerebral edema (Edwards et al, 1983; Reeves et al, 1998). If slower water repletion is undertaken brain cells lose the accumulated intracellular solutes and osmotic equilibrium can occur without cell swelling.

The initial priority is to restore the ECF volume to normal. The choice of fluid to be administered depends on whether circulatory collapse is present, the rate at which hypernatremia developed, and the magnitude of the hypernatremia. In patients with modest volume contraction (e.g., tachycardia, dry mucous membranes, slow skin turgor), fluid deficits should be corrected with 0.9% saline supplemented with an appropriate amount of potassium. In replacing deficits, rapid administration of fluids is contraindicated unless there are signs of significant hypovolemia. Any fluid should be administered in a volume only large enough to correct hypovolemia. Serum sodium concentration should be measured frequently (every 4 to 6 hours) to assess response to treatment and status of the CNS evaluated frequently for change in clinical signs. Worsening neurologic status or sudden onset of seizures during fluid therapy is generally indicative of cerebral edema and the need for hypertonic saline solution or mannitol therapy.

Once ECF deficits have been replaced, the serum sodium concentration should be reevaluated and water deficits corrected if hypernatremia persists. An approximation of the free water deficit in liters may be calculated using the following formula:

$$(\text{current } [Na^+] \div \text{normal } [Na^+] - 1) \times (0.6 \times \text{body weight in kg})^2$$

Oral fluid administration is preferable for correcting water deficits, with fluid administered through an IV route if oral administration is not possible. Maintenance crystalloid solutions (e.g., half-strength [0.45%] saline solution with 2.5% dextrose or half-strength lactated Ringer's solution with 2.5% dextrose) should be used to correct the water deficit in hypernatremic animals with normal perfusion and hydration and should also be used in dehydrated animals with persistent hypernatremia after the correction of fluid deficits. Dextrose 5% in water (D5W) solution can be substituted for maintenance crystalloid solutions if the hypernatremia does not abate after 12 to 24 hours of fluid therapy.

The water deficit should be replaced slowly. Approximately 50% of the water deficit should be corrected in the first 24 hours, with the remainder corrected over the ensuing 24 to 48 hours. The serum sodium concentration should decline slowly, preferably at a rate of less than 1 mEq/L/hr. The rate of fluid administration should be adjusted as needed to ensure an appropriate decrease in the serum sodium concentration. A gradual reduction in the serum sodium concentration minimizes the fluid shift from the extracellular to the intracellular compartment, thereby minimizing neuronal cell swelling and cerebral edema and increasing intracranial pressure. A deterioration in CNS status after the start of fluid therapy indicates the presence of cerebral edema and the immediate need to reduce the rate of fluid administration. Frequent monitoring of serum electrolyte concentrations, with appropriate adjustments in the type of fluid administered and rate of fluid administration, is important in the successful management of hypernatremia. It is much simpler to avoid these complications by careful monitoring during water deprivation.

Plasma Vasopressin Determinations

The direct assay of plasma AVP substantially improves the accuracy of conventional tests used in the differential diagnosis of polyuria in humans (Zerbe and Robertson, 1981). The modified water deprivation test alone is consistently correct in establishing a diagnosis of *severe* CDI, because direct measure of AVP concentrations does not alter the results of tests in which a patient did not concentrate urine during dehydration. However, inaccuracies may occur in differentiating patients with partial CDI from those with primary polydipsia and primary NDI; incorporating plasma AVP determinations into the modified water deprivation test helps differentiate these disorders.

Reports incorporating plasma AVP measurements into the modified water deprivation test are sporadic in the veterinary literature. Plasma AVP concentrations failed to increase after 5% loss of body weight by water deprivation in two dogs with primary

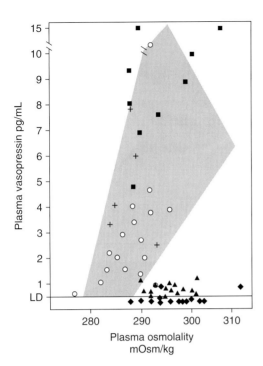

FIGURE 1-26 Relationship of plasma arginine vasopressin (AVP) to plasma osmolality after dehydration in human beings with diabetes insipidus and primary polydipsia. Note that values from patients with central diabetes insipidus (CDI) fall below the normal range *(shaded area)*, whereas those from patients with nephrogenic diabetes insipidus (NDI) and primary polydipsia are almost always within or above the normal range. (From Robertson GL: Posterior pituitary. In Felig P, et al., editors: *Endocrinology and metabolism*, ed 2, New York, 1987, McGraw Hill, p. 338.) *LD,* Limit of detection.

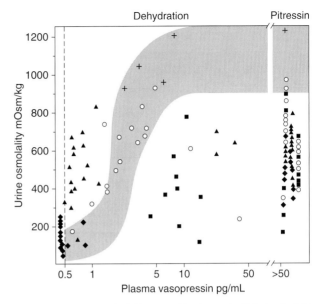

◆ = Severe diabetes insipidus   ■ = Nephrogenic diabetes insipidus
▲ = Partial diabetes insipidus   ○ = Primary polydipsia
+ = Normal subjects

FIGURE 1-27 Relationship of urine osmolality to plasma vasopressin in human beings with diabetes insipidus and primary polydipsia. Note that values obtained during dehydration in humans with central diabetes insipidus (CDI) almost always fall within or above the normal range, whereas those from patients with nephrogenic diabetes insipidus (NDI) fall uniformly below normal. Values in most humans with primary polydipsia are normal, but a few may be subnormal, presumably as a consequence of washout of the medullary concentration gradient. (From Robertson GL: Posterior pituitary. In Felig P, et al., editors: *Endocrinology and metabolism,* ed 2, New York, 1987, McGraw Hill, p. 338.)

CDI compared with normal dogs (Post et al, 1989). Plasma AVP concentration was 3.3 and 3.7 pg/mL in these two dogs versus a mean of 31.3 pg/mL in three healthy dogs after water deprivation. A similar deficiency in plasma AVP after water deprivation was identified in a cat with CDI (plasma AVP, 1.3 pg/mL versus a mean of 84.6 pg/mL in eight healthy cats) (Brown et al, 1993). Plasma AVP concentrations remained within or below the reference range (i.e., less than 7 pg/mL) during water deprivation in four dogs with suspected primary polydipsia that were subsequently identified with a disturbance in the regulation of AVP secretion (van Vonderen et al, 1999).

When measurement of plasma AVP is incorporated into the modified water deprivation test, plasma for AVP determination should be obtained after 3% loss of body weight is caused by water deprivation but before exogenous AVP is administered (i.e., at the end of phase I). Plasma for AVP determination can also be obtained prior to water deprivation, although this may not be necessary. Commercially available canine and feline plasma AVP assays are not widely available in the United States, but this may change in the near future. Recently a commercially available human enzyme immunoassay kit for measurement of plasma AVP concentration was validated for use in dogs and the plasma concentration of AVP was significantly higher in dogs with congestive heart failure, compared with healthy dogs; results that suggest the assay may be diagnostically useful in dogs with suspected diabetes insipidus (Scollan et al, 2013).

In humans, the plasma AVP value is interpreted in conjunction with the concurrent plasma and urine osmolality. When evaluating plasma AVP and plasma osmolality *concurrently* after dehydration, values from humans with severe or partial CDI fall below the normal range, whereas those from humans with NDI or primary polydipsia are almost always within or above the normal range (Fig. 1-26; Robertson, 1988). When plasma AVP and urine osmolality are evaluated *concurrently* after dehydration, values from humans with severe or partial CDI almost always fall within or above the normal range, whereas those from humans with NDI fall uniformly below normal (Fig. 1-27). In most cases, the values from humans with primary polydipsia are normal, but a few may be subnormal, presumably as a consequence of renal medullary solute washout. The AVP response to IV infusion of 20% saline was evaluated in conjunction with plasma and urine osmolality and results did not consistently distinguish between CDI, NDI, and primary polydipsia in 18 young dogs with polyuria and polydipsia suspected to have one of the these three disorders (van Vonderen et al, 2004). The authors speculated that the results of the study raise doubt about the generally accepted notion that AVP measurements during hypertonic saline infusion are the "gold standard" for the diagnostic interpretation of polyuria in dogs.

Until more extensive studies have been completed, we interpret plasma AVP concentrations after dehydration as follows: patients with severe or partial CDI should have AVP deficiencies, and those with primary NDI or primary/psychogenic polydipsia should have normal or excessive concentrations of AVP in the face of dehydration and subnormal urine osmolality (Table 1-5).

TABLE 1-5   RESULTS OF DIAGNOSTIC STUDIES IN DOGS WITH CENTRAL DIABETES INSIPIDUS, NEPHROGENIC DIABETES INSIPIDUS, AND PSYCHOGENIC POLYDIPSIA

TEST	CENTRAL DIABETES INSIPIDUS	NEPHROGENIC DIABETES INSIPIDUS	PSYCHOGENIC POLYDIPSIA
Random plasma osmolality	Normal or ↑	Normal or ↑	Normal or ↓
Random urine osmolality	↓	↓	↓
Urine osmolality after water deprivation (≥ 3% loss of body weight)	No change	No change	↑
Urine osmolality during hypertonic saline infusion	No change	No change	↑
Urine osmolality after vasopressin administration	↑	No change	No change or mild ↑
Plasma vasopressin after water deprivation (≥ 3% loss of body weight)	Low	Normal or high	Normal or high

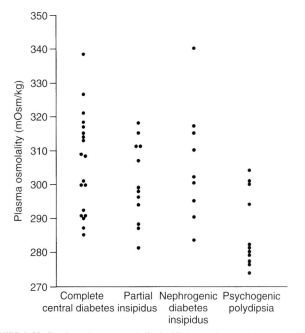

 FIGURE 1-28 Random plasma osmolality in 19 dogs with complete central diabetes insipidus (CDI), 12 dogs with partial CDI, 9 dogs with primary nephrogenic diabetes insipidus (NDI), and 11 dogs with primary (psychogenic) polydipsia. Note the overlap in values between groups of dogs.

RANDOM PLASMA OSMOLALITY AS A DIAGNOSTIC TOOL

Measurement of random plasma osmolality may help identify primary or psychogenic polydipsia and should be done while the dog or cat has unrestricted access to water. Plasma osmolality in normal dogs and cats is approximately 280 to 300 pOsm. Dogs and cats with CDI and NDI have a primary polyuric disorder with secondary compensatory polydipsia; that is, they drink excessively because they urinate excessively. The stimulation for water intake in CDI and NDI is loss of free water through the kidneys, resulting in decreased blood volume and increased serum osmolality. Thus, patients with CDI and NDI should have high normal or high plasma osmolalities (Fig. 1-28). In contrast, dogs with primary or psychogenic polydipsia have a primary polydipsic disorder with secondary compensatory polyuria; that is, they urinate

excessively because they drink excessively. In these dogs, uncontrollable fluid intake raises blood volume and decreases plasma osmolality, which in turn causes decreased secretion of AVP and a decreased renal medullary concentration gradient, resulting in large urine volumes. Dogs with psychogenic polydipsia, in theory, should have plasma osmolalities on the low end of or below the reference interval.

It should be pointed out that the above discussion applies to the "classic" situation. Unfortunately, nature rarely provides us with "classic" patients. This is illustrated in a study of polyuric humans, in whom the serum osmolality varied from 281 to 298 sOsm in CDI, 285 to 292 in NDI, and 275 to 291 in primary polydipsia (Zerbe and Robertson, 1981). In our series of dogs, as well as those reported in the literature, plasma osmolality varied from 281 to 339 pOsm in CDI, 283 to 340 in NDI, and 274 to 304 in psychogenic polydipsia (see Fig. 1-28). Based on our experiences, a random plasma osmolality of less than 280 pOsm obtained while the dog or cat has free access to water suggests primary or psychogenic polydipsia, whereas a plasma osmolality greater than 280 pOsm is consistent with CDI, NDI, or psychogenic polydipsia.

 ## ADDITIONAL DIAGNOSTIC TESTS: COMPUTED TOMOGRAPHY AND MAGNETIC RESONANCE IMAGING

Neoplasia in the region of the pituitary and hypothalamus should be considered in the older dog or cat in which CDI develops. A complete neurologic evaluation, including CT or MRI may be warranted before idiopathic CDI is arbitrarily diagnosed, especially if the client is willing to consider radiation therapy or chemotherapy should a tumor be identified (see Fig. 1-9).

MRI has been used to identify the presence of vasopressin in the posterior pituitary in humans. On T1-weighted images, MRI produces a bright spot in the sella caused by stored hormone in the neurosecretory granules in the posterior pituitary (Moses et al, 1992; Kurokawa et al, 1998). The bright spot is present in approximately 80% of normal humans and is absent in patients with CDI, although some studies have identified a bright spot in patients with clinical evidence of CDI (Maghnie et al., 1997; Saeki et al., 2003). The bright spot decreases with a prolonged stimulus for vasopressin secretion and has been variably reported in other polyuric disorders (Fujisawa et al, 2004). A bright spot in the region of the posterior pituitary has also been identified in dogs and presumably represents vasopressin stored in neurosecretory

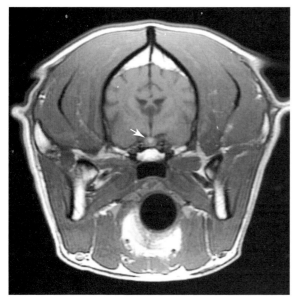

FIGURE 1-29 Magnetic resonance imaging (MRI) T1-weighted transverse image of the pituitary gland in a healthy adult dog illustrating the hyperintense "bright spot" *(arrow)* in the sella. In humans, the bright spot is caused by stored arginine vasopressin (AVP) in the neurosecretory granules in the posterior pituitary. Presumably the same is true in dogs.

granules (Fig. 1-29). Studies evaluating changes in the presence and intensity of the bright spot in dogs with polyuric disorders have not yet been reported.

 TREATMENT

Therapeutic options for dogs and cats with diabetes insipidus are listed in Box 1-5.

Vasopressin Analogues (Used in Central Diabetes Insipidus and Partial Central Diabetes Insipidus)

The synthetic analogue of vasopressin, DDAVP (see Fig. 1-1), is the standard therapy for CDI. DDAVP has almost three times the antidiuretic action of AVP with minimal-to-no vasopressor or oxytocic activity (Robinson, 1976). Several extrarenal actions of DDAVP have also been described: release of two coagulation factors (Factor VIIIc and von Willebrand factor (Richardson and Robinson, 1985); a decrease in blood pressure and peripheral resistance; and an increase in plasma renin activity (Schwartz et al, 1985).

The metabolism of DDAVP in humans follows a bi-exponential curve with first and second half-lives of 7.8 and 75.5 minutes, respectively. Similar findings are noted in experiments with normal dogs (Ferring, 1985) and in spontaneous canine cases of CDI. Additionally, blood chemistry studies and necropsies on treated dogs (Ferring, 1985) and clinical experience in dogs and cats with CDI (Kraus, 1987; Harb et al, 1996; Oliveira et al, 2013) indicate that the drug is safe for use in dogs and cats.

The intranasal DDAVP preparation (DDAVP nasal, 2.5- and 5.0-mL bottles containing 100 μg DDAVP/mL) is used most commonly for treating CDI in humans and is effective for the treatment of CDI in dogs and cats (Harb et al, 1996). Administration of DDAVP nasal to dogs and cats via the intranasal route is possible but not recommended. DDAVP nasal should be

---

BOX 1-5 **Therapies Available for Polydipsic/Polyuric Dogs with Central Diabetes Insipidus, Nephrogenic Diabetes Insipidus, or Primary (Psychogenic) Polydipsia**

A. CDI (severe)
  1. DDAVP
    a. Effective
    b. Expensive
    c. Oral tablets or drops of nasal solution in conjunctival sac
    d. DDAVP injection SC once or twice a day
  2. LVP (lypressin [Diapid])
    a. Short duration of action; less potent than DDAVP
    b. Expensive
    c. Requires drops into nose or conjunctival sac
  3. No treatment—provide continuous source of water
B. CDI (partial)
  1. DDAVP
  2. LVP
  3. Chlorpropamide
    a. 30% to 70% effective
    b. Inexpensive
    c. Pill form
    d. Takes 1 to 2 weeks to obtain effect of drug
    e. May cause hypoglycemia
  4. Thiazide diuretics
    a. Mildly effective
    b. Inexpensive
    c. Pill form
    d. Should be used with low-sodium diet
  5. Low-sodium diet
  6. No treatment—provide continuous source of water
C. NDI
  1. Thiazide diuretics—as described earlier
  2. Low sodium diet
  3. No treatment—provide continuous source of water
D. Primary (psychogenic) polydipsia
  1. Water restriction at times
  2. Water limitation
  3. Behavior modification
    a. Change environment
    b. Change in daily routine
    c. Increase daily exercise
    d. Increase contact with humans or dogs

CDI, Central diabetes insipidus; *DDAVP*, desmopressin acetate; *LVP*, lysine vasopressin; *NDI*, nephrogenic diabetes insipidus; *SC*, subcutaneous.

---

transferred to a sterile eye dropper bottle and drops placed into the conjunctival sac of the dog or cat. Although the solution is acidic, ocular irritation rarely occurs. One drop of DDAVP nasal contains 1.5 to 4 μg of DDAVP, and a dosage of one to two drops administered once or twice daily controls signs of CDI in most dogs and cats.

Because of the expense of DDAVP nasal and loss of DDAVP drops from the conjunctival sac with head shaking, blinking, and inadvertent application of excessive amounts, our preference is to initially use DDAVP tablets (0.1 and 0.2 mg) when using response to DDAVP to establish the diagnosis of CDI and for long-term treatment of CDI. Clinical response in humans is variable, in part, because the bioavailability of DDAVP tablets is approximately 5% to 15% of the intranasal dose in humans. Similar information is not available for dogs and cats. Our initial dose for DDAVP tablets is 0.05 mg for dogs weighing less than 5 kg and for cats, 0.1 mg for dogs weighing 5 to 20 kg, and 0.2 mg for dogs weighing more than 20 kg given every 12 hours. The frequency of administration is increased to every 8 hours if unacceptable polyuria and polydipsia persist 1 week after therapy is initiated. Treatment should be switched to DDAVP nasal if there is minimal to no response to oral DDAVP administered three times a day. Decreasing the frequency of administration of the tablets, decreasing the dose of DDAVP, or both can be tried once clinical response has been documented. To date, most dogs and cats have required 0.1 to 0.2 mg and 0.025 to 0.05 mg, respectively, of oral DDAVP two to three times a day to control polyuria and polydipsia (Aroch et al, 2005).

DDAVP parenteral (2 mL vials containing 4 μg/mL) can be used in lieu of the nasal formulation or oral tablets. In humans, parenteral administration of DDAVP is 5 to 20 times as potent as DDAVP nasal (Richardson and Robinson, 1985). The initial parenteral dosage of DDAVP is 0.5 to 1.0 μg administered SC once a day. Subsequent adjustments in the dose and frequency of administration are based on improvement in polyuria and polydipsia, duration of clinical response, and changes in serum sodium concentration. Hyponatremia is more apt to develop with parenteral DDAVP than with tablets or nasal spray and can mimic the syndrome of inappropriate vasopressin secretion.

In humans with CDI, a decrease in urine volume usually occurs within 2 hours after administration of DDAVP, regardless of the route of administration, and the total duration of action varies from 6 to 18 hours (Lam et al, 1996). Larger doses of DDAVP appear both to increase its antidiuretic effects and to prolong its duration of action; however, expense becomes a limiting factor. The medication may be administered exclusively in the evening as insurance against nocturia.

We have had excellent results in dogs and cats receiving daily medication for longer than 5 years. Owners of dogs and cats with CDI have reported that their pets become accustomed to receiving eye drops, mentioning eye or conjunctival irritation as an infrequent complication. If polyuria and polydipsia recur despite DDAVP therapy, several possibilities should be considered, including problems with owner compliance or administration technique, inadequate dose, outdated or inactivated DDAVP, or development of a concurrent disorder causing polyuria and polydipsia. Hyperadrenocorticism is the primary differential diagnosis when polyuria and polydipsia recur despite DDAVP treatment in a dog with CDI.

DDAVP was effective in Husky puppies with familial NDI caused by a defect in V_2 receptor binding affinity for AVP (Luzius et al, 1992). However, extremely high dosages (0.33 U/kg body weight intramuscularly three times a day) of DDAVP were required to obtain improvement in polyuria and polydipsia, dosages that most owners would consider cost-prohibitive. For practical purposes, DDAVP is considered ineffective in the treatment of NDI.

Oral Agents (Used in Central Diabetes Insipidus, Partial Central Diabetes Insipidus, Nephrogenic Diabetes Insipidus, and Primary Polydipsia)

Chlorpropamide

Chlorpropamide (Diabinese) is an oral sulfonylurea drug used for the treatment of hyperglycemia in humans. Largely by chance, chlorpropamide has also been found to be efficacious in treating humans with CDI and has been found to reduce urine output 30% to 70% in humans afflicted with partial CDI. This reduction

is associated with a proportional rise in urine osmolality, correction of dehydration, and a reduction in fluid consumption similar to that observed with small doses of vasopressin (Robertson, 1981).

The exact mechanism of the potentiating effect of chlorpropamide on the action of AVP in the kidney is not known. Chlorpropamide may enhance AVP stimulation of renal medullary cAMP by augmenting adenylate cyclase sensitivity to AVP or by inhibiting phosphodiesterase (Reeves et al, 1998). Inhibition of prostaglandin E_2 (PGE_2) synthesis, thereby removing an antagonist of AVP, has also been proposed as a mechanism for chlorpropamide potentiation. Finally, chlorpropamide treatment may augment AVP dependent NaCl absorption by the medullary thick ascending loop of Henle, thereby increasing the driving force for water absorption in collecting ducts (Kusano et al, 1983). Like DDAVP, chlorpropamide is ineffective in treating patients with NDI. Other drugs of the sulfonylurea class do not have a significant antidiuretic effect in CDI and, in some humans, may actually be mildly diuretic.

The effectiveness of chlorpropamide in the treatment of canine CDI is a matter unresolved in the literature. As in humans, use of the drug in dogs requires the presence of some endogenous AVP. Some veterinarians have had little or no success using chlorpropamide, citing a reduction in urine volume of only 18% during 7 days of therapy (Schwartz Porsche, 1980). Other veterinarians have claimed a 50% reduction in urine volume after 5 days of therapy. The drug has also had mixed results when used in cats with CDI (Kraus, 1987).

An effective dosage of chlorpropamide for the treatment of partial CDI has not been determined in the dog or cat, although 10 to 40 mg/kg/day has been suggested (Hardy, 1982). The dose of chlorpropamide used in the unsuccessful study in dogs was 250 mg twice daily (Schwartz Porsche, 1980) and was approximately 30 mg/kg/day in one cat that failed to respond (Kraus, 1987). The dosage was not mentioned in the dog study and was approximately 10 mg/kg/day in one cat in which chlorpropamide improved polyuria and polydipsia.

The primary adverse effect of chlorpropamide is hypoglycemia caused by chlorpropamide-induced insulin secretion. Regular feeding schedules should be adhered to if hypoglycemic problems are to be avoided. We have had little experience with chlorpropamide simply because our success with DDAVP has been excellent, and our owners have accepted the cost and difficulties encountered in treating their pets with this drug. If successful in a trial administration period, chlorpropamide may prove to be a valid alternative in treating partial CDI.

Thiazide Diuretics

The thiazide diuretics may reduce the polyuria in animals with diabetes insipidus (Breitschwerdt et al, 1981). This seemingly paradoxic effect is seen in NDI, as well as in CDI, suggesting that this therapeutic agent has a mode of action distinct from that of chlorpropamide. By inhibiting sodium reabsorption in the ascending limb of the loop of Henle, the thiazides reduce total body sodium concentrations, thus contracting the ECF volume and increasing salt and water resorption in the proximal renal tubule. This results in lower sodium concentrations in the distal renal tubule and less osmotic effect to maintain tubular volume, resulting in a reduction in urine volume. The net effect in diabetes insipidus is to cause a slight rise in urine osmolality and a proportionate reduction in urine volume. Depending on sodium intake, polyuria can be reduced 30% to 50% in humans with NDI or CDI. Apart from occasional hypokalemia, significant side effects are uncommon. The thiazides reduce the ability to excrete a water load and, if given to a patient with primary polydipsia, may precipitate water intoxication (Robertson, 1981).

Chlorothiazides are recommended at a dose of 20 to 40 mg/kg twice daily, in concert with low-sodium diets. Periodic serum electrolyte determinations (every 2 to 3 months) should aid in avoiding iatrogenic problems.

Sodium Chloride (Salt) Restriction

Restricting salt intake, as the sole therapy in diabetes insipidus, reduces urine output by increasing the volume of filtrate absorbed isosmotically in the proximal nephron. This simple therapy may be helpful in the treatment of both CDI and NDI. Salt content of commercial dog and cat foods is quite variable, ranging from 0.14 to 3.27 g Na/Mcal for dog foods and 0.3 to 4.0 g Na/Mcal for cat foods. In general, diets considered lower in sodium content contain less than 1.0 g Na/Mcal.

No Treatment

Therapy for diabetes insipidus (CDI and NDI) and primary polydipsia is not mandatory as long as the dog or cat has unlimited access to water and is maintained in an environment where polyuria does not create problems. In most instances, untreated pets are outdoor animals. Some of our owners have elected not to treat their pets after the diagnosis is established. More commonly, owners have discontinued DDAVP treatment after 1 or 2 months of therapy, primarily because of the expense. Still others treat their pet with DDAVP periodically, when it is undesirable for the dog or cat to be exhibiting severe polyuria and polydipsia (e.g., relatives staying at the house). If an owner elects not to treat his or her pet, it is imperative that the dog or cat have access to a constant water supply because relatively short periods of water restriction can have catastrophic results, such as the development of hypernatremic, hypertonic dehydration, and neurologic signs; a complication that would occur with CDI and primary NDI but not psychogenic polydipsia.

Behavior Modification (Used in Psychogenic Polydipsia)

Water Restriction

Gradually limiting water intake to amounts in the high normal range (60 to 80 mL/kg/24 h) improves and may resolve polyuria and polydipsia in dogs with psychogenic polydipsia. In some dogs, rapid water restriction results in bizarre behavior, excessive barking, urine consumption, and dehydration. Therefore, we prefer to have the owner first calculate the dog's approximate water intake per 24 hours while free-choice water is allowed. This volume of water is then reduced by 10% per week until water volumes of 60 to 80 mL/kg/24 h are reached. The total 24-hour volume of water should be divided into several aliquots, with the last aliquot given at bedtime. Oral salt (1 g/30 kg twice a day) and/or oral sodium bicarbonate (0.6 g/30 kg twice a day) may also be administered for 3 to 5 days, to reestablish the medullary concentration gradient. We have had excellent success with gradual water restriction and do not routinely use oral salt or sodium bicarbonate.

Change in Environment

Changes in the dog's environment or daily routine should also be considered for dogs with psychogenic polydipsia, such as initiating a daily exercise routine, bringing a second pet into the home, providing some distraction (e.g., a radio playing when the clients are not home), or moving the dog to an area with an increased amount of contact with humans.

PROGNOSIS

Dogs and cats with idiopathic or congenital CDI usually become asymptomatic with appropriate therapy, and with proper care these animals have an excellent life expectancy. Unfortunately, many owners discontinue DDAVP therapy or elect euthanasia of their pet after a few months because of the expense of DDAVP. Without therapy, these animals often lead acceptable lives as long as water is constantly provided and they are housed in an environment that cannot be damaged by severe polyuria. However, the untreated animal is always at risk for developing life-threatening dehydration if water is withdrawn for longer than a few hours. Additionally, even mild illness that causes vomiting or reduces water intake can develop into one associated with severe dehydration. Thus, untreated dogs and cats carry a guarded prognosis.

In one study, long-term follow-up of 19 dogs with CDI found 7 of 19 dogs still alive a mean of 29 months (median, 30 months) from the time of diagnosis of CDI (Harb et al, 1996). Six of these seven dogs were 3 years of age or younger at the time CDI was diagnosed. Of the original 19 dogs, 12 had died within an average of 6 months (median, 2 months) after diagnosis of CDI. Three dogs died from unrelated or unknown causes, two dogs were euthanized shortly after the diagnosis of CDI was established, and seven dogs died or were euthanized because of development of neurologic disease. In these later seven dogs, neurologic signs developed 2 months (median, 1 month; range, 0.5 to 5 months) and the dogs were dead 3.3 months (median, 1.5 months; range, 1 to 7 months) after CDI was diagnosed (Harb et al, 1996). A mass in the region of the pituitary gland was identified by CT scan or at necropsy in six of the dogs in which these procedures were performed. The seven dogs that developed neurologic signs were older than 6 years of age.

Obviously, dogs with aggressive hypothalamic or pituitary problems, such as a growing tumor, have a grave prognosis. Treatment of tumors in the region of the hypothalamus and pituitary, using either irradiation (see Chapter 10) or chemotherapy (e.g., bis-chloroethylnitrosourea [BCNU]), can be tried; however, results are unpredictable. Polyuria and polydipsia typically persists despite radiation therapy, in part, because clinical signs of CDI do not develop until 90% of the magnocellular neurons are destroyed (Robinson and Verbalis, 2011). Based on experience with pituitary macrotumors, successful response to radiation therapy is more likely when the tumor is small and before neurologic clinical signs develop. CT or MRI scan is warranted at the time of diagnosis of CDI, especially when CDI is acquired in an older dog or cat.

The prognosis for dogs and cats with primary NDI is guarded to poor because of limited therapeutic options, the generally poor response to therapy, and the risk for developing severe dehydration and hypernatremia. The prognosis with acquired NDI depends on the prognosis of the primary problem.

The prognosis in psychogenic polydipsia is usually excellent. Water restriction and some form of behavior modification help most of these animals to become asymptomatic, although relapses do occur.

SYNDROME OF INAPPROPRIATE VASOPRESSIN SECRETION: EXCESS VASOPRESSIN

A primary excess of AVP occurs in two clinical settings—in the syndrome of inappropriate antidiuretic hormone (SIADH) and as a consequence of drugs that stimulate AVP secretion, activate renal V_2 receptors, or potentiate the antidiuretic effect of AVP (Box 1-6). In SIADH, sustained release of AVP occurs in

---

BOX 1-6   Drugs and Hormones Reported to Affect Vasopressin Secretion or Action

Secretion

Stimulate AVP release	Inhibit AVP release
Acetylcholine	α-Adrenergic drugs
Anesthetic agents	ANP
Angiotensin II	Glucocorticoids
Apomorphine	Haloperidol
β-Adrenergic drugs	Oxilorphan
Barbiturates	Phenytoin
Carbamazepine	Promethazine
Clofibrate	
Cyclophosphamide	
Histamine	
Insulin	
Metoclopramide	
Morphine and narcotic analogues	
PGE_2	
Vincristine	

Renal

Potentiate AVP action	Inhibit AVP action
Aspirin	α-Adrenergic drugs
Carbamazepine	ANP
Chlorpropamide	Barbiturates
Nonsteroidal anti-inflammatory agents	Demeclocycline
Thiazides	Glucocorticoids
	Hypercalcemia
	Hypokalemia
	Methoxyflurane
	PGE_2
	Protein kinase C
	Tetracyclines
	Vinca alkaloids

ANP, Atrial natriuretic peptide; *AVP,* arginine vasopressin; PGE_2, prostaglandin E_2.

BOX 1-7   Conditions Associated with Syndrome of Inappropriate Antidiuretic Hormone in Humans

Malignant Neoplasia
Carcinoma; bronchogenic, pancreatic, prostatic, bladder
Lymphoma and leukemia
Thymoma and mesothelioma

Drug-Induced
ACE inhibitors
Chlorpropamide
Clofibrate
Clozapine
Cyclophosphamide
Omeprazole
Serotonin reuptake inhibitors
Thiazides
Vincristine
Others

Central Nervous System Disorders
Degenerative/demyelinating diseases
Head trauma
Infection
Inflammatory diseases
Porphyria
Tumors

Endocrine Diseases
Adrenal insufficiency
Pituitary insufficiency
Hypothyroidism

Pulmonary Disorders
Acute respiratory failure
Aspergillosis
Bacterial and viral pneumonia
Tuberculosis

Adapted from Ramsay DJ: Posterior pituitary gland. In Greenspan FS, Fosham PH, editors: *Basic and clinical endocrinology,* Los Altos, CA, 1983, Lange Medical Publications, p. 120.
ACE, Angiotensin converting enzyme.

---

the absence of either osmotic or nonosmotic stimuli. In humans, SIADH has been observed in a variety of disorders, particularly pulmonary, CNS, and neoplastic disorders (Box 1-7) (Robinson and Verbalis, 2011). The most common association of SIADH is with tumors, most notably bronchogenic carcinomas. Vasopressin or a peptide having comparable biologic activity is produced by tumors. SIADH is rare in the dog and cat and has been reported in one dog with heartworm disease, one dog with liver disease, one dog with an undifferentiated carcinoma, one dog with a tumor in the region of the hypothalamus, one cat following anesthesia, laparoscopy and metoclopramide treatment, and was considered idiopathic in two dogs (Rijnberk et al, 1988; Houston et al, 1989; Cameron and Gallagher, 2010; Kang and Park, 2012).

As a result of sustained release of AVP or AVP-like peptides, patients retain ingested water and become hyponatremic and modestly volume-expanded and generally gain body weight (Robinson and Verbalis, 2011). This volume expansion results in reduced rates of proximal tubular sodium absorption and, consequently, natriuresis. Increased levels of ANP also contribute to the natriuresis. The diagnostic features that characterize this syndrome include hyponatremia, clinical euvolemia as defined by the absence of signs of hypovolemia (e.g., decreased skin turgor, tachycardia) and hypervolemia (e.g., subcutaneous edema,

ascites), plasma hyposmolality (< 275 pOsm), urine osmolality greater than that appropriate for the concomitant osmolality of plasma, and increased renal sodium excretion despite hyponatremia. A similar clinical picture can be produced experimentally by giving high doses of AVP to a normal subject who receives a normal to increased fluid intake, with subcutaneous administration of high doses of parenteral DDAVP to dogs with CDI, and theoretically with administration of DDAVP to dogs with psychogenic polydipsia. Water restriction results in the plasma osmolality and serum sodium concentrations returning to normal (Aron et al, 2001; Cameron and Gallagher, 2010).

Four patterns of plasma AVP secretion have been described in humans with SIADH, suggesting four patterns of osmoregulatory defects in this syndrome. The most common derangement is random hypersecretion of AVP independent of osmotic and nonosmotic control (Robinson and Verbalis, 2011). This erratic and irregular secretion of AVP can be associated with both malignant and nonmalignant disease. Others include a "reset osmostat" system in which the threshold for AVP secretion is abnormally low but there is an appropriate response to changes in osmolality, an "AVP leak" pattern characterized by inappropriate nonsuppressible basal AVP secretion but normal secretion in response to osmolar changes above plasma osmolality, and low to undetectable AVP concentrations despite classic clinical characteristics of SIADH. The pattern of SIADH that occurs without measureable AVP secretion may represent increased renal sensitivity to low circulating AVP concentrations, which is possibly a result of an activating mutation of the V_2 receptor (Kamoi, 1997; Feldman et al, 2005). Thus far, it has not been possible to correlate the pattern of AVP abnormality with the pathology of the syndrome. The threshold and sensitivity of vasopressin secretion were studied by infusion of hypertonic saline in two dogs with idiopathic SIADH (Rijnberk et al, 1988). One dog demonstrated a pattern of reset osmostat and the other, a pattern consistent with vasopressin leak.

Clinical signs of hyponatremia include lethargy, anorexia, vomiting, weakness, muscle fasciculations, obtundation, disorientation, seizures, and coma. CNS signs are the most worrisome, occur when hyponatremia is severe (< 120 mEq/L), and develop as changes in plasma osmolality cause fluid to shift from the extracellular to the intracellular space, resulting in neuronal swelling and lysis. The onset and severity of clinical signs depend on the rapidity with which the hyponatremia develops as well as on the degree of hyponatremia. The more chronic the hyponatremia and the more slowly it develops, the more capable the brain is of compensating for changes in osmolality through the loss of potassium and organic osmolytes from cells. Clinical signs develop when the decrease in plasma osmolality occurs faster than the brain's defense mechanisms can counter the influx of water into neurons.

The diagnosis of SIADH is made by excluding other causes of hyponatremia (see Chapter 12) and meeting the following criteria: hyponatremia with plasma hyposmolality; inappropriately high urine osmolality in the presence of plasma hyposmolality; normal renal and adrenal function; presence of natriuresis despite hyponatremia; no evidence of hypovolemia (e.g., decreased skin turgor, tachycardia), ascites or edema; and correction of hyponatremia with fluid restriction (Reeves et al, 1998). Another supportive criterion is an inappropriately increased plasma AVP concentration in relation to plasma osmolality. However, plasma AVP concentrations are often in the reference range in humans with SIADH and are abnormal only in relation to plasma osmolality (Fig. 1-30), some patients do not have measurably increased plasma AVP concentrations, and most disorders causing solute and volume depletion are associated with appropriately increased plasma AVP concentrations (Robinson and Verbalis, 2011).

Treatment is directed toward alleviation of hyponatremia and elimination of the underlying disease causing SIADH. The goal of treatment directed at the hyponatremia is to correct body water osmolality and restore cell volume to normal by raising the ratio of sodium to water in ECF using IV fluid therapy, water restriction, or both. The increase in ECF osmolality draws water from cells and therefore reduces their volume. Rapid correction of severe hyponatremia can result in demyelination in white matter areas of the brain, a syndrome referred to as osmotic demyelination syndrome, and must be avoided (Verbalis and Martinez, 1991). This pathologic disorder is believed to be precipitated by brain dehydration that occurs after correction of serum sodium concentration towards normal (Sterns et al, 1989). Because loss of brain idiogenic osmoles represents one of the compensatory mechanisms for preserving brain cell volume during dilutional states, an increase in serum sodium concentration toward normal (greater than 140 mEq/L) is relatively hypertonic to brain cells that are partially depleted of idiogenic osmoles as a result of hyponatremia (Sterns et al, 1989; Sterns et al, 1993). Consequently, raising the serum

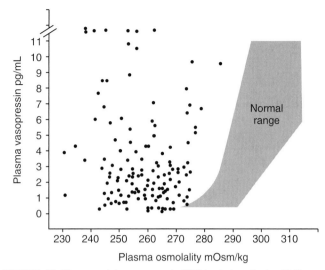

FIGURE 1-30 Plasma arginine vasopressin (AVP) levels in patients with the syndrome of inappropriate antidiuretic hormone (SIADH) secretion as a function of plasma osmolality. Each point depicts one patient at a single point in time. The *shaded area* represents AVP levels in normal subjects over physiologic ranges of plasma osmolality. (Modified from Zerbe RL, Stropes L, Robertson GL: Vasopressin function in the syndrome of inappropriate antidiuresis, *Annu Rev Med* 31:315-327, 1980. In Robertson GL, et al: Neurogenic disorders of osmoregulation, *Am J Med* 72: 339, 1982.)

sodium concentration rapidly to greater than 125 mEq/L can cause demyelination in the CNS (Ayus et al, 1987; Sterns et al, 1994).

Humans and presumably dogs and cats with SIADH are assumed to have chronic hyponatremia, arbitrarily defined as the presence of hyponatremia of less than 130 mEq/L for 48 hours or longer. The current recommendation for correcting severe chronic hyponatremia is to increase the serum sodium concentration slowly at a rate of approximately 0.5 to 1.0 mEq/L per hour using intravenously administered normal (0.9%) or hypertonic (3% to 5%) saline. Adjustments in the rate of fluid administration or composition of the fluid should be based on results of frequent assessment of serum electrolyte concentrations and the patient's CNS status. Once the serum sodium concentration is greater than 125 mEq/L, further correction of hyponatremia is accomplished by restricting water intake. Reduction of fluid intake to the point at which urinary and insensible losses induce a negative water balance leads to restoration of normal body fluid volume, reduction in urinary sodium excretion, and increased serum sodium concentration.

Long term treatment of SIADH includes discontinuation of any drugs known to be associated with SIADH and daily restriction of water intake. The approach to water restriction is similar to that used to treat dogs with psychogenic polydipsia (see Psychogenic Polydipsia under Responses to the Modified Water Deprivation Test earlier in this chapter). However, the goal of water restriction for SIADH is to identify a daily water intake that maintains the serum sodium concentration near the lower end of the reference range. Additional treatments for SIADH in humans include agents that interfere with AVP signaling (e.g., demeclocycline) and AVP receptor antagonists (e.g., tolvaptan). There are no reports on the use of demeclocycline for SIADH in dogs or cats. Treatment of a dog with SIADH with tolvaptan (Otsuka Pharmaceuticals) at a dose of 3 mg/kg orally every 12 hours resulted in a marked increase in free-water excretion and significant palliation of clinical signs with no discernible side effects detected over a 3-year treatment period (Fleeman et al, 2000).

HYPODIPSIC HYPERNATREMIA

Hypodipsic hypernatremia is a neurologic disorder causing diminished sensation of thirst and diminished release of AVP in response to osmotic stimulation. Hypodipsic hypernatremia is characterized by chronic hypernatremia in a setting of euvolemia, normal renal function, decreased thirst perception, and a normal renal response to exogenous AVP (Reeves et al, 1998). Despite elevations of serum sodium concentration and ECF osmolalities, affected patients exhibit hypodipsia and an inappropriately dilute urine for the corresponding plasma osmolality. The primary defect in human patients with hypodipsic hypernatremia appears to be an insensitivity of thirst centers and osmoreceptors to osmotic stimuli. Affected patients have a normal response of AVP release, measured either as a rise in urine osmolality or as an increase in plasma AVP levels, to baroreceptor stimulation following volume contraction.

Given the association of a diminished sensation of thirst and a diminished release of AVP in response to osmotic stimulation, it is likely that hypodipsic hypernatremia represents a more or less specific ablation of hypothalamic osmoreceptor function. In humans, hypodipsic hypernatremia has been reported in children as a congenital disease and in adults in association with CNS histiocytosis, pineal tumors, surgery for craniopharyngioma, head trauma, and vascular disturbances (e.g., ischemia, hemorrhage). Necropsy has been performed in six dogs with hypodipsic hypernatremia and revealed hypothalamic dysplasia in a 4½-month-old Dalmatian (Bagley et al, 1993); hydrocephalus in an adult mixed-breed dog (DiBartola et al, 1994); astrogliosis and neuronal degeneration in the region of the hypothalamus and thalamus in a 7-month-old Miniature Schnauzer (Crawford et al, 1984); focal, severe meningoencephalitis in the hypothalamus in a 7-year-old Doberman Pinscher (Mackay and Curtis, 1999); lobar holoprosencephaly in a 9-month-old Miniature Schnauzer (Sullivan et al, 2003); and no identifiable lesions in the anterior, third cerebral ventricular area, hypothalamus or pituitary gland in a 5-month-old Great Dane (Hawks et al, 1991). Results of an MRI of the CNS in a 6-month-old Miniature Schnauzer with hypodipsic hypernatremia revealed dysgenesis of the corpus callosum and other forebrain structures (Miyama et al, 2009). Hypodipsic hypernatremia has also been described in a 14-month-old Miniature Schnauzer (Hoskins and Rothschmitt, 1984), but the dog was still alive at the time of the report. Hypodipsic hypernatremia was also reported in a 7-month-old Domestic Short-Haired cat in which hydrocephalus was identified with CT imaging (Dow et al, 1987).

Interestingly, congenital hypodipsic hypernatremia has been identified most commonly in Miniature Schnauzers.

Dogs and cats typically present to the veterinarian with signs related to hypernatremia (i.e., lethargy, inappetence, weakness, neurologic signs). Consistent findings on physical examination and initial clinical pathology include dehydration, hypernatremia, hyperchloridemia, prerenal azotemia, and urine specific gravities greater than 1.030. Serum sodium concentrations ranged from 168 to 215 mEq/L; consequently, serum osmolalities were markedly increased. The dogs and cat were conscious and adipsic or hypodipsic despite severe hypernatremia and hyperosmolality, findings that strongly support the diagnosis of hypodipsic hypernatremia. The diagnosis was confirmed in one dog by documenting lack of endogenous AVP secretion with worsening hyperosmolality induced by hypertonic saline infusion and marked AVP secretion in response to conjunctival administration of apomorphine (DiBartola et al, 1994).

Treatment is directed toward alleviation of the hypernatremia and, if possible, elimination of the underlying disease. Rapid correction of hypernatremia by administration of hypotonic fluids intravenously is not recommended, because hypernatremia typically has been developing for more than a week and intracellular idiogenic osmoles have been produced within neurons in response to the increased osmolality of the ECF. Rapid reduction of plasma osmolality can result in an intracellular influx of water into neurons, thereby worsening neurologic signs (see Complications of the Modified Water Deprivation Test: Hypertonic Dehydration and Hypernatremia). Forced oral hydration is recommended in humans, but it does not consistently correct the hypernatremia. Addition of water to the food in excess of maintenance requirements and/or forced oral administration of water was beneficial in most, but not all, dogs and the cat with hypodipsic hypernatremia. One dog was clinically healthy 3 years after establishing the diagnosis and initiating water supplementation with food (Miyama et al, 2009). Chlorpropamide, a sulfonylurea drug that augments the antidiuretic effect of low levels of circulating AVP (see Chlorpropamide under Oral Agents (Used in Central Diabetes Insipidus, Partial Central Diabetes Insipidus, Nephrogenic Diabetes Insipidus, and Primary Polydipsia earlier in this chapter), has been useful in restoring osmotic homeostasis in humans with hypodipsic hypernatremia (Reeves et al, 1998). Chlorpropamide (33 mg/kg/day for 2 weeks) was ineffective in stimulating thirst or correcting hypernatremia in one dog (Crawford et al, 1984). Patients with neurologic signs induced by severe hypernatremia may require intensive fluid therapy to initially control the hypernatremia.

REFERENCES

Abe T: Lymphocytic infundibulo-neurohypophysitis infundibulopanhypophysitis regarded as lymphocytic hypophysitis variant, *Brain Tumour Pathol* 25(2):59, 2008.

Aroch I, et al.: Central diabetes insipidus in five cats: clinical presentation, diagnosis and oral desmopressin therapy, *J Fel Med Surg* 7:333, 2005.

Aron DC, et al.: Hypothalamus and pituitary. In Greenspan FS, Gardner DG, editors: *Basic and clinical endocrinology*, New York, 2001, McGraw Hill, p 100.

Authement JM, et al.: Transient, traumatically induced, central diabetes insipidus in a dog, *J Am Vet Med Assoc* 194:683, 1989.

Ayus JC, et al.: Treatment of symptomatic hyponatremia and its relation to brain damage: a prospective study, *N Engl J Med* 317:1190, 1987.

Bagley RS, et al.: Hypernatremia, adipsia, and diabetes insipidus in a dog with hypothalamic dysplasia, *JAAHA* 29:267, 1993.

Barsanti JA, et al.: Diagnostic approach to polyuria and polydipsia. In Bonagura JD, editor: *Current veterinary therapy XIII*, Philadelphia, 2000, WB Saunders, p 831.

Baylis PH, Robertson GL: Vasopressin function in familial cranial diabetes insipidus, *Postgrad Med J* 57:36, 1981.

Baylis PH, Thompson CJ: Osmoregulation of vasopressin secretion and thirst in health and disease, *Clin Endocrinol* 29(5):549, 1988.

Bhan GL, O'Brien TD: Autoimmune endocrinopathy associated with diabetes insipidus, *Postgrad Med J* 58:165, 1982.

Bichet DG: Nephrogenic diabetes insipidus, *Semin Nephrol* 26:224, 2006.

Biewenga WJ, et al.: Osmoregulation of systemic vasopressin release during long-term glucocorticoid excess: a study in dogs with hyperadrenocorticism, *Acta Endocrinol* 124:583, 1991.

Block LH, et al.: Changes in tissue sensitivity to vasopressin in hereditary hypothalamic diabetes insipidus, *Klin Wochenschr* 59:831, 1981.

Breitschwerdt EB, et al.: Nephrogenic diabetes insipidus in three dogs, *J Am Vet Med Assoc* 179:235, 1981.

Brown BA, et al.: Evaluation of the plasma vasopressin, plasma sodium, and urine osmolality response to water restriction in normal cats and a cat with diabetes insipidus [abstract], *J Vet Intern Med* 7:113, 1993.

Burnie AG, Dunn JK: A case of central diabetes insipidus in the cat: diagnosis and treatment, *J Small Anim Pract* 23:237, 1982.

Cameron K, Gallagher A: Syndrome of inappropriate antidiuretic hormone secretion in a cat, *J Am Anim Hosp Assoc* 46:425, 2010.

Capen CC, Martin SL: Diseases of the pituitary gland. In Ettinger SJ, editor: *Textbook of veterinary internal medicine*, ed 2, Philadelphia, 1983, WB Saunders, p 1523.

Crawford MA, et al.: Hypernatremia and adipsia in a dog, *J Am Vet Med Assoc* 184:818, 1984.

Cronin RE: Psychogenic polydipsia with hyponatremia: report of eleven cases, *Am J Kidney Dis* 4:410, 1987.

Davenport DJ, et al.: Diabetes insipidus associated with metastatic pancreatic carcinoma in a dog, *J Am Vet Med Assoc* 189:204, 1986.

Deppe TA, et al.: Glomerular filtration rate and renal volume in dogs with congenital portosystemic vascular anomalies before and after surgical ligation, *J Vet Int Med* 13:465, 1999.

DiBartola SP, et al.: Hypodipsic hypernatremia in a dog with defective osmoregulation of antidiuretic hormone, *J Am Vet Med Assoc* 204:922, 1994.

Dillingham MA, Anderson RJ: Inhibition of vasopressin action by atrial natriuretic factor, *Science* 231:1572, 1986.

Dow SW, et al.: Hypodipsic hypernatremia and associated myopathy in a hydrocephalic cat with transient hypopituitarism, *J Am Vet Med Assoc* 191:217, 1987.

Edwards DF, et al.: Hypernatremic, hypertonic dehydration in the dog with diabetes insipidus and gastric dilatation volvulus, *J Am Vet Med Assoc* 182:973, 1983.

Feldman BJ, et al.: Nephrogenic syndrome of inappropriate antidiuresis, *N Engl J Med* 352:1884, 2005.

Ferring AB: *Product Information, DDAVP*, Malmo, 1985, Sweden.

Fleeman LM, et al.: Effects of an oral vasopressin receptor antagonist (OPC-31260) in a dog with syndrome of inappropriate secretion of antidiuretic hormone, *Aust Vet J* 78:825, 2000.

Fujisawa I: Magnetic resonance imaging of the hypothalamic-neurohypophyseal system, *J Neuroendocrinol* 16:297, 2004.

Goldman MB, et al.: Mechanisms of altered water metabolism in psychotic patients with polydipsia and hyponatremia, *N Engl J Med* 318:397, 1988.

Goossens MMC, et al.: Central diabetes insipidus in a dog with a pro-opiomelanocortin-producing pituitary tumor not causing hyperadrenocorticism, *J Vet Int Med* 9:361, 1995.

Grunbaum EG, Moritz A: Zur diagnostik des diabetes insipidus renalis beim hund, *Tierarztliche Praxis* 19:539, 1991.

Grunbaum EG, et al.: Genetisch bedingter diabetes insipidus renalis beim hund. 35th Annual Meeting, Deutsche Veterinarmedizinische Gesellschaft DVG, Fachgeruppe Kleintierkrankheiten (ed. DVG), DVG, GieBen FRG, 1990, p. 126.

Hanson JM, et al.: Efficacy of transsphenoidal hypophysectomy in treatment of dogs with pituitary-dependent hyperadrenocorticism, *J Vet Intern Med* 19: 687, 2005.

Harb M, et al.: Central diabetes insipidus: 20 dogs (1986-1995), *J Am Vet Med Assoc* 209:1884, 1996.

Hardy RM: Disorders of water metabolism, *Vet Clin North Am Small Anim Pract* 12(3):353, 1982.

Hardy RM, Osborne CA: Water deprivation test in the dog: maximal normal values, *J Am Vet Med Assoc* 174:479, 1979.

Hawks D, et al.: Essential hypernatremia in a young dog, *J Small Anim Pract* 32:420, 1991.

Heiene R, et al.: Vasopressin secretion in response to osmotic stimulation and effects of desmopressin on urinary concentrating capacity in dogs with pyometra, *Am J Vet Res* 65(4):404, 2004.

Hoskins JD, Rothschmitt J: Hypernatremic thirst deficiency in a dog, *Vet Med* 79:489, 1984.

Houston DM, et al.: Syndrome of inappropriate antidiuretic hormone secretion in a dog, *Can Vet J* 30:423, 1989.

Kamoi K: Syndrome of inappropriate antidiuresis without involving inappropriate secretion of vasopressin in an elderly woman: effect of intravenous administration of the nonpeptide vasopressin V_2 receptor antagonist OPC-31260, *Nephron* 76:111, 1997.

Kang MH, Park HM: Syndrome of inappropriate antidiuretic hormone secretion concurrent with liver disease in a dog, *J Vet Med Sci* 74:645, 2012.

Kaplowitz PB, et al.: Radioimmunoassay of vasopressin in familial central diabetes insipidus, *J Pediatr* 100:76, 1982.

Kraus KH: The use of desmopressin in diagnosis and treatment of diabetes insipidus in cats, *Compend Cont Educ Small Anim Pract* 9:752, 1987.

Kurokawa H, et al.: Postserior lobe of the pituitary gland: correlation between signal intensity on T1-weighted M images and vasopressin concentration, *Radiology* 207:79, 1998.

Kusano E, et al.: Chlorpropamide action on renal concentrating mechanism in rats with hypothalamic diabetes insipidus, *J Clin Invest* 72:1298, 1983.

Lam KS, et al.: Pharmacokinetics, pharmacodynamics, long-term efficacy and safety of oral 1-deamino-8-D-arginine vasopressin in adult patients with central diabetes insipidus, *Br J Clin Pharmacol* 42(3):379, 1996.

Lantz GC, et al.: Transsphenoidal hypophysectomy in the clinically normal dog, *Am J Vet Res* 49:1134, 1988.

Lee J, et al.: Atrial natriuretic factor inhibits vasopressin secretion in conscious sheep, *Proc Soc Exp Biol Med* 185:272, 1987.

Luzius H, et al.: A low affinity vasopressin V_2 receptor in inherited nephrogenic diabetes insipidus, *J Receptor Res* 12:351, 1992.

Mackay BM, Curtis N: Adipsia and hypernatremia in a dog with focal hypothalamic granulomatous meningoencephalitis, *Aust Vet J* 77:14, 1999.

Maghnie M, et al.: Persistent high MR signal of the posterior pituitary gland in central diabetes insipidus, *J Neuroradiol* 18:1749, 1997.

Marver D: Evidence of corticosteroid action along the nephron, *Am J Physiol* 246:F111, 1984.

Meij BP, et al.: Lymphocytic hypophysitis in a dog with diabetes insipidus, *J Comp Path* 147:503, 2012.

Miyama TS, et al.: Magnetic resonance imaging and clinical findings in a Miniature Schnauzer with hypodipsic hypernatremia, *J Vet Med Sci* 71:1387, 2009.

Moses AM, Clayton B: Impairment of osmotically stimulated AVP release in patients with primary polydipsia, *Am J Physiol* 265:R1247, 1993.

Moses AM, et al.: Use of T1-weighted MR imaging to differentiate between primary polydipsia and central diabetes insipidus, *Am J Neuroradiol* 13(5):1373, 1992.

Neer TM, Reavis DU: Craniopharyngioma and associated central diabetes insipidus and hypothyroidism in a dog, *J Am Vet Med Assoc* 182:519, 1983.

Oliveira KM, et al.: Head trauma as a possible cause of central diabetes insipidus in a cat, *J Fel Med Surg* 15:155, 2013.

Papanek PE, Raff H: Chronic physiological increases in cortisol inhibit the vasopressin response to hypertonicity in conscious dogs, *Am J Physiol* 267:R1342, 1994.

Papanek PE, et al.: Corticosterone inhibition of osmotically stimulated vasopressin from hypothalamic-neurohypophysial explants, *Am J Physiol* 272:R158, 1997.

Peterson ME, et al.: Acromegaly in 14 cats, *J Vet Intern Med* 4:192, 1990.

Pittari JM: Central diabetes insipidus in a cat, *Feline Pract* 24:18, 1996.

Pollock AS, Arieff AI: Abnormalities of cell volume and their functional consequence, *Am J Physiol* 239:F195, 1980.

Post K, et al.: Congenital central diabetes insipidus in two sibling Afghan Hound pups, *J Am Vet Med Assoc* 194:1086, 1989.

Quinkler M, Stewart PM: Hypertension and the cortisol-cortisone shuttle, *J Clin Endocrinol Metab* 88:2384, 2003.

Ramsay DJ: Posterior pituitary gland. In Greenspan FS, Forsham PH, editors: *Basic and clinical endocrinology*, Los Altos, CA, 1983, Lange Medical Publications, p 120.

Reeves WB, et al.: The posterior pituitary and water metabolism. In Wilson JD, Foster DW, Kronenberg HM, Larsen PR, editors: *Williams textbook of endocrinology*, ed 9, Philadelphia, 1998, WB Saunders, p 341.

Reidarson TH, et al.: Extreme hypernatremia in a dog with central diabetes insipidus: a case report, *JAAHA* 26:89, 1990.

Richardson DW, Robinson AG: Desmopressin, *Ann Intern Med* 103:228, 1985.

Rijnberk A, et al.: Inappropriate vasopressin secretion in two dogs, *Acta Endocrinol* 117:59, 1988.

Rijnberk A, et al.: Aldosteronoma in a dog with polyuria as the leading symptom, *Domest Anim Endocrinol* 20:227, 2001.

Robben JH, et al.: Cell biological aspects of the vasopressin type-2 receptor and aquaporin 2 channel in nephrogenic diabetes insipidus, *Am J Physiol Renal Physiol* 291:F257, 2006.

Robertson GL: Diseases of the posterior pituitary. In Felig P, et al.: *Endocrinology and metabolism*, New York, 1981, McGraw Hill, p 251.

Robertson GL: Differential diagnosis of polyuria, *Ann Rev Med* 39:425, 1988.

Robertson GL, Scheidler JA: A newly recognized variant of familial nephrogenic diabetes insipidus distinguished by partial resistance to vasopressin (type 2) [abstract], *Clin Res* 29:555A, 1981.

Robinson AG: DDAVP in the treatment of central diabetes insipidus, *N Engl J Med* 294:507, 1976.

Robinson AG, Verbalis G: Posterior pituitary. In Melmed S, Polonsky K, Larsen PR, Kronenberg HM, editors: *Williams textbook of endocrinology*, ed 12, Philadelphia, 2011, Elsevier, p 291.

Saeki N, et al.: MRI of ectopic posterior pituitary bright spot with large adenomas: appearances and relationship to transient postoperative diabetes insipidus, *Neuroradiology* 45:713, 2003.

Salvi M, et al.: Role of autoantibodies in the pathogenesis and association of endocrine autoimmune disorders, *Endocr Rev* 9:450, 1988.

Sands JM, Bichet DG: Neprogenic diabetes insipidus, *Ann Intern Med* 144:186, 2006.

Scherbaum WA: Role of autoimmunity in hypothalamic disorders, *Bailliere's Clin Immunol* 1:237, 1987.

Scherbaum WA, et al.: Autoimmune cranial diabetes insipidus: its association with other endocrine diseases and with histiocytosis X, *Clin Endocrinol* 25:411, 1986.

Schwartz J, et al.: Hemodynamic effects of neurohypophyseal peptides with antidiuretic activity in dogs, *Am J Physiol* 249:H1001, 1985.

Schwartz Porsche D: Diabetes insipidus. In Kirk RW, editor: *Current veterinary therapy VII*, Philadelphia, 1980, WB Saunders, p 1005.

Scollan KF, et al.: Validation of a commercially available enzyme immunoassay for measurement of plasma antidiuretic hormone concentration in healthy dogs and assessment of plasma antidiuretic hormone concentration in dogs with congestive heart failure, *Am J Vet Res* 74:1206, 2013.

Spanakis E, et al.: AVPR2 variants and mutations in nephrogenic diabetes insipidus: review and missense mutation significance, *J Cell Physiol* 217:605, 2008.

Sterns RH, et al.: Brain dehydration and neurologic deterioration after rapid correction of hyponatremia, *Kidney Int* 35:69, 1989.

Sterns RH, et al.: Organic osmolytes in acute hyponatremia, *Am J Physiol* 264:F833, 1993.

Sterns RH, et al.: Neurologic sequelae after treatment of severe hyponatremia: a multicenter perspective, *J Am Soc Nephrol* 4:1522, 1994.

Stocker SD, et al.: Role of renin-angiotensin system in hypotension-evoked thirst: studies with hydralazine, *Am J Physiol Regul Integr Comp Physiol* 279:R576, 2000.

Sullivan SA, et al.: Lobar holoprosencephaly in a Miniature Schnauzer with hypodipsic hypernatremia, *J Am Vet Med Assoc* 223:1783, 2003.

Teshima T, et al.: Central diabetes insipidus after transsphenoidal surgery in dogs with Cushing's disease, *J Vet Med Sci* 73:33, 2011.

Thrasher TN: Baroreceptor regulation of vasopressin and renin secretion: low-pressure versus high-pressure receptors, *Front Neuroendocrinol* 15(2):157, 1994.

van Lieburg AF, et al.: Clinical presentation and follow-up of 30 patients with congenital nephrogenic diabetes insipidus, *J Am Soc Nephrol* 10:1958, 1999.

van Vonderen IK, et al.: Polyuria and polydipsia and disturbed vasopressin release in two dogs with secondary polycythemia, *J Vet Int Med* 11:300, 1997a.

van Vonderen IK, et al.: Intra- and interindividual variation in urine osmolality and urine specific gravity in healthy pet dogs of various ages, *J Vet Int Med* 11:30, 1997b.

van Vonderen IK, et al.: Disturbed vasopressin release in four dogs with so-called primary polydipsia, *J Vet Int Med* 13:419, 1999.

van Vonderen IK, et al.: Vasopressin response to osmotic stimulation in 18 young dogs with polyuria and polydipsia, *J Vet Intern Med* 18:800, 2004.

Verbalis JG, Martinez AJ: Neurological and neuropathological sequelae of correction of chronic hyponatremia, *Kidney Int* 39:1274, 1991.

Victor W, et al.: Failure of antipsychotic drug dose to explain abnormal diurnal weight gain among 129 chronically psychotic inpatients, *Prog Neuropsychopharmacol Biol Psychiatry* 13:709, 1989.

Winterbotham J, Mason KV: Congenital diabetes insipidus in a kitten, *J Small Anim Pract* 24:569, 1983.

Zerbe RL, Robertson GL: A comparison of plasma vasopressin measurements with a standard indirect test in the differential diagnosis of polyuria, *N Engl J Med* 305:1539, 1981.

CHAPTER 2 | Disorders of Growth Hormone

Claudia E. Reusch

CHAPTER CONTENTS

 PITUITARY DEVELOPMENT

The pituitary gland plays a central role in the regulation of growth. The organ is composed of two main parts, the adenohypophysis and the neurohypophysis, which have different embryonic origin. The adenohypophysis, which is also known as the anterior lobe of the pituitary, consists of the pars distalis, the pars intermedia, and the pars infundibularis. The structure, which gives rise to the adenohypophysis, was first described by Rathke, a German anatomist, embryologist, and zoologist in 1838 and was named after him. During embryogenesis the adenohypophysis develops from Rathke's pouch, which is an upward protuberance of a single-cell-thick layer of ectoderm of the roof of the primitive mouth. This layer migrates to join the neuroectoderm of the primordium of the ventral hypothalamus; the contact is important, because inductive signals from the hypothalamus are essential for normal development of the anterior pituitary gland. Subsequently, Rathke's pouch separates by constriction from the oral cavity, and the anterior wall thickens and forms the pars distalis of the adenohypophysis. The posterior wall of Rathke's pouch forms the pars intermedia, which remains separated from the pars distalis by the hypophyseal cleft, the former lumen of Rathke's pouch. The neurohypophysis originates of the neural ectoderm as extension of the ventral hypothalamus. In the dog and cat, the adenohypophysis forms a collar around the proximal neurohypophysis and also surrounds part of the median eminence (Meij, 1997; Kooistra, 2000; Meij et al, 2010a; Fig. 2-1).

The development of the pituitary gland and the determination of the specific cell types from common primordial cells follow a distinct, well-regulated order. These processes are under the control of a complex cascade of transcription factors and signaling molecules. After proliferation, the different cell types arise in a temporal and spatial manner and undergo a highly selective differentiation. The corticotrophs are the first distinct cell type in the maturating anterior pituitary gland (Kooistra et al, 2000a; Kelberman et al, 2009; Javorsky et al, 2011; Fig. 2-2). In humans, abnormalities in these processes and pathways are associated with a large spectrum of diseases, and the topic is an area of intensive research; in dogs and cats, exploration of potential mutations has only recently begun.

The cells of the anterior lobe were originally described by their reactions with different colored stains as acidophils, basophils, and chromophobes. Today, immunolabeling techniques allow us to classify pituitary cells by their specific secretory products (Childs, 2009). There are five distinct types of endocrine cells: corticotrophs (secreting adrenocorticotropic hormone [ACTH] and related peptides), thyrotrophs (secreting

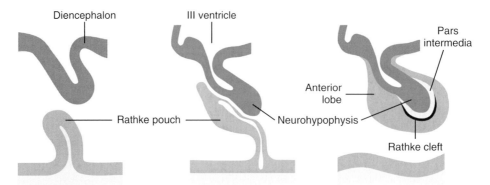

FIGURE 2-1 Simplified illustration of the pituitary ontogenesis. (Reproduced with permission from Meij BP, et al.: Hypothalamus-pituitary system. In Rijnberk A, Kooistra HS, editors: *Clinical endocrinology of dogs and cats,* ed 2, Hannover, 2010, Schlütersche.)

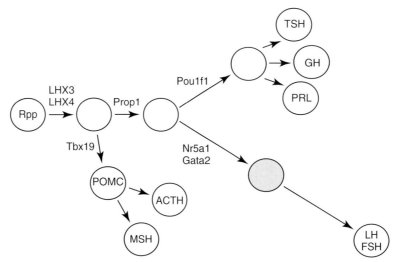

FIGURE 2-2 Simplified, schematic representation of the differentiation of pituitary cell lineages. The final endocrine cell types are labeled with the hormone synthesized by them. Various transcription factors are involved in the process of cellular differentiation. Some of the best known factors are given. (Redrawn and modified from Kelberman D, et al.: Genetic regulation of pituitary gland development in human and mouse, *Endocr Rev* 30[7]:790-829, 2009; and Metherell LA, et al.: Genetic defects of the human somatotropic axis. In Wass JAH, Stewart PM, Amiel SA, Davies MJ, editors: *Oxford textbook of endocrinology and diabetes,* ed 2, Oxford, 2011, Oxford University Press.) *ACTH,* Adrenocorticotropic hormone; *FSH,* follicle-stimulating hormone; *Gata2,* gata binding protein 2; *GH,* growth hormone; *LH,* luteinizing hormone; *LHX3/LHX4,* LIM-domain transcription factor ¾; *MSH,* melanocyte-stimulating hormone; *Nr5a1,* nuclear receptor subfamily 5, group A, member 1 (also termed *steroidogenic factor-1 [SF1]*); *POMC,* proopiomelanocortin; *Pou1f1* (also termed *PIT1*), pituitary-specific positive transcription factor 1; *PRL,* prolactin; *Prop1,* prophet of PIT1 transcription factor; *Rpp,* Rathke pouch progenitor; *Tbx19;* T-box transcription factor 19 (previously termed *T-box pituitary transcription factor [TPIT]*), *TSH,* thyroid-stimulating hormone.

thyroid stimulating hormone [TSH]), gonadotrophs (secreting luteinizing hormone [LH] and follicle-stimulating hormone [FSH]), somatotrophs (secreting growth hormone [GH]) and lactotrophs (secreting prolactin). Somatotrophs and lactotrophs are acidophil-staining cells, and thyrotrophs and gonadotrophs are basophil-staining cells. Chromophobic cells include corticotrophs, nonsecretory follicular (stellate) cells, degranulated chromophils, and undifferentiated stem cells (Capen, 2007). Somatotrophs are the most abundant cells and account for approximately 50% of the cells of the anterior lobe. The percentage of the other cell types ranges between 10% and 15%. The distribution of the different cell types is not random, but it follows a topological and numeric organization. Somatotrophs are mostly located in the dorsal region of the pars distalis close

to the pars intermedia (Meij et al, 2010b). During the last two decades, however, it has become obvious that the traditional concept that each cell type in the pituitary stores and secretes only a single hormone and is regulated by its specific hypothalamic releasing factor, is too narrow and that additional mechanisms exist (Childs, 2009; Meij et al, 2010b). There are subpopulations within the same endocrine cell type that synthesize several hormones and that may be activated by several releasing hormones. Examples are mammosomatotropes that can store and release GH and prolactin, somatogonadotropes that can store and release GH and LH/FSH, thyrosomatotropes that contain TSH and GH. Those cells may undergo a phenotypic switch between the two respective mature cell types depending on the body's need, which is a phenomenon called *transdifferentiation*

(Kineman et al, 1992; Childs, 2000; Vidal et al, 2000; Villalobos et al, 2004; Childs, 2009). Most of the studies have been performed in experimental animals, cell cultures, or in biopsy specimens from humans, and knowledge on potential transdifferentiation of pituitary cells in dogs and cats is scarce. A recent study suggests, however, the existence of similar mechanisms. A group of Beagle dogs was followed for 3 years after the induction of primary hypothyroidism. Basal plasma GH levels increased during this time, and there was a paradoxical hyperresponsiveness to thyrotropin-releasing hormone (TRH) stimulation. Histomorphology and immunohistochemistry of the pituitary gland revealed thyrotroph hyperplasia, large vacuolated thyroid deficiency cells, and pituitary cells that double stained for both GH and TSH, the latter being indicative for transdifferentiation of somatotrophs into thyrotrophs (Diaz-Espiñeira et al, 2008).

BIOSYNTHESIS OF GROWTH HORMONE AND INSULIN-LIKE GROWTH FACTOR-1

Pituitary Growth Hormone and Insulin-like Growth Factor-1

GH, also known as *somatotropin,* is a rather large, single chain polypeptide. The hormone has a molecular weight of approximately 22 kDa and contains 191 amino acids with two intrachain disulfide bridges. It is produced in the somatotropic cells, which represent the most abundant cells of the anterior pituitary (Rijnberk, 1995; Javorsky et al, 2011). The amino acid sequence of canine GH is identical to the sequence of porcine GH; feline GH differs from canine GH by only one amino acid. GH of humans (and other primates) differs considerably (i.e., there is a difference of approximately 33%) (Ascacio-Martínez and Barrera-Saldaña, 1994; Castro-Peralta and Barrera-Saldaña, 1995; Warren et al, 1996; Liu et al, 2001; Wallis, 2008).

In most mammalian species, GH is encoded by a single gene, in humans (and other primates), a cluster of five genes encode pituitary GH and human chorionic somatomammotropin (GH-hCs cluster). The hGH-N gene codes for the 22 kDa (191 amino acids) protein, and transcription is selectively in the somatotrophs of the pituitary. Other genes are expressed in various structures of the placenta. In humans, it is known that the pituitary somatotrophs secrete a mixture of several different forms of GH, which derive from the 22 kDa form by posttranslational modifications. The "normal" 22 kDa, 191 amino acid protein is the major physiological form and accounts for 75% of the pituitary GH secretion (Melmed et al, 2011; Barret et al, 2012).

GH is secreted in a pulsatile fashion in mammalians, as are the other hormones of the anterior pituitary gland. The pulses are mainly induced by the effect of GH-releasing hormone (GHRH), whereas the intervening troughs are primarily generated by somatostatin (Melmed et al, 2011). The number of GH pulses demonstrated in healthy dogs differs slightly between studies: 1 to 3 pulses/6 h, 1 pulse/4.5 h, 2 to 7 pulses/12 h (Cowan et al, 1984; French et al, 1987; Beijerink et al, 2011). In humans, the onset of sleep is a strong stimulus for GF secretion. In dogs, however, no difference was found between awake or asleep phases (French et al, 1987). In various mammalian species, age and gender-related differences in GH secretion have been demonstrated. In dogs, however, GH secretion does not differ between females (in anestrus) and males; aging, however, is associated with a reduction in GH secretion in dogs (Gobello et al, 2002; Lee, 2004). GH secretion in intact female dogs changes during the luteal phase of the cycle, because basal GH secretion is higher and GH secretion in

pulses is lower during times when plasma progesterone concentration is high. This has been explained by the partial suppression of pituitary GH secretion by progesterone-induced GH synthesis in the mammary gland (see later) (Kooistra et al, 2000b). Systematic evaluation of GH secretion patterns in cats has not yet been performed. In the circulation, GH is to some extent bound to GH-binding proteins, which reduces fluctuations in GH levels and prolongs plasma half-life. The canine GH receptor has been characterized at a molecular level and its coding sequence shows extensive homology with the GH receptor of several other species. After binding GH, the receptor dimerizes and activates cytosolic tyrosine kinases of the Janus kinases (Jak) family (van Garderen et al, 1999).

Originally, it was believed that the actions of GH are mediated by the direct effect of the hormone on tissues. In 1957, growth factors, which were termed *sulfation factors,* were discovered by Salmon and Daughaday and were renamed to *somatomedins* by Daughaday et al. (1972). After their isolation by Rinderknecht and Humble (1978a, b), they were then called *insulin-like growth factors (IGFs),* a term that is used today. There are two main IGFs, IGF-1 (previously somatomedin-C) being the most important and IGF-2. Initially it was proposed that GH induces IGF-1 synthesis in the liver, which then acts on target tissues to promote growth. Currently, it is supposed that GH and IGF-1 act in fact in concert as well as independently to stimulate pathways that lead to growth and that regulate many metabolic processes. It has also become clear that IGF-1 is not only produced in the liver, but in almost all tissues of the body where it acts in an autocrine/paracrine manner. Circulating IGF-1 levels, which are mainly derived from the liver, parallel those of GH (i.e., in conditions in which GH is low, IGF-1 levels are also reduced and vice versa) (Le Roith et al, 2001). Liver disease also has an influence on IGF-1, because its level decreases with decreasing functional liver mass (Styne, 2011).

IGF-1 is a basic, single chain polypeptide of 70 amino acids with three intrachain disulfide bridges and a molecular weight of approximately 7.5 kDa. Its structure displays substantial homology to proinsulin (Rinderknecht and Humble, 1978a; Cooke et al, 2011; Frystyk, 2012). The IGF-1 molecule seems to be well conserved between species, including dog and cat (Zangger et al, 1987; Delafontaine et al, 1993). Different to insulin, IGF-1 is bound by a group of six high-affinity proteins (IGF-binding protein-1 [IGFBP-1] to IGFPB-6), and less than 1% of the circulating IGF-1 is present as free form. IGFBP-3 is the most important binding protein that binds most of the IGF-1 (approximately 80% to 85%) in conjunction with an acid-labile subunit (ALS). A similar, less abundant complex is also formed with IGFBP-5. These three molecules (IGF-1, IGFBP-3/IGFBP-5, ALS) form large 150 kDa ternary complexes. (Le Roith et al, 2001; Cooke et al, 2011). ALS is an 85 kDa glycoprotein, almost exclusively produced in the liver under the control of GH, from where it is secreted into the circulation. Its main function is to prolong the half-life of the ternary complexes, which cannot cross the vascular endothelium. This is in contrast to the small amount of IGF-1 that binds to the other IGFBPs, resulting in 50 kDa binary complexes, and that may cross the endothelial barrier more easily. The half-life of free IGF-1 is approximately 10 minutes, and it extends to more than 12 hours in case of the ternary complexes. Half-life of the binary complexes has been described to be 30 minutes (Guler et al, 1989a; Boisclair et al, 2001; Cooke et al, 2011). The binding of most of the IGF-1 in the large ternary complexes allows "storage" of high concentrations of IGF-1 in the circulation by preventing their insulin-like activity, which would otherwise cause hypoglycemia (Zapf et al, 1995). In sum, IGFBPs can be

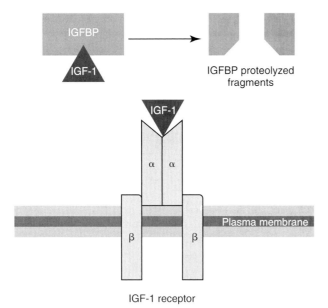

FIGURE 2-3 Simplified, schematic representation of the dissociation of insulin-like growth factor-1 (IGF-1) from IGF-binding protein (IGFBP) and the binding of free IGF-1 to its receptor. (Redrawn and modified from Cooke DW, et al.: Normal and aberrant growth. In Melmed S, Polonsky KS, Larsen PR, Kronenberger HM, editors: *Williams' textbook of endocrinology*, ed 12, Philadelphia, 2011, Saunders/Elsevier.)

regarded as carrier proteins for IGF-1 and as regulators of IGF-1 actions by modulating IGF-1 availability. Interestingly, IGFBPs may also have intrinsic bioactivity independent of IGF-1 (Firth and Baxter, 2002). IGF-1 dissociates from IGFBP by proteolysis, mass action, or other so far unknown mechanisms; thereafter, free IGF-1 binds and activates its ubiquitously expressed cell surface receptor (Fig. 2-3). The IGF-1 receptor is very similar to the insulin receptor; both belong to the transmembrane tyrosine kinase family. Structurally, they are tetramers consisting of two extracellular α-subunits with binding sites for the ligand and two mainly intracellular β-subunits. The latter contains the tyrosine kinase activity that upon activation of the receptor initiates multiple signaling pathways (Le Roith et al, 2001; Cooke et al, 2011; Frystyk, 2012). The IGF-1 receptor binds IGF-1 with high affinity; it also binds insulin, however, with hundredfold less affinity. IGF-1 may bind to the insulin receptor as well, however, with low affinity (Cooke et al, 2011; Bach et al, 2013). In dogs, IGFBP profiles have been shown to be similar to other species and IGFBP-3 also is the most abundant binding protein (Maxwell et al, 1998). Cats seem to have less IGFBP-3 ternary complex formation, and it is suggested that ALS is the limiting factor (Lewitt et al, 2000).

IGF-2 is a single chain polypeptide with 67 amino acids and a molecular weight of approximately 7.5 kDa. Like IGF-1, it is structurally similar to proinsulin, and it circulates in plasma complexed to the six high-affinity IGFBP (Frystyk, 2012). However, the IGF-2 receptor has no structural homology with either the IGF-1 receptor or the insulin receptor. Whereas the IGF-1 receptor binds both IGFs with high affinity, the IGF-2 receptor binds only IGF-2 with high affinity. IGF-1 binds to the IGF-2 receptor with lower affinity, and insulin does not bind at all (Cooke et al, 2011).

Mammary Growth Hormone

In dogs, circulating GH not only derives from the adenohypophysis but can also originate from the mammary gland. In the 1970s, it was described that administration of progestagens could lead to

acromegalic features, glucose intolerance, and mammary tumors in dogs (Sloan and Oliver, 1975; Owen and Briggs, 1976; Gräf and El Etreby, 1979). Subsequent investigations revealed that the phenomenon was due to the induction of high amounts of GH by the progestagens (Concannon et al, 1980; Rijnberk et al, 1980; Eigenmann and Rijnberk, 1981; Eigenmann and Eigenmann, 1981a). The increase in GH was higher when the bitches were estradiol-primed before the administration of progestagens (Eigenmann and Eigenmann, 1981b), and the increase was more pronounced in older than in younger bitches (McCann et al, 1987). At that time it was also realized that GH excess and acromegaly as well as diabetes mellitus do not only develop after the exposure to exogenous progestagens but may also occasionally occur in middle-aged to elderly bitches during the luteal phase of the estrus cycle (i.e., when endogenous progestagen levels are high) (Eigenmann et al, 1983). GH overproduction, acromegalic features as well as diabetes mellitus were shown to be reversible after withdrawal of exogenous progesterone or ovariohysterectomy, respectively (Rijnberk et al, 1980; Eigenmann et al, 1983). The GH excess was associated with marked increase in IGF-1, which also declined after treatment (Eigenmann, 1984). It was recognized thereafter, that progestagen-induced GH does not show a pulsatile secretion pattern and is unresponsive to the stimulation with GHRH or clonidine and to the suppression with a somatostatin analogue (Rutteman et al, 1987; Watson et al, 1987; Selman et al, 1991). The additional discovery that hypophysectomy did not lead to a significant decrease in GH levels gave rise to the assumption that progestagen-induced GH is produced at an extra-pituitary site. The analysis of homogenates of various tissues from progestagen-treated dogs revealed that GH immunoreactivity was by far highest in the mammary gland. GH immunoreactivity was localized primarily in hyperplastic ductular epithelium, as well as in ductular epithelium of mammary adenomas that had developed in some dogs during treatment. Mammary gland origin of the GH excess was confirmed by the finding that GH levels normalized within 2 hours after complete mammectomy (Selman et al, 1994a). Sequence analysis revealed 100% homology between the mammary- and the pituitary-expressed GH gene (Mol et al, 1995). Different to pituitary GH, however, mammary GH expression takes place in the absence of the transcription factor Pou1f1, previously known as pituitary-specific positive transcription factor (*PIT-1*) (Lantinga-van Leeuwen et al, 1999; see Fig. 2-2). Abnormally increased secretion of mammary GH occurs after prolonged exposure to exogenous progestagens or endogenously in some elderly to old intact bitches. However, GH secretion from the mammary gland is also a physiological event and occurs in all cyclic bitches. During the luteal phase in which plasma progesterone concentration is high, basal GH concentration is also increased and less GH is secreted in pulses compared to anestrus. As already mentioned earlier, the loss of pulsatility is thought to be due to suppression of pituitary GH by the progestagen-induced mammary GH (Kooistra et al, 2000b). Mammary GH seems to act in an autocrine and/or paracrine fashion and is important for normal mammary gland development (van Garderen et al, 1997). The growth-promoting effects are achieved by direct effects of GH as well as indirectly by stimulating the synthesis of IGF-1. The effects of the latter are modulated by the local production of IGF-binding proteins (Mol et al, 1997; Mol et al, 1999). The progesterone-GH-IGF-1 system also seems to play an important role in mammary tumorigenesis. It is known that treatment of female dogs with progestagens leads to the development of mammary tumors in a dose-dependent manner. Many of those tumors are benign; however, malignant tumors have also been documented (Mol et al, 1995). Spontaneous mammary tumors are also very common in dogs, and it is assumed that the long exposure to high progesterone concentrations during the long luteal phase is a key factor in their formation (Rao et al, 2009). The link seems to be the progesterone-induced local GH production, because GH has been documented in the vast majority of benign and malignant mammary tumors (Mol et al, 1995; van Garderen et al, 1997). Tissue and plasma GH and IGF-1 are significantly higher in malignant than in benign tumors (Queiroga et al, 2008; Queiroga et al, 2010). Gene expression profiles of progestagen-induced mammary hyperplasia and spontaneous mammary tumors of dogs identified altered expression of various genes involved in tumor development and progression and confirmed the role of progesterone in the process of cell proliferation (Rao et al, 2009). In cats, the gene encoding GH is also expressed in the mammary gland. The highest expression was demonstrated in fibroadenomatous hyperplasia induced by the administration of progestagens (Mol et al, 1995; Rijnberk and Mol, 1997). However, in cats, mammary GH does not seem to be secreted into the systemic circulation (Peterson, 1987).

REGULATION OF GROWTH HORMONE SECRETION FROM THE PITUITARY GLAND

Synthesis and secretion of pituitary GH is regulated by a complex network of stimulating and inhibiting factors. The integration of all those factors results in the pulsatile release of GH from the somatotropic cells of the anterior pituitary gland (Mol and Meij, 2008). GHRH and somatostatin (also termed *somatotropin-release inhibiting factor [SRIF]*) thereby play a predominant role and are the best known regulators. Both hormones derive from hypothalamic neurons, from where they are transported by nerve fibers to the outer lamina of the median eminence. By subsequent release into the capillaries of the hypothalamic-hypophyseal portal system, they reach the anterior pituitary gland (Meij et al, 2010a). GHRH is a peptide consisting of 44 amino acids and arises from posttranslational modification of a larger prohormone. Its structure varies somewhat between species. The GHRH receptor belongs to a subfamily of G-protein coupled receptors and activates the somatotrophs through activation of the adenylate cyclase/cyclic adenosine monophosphate (cAMP) pathways. The activation of the receptors leads to the release of preformed GH as well as to stimulation of gene transcription and synthesis of new GH (Mayo et al, 2000; Low, 2011). The pituitary actions of GHRH are almost completely specific for GH secretion, and there appears to be no relevant interaction between GHRH and other hypothalamic releasing hormones (Giustina and Veldhuis, 1998; Low, 2011). Half-life of GHRH is short (e.g., in humans between 2 to 4 minutes) (Javorsky et al, 2011).

Somatostatin is a potent inhibitor of GH and suppresses both basal and GHRH-stimulated pulse amplitude and frequency. It does not affect the synthesis of GH. Although many other factors are involved, it is currently believed that GH pulses predominantly reflect the pulsatile secretion of GHRH, whereas the GH troughs are mainly controlled by somatostatin. The high level of somatostatin during a GH trough period probably primes the somatotropic cells to maximally respond to subsequent GHRH pulses (Melmed et al, 2011). Somatostatin not only occurs in the hypothalamus, but in various other regions of the central and peripheral nervous system as well as in the gastrointestinal tract, pancreas, and other tissues. Consequently, additionally to its profound inhibition of GH, it also displays inhibitory effects

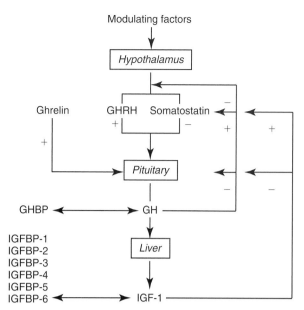

FIGURE 2-4 Simplified, schematic representation of the hypothalamus-pituitary-growth hormone (GH)/insulin-like growth factor-1 (IGF-1) axis. See Box 2-1 for details on modulating factors. *GHBP,* Growth hormone-binding protein; *GHRH,* GH-releasing hormone; *IGFBP,* IGF-binding protein.

on other hormones (e.g., TSH, insulin glucagon, gastrin) and on immune functions and tumor growth, and it has important impact on the gastrointestinal tract and other organ functions (Reichlin, 1983; Giustina and Veldhuis, 1998). Somatostatin derives from prohormone cleavage, resulting in the generation of the tetradecapeptide somatostatin 14 and a somatostatin molecule containing 28 amino acids, termed *somatostatin 28.* Somatostatin 14 is the major form in the brain, including the hypothalamus and is identical in all vertebrates; somatostatin 28 is the main form in the gastrointestinal tract (Low, 2011). Five somatostatin receptors (SSTR1 to SSTR5) have been identified and all of them are expressed in the pituitary gland (Giustina and Veldhuis, 1998). Binding to the somatostatin receptor leads to activation of membrane-bound inhibitory G-protein and inhibition of adenyl cyclase activity and decrease of intracellular cAMP (Low, 2011). Half-life of somatostatin is approximately as short as of GHRH (Javorsky et al, 2011).

A complex interplay of feedback signals involves the four peptides GH, IGF-1, GHRH, and somatostatin (Fig. 2-4). GH itself stimulates hypothalamic somatostatin release, inhibits GHRH, and has a direct inhibitory effect on somatotropic cells. GHRH and somatostatin can each negatively regulate its own secretion and reciprocally controls secretion of its counterpart (Giustina and Veldhuis, 1998). IGF-1 inhibits GH secretion on the hypothalamic levels by increasing somatostatin release as well as directly on the pituitary level (Melmed et al, 2011).

The actions of GHRH and somatostatin do not completely account for all pulses of GH secretion. A complex array of external and internal stimuli (e.g., body composition and nutritional status, age, gender, sleep, exercise, fasting, genetic background, disease status, and many others) regulate GH amplitude and frequency. The importance of those factors may differ between species; for instance GH secretion does not seem to be related to sleep or day-night cycles, and insulin-induced hypoglycemia does not consistently result in GH secretion in dogs (French et al, 1987; Bhatti et al, 2006a; Mol and Meij, 2008; Box 2-1).

BOX 2-1 Factors Modulating Growth Hormone Release in Humans

Stimulatory Factors	Inhibitory Factors
Physiologic	**Physiologic**
Sleep	Postprandial hyperglycemia
Exercise	Rise in free fatty acids
Stress	Aging
Postprandial decline of blood glucose	
Pathologic	**Pathologic**
Protein depletion	Obesity
Starvation	Hypothyroidism
Chronic renal failure	Hyperthyroidism
Liver cirrhosis	Hyperadrenocorticism
Type 1 diabetes	
Interleukins 1,2,6	
Pharmacologic	**Pharmacologic**
Insulin-induced hypoglycemia	Somatostatin
Amino acid infusion (arginine, lysine)	IGF-1, IGF-2
GHRH	Glucocorticoids (chronic
Ghrelin	administration)
ACTH, α-MSH, vasopressin	α-adrenergic antagonists
Estrogen	β-adrenergic agonists
α-adrenergic agonists (e.g., clonidine)	Serotonin antagonists
β-adrenergic antagonists	Dopamine antagonists
Dopamine agonists	
Serotonin precursors	
GABA agonists	
Potassium infusion	

Modified from Javorsky BR, et al.: Hypothalamus and pituitary gland. In Gardner DG, Shoback D, editors: *Greenspan's basic & clinical endocrinology,* ed 9, San Francisco, 2011, McGraw Hill; and Low MJ: Neuroendocrinology. In Melmed S, Polonsky KS, Larsen PR, Kronenberger HM, editors: *Williams' textbook of endocrinology,* ed 12, Philadelphia, 2011, Saunders Elsevier.

α-MSH, α-Melanocyte-stimulating hormone; *ACTH,* adrenocorticotropic hormone; *GABA,* gamma aminobutyric acid; *GHRH,* GH-releasing hormone; *IGF,* insulin-like growth factor.

Please note that there is variability between species, e.g., hypothyroidism in dogs is associated with increased GH release and GH secretion in dogs does not seem to be related to sleep or day-night cycles.

Approximately 15 years ago, ghrelin, another major factor in the complex regulation network, was identified (Kojima et al, 1999). *Ghre* is the Indo-European root of the word *grow,* and *relin* means release (Bhatti et al, 2006a). Ghrelin is a 28-amino acid peptide with a high degree of structural similarity between species. It circulates in the blood in a non-acylated and an acylated form; acylation is mandatory for its biological effects (Nass et al, 2011). The main site of ghrelin synthesis is the fundus of the stomach, but synthesis has also been demonstrated in the small intestinal tract and many other tissues, including pancreas, pituitary, and hypothalamus (Nass et al, 2011; Sato et al, 2012). Ghrelin acts through a receptor separate from the GHRH receptor, called the *GH secretagogue receptor (GHS-R),* or *ghrelin receptor.* It is a typical G-protein coupled receptor and highly expressed in the anterior pituitary gland, hypothalamus, hippocampus, and other areas in the brain; its structure is well conserved across vertebrate species (Sato et al, 2012). Interestingly, the GHS-R was identified several years before the discovery of its natural ligand ghrelin and was therefore also called "orphan" GHS-R. Initially, it was found that enkephalins reveal GH-releasing properties, which then lead to the development of synthetic compounds inducing GH secretion

(GH secretagogues, GHS). After the identification of the GHS receptor (GHS-R), an active search for its endogenous ligand was undertaken (Koijma et al, 1999; Sato et al, 2012).

Ghrelin acts directly at the level of the pituitary gland to stimulate the release of GH (see Fig. 2-4). The effect is greater in vivo than in vitro, suggesting a synergistic action of ghrelin and GHRH (i.e., GHRH is necessary to induce a maximal GH release) (Sato et al, 2012). With regard to potency and effect on other pituitary hormones, species specific differences have been demonstrated. In humans, GH release after ghrelin administration is more pronounced than after GHRH administration, and the effect is not absolutely specific, because ghrelin also increases the secretion of prolactin, ACTH, and cortisol (Bhatti et al, 2006a). In dogs, ghrelin release appears to be age-related (Yokoyama et al, 2005; Bhatti et al, 2006b). In young dogs (13 to 17 months), ghrelin exhibited more powerful GH-releasing effects than GHRH, whereas in older dogs (7 to 12 years), GH secretion was significantly higher after GHRH than after ghrelin application (Bhatti et al, 2006b). In dogs, ghrelin neither activates the pituitary-adrenocortical axis nor stimulates the release of prolactin, TSH, and LH (Bhatti et al, 2002). In cats, ghrelin also stimulates GH release in a dose-dependent manner (Ida, 2012). So far, its potency, age-dependency, and specificity for somatotrophs have not been evaluated in the cat. Ghrelin has various additional physiological functions, such as appetite regulation (induction of hunger), stimulation of gastric motility and gastric acid secretion, decrease of insulin secretion, and also has cardiovascular and antiproliferative effects (Sato et al, 2012).

Finally, GH synthesis and release is modulated by other hormones, such as thyroid hormones, glucocorticoids, and sex hormones. In humans, primary hypothyroidism is associated with attenuated GH secretion. In hypothyroid dogs, however, basal GH and IGF-1 concentrations are increased (Lee et al, 2001). In dogs with pituitary-dependent hyperadrenocorticism, basal GH concentrations are normal, but pulse frequency is lower and less GH is secreted in pulses. The inhibitory effect of prolonged glucocorticoid excess is also seen in humans and may in part be mediated by enhancement of somatostatin release (Lee et al, 2003).

METABOLIC ACTIONS OF GROWTH HORMONE AND INSULIN-LIKE GROWTH FACTOR-1

The actions of GH and IGF-1 are usually described as separate entities (i.e., rapid, direct actions are attributed to GH, and slow, indirect actions are attributed to IGF-1). However, understanding has evolved, and it is now recognized that there is a tight and much more complex interplay between the two hormones. Several studies have shown the existence of so-called crosstalk between the pathways activated by GH, IGF-1, and insulin (Vijayakumar et al, 2010). Roughly, GH exerts its effects by binding to the GH receptor, which is expressed abundantly in the liver but also in other tissues. Many of its effects are mediated through subsequent production of IGF-1 (Fig. 2-5). The liver is the predominant source of IGF-1, although it is also synthesized in many other tissues, where it acts in an autocrine/paracrine manner (Aragon-Alonso et al, 2011). Circulating IGF-1 is stimulated by GH when nutrient intake is sufficient and insulin concentration in the portal vein is high, whereas IGF-1 concentration decreases during fasting (Møller and Jørgensen, 2009). In adults, GH is a major metabolic hormone and functions by optimizing body composition and physical function as well as by regulating energy and substrate metabolism. It interacts closely with insulin to control fat, protein and carbohydrate metabolism during fasting and fed states (Melmed et al, 2011). GH stimulates lipolysis and fatty acid oxidation, which is of particular importance

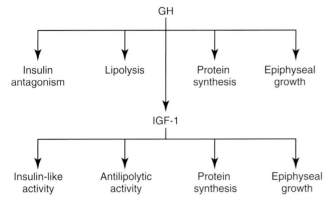

FIGURE 2-5 Simplified scheme of the major metabolic actions of growth hormone (GH) and insulin-like growth factor-1 (IGF-1).

in the fasted state to provide energy without protein degradation. The latter (protein-sparing) effect is an important mechanism by which GH promotes growth and development (Melmed et al, 2011; Javorsky et al, 2011). GH also plays a role in adipocyte differentiation; the generation of large mature adipocytes is associated with an increased capacity to store triglyceride and higher lipophilic activity (Vijayakumar et al, 2010). GH increases protein synthesis (directly and via IGF-1), by enhancing all facets of amino acid uptake and incorporation into protein while suppressing proteolysis. The carbohydrate metabolism is affected by GH both directly and indirectly. The direct, anti-insulin actions of GH are of particular importance during starvation and include decrease of glucose uptake in extrahepatic tissues, increase in hepatic glucose output, and increase of plasma glucose concentration (Sjaastad et al, 2010; Javorsky et al, 2011). IGF-1 has very different effects on carbohydrate metabolism. They are insulin-like and include increase of glucose uptake in extrahepatic tissues, decrease of hepatic glucose output, and decrease of plasma glucose concentration (Mauras and Haymond, 2005; Javorsky et al, 2011). In case of GH excess, its anti-insulin or "diabetogenic" effect may lead to overt diabetes, which may become insulin-resistant.

In the growing individual, normal GH secretion and the functional integrity of the GH-IGF-1 axis is mandatory for normal linear growth and skeletal development. In human medicine, the respective roles of GH, IGF-1, their binding proteins and receptors, as well as the influence of other factors (e.g., cytokines) are an area of intensive research, and an impressive number of genetic defects have so far been described (Savage et al, 2011). GH is thought to act on the precursors of the growth plate to stimulate the differentiation of chondrocytes and stimulate local IGF-1 synthesis, which in turn acts in an autocrine/paracrine manner and induces clonal expansion and hypertrophy of chondrocytes. GH may also have an additional direct effect on proliferation and hypertrophy of the chondrocytes (Zezulak and Green, 1986; Gevers et al, 2002). Part of the growth-promoting effect is also mediated by the circulating, liver-derived IGF-1 (Stratikopoulos et al, 2008).

The dog is unique among mammalian species, because body weight at the opposite end of the scale (e.g., Chihuahua and St. Bernard) may differ nearly hundredfold (Favier et al, 2001; Rijnberk et al, 2003). Initial studies showed that circulating IGF-1 levels were different between adult dogs of different breeds; smaller breed dogs had lower IGF-1 levels than middle sized dogs, and the latter had lower levels than large breed dogs (Eigenmann et al, 1984a). Similarly, IGF-1 levels paralleled body size among genetic subgroups within one breed, because Standard Poodles had much higher IGF-1 levels than Toy Poodles, whereas GH levels were similar (Eigenmann

et al, 1984c). Another study investigating a large number of dogs of many different breeds confirmed the relation between IGF-1 and body size, because IGF-1 increased with increasing weight (Greer et al, 2011). Evaluation of young, growing dogs, however, raised doubts on the assumption that the circulation level of IGF-1 is the major determinant of body size in dogs (Rijnberk et al, 2003). Prolonged treatment of Toy Poodle puppies with recombinant human IGF-1, although associated with substantial rise in circulating IGF-1 levels, did not increase body size in comparison to controls (Guler et al, 1989b). No correlation was found between IGF-1 levels and growth rate in Standard and Toy Poodle puppies (Bürki, 2000).

The issue of IGF-1 and body size was further investigated by genetic studies. The IGF-1 gene, as a candidate gene for body size, was shown to be a major gene to contribute to the size diversity in dogs. The IGF-1 gene and the associated gene regions account for approximately 50% of the genetic variations in dog size (Sutter et al, 2007; Boyko, 2011; Wayne and vonHoldt, 2012). Small breed dogs have IGF-1 haplotypes that are closely related to those of wolves from the Middle East, suggesting an early evolution of small dog size there (Gray et al, 2010; Wayne and vonHoldt, 2012). It is obvious that additional factors are involved, and it is likely that GH plays an important role. Basal GH concentrations as well as GH release during pulses in Great Dane puppies were shown to be significantly higher than the corresponding levels of Beagles of the same age. In the Beagles, GH decreased into the range of adults already by week 7, whereas the decrease was much slower in the Great Danes in which GH stayed elevated throughout the observation period of 24 weeks. The authors therefore assumed that the different duration of GH elevation may be responsible for the differences in body size between medium and large breed dogs (Favier et al, 2001).

CAUSES OF GROWTH FAILURE

Humans

Decreased growth during childhood and short adult height may be due to a large number of non-endocrine and endocrine causes. Non-endocrine causes include constitutional short stature (which is not considered a disease but a variation from normal for the population) as a familial pattern and as a characteristic pattern of various syndromes (e.g. Turner syndrome). Malnutrition, severe chronic diseases and dysfunction of many organ systems are additional important causes. Main endocrine disorders include GH deficiency, GH insensitivity, hypothyroidism, endogenous or exogenous glucocorticoid excess, disorders of vitamin D metabolism and poorly-regulated diabetes mellitus (Styne, 2011). GH deficiency in turn may be due to various abnormalities at the hypothalamic or pituitary level; additional defects are known at the level of IGF-1 and its receptor (Box 2-2). In cases of isolated GH deficiency at the pituitary level, often no cause can be identified (so-called idiopathic GH deficiency); however, there is increasing recognition of genetic defects (e.g., mutations in the GHRH receptor gene or in the gene encoding GH, or synthesis of mutant GH with reduced bioactivity) (Cooke, 2011). As discussed at the beginning of the chapter pituitary development and the determination of specific cell types follows a distinct, well-regulated order under the control of transcription factors and signaling molecules (Kelberman et al, 2009; Javorsky et al, 2011; see Fig. 2-2). Multiple genetic defects have been identified within this complex cascade leading to combined pituitary hormone deficiencies. Mutations in the prophet of PIT1 (PROP1) gene result in GH, TSH, prolactin, FSH, and LH deficiencies. Mutations in the POU1F1 (or PIT1) gene lead to GH, TSH, and prolactin deficiencies (Kelberman et al, 2009). In humans, mutations in the POU1F1 or PROP1 gene are

BOX 2-2   **Causes for Growth Hormone and Insulin-Like Growth Factor-1 Deficiency in Humans**

1. Hypothalamic dysfunction (GHRH deficiency)
   a) Congenital
   b) Acquired (e.g., tumors, trauma, inflammation)
2. Anterior pituitary dysfunction
   a) Congenital
   - Isolated GH deficiency
   - Combined pituitary hormone deficiency
   b) Acquired (e.g., tumors, trauma, inflammation)
3. GH dysfunction or GH insensitivity
   a) Defects of GH receptor or postreceptor signaling pathways (Laron syndrome and its variants)
4. Abnormalities of IGF-1 and IGF-1 receptor and signaling pathways

Modified from Cooke DW, Divall SA, Radovick S: Normal and aberrant growth. In Melmed S, Polonsky KS, Larsen PR, Kronenberger HM, editors: *Williams' textbook of endocrinology*, ed 12, Philadelphia, 2011, Saunders Elsevier; and Styne D: Growth. In Gardner DG, Shoback D, editors: *Greenspan's basic & clinical endocrinology*, ed 9, San Francisco, 2011, McGraw Hill.
GH, Growth hormone; *GHRH*, GH-releasing hormone; *IGF-1*, insulin-like growth factor-1.

the most common causes for combined pituitary hormone deficiency. LIM-domain transcription factor 3 (LHX3) belongs to a family of transcription factors that are essential for the development of the pituitary gland and the nervous system. Mutations in the LHX3 gene (recently shown to be associated with pituitary dwarfism in German Shepherds) are a rare cause of hypopituitarism in humans; affected individuals have GH, TSH, prolactin, FSH, and LH deficiencies, whereas ACTH synthesis is most often normal. The phenotypes with LHX3 mutations are similar to those of the PROP1 defect; however, short rigid cervical spine with limited head rotation is an additional feature. The genetic defects may be associated with structural defects of the pituitary and other parts of the brain as well as in other parts of the body (Kelberman et al, 2009; Cooke et al, 2011; Metherell et al, 2011). Dysfunction of the GH-IGF-1 axis may also be caused by GH insensitivity and IGF-1 associated abnormalities. GH insensitivity, referred to as *primary IGF-1 deficiency*, comprises a variety of genetic syndromes characterized by high GH levels and very low IGF-1 levels. Those findings have been first described by Laron. The abnormalities are therefore also collectively known as *Laron syndrome*. The disorders reflect defects at the GH receptor or in postreceptor signaling pathways (Cooke et al, 2011). For more details on transcriptional control of pituitary development and genetic defects in the human GF-IGF-1 axis, see Savage, et al. (2003), Kelberman, et al. (2009), and Savage, et al. (2011).

Dogs and Cats

As in humans, failure to grow in dogs and cats may be caused by non-endocrine and endocrine disorders (Box 2-3). Non-endocrine causes comprise malnutrition, dysfunction of nearly any organ in the body, as well as any chronic disease. In dogs and cats, there is also a counterpart to human constitutional and familial short stature, because individual dogs or cats may be somewhat smaller than their littermates, and certain dog families within a breed may also be smaller than other families of the same breed. Congenital hyposomatotropism and congenital hypothyroidism are endocrinopathies usually causing serious growth failure. Early development of other endocrinopathies such as diabetes mellitus, hyperadrenocorticism, hypoadrenocorticism, and disorders of vitamin D metabolism may also be associated with impaired growth.

BOX 2-3   **Nonendocrine and Endocrine Causes of Growth Failure in Dogs and Cats**

Non-Endocrine Causes of Growth Failure	Endocrine Causes of Growth Failure
Constitutional*	GH/IGF-1 deficiency
Familial*	Hypothyroidism
Malnutrition	Glucocorticoid excess
Any severe chronic disease including chronic infection	(endogenous and exogenous)
Cardiac disorders (e.g., left-to-right shunt)	Diabetes mellitus
Pulmonary disorders	Hypoadrenocorticism
Disorders of swallowing (e.g., vascular ring anomaly, megaesophagus)	Disorders of vitamin D metabolism
Gastrointestinal and pancreatic disorders (e.g., parasites, malabsorption, exocrine pancreatic insufficiency)	
Hepatic disorders (e.g., portosystemic shunt, glycogen storage disease)	
Hematological disorders	
Renal disorders	
Immunological disorders	
CNS disorders	
Abnormal bone growth (e.g., chondrodystrophy)	

Modified from Ihle SL: Failure to grow. In Ettinger SJ, Feldman EC, editors: *Textbook of veterinary internal medicine*, ed 7, St. Louis, 2010, Saunders Elsevier; and Styne D: Growth. In Gardner DG, Shoback D, editors: *Greenspan's basic & clinical endocrinology*, ed 9, San Francisco, 2011, McGraw Hill.
CNS, Central nervous system; *GH*, growth hormone; *IGF-1*, insulin-like growth factor-1.
* Terms adapted from human medicine (Styne, 2011).

 CONGENITAL HYPOSOMATOTROPISM (PITUITARY DWARFISM) IN DOGS AND CATS

Etiopathogenesis

Any defect in the hypothalamus-anterior pituitary axis and in pituitary organogenesis may result in isolated or combined pituitary hormone deficiency. Congenital hyposomatotropism is certainly the most striking example of pituitary hormone deficiency (Kooistra, 2010). Congenital hyposomatotropism or pituitary dwarfism is long known as autosomal recessive disorder in the German Shepherd dog and the Karelian Bear dog (Andresen and Willeberg, 1976 and 1977). Genealogical investigations by Andresen in 1978 indicated that the mutation evolved around 1940 or even before. Several champion dogs were shown to be carriers of the genetic defect, which was certainly one of the reasons why the disease spread all around the world (Andresen, 1978; Nicholas, 1978; Voorbij and Kooistra, 2009; Kooistra, 2010). It is assumed that the genetic defect in the Karelian Bear dog is the same as in the German Shepherds, because both breeds were crossed in Finland in the 1940s (Andresen and Willeberg, 1976). The situation is similar for the Saarloos Wolfhound and the Czechoslovakian Wolfdog, in which pituitary dwarfism is also known, and the German Shepherd has been used for breeding. It is possible that the defect is also present in other breeds in which a German Shepherd carrier has been used. For instance, GH deficiency was described in a litter of Weimaraner dogs; however, three generations previously, a mismating to a German Shepherd had occurred (Roth et al, 1980).

Initially, it was assumed that the hormone deficiency was the result of pressure atrophy of the anterior pituitary gland by pituitary cysts. Those cysts may develop from remnants of the distal craniopharyngeal duct (Rathke pouch), which normally disappears at birth. Occasionally, they may become large, exert pressure on the infundibular stalk, the hypophyseal portal system, median eminence, or pars distalis and cause pituitary atrophy due to compression and impaired blood supply. Rupture of large cysts and escape of their proteinaceous content may lead to inflammation, subsequent fibrosis, and reduced pituitary function. Cystic remnants are relatively common and occur in many breeds. Most often they are small and clinically insignificant (Capen, 2007). Further research indicated that the developmental defect in German Shepherd dwarfs is different from those craniopharyngeal remnants. Severe hypoplasia of the anterior pituitary has been found in German Shepherds with very small cysts, which were considered unlikely to be responsible for pressure atrophy. In some dwarfs, there may even be no cysts at all (Kooistra et al, 1998; Hamann et al, 1999; Kooistra et al, 2000a). According to current knowledge, pituitary dwarfism in the German Shepherd dog (and Karelian Bear dog and Saarloos Wolfhound) is caused by a failure of the oropharyngeal ectoderm of the Rathke pouch to differentiate into normal trophic-hormone-secreting cells of the pars distalis. Accumulation of proteinaceous material may follow, which may lead to cystic changes attracting water. This assumption is compatible with the observation that cysts may enlarge with time (Fig. 2-6). Cyst formation therefore is most likely a consequence and not the cause of pituitary dwarfism (Kooistra et al, 1998; Kooistra et al, 2000a; Capen, 2007).

In line with the assumption of complex failure of cell differentiation is the finding that the secretory capacity of other pituitary cells than the somatotrophs is also impaired. Kooistra, et al. (2000a) studied the release of GH, TSH, prolactin, FSH, LH, and ACTH in a combined pituitary function test using four releasing hormones (GHRH, TRH, gonadotropin-releasing hormone [GnRH], and corticotropin-releasing hormone [CRH]) in a group of eight German Shepherd dwarfs. Basal GH, TSH, and prolactin were significantly lower than those of healthy controls and did not respond to stimulation. Basal LH was not different from basal LH of controls; however, stimulation was significantly less. With regard to FSH, a gender difference was obvious. In male dwarfs, basal and stimulated FSH concentrations were undetectably low; in female dwarfs, basal FSH levels were measurable, however, somewhat lower than in age-matched female controls, and there was only a slight increase after stimulation. Basal ACTH and ACTH concentrations after stimulation were not different to controls (Fig. 2-7 and Fig. 2-8). In summary, German Shepherds were shown to have a combined deficiency of GH, TSH, and prolactin, together with impaired release of gonadotropins. In contrast, ACTH secretion is preserved (Kooistra et al, 2000a).

During the last decade, an extensive search was performed, mostly at the University of Utrecht, to identify the causative defect. Please see Fig. 2-2 for the differentiation of pituitary cell lineages and the main important transcription factors involved. As mentioned earlier, mutations in the POU1F1 (or PIT1) and PROP1 genes are the most common defects associated with pituitary hormone deficiency in humans. It was, therefore, reasonable to explore potential defects in those two genes also in the German Shepherd. However, the gene encoding for transcription factor POU1F1 (or PIT1) was the first one to be excluded as a candidate gene for pituitary dwarfism. This was in agreement with the hormone studies described earlier, because a defect in the POU1F1 gene would only cause GH, TSH, and prolactin deficiency, whereas LH, FSH, and ACTH would not be affected (Lantinga-van Leeuwen et al, 2000a; Kooistra et al, 2000a). PROP1 gene mutation would

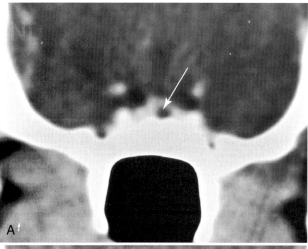

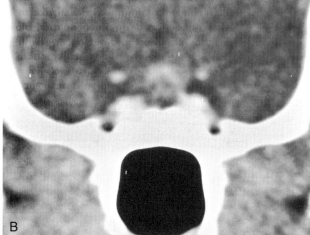

FIGURE 2-6 A, Contrast-enhanced computed tomography (CT) images of a 6-month-old German Shepherd dwarf with a pituitary of normal size (height 3.6 mm, width 4.3 mm) but having a radiolucent area due to a cyst *(arrow).* **B,** At the age of 3 years, the pituitary is enlarged (height 6.5 mm, width 5.4 mm), and the greater part of it lacks contrast enhancement due to the cyst. (Reproduced with permission from Meij BP, et al.: Hypothalamus-pituitary system. In Rijnberk A, Kooistra HS, editors: *Clinical endocrinology of dogs and cats,* ed 2, Hannover, 2010, Schlütersche.)

in principle fit with the phenotype in German Shepherd dwarfs because a defect results in combined deficiency of GH, TSH, prolactin, LH, and FSH. However, PROP1 was also excluded as a candidate gene (Lantinga-van Leeuwen et al, 2000b). Thereafter, factors acting at earlier stages of the pituitary development were investigated. The LHX4 gene was also excluded as a candidate gene, as well as the leukemia inhibiting factor receptor gene. Leukemia inhibitor factor (LIF) is a pleiotropic cytokine that plays an important role in the ontogeny of the anterior pituitary gland (Van Oost et al, 2002; Hanson et al, 2006). More recently, the search was successful, and the genetic defect could be located in the LHX3 gene (Voorbij et al, 2011). LHX3 is a member of a family of transcription factors (the LIM homeodomain family) that are critical for cell specialization during embryonic development and essential for the development of the pituitary gland and the nervous system. In humans, defects in the LHX3 gene are associated with combined pituitary hormone deficiency (usually ACTH secretion is preserved); this is very similar to the findings in the German Shepherd dwarfs. A genetic test is now available through the University of Utrecht and several other

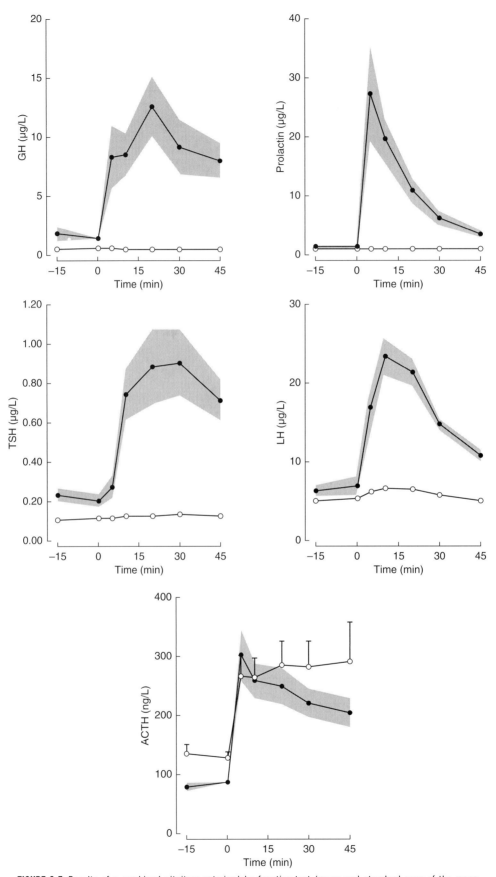

FIGURE 2-7 Results of a combined pituitary anterior lobe function test (mean and standard error of the mean [SEM]) in eight German Shepherd dogs with dwarfism (○) and in eight adult healthy Beagle dogs (●). The bars indicating the SEM in the German Shepherd dwarfs are only depicted when they exceed the size of the symbols. (Reproduced with permission from Kooistra HS, et al.: Combined pituitary hormone deficiency in German Shepherd dogs with dwarfism, *Domest Anim Endocrinol* 19[3]:177-190, 2000.) *ACTH*, Adrenocorticotropic hormone; *GH*, growth hormone; *LH*, luteinizing hormone; *TSH*, thyroid-stimulating hormone.

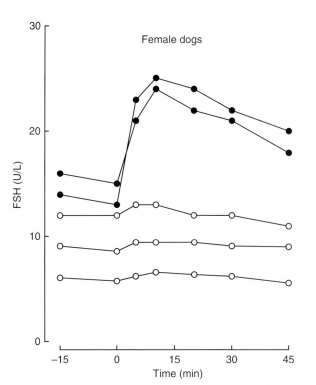
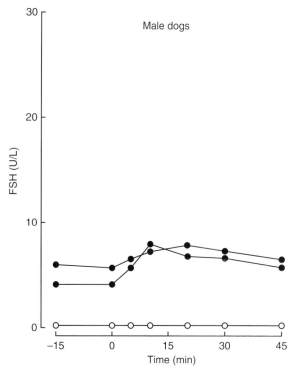

FIGURE 2-8 Basal and stimulated plasma follicle-stimulating hormone (FSH) concentrations in three female and four male German Shepherd dogs with dwarfism (○) and in two healthy female and two healthy male Beagle dogs of the same age (●). *FSH,* Follicle-stimulating hormone. (Reproduced with permission from Kooistra HS, et al.: Combined pituitary hormone deficiency in German Shepherd dogs with dwarfism, *Domest Anim Endocrinol* 19[3]:177-190, 2000.)

laboratories, which enables the diagnosis of pituitary dwarfism and the identification of carriers of the mutation.

There may be additional abnormalities in the GHRH-GH-IGF-1 axis in dogs; however, no studies have been performed. Randolph, et al. (1990) reported on two German Shepherd littermates showing stunted growth during the first weeks to months but thereafter growing at steady rate and reaching normal height at 1 year of age. Functional testing did not reveal any hormonal abnormalities. Interestingly, two other littermates were euthanized at early age, and hypoplasia of the anterior pituitary gland as well as reduced number of cells was demonstrated. The authors hypothesized that the delayed growth of the two surviving dogs may represent one end of a clinical spectrum associated with pituitary dwarfism in German Shepherd dogs. Müller-Peddinghaus, et al. (1980) described a German Shepherd dwarf with high GH concentration and very low IGF-1 concentration, which is a constellation typically seen in Laron disease (GH insensitivity) in humans. So far, similar cases have not been reported.

Congenital hyposomatotropism has also been described in cats (Donaldson et al, 2008); however, it seems to be extremely rare.

Signalment

Pituitary dwarfism occurs primarily in the German Shepherd dog, although it is also seen in the Karelian Bear dog, the Saarloos Wolfdog, and the Czechoslovakian Wolfdog. In the German Shepherd dog the genetic defect has recently been identified (Voorbij et al, 2011), and it seems that the defect is identical in the Karelian Bear dog and the Wolfhound breeds in which the German Shepherd has been used for breeding. In the German Shepherd and the Karelian Bear dog, the disease has been known for many years to be transmitted through autosomal recessive

inheritance (Andresen and Willeberg, 1976 and 1977). Pituitary dwarfism has also been seen in the Weimaraner, Spitz, Miniature Pinscher, Golden Retriever, Labrador Retriever, and cats. No studies with regard to genetic defects have been performed in those breeds. There does not seem to be a gender predilection.

Clinical Manifestations

The clinical manifestations of pituitary dwarfism are the result of hormone deficiency, in particular lack of GH and TSH. Normal GH levels (and normal IGF-1 levels) in concert with normal thyroid function are essential for linear growth and physiological bone development. Lack of gonadotropins leads to hypogonadism and infertility.

Pituitary dwarfs are most often presented to the veterinarian at the age of 3 to 5 months due to growth retardation and skin and hair coat abnormalities. During the first 1 to 2 months, the affected animals are usually normal in size; thereafter, their growth rate is slower than that of their normal littermates. By the age of 3 to 4 months, they are obviously undersized, and they usually never attain full adult height (Feldman and Nelson, 2004). The growth failure in pituitary dwarfism is proportionate (i.e., the patient has normal body contour and just looks like the miniature version of the same breed) (Fig. 2-9 and Fig. 2-10). In contrast, in congenital hypothyroidism growth failure is disproportionate (i.e., the affected animals have thick broad heads and short limbs). The pituitary dwarfs often have a pointed muzzle, resembling that of a fox (Meij et al, 2010a). Closure of the growth plates is usually delayed, fontanelles of the skull may remain open, and there may be some delay in dental eruption, but dentition is otherwise normal.

The most obvious dermatological sign is a soft and wooly hair coat because the puppy coat of secondary hairs is retained. Primary or

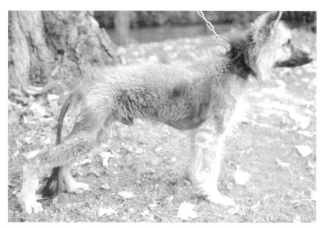

FIGURE 2-9 A 12-month-old male German Shepherd with pituitary dwarfs. There is obvious growth failure with normal body contours, foxlike face expression, alopecia, and hyperpigmentation.

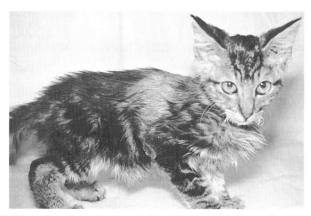

FIGURE 2-10 An 8-month-old male Domestic Short-Haired cat with pituitary dwarfism. The cat's size was similar to that of an 8-week-old kitten; body contours were normal. (Reproduced from Feldman EC, Nelson RW: Disorders of growth hormone. In Feldman EC, Nelson RW, editors: *Canine and feline endocrinology and reproduction,* St Louis, 2004, Saunders.)

guard hair does not develop or is often only present on the face and distal extremities. The stagnant development of skin and hair coat leads to increasing hair loss; initially, hair loss is confined to the areas of wear, such as the neck (from collar) and posterolateral aspects of the thighs (from sitting). With time, the entire trunk, neck, and proximal limbs become alopecic with primary hairs remaining only on the face and distal extremities (Feldman and Nelson, 2004; Meij et al, 2010a; Miller et al, 2013). The skin is initially normal, but it becomes progressively hyperpigmented, scaly, thin and wrinkled; comedones, papules, and pyoderma are common with increasing age (Feldman and Nelson, 2004). In the male dwarf, uni- or bilateral cryptorchidism, testicular atrophy, flaccid penile sheath, and azoospermia are typical manifestations of the gonadotropin deficiency, which is part of the combined pituitary deficiency. In the female dwarf, persistent anestrus is common, or estrus is irregular. Most dwarfs continue to have a puppy-like, shrill bark. They are usually lively and alert as long as they are young; however, at approximately 2 to 3 years of age, they start to become lethargic, inactive, dull, and lose appetite. These changes may reflect the deficiency of TSH (i.e., secondary hypothyroidism), the progressive enlargement of the pituitary cysts, and the development of renal insufficiency (Andresen, 1978; Feldman and Nelson, 2004; Meij et al, 2010b; Box 2-4).

The degree of growth failure is variable. Adult dogs with pituitary dwarfism may be as small as 2 kg of body weight or up to nearly half

BOX 2-4   Clinical Signs Associated with Pituitary Dwarfism

Musculoskeletal
Stunted growth (proportionate, normal body contours)
Fox-like facial features
Thin skeleton
Changes in ossification centers
Delayed closure of growth plates
Delayed dental eruption
Muscle atrophy

Dermatologic
Soft, wooly hair coat
Retention of secondary hair
Lack of primary, guard hair
Bilateral symmetrical alopecia (neck, trunk, proximal extremities)
Hyperpigmentation of skin
Thin, wrinkled skin
Scales
Comedones
Papules
Pyoderma

Reproduction
Uni- or bilateral cryptorchidism
Testicular atrophy
Flaccid penile sheath
Persistent anestrus

Other signs
Puppy-like, shrill bark
Lethargy
Listlessness
Inappetence
Mental dullness
Signs of secondary hypothyroidism

Modified from Feldman EC, Nelson RW: Disorders of growth hormone. In Feldman EC, Nelson RW, editors: *Canine and feline endocrinology and reproduction,* St. Louis, 2004, Saunders; and Voorbij AMWY, Kooistra HS: Pituitary dwarfism in German Shepherd dogs, *J Vet Clin Sci* 1:4, 2009.

of normal size. Likewise, the severity of the other clinical signs may also vary. The variation in severity as well as time of onset and rapidity of deterioration is probably related to the degree of penetrance of the defect. The degree to which the oropharyngeal ectoderm fails to develop into normal trophic-hormone cells is variable, and the rapidity with which the pituitary cysts enlarge and exert pressure atrophy is also different between individuals (Capen, 2007).

Clinical Pathology

Results of hematology, serum biochemistry profile, and urinalysis are often normal. There may be mild anemia, hypophosphatemia, and hypoalbuminemia (Eigenmann, 1982a). Azotemia may be present as a result of abnormal glomerular development and decreased glomerular filtration associated with GH and thyroid hormone deficiencies (Kooistra, 2010). Hypercholesterolemia may be seen as a result of secondary hypothyroidism.

Dermatohistopathology

The histopathological abnormalities in dogs with pituitary dwarfism are consistent with an endocrine disorder and similar to findings in many other endocrinopathies. They include varying degrees of orthokeratotic hyperkeratosis, follicular hyperkeratosis, follicular dilatation, follicular atrophy, hair follicles predominantly in telogen phase, excessive trichilemmal keratinization, sebaceous gland atrophy, epidermal melanosis, and thinning of the dermis. A decreased amount and size of dermal elastin fibers have been considered a highly suggestive finding; however, this issue is controversial. In case of secondary hypothyroidism, vacuolated or hypertrophied arrector pili muscles may be present (Miller et al, 2013).

Differential Diagnosis

Stunted growth may be due to various non-endocrine and endocrine disorders (see Box 2-3). The possibility should also be considered that the patient is just a small individual within the normal biological variation, or that the small stature is the result of an unrecognized mating with a small sire (Meij et al, 2010b). The cause of growth failure may also be feeding a low-caloric or poorly composed diet, heavy intestinal parasitism, or the administration of glucocorticoids at an early age. A detailed history (including dietary history and deworming program), physical examination, and routine laboratory evaluation (hematology, serum biochemistry profile, urinalysis, and fecal evaluation for parasites) helps to narrow the list of differential diagnosis. Depending on the results, further step-by-step work-up should be pursued, including tests such as liver function tests, measurement of circulating trypsinlike immunoreactivity (TLI), radiology of skeletal abnormalities, ultrasonography, and echocardiography. Congenital hypothyroidism may be the most important differential diagnosis, although the dogs look quite different. Congenital hyposomatotropism is associated with proportionate dwarfism, whereas animals with congenital hypothyroidism are disproportionate dwarfs. Usually, congenital hypothyroidism is a primary thyroid disease (i.e., the defect lies within the thyroid gland; e.g., thyroid dysgenesis, defective thyroid hormone synthesis) or is due to iodine deficiency. Secondary hypothyroidism (i.e., hypothyroidism due to TSH deficiency) has been described, but it seems to be extremely rare. See Chapter 3 for further details on etiopathogenesis and diagnostic work-up. It is important to note that hyposecretion of TSH is usually part of the combined pituitary hormone deficiency, which is typically seen in pituitary dwarfism in the German Shepherd dog. In these dogs, the clinical manifestations of hypothyroidism are overshadowed by the pronounced deficiency of GH; this is in part because a small but significant fraction of thyroid function is independent of TSH (Meij et al, 2010b; Brent and Davies, 2011).

Endocrinological Evaluation and Diagnosis

History and physical changes are often typical and highly suggestive for pituitary dwarfism. As discussed earlier, pituitary dwarfism in the German Shepherd dog (and related breeds such as the Karelian Bear dog, Saarloos Wolfhound, and Czechoslovakian Wolfdog) is due to a mutation in the LHX3 gene (Voorbij et al, 2011). A dwarf with this mutation has combined pituitary hormone deficiency, because this gene is important for the differentiation of all endocrine cells in the anterior pituitary, except for the corticotrophs.

Genetic Testing

A genetic test for the LHX3 gene mutation is now available through the University of Utrecht and several other laboratories. If a dwarf is tested positive for the mutation, further endocrinological evaluations (including measurement of GH) are unnecessary.

All German Shepherd dwarfs tested at the University of Utrecht during the last 3 years (i.e., since the availability of the genetic test) had the LHX3 mutation (H.S. Kooistra, personal communication, 2013). The test requires 2 mL of randomly sampled ethylenediaminetetraacetic acid (EDTA) plasma.

Pituitary dwarfism in other breeds than the German Shepherd (and related breeds) and in cats is extremely rare. This means that in most cases the disease can be diagnosed by genetic testing. In the very few cases in which genetic testing is negative or testing is inappropriate (e.g., cats) measurement of GH after stimulation with GHRH, clonidine, or xylazine is the test of choice. Unfortunately, GH measurement is only done in very few laboratories (e.g., University of Utrecht). If GH measurement is unavailable, the veterinarian should first exclude the various endocrine and non-endocrine causes for growth failure (see Box 2-3). In disproportionate dwarfs, evaluation of thyroid function should primarily be pursued (see Chapter 3). Thereafter, measurement of IGF-1 may be pursued as a surrogate for GH measurement. False positive results (i.e., low IGF-1 due to other reasons) may occur, and therefore test results need to be interpreted with care (see "Hormonal Evaluation").

Basal Growth Hormone

Similar to the situation in many other endocrinopathies, measurement of circulating basal hormone values is of little diagnostic relevance in the work-up of animals with suspected pituitary dwarfism. Various studies showed that random basal GH concentrations of pituitary dwarfs overlap largely with those of healthy dogs. Healthy dogs may at times have low to undetectable GH levels, because GH is secreted in pulses and GH may be very low between the normal pulses (Eigenmann, 1982b; Eigenmann et al, 1984d; Kooistra et al, 2000a; Bhatti et al, 2006c). Eigenmann, et al. (1984d) reported basal GH levels of 0.48 ± 0.09 μg/L in German Shepherd dwarfs and of 1.5 ± 1.2 μg/L in healthy dogs. In the study of Kooistra, et al. (2000a), basal GH levels ranged between 0.3 to 1.5 μg/L (mean 0.5) in the German Shepherd dwarfs and between 0.6 to 5.2 μg/L (mean 1.8) in healthy Beagle dogs. Bhatti, et al. (2006c) found basal GH levels in German Shepherd dwarfs to be between 0.4 to 1.2 μg/L (mean 0.7) and 0.2 to 1.0 μg/L (mean 0.6) in healthy Beagle dogs. Basal GH concentrations in healthy cats were reported to be 3.2 ± 0.7 μg/L (Eigenmann et al, 1984b) and 1.2 ± 1.0 μg/L (Peterson et al, 1990).

Growth Hormone Stimulation Tests

A general rule for the work-up of endocrine disease is that the confirmation of a hypofunctional state requires a stimulation test, and confirmation of a hyperfunctional test requires a suppression test (Eigenmann, 1982b). Consequently, confirmation of hyposomatotropism requires the use of a stimulation test. Isolated GH deficiency may be documented by a stimulation test using GHRH, clonidine, or xylazine. Stimulation with ghrelin has also been described (Table 2-1). For the diagnosis of combined pituitary hormone deficiency, the combined pituitary function test, using four releasing hormones, is an appropriate test. Circulating GH concentrations are measured in blood samples taken at several time points after the application of the stimulating substance. GH deficiency is diagnosed if GH does not increase above a certain cut-off value. A few important factors have to be considered with regard to test interpretation. First, GH deficiency may be complete or only partial. In case of complete GH deficiency, there is absence of GH increase after stimulation. In case of partial GH deficiency, however, mild to moderate response may be seen, which may overlap with the response of healthy animals. The problem of overlapping GH levels also exists in human medicine, where the cut-off between normal and abnormal is matter of great debate and at least two provocative tests of assessing

TABLE 2-1	PROTOCOLS FOR GROWTH HORMONE STIMULATION TESTS			
TEST	**SUBSTANCE, DOSE, ROUTE OF ADMINISTRATION**	**TIME OF BLOOD SAMPLING (MINUTES)**	**NORMAL RESULTS**	**ADVERSE REACTIONS**
GHRH stimulation test	Human GHRH, 1 µg/kg, IV	0*, 5, 10, 20*, 30*, 45	GH > 5 µg/L (poststimulation)	None reported
Clonidine stimulation test	Clonidine, 10 µg/kg, IV	0*, 15*, 30*, 45, 60, 90	GH > 10 µg/L (poststimulation)	Sedation, bradycardia, hypotension, dizziness, aggressive behavior
Xylazine stimulation test	Xylazine, 100 µg/kg, IV	0*, 15*, 30*, 45, 60, 90	GH > 10 µg/L (poststimulation)	Sedation, bradycardia, hypotension, dizziness, aggressive behavior
Ghrelin stimulation test	Human ghrelin, 2 µg/kg, IV	0*, 5, 10, 20*, 30*, 45	GH > 5 µg/L (poststimulation)	None reported

GH, Growth hormone; *GHRH*, GH-releasing hormone; *IV*, intravenous. The reader should note that the original protocols include frequent blood sampling; not all of the blood samples are required to decide if GH response is normal or insufficient. Blood samples should be taken at the time of peak GH response. Sampling may therefore be limited to times labeled with *. Please see text for further details on handling of the blood samples. Also see text for discussion on the combined pituitary function test.

GH reserve are necessary before the diagnosis of GH deficiency should be made (Cooke et al, 2011).

Secondly, availability of GH measurement in dogs is extremely limited, because a species-specific, homologous assay has to be used. Feline GH can reliably be measured in a radioimmunoassay (RIA) developed for dogs (Kooistra, 2010). So far, no comparison studies have been performed between different GH assays in veterinary medicine. In human medicine, one of the biggest confounders in the evaluation of GH secretion is the variability of the measured GH levels across different assays (Cooke et al, 2011). It is therefore of utmost importance that any GH assay used in dogs (and cats) has been validated for the species and that assay-specific reference ranges are available.

Thirdly, GH response to stimulation is known to be influenced by various factors; their relevance, however, has not yet been thoroughly investigated in dogs and cats. In humans (i.e., children with suspected GH deficiency), GH stimulation tests should only be performed after an overnight fast, because carbohydrates and fat suppress GH secretion. Obesity also leads to an attenuated GH response. Testing should not be performed if the patient takes supraphysiological doses of glucocorticoids, because these drugs suppress GH release (Cooke et al, 2011; Styne, 2011). Glucocorticoids are also known to have a negative impact on GH release in dogs. In dogs with pituitary-dependent hyperadrenocorticism, GH release is suppressed after GHRH, clonidine, or xylazine (Peterson and Altszuler, 1981; Regnier and Garnier, 1995; Meij et al, 1997). It appears likely, that GH response may also be impaired in animals receiving exogenous glucocorticoids. Taken together, GH stimulation testing should routinely be performed after an overnight fast in an otherwise adequately nourished animal who has not received glucocorticoids. None of the tests discussed below has been investigated in the cat.

GH-Releasing Hormone Test

The GHRH test using human GHRH has been shown to be a suitable test for the diagnosis of GH deficiency in dogs. Initial studies in healthy dogs using varying doses of GHRH showed that GH rises within a few minutes after application of GHRH without any apparent clinical side effects. The use of 1 µg/kg GHRH is similar effective as the standard clonidine test (10 µg/kg clonidine) (Abribat et al, 1989). After collection of a zero blood sample, 1 µg/kg of human GHRH is injected intravenously and further blood samples are taken at 5, 10, 20, 30, and 45 minutes (Rijnberk and Kooistra, 2010). In some of the initial protocols, additional samples were taken after 60, 90, and 120 minutes; however, as the GH peak occurs early (between 10 and

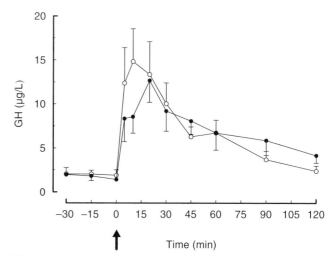

FIGURE 2-11 Plasma growth hormone (GH) response (mean ± standard error) in eight healthy Beagle dogs after rapid (30-second) intravenous injection *(arrow)* of a combination of four hypothalamic releasing hormones (●) compared with single stimulation with 1 µg/kg GH-releasing hormone (GHRH) (○). The area under the curve (AUC) and the increment (peak basal level at 0 min) in GH concentrations were not significantly different between combined and single stimulation test. (Reproduced with permission from Meij BP, et al.: Assessment of a combined anterior pituitary function test in beagle dogs: rapid sequential intravenous administration of four hypothalamic releasing hormones, *Domest Anim Endocrinol* 13[2]:161-170, 1996.)

30 minutes), those samples are deemed unnecessary. Samples for GH measurement have to be handled carefully because rapid proteolytic degradation of the hormone may occur. We routinely collect blood samples in EDTA-coated ice-chilled tubes and centrifuge them immediately; the use of a cooled centrifuge is advantageous. Samples are stored at or below –20° C and are shipped to the laboratory on dry ice with express service (Rijnberk and Kooistra, 2010). There is a great inter-individual variability of the normal GH response to GHRH. Meij, et al. (1996a) investigated the GH response in eight healthy Beagle dogs after the single administration of GH and compared it to the response after the combined administration of four releasing hormones. Single GHRH application resulted in maximum GH concentrations between 4.9 and 27.5 µg/L (mean 14.7 ± 3.7) after 10 minutes. Application of the combined stimulation test (see also later) leads to maximum GH concentrations of 5.4 to 24.8 µg/L (12.6 ± 2.5) after 20 minutes. The GH responses did not differ between the single and the combined test (Fig. 2-11). The study by Meij, et al.

(1996a) was performed in 1- to 6-year-old dogs (median 2 years). In elderly Beagle dogs (7 to 12 years, median 10 years), the GH response was considerably lower, confirming that GH responsiveness to GHRH stimulation decreases with age (Bhatti et al, 2006b). In German Shepherd dwarfs, basal GH was shown to be low and did not respond to stimulation with GHRH (Hamann et al, 1999; Kooistra et al, 2000a; see Fig. 2-7). As already mentioned earlier, it may be difficult to differentiate partial GH deficiency from normal because GH concentrations may overlap. A normal response would be a poststimulation GH concentration above 5 µg/L. GHRH may not be available in some countries.

Stimulation with Ghrelin

Ghrelin is a GH secretogogue that stimulates GH release from pituitary somatotrophs through the GHS-R. In contrast to humans, administration of ghrelin does not stimulate the release of other pituitary hormones in dogs (e.g., the effect is specific for GH). GH responsiveness to ghrelin also decreases with age, which is similar to the somatotrophic response to GHRH (Bhatti et al, 2002; Bhatti et al, 2006b). In eight healthy young Beagle dogs (age 13 to 17 months, median 10), maximum GH concentration after ghrelin ranged from 0.2 to 124 µg/L (median 52). In six German Shepherd dwarfs (age 9 to 21 months, median 12) maximum GH increase after ghrelin was 0.7 to 4.1 µg/L (median 1.9), which was significantly lower compared to the healthy dogs. None of the dwarfs had a GH release greater than 5 µg/L; however, this was also true for three of the healthy dogs (Bhatti et al, 2006c). Due to the relatively high number of false positive test results, the ghrelin test appears to be inferior to the GHRH test and the clonidine or xylazine test.

The ghrelin test was performed in all studies mentioned earlier by intravenous (IV) injection of 2 µg/kg human ghrelin and sampling blood for GH measurement before injection and 5, 10, 20, 30, and 45 minutes thereafter. Sample handling was done as described for the GHRH test.

Clonidine Stimulation Test

Clonidine is a centrally-acting α_2-adrenergic agonist that stimulates the release of GHRH and GH. The test was established for use in dogs more than 30 years ago (Hampshire and Altszuler, 1981; Eigenmann and Eigenmann, 1981a). It can still be considered a suitable test for the diagnosis of GH deficiency. Clonidine doses ranging from 3 to 30 µg/kg have been used by different investigators. A dose of 10 µg/kg is usually considered to be the standard dose (Roth et al, 1980; Hampshire and Altszuler, 1981; Eigenmann and Eigenmann, 1981a; Feldman and Nelson, 2004). GH increases within 10 to 15 minutes and reaches its peak 15 to 30 minutes after the administration of clonidine; as seen after stimulation with GHRH, there is great inter-individual variability with regard to GH response. It is not clear if administration of clonidine to healthy dogs results in a more pronounced GH release than GHRH. Abribat, et al. (1989) found no difference between the GH response when 1 µg/kg GHRH and 10 µg/kg clonidine were compared. Eigenmann, et al. (1984d) found a maximum GH release after clonidine of 44.4 ± 13.9 µg/L, whereas in a study by Meij, et al. (1996a) GHRH resulted in a maximum GH release of 14.7 ± 3.7 µg/L (see Fig. 2-11; Fig. 2-12). Adverse reactions to clonidine are possible, but they are more likely and more severe with doses above 10 µg/kg. They include sedation, bradycardia, hypotension, dizziness, or aggressive behavior and may last 15 to 60 minutes. If necessary, atropine can be used to combat bradycardia, IV fluids are indicated if hypotension is severe, and yohimbine or atipamezole may be used as α antagonists. The test

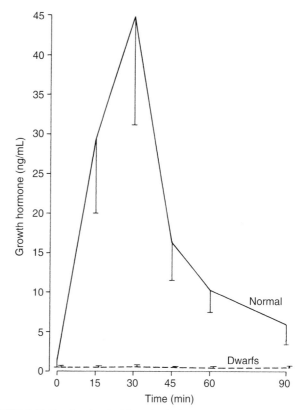

FIGURE 2-12 Results of a clonidine stimulation test in normal dogs and nine German Shepherd dogs with pituitary dwarfism. Clonidine, 10 µg/kg body weight was given intravenously at time 0. (Graph redrawn from data in Eigenmann JE, et al.: Growth hormone and insulin-like growth factor I in German Shepherd dwarf dogs, *Acta Endocrinol* 105[3]:289-293, 1984. Reproduced from Feldman EC, Nelson RW: Disorders of growth hormone. In Feldman EC, Nelson RW, editors: *Canine and feline endocrinology and reproduction,* St Louis, 2004, Saunders.)

protocol as described by Eigenmann, et al. (1984d) includes the IV administration of 10 µg/kg clonidine and sampling blood for GH measurement before injection and 15, 30, 45, 60, and 90 minutes thereafter. Sample handling should be done as described for the GHRH test. An increase in GH above 10 µg/L is considered a normal response (Eigenmann et al, 1984d).

Xylazine Stimulation Test

Xylazine is a sedative analgesic that is structurally related to clonidine. Xylazine administration to healthy dogs results in GH release similar to the actions of clonidine (Hampshire and Altszuler, 1981), rendering the xylazine stimulation test a suitable test for the diagnosis of GH deficiency. Adverse effects and their treatments are also similar to clonidine (see earlier). After taking a zero sample, 100 µg/kg xylazine are injected intravenously and further blood samples are taken as described for the clonidine stimulation test. Test interpretation is similar to the clonidine stimulation test (i.e., a GH increase greater than 10 µg/L is considered a normal response).

Combined Pituitary Function Testing and Evaluation of Thyroid Function

Lack of GH can occur as isolated GH deficiency, or in concert with deficiencies of other pituitary hormones, called *combined pituitary hormone deficiency*. The latter is present in the German Shepherd dwarfs (and related breeds) and includes a lack of GH, TSH, and prolactin together with impaired release of gonadotropins, whereas secretion of ACTH is preserved. The complexity of deficiencies was revealed by studies employing the combined pituitary function test (Kooistra et al, 2000a). The disease is due to a mutation in the LHX3 gene, and nowadays, a genetic test replaces the combined pituitary function tests in the German Shepherd (and related breeds). Pituitary dwarfism also occurs sporadically in other breeds, although very rarely. Because combined pituitary function tests have not been used in those cases, it is not known how many of those have isolated GH deficiency versus combined pituitary hormone deficiency. The original protocol of combined pituitary function tests consists of rapid (within 30 seconds) sequential IV injections of four releasing hormones: CRH (1 µg/kg), GHRH (1 µg/kg), GnRH (10 µg/kg) and TRH (10 µg/kg). Blood samples are collected for the measurement of ACTH, GH, LH, TSH, and prolactin prior to the administration and 5, 10, 20, 30, 45, 60, 90, and 120 min thereafter. Handling and storage of blood samples is done as described with the GHRH test. When the combined test was compared with the separate administration of the four releasing hormones, there was no apparent inhibition or synergism with regard to ACTH, GH, and prolactin concentrations. LH and TSH responses were less in the combined test; however, the difference in TSH secretion was minor. Adverse effects of the combined test included vomiting, hypersalivation, and restlessness in a few dogs, which disappeared within 5 minutes after the injection (Meij et al, 1996a; Meij et al, 1996b). The test has been modified slightly as sampling at 60, 90, and 120 minutes was omitted (Kooistra et al, 2000a). Performance of the combined pituitary function test is time consuming, expensive, and availability of some of the hormone analysis is limited. To be considered normal, GH should increase above 5 µg/L. However, this cut-off as well as the cut-offs of the other hormones are assay-dependent. It should be noted that combined pituitary hormone deficiency is most likely more common than isolated GH deficiency. An alternative approach to the performance of the combined pituitary hormone deficiency would be to first document that the patient has GH deficiency by using one of the tests described earlier (stimulation with GHRH, clonidine, or xylazine). Thereafter, a search for further hormone deficiencies may be limited to the evaluation of thyroid function. TSH deficiency is a common component of the combined pituitary hormone deficiency complex, and its documentation is of great importance, because normal thyroid function is required for physiological growth and development. Finding low basal thyroxine (T_4) and free T_4 concentrations, however, is not sufficient to confirm that there is a lack of TSH. Basal T_4 and free T_4 overlap between healthy and hypothyroid dogs, and low thyroid hormone levels may be caused by various factors, such as nonthyroidal illness and drugs. Some dwarfs may have basal T_4 in the lower range of normal and may even show some increase when the TSH stimulation test is applied (Kooistra et al, 1998). A low endogenous TSH level also does not confirm that there is a lack of pituitary TSH production, because low levels are also seen in healthy dogs. For these reasons, evaluation of TSH deficiency requires performance of the TRH stimulation test. For a complete discussion of the TRH stimulation test, see Chapter 3. In the study by Meij, et al. (1996b), basal TSH ranged between 0.07 to 0.27 µg/L in healthy dogs, and the injection of 10 µg/kg TRH resulted in a rapid increase in plasma TSH levels. In the single TRH test, maximum TSH concentration was 1.26 ± 0.22 µg/L at 10 minutes. In the combined pituitary function test, maximum TSH was 0.85 ± 0.17 µg/L at 30 minutes. The TRH test should be normal in cases with isolated GH deficiency. In the German Shepherd dwarfs with combined pituitary hormone deficiency,

basal TSH concentrations were very low and did not increase after stimulation (Hamann et al, 1999; Kooistra et al, 2000a).

Corticotroph function is usually normal in pituitary dwarfism. Performance of a CRH stimulation test with measurement of ACTH may be warranted in dwarfs that develop signs of cortisol deficiency (e.g., lethargy, inappetence, vomiting, weight loss) (Feldman and Nelson, 2004).

Growth Hormone Stimulation by Amino Acid Administration and Insulin-Induced Hypoglycemia

In humans, administration of arginine or insulin-induced hypoglycemia is used (amongst others) as tests to provoke GH secretion. In dogs, however, the GH response after those stimuli is inconsistent, rendering the tests of limited use (Eigenmann and Eigenmann, 1981a).

Measurement of Insulin-like Growth Factor-1 Concentration

A deficiency in GH is associated with a low concentration of IGF-1. Different to GH concentrations, which rise and fall due to their pulsatile secretion, circulating IGF-1 is stable throughout the day. In human medicine, measurement of IGF-1 and IGF-binding protein-3 (IGFBP-3) are used as additional tools to evaluate patients for GH deficiency. The IGF-1 test, however, is known to have substantial limitations, because IGF-1 levels are influenced by various factors including age, degree of sexual maturation, and nutritional status. Starvation lowers IGF-1 levels into ranges seen in children with GH deficiency (Cooke et al, 2011). IGFBP-3 levels vary less with age and are less dependent on nutritional status; however, sensitivity for GH deficiency in humans is only moderate (Styne, 2011). Eigenmann, et al. (1984d) reported mean IGF-1 levels in German Shepherd dwarfs of 11 ± 2 µg/L, in healthy adult German Shepherds of 280 ± 23 µg/L, and in healthy immature German Shepherd of 345 ± 50 µg/L. Very low IGF-1 levels in German Shepherd dwarfs were also found in other studies (Rijnberk et al, 1993; Kooistra et al, 1998; Kooistra et al, 2000a; Knottenbelt and Herrtage, 2002). However, a low IGF-1 concentration should not be used as a sole criterion to diagnose GH deficiency. Starvation and illness may also lead to low IGF-1 concentrations; and it should be remembered that specific reference ranges are required because IGF-1 is age-dependent and correlates with body weight. Measurement of IGFBP-3 has not yet been described in pituitary dwarfs.

See the section Hypersomatotropism (Acromegaly) in Cats for more details on IGF-1 measurement.

Diagnostic Imaging

Computed tomography (CT) or magnetic resonance imaging (MRI) of the pituitary gland often reveals the presence of pituitary cysts in dogs with pituitary dwarfism. In young dwarfs, the cysts are usually small; however, their size gradually increases with age. Because healthy dogs may also have pituitary cysts, diagnosis of pituitary dwarfism should not be based on pituitary imaging (Kooistra, 2010).

Treatment

In humans, GH of non-primate origin is not biologically active. For many years, replacement therapy was therefore performed by using GH derived from human cadavers. In the 1980s distribution of human growth hormone (hGH) was ceased due to the concern of a causal relationship with Creutzfeldt-Jakob disease. At that time, recombinant human growth hormone (rhGH) became available, which is now the accepted treatment for children with GH deficiency (Cooke et al, 2011). In dogs, the use of hGH, rhGH, porcine, ovine, and bovine GH has been reported (Eigenmann, 1981a; Eigenmann and Patterson, 1984; Scott and Walton, 1986; Schmeitzel and Lothrop, 1990; Van Herpen et al, 1994). The clinical response varied, which, however, may in several of the cases not have been due to the substance itself, but due to an erroneous assumption. Most of the studies were performed in dogs with adult onset alopecia, previously thought to be caused by acquired GH deficiency. However, there is now strong evidence that the phenomenon in fact is not due to a lack in GH (see later). It is therefore not surprising that response to GH administration was poor. Reports on GH treatment in congenital GH deficiency (i.e., in German Shepherds dwarfs) is limited to a low number of cases. In one study, use of rhGH had to be discontinued in a dwarf (and an adult Poodle with alopecia) after 1 month, because they collapsed and developed pale mucus membranes shortly after the injection. Further investigations revealed the presence of antibodies to the human GH (Van Herpen et al, 1994). Porcine GH is considered to be the better choice for treatment of congenital GH deficiency in dogs, because the amino acid sequences of porcine and canine GH are identical. Biosynthetic porcine GH has been developed; however, at times availability may be a problem. Due to the rarity of pituitary dwarfism, no studies have been performed comparing different treatment regimens. The currently recommended initial dose for porcine GH is 0.1 IU/kg body weight administered subcutaneously three times a week. Dose adjustments should be based on clinical response and circulating IGF-1 levels. The goal is to have the IGF-1 levels increase into the normal range; because IGF-1 levels correlate with body weight and are age-dependent, specific reference ranges have to be used (Feldman and Nelson, 2004). GH administration may lead to glucose intolerance and possibly to overt diabetes mellitus, requiring cessation of treatment or dose reduction. Hypersensitivity reactions are also possible. Reevaluation of the patient should be scheduled approximately every 4 to 6 weeks and should include physical examination, measurement of blood glucose, and IGF-1 concentrations; T_4 concentrations should also be evaluated regularly in dogs treated for secondary hypothyroidism. Improvement in hair coat and skin is usually seen within 6 to 8 weeks of treatment. Regrowth of secondary hair growth is relatively consistent, whereas regrowth of primary hair is more variable. Some dogs develop a full hair coat (Fig. 2-13). The status of the growth plates at the time of initiation of GH therapy determines if linear growth

will be possible; usually, however, there is only a slight increase in height. After a few months, the maximum possible treatment success is usually achieved, allowing reduction in GH dose and frequency of application. Long-term dose rates depend on the IGF-1 levels, which should be maintained in the normal range for age and breed. Because GH is not only essential for linear growth but is also important during adulthood, life-long treatment (albeit at a lower dose) is recommended.

In children with GH deficiency, treatment is more successful when the same weekly GH doses are administered in seven daily doses, instead of a 6 day/week or 3 day/week schedule (Cooke et al, 2011). A similar protocol has not been published for dogs yet. However, it may be a consideration to split the aforementioned dose into smaller daily portions.

The application of synthetic progesterone has been reported as an alternative treatment option to GH supplementation. In dogs, progesterone induces synthesis of GH in the mammary gland; as discussed in "Mammary Growth Hormone," this is a physiological event in intact bitches and important for normal mammary gland development (van Garderen et al, 1997). Treatment of two young German Shepherd dwarfs (one male, one female) with medroxyprogesterone acetate (MPA) was described by Kooistra, et al. (1998). The dogs were injected with 2.5 to 5.0 mg/kg MPA subcutaneously (starting dose of 5 mg/kg MPA), initially at 3 week intervals and subsequently at 6 weeks interval. Primary hair started to grow after 9 weeks of treatment, and both dogs developed a full hair coat within 6 months, body weight increased substantially, and body size increased only slightly. Circulating GH and IGF-1 concentrations increased during treatment. Although GH never exceeded the upper limit of the reference range, one of the two dogs developed acromegalic features (soft tissue swelling of the muzzle, the abdomen, and the feet), suggesting that there was an excessive exposure to GH. The most likely explanation is that progesterone-induced GH secretion lacks the physiological pulsatility of the pituitary GH. The daily secretion of GH may have been too high despite normal plasma levels. Measurement of circulating IGF-1 levels may be a better parameter to monitor treatment and to assess if the dose of MPA is correct. Further adverse effects were recurrent episodes of pruritic pyoderma in both dogs and cystic endometrial hyperplasia with mucometra in the female dog. The latter complication leads to the recommendation that female dogs should be ovariohysterectomized before the start of progestin treatment. The dogs stayed otherwise healthy for at least 3 to 4 years (Kooistra et al, 1998). A similar approach was taken by Knottenbelt and Herrtage (2002) who treated three German Shepherd dwarfs (two female, one male) with proligestone (PROL), 10 mg/kg every 3 weeks subcutaneously. Two dwarfs were also supplemented with T_4. Treatment resulted in a substantial increase in IGF-1 levels, increase in body weight, and development of a full hair coat in all three. Two of the dogs developed acromegalic features, requiring temporary cessation of PROL. Recurrent pyoderma and cystic endometrial hyperplasia occurred in one dog each. None of the dogs in the two studies developed hyperglycemia; it should, however, be kept in mind that diabetes mellitus is a potential complication of progestin (and GH) therapy. Development of mammary tumors is another potential side-effect of progestin administration.

Treatment with progestins may be a suitable alternative to porcine GH administration if the latter is unavailable. Both protocols certainly need refinement. As with GH treatment, regular reevaluations are mandatory, and they should at least include physical examination and measurement of blood glucose, IGF-1, and T_4 concentrations.

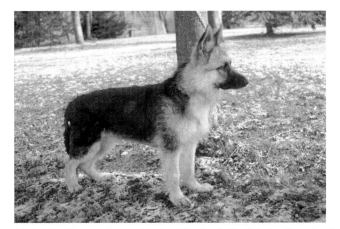

FIGURE 2-13 The same German Shepherd dwarf as in Fig. 2-9 after 4 months of treatment with porcine growth hormone (GH) and thyroxine (T_4). The dog developed a full hair coat and the foxlike facial expression disappeared. Linear growth was not achieved.

German Shepherd dwarfs and dwarfs of related breeds suffer from combined pituitary hormone deficiency. The lack of GH and TSH constitutes the biggest problem for normal growth and development. In those dogs, treatment with GH or progestins should always be accompanied by life-long T_4 administration. The same accounts for dwarfs of other breeds with combined pituitary hormone deficiency. Dwarfs with isolated GH deficiency (i.e., normal TSH response after TRH application) do not need T_4 supplementation. See Chapter 3 for details on dose and treatment monitoring. No treatment protocols have been described for congenital hyposomatotropism in cats.

Prognosis

Dogs that are left untreated develop severe hair coat and skin abnormalities and become increasingly thin, lethargic, and dull. They usually die or are euthanized between 3 and 5 years of age. The poor condition is due to progressive loss of pituitary functions, expansion of pituitary cysts, renal failure, or infections. Dogs that are treated with GH or progestins and T_4 can live a relatively healthy life for several years, provided that complications (e.g., acromegaly, diabetes mellitus, pyometra, and pyoderma) are avoided. The long-term prognosis, however, remains guarded; pituitary dwarfs usually do not have a normal life-expectancy (Feldman and Nelson, 2004; Meij et al, 2010b).

 ACQUIRED HYPOSOMATOTROPISM

Humans

In humans, acquired GH deficiency is a well-recognized albeit rare clinical entity. The partial or complete lack of GH has negative effects on multiple organs systems. The most important of which are abnormal body composition (e.g., increased central fat deposition, reduced skeletal muscle and lean body mass), increase of cardiovascular risk factors (e.g., abnormal lipid profile, endothelial dysfunction, microvascular abnormalities, change in cardiac size and function) and reduced bone mass. It also has a negative impact on quality of life (i.e., due to a low energy level and emotional liability) (Doga et al, 2006; Aragon-Alonso et al, 2011; Melmed et al, 2011). The most common causes of acquired GH deficiency are pituitary-hypothalamic tumors. In affected patients, GH deficiency may develop either before or after neurosurgery or radiation therapy. These scenarios account for more than 80% of cases. Other conditions associated with the risk of acquired GH deficiency are traumatic brain injury and acute vascular injuries (e.g., subarachnoid hemorrhage and inflammatory/infectious disorders) (Ghigo et al, 2008; Melmed, 2013; Box 2-5). Acquired GH deficiency may occur as isolated deficit. It is, however, often associated with the failure of other cell types in the anterior pituitary gland. Because somatotrophs are the most sensitive cells to pituitary insults, GH deficiency usually precedes the development of multiple failure (Melmed, 2013). There is some controversy on the topic of so-called idiopathic adult GH deficiency. The GH Deficiency Consensus Workshop states that idiopathic isolated GH deficiency is not a recognized diagnosed entity (Ho, 2007). Nevertheless, about 15% of humans with adult GH deficiency are reported as suffering from an idiopathic cause. Those patients, however, may at least in part reflect a group of individuals with unclear or incomplete medical history (e.g., forgotten past sports head injury or car accident) and incomplete work-up, inadequate biochemical testing, or with a yet to be defined occult defect (Melmed, 2013).

See the Consensus guidelines for the diagnosis and treatment of adults with GH deficiency for more details (Ho, 2007).

Dogs and Cats

The categories listed in Box 2-5 as causes for acquired GH deficiency in humans in principle also account for dogs and cats. It should be noted, however, that knowledge on acquired GH deficiency in dogs and cats is extremely scarce.

Neoplastic, traumatic, vascular, inflammatory, and infectious disorders may result in pituitary destruction including the somatotrophic cells. Depending on the extent of the destruction, other endocrine cell types of the pituitary gland may also be involved, resulting in the deficiency of several pituitary hormones. In those cases, the clinical signs of GH deficiency are usually overshadowed by the signs caused by the deficiency of ACTH, TSH, and vasopressin or by neurological dysfunction in case of large masses. This statement is illustrated by two case reports on lymphocytic and lymphoplasmacytic hypophysitis (Wolfesberger et al, 2011; Meij et al, 2012a). One of the two dogs was presented

---

BOX 2-5   Causes of Acquired Growth Hormone Deficiency in Adult Humans

Traumatic
Surgical damage
Radiation damage
Traumatic brain injury

Neoplastic
Pituitary tumor
Craniopharyngioma
Hypothalamic tumor
Metastasis into pituitary
Hematological malignancy
Parasellar mass (Rathke cyst, dermoid cyst, meningioma, and other brain tumors)

Vascular
Subarachnoidal hemorrhage
Pregnancy-related
Aneurysm
Apoplexy
Arteritis

Inflammatory/Infiltrative
Primary hypophysitis (lymphocytic, granulomatous, xanthomatous)
Secondary hypophysitis (sarcoidosis, histiocytosis X)
Hemochromatosis
Immune-mediated (Pit-1 antibodies)

Infection
Tuberculosis
Fungal (histoplasmosis, aspergillosis, pneumocystis)
Parasitic (toxoplasmosis)
Viral (cytomegalovirus)

Hormonal
Hyperparathyroidism
Glucocorticoids
Somatostatin analogs

Idiopathic?

Modified from: Melmed S: Update: idiopathic adult growth hormone deficiency, *J Clin Endocrin Metabol* 98:2187, 2013.

with progressive anorexia, weight loss, and cachexia. Histopathology and immunohistochemistry of the pituitary gland revealed severe lymphoplasmacytic adenohypophysitis and marked reduction of ACTH- and GH-positive cells, as well as some reduction of prolactin-positive cells. The zona fasciculata and reticularis of the adrenal cortex were atrophied, and the dog's sudden death was attributed to secondary adrenocortical insufficiency resulting from the ACTH deficiency (Wolfesberger et al, 2011). The other dog suffered from polyuria and polydipsia, exercise intolerance, and a dull hair coat. Central diabetes insipidus, secondary hypothyroidism, and hyposomatotropism were diagnosed during endocrinological work-up. The dog was finally euthanized, and the histological diagnosis was lymphocytic hypophysitis (Meij et al, 2012a). It remains unclear whether GH deficiency contributed to the clinical signs of lethargy and dull hair coat, because both symptoms may have also been exclusively caused by secondary hypothyroidism.

Multiple hormone deficiency including lack of GH has been demonstrated to occur in dogs after transsphenoidal hypophysectomy. Those dogs are cured from their pituitary-dependent hypercortisolism (which was the reason for surgery) and are supplemented with T_4 and glucocorticoids; however, some of them do not regain normal liveliness, muscle mass, or hair coat. It has been assumed, that these signs may reflect GH deficiency and that treatment with porcine GH or progestins may bring improvement (Meij et al, 2010a). The possibility of radiation therapy of pituitary masses leading to GH deficiency in dogs has not yet been investigated.

For many years, veterinarians have hypothesized that in some breeds acquired GH deficiency may be the cause of bilateral symmetrical alopecia and hyperpigmentation. The affected breeds include those with double coat and dense undercoat, such as Pomeranian, Alaskan Malamute, Chow Chow, and Keeshond. It has also been seen in Miniature and Toy Poodles. For some time, imbalance within the steroid biosynthesis pathway in the adrenal cortex (i.e., partial deficiency of the 21-hydroxylase enzyme) was favored as an alternative cause.

Over time, the disorder has been termed *adult-onset GH deficiency, GH-responsive alopecia, castration-responsive alopecia, biopsy-responsive alopecia, black skin disease,* and *congenital adrenal hyperplasia-like syndrome.* More recently, the term *Alopecia X* was created, reflecting the mystery of the disease. The theory of an acquired GH deficiency was discarded when various studies revealed normal GH response after stimulation and normal IGF-1 levels in many of the affected dogs. Similarly, abnormal adrenal steroid precursor or sex hormone production turned out to be highly unlikely. The reason, why some of the affected dogs show suppressed GH response remains speculative. Glucocorticoids are known to increase somatostatin release, thereby interfering with GH release. It may be that some of those dogs had received exogenous glucocorticoids before referral for further work-up, in others, ACTH stimulation test and low-dose dexamethasone (resulting in increased steroid concentrations) test may have been performed prior to GH testing. Recently, mild hypercortisolism has been proposed as cause of the disease in Miniature Poodles and Pomeranians. The age of onset of the disease is usually between 9 months and 2 years; however, it may also occur much later in life. The initial signs are hair loss in areas of wear (collar, caudal thighs) slowly progressing to nearly complete alopecia of the trunk, neck, and proximal legs, sparing head, distal legs, and distal tail. In some animals, a sparse, wooly hair coat remains. An interesting finding is the very focal regrowth of hair after skin biopsy or focal trauma in some cases. Hyperpigmentation develops at the same time as alopecia; however, it may be absent, in particular in white poodles.

The affected dogs are otherwise clinically unremarkable. Diagnosis is by exclusion of endocrinopathies, such as hypercortisolism, hypothyroidism, hyperestrogenism, hyperprogesteronism (a very rare event in some adrenocortical or testicular tumors), and conditions such as cyclic flank alopecia, follicular dysplasia, or sebaceous adenitis. Skin biopsies show changes typically seen in endocrinopathies. A 100% reliable discrimination of Alopecia X from the other disorders is not possible. However, so-called flame follicles appear to be more prominent and abundant than in the other dermatopathies. They are sometimes diffusely interspersed in a biopsy specimen. Flame follicles are characterized by large spikes of fused keratin appearing to protrude through the outer root sheath to the vitreous layer, creating a fiery effect (Gross et al, 2005).

Various treatments have been used in those dogs, including GH, castration, melatonin, mitotane, and trilostane. They are not always effective, and because hair cycle arrest is a "cosmetic" disease, the risk of treatment has to weigh against the benefit. See the comprehensive review of Frank (2005) and the section on hair cycle arrest in the latest edition of *Muller and Kirk's Small Animal Dermatology* (Miller et al, 2013) for more details, as well as the previous edition of this textbook for the references of the multiple studies performed on this topic. The earlier section is a summary of the text of Frank (2005) and Miller, et al. (2013). The study of Cerundolo, et al. (2007) on assumed mild hypercortisolism as the cause of the disorder might also be interesting for the reader. The strong predilection and familial accumulation suggests a hereditary background (Mausberg et al, 2007a). Genetic studies have been initiated and a few candidate genes have already been excluded (Mausberg et al, 2007b; Mausberg et al, 2008).

In summary, there is no evidence that the alopecic disorder in the breeds listed earlier is due to acquired GH deficiency. Until further studies bring light into the issue, the disorder might continue to be termed *Alopecia X,* which is a term used by many dermatologists.

 ## HYPERSOMATOTROPISM (ACROMEGALY) IN HUMANS

In 1886, Pierre Marie, a French neurologist published the first description of GH excess and proposed the name "acromegaly" (Melmed and Kleinberg, 2011). The term derives from the Greek words *akron* (extreme or extremity) and *megas* (large) and is used until today to describe the disease in adults, in which there is local overgrowth of bone. GH excess in childhood and adolescence leads to linear growth and large stature, which is termed *gigantism.*

Acromegaly was traditionally considered to be a rare disorder with an estimated prevalence of 30 to 40 individuals per million. More recently, it is assumed that the prevalence is much higher, ranging between 100 to 130 cases or being even up to 1000 cases per million (Chanson et al, 2009). In more than 95% of affected humans, the disease is due to a GH-producing adenoma in the anterior pituitary gland. Acromegaly may also be induced by extra-pituitary disorders, but these are rare events (Melmed and Kleinberg, 2011). Approximately 60% of the pituitary adenomas are pure GH-secreting adenomas of the somatotrophic cells, which are histologically classified into two variants: they contain either densely granulated or sparsely granulated staining cytoplasmic GH vesicles. Biological behavior differs because sparsely granulated GH adenomas are more likely to be locally invasive and grow faster than their densely granulated counterpart; they also occur at younger age (Lopes, 2010). Most of the remaining pituitary adenomas secrete GH and prolactin and occur as three different tumor types: mixed GH cell/prolactin cell adenoma, mammosomatotroph cell adenoma, and acidophilic stem cell adenoma. Mixed GH cell/prolactin cell adenomas resemble

GH-secreting adenomas, but are bimorphous tumors with two separate cell populations, GH cells and prolactin cells. Mammosomatotroph adenomas contain monomorphous cell populations, and GH and prolactin is present in the same tumor cell. Acidophilic stem cell adenomas are very rare and are composed of a single population of immature cells with features reminiscent of GH cells and prolactin cells. In affected patients, symptoms of hyperprolactinemia dominate the clinical picture (Lopes, 2010). Mixed GH- and TSH-secreting adenomas, or adenomas also secreting ACTH, are rare (Chanson et al, 2009). The large majority of GH-producing tumors are adenomas. GH secreting pituitary carcinomas are the exception. The origin of the somatotroph adenoma is not yet clear. The fact that the adenomas are monoclonal in nature and usually do not relapse after surgical removal point to a pituitary etiology (Chanson et al, 2009). It is assumed, that they result from a multistep and multicausal process in which a genetic disposition, endocrine factors, and specific somatic mutations play a role (Lopes, 2010). The most common genetic defect, found in approximately 40% of sporadic cases, is a mutation in the gene for the α-subunit of the stimulatory G-protein (GNAS), which is a stimulatory protein of adenylate cyclase at the membrane level. The GNAS protein is coupled to the GHRH receptor, and the mutation mimics the effects of GHRH on hormone signaling (Freda et al, 2007; Chanson et al, 2009; Lopes, 2010). Less than 5% of cases are due to extrapituitary acromegaly or are part of genetic syndromes. Extrapituitary GH excess can result from an ectopic pituitary adenoma (e.g., in sphenoidal sinus, nasopharyngeal cavity) or from peripheral tumors, such as islet cell tumors or lymphoma. Another category of causes is hypersecretion of GHRH that leads to hyperplasia of the somatotrophic cells and consequently GH excess. GHRH hypersecretion either results from a hypothalamic tumor or more often from peripheral tumors, including bronchial carcinoid, islet cell tumors, and various other endocrine tumors (Chanson et al, 2009; Box 2-6).

 HYPERSOMATOTROPISM (ACROMEGALY) IN CATS

Prevalence and Etiology

In 1976, Gembardt and Loppnow described the first two cats with diabetes mellitus and acidophilic pituitary adenomas. Although GH was not measured, the authors proposed that GH excess from these tumors was responsible for the diabetes. During the following 30 years, further cases were only published sporadically or in a few case series, and feline acromegaly was considered a rare disease. The rareness started to be questioned in 2007 when two larger studies accompanied by an editorial were published in the same issue of the *Journal of Veterinary Internal Medicine* (Berg et al, 2007; Niessen et al 2007a; Peterson, 2007). The study of Berg, et al. (2007), however, was not designed to evaluate the prevalence of acromegaly, but compared circulating IGF-1 levels in diabetic cats known to have acromegaly with levels in cats without acromegaly. Unfortunately, this study is often quoted in discussions on prevalence of feline acromegaly, something that seems inappropriate. Niessen, et al. (2007a) screened blood samples from diabetic cats in the United Kingdom for the possible presence of acromegaly by measuring circulating IGF-1 levels. IGF-1 was found to be markedly increased (> 1000 ng/mL, reference range 208 to 443) in 59 of 184 (32%) variably controlled diabetic cats. Further work-up was possible in 18 cats, and acromegaly was diagnosed in 17 of them. More recently, the same research group confirmed the relatively high percentage of increased IGF-1 levels in diabetic cats by doing an extensive screening project: IGF-1 levels were measured in 1222 diabetic cats and found to be elevated

---

BOX 2-6   Causes of Acromegaly in Humans

Growth Hormone–Producing Pituitary Tumor
Adenoma
  GH-secreting (densely and parsley granulated)
  Mixed GH cell/prolactin cell adenoma
  Mammosomatotroph adenoma
  Acidophilic stem cell adenoma
  GH-/TSH-secreting adenoma
  Other plurihormonal adenoma
Carcinoma

Extra-Pituitary Growth Hormone–Producing Tumor
Ectopic pituitary adenoma
Peripheral tumor
  Islet cell tumor
  Lymphoma

Growth Hormone–Releasing Hormone Hypersecretion
Hypothalamic tumor
  Gangliocytoma
  Hamartoma
  Choristoma
  Glioma
Peripheral tumor
  Bronchial carcinoid
  Islet cell tumor
  Adrenal adenoma
  Medullary thyroid carcinoma
  Pheochromocytoma

Genetic Syndromes Associated with Acromegaly
McCune-Albright syndrome
Carney complex
Multiple endocrine neoplasia type 1
Familial isolated pituitary adenoma

Modified from Melmed S, Kleinberg D: Pituitary masses and tumors. In Melmed S, Polonsky KS, Larsen PR, Kronenberger HM, editors: *Williams' textbook of endocrinology,* ed 12, Philadelphia, 2011, Saunders Elsevier.
GH, Growth hormone; *TSH,* thyroid-stimulating hormone.

---

in 334 of them (27.3%) (Niessen et al, 2013a). Similar screenings in Switzerland and the Netherlands resulted in somewhat lower prevalence: 36 of 202 diabetic cats (17.8%) had IGF-1 levels less than 1000 ng/mL (Schäfer et al, 2013). It is very important to note that a high IGF-1 level does not automatically mean that the cat suffers from acromegaly. There are several reasons why IGF-1 may be falsely increased (e.g., methodological problems with the various IGF-1 assays). See the Hormonal Evaluation, Cats section later for more details. The studies mentioned earlier may also be confounded by selection bias. Poorly regulated diabetic cats (which are more likely to harbor acromegaly) are usually presented to the veterinarian more often than well regulated cats and, therefore, the likelihood of sampling those cats is higher. On the other hand, it is possible that the IGF-1 cut-off value of 1000 ng/mL is too high and cats with acromegaly are missed (Niessen et al, 2013a). The definitive prevalence of acromegaly in diabetic cats is unknown so far. In the author's hospital, screening for acromegaly is routinely done in all diabetic cats for many years. From those data, it is estimated, that the prevalence of acromegaly in the "normal" diabetic cat population is 10% to 15%; in the population of cats that are difficult to regulate, the percentage is substantially higher and may be 30% or more.

In the vast majority of cats, acromegaly is caused by a GH-producing acidophil pituitary adenoma. Capen (2007) mentions densely granulated and sparsely granulated cells in the adenomas; it is, however, unknown so far if those findings represent different variants of the disease as known in humans (see earlier). It is also not yet known how many of those tumors exclusively secrete GH and how many are mixed or plurihormonal tumors. Such an investigation would require immunohistochemical staining for the various pituitary hormones, which has only been reported for a small number of cases (Middleton et al, 1985; Heinrichs et al, 1989; Allgoewer et al, 1998; Meij et al, 2004; Meij et al 2010b; Sharman et al, 2013). The pituitary tumors of three acromegalic cats only stained positive for GH (Heinrichs et al, 1989; Meij et al, 2004; Meij et al, 2010b), the tumors of three other cats mainly stained positive for GH, but also had some positive staining for prolactin, ACTH and prolactin, and β-endorphin, FSH, and TSH respectively (Middleton et al, 1985; Allgoewer et al, 1998; Sharman et al, 2013). Those mixed tumors, in which several hormones are synthesized within the same mass are different from so-called double adenoma. Meij, et al. (2004) reported the concurrent existence of a somatotroph and a corticotroph adenoma in a cat with diabetes mellitus. Immunohistochemistry confirmed that the GH-cell adenoma and the ACTH-cell adenoma were separated by unaffected adenohypophyseal tissue. The clinical picture was dominated by insulin-resistant diabetes mellitus and hyperadrenocorticism; physical changes of acromegaly were not obvious. Very recently, another case of double adenoma was reported (Sharman et al, 2013). The cat was referred for insulin-resistant diabetes mellitus and physical changes consistent with acromegaly; 16 months later, the cat developed additional signs consistent with hyperadrenocorticism. The presence of double adenoma was confirmed by necropsy: one acidophilic adenoma stained strongly positive for GH, with some positivity for β-endorphin, FSH, and TSH and was considered consistent with a somatotroph adenoma; the other chromophobe adenoma stained positive for ACTH, melanocyte-stimulating hormone (MSH), FSH, and β-endorphin consistent with a plurihormonal pituitary tumor. In summary, most cats with acromegaly have acidophil pituitary tumors, which predominantly secrete GH. Some of them also secrete other pituitary hormones albeit in small amounts. In the latter cases, the clinical picture is usually dominated by the excessive secretion of GH. On rare occasions, cats may have double adenomas. The clinical manifestations depend on their secretory products. Interestingly, in a few cats with acromegaly the histological diagnosis was pituitary acidophilic hyperplasia instead of acidophilic adenoma (Norman and Mooney, 2000; Niessen et al, 2007a). Because hyperplasia of the somatotropic cells is difficult to distinguish from GH-cell adenoma (Melmed and Kleinberg, 2011), it may be that the lesions in fact were adenomas. However, the possibility of true hyperplasia has to be taken into account, which points to a different etiology. In acromegalic humans, hyperplasia usually results from excessive GHRH, either caused by hypothalamic or peripheral tumors (see Box 2-6). It is important to be aware of somatotroph hyperplasia, as in those cats, pituitary imaging by CT/MRI may be negative (Niessen et al, 2007a).

Pathophysiology

In acromegaly, circulating GH concentrations are chronically increased, although secretion remains episodic. GH has direct and indirect metabolic effects; the latter are mediated through the stimulation of IGF-1 synthesis in the liver and in other tissues. See the section Metabolic Actions of Growth Hormone and Insulin-like Growth Factor 1 and Fig. 2-5 for more details. The growth promoting effects of increased GH and IGF-1 result in the proliferation of bone, cartilage, soft tissues, and increase in size of various organs, leading to the characteristic physical ("acral") changes of acromegaly. GH and IGF-1 also have profound effects on carbohydrate metabolism. GH, IGF-1, and insulin can directly interact with each other by signaling crosstalk (Vijayakumar el at, 2010). Consequently, disturbance of the GH and IGF-1 system has impact on insulin action and vice versa. GH has anti-insulin actions that include increase in hepatic glucose production and decrease of glucose uptake in extrahepatic tissues. Chronic GH excess is associated with defects in both, hepatic and extrahepatic insulin actions (Hansen et al, 1986). Recent studies suggest that GH excess reduces insulin sensitivity by multiple mechanisms involving the insulin receptor as well as various steps in the postreceptor pathways (Dominici et al, 2005; Xu and Messina, 2009; Clemmons, 2012). In contrast to GH, IGF-1 enhances insulin sensitivity in hepatic and extrahepatic tissues. However, in acromegaly, increased IGF-1 levels are unable to counteract the insulin-resistance induced by the excessive GH concentrations (Resmini et al, 2009). In normal individuals, insulin resistance is compensated by an increased insulin production from the β-cells and normoglycemia is maintained. Diabetes mellitus only develops in individuals in which β-cells with time fail to maintain high insulin synthesis to meet the increased demand. Various mechanisms have been proposed to explain β-cell failure. See Chapter 7 for details. So far, the cause for β-cell failure in acromegaly is unknown. The vast majority of acromegalic cats suffer from diabetes mellitus. In many but not all diabetic cats, insulin-resistance is pronounced at the time of diagnosis. Acromegaly in cats is almost always due to a GH-producing pituitary tumor. Neurological signs may develop as a result of a large tumor involving the hypothalamus and further areas of the brain.

Signalment

Acromegaly is typically diagnosed in elderly cats. Most cats are 8 years and older. The average age is 10 to 11 years with a range between 4 and 17 years (Feldman and Nelson, 2004). Pedigree cats are rarely affected; the vast majority of acromegalic cats are Domestic Short-Haired and some are Domestic Long-Haired. There appears to be a clear male predisposition, because approximately 88% of the cats described during the last decades were male or male-castrated. It should be noted that there is also a male predisposition for diabetes in general (i.e., 70% to 80% of diabetic cats are male). Interestingly, however, in one study, only 50% of acromegalic cats were male (Fischetti et al, 2012). Body weight ranges between 4 kg and 9 kg; most affected cats weigh between 5 kg and 7 kg.

Clinical Manifestations

Clinical signs mainly result from the diabetogenic effect of GH and the effects of GH and IGF-1 with regard to acral enlargement and on growth of soft tissues and organs. In some cats, expansion of the pituitary tumor causes additional neurological signs (Table 2-2; Fig. 2-14 and Fig. 2-15).

The earliest and most common clinical signs usually are polyuria, polydipsia, and polyphagia associated with GH-induced diabetes mellitus. Polyphagia may also develop as a direct effect of the GH excess and can become extreme. Weight loss may or may not be present during the initial phases. Often, initial weight loss is followed by a period of stabilization and thereafter slow and progressive weight gain develops. Weakness, ataxia, and a

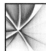

TABLE 2-2	CLINICAL SIGNS AND PHYSICAL EXAMINATION FINDINGS IN CATS WITH ACROMEGALY

CLINICAL FINDINGS	PERCENT OF OCCURRENCE
Diabetes mellitus (usually poorly controlled)	96% – 100%
Polyuria/polydipsia	83% – 100%
Polyphagia	78% – 100%
Enlargement of head, abdomen, paws	50% – 83%
Prognathia inferior	35% – 71%
Weight gain	35% – 59%
Hepatomegaly and/or renomegaly	26% – 100%
Heart murmur and/or gallop rhythm	17% – 64%
Weight loss	9% – 57%
CNS signs	9% – 14%
Diabetic neuropathy (plantigrade stance)	6% – 26%
Enlargement of tongue	6% – 21%
Lameness or degenerative arthropathy	5% – 43%
Respiratory stridor	4% – 53%

Data are compiled from Feldman EC, Nelson RW: Disorders of growth hormone. In Feldman EC, Nelson RW, editors: *Canine and feline endocrinology and reproduction*, St. Louis, 2004, Saunders; Niessen SJM, et al: Feline acromegaly: an underdiagnosed endocrinopathy? *J Vet Intern Med* 21:899, 2007a; and Peterson ME, et al: Acromegaly in 14 cats, *J Vet Intern Med* 4:192, 1990. *CNS*, Central nervous system.

plantigrade stance caused by diabetic neuropathy may be seen in some cats. A poor unkempt hair coat is another albeit unspecific possible finding (Feldman and Nelson, 2004). During the first few weeks or months after initiating therapy, insulin requirement may be relatively low (i.e., 1 to 3 units per cat b.i.d. [bis in die; twice a day]) and then starts to increase as the insulin resistance worsens. Insulin requirement may easily exceed 1.5 to 2.0 U/kg body weight b.i.d., and the use of 30 units b.i.d. and more has been reported (Peterson et al, 1990; Norman and Mooney 2000; Niessen et al, 2007a). The possibility of an underlying endocrinopathy (e.g., acromegaly) is often considered only after the diabetes becomes difficult to control or high insulin doses are needed to decrease blood glucose concentrations into an acceptable range. A cat with difficult to regulate diabetes and weight gain at the same time should alert the clinician to consider the possibility of acromegaly. Poor glycemic control is usually associated with weight loss, whereas weight gain is seen in cases with insulin overdose (because insulin is an anabolic hormone) and with acromegaly. It is important to note that not all acromegalic cats are (severely) insulin resistant. In some cats "normal" insulin doses (1 to 3 units per cat b.i.d.) are sufficient for long-term adequate glycemic control. It has been the impression of the author and other investigators that in some cases, even diabetic remission may occur in acromegalic cats without the treatment of the GH excess. This, however, would be an extremely rare event, and further studies are needed to confirm the observation. Interestingly, in human medicine, only

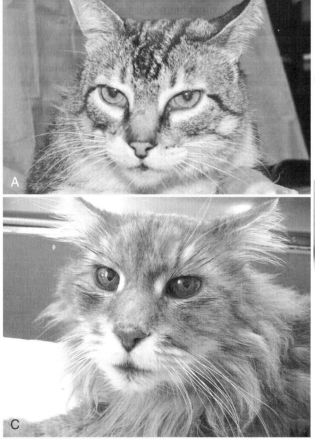

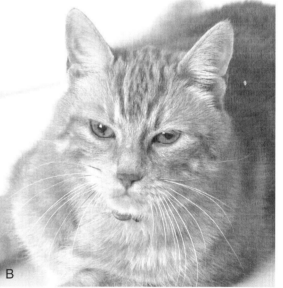

FIGURE 2-14 Three cats with diabetes mellitus and acromegaly revealing different degrees of physical changes. **A,** Domestic Short-Haired (mc, 8 y) with nearly normal facial features. The chin may be slightly prominent. **B,** Domestic Short-Haired (mc, 11 y) with more obvious prognathia inferior than in cat A. **C,** Domestic Short-Haired (mc, 12 y) with the "typical" broad head and prognathia inferior in more advanced acromegaly.

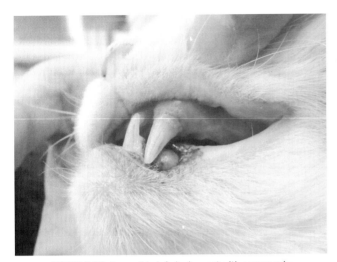

FIGURE 2-15 Prognathia inferior in a cat with acromegaly.

approximately one-third of patients with acromegaly develop overt diabetes mellitus (Wass et al, 2011). So far, all acromegalic cats described in case reports and case series had concurrent diabetes mellitus, and the majority of them were difficult to regulate due to GH-induced insulin resistance. It may be possible that in the beginning of the acromegalic disease or in cats with very mild GH excess, glucose tolerance is maintained. It is also possible that cats suffer from acromegaly without ever developing diabetes; however, this is extremely uncommon. The physical changes of acromegaly are induced by the anabolic effects of GH and IGF-1; they have an insidious onset and progress very slowly. Clinical signs may be obvious at the time diabetes is diagnosed or may become apparent during the following weeks to months. Because of the slow progression, the owners often do not notice the subtle changes in the appearance of their cat until they are specifically questioned. It is important to note that a cat with acromegaly may initially be unremarkable during physical examination and may be indistinguishable from other diabetic cats (Niessen et al 2007a; Niessen, 2010). The soft tissue overgrowth and the osseous changes cause weight gain, enlargement (broadening) of the head, enlargement of the mandible (prognathia inferior), widening of the interdental spaces, and sometimes a large tongue. Diffuse thickening of oropharyngeal tissue can lead to respiratory stridor and respiratory distress. Enlargement of the abdomen and the paws ("clubbed" paws) are also identified regularly. The general impression is that of a large cat. Degenerative arthropathy due to proliferation of chondrocytes and disruption of joint geometry is common and involves shoulder, elbow, carpus, digits, stifle, and spine. Those lesions may result in lameness; however, they may also be clinically silent and just be detected radiographically (Peterson et al, 1990; Feldman and Nelson, 2004; Niessen et al, 2007a; Niessen et al, 2013a). Systolic heart murmur is common, and further work-up may reveal cardiomegaly and echocardiographic abnormalities. Cardiomegaly has been reported to worsen over time, and congestive heart failure may develop during later stages of the acromegalic disease. Electrocardiography is usually unremarkable (Peterson et al, 1990; Niessen et al, 2007a). Cardiomyopathy may be the result of the GH excess. In some cases, however, there may have been pre-existing cardiomyopathy that worsens during the course of acromegaly. In humans, cardiac involvement and a specific cardiomyopathy is a consistent feature of acromegaly (Chanson and Salenave, 2008). Blood pressure is usually normal or only slightly increased. Organomegaly not only involves the heart but also liver, kidney, spleen, and pancreas as well as other endocrine organs, such as adrenal glands, thyroid, and parathyroid glands. Hepatomegaly, renomegaly, and thyroid/parathyroid enlargement may be evident during physical examination. Central nervous system (CNS) signs as a result of pituitary tumor growth are seen in approximately 10% to 15% of cats and include lethargy, behavioral changes, impaired vision, adipsia, anorexia, temperature dysregulation, circling, somnolence, stupor, and seizures.

Clinical Pathology

The (often poorly) controlled diabetes mellitus is responsible for most of the abnormalities identified on the complete blood count (CBC), biochemistry profile, and urinalysis. Hyperglycemia, glucosuria, and increased serum fructosamine is almost always present. In a recent study, a trend toward blood glucose and fructosamine being more elevated in diabetic cats with than without acromegaly has been found; however, there was considerable overlap (Niessen, 2010). Hyponatremia, hypercholesterolemia, and a mild increase in alanine aminotransferase (ALT) and alkaline phosphatase (ALP) activities are seen in some cats. Ketonuria is usually absent. A substantial percentage of acromegalic cats reveal hyperproteinemia or total protein concentrations in the upper range of normal, reflecting either increased protein synthesis induced by the GH excess and/or dehydration associated with poorly regulated diabetes. Hyperproteinemia was the only parameter being more frequently present in acromegalic compared to non-acromegalic diabetic cats (Niessen, 2010). Hyperphosphatemia (without azotemia) has occasionally been seen and is due to the GH/IGF-1 mediated increased renal tubular resorption (Peterson et al, 1990; Javorsky et al, 2011). There is some controversy as to which chronic renal failure develops more frequently in acromegalic cats. Peterson, et al. (1990) reported the development of chronic renal failure in 50% of acromegalic cats within 8 to 36 months after initial examination, whereas the prevalence of azotemia was low (12%) in the study by Niessen, et al. (2007a). Chronic renal failure is very common in the elderly cat population, and further studies are needed to investigate the potential role of GH excess. Other occasional findings include erythrocytosis, leukocytosis, and proteinuria; the latter is often associated with azotemia. In summary, acromegalic cats show various abnormalities. However, the findings are not helpful to distinguish acromegalic from non-acromegalic diabetic cats.

Diagnostic Imaging

Conventional Radiography

Abdominal radiographs most often reveal hepatomegaly, which is also seen in non-acromegalic diabetic cats. Further findings may include renomegaly and rarely splenomegaly. Thoracic radiographs may show mild to moderate cardiomegaly and pulmonary edema or pleural effusion if congestive heart failure is present. Findings of radiographs of skull, joints, and spine include diffuse increase of soft tissue in the oropharyngeal region, enlargement of the mandible, hyperostosis of the bony calvarium and nasal bones, degenerative arthropathy of shoulder, elbow, stifle, carpus, digits, and spondylosis deformans of the spine. Radiography may also be completely normal or reveal only very mild abnormalities. The presence and severity of the changes depend on the severity and duration of the GH excess (Peterson et al, 1990; Feldman and Nelson, 2004; Fig. 2-16).

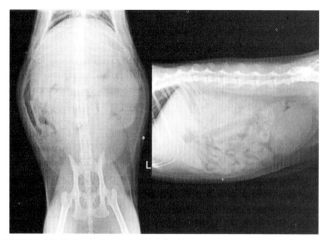

FIGURE 2-16 Abdominal radiographs of a 7-year-old male-castrated Domestic Short-Haired cat with diabetes mellitus and acromegaly. Note the enlargements of liver and kidneys. (Courtesy Dr. Matthias Dennler and Prof. Patrick Kircher, Division of Diagnostic Imaging, Vetsuisse Faculty, Zurich, Switzerland.)

Abdominal Ultrasonography

Hepatomegaly is the most consistent finding, as mentioned earlier, and it is also the most frequent finding in non-acromegalic diabetic cats. Further abnormalities include renal enlargement with or without reduced corticomedullary definition and/or mild pelvic dilation, enlarged pancreas, splenomegaly, and bilateral adrenomegaly (Posch et al, 2011). The width (or thickness) of the adrenal glands is the most important parameter to determine their size by ultrasonography. In healthy cats, width of the left and right adrenal gland ranged between 0.3 to 0.53 cm and 0.29 to 0.45 cm, respectively (Zimmer et al, 2000). In cats with diabetes mellitus (without acromegaly), left and right adrenal gland width ranged between 0.24 to 0.46 cm and 0.26 to 0.48 cm, respectively, and it was not different to the width in healthy cats (Kley et al, 2007). Both studies were performed in the institution of the author and are therefore comparable, because the same measuring approach was used. A typical finding in our diabetic cats with acromegaly is a slight bilateral symmetrical enlargement of the adrenal glands; the width often is between 0.5 and 0.65 cm. Adrenomegaly is not pathognomonic for acromegaly, because it is also found in cats with pituitary-dependent hypercortisolism. Adrenomegaly in conjunction with enlargement of other abdominal organs, in particular the kidney, however, should raise suspicion for the presence of acromegaly (Fig. 2-17).

Echocardiography

Echocardiography findings include generalized or focal (septal, basal, free wall) left ventricular hypertrophy with or without left atrial dilation. In some cats, right heart disease with right-sided heart failure may predominate. Echocardiography, however, can also be unremarkable.

Computed Tomography and Magnetic Resonance Imaging

Pituitary imaging plays a major role in the work-up of cats with suspected acromegaly. The demonstration of a pituitary mass is important to establish the final diagnosis of acromegaly in concert with the clinical findings and the results of the hormonal evaluations. Determination of the exact size of the mass is also required for the discussion on treatment options with the owner. CT/MRI studies should always include post-contrast images, because the mass may not be visualized on native studies. In the vast majority of cats, the disease is caused by an adenoma

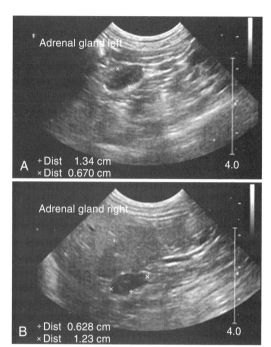

FIGURE 2-17 Ultrasonographic images of the left and right adrenal gland of a 13-year-old male-castrated Domestic Short-Haired cat with diabetes mellitus and acromegaly. Note the slight to moderate bilateral symmetrical enlargement of the glands with maintained shape. **A,** The width of the left adrenal gland measured 0.67 cm. **B,** The width of the right adrenal gland 0.63 cm. Adrenal gland width in healthy cats ranges between 0.3 to 0.53 cm. (Courtesy Dr. Matthias Dennler and Prof. Patrick Kircher, Division of Diagnostic Imaging, Vetsuisse Faculty, Zurich, Switzerland.)

of the somatotrophic cells, which is usually visible by the time of presentation. In fact, the masses can become quite large, and suprasellar extension with involvement of the diencephalon is a frequent finding (Posch et al, 2011). However, if pituitary imaging is performed in early stages of the disease, the mass may still be small and difficult to visualize. MRI with adequate resolution is superior to conventional CT to detect small masses. If dynamic CT is available, the evaluation and displacement of the so-called "pituitary flush" is helpful for the documentation of small pituitary tumors (Meij et al, 2010b; Hecht and Schwarz, 2011). On rare occasions, CT/MRI imaging of the pituitary gland is unremarkable. Potential causes are a very small size of the tumor or a different etiology of the acromegalic disease. In approximately 2% of human patients with acromegaly, the disease is due to somatotrophic hyperplasia caused by hypersecretion of GHRH, which either derives from a hypothalamic or a peripheral tumor (Melmed and Kleinberg, 2011). Such an etiology has not yet been demonstrated in cats; however, in one cat with normal CT and MRI studies, histopathology revealed acidophilic proliferation, not adenoma in the pituitary gland (Niessen et al, 2007a; Fig. 2-18, Fig. 2-19, and Fig. 2-20).

Hormonal Evaluation

Acromegaly should be considered in cats with difficult to regulate diabetes in which problems associated with the insulin and the insulin administration, short duration of insulin effect, and other common concurrent problems (e.g., glucocorticoid administration, severe stomatitis/gingivitis, urinary tract infection) have been excluded. See Chapter 7 for more details.

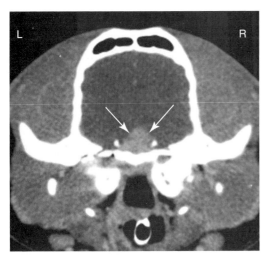

FIGURE 2-18 Computed tomography (CT) image of the pituitary region in a 7-year-old male castrated Domestic Short-Haired cat with diabetes mellitus and acromegaly. A large mass was identified *(arrows)*. (Courtesy Dr. Matthias Dennler and Prof. Patrick Kircher, Division of Diagnostic Imaging, Vetsuisse Faculty, Zurich, Switzerland.)

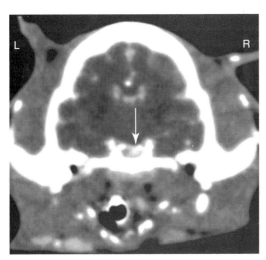

FIGURE 2-19 Selected image of the transverse dynamic computed tomography (CT) study of the pituitary region in a 6-year-old cat with diabetes mellitus and acromegaly. The pituitary gland is not enlarged; however, the pituitary flush (corresponding to the neurohypophysis) is displaced to the right indicating a small space occupying lesion of the adenohypophysis on the left side *(arrow)*. (Courtesy Dr. Matthias Dennler and Prof. Patrick Kircher, Division of Diagnostic Imaging, Vetsuisse Faculty, Zurich, Switzerland.)

Human Medicine

The diagnosis is traditionally based on the demonstration of GH hypersecretion and increased IGF-1 levels (Ribeiro-Oliveira and Barkan, 2012). The episodic nature of GH secretion renders the measurement of basal GH levels unreliable, because ranges of acromegalic and healthy humans overlap. Even if multiple samples for GH measurement are taken throughout the day, a reliable differentiation between individuals with and without acromegaly is not possible. The standard procedure is to evaluate GH concentrations during an oral glucose tolerance test. After an overnight fast, blood samples are usually taken at baseline and at several times after ingestion of a glucose drink. The protocols may vary slightly between different institutions. In healthy humans, the sudden increase in blood glucose suppresses GH secretion

from the pituitary gland below a certain threshold. In contrast, in patients with acromegaly, GH levels remain either unchanged, show a paradoxical increase, or decrease slightly. The threshold (also called the *GH nadir*) has been lowered over time with the development of more sensitive GH assays. Nevertheless, some patients (in particular those with mild disease) may suppress GH below the threshold and diagnosis may be missed. The GHRH test has no diagnostic value (Dimaraki et al, 2002; Freda, 2003; Ribeiro-Oliveira and Barkan, 2012).

IGF-1 directly reflects GH activity as it is synthesized in the liver (and other tissues) under the control of GH. Blood levels are relatively stable throughout the day, and measurement requires only a single randomly-obtained blood sample. Measurement of IGF-1 is routinely used to screen for acromegaly in humans, and high IGF-1 levels are sensitive markers for GH excess. IGF-1 levels correlate with the mean 24-hour GH output; if mean GH levels are very high, IGF-1 levels, however, reach a plateau due to the limited capacity of the liver to synthesize the polypeptide (Freda, 2003; Ribeiro-Oliveira and Barkan, 2012). The drawbacks of the test are the requirement for age- and sex-adjusted reference ranges and the possibility of biological and technical problems. Various conditions, including malnutrition, liver and renal failure, hypothyroidism, poorly controlled diabetes, and oral estrogen intake may lower IGF-1 levels and therefore mask acromegaly. Technical problems are mainly due to the interference of the IGF-1 binding proteins (IGFBPs) with the IGF-1 measurement. For correct IGF-1 measurement, the binding proteins need to be removed by a separate step; however, assays differ in the quality of this removal (Freda, 2003; Ribeiro-Oliveira and Barkan, 2012).

Cats

As in humans, diagnosis of acromegaly in cats requires the demonstration of GH excess and/or high IGF-1 concentrations. Feline GH can be measured in heterologous canine and ovine radioimmunoassays (Eigenmann et al, 1984b; Niessen et al, 2007b). However, availability of the assays may be a problem.

Eigenmann, et al. (1984b) described extremely elevated GH levels in an acromegalic cat that did not decrease during an intravenous glucose tolerance test (IVGTT). This test can, in principle, be regarded as the pendent to the aforementioned oral glucose tolerance test, which is routinely used in humans. However, suitability of the IVGTT is limited because glucose infusions in healthy cats also do not result in a GH decrease (Kokka et al, 1971). Random GH concentrations were measured in several studies. So far, all acromegalic cats had increased GH concentrations. In some cats, GH was highly elevated; in others, the increase above normal was only small (Table 2-3). The cats of those studies most likely were in an advanced stage of the disease. With increased awareness, however, milder cases of acromegaly of cats at an earlier stage of the disease will be worked-up, and due to the episodic nature of GH secretion, random GH levels may at times be in the normal range. It is also important to note, that a single elevated GH level is not diagnostic for acromegaly, because it may be the result of a secretory pulse in a non-acromegalic cat. Mildly increased GH levels have been seen in diabetic cats without acromegaly (Reusch et al, 2006; Niessen et al, 2007a). It is currently recommended to collect three to five samples for GH measurement at 10-minute intervals (Meij et al, 2010a). The more of those samples that reveal an increased GH level and the higher those levels are, the more likely the cat has acromegaly.

Blood samples should be handled carefully to avoid degradation of the hormone. We routinely collect the samples into EDTA-coated ice-chilled tubes. After immediate centrifugation, they are stored at –20° C until shipping to the laboratory on dry ice with express

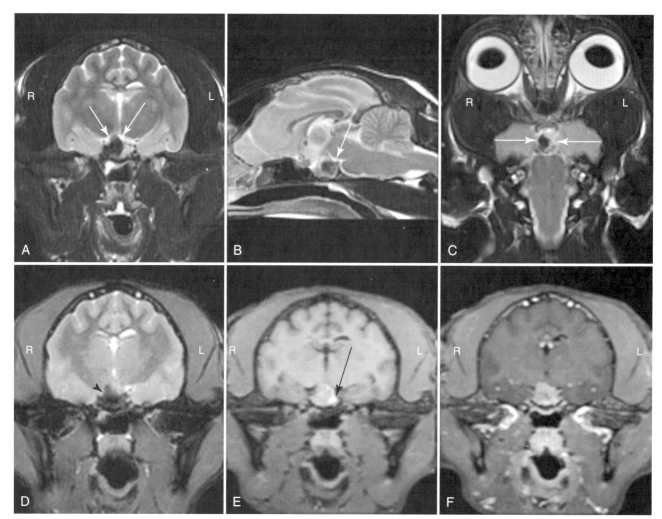

FIGURE 2-20 Magnetic resonance imaging (MRI) images of the pituitary region of a 12-year-old Domestic Short-Haired cat with acromegaly. Transverse **(A)**, sagittal **(B)**, and dorsal **(C)** T2 weighted images show a space-occupying lesion *(white arrows)*, hypointense in comparison to white matter, which originates from the right aspect of the pituitary gland. **D**, Transverse T2: The sequence reveals susceptibility artifact *(black arrowhead)* in the center of the space-occupying lesion, which is highly suspicious for pituitary apoplexy. This is a hemorrhagic insult and occurs often in pituitary tumors and may be responsible for an acute deterioration of the clinical signs. **E**, T1 3D turbo field echo (TFE): The described space occupying lesion is isointense to white matter. The pituitary lesion causes distortion and displacement of the normally rounded and centrally located T1W-hyperintensity of the neurohypophysis *(black arrow)*. **F**, T1 3D TFE in the equilibrium phase after intravenous-administration of gadodiamide (Omniscan; 0.3 mmol/kg): The space occupying lesion exhibits moderate contrast medium uptake with a hypointense center. (Courtesy Dr. Matthias Dennler and Prof. Patrick Kircher, Division of Diagnostic Imaging, Vetsuisse Faculty, Zurich, Switzerland.)

service. In a recent study, GH was stable with less strict sampling and storage conditions (Niessen et al, 2007b). It is important to contact the laboratory prior to sampling for the specific details.

Measurement of IGF-1 has become a popular test for feline acromegaly during the last years. IGF-1 reflects the 24-hour GH secretion (see the section Hormonal Evaluation, Human Medicine) and its measurement has several advantages over the measurement of GH (IGF-1 flyer, Dechra Specialist Laboratories UK, www.thehormonelab.com; IGF-1 Collection Protocol, Diagnostic Center for Population and Animal Health, Michigan State University, www.dcpah.msu.edu):

1. IGF-1 is not secreted in pulses, and its concentration is constant throughout the day, requiring just a single random blood sample (Fig. 2-21).
2. Its structure is conserved across species, and it can be measured in assays designed for humans.

3. It is stable, and a serum sample can be sent by regular mail.

IGF-1 concentrations have been measured in several of the studies published during the past years and found to be increased in the vast majority of acromegalic cats. Normal IGF-1 levels have been seen in a few cases, which may reflect an early stage of the disease. Some of those cats were retested after some time, and IGF-1 was then found to be increased (Norman and Mooney, 2000; Berg et al, 2007). Several other potential causes should be considered if a normal IGF-1 level is found in a cat with suspected acromegaly. First, in humans, various concurrent problems are known to decrease IGF-1 concentrations (see earlier). Not all of them have been evaluated in cats yet; however, serious disease (e.g., lymphoma) was shown to drastically decrease IGF-1 concentrations (Tschuor et al, 2012; Fig. 2-22).

Second, IGF-1 level may be normal in acromegalic cats if the measurement is performed prior to the start of insulin therapy.

TABLE 2-3	**GH CONCENTRATIONS IN PUBLISHED CASES OF CATS WITH ACROMEGALY**		
NUMBER OF CATS WITH ACROMEGALY	**GH CONCENTRATION (µG/L)**	**REFERENCE RANGE**	**REFERENCE**
1	335	3.2 ± 0.7	Eigenmann et al, 1983
1	100	1.2 ± 0.14	Morrison et al, 1989
14	22 – 131	< 1 – 8.5	Peterson et al, 1990
3	14, 41, 42	1.5 – 7.9	Goosens et al, 1998
4	> 29.7	1.5 – 7.9	Elliott et al, 2000
4	9.5, > 17, > 18, 158	2 – 5	Norman and Mooney, 2000
1	24	< 6	Meij et al, 2004
7	8, 10.4, 11, 16, 21.9, 32, 40	1.5 – 7.9	Reusch et al, 2006
2	8, 23	1.5 – 7.9	Berg et al, 2007
9	9 – 33.7	1.9 – 6.3	Niessen et al, 2007a
5	16/16, 18/16, 20/22, 35/25, 415/230*	0.8 – 7.2	Slingerland et al, 2008
1	51	0.8 – 7.2	Meij et al, 2010b

*In each cat, GH was measured in 2 separate samples taken within a 15 min interval.

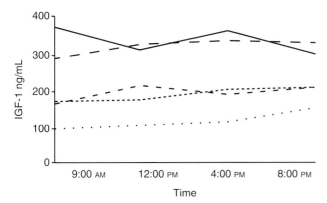

FIGURE 2-21 Insulin-like growth factor-1 (IGF-1) concentrations in five cats with diabetes mellitus measured at four different times, demonstrating that the blood levels are stable throughout the day. (Modified from Reusch CE, et al.: Measurement of growth hormone and insulin-like growth factor 1 in cats with diabetes mellitus, *Vet Rec* 158:195, 2006.)

IGF-1 has been shown to be significantly lower in untreated diabetic cats (without acromegaly) compared to healthy controls; after the start of insulin treatment, IGF-1 increased and was not different from levels in controls after a few weeks (Fig. 2-23). The same observation was made in a small number of diabetic cats with acromegaly in which the initially low IGF-1 levels increased markedly after insulin therapy was started (Reusch et al, 2006). Insulin deficiency is also known to decrease IGF-1 levels in humans, dogs, and rats. This phenomenon is explained by the fact that high insulin concentrations are needed in the portal vein for the expression and function of GH receptors on hepatocytes and that this mechanism is disturbed in insulin-deficient states (Eigenmann et al, 1977; Yang et al, 1990; Bereket et al, 1999; Ekmann et al, 2000; Reusch et al, 2001; Reusch et al, 2006; Lim et al, 2007). In our institution, diabetic cats that are suspected to suffer from acromegaly are therefore treated with insulin for approximately 6 to 8 weeks before IGF-1 is measured (Reusch, 2010). Cats in advanced stages of the acromegalic disease may have high IGF-1 levels already at initial presentation. However, if we find a normal or borderline IGF-1 result, we repeat the testing after several weeks of insulin therapy.

A third reason why the diagnosis of acromegaly may be missed is the currently used cut-off values, which may be too high to detect milder or early stages of the disease. For instance, for many of the currently available assays, IGF-1 concentrations greater than 1000 ng/mL are considered to be suspicious of acromegaly. However, IGF-1 levels in healthy cats and non-acromegalic cats usually are less than 800 ng/mL. The range between 800 and 1000 ng/mL should be considered as grey zone. If the suspicion of acromegaly is strong, pituitary imaging would be a logical next step. In other cases, IGF-1 measurement should be repeated after a few weeks. An increasing level would then strengthen the suspicion of acromegaly. Reference ranges may differ depending on the methodology; therefore, interpretation of IGF-1 results should be based on the reference range established in cats by the laboratory.

As with any other test, IGF-1 measurement may also be false positive. Lewitt, et al. reported in 2000 that IGF-1 concentrations in eight non-acromegalic diabetic cats were significantly higher than those of healthy cats. Those results were surprising because it was already known from humans, dogs, and rats that insulin deficiency reduces IGF-1 levels. As mentioned earlier, the same mechanism was then also shown to exist in cats (Reusch et al, 2001; Reusch et al, 2006; see Fig. 2-23). Insulin treatment increases IGF-1 levels, and it was hypothesized that the high IGF-1 levels found by Lewitt, et al. (2000) had been due to long-term insulin therapy (Starkey et al, 2004). However, it is important to note, that technical issues may also contribute to false increase in IGF-1 levels. Circulating IGF-1 is nearly completely bound to binding proteins, which are known to interfere with the measurement; depending on the assay, they lead to spuriously high or low IGF-1 values. Most immunoassays are therefore preceded by methods that remove those binding proteins. Unfortunately, they are not equally effective and constitute a notorious source of error (Chestnut and Quarmby, 2002; Frystyk et al, 2010). Recently, three assays preceded by different sample preparation methods were compared against an assay using acid chromatography for removal of binding proteins (which is considered to be the gold standard) in groups of healthy and non-acromegalic diabetic cats as well as cats with various medical problems. The most remarkable finding was, that with one of the assays, 8 of the 60 cats (amongst them two healthy and one non-acromegalic diabetic cat) had IGF-1 concentrations more than 1000 ng/mL, whereas their concentrations were clearly below 1000 ng/mL with all the other assays (see Fig. 2-22). It

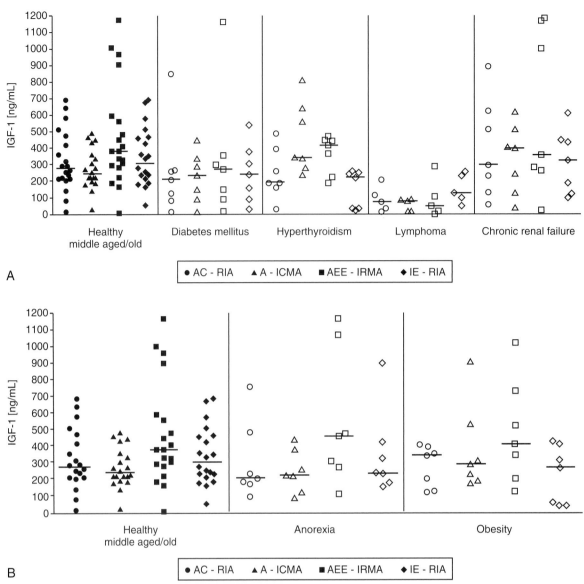

FIGURE 2-22 Scatterplots of plasma insulin-like growth factor-1 (IGF-1) concentrations in healthy middle-aged to older cats and cats with diabetes mellitus, hyperthyroidism, lymphoma, and with chronic renal failure **(A)**, as well as in cats with anorexia of 3-days duration and obesity **(B)**. IGF-1 concentrations were measured with four different assays with different methods of removal of IGF-1 binding proteins. *AC-RIA*, Acid chromatography radioimmunoassay; *A-ICMA*, acidification immunochemiluminescence assay, *AEE-IRMA*, acid-ethanol extraction immunoradiometric assay, *IE-RIA*, insulin-like growth factor-2 excess radioimmunoassay. (Modified from Tschuor F, et al.: Evaluation of four methods used to measure plasma insulin-like growth factor 1 concentrations in healthy cats and cats with diabetes mellitus or other diseases, *Am J Vet Res* 73[12]:1925-1931, 2012.)

is likely, that the high levels were due to incomplete removal of binding proteins by the acid/ethanol extraction (Tschuor et al, 2012). It is certainly worthwhile to use one of the other assays. We have seen IGF-1 more than 1000 ng/mL in several diabetic cats in which further work-up and follow-up examinations did not reveal any signs of acromegaly. When aliquots of the serum samples were measured with different assays, including the "gold standard assay," IGF-1 levels continued to stay high, rendering interference with binding proteins as cause highly unlikely. So far, the reason is unknown; it may be that vigorous and/or long-term insulin treatment plays a role (Box 2-7).

In human patients, IGF-1 levels are compared to age- and sex-dependent normative data. In cats, no difference was found between males and females, and there was no correlation between

IGF-1 and the cats' bodyweight (Reusch et al, 2006). In the study by Tschuor, et al. (2012), IGF-1 levels of younger cats (2 to 4½ years) were higher than those of elderly cats (6 to 14 years). However, the difference was significant only for one of the four assays. Ideally, laboratories offering IGF-1 measurements should establish assay-specific reference ranges for different age-groups.

Establishing the Diagnosis

Most cats with acromegaly are presented to the veterinarian because of poorly controlled diabetes mellitus. Physical changes typical of acromegaly may be obvious. However, a substantial number of acromegalic cats reveal only very minor alterations or may even look like any other diabetic cat. If typical changes are

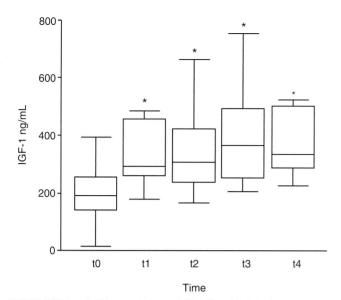

FIGURE 2-23 Insulin-like growth factor-1 (IGF-1) in 11 diabetic cats (without acromegaly) before they were treated with insulin (t0) and 1 to 3 weeks (t1), 4 to 8 weeks (t2), 9 to 12 weeks (t3), and 13 to 16 weeks (t4) after the treatment with insulin was started. * Significantly different ($P > 0.05$) from t0. Box and whisker plots are used to show the distribution of data. In the same study, IGF-1 levels in healthy cats ranged between 196.0 and 791.0 ng/mL. (Modified from Reusch CE, et al.: Measurement of growth hormone and insulin-like growth factor 1 in cats with diabetes mellitus, *Vet Rec* 158:195, 2006.)

BOX 2-7   Potential Causes for False Negative and False Positive Insulin-Like Growth Factor-1 Results

Potential Causes for Normal Insulin-like Growth Factor-1 Concentrations in Cats with Acromegaly
- Early stage of the acromegalic disease
- Currently used cut-off values too high to detect milder or early stages of the acromegalic disease
- Serious concurrent disease
- Starvation
- Lack of insulin (i.e., measurement performed prior to insulin therapy)
- Poorly controlled diabetes

Potential Causes for Increases Insulin-like Growth Factor-1 Levels in Cats without Acromegaly
- Incomplete removal of IGF-1 binding proteins prior to measurement and interference with assay
- Vigorous and/or long-term insulin treatment

IGF-1, Insulin-like growth factor-1.

---

present, the next step would be to measure GH (3 to 5 samples at 10-minute intervals) or IGF-1 concentrations (one random sample). Different to the very limited availability of the GH assay, most laboratories offer IGF-1 measurements. A high IGF-1 level, however, does not by itself confirm the diagnosis, because false positive test results may occur. The finding of a high IGF-1 level would, however, support the suspicion of acromegaly and provide justification for imaging of the pituitary gland by CT or MRI (Berg et al, 2007). A pituitary mass is visible in the vast majority of cases at the time of presentation. The finding of a normal IGF-1 concentration, on the other hand, does not rule out acromegaly. IGF-1 measurement should be repeated after a few more weeks of insulin therapy (or 6 to 8 weeks after insulin therapy has been initiated). Alternatively, GH concentrations may be measured (if available) or an immediate search for a pituitary mass by CT/MRI may be considered.

In cats without typical physical changes of acromegaly, other more common causes of poor glycemic control should be considered, and a systematic work-up should be pursued. See Chapter 7 for more details. Hyperadrenocorticism is among the many differential diagnosis for poor glycemic control. It is often also associated with insulin resistance and is also caused by a pituitary tumor in many cases. Clinical signs, however, differ between the two diseases. Hyperadrenocorticism is a debilitating disease that results in weight loss, potentially leading to cachexia, and it is often associated with obvious hair coat and skin abnormalities (hair loss, change in coat color, thin skin, and fragile skin). In contrast, cats with acromegaly usually do not show relevant hair coat and skin abnormalities. They often have physical changes (e.g., broad head and prognathia inferior), and they may gain weight despite poorly regulated diabetes (Feldman and Nelson, 2004). It is important to note, however, that typical changes may be lacking in early stages or mild forms of both diseases. Diagnostic imaging findings in both diseases may include hepatomegaly, mild to

moderate adrenomegaly, and a pituitary mass. Ultimately, differentiation of the two diseases is based on the results of GH and/or IGF-1 measurements and tests of the pituitary-adrenocortical axis (see Chapter 11).

Not all acromegalic cats are (severely) insulin-resistant. In some cats, a more or less adequate glycemic control can be achieved with insulin doses less than 1 U/kg body weight b.i.d. (e.g., with doses of 1 to 3 U per cat b.i.d.). In some of those cases, the disease progresses and work-up usually becomes necessary at a later stage.

Treatment

Humans

The aims of treatment are to relieve symptoms, to reduce the size of the pituitary tumor, to avoid tumor relapse, and to improve long-term morbidity and mortality. Several consensus documents have been published on disease management and on the criteria to define good control of acromegaly. Both, GH and IGF-1 have to be measured as biochemical markers of response. GH concentrations must return to less than 1.0 µg/L if measured in a random sample, or to a GH nadir of less than 0.4 µg/L during an oral glucose tolerance test; IGF-1 levels also must return into the normal range (Chanson and Salenave, 2008; Melmed et al, 2009; Giustina et al, 2010). The three approaches to therapy are neurosurgery, medical management, and radiation therapy. Transsphenoidal surgery is generally the first line treatment for small pituitary tumors, non-invasive macroadenomas, and when the tumor is causing compression symptoms. Success rates range between 75% to 95% in patients with microadenomas and decrease to 40% to 68% in patients with non-invasive macroadenomas. Expertise of the neurosurgeon is known to be of utmost importance (Melmed et al, 2009). When surgery fails to achieve adequate control of the disease or when surgery is impossible or contraindicated, medical therapy and/or radiation therapy are offered. Medical therapy is usually considered the second line approach. Currently, three classes of drugs are available: somatostatin receptor ligands, dopamine agonists, and GH receptor antagonists.

Somatostatin inhibits GH secretion as well as secretion of many other hormones in the body. It also reduces proliferation of various normal and tumoral cells. Those actions are mediated through interaction with five different somatostatin receptors

(SSTR 1-5), GH release is mediated through SSTR 2 and 5. Somatotroph adenomas are characterized by a higher density of SSTR 2 and SSTR 5; however, they can express multiple SSTR, explaining the variable response to somatostatin therapy. The very short half-life of somatostatin leads to the development of somatostatin receptor ligands, also called *somatostatin analogs.* They are the first-line medical treatment option for human patients with acromegaly. Octreotide (Sandostatin) was the first analog to be marketed and has to be injected 2 to 3 times daily. During the recent years, a sustained release version of octreotide (Sandostatin LAR) for once a month injection became available. Lanreotide is another somatostatin analog, coming as two long-acting formulations (Somatuline LA every 10 to 14 days, Somatuline Depot or Autogel once a month). The main limitation of octreotide and lanreotide is their selective binding to the SSTR subtypes, because their binding affinity is high for SSRT 2 but only moderate for SSTR 5 and SSTR 3 and very low for the other two. Reported efficacy with regard to normalization of GH and IGF-1 differs largely between studies and ranges between 20% and 80%. Tumor shrinkage, defined as 20% to 25% decrease in tumor volume, has been seen in up to 82% of human patients (Jallad and Bronstein, 2013). Common adverse effects consist of gastrointestinal signs. They usually decrease over the first few months of treatment (Melmed et al, 2009). Pasireotide (Signifor) is a new somatostatin analog with high affinity for SSTR 2 and SSTR 5, as well as for SSTR 1 and SSTR 3. Due to the improved binding profile, it has the potential to be more effective in patients with acromegaly than octreotide and lanreotide (Jallad and Bronstein, 2013; Petersenn et al, 2013).

The use of pegvisomant (Somavert), which is the only currently available GH receptor antagonist, is another treatment modality. It reduces the synthesis of IGF-1; however, it does not suppress GH secretion and does not have any inhibitory effect on the pituitary tumor growth (Jallad and Bronstein, 2013). The drug usually has to be injected daily. Adverse effects include gastrointestinal signs and increase in liver enzymes. Pegvisomant is currently mainly reserved for patients who have failed therapy with surgery and somatostatin receptor ligands (Javorsky et al, 2011). The dopamine agonist cabergoline is effective in less than 10% of patients with acromegaly, and its use is limited to a few particular clinical situations (patient prefers oral medication, or drug is used as part of a combination therapy) (Melmed et al, 2009). Medical treatment options are an area of intensive research and novel treatment modalities are currently in development (Jallad and Bronstein, 2013).

Radiation therapy is generally considered for third-line treatment and occasionally as second line treatment. It is currently proposed to a subset of patients with persistent active disease after surgery and/or during medical therapy (Minniti et al, 2011). With conventional radiation therapy, normalization of GH and IGF-1 levels is seen in 5% to 60% of human patients after a median follow-up of 7 years. Longer follow-up studies revealed hormone normalization in more than 70% of patients after 10 to 15 years. The long latency period to hormonal normalization of up to several years is one of the major disadvantages of radiotherapy, usually requiring additional medical treatment. Further limitations are the possible side effects of conventional radiation therapy, including impairment in neurocognitive function, visual dysfunction caused by optic neuropathy, and radiation induced secondary malignancy (Jagannathan et al, 2009). A major additional concern is hypopituitarism, which occurs in up to 60% of patients within 10 years after treatment. Stereotactic radiotherapy is a refinement of conventional radiotherapy with the principle aim to deliver more localized irradiation, possibly minimizing the long-term adverse consequences. It may produce beneficial effects on GH and IGF-1 sooner than conventional radiation therapy, but this assumption needs confirmation by further studies (Melmed et al, 2009; Minniti et al, 2011).

Cats

The aims of therapy in cats are twofold: treatment of the acromegalic condition itself and treatment of the concurrent diabetes mellitus. In some of the cats, treatment is limited to the latter because the owner denies treatment of the acromegalic condition. See Chapter 7 for management guidelines. Insulin resistance varies widely between acromegalic cats. In some cats, glycemic control may be achieved with "normal" insulin doses (1 to 3 U/cat b.i.d.); in others, much higher doses are required. We usually increase the insulin dose in steps of 0.5 to 1.0 U/cat b.i.d. approximately every 5 to 7 days until glycemic control is acceptable (e.g., most blood glucose levels throughout the day are between approximately 100 to 300 mg/dL [5.6 to 17.0 mmol/L]). Close monitoring of the cats is mandatory, and we highly recommend home-monitoring of glucose by the owners in those patients. Unfortunately, insulin resistance also varies within a given patient, and severe hypoglycemia is possible in particular in conjunction with anorexia. Whenever possible, we do not increase the insulin dose above 12 to 15 U/cat b.i.d.

As in humans, specific treatment modalities for acromegaly in cats include pituitary surgery, medical therapy, and radiation therapy. See the section Treatment, Humans for some principal explanations. Pituitary surgery has the potential to become the treatment of choice also in cats. The procedure, however, is technically highly demanding and currently only offered in very few specialized centers. So far, only a few case reports have been published (Abrams-Ogg et al, 1993; Blois and Holmberg, 2008; Meij et al, 2010b). Transsphenoidal cryohypophysectomy resulted in a decrease in insulin requirement, well-controlled diabetes mellitus, and no signs of acromegaly during an observation period of 18 months in one cat (Blois and Holmberg, 2008). In another cat, transsphenoidal hypophysectomy led to a decrease in insulin requirement by 95% during the first days after surgery and to diabetic remission after 3 weeks. The cat was followed up for 18 months after surgery, GH and IGF-1 levels normalized, and the cat was doing well without the need of exogenous insulin (Meij et al, 2010b). Recently, the same group reported three more cases with favorable outcome after transsphenoidal hypophysectomy. In all three cats, diabetic remission occurred within the first 4 weeks after surgery, and GH as well as IGF-1 levels normalized (Meij et al, 2012b). The latter cases demonstrate that β-cells have the potential for recovery in acromegalic cats with appropriate treatment. Very close monitoring of blood glucose is essential to avoid life-threatening hypoglycemia.

So far, medical treatment has shown very little to no effect. The number of treated cats, however, is small, and no systematic evaluations of dose-responses have been performed. One cat was treated with the dopamine agonist L-deprenyl (initial dose 5 mg s.i.d. [semel in die; once a day], increased to 10 mg s.i.d. after 1 month) for 9 months without any improvement in clinical signs and insulin requirement (Abraham et al, 2002). The use of somatostatin receptor ligand octreotide has been reported in five acromegalic cats (Morrison et al, 1989; Peterson et al, 1990). Doses ranged between 5 and 100 μg given two or three times daily for up to 4 weeks without improvement of glycemic control and GH hypersecretion. We have used the sustained release octreotide in a few cats during the last years. The effect on insulin requirement, however, was small. As mentioned earlier, the main limitations of the somatostatin analogs octreotide and lanreotide in humans is their selective binding to the SSTR subtypes because their density and distribution pattern varies in acromegalic patients. The same may hold true for acromegalic cats. A recent study investigated if a single application of octreotide to acromegalic cats would be useful as a pre-entry test for treatment with somatostatin analogs. GH concentrations were measured prior to and 15, 30, 60, 90, and 120 minutes after the intravenous administration of octreotide (5 μg/kg bodyweight). Two of the five acromegalic cats showed a clear-cut decrease in GH concentrations, whereas the decrease in the other three cats was small (Slingerland et al, 2008). Further studies are needed to evaluate if the responders of the octreotide test will also show favorable treatment response. A recently presented study showed promising results by using the new somatostatin analog pasireotide in eight cats with acromegaly. All cats showed a significant decrease in blood glucose and IGF-1 concentrations (Niessen et al, 2013b). No information on the use of pegvisomant, a GH receptor antagonist, is available at this time.

Radiation therapy is currently the most frequently used treatment modality in acromegalic cats. In the studies described in the past, types and techniques of radiation (Cobalt-60, betatron, linear accelerator), treatment planning (manual or computerized), as well treatment protocols (number of fractions, total radiation dose) varied considerably (Goossens et al, 1998; Peterson et al, 1990; Kaser-Hotz et al, 2002; Brearley et al, 2006; Littler et al, 2006; Mayer et al, 2006; Dunning et al, 2009; Sellon et al, 2009). Additionally, follow-up periods and parameters to evaluate treatment outcome also differed, rendering direct comparison between the studies impossible. Many of the treatments are not state-of-the-art anymore and, therefore, results have to be interpreted with care. The most consistent effect of radiotherapy is improvement or resolution of neurological signs. In cats with large pituitary tumors, improvement is often seen during or soon after radiation therapy. If tumor size is reevaluated by CT or MRI a few months after completion of radiation therapy, considerable size reduction (e.g., partial or complete remission) may be seen. Improvement of clinical signs of diabetes is more variable and difficult to predict. Insulin requirement may start to decrease already during radiation therapy or soon thereafter. In a recent study, the mean time to improved glycemic control was 5 weeks after the completion of radiotherapy, with a range of 0 to 20 weeks. In 6 of 14 cats, diabetic remission was achieved after a mean time of 3.6 months with a range of 0 to 6 months (Dunning et al, 2009). It is important to note that diabetic remission may occur as late as 1 year after radiation. The unpredictable course of the diabetes is one of the challenging problems because it requires close monitoring of the cat's blood glucose concentrations. Failure to identify improvement or resolution of insulin resistance may result in hypoglycemia and death. As already mentioned earlier, we highly recommend home-monitoring of blood glucose in cats with acromegaly—in particular after they have undergone surgical or radiation therapy. In some cats, diabetic remission is transient, and insulin therapy has to be re-introduced. Based on the currently available data, improvement of the clinical signs of diabetes is possible in approximately 70% to 80% of cases; in approximately 50% of cases, diabetic remission may be achieved. However, the physical changes of acromegaly usually persist or improve only slightly. In human medicine, the goal of any therapy in acromegalic patients is a normalization of GH and IGF-1 concentrations. After radiation therapy, hormone levels in humans decrease only slowly, and it may take many years until they are within the normal range. In cats GH is rarely measured, and

IGF-1 is often not followed long-term after radiation therapy. It is therefore unknown if resolution of the GH excess is ever achieved. Persistently high IGF-1 levels have been reported in some cats after radiation. Interestingly, in several of those cases, diabetes was well controlled or even in remission (Littler et al, 2006; Dunning et al, 2009). In a few other studies, a decrease of GH concentrations was demonstrated in some of the cats (Goosens et al, 1998; Peterson et al, 1990). It is likely that radiation therapy results in a substantial decrease in GH production, which is sufficient to restore β-cell function. However, GH levels (or pulses) may not be completely normal and still high enough to stimulate excessive IGF-1 production. So far, measurement of IGF-1 levels after radiation does not appear to be helpful to predict the course of diabetes. Radiation therapy is well tolerated in the vast majority of cats. Late radiation side effects (e.g., hearing impairment or ischemic brain necrosis) are rare and can be avoided with the use of appropriate fractionation protocol; hypopituitarism, a common adverse effect in humans, has not yet been reported in cats. The disadvantages of radiation therapy are limited availability, expense, need for frequent anesthesia, as well as the unpredictable outcomes in terms of hormonal control. Some of those disadvantages may potentially be overcome with the use of more sophisticated radiation techniques and radiation protocols (e.g., hypofractionated stereotactic [image-guided] radiation therapy, and stereotactic radiosurgery), allowing more precise radiation fields and less exposure of normal tissue. In cats with favorable response to radiation therapy, survival times for up to 5 years have been reported (Dunning et al, 2009; Fig. 2-24).

Histopathology

In most cases, histopathology reveals an acidophil adenoma of the pituitary gland with or without involvement (compression or invasion) of the pars intermedia, pars distalis, hypothalamus, and thalamus. On rare occasions, no tumor but proliferation of

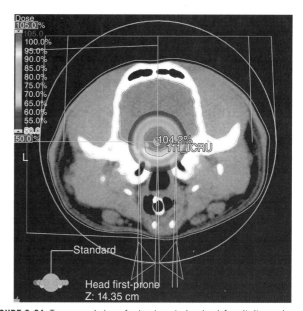

FIGURE 2-24 Transversal view of a treatment plan (arc) for pituitary adenoma. The colors represent the dose distribution within the planning target volume *(red line surrounding the tumor)* with red and orange colors representing the high-dose area (90% to 105% of the prescribed dose) and blue and green colors displaying the rapid fall-off of dose outside the target structure. (Courtesy of Dr. Carla Rohrer Bley, Division of Radiation Oncology, Vetsuisse Faculty, University of Zurich.)

the acidophilic cells is found (Niessen et al, 2007a). Microscopic findings of other organs include adenomatous hyperplasia of the thyroid and the parathyroid glands, multinodular hyperplasia of the adrenal cortices, multifocal or disseminated nodular hyperplasia of the pancreas with ductal fibrosis, interstitial lymphocytic or lymphocytic-plasmacytic infiltration, hyalinization of the islets, and amyloid deposition. Kidneys usually reveal findings consistent with glomerulopathy/glomerulonephritis and interstitial nephritis, including thickening of the glomerular basement membrane, thickening of the Bowman capsule, expansion of the mesangial matrix, periglomerular fibrosis, interstitial fibrosis with lymphocytic-plasmacytic infiltration, and renal tubular degeneration. Steatosis and lymphocytic-plasmacytic cholangiohepatitis are typical liver abnormalities. Myocardial lesions are characterized by myofiber hypertrophy, myocytolysis, interstitial fibrosis, and arteriosclerosis. Microscopic joint alterations include erosion and ulceration of cartilage with chondroid hyperplasia and fissure formation (Middleton et al, 1985; Peterson et al, 1990; Abrams-Ogg et al, 1993; Abraham et al, 2002; Niessen et al 2007a; Greco, 2012).

Prognosis

If the cat is not treated for acromegaly, the prognosis is guarded to poor. In most cats, clinical signs and insulin resistance are progressive, rendering insulin treatment increasingly difficult. Most cats are euthanized within a few months after diagnosis, because the owner becomes frustrated by the poor control of the diabetes and the increasing or fluctuating insulin requirement. Other cats are euthanized or die because of the development of congestive heart failure, renal failure, respiratory distress, or neurological signs associated with expansion of the pituitary tumor. Cats in which the GH excess is treated with either pituitary surgery or radiation therapy may have a favorable outcome. Glycemic control often improves, and diabetic remission is possible; survival for several years has been seen.

HYPERSOMATOTROPISM (ACROMEGALY) IN DOGS

The etiopathogenesis of acromegaly is quite different in dogs and cats. In dogs, acromegaly is almost always induced by endogenous or exogenous progestagens giving rise to GH hypersecretion from the mammary gland. Acromegaly, due to a GH-producing tumor in the pituitary gland, which is the cause of feline acromegaly, is an extremely rare event in the dog (Kooistra, 2010).

Etiology

Pituitary Neoplasia

So far, the occurrence of a somatotrophic adenoma has only been described in two dogs. Van Keulen, et al. (1996) reported a 9-year-old male Doberman Pinscher with difficult to regulate diabetes mellitus but without obvious physical changes of acromegaly. Necropsy revealed an acidophilic adenoma with strong positive immunohistochemical staining for GH. More recently, Fracassi, et al. (2007) described a 10-year-old Dalmatian dog with typical acromegalic features, including polyphagia, weight gain, inspiratory stridor, enlargement of head and tongue, widening of interdental spaces, thickening of the skin particularly of head and neck with redundant skin folds, panting, and chronic progressive stiffness and neck rigidity. The dog also suffered from polyuria and polydipsia. His insulin levels were increased and glucose intolerance was demonstrated during a glucose tolerance

test; however, he was not overtly diabetic as basal blood glucose concentrations were measured repetitively and found to be normal. GH and IGF-1 levels were increased, and CT imaging revealed a pituitary mass. The dog was left untreated and was euthanized after a few months because of progressive worsening of the clinical signs. Histology and immunohistochemistry confirmed the presence of an acidophilic adenoma that stained positive for GH. It is interesting to note, that in one of the two dogs the insulin-antagonistic actions occurred; in the other dog, however, the anabolic effects of GH excess dominated the clinical picture. In our institution, we recently diagnosed another case in a 7-year-old male castrated Labrador Retriever with both difficult to regulate diabetes mellitus and typical physical features of acromegaly.

Endogenous and Exogenous Progestagens

In dogs, circulating GH does not only derive from the anterior pituitary but also originates from the mammary gland. Mammary GH is stimulated by progesterone, which is a physiological event and occurs in all intact bitches. See "Mammary Growth Hormone" at the beginning of the chapter for more details. Administration of synthetic progestagens for estrus prevention may result in excessive GH secretion and increased IGF-1 synthesis and potentially acromegaly and diabetes mellitus. Treatment in male dogs (e.g., for benign prostatic hyperplasia) may have the same effect. GH excess may also occur in some middle-aged to elderly bitches during the luteal phase of the estrus cycle (Kooistra, 2013).

The phenomenon of progestagen-induced GH excess was discovered in the 1970s and 1980s. Rijnberk, et al. (1980) described acromegalic features and increased GH concentrations in a dog that had received twelve injections of MPA for estrus prevention over the course of 4 years. The dog was not overtly diabetic but revealed glucose intolerance during an oral glucose tolerance test. After cessation of MPA application, physical changes gradually improved; GH and insulin concentrations as well as glucose intolerance normalized with time. Soon thereafter, Eigenmann and Venker-van Haagen (1981) reported on another fifteen dogs that had received MPA injections twice yearly for estrus prevention. All dogs had typical physical features of acromegaly, and thirteen of the fifteen dogs showed hyperglycemia. The latter was mild (blood glucose ≤ 180 mg/dL, 10 mmol/L) in eight dogs and severe (blood glucose more than 180 mg/dL, 10 mmol/L) in five dogs. GH concentrations were increased in all fifteen dogs with marked variation from dog to dog (11 to 178 µg/L, median 34.2; normal dogs less than 5 µg/L). Clinical signs and hyperglycemia improved after cessation of MPA administration. Experimental studies confirmed the causal relationship between the application of progestagens and the development of acromegaly, glucose intolerance, and diabetes mellitus (Concannon et al, 1980; Eigenmann and Rijnberk, 1981; Eigenmann and Eigenmann 1981a, Scott and Concannon, 1983; Selman et al 1994b; Selman et al, 1997).

Selman et al (1994b) administered 10 mg/kg MPA and 50 mg/kg PROL to castrated Beagle bitches at intervals of 3 weeks for a total of eight injections. The doses were twice as high as recommended for estrus prevention, and application frequency was much higher (for estrus prevention only once every 6 months). GH levels were significantly higher compared to the initial levels already after the second injection and increased steadily, with considerable inter-individual variation. IGF-1 concentrations increased simultaneously, and large increases in GH were associated with large increases in IGF-1 levels. Both progestagen preparations resulted in similar increases. Insulin levels also increased and were significantly higher compared with pre-treatment levels after the third injection but did not increase further. After six injections, glucose intolerance became apparent, and one dog in each group developed severe diabetes mellitus. During the recovery period of 30 weeks after the last injection, neither GH nor IGF-1 returned to normal, and glucose tolerance remained impaired.

In summary, application of progestagens to dogs results in increase in GH and IGF-1 concentrations, albeit with large inter-individual differences. The increases appear to be dose-related: higher doses, and more frequent applications lead to more pronounced increase. The effects are similar with different progestagen preparations. The hormone excess is associated with the development of acromegalic features; their severity also varies between individuals. Initially, glucose tolerance is maintained by increased insulin production. With time, however, further insulin increase is not possible, resulting in glucose intolerance. Some dogs may develop overt diabetes mellitus. The abnormalities are potentially reversible after weeks to months; however, bone lesions usually persist. Progesterone-induced GH excess may also occur in some middle-aged to elderly intact bitches associated with the luteal phase of their estrus cycle. The increase in GH and IGF-1 is a physiological event (e.g., it occurs also in healthy intact bitches). Basal GH levels are highest during the first part of the luteal phase (luteal phase 1), when progesterone levels are also highest, both hormones decrease in parallel and are lowest in anestrus. GH concentrations were shown to be 2.2 ± 0.3 in luteal phase 1 and 1.4 ± 0.2 µg/L in anestrus; progesterone concentrations were 123 ± 15 and 0.9 ± 0.2 nmol/L, respectively (Kooistra et al, 2000b). In bitches developing spontaneous acromegaly, progesterone levels are within the range of normal dogs, whereas GH concentrations are increased (Eigenmann, 1986). As seen after exogenous progesterone application, GH levels vary markedly between individual dogs, ranging between 11.8 to 1476 µg/L (median 31.7; normal dogs less than 5 µg/L) in seven bitches with spontaneous GH excess (Eigenmann and Venker-van Haagen, 1981). Dogs with spontaneous GH excess may be overtly diabetic or reveal glucose intolerance during a glucose tolerance test, and insulin levels are usually high (Eigenmann, 1981b; Eigenmann et al, 1983). Recovery is potentially possible after ovariohysterectomy. The reason why some intact bitches develop diestrus-associated acromegaly and diabetes has not yet been clarified. Gestational diabetes mellitus has been reported several times (Norman et al, 2006; Fall et al, 2008; Fall et al, 2010; Armenise et al, 2011). Usually, the signs associated with diabetes mellitus dominate the clinical picture; obvious acromegalic features have only been seen in one dog (Norman et al, 2006).

Of note, circulating GH may not only originate from normal mammary tissue but also from mammary tumors. There is an association with tumor characteristics, because GH and IGF-1 levels in plasma and tumor tissue were shown to be significantly higher in dogs with malignant tumors than in dogs with benign tumors (Queiroga et al, 2008; Queiroga et al, 2010). Very recently, acromegalic features were described in two dogs with mammary tumors staining positive for GH (Murai et al, 2012). Mammary tumor-induced acromegaly, however, is generally rare.

Hypothyroidism

Dogs with primary hypothyroidism were shown to have elevated basal GH concentrations and increased IGF-1. It is suggested that some of the physical changes seen in hypothyroidism (thick skin, skin folds) are, at least in part, due to increased GH and IGF-1 levels (Lee et al, 2001).

Pathophysiology

See the section Metabolic Actions on Growth Hormone and Insulin-like Growth Factor-1 and the section Hypersomatotropism (Acromegaly) in Cats, Pathophysiology.

Signalment

GH-secreting pituitary tumors have so far only been seen in male dogs of large breeds (Doberman Pinscher, Dalmatian, Labrador Retriever), with age ranges between 7 and 10 years (Van Keulen et al, 1996; Fracassi et al, 2007).

GH-excess due to exogenous progestagen application has been seen by us and others in numerous breeds of different sizes, including Dachshund, French Bulldog, Scottish Terrier, English Cocker Spaniel, American Cocker Spaniel, Springer Spaniel, Standard Poodle, English Setter, Dalmatian, Belgian Shepherd, and mixed breed dogs. The dogs were intact females and developed the disorder after receiving progestagens for estrus prevention, with age ranges between 4 and 11 years. Similarly, GH excess associated with the luteal phase of the estrus cycle has been seen in various breeds; the bitches were usually middle-aged to elderly (6 to 13 years). The breeds included Dachshund, Beagle, English Cocker Spaniel, Dalmatian, Golden Retriever, German Shepherd, Bouvier, and mixed breed dogs (Rijnberk et al, 1980; Eigenmann, 1981b; Eigenmann and Venker-van Haagen, 1981). A study undertaken in Sweden showed that in some breeds (e.g., Swedish and Norwegian Elkhounds, Border Collies, and Beagles), diabetes mellitus occurs almost exclusively in intact females, and it was assumed that in many of the dogs the disease is diestrus-associated (Fall et al, 2007). Gestational diabetes was reported in Elkhounds, Alaskan Malamute, Siberian Husky, Drever, Border Collie, Labrador Retriever, and Yorkshire Terrier, with age ranges between 6 to 8 years (Norman et al, 2006; Fall et al, 2007; Fall et al, 2008; Fall et al, 2010; Armenise et al, 2011).

The two dogs with assumed mammary-tumor derived GH-excess were a 10-year-old Miniature Dachshund and a 13-year-old Papillon, both were female-intact (Murai et al, 2012).

Clinical Manifestations

The clinical signs of GH excess tend to develop slowly. In cases, in which the disorder is induced by exogenous progestagens, the onset is variable and depends in part on dosage and frequency of application of the compound (Feldman and Nelson, 2004). In case of diestrus-associated hypersecretion of GH, dogs are often presented 3 to 5 weeks after estrus. The owner may report, however, that similar signs (e.g., inspiratory dyspnea, polyuria/polydipsia) had already been apparent after the previous estrus, albeit milder and improved during anestrus. Although the increase of GH during the luteal phase is a physiological event, it should be remembered that only very few intact bitches develop pathological GH hypersecretion (Fig. 2-25).

Clinical signs mainly result from the anabolic, growth-promoting effect of GH and IGF-1 and the diabetogenic effects of GH. Cats with acromegaly are almost always presented because of diabetes mellitus, which is difficult to regulate in many cases. Acromegalic features often only become obvious with time. In dogs, manifestations, however, are more variable. Some dogs only reveal the typical physical changes of acromegaly, some predominantly show clinical signs of diabetes mellitus, and others have both categories of symptoms. Part of the variability may be breed-related. As for instance in Elkhound dogs, diestrus-associated

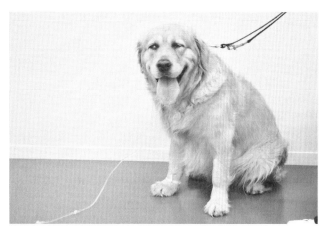

FIGURE 2-25 Female 9-year-old intact Golden Retriever with diestrus-associated acromegaly. The dog was presented with inspiratory stridor, dyspnea, lethargy, thickening of the skin, excessive skin folds in the head and neck area, and coarse facial features. Blood glucose concentration was normal. The circulating proges- terone concentration was 13.5 ng/mL and consistent with diestrus, the insulin- like growth factor-1 (IGF-1) concentration was 1600 ng/mL and severely increased (normal < 800). Two weeks after ovariohysterectomy, the progesterone concentra- tion was 1.9 ng/mL, and IGF-1 had decreased to 383 ng/mL. The acromegalic features resolved with time.

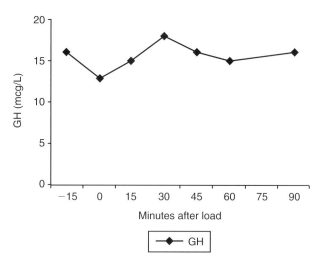

FIGURE 2-26 Serum growth hormone (GH) concentrations at −15, 0, 15, 30, 45, 60, and 90 minutes after the intravenous administration of 10 µg/kg somatosta- tin per kg body weight in a 10-year-old male Dalmatian dog with acromegaly due to a somatotroph adenoma. Basal GH concentration was markedly elevated (reference range: 2 to 5 µg/L) and did not decrease after somatostatin. (Repro- duced with permission from Fracassi F, et al.: Acromegaly due to a somatotroph adenoma in a dog, *Domest Anim Endocrinol* 32[1]:43-54, 2007.)

diabetes, but no physical changes of acromegaly have been reported (Fall et al, 2010). In dogs, typical and early signs are inspiratory stridor and possibly dyspnea, panting, and exercise intolerance due to an increase in soft tissue mass in the oropharyngeal region. Further physical changes include enlargement of the tongue, prognathia inferior, widening of interdental spaces, broadening of the head, increased skin thickness and excessive skin folds mainly in the head and neck area and distal extremities, enlargement of abdomen due to visceromegaly, enlargement of paws, weight gain, thickened hair coat with long and curly hair, difficulties to rise or walk due to degenerative arthropathy, and mammary tumors (Rijnberk et al, 1980; Eigenmann and Venker-van Haagen, 1981; Scott and Concannon, 1983; Feldman and Nelson, 2004; Norman et al, 2006; Fracassi et al, 2007; Meij et al, 2010a; Murai et al, 2012). Overt diabetes mellitus develops in a substantial percentage of dogs and is associated with polyuria and polydipsia. However, mild to moderate polyuria and polydipsia may also be present without diabetes and is probably related to either exogenous progestagens and/or the GH excess. In the very rare event of GH excess caused by a pituitary tumor, additional neurological signs may be present.

Clinical Pathology

Blood glucose concentrations may be normal, or range from mildly to severely increased. Depending on the degree of hyperglycemia, glucosuria may or may not be present. Similarly, serum fructosamine concentrations may be normal or increased. Ketonuria and diabetic ketoacidosis have been seen in diestrus-associated diabetes, but they are rare. In case of overt diabetes mellitus, additional abnormalities (e.g., increased cholesterol, increased ALT and ALP) may be found.

Diagnostic Imaging

Potential radiological and/or ultrasonographic abnormalities include increase in soft tissue in the oropharyngeal region, degenerative arthropathy, spondylosis, and organomegaly. In

the very rare event of GH hypersecretion due to a tumor of the somatotrophic cells, CT/MRI will reveal a pituitary mass.

Hormonal Evaluation

Circulating GH and IGF-1 levels are usually increased in dogs with acromegaly. As GH is secreted in pulses, a single measurement is often not sufficient for the diagnosis. A high GH level may just be the result of a secretory pulse. The exception would be a dog with several-fold increase from normal. On the other hand, in dogs with mild or beginning acromegaly, basal GH levels may still be within the normal range. There are several options to increase the diagnostic accuracy:
1. Measurement of GH in three to five samples taken at 10 minute intervals. The more of those samples that reveal an increased GH level and the higher those levels are, the more likely the dog has acromegaly.
2. Measurement of GH during a somatostatin suppression test. The latter is performed by collecting blood samples for GH determi- nation before and 15, 30, 45, 60, and 90 minutes after the intra- venous application of 10 µg/kg body weight somatostatin. GH should show minimal or no decrease in dogs with acromegaly.
3. Measurement of GH during an IVGTT. The additional mea- surement of the insulin concentrations allows evaluation of the degree of glucose intolerance. The test is, therefore, suitable for dogs with normal or only mildly increased blood glucose concentrations. Blood samples for determination of GH, in- sulin, and glucose are taken before and 15, 30, 60, and 90 minutes after the IV administration of 1 g/kg body weight of a 50% glucose solution. GH concentrations should show no or minimal decrease in the case of acromegaly. Basal insulin con- centrations are often very high without further increase after the glucose load, more moderately increased basal insulin levels may show some increase; despite high insulin levels, glucose tolerance is impaired (i.e., delayed return to normal).

GH should be determined in a canine-specific radioimmunoas- say. Unfortunately availability is often limited (Eigenmann et al, 1983; Feldman and Nelson, 2004; Fracassi et al, 2007; Kooistra 2010, 2013; Fig. 2-26 and Fig. 2-27). Sample handling for GH

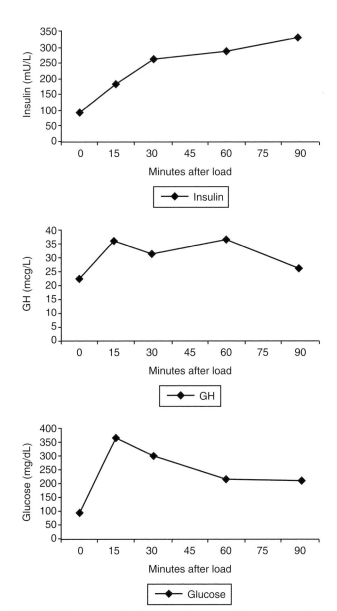

FIGURE 2-27 Serum concentrations of growth hormone (GH), insulin, and glucose at 0, 15, 30, 60, and 90 minutes after the intravenous administration of 1g/kg body weight of a 50% glucose solution in a 10-year-old male Dalmatian dog with acromegaly due to a somatotroph adenoma. Basal insulin concentration was high and increased considerably after the glucose load. Glucose concentrations, however, did not return to normal, indicating glucose intolerance. Basal GH concentration was markedly elevated (reference range; 2 to 5 μg/L) and did not decrease after the glucose load. (Reproduced with permission from Fracassi F, et al.: Acromegaly due to a somatotroph adenoma in a dog, *Domest Anim Endocrinol* 32[1]:43-54, 2007.)

determination is critical, and the laboratory should be contacted prior to performing the test.

Measurement of IGF-1 is a suitable alternative test. Because IGF-1 is not secreted in pulses, one single random blood sample is required. It can be measured with assays designed for humans, and the sample can be sent by regular mail. In acromegalic dogs, IGF-1 levels are often highly increased (e.g., two to three times the upper limit of normal is no exception). As with any other disease, however, in mild or beginning disease, there may be overlap between healthy and affected dogs. IGF-1 levels correlate with body size; therefore, size-dependent reference ranges should be

used. IGF-1 measurement may be associated with some biological and technical problems; see the discussion on IGF-1 in the section Hypersomatotropism in Cats, Hormonal Evaluation.

Baseline T_4 and TSH concentrations are usually normal in dogs with acromegaly. Conversely, in dogs with primary hypothyroidism, basal GH and IGF-1 levels are increased.

The intrinsic glucocorticoid-activity of exogenous progestagens may suppress endogenous ACTH secretion, causing low basal cortisol concentration and impaired cortisol response after ACTH administration (Concannon et al, 1980; Court et al, 1998).

Establishing the Diagnosis

A tentative diagnosis of acromegaly is based on the presence of typical physical changes of acromegaly and/or diabetes mellitus in association with the history of chronic progestagen administration or diestrus. In case of diestrus-associated GH hypersecretion, dogs are often presented 3 to 5 weeks after estrus. Careful questioning of the owner often reveals that milder signs had already been apparent after the previous estrus and improved during anestrus. The definitive diagnosis requires the documentation of increased GH (and impaired suppression after somatostatin or glucose) or increased IGF-1 concentrations. The most important differential diagnosis for a dog with physical changes of acromegaly is hypothyroidism. The latter disease may also be associated with clinical signs (e.g., thickening of the skin, abundant skin folds particular in the head area, lethargy and weight gain) and therefore, dogs with acromegaly and hypothyroidism may look alike. It is very important to realize that dogs with primary hypothyroidism have elevated GH and IGF-1 concentrations (Lee et al, 2001). Dogs with acromegaly typically have normal T_4 and TSH levels. In male dogs with no history of progestagen administration, the possibility of a pituitary tumor should be explored by CT or MRI imaging. In dogs with polyuria and polydipsia (without diabetes mellitus and without acromegalic features) various diagnoses have to be considered (see Chapters 1 and 3).

Treatment

In bitches with diestrus-associated acromegaly, ovariohysterectomy should be performed as soon as possible. GH and IGF-1 concentrations return to normal very soon thereafter. In case of diabetes mellitus, immediate measures are highly recommended to limit the deleterious effects of glucose toxicity on β-cell function, thereby improving the chance of diabetic remission. We usually do not wait until we receive the results of the GH/IGF-1 measurements. Insulin therapy is initiated immediately in all dogs with moderate to highly increased blood glucose concentrations (>140 mg/dL, 8 mmol/L); the insulin dose depends on the severity of hyperglycemia and ranges between approximately 0.05 to 0.25 U/kg b.i.d. If ovariohysterectomy has to be delayed for more than one day, we routinely administer the progesterone receptor aglépristone (Alizin, Virbac) in a dose of 10 mg/kg subcutaneously and repeat the same dose after 24 hours. During surgery and during the following days to weeks, blood glucose concentrations should be monitored closely. Insulin requirements may decrease rapidly due to the cessation of insulin resistance, and hypoglycemia may occur if insulin doses are not amended. In dogs with acromegaly due to exogenous progestagens, their administration should be discontinued immediately. Insulin treatment is initiated as described earlier if diabetes is present. Usually, those dogs were treated with depot progestagen preparations with long lasting effects. In dogs with severe signs of acromegaly and in all dogs which are diabetic, we administer aglépristone (Alizin, Virbac) in a dose of 10 mg/kg subcutaneously twice at 24-hour intervals. Because the progestagen effect is usually much longer lasting than the effect of aglépristone, the administration of the latter is repeated approximately once a week. This approach is empirical and based on the study of Bhatti, et al. (2006d) and our own experience. The optimal protocol has not yet been established. Mammary tumors should be removed surgically, because they may be a source of GH/IGF-1 production.

In dogs with acromegaly due to a pituitary tumor, either radiation therapy or hypophysectomy should be considered; due to the rarity of cases, experience with regard to outcome, however, is lacking.

Prognosis

The prognosis of progestagen-induced acromegaly is usually good. The soft-tissue changes usually resolve over weeks to months, and the dog may regain a more or less normal appearance. If the bony changes persist, usually they do not cause clinical problems (Kooistra, 2013). The course of the diabetes mellitus is more variable and depends on the degree of β-cell damage. Diabetic remission may occur within a few weeks (1 to 8 weeks after ovariohysterectomy) if treatment is instituted early; however, persistence of diabetes is also possible.

REFERENCES

Abraham LA, et al.: Treatment of an acromegalic cat with the dopamine agonist L-deprenyl, *Aus Vet J* 80:479, 2002.

Abrams-Ogg ACG, et al.: Acromegaly in a cat: diagnosis by magnetic resonance imaging and treatment by cryohypophysectomy, *Can Vet J* 34:682, 1993.

Abribat T, et al.: Growth hormone response induced by synthetic human growth hormone-releasing factor (1-44) in healthy dogs, *J Vet Med* 36:367, 1989.

Allgoewer I, et al.: Somatotropes Hypophysenadenom mit Läsion des n. oculomotorius bei einer Katze, *Tierärztl Prax* 26:267, 1998.

Andresen E: Herkunft und Verbreitung von hypophysärem Zwergwuchs beim Hund und Grundlage zur Ermittlung von Anlageträgern verschiedener genetisch bedingter Krankheiten unter Anwendung biochemischer Methoden, *Kleintierpraxis* 23:65, 1978.

Andresen E, Willeberg P: Pituitary dwarfism in German shepherd dogs: additional evidence of simple, autosomal recessive inheritance, *Nord Vet Med* 28:481, 1976.

Andresen E, Willeberg P: Pituitary dwarfism in Carelian bear-dogs: evidence of simple, autosomal recessive inheritance, *Hereditas* 84:232, 1977.

Aragon-Alonso A, et al.: Adult growth hormone deficiency. In Wass JAH, Stewart PM, Amiel SA, Davies MJ, editors: *Oxford textbook of endocrinology and diabetes*, ed 2, Oxford, 2011, Oxford University Press.

Armenise A, et al.: Gestational diabetes mellitus with diabetes ketoacidosis in a Yorkshire Terrier bitch, *J Am Anim Hosp Assoc* 47:285, 2011.

Ascacio-Martinez JA, Barrera-Saldaña HA: A dog growth hormone cDNA codes for a mature protein identical to pig growth hormone, *Gene* 143:277, 1994.

Bach LA, et al.: Insulin-like growth factor-binding protein-6 and cancer, *Clin Sci* 124:215, 2013.

Barrett KE, et al.: The pituitary gland. In Barrett KE, Barman SM, Boitano S, Brooks HL, editors: *Ganongs review of medical physiology*, ed 24, McGraw-Hill Companies, 2012.

Beijerink NJ, et al.: Evaluation of pulsatile plasma concentrations of growth hormone in healthy dogs and dogs with dilated cardiomyopathy, *Am J Vet Res* 72:59, 2011.

Bereket A, et al.: Alterations in the growth hormone-insulin-like growth factor axis in insulin dependent diabetes mellitus, *Horm Metab Res* 31:172, 1999.

Berg RIM, et al.: Serum insulin-like growth factor-I concentrations in cats with diabetes mellitus and acromegaly, *J Vet Intern Med* 21:892, 2007.

Bhatti SF, et al.: Effects of growth hormone-releasing peptides in healthy dogs and in dogs with pituitary-dependent hyperadrenocorticism, *Mol Cell Endocrinol* 197:97, 2002.

Bhatti SF, et al.: Ghrelin, an endogenous growth hormone secretagogue with diverse endocrine and nonendocrine effects, *Am J Vet Res* 67:180, 2006a.

Bhatti SF, et al.: Effects of growth hormone secretagogues on the release of adenohypophyseal hormones in young and old healthy dogs, *Vet J* 172:515, 2006b.

Bhatti SF, et al.: Ghrelin-stimulation test in the diagnosis of canine pituitary dwarfism, *Res Vet Sci* 81:24, 2006c.

Bhatti SF, et al.: Treatment of growth hormone excess in dogs with the progesterone receptor antagonist aglépristone, *Theriogenology* 66:797, 2006d.

Blois SL, Holmberg DL: Cryohypophysectomy used in the treatment of a case of feline acromegaly, *J Small Anim Pract* 49:596, 2008.

Boisclair YR, et al.: The acid-labile subunit (ALS) of the 150 kDa IGF-binding protein complex: an important but forgotten component of the circulating IGF system, *J Endocrinol* 170:63, 2001.

Boyko AR: The domestic dog: man's best friend in the genomic era, *Genome Biol* 12:216, 2011.

Brearley MJ, et al.: Coarse fractionated radiation therapy for pituitary tumours in cats: a retrospective study of 12 cases, *Vet Comparat Oncol* 4:209, 2006.

Brent GA, Davies TF: Hypothyroidism and thyroiditis. In Melmed S, Polonsky KS, Larsen PR, Kronenberg HM, editors: *Williams textbook of endocrinology*, ed 12, Philadelphia, 2011, Saunders Elsevier.

Bürki CD: Wachstumshormon (GH) und Insulin-ähnliche Wachstumsfaktoren (IGF) beim wachsenden Hund in Relation zur Körpergrösse am Modell des Pudels, Inaugural-Dissertation, Departement für Veterinärphysiologie und Tierernährung der Universität Zürich, *Zürich*, 2000.

Capen CC: Endocrine glands. In ed 5, Maxie MG, editor: *Jubb, Kennedy, and Palmer's pathology of domestic animals*, Vol 3. St Louis, 2007, Saunders Elsevier.

Castro-Peralta F, Barrera-Saldaña HA: Cloning and sequencing of cDNA encoding the cat growth hormone, *Gene* 160:311, 1995.

Cerundolo R, et al.: Alopecia in pomeranians and miniature poodles in association with high urinary corticoid:creatinine ratios and resistance to glucocorticoid feedback, *Vet Rec* 160:393, 2007.

Chanson P, Salenave S: Acromegaly, *Orphanet J Rare Dis* 3:17, 2008.

Chanson P, et al.: Acromegaly, *Best Pract Res Clin Endocrinol Metab* 23:555, 2009.

Chestnut RE, Quarmby V: Evaluation of total IGF-I assay methods using samples from type I and type II diabetic patients, *J Immunol Methods* 259:11, 2002.

Childs GV: Growth hormone cells as cogonadotropes: partners in the regulation of the reproductive system, *Trends Endocrinol Metab* 11:168, 2000.

Childs GV: Pituitary gland (cell types, mediators, development). In Larry R, Squire LR, editors: *Encyclopedia of neuroscience*, University of Arkansas for Medical Sciences, 2009. Elsevier

Clemmons DR: Metabolic actions of insulin-like growth factor-I in normal physiology and diabetes, *Endocrinol Metab Clin N Am* 41:425, 2012.

Concannon P, et al.: Growth hormone, prolactin, and cortisol in dogs developing mammary nodules and an acromegaly-like appearance during treatment with medroxyprogesterone acetate, *Endocrinol* 106:1173, 1980.

Cooke DW, et al.: Normal and aberrant growth. In Melmed S, Polonsky KS, Larsen PR, Kronenberger HM, editors: *Williams textbook of endocrinology*, ed 12, Philadelphia, 2011, Saunders Elsevier.

Court EA, et al.: Effects of delmadinone acetate on pituitary-adrenal function, glucose tolerance and growth hormone in male dogs, *Aust Vet J* 76:555, 1998.

Cowan JS, et al.: Secretory bursts of growth hormone secretion in the dog may be initiated by somatostatin withdrawal, *Can J Physiol Pharmacol* 62:199, 1984.

Daughaday WH, et al.: Somatomedin: proposed designation for sulphation factor, *Nature* 14:107, 1972.

Delafontaine P, et al.: Sequence of a cDNA encoding dog insulin-like growth factor I, *Gene* 130:305, 1993.

Diaz-Espiñeira MM, et al.: Functional and morphological changes in the adenohypophysis of dogs with induced primary hypothyroidism: loss of TSH hypersecretion, hypersomatotropism, hypoprolactinemia, and pituitary enlargement with transdifferentiation, *Domest Anim Endocrinol* 35:98, 2008.

Dimaraki EV, et al.: Acromegaly with apparently normal GH secretion: implications for diagnosis and follow-up, *J Clin Endocrinol Metab* 87:3537, 2002.

Doga M, et al.: Growth hormone deficiency in the adult, *Pituitary* 9:305, 2006.

Dominici FP, et al.: Influence of the crosstalk between growth hormone and insulin signalling on the modulation of insulin sensitivity, *Growth Horm IGF Res* 15:324, 2005.

Donaldson D, et al.: Congenital hyposomatotropism in a domestic shorthair cat presenting with congenital corneal oedema, *J Small Anim Pract* 49:306, 2008.

Dunning MD, et al.: Exogenous insulin treatment after hypofractionated radiotherapy in cats with diabetes mellitus and acromegaly, *J Vet Intern Med* 23:243, 2009.

Eigenmann JE: Diagnosis and treatment of dwarfism in a german shepherd dog, *J Am Anim Hosp Assoc* 17:798, 1981a.

Eigenmann JE: Diabetes mellitus in elderly female dogs: recent findings on pathogenesis and clinical implications, *J Am Anim Hosp Assoc* 17:805, 1981b.

Eigenmann JE: Diagnosis and treatment of pituitary dwarfism in dogs, *Proceedings of the 6th Kal Kan Symposium* 107–110, 1982a.

Eigenmann JE: Diabetes mellitus in dogs and cats, *Proceedings of the 6th Kal Kan Symposium*, 51–58, 1982b.

Eigenmann JE: Acromegaly in the dog, *Vet Clin North Am Small Anim Pract* 14:827, 1984.

Eigenmann JE: Disorders associated with growth hormone oversecretion: diabetes mellitus and acromegaly. In Kirk RW, editor: *Current veterinary therapy IX, small animal practice*, Philadelphia, 1986, Saunders Elsevier.

Eigenmann JE, Eigenmann RY: Influence of medroxyprogesterone acetate (Provera) on plasma growth hormone levels and on carbohydrate metabolism, *Acta Endocrinol* 98:603, 1981a.

Eigenmann JE, Eigenmann RY: Radioimmunoassay of canine growth hormone, *Acta Endocrinol* 98:514, 1981b.

Eigenmann JE, Patterson DF: Growth hormone deficiency in the mature dog, *J Am Anim Hosp Assoc* 20:741, 1984.

Eigenmann JE, Rijnberk A: Influence of medroxyprogesterone acetate (Provera) on plasma growth hormone levels and on carbohydrate metabolism, *Acta Endocrinol* 98:599, 1981.

Eigenmann JE, Venker-van Haagen AJ: Progestagen-induced and spontaneous canine acromegaly due to reversible growth hormone overproduction: clinical picture and pathogenesis, *J Am Anim Hosp Assoc* 17:813, 1981.

Eigenmann JE, et al.: Decrease of non-suppressible insulin-like activity after pancreatectomy and normalization by insulin therapy, *Acta Endocrinol* 85:818, 1977.

Eigenmann JE, et al.: Progesterone-controlled growth hormone overproduction and naturally occurring canine diabetes and acromegaly, *Acta Endocrinol* 104:167, 1983.

Eigenmann JE, et al.: Insulin-like growth factor I in the dog: a study in different dog breeds and in dogs with growth hormone elevation, *Acta Endocrinol (Copenh)* 105:294, 1984a.

Eigenmann JE, et al.: Elevated growth hormone levels and diabetes mellitus in a cat with acromegalic features, *J Am Anim Hosp Assoc* 20:747, 1984b.

Eigenmann JE, et al.: Body size parallels insulin-like growth factor I levels but not growth hormone secretory capacity, *Acta endocrinol (Copenh)* 106:448, 1984c.

Eigenmann JE, et al.: Growth hormone and insulin-like growth factor I in German Shepherd dwarf dogs, *Acta Endocrinol* 105:289, 1984d.

Ekman B, et al.: Circulating IGF-I concentrations are low and not correlated to glycaemic control in adults with type 1 diabetes, *Europ J Endocrinol* 143:505, 2000.

Elliott DA, et al.: Prevalence of pituitary tumors among diabetic cats with insulin resistance, *J Am Vet Med Assoc* 216:1765, 2000.

Fall T, et al.: Diabetes mellitus in a population of 180,000 insured dogs: incidence, survival, and breed distribution, *J Vet Intern Med* 21:1209, 2007.

Fall T, et al.: Gestational diabetes mellitus in 13 dogs, *J Vet Intern Med* 22:1296, 2008.

Fall T, et al.: Diabetes mellitus in elkhounds is associated with diestrus and pregnancy, *J Vet Intern Med* 24:1322, 2010.

Favier RP, et al.: Large body size in the dog is associated with transient GH excess at a young age, *J Endocrinol* 170:479, 2001.

Feldman EC, Nelson RW: Disorders of growth hormone. In Feldman EC, Nelson RW, editors: *Canine and feline endocrinology and reproduction*, St Louis, 2004, Saunders.

Firth SM, Baxter RC: Cellular actions of the insulin-like growth factor binding proteins, *Endocr Rev* 23:824, 2002.

Fischetti AJ, et al.: CT and MRI evaluation of skull bones and soft tissues in six cats with presumed acromegaly versus 12 unaffected cats, *Vet Radiol Ultrasound* 53:535, 2012.

Fracassi F, et al.: Acromegaly due to a somatroph adenoma in a dog, *Domest Anim Endocrinol* 32:43, 2007.

Frank LA: Growth hormone-responsive alopecia in dogs, *J Am Vet Med Assoc* 226:1494, 2005.

Freda PU: Current concepts in the biochemical assessment of the patient with acromegaly, *Growth Horm IGF Res* 13:171, 2003.

Freda PU, et al.: Analysis of GNAS mutations in 60 growth hormone secreting pituitary tumors: correlation with clinical and pathological characteristics and surgical outcome based on highly sensitive GH and IGF-I criteria for remission, *Pituitary* 10:275, 2007.

French MB, et al.: Secretory pattern of canine growth hormone, *Am J Physiol* 252:E268, 1987.

Frystyk J: Quantification of the GH/IGF-axis components: lessons from human studies, *Domestic Animal Endocrinol* 43:186, 2012.

Frystyk J, et al.: The current status of IGF-I assays—a 2009 update, *Growth Horm IGF Res* 20:8, 2010.

Gembardt C, Loppnow H: Pathogenesis of spontaneous diabetes mellitus in the cat. II. Acidophilic adenoma of the pituitary gland and diabetes mellitus in 2 cases, *Berl Munch Tierarztl Wochenschr* 89:336, 1976.

Gevers EF, et al.: Localization and regulation of the growth hormone receptor and growth hormone-binding protein in the rat growth plate, *J Bone Miner Res* 17:1408, 2002.

Ghigo E, et al.: Diagnosis of adult GH deficiency, *Growth Horm IGF Res* 18:1, 2008.

Giustina A, Veldhuis JD: Pathophysiology of the neuroregulation of growth hormone secretion in experimental animals and the human, *Endocrine Reviews* 19:717, 1998.

Giustina A, et al.: A consensus on criteria for cure of acromegaly, *J Clin Endocrinol Metab* 95:3141, 2010.

Gobello C, et al.: Secretory patterns of growth hormone in dogs: circannual, circadian, and ultradian rhythms, *Canad J Vet Res* 66:108, 2002.

Goossens MM, et al.: Cobalt 60 irradiation of pituitary gland tumors in three cats with acromegaly, *J Am Vet Med Assoc* 213:374, 1998.

Gräf KJ, El Etreby MF: Endocrinology of reproduction in the female beagle dog and its significance in mammary gland tumorigenesis, *Acta Endocrinol Suppl (Copenh)* 222:1, 1979.

Gray MM, et al.: The *IGF1* small dog haplotype is derived from Middle Eastern grey wolves, *BMC Biology* 8:16, 2010.

Greco DS: Feline acromegaly, *Topics in Compan An Med* 27:31, 2012.

Greer KA, et al.: Connecting serum IGF-1, body size, and age in the domestic dog, *AGE* 33:475, 2011.

Gross TL, et al.: Atrophic diseases of the adnexa. In Gross TL, Ihrke PJ, Walder EJ, Affolter VK, editors: *Skin diseases of the dog and cat, clinical and histopathologic diagnosis*, Oxford, 2005, Blackwell Science Ltd.

Guler HP, et al.: Insulin-like growth factors I and II in healthy man. Estimations of half-lives and production rates, *Acta Endocrinol (Copenh)* 121:753, 1989a.

Guler HP, et al.: Small stature and insulin-like growth factors: prolonged treatment of mini-poodles with recombinant human insulin-like growth factor I, *Acta Endocrinol (Copenh)* 121:456, 1989b.

Hamann F, et al.: Pituitary function and morphology in two German shepherd dogs with congenital dwarfism, *Vet Rec* 144:644, 1999.

Hampshire J, Altszuler N: Clonidine or xylazine as provocative tests for growth hormone secretion in the dog, *Am J Vet Res* 42:1073, 1981.

Hansen I, et al.: Insulin resistance in acromegaly: defects in both hepatic and extrahepatic insulin action, *Am J Physiol* 250:269, 1986.

Hanson JM, et al.: The leukemia inhibitory factor receptor gene is not involved in the etiology of pituitary dwarfism in German shepherd dogs, *Res Vet Sci* 81:316, 2006.

Hecht S, Schwarz T: Pituitary gland. In Schwarz T, Saunders J, editors: *Veterinary computed tomography*, Wiley-Blackwell, 2011.

Heinrichs M, et al.: Immunocytochemical demonstration of growth hormone in an acidophilic adenoma of the adenohypophysis in a cat, *Vet Pathol* 26:179, 1989.

Ho KK: Consensus guidelines for the diagnosis and treatment of adults with GH deficiency II: a statement of the GH research society in association with the European Society for Pediatric Endocrinology, Lawson Wilkins Society, European Society of Endocrinology, Japan Endocrine Society, and Endocrine Society of Australia, *Eur J Endocrinol* 157:695, 2007. Kooistra H.S., personal communication, 2013.

Ida T: Variety of acyl modifications in mammalian ghrelins, *Methods Enzymol* 514:63, 2012.

Jagannathan J, et al.: Gamma knife radiosurgery to the surgical cavity following resection of brain metastasis, *J Neurosurg* 111:431, 2009.

Jallad RS, Bronstein MD: The place of medical treatment of acromegaly: current status and perspectives, *Expert Opin Pharmacother* 14:1001, 2013.

Javorsky BR, et al.: Hypothalamus and pituitary gland. In Gardner DG, Shoback D, editors: *Greenspan's basic & clinical endocrinology*, ed 9, San Francisco, 2011, McGrawHill.

Kaser-Hotz B, et al.: Radiotherapy of pituitary tumours in five cats, *J Small Anim Pract* 43:303, 2002.

Kelberman D, et al.: Genetic regulation of pituitary gland development in human and mouse, *Endocr Rev* 30:790, 2009.

Kineman RD, et al.: Steroids can modulate transdifferentiation of prolactin and growth hormone cells in bovine pituitary cultures, *Endocrinol* 130:3289, 1992.

Kley S, et al.: Evaluation of the low-dose dexamethasone suppression test and ultrasonographic measurements of the adrenal glands in cats with diabetes mellitus, *Schweiz Arch Tierheilk* 149:493, 2007.

Knottenbelt CM, Herrtage ME: Use of proligestone in the management of three German shepherd dogs with pituitary dwarfism, *J Small Anim Pract* 43:164, 2002.

Kojima M, et al.: Ghrelin is a growth-hormone-releasing acylated peptide from stomach, *Nature* 402:656, 1999.

Kokka N, et al.: Immunoassay of plasma growth hormone in cats following fasting and administration of insulin, arginine, 2-deoxyglucose and hypothalamic extract, *Endocrinol* 88:359, 1971.

Kooistra HS: Adenohypophyseal function in healthy dogs and in dogs with pituitary disease, *Thesis Universiteit Utrecht*, 2000.

Kooistra HS: Growth hormone disorders: acromegaly and pituitary dwarfism. In Ettinger SJ, Feldman EC, editors: *Textbook of veterinary internal medicine*, ed 7, St Louis, 2010, Elsevier Saunders.

Kooistra HS: Acromegaly in dogs. In Rand J, editor: *Clinical endocrinology of companion animals*, Ames, IA, 2013, Wiley-Blackwell.

Kooistra HS, et al.: Progestin-induced growth-hormone (GH) production in the treatment of dogs with congenital GH deficiency, *Domest Anim Endocrinol* 15:93, 1998.

Kooistra HS, et al.: Combined pituitary hormone deficiency in German shepherd dogs with dwarfism, *Domest Anim Endocrinol* 19:177, 2000a.

Kooistra HS, et al.: Pulsatile secretion pattern of growth hormone during the luteal phase and mid-anoestrus in beagle bitches, *J Reprod Fertil* 119:217, 2000b.

Lantinga-van Leeuwen IS, et al.: Canine mammary growth hormone gene transcription initiates at the pituitary-specific start site in the absence of Pit-1, *Mol Cell Endocrinol* 150:121, 1999.

Lantinga-van Leeuwen IS, et al.: Cloning of the canine gene encoding transcription factor Pit-1 and its exclusion as candidate gene in a canine model of pituitary dwarfism, *Mamm Genome* 11:31, 2000a.

Lantinga-van Leeuwen IS, et al.: Cloning, characterization, and physical mapping of the canine Prop-1 gene (PROP1): exclusion as a candidate for combined pituitary hormone deficiency in German Shepherd dogs, *Cytogenet Cell Genet* 88:140, 2000b.

Lee WM: Growth hormone secretion in healthy and diseased dogs, *Thesis Universiteit Utrecht*, 2004.

Lee WM, et al.: Primary hypothyroidism in dogs is associated with elevated GH release, *J Endocrinol* 168:59, 2001.

Lee WM, et al.: Pulsatile secretion pattern of growth hormone in dogs with pituitary-dependent hyperadrenocorticism, *Domest Anim Endocrinol* 24:59, 2003.

Le Roith D, et al.: The somatomedin hypothesis: 2001, *Endocrine Rev* 22:53, 2001.

Lewitt MS, et al.: Regulation of insulin-like growth factor-binding protein-3 ternary complex in feline diabetes mellitus, *J Endocrinol* 166:21, 2000.

Lim DJ, et al.: Acromegaly associated with type 2 diabetes showing normal IGF-1 levels under poorly controlled glycemia, *Endocrine J* 54:537, 2007.

Littler RM, et al.: Resolution of diabetes mellitus but not acromegaly in a cat with pituitary macroadenoma treated with hypofractionated radiation, *J Small Anim Pract* 47:392, 2006.

Liu JC, et al.: Episodic evolution of growth hormone in primates and emergence of the species specificity of human growth hormone receptor, *Mol Biol Evol* 18:945, 2001.

Lopes MBS: Growth hormone-secreting adenomas: pathology and cell biology, *Neurosurg Focus* 29:1, 2010.

Low MJ: Neuroendocrinology. In Melmed S, Polonsky KS, Larsen PR, Kronenberger HM, editors: *Williams textbook of endocrinology*, ed 12, Philadelphia, 2011, Saunders Elsevier.

Mauras N, Haymond MW: Are the metabolic effects of GH and IGF-I separable? *Growth Horm IGF Res* 15:19, 2005.

Mausberg EM, et al.: Inherited alopecia X in Pomeranians, *Dtsch Tierarztl Wochenschr* 114:129, 2007a.

Mausberg EM, et al.: Evaluation of the CTSL2 gene as a candidate gene for alopecia X in pomeranians and keeshonden, *Anim Biotechnol* 18:291, 2007b.

Mausberg EM, et al.: Exclusion of patched homolog 2 *(PTCH2)* as a candidate gene for alopecia X in pomeranians and keeshonden, *Vet Rec* 163:121, 2008.

Maxwell A, et al.: Nutritional modulation of canine insulin-like growth factors and their binding proteins, *J Endocrinol* 158:77, 1998.

Mayer MN, et al.: Outcomes of pituitary tumor irradiation in cats, *J Vet Intern Med* 20:1151, 2006.

Mayo KE, et al.: Regulation of the pituitary somatotroph cell by GHRH and its receptor, *Recent Prog Horm Res* 55:237, 2000.

McCann JP, et al.: Growth hormone, insulin, glucose, cortisol, luteinizing hormone, and diabetes in beagle bitches treated with medroxyprogesterone acetate, *Acta Endocrinol (Copenh)* 116:73, 1987.

Meij BP: Transsphenoidal hypophysectomy for treatment of pituitary-dependent hyperadrenocorticism in dogs, *Thesis Universiteit Utrecht*, 1997.

Meij BP, et al.: Assessment of a combined anterior pituitary function test in beagle dogs: rapid sequential intravenous administration of four hypothalamic releasing hormones, *Domest Anim Endocrinol* 13:161, 1996a.

Meij BP, et al.: Thyroid-stimulating hormone responses after single administration of thyrotropin-releasing hormone and combined administration of four hypothalamic releasing hormones in beagle dogs, *Domest Anim Endocrinol* 13:465, 1996b.

Meij BP, et al.: Alterations in anterior pituitary function of dogs with pituitary-dependent hyperadrenocorticism, *J Endocrinol* 154:505, 1997.

Meij BP, et al.: Somatotroph and corticotroph pituitary adenoma (double adenoma) in a cat with diabetes mellitus and hyperadrenocorticism, *J Comp Path* 130:209, 2004.

Meij BP, et al.: Hypothalamus-pituitary system. In Rijnberk A, Kooistra HS, editors: *Clinical endocrinology of dogs and cats*, ed 2, Hannover, 2010a, Schlütersche.

Meij BP, et al.: Successful treatment of acromegaly in a diabetic cat with transsphenoidal hypophysectomy, *J Feline Med Surg* 12:406, 2010b.

Meij BP, et al.: Lymphocytic hypophysitis in a dog with diabetes insipidus, *J Comp Path* 147:503, 2012a.

Meij BP, et al.: Surgical treatment of acromegaly in cats, Abstracts European Veterinary Conference Voorjaarsdagen, Amsterdam, The Netherlands, p. 232-233, 2012b.

Melmed S: Update: idiopathic adult growth hormone deficiency, *J Clin Endocrin Metab* 98:2187, 2013.

Melmed S, et al.: Guidelines for acromegaly management: an update, *J Clin Endocrinol Metab* 94:1509, 2009.

Melmed S, et al.: Pituitary physiology and diagnostic evaluation. In Melmed S, Polonsky KS, Larsen PR, Kronenberg HM, editors: *Williams textbook of endocrinology*, ed 12, Philadelphia, 2011, Saunders Elsevier.

Melmed S, Kleinberg D: Pituitary masses and tumors. In Melmed S, Polonsky KS, Larsen PR, Kronenberger HM, editors: *Williams textbook of endocrinology*, ed 12, Philadelphia, 2011, Saunders Elsevier.

Metherell LA, et al.: Genetic defects of the human somatotropic axis. In Wass JAH, Stewart PM, Amiel SA, Davies MJ, editors: *Oxford textbook of endocrinology and diabetes*, ed 2, Oxford, 2011, Oxford University Press.

Middleton DJ, et al.: Growth hormone-producing pituitary adenoma, elevated serum somatomedin C concentration and diabetes mellitus in a cat, *Can Vet J* 26:169, 1985.

Miller WH, et al.: Endocrine and metabolic diseases. In Miller WH, Griffin CE, Campbell KL, editors: *Muller and Kirk's small animal dermatology*, ed 7, Saunders, 2013.

Minniti G, et al.: Radiation techniques for acromegaly, *Radiat Oncol* 6:167, 2011.

Møller N, Jørgensen OL: Effects of growth hormone on glucose, lipid, and protein metabolism in human subjects, *Encocr Rev* 30:152, 2009.

Mol JA, et al.: Growth hormone mRNA in mammary gland tumors of dogs and cats, *J Clin Invest* 95:2028, 1995.

Mol JA, et al.: The role of progestins, insulin-like growth factor (IGF) and IGF-binding proteins in the normal and neoplastic mammary gland of the bitch: a review, *J Reprod Fertil Suppl* 51:339, 1997.

Mol JA, et al.: Mammary growth hormone and tumorigenesis—lessons from the dog, *Vet Q* 21:111, 1999.

Mol JA, Meij BP: Pituitary function. In Kaneko JJ, Harvey JW, Bruss ML, editors: *Clinical biochemistry of domestic animals*, ed 6, San Diego, 2008, Elsevier Saunders.

Morrison SA, et al.: Hypersomatotropism and insulin-resistant diabetes mellitus in a cat, *J Am Vet Med Assoc* 194:91, 1989.

Müller-Peddinghaus R, et al.: Hypophysärer Zwergwuchs beim Deutschen Schäferhund, *Vet Pathol* 17:406, 1980.

Murai A, et al.: GH-producing mammary tumors in two dogs with acromegaly, *J Vet Med Sci* 74:771, 2012.

Nass R, et al.: The role of ghrelin in GH secretion and GH disorders, *Mol Cell Endocrinol* 340:10, 2011.

Nicholas F: Pituitary dwarfism in German Shepherd dogs: a genetic analysis of some Australian data, *J Small Anim Pract* 19:167, 1978.

Niessen S: Feline acromegaly, an essential differential diagnosis for the difficult diabetic, *J Feline Med Surg* 12:15, 2010.

Niessen SJM, et al.: Feline acromegaly: an underdiagnosed endocrinopathy? *J Vet Intern Med* 21:899, 2007a.

Niessen SJM, et al.: Validation and application of a radioimmunoassay for ovine growth hormone in the diagnosis of acromegaly in cats, *Vet Rec* 160:902, 2007b.

Niessen SJM, et al.: Hypersomatotropism, acromegaly, and hyperadrenocorticism and feline diabetes mellitus, *Vet Clin Small Anim* 43:319, 2013a.

Niessen SJM, et al.: Pasireotide (som230) opens doors to medical management of feline hypersomatotropism, *J Vet Intern Med* 27:685, 2013b. abstract.

Norman EJ, Mooney CT: Diagnosis and management of diabetes mellitus in five cats with somatotrophic abnormalities, *J Feline Med Surg* 1:183, 2000.

Norman EJ, et al.: Pregnancy-related diabetes mellitus in two dogs, *New Zealand Vet J* 54:360, 2006.

Owen LN, Briggs MH: Contraceptive steroid toxicology in the Beagle dog and its relevance to human carcinogenicity, *Curr Med Res Opin* 4:309, 1976.

Petersenn S, et al.: Long-term efficacy and safety of subcutaneous pasireotide in acromegaly: results from an open-ended-multicenter, Phase II extension study, *Pituitary* 17:132, 2014.

Peterson ME, Altszuler N: Suppression of growth hormone secretion in spontaneous canine hyperadrenocorticism and its reversal after treatment, *Am J Vet Res* 42:1881, 1981.

Peterson ME: Effects of megestrol acetate on glucose tolerance and growth hormone secretion in the cat, *Res Vet Sci* 42:354, 1987.

Peterson ME: Acromegaly in cats: are we only diagnosing the tip of the iceberg? *J Vet Intern Med (editorial)* 21:889, 2007.

Peterson ME, et al.: Acromegaly in 14 cats, *J Vet Intern Med* 4:192, 1990.

Posch B, et al.: Magnetic resonance imaging findings in 15 acromegalic cats, *Vet Radiol Ultrasound* 52:422, 2011.

Queiroga FL, et al.: Crosstalk between GH/IGF-I axis and steroid hormones (progesterone, 17beta-estradiol) in canine mammary tumours, *J Steroid Biochem Mol Biol* 110:76, 2008.

Queiroga FL, et al.: Serum and intratumoural GH and IGF-I concentrations: prognostic factors in the outcome of canine mammary cancer, *Res Vet Sci* 89:396, 2010.

Randolph JF, et al.: Delayed growth in two German Shepherd dog littermates with normal serum concentrations of growth hormone, thyroxine, and cortisol, *J Am Vet Med Assoc* 196:77, 1990.

Rao NAS, et al.: Gene expression profiles of progestin-induced canine mammary hyperplasia and spontaneous mammary tumors, *J Physiol Pharmacol* (Suppl 1)73, 2009.

Rathke M: Über die Entstehung der Glandula pituitaria, Archiv für Anatomie, Physiologie und wissenschaftliche, *Medicin, Berlin,* S482–485, 1838.

Regnier A, Garnier F: Growth hormone responses to growth hormone, *Vet Sci* 58:169, 1995.

Reichlin S: Medical progress—somatostatin, *N Engl J Med* 309:1495, 1983.

Resmini E, et al.: Secondary diabetes associated with principal endocrinopathies: the impact of new treatment modalities, *Acta Diabetol* 46:85, 2009.

Reusch CE: Feline diabetes mellitus. In Ettinger SJ, Feldman EC, editors: *Textbook of veterinary internal medicine*, ed 7, St Louis, 2010, Saunders Elsevier.

Reusch CE, et al.: Alteration in the growth hormone-insulin-like growth factor axis in cats with diabetes mellitus, *J Vet Intern Med* 15:297, 2001.

Reusch CE, et al.: Measurements of growth hormone and insulin-like growth factor 1 in cats with diabetes mellitus, *Vet Rec* 158:195, 2006.

Ribeiro-Oliveira A, Barkan A: The changing face of acromegaly—advances in diagnosis and treatment, *Nat Rev Endocrinol* 8:605, 2012.

Rijnberk A: Growth hormone: its clinical relevance, *Vet Q* 17:17, 1995.

Rijnberk A, Kooistra HS: Protocols for function tests. In Rijnberk A, Kooistra HS, editors: *Clinical endocrinology of dogs and cats: an illustrated text*, ed 2, Hannover, 2010, Schlütersche.

Rijnberk A, Mol JA: Progestin-induced hypersecretion of growth hormone: an introductory review, *J Reprod Fertil Suppl* 51:335, 1997.

Rijnberk A, et al.: Acromegaly associated with transient overproduction of growth hormone in a dog, *J Am Vet Med Assoc* 177:534, 1980.

Rijnberk A, et al.: Disturbed release of growth hormone in mature dogs: a comparison with congenital growth hormone deficiency, *Vet Rec* 133:542, 1993.

Rijnberk A, et al.: Endocrine diseases in dogs and cats: similarities and differences with endocrine diseases in humans, *Growth Horm IGF Res* 13:S158, 2003.

Rinderknecht E, Humbel RE: The amino acid sequence of human insulin-like growth factor I and its structural homology with pro-insulin, *J Biol Chem* 253:2769, 1978a.

Rinderknecht E, Humbel RE: Primary structure of human insulin-like growth factor II, *FEBS Lett* 89:283, 1978b.

Roth JA, et al.: Thymic abnormalities and growth hormone deficiency in dogs, *Am J Vet Res* 41:1256, 1980.

Rutteman GR, et al.: Medroxy-progesterone acetate administration to ovariohyster-ectomized, oestradiol-primed beagle bitches, *Acta Endocrinol (Copenh)* 114:275, 1987.

Salmon WD, Daughaday WH: A hormonally controlled serum factor which stimulates sulfate incorporation by cartilage in vitro, *J Lab Clin Med* 49:825, 1957.

Sato T, et al.: Structure, regulation and function of ghrelin, *J Biochem* 151:119, 2012.

Savage JJ, et al.: Transcriptional control during mammalian anterior pituitary development, *Gene* 319:1, 2003.

Savage MO, et al.: Genetic defects in the growth hormone-IGF-I axis causing growth hormone insensitivity and impaired linear growth, *Front Endocrinol* 2:95, 2011.

Schäfer S, et al.: *Evaluation of insulin-like growth factor (IGF-1), T4, feline pancreatic lipase immunoreactivity (FPLI) and urinary corticoid creatinine ratio (UCCR) in cats with diabetes mellitus in Switzerland and the Netherlands*, Liverpool, UK, 2013, abstr ECVIM. 12.-14.09.

Schmeitzel LP, Lothrop CD: Hormonal abnor-malities in Pomeranians with normal coat and in Pomeranians with growth hormone-responsive dermatosis, *J Am Vet Med Assoc* 197:1333, 1990.

Scott DW, Concannon PW: Gross and micro-scopic changes in the skin of dogs with progestagen-induced acromegaly and el-evated growth hormone levels, *J Am Anim Hosp Assoc* 19:524, 1983.

Scott DW, Walton DK: Hyposomatotropism in the mature dog: a discussion of 22 cases, *J Am Anim Hosp Assoc* 22:467, 1986.

Sellon RK, et al.: Linear-accelerat or-based modified radiosurgical treatment of pituitary tumors in cats: 11 cases (1997-2008), *J Vet Intern Med* 23:1038, 2009.

Selman PJ, et al.: Progestins and growth hor-mone excess in the dog, *Acta Endocrinol* 125:42, 1991.

Selman PJ, et al.: Progestin-induced growth hormone excess in the dog originates in the mammary gland, *Endocrinol* 134:287, 1994a.

Selman PJ, et al.: Progestin treatment in the dog. I. Effects on growth hormone, insulin-like growth factor I and glucose homeosta-sis, *Europ J Endocrinol* 131:413, 1994b.

Selman PJ, et al.: Effects of progestin adminis-tration on the hypothalamic-pituitary-adrenal axis and glucose homeostasis in dogs, *J Reprod Fertil Suppl* 51:345, 1997.

Sharman M, et al.: Concurrent somatotroph and plurihormonal pituitary adenomas in a cat, *J Feline Med Surg* 15:945, 2013.

Sjaastad OV, et al.: The endocrine system. In Sjaastad OV, Sand O, Hove K, editors: *Physiology of domestic animals*, Oslo, 2010, Scandinavian Veterinary Press.

Slingerland LI, et al.: Growth hormone excess and the effect of octreotide in cats with diabetes mellitus, *Domest Anim Endocri-nol* 35:352, 2008.

Sloan JM, Oliver IM: Progestogen-induced dia-betes in the dog, *Diabetes* 24:337, 1975.

Starkey SR, et al.: Investigation of serum IGF-I levels amongst diabetic and non-diabetic cats, *J Feline Med Surg* 6:149, 2004.

Stratikopoulos E, et al.: The hormonal action of IGF1 in postnatal mouse growth, *PNAS* 105:19378, 2008.

Styne D: Growth. In Gardner DG and Shoback D, editors: Greenspan's basic & clinical endocrinology, ed 9, San Francisco, 2011.

Sutter NB, et al.: A single IGF1 allele is a major determinant of small size in dogs, *Science* 316:112, 2007.

Tschuor F, et al.: Evaluation of four methods used to measure plasma insulin-like growth factor 1 concentrations in healthy cats and cats with diabetes mellitus and other diseases, *Am J Vet Res* 73:1925, 2012.

van Garderen E, et al.: Expression of growth hormone in canine mammary tissue and mammary tumors, evidence for a potential autocrine/paracrine stimulatory loop, *Am J Pathol* 150:1037, 1997.

van Garderen E, et al.: Expression and molecu-lar characterization of the growth hormone receptor in canine mammary tissue and mammary tumors, *Endocrinol* 140:5907, 1999.

Van Herpen H, et al.: Production of antibodies to biosynthetic human growth hormone in the dog, *Vet Rec* 134:171, 1994.

Van Keulen LJM, et al.: Diabetes mellitus in a dog with a growth hormone-producing aci-dophilic adenoma of the adenohypophysis, *Vet Pathol* 33:451, 1996.

Van Oost BA, et al.: Exclusion of the lim home-odomain gene LHX4 as a candidate gene for pituitary dwarfism in German shepherd dogs, *Mol Cell Endocrinol* 197:57, 2002.

Vidal S, et al.: Transdifferentiation of somato-trophs to thyrotrophs in the pituitary of patients with protracted primary hypothy-roidism, *Virchows Arch* 436:43, 2000.

Vijayakumar A, et al.: Biological effects of growth hormone on carbohydrate and lipid metabolism, *Growth Horm IGF Res* 20:1, 2010.

Villalobos C, et al.: Anterior pituitary thyro-tropes are multifunctional cells, *Am J Physiol Endocrinol Metab* 287:E1166, 2004.

Voorbij MWY, Kooistra HS: Pituitary dwarfism in German Shepherd dogs, *JVCS* 2:4, 2009.

Voorbij AM, et al.: A contracted DNA repeat in LHX3 intron 5 is associated with aberrant splicing and pituitary dwarfism in German Shepherd dogs, *PLoS One* 6(11):1, 2011.

Wallis M: Mammalian genome projects reveal new growth hormone (GH) sequences. Characterization of the GH-encoding genes of armadillo (Dasypus novemcinctus), hedgehog (Erinaceus europaeus), bat (Myotis lucifugus), hyrax (Procavia capen-sis), shrew (Sorex araneus), ground squirrel (Spermophilus tridecemlineatus), elephant (Loxodonta africana), cat (Felis catus) and opossum (Monodelphis domestica), *Gen Comp Endocrinol* 155:271, 2008.

Warren WC, et al.: Cloning of the cDNAs coding for cat growth hormone and prolactin, *Gene* 168:247, 1996.

Wass JAH, et al.: Acromegaly. In Wass JAH, Stewart PM, Amiel SA, Davies MC, editors: *Oxford textbook of endocrinology and diabetes*, ed 2, Oxford, 2011, Oxford University Press.

Watson ADJ, et al.: Effect of somatostatin analogue SMS 201-995 and antiproges-tin agent RU 486 in canine acromegaly. In Rijnberk A, van Wimersma Greidanus TB, editors: *Front horm res, comparative pathophysiology of regulatory peptides*, ed 17, Basel, 1987, Karger.

Wayne RK, vonHoldt BM: Evolutionary genom-ics of dog domestication, *Mamm Genome* 23:3, 2012.

Wolfesberger B, et al.: Sudden death in a dog with lymphoplasmacytic hypophysitis, *J Comp Path* 145:231, 2011.

Xu J, Messina JL: Crosstalk between growth hormone and insulin signaling, *Vitam Horm* 80:125, 2009.

Yang H, et al.: Effects of streptozotocin-induced diabetes mellitus on growth and hepatic insulin-like growth factor I gene expression in the rat, *Metabol* 39:295, 1990.

Yokoyama M, et al.: Relationship between growth and plasma concentrations of ghrelin and growth hormone in juvenile beagle dogs, *J Vet Med Sci* 67:1189, 2005.

Zangger I, et al.: Insulin-like growth factor I and II in 14 animal species and man as determined by three radioligand assays and two bioassays, *Acta Endocrinol (Co-penh)* 114:107, 1987.

Zapf J, et al.: Intravenously injected insulin-like growth factor (IGF) I/IGF binding protein-3 complex exerts insulin-like effects in hy-pophysectomized, but not in normal rats, *J Clin Invest* 95:179, 1995.

Zezulak KM, Green H: The generation of insulin-like growth factor-I—sensitive cells by growth hormone action, *Science* 233:551, 1986.

Zimmer C, et al.: Ultrasonographic examination of the adrenal gland and evaluation of the hypophyseal-adrenal axis in 20 cats, *J Small Anim Pract* 41:156, 2000.

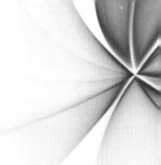

CHAPTER 3 | Hypothyroidism

J. Catharine Scott-Moncrieff

CHAPTER CONTENTS

ANATOMY AND PHYSIOLOGY OF THE THYROID GLAND

The thyroid gland was first described in detail by Vesalius in the sixteenth century. Thomas Wharton (1614-1673) named the gland from the Greek word *thyreos,* or shield, based on its physical appearance. One of the first described thyroid disorders was an association between iodine deficiency and enlargement of the thyroid (goiter), which was initially suspected in the 1500s to be a possible cause of cretinism. This description also represents the

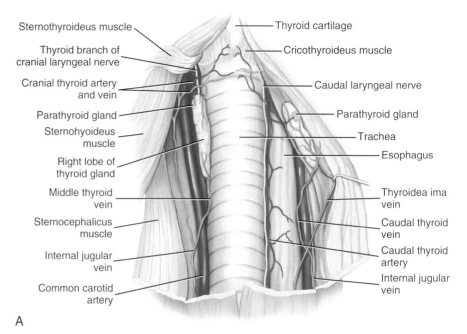

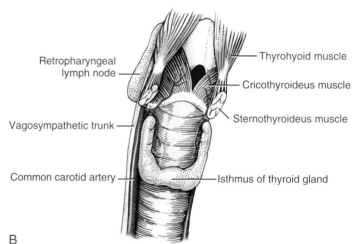

FIGURE 3-1 A and **B,** Thyroid anatomy of the dog and cat. (From Hullinger RL: The endocrine system. In Evans HE, de Lahunta A, editors: *Miller's anatomy of the dog,* ed 4, St Louis, 2013, Elsevier.)

first mention of thyroid gland enlargement. Endemic cretinism in the region around Salzburg, Austria, was described by the Swiss-German physician Paracelsus (1493-1541).

The thyroid gland develops in the embryo in close association with the gastrointestinal tract, which explains why both the gastric and salivary glands concentrate iodide in their secretions. In dogs and cats the thyroid gland is comprised of two lobes in the mid-cervical region that lie to either side of the trachea. The lobes are elongated dark red structures adjacent to the right and left lateral surfaces of the proximal trachea (Fig. 3-1) and are not normally palpable. The thyroid gland has an extensive vascular supply primarily from the cranial and caudal thyroid arteries. The functional unit of the thyroid gland is the follicle, a sphere of cells with a lumen containing a clear proteinaceous colloid (Fig. 3-2). The colloid contains primarily thyroglobulin (Tg), a large glycoprotein dimer that serves as a reservoir for thyroid hormone. Parafollicular cells (C cells) lie in the interstitium between the follicles and synthesize and secrete calcitonin.

Thyroid Hormone Synthesis

Thyroxine (T_4) and 3,5,3′-triiodothyronine (T_3) are iodine–containing amino acids. Thyroid hormone synthesis requires iodine and is dependent upon ingestion of adequate iodide from the diet. Iodide is actively transported from the extracellular fluid into the thyroid follicular cell by the sodium-iodine symporter (NIS), where it is rapidly oxidized by thyroid peroxidase (TPO) into a reactive intermediate (Fig. 3-3). At the apical membrane, iodine is incorporated into the tyrosine residues of Tg (Salvatore et al, 2011). TPO also catalyzes the coupling of the non-biologically active iodinated tyrosine residues (monoiodotyrosine [MIT], and diiodotyrosine [DIT]) to form the biologically active iodothyronines—T_4 and T_3 (Fig. 3-4). These iodination reactions are referred to as *organification* and occur within Tg rather than on the free amino acids.

Tg is stored extracellularly in the follicular lumen. As a prerequisite for thyroid hormone secretion into the blood, Tg must first reenter the thyroid cell and undergo proteolysis. Pseudopods from the apical cell surface extend into the colloid in the follicular lumen, and large colloid droplets enter the cytoplasm by endocytosis (Salvatore et al, 2011). Each colloid droplet is enclosed in a membrane derived from the apical cell border. Electron-dense lysosomes then fuse with the colloid droplets to produce phagolysosomes. These phagolysosomes migrate toward the basal aspect of the cell, while lysosomal proteases hydrolyze Tg. T_4 and, to a much lesser degree, T_3 liberated from Tg by the proteolytic process pass from the phagolysosome into the

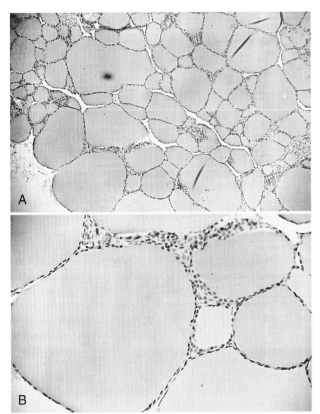

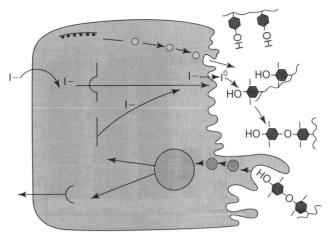

FIGURE 3-3 Thyroid hormone synthesis. Thyroglobulin (Tg) is synthesized within thyroid follicular cells and secreted into the colloid. Iodide is oxidized and bound to tyrosine residues on the Tg molecule by thyroid peroxidase (TPO). Iodinated tyrosine residues (monoiodotyrosine [MIT] and diiodotyrosine [DIT]) within the Tg molecule then undergo oxidative condensation to form the iodothyronines (T_3 and T_4), which remain bound to Tg until secreted. Tg is ingested by endocytosis from the colloid; the peptide bonds between the iodinated residues and the Tg are hydrolyzed; and MIT, DIT, T_4, and T_3 are released into the cytoplasm. MIT and DIT are de-iodinated and the iodine is recycled, whereas T_4 and T_3 are released into the bloodstream. (Modified from Mountcastle VB: *Medical physiology*, ed 14, vol 2, St Louis, 1980, Mosby.)

FIGURE 3-2 A and **B**, Histologic section of a thyroid gland from a healthy dog, illustrating variable-sized follicles, each lined by follicular epithelial cells with a lumen containing colloid. The follicle is surrounded by a basement membrane which separates the follicular cells from a capillary bed. The wall of the follicle is a single layer of follicular epithelial cells, which are cuboidal when quiescent and columnar when active. (**A**, H&E ×40; **B**, H&E ×160.)

blood by diffusion. Most of the liberated iodotyrosines (MIT, DIT) are de-iodinated, releasing iodide, which can be reused for Tg iodination or diffuse out into the circulation. A small quantity of intact Tg also enters the circulation. This leakage is increased when the thyroid cells are damaged, such as in lymphocytic thyroiditis.

Regulation of Thyroid Function

Thyroid hormone synthesis and secretion are regulated by extrathyroidal (thyrotropin) and intrathyroidal (autoregulatory) mechanisms. Thyroid-stimulating hormone (also known as thyrotropin; TSH) increases both synthesis and secretion of T_4 and T_3 and is the major modulator of thyroid hormone concentration (Fig. 3-5). TSH secretion by the pituitary is modulated by thyroid hormone in a negative feedback regulatory mechanism. At the pituitary, it is primarily T_3, produced locally by the monodeiodination of T_4 that inhibits TSH secretion (Salvatore et al, 2011). TSH secretion from the pituitary gland is modulated by thyrotropin-releasing hormone (TRH) from the hypothalamus (see Fig. 3-4). Hypothalamic production and release of TRH are controlled by poorly understood neural pathways from higher brain centers.

Autoregulatory intrathyroidal mechanisms also regulate iodide uptake and thyroid hormone synthesis. Examples of autoregulatory mechanisms include the Wolff-Chaikoff block (decrease in Tg iodination and thyroid hormone synthesis with increasing iodide intake), intrathyroidal alterations in thyroid sensitivity to TSH stimulation, and increased ratio of T_3 to T_4 secretion by the thyroid gland during periods of iodide insufficiency.

Thyroid Hormones in Plasma

T_4 is the major secretory product of the normal thyroid gland. Thyroid hormones in plasma are highly protein bound with T_4 more highly bound than T_3. Less than 1% of T_4 and T_3 circulate in the unbound "free" state. In the dog, the thyroid binding proteins are thyroxine-binding globulin (TBG), thyroxine-binding prealbumin (TBPA), albumin, and certain plasma lipoproteins. TBG is the major binding protein in the dog but is absent in the cat. The lower concentration of TBG and differences in structure between species may explain the low serum T_4 levels and rapid T_4 metabolism seen in dogs compared to humans. Only free or unbound thyroid hormones enter cells to produce a biologic effect or regulate pituitary TSH secretion. Protein-bound thyroid hormones serve as a large reservoir that is slowly drawn upon as the free hormone dissociates from the binding proteins and enters the cells.

Thyroid hormone entry into cells is mediated by transporter proteins. T_3 enters cells more rapidly, has a more rapid onset of action, and is three to five times more potent than T_4. Thyroid hormones bind to receptors in the nuclei; the hormone receptor complex then binds to DNA and influences the expression of many genes coding for regulatory enzymes. Thyroid hormone is also believed to have some non-genomic effects mediated by receptors in the plasma membrane and the cytoplasm (Yen and Brent, 2013).

Physiologic Functions of Thyroid Hormones

Thyroid hormones regulate many metabolic processes, influencing the concentration and activity of numerous enzymes; the metabolism of substrates, vitamins, and minerals; the secretion and degradation rates of virtually all other hormones; and the response of their target tissues to those hormones. Thyroid hormones are critically important in fetal development, particularly of the neural and skeletal systems. Thyroid hormones stimulate calorigenesis,

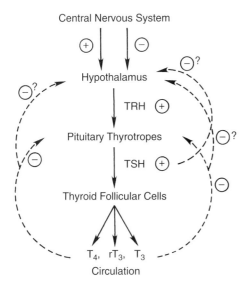

FIGURE 3-4 Structure of the thyroid hormones and their precursors.

FIGURE 3-5 Regulation of thyroid hormone concentration by the hypothalamic-pituitary-thyroid axis. Thyroid hormone concentrations are controlled by the hypothalamic-pituitary-thyroid axis, which operates as a negative feedback loop. Thyrotropin *(TSH)* causes synthesis and release of thyroxine *(T$_4$)* and lesser amounts of 3,5,3'-triiodothyronine *(T$_3$)* from the thyroid gland. Intracellular T$_3$, derived from de-iodination of T$_4$ within the pituitary gland, causes decreased TSH synthesis and secretion and is the main determinant of TSH concentration. Thyrotropin-releasing hormone *(TRH)*, secreted by the hypothalamus, modulates TSH release from the pituitary gland. Increased thyroid hormone concentrations are also believed to decrease TRH synthesis and secretion. Hormones that inhibit TSH secretion include dopamine, somatostatin, serotonin, and glucocorticoids. TRH, prostaglandins, and alpha-adrenergic agonists increase TSH secretion. *rT$_3$,* Reverse 3,3',5'-triiodothyronine; +, stimulation; –, inhibition.

protein and enzyme synthesis, and virtually all aspects of carbohydrate and lipid metabolism, including synthesis, mobilization, and degradation (Yen and Brent, 2013). Furthermore, thyroid hormones have marked chronotropic and inotropic effects on the heart; increase the number and affinity of beta-adrenergic receptors; enhance the response to catecholamines; are necessary for normal hypoxic and hypercapnic drive to the respiratory centers; stimulate erythropoiesis; and stimulate bone turnover, increasing

both formation and resorption of bone (Greenspan, 2001). In essence, no tissue or organ system escapes the adverse effects of thyroid hormone excess or insufficiency.

Thyroid Hormone Metabolism

The major pathway of T$_4$ metabolism is the progressive deiodination of the molecule. The initial deiodination of T$_4$ may occur in the outer ring, producing T$_3$, or in the inner ring, producing reverse T$_3$ (rT$_3$; see Fig. 3-4). Because conversion of T$_4$ to T$_3$ increases biologic activity, whereas conversion of T$_4$ to rT$_3$ has the opposite effect, the conversion of T$_4$ to T$_3$ or rT$_3$ by outer or inner ring iodothyronine deiodinase is a pivotal regulatory step in determining thyroid hormone biologic activity. Three unique deiodinases (D1, D2, and D3) with different tissue distributions, and different affinity for inner or outer ring deiodination, play a major regulatory role in thyroid hormone homeostasis by influencing the concentration of intracellular T$_3$. The integration of plasma T$_3$ and local deiodinase produced T$_3$ together with local inactivation of thyroid hormone, ultimately determines nuclear T$_3$ concentration and the thyroid status of the cell (Bianco and Kim, 2013). In dogs approximately 40% to 60% of T$_3$ is believed to be derived from outer ring monodeiodination of T$_4$ in peripheral tissues. Conjugation of thyroid hormone to soluble glucuronides and sulfates with subsequent excretion in the bile and urine represents another major metabolic pathway for thyroid hormone.

CANINE HYPOTHYROIDISM

 ## CLASSIFICATION

Canine hypothyroidism may occur due to thyroid gland destruction, decreased stimulation by TSH from the pituitary gland, or failure in any of the steps of thyroid hormone synthesis. Hypothyroidism is the most common thyroid disorder in dogs and may be acquired or congenital. Hypothyroidism is classified as primary if it is due to an abnormality at the level of the thyroid gland, secondary if it is due to decreased TSH secretion, and tertiary if it is due to TRH deficiency. Primary hypothyroidism is the most

BOX 3-1   Potential Causes of Hypothyroidism in the Dog

Primary Hypothyroidism
Lymphocytic thyroiditis*
Idiopathic atrophy*
Neoplastic destruction*
Iodine deficiency*
Goitrogen ingestion
Iatrogenic*
    Surgical removal*
    Anti-thyroid medications/potentiated sulfonamides*
    Radioactive iodine treatment*

Congenital*
Thyroid gland dysgenesis*
Dyshormonogenesis*
Defective thyroid hormone transporters/receptors
Iodine deficiency
Maternal antibodies
Maternal medications

Secondary Hypothyroidism
Pituitary malformation*
Pituitary cyst
    Pituitary hypoplasia
Pituitary destruction*
    Neoplasia
Defective TSH molecule
Defective TSH-follicular cell receptor interaction
Iatrogenic*
    Drug therapy, most notably glucocorticoids
    Radiation therapy
    Hypophysectomy

Tertiary Hypothyroidism
Congenital hypothalamic malformation
Acquired destruction of hypothalamus
    Neoplasia*
    Hemorrhage
    Abscess
    Granuloma
    Inflammation
Deficient/defective TRH molecule
Defective TRH-thyrotroph receptor interaction

TRH, Thyrotropin-releasing hormone; *TSH,* thyroid-stimulating hormone (also known as thyrotropin).
* Established etiology in the dog

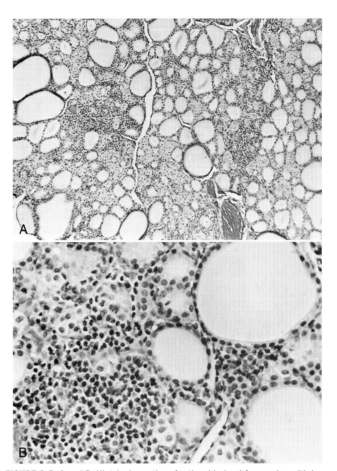

FIGURE 3-6 A and **B,** Histologic section of a thyroid gland from a dog with lymphocytic thyroiditis and hypothyroidism. Note the mononuclear cell infiltration, disruption of the normal architecture, and loss of colloid-containing follicles. (**A,** H&E ×63; **B,** H&E ×250.)

include iodine deficiency, goitrogen ingestion, congenital hypothyroidism, thyroid gland destruction by neoplasia, drug therapy, surgical thyroidectomy, and treatment with radioactive iodine.

Lymphocytic Thyroiditis

Lymphocytic thyroiditis is characterized histologically by diffuse infiltration of lymphocytes, plasma cells, and macrophages into the thyroid gland, resulting in progressive destruction of follicles and secondary fibrosis (Gosselin et al, 1981b; Fig. 3-6). Destruction of the thyroid gland is progressive, and clinical signs do not become evident until at least 80% of the gland has been destroyed. Studies suggest that the onset of clinical signs and development of decreased serum thyroid hormone and increased serum TSH concentrations occurs over a prolonged time period of 1 to 3 years, suggesting a slowly progressive destructive process (Nachreiner et al, 2002; Graham et al, 2007). Graham, et al. (2007) have proposed four stages in the development of lymphocytic thyroiditis in dogs. The first stage (subclinical thyroiditis) is characterized by focal lymphocytic thyroid gland infiltration and positive Tg and thyroid hormone autoantibody tests. In stage 2 (antibody positive subclinical hypothyroidism) loss of greater than 60% to 70% of thyroid mass results in a compensatory increase in TSH, which stimulates the thyroid gland to maintain normal T_4 concentrations. In stage 3 (antibody positive overt hypothyroidism) most functional thyroid tissue is destroyed, and decreased serum thyroid hormone concentrations and increased TSH concentration are present (Table 3-1). Stage 4 (noninflammatory atrophic

common cause of hypothyroidism in dogs. Secondary hypothyroidism due to impaired secretion of TSH is rare in dogs, and tertiary hypothyroidism is presumed to be extremely rare.

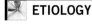 **ETIOLOGY**

Primary Hypothyroidism

Acquired primary hypothyroidism is the most common cause of naturally occurring thyroid failure in the adult dog, accounting for more than 95% of cases. Two histologic forms of primary hypothyroidism are recognized in dogs; lymphocytic thyroiditis and idiopathic atrophy (Box 3-1). It is likely that some cases of idiopathic atrophy are the end result of severe lymphocytic thyroiditis. Other much more rare causes of primary hypothyroidism

TABLE 3-1   PROPOSED FUNCTIONAL STAGES OF LYMPHOCYTIC THYROIDITIS IN DOGS

STAGE OF THYROIDITIS	CLINICAL SIGNS OF HYPOTHYROIDISM	SERUM THYROXINE AND FREE THYROXINE	SERUM THYROTROPIN	ANTI-THYROGLOBULIN ANTIBODY
I: Subclinical thyroiditis	Not present	Normal	Normal	Positive
II: Subclinical hypothyroidism	Not present	Normal	Increased	Positive
III: Overt hypothyroidism	Present	Decreased	Increased	Positive
IV: Noninflammatory atrophic hypothyroidism	Present	Decreased	Increased	Negative

Adapted from Graham PA, et al.: Lymphocytic thyroiditis, *Vet Clin North Am Small Anim Pract* 37(4):617, 2007.

hypothyroidism) is characterized by replacement of thyroid tissue by fibrous and adipose tissue and disappearance of inflammatory cells and circulating antibodies. What proportion of cases of antibody negative idiopathic thyroid atrophy is actually due to stage 4 thyroiditis has not been determined. Analysis of age distributions of dogs with laboratory test results (i.e., Tg antibody, T_4, and TSH) consistent with the different stages or classifications of lymphocytic thyroiditis suggests that the age of peak prevalence progresses by 1 to 2 years through each of the classifications (Graham et al, 2001; Fig. 3-8). Studies also suggest that there are breed-specific differences in the progression rate and likelihood of progression of thyroiditis.

Lymphocytic thyroiditis is an immune-mediated disorder, and both humoral and cell mediated immunity play a role in pathogenesis. The major thyroid antigens that initiate an immune response in the thyroid gland are Tg and TPO. Tg is the main antigen in colloid, and anti-thyroglobulin antibodies (ATAs) are a sensitive indicator of canine thyroiditis (Gosselin et al, 1980; Nachreiner et al, 1998). TPO is a membrane bound glycosylated hemoprotein that catalyzes the biosynthesis of thyroid hormones. Despite being the most prevalent anti-thyroid antibody in humans with Hashimoto thyroiditis, anti-TPO antibodies are found in only 17% of dogs with thyroiditis (Skopek et al, 2006). Evidence for humoral mechanisms in the pathogenesis of canine thyroiditis is the presence of circulating autoantibodies to thyroid antigens; identification by electron microscopy of thickened basement membranes containing electron-dense deposits that are believed to be antigen-antibody complexes in thyroid follicles; and the induction of lesions similar to lymphocytic thyroiditis in dogs following the intrathyroidal injection of Tg antibodies (Gosselin et al, 1980; 1981a; 1981b; 1981c; Gaschen et al, 1993). Antibody binding to the follicular cell, colloid, or Tg antigens is believed to activate the complement cascade, antibody-dependent cell-mediated cytotoxicity, or both, causing follicular cell destruction. In humans anti-TPO antibodies but not ATAs have been demonstrated to fix complement. The cell-mediated immune system may also play an important, and possibly primary, role in the development and perpetuation of lymphocytic thyroiditis. Canine peripheral blood mononuclear cells in hypothyroid dogs that are positive for ATAs show proliferation in response to canine Tg. There was a positive correlation between the number of CD4+ cells and the concentration of Tg in the cultures, suggesting that a loss of self-tolerance of CD4 + cells is important in the pathogenesis of canine thyroiditis (Tani et al, 2005).

The initiating factors involved in the development of lymphocytic thyroiditis are poorly understood. Genetics undoubtedly plays a major role, especially given the increased incidence of this disorder in certain breeds. Lymphocytic thyroiditis is an inherited disorder in colony-raised Beagles, with a polygenic mode of inheritance, and

was identified as an autosomal-recessive trait in a family of Borzoi dogs (Conaway et al, 1985a). An increased prevalence of circulating thyroid hormone autoantibodies has also been found in certain breeds, and the progression rate is different for different breeds (Nachreiner et al, 2002; Graham et al, 2007; Ferm et al, 2009; Table 3-2). A strong association between thyroiditis and certain major histocompatibility complex DLA class II haplotypes has been demonstrated in Doberman Pinchers, English Setters, Rhodesian Ridgebacks, and Giant Schnauzers (Kennedy et al, 2006a; 2006b; Wilbe et al, 2010). Environmental risk factors for canine thyroiditis have not been well defined. Infection-induced damage to the thyroid gland, causing release of antigens into the circulation and their subsequent exposure to the host's immune system, or antigenic mimicry of thyroid antigens by viral or bacterial agents could initiate the immune-mediated inflammatory process. The proportion of euthyroid dogs with evidence of thyroiditis is highest in the summer and lowest in the winter months (Graham et al, 2007). The significance of this finding is unclear, but it could indicate a relationship between infection and thyroiditis. Vaccine administration has also been hypothesized to be a contributing factor for development of lymphocytic thyroiditis. A significant increase in ATAs was documented in Beagles after repeated vaccination beginning at 8 weeks of age (Scott-Moncrieff et al, 2002; 2006); however further research did not document an increased prevalence of thyroiditis in the vaccinated beagles at necropsy after 5½ years of follow-up.

Lymphocytic Thyroiditis and Polyglandular Autoimmune Syndromes

Because autoimmune mechanisms play an important role in the pathogenesis of lymphocytic thyroiditis, it is not surprising that lymphocytic thyroiditis may sometimes occur together with other immune-mediated endocrine deficiency syndromes. Combinations of immune-mediated endocrine deficiency disorders such as hypothyroidism and diabetes mellitus, and hypothyroidism and hypoadrenocorticism have been documented in dogs (Hargis et al, 1981; Haines and Penhale, 1985; Bowen et al, 1986; Ford et al, 1993; Kooistra et al, 1995; Greco, 2000; Blois et al, 2011). These combined disorders are rare, occurring in less than 2% of dogs with immune-mediated endocrinopathies (Blois et al, 2011). In a retrospective study of 225 dogs with hypoadrenocorticism, 4% of the dogs also had hypothyroidism, 0.5% had concurrent diabetes mellitus, and one dog had concurrent hypothyroidism, diabetes mellitus, and hyperparathyroidism (Peterson et al, 1996). In a retrospective study of multiple endocrine disease in 35 dogs, the most common combination of immune-mediated endocrine disorders were hypothyroidism and diabetes mellitus in 10 dogs and hypothyroidism and hypoadrenocorticism in 8 dogs (Blois et al, 2011). Concurrent thyroiditis and orchitis have been documented in a colony of related Beagles and both disorders are highly heritable (Fritz et al, 1976). In humans, two polyglandular

TABLE 3-2	NINETEEN BREEDS WITH THE HIGHEST AND TWENTY BREEDS WITH THE LOWEST PREVALENCE OF THYROGLOBULIN ANTIBODY IN 140,821 SERUM SAMPLES SUBMITTED FOR INVESTIGATION OF THYROID DISEASE*

NAME	TOTAL SERA	THYROGLOBULIN AUTOANTIBODY– POSITIVE	PREVALENCE
English Setter	585	184	31%
Old English Sheepdog	368	86	23%
Boxer	2642	496	19%
Giant Schnauzer	263	49	19%
American Pit Bull Terrier	345	64	19%
Beagle	2452	449	18%
Dalmatian	1372	246	18%
German Wirehaired Pointer	112	20	18%
Maltese Dog	594	105	18%
Rhodesian Ridgeback	626	107	17%
Siberian Husky	1129	164	15%
American Staffordshire Terrier	151	24	16%
Cocker Spaniel	8576	1305	15%
Chesapeake Bay Retriever	509	74	15%
Tibetan Terrier	106	15	14%
Shetland Sheepdog	5765	813	14%
Golden Retriever	17782	2397	13%
Borzoi	266	35	13%
Brittany Spaniel	556	71	13%
Dachshund	3612	115	3%
Basset Hound	699	22	3%
Cairn Terrier	590	18	3%
Schnauzer (unspecified)	1257	38	3%
Wirehaired Fox Terrier	170	5	3%
Cavalier King Charles Spaniel	274	8	3%
Welsh Corgi (undetermined)	457	13	3%
Yorkshire Terrier	1178	33	3%
Norwegian Elkhound	263	7	3%
Belgian Tervuren	235	6	3%
Chihuahua	611	15	2%
Greyhound	1409	32	2%
Pekingese	407	9	2%
Boston Terrier	500	11	2%
Pomeranian	1301	26	2%
Irish Wolfhound	210	4	2%
Whippet	114	2	2%
Soft-coated Wheaten Terrier	214	3	1%
Bichon Frise	657	8	1%
Miniature Schnauzer	828	10	1%

From Graham PA, et al.: Etiopathologic findings of canine hypothyroidism, *Vet Clin North Am Small Anim Pract* 37(4):617-631, 2007; with permission.

*Overall thyroglobulin autoantibody prevalence in this study was 10%.

autoimmune syndromes, type I and type II, have been described. In polyglandular autoimmune syndrome type II (Schmidt syndrome), which is the most common of the immunoendocrinopathy syndromes in humans, there is primary adrenal insufficiency in combination with autoimmune thyroiditis, insulin-dependent diabetes mellitus, or both; whereas in type I the components are more variable (Eisenbarth et al, 2004).

Polyglandular autoimmune syndromes should be suspected when multiple endocrine gland failure is identified in a dog. Hypoadrenocorticism, hypothyroidism, and diabetes mellitus are the most common disorders involved, and the time between diagnosis of the first and second disorder ranges from 0 to 53 months (median 4 months). Diagnosis and treatment are directed at each disorder as it becomes recognized, because it is not possible to reliably predict or prevent any of these disorders. It is important to recognize that the clinician must consider the effects that one endocrine disorder may have on the tests used to diagnose another disorder (e.g., untreated diabetes mellitus suppresses circulating thyroid hormone concentrations) and the effects that treating one endocrine disorder may have on the treatment of concurrent endocrine disorders (e.g., initiation of thyroid supplementation may dramatically improve insulin sensitivity in a diabetic animal; thyroid supplementation may precipitate an Addisonian crisis in hypoadrenocorticism). Immunosuppressive drug therapy is not indicated in these syndromes and may actually create problems (e.g., insulin resistance or thyroid suppression with high-dose glucocorticoid therapy).

Idiopathic Atrophy

Idiopathic atrophy of the thyroid gland is characterized microscopically by progressive reduction in the size of the thyroid follicles, and replacement of the degenerating follicles with adipose tissue (Fig. 3-7). An inflammatory infiltrate is absent, even in areas in which small follicles or follicular remnants are present (Gosselin et al, 1981b) and tests for lymphocytic thyroiditis are negative. The parathyroid glands are not affected, and variable numbers of parafollicular cells remain.

Idiopathic thyroid atrophy may be either a primary degenerative disorder (Gosselin et al, 1981b), or an end stage of lymphocytic thyroiditis. Evaluation of the morphologic changes involved in lymphocytic thyroiditis in a colony of related Borzoi dogs revealed initial degenerative thyroidal parenchymal changes, which progressed to progressively worsening inflammation, subsequent fibrosis, and thyroid gland destruction, that was histologically similar to idiopathic follicular atrophy (Conaway et al, 1985b). However, residual inflammation was still evident. Idiopathic atrophy can be distinguished from the atrophy associated with decreased TSH secretion (i.e., secondary hypothyroidism), because in secondary degeneration, the follicles are lined by low cuboidal epithelial cells with no indication of degeneration.

In one study, the mean age at the time of diagnosis of hypothyroidism was older in dogs with suspected idiopathic atrophy when compared with dogs diagnosed with lymphocytic thyroiditis; a finding that supports the theory that idiopathic atrophy may be an end stage of lymphocytic thyroiditis (Graham et al, 2001). Results for serum Tg and thyroid hormone autoantibody tests also progress from positive to negative with time in dogs with lymphocytic thyroiditis, suggesting that the inciting antigens for lymphocytic thyroiditis disappear with time. Although idiopathic atrophy may represent an end-stage form of autoimmune lymphocytic thyroiditis, the inability to demonstrate an inflammatory cell infiltrate, even when follicles are still present, suggests that there may be more than one etiology for thyroid atrophy in the dog. Unlike for

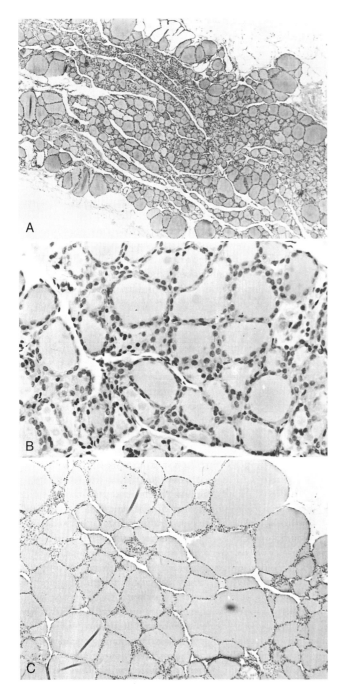

FIGURE 3-7 A and **B**, Histologic section of a thyroid gland from a dog with idiopathic atrophy of the thyroid gland and hypothyroidism. Note the small size of the gland (compare with **C**), decrease in follicular size and colloid content, and lack of a cellular infiltration. (**A**, H&E ×40; **B**, H&E ×250.) **C**, Histologic section of a normal thyroid gland at the same magnification as **A**. Note the increased size of the gland, the follicles, and the colloid content compared with the gland in **A**. (**C**, H&E ×40.)

lymphocytic thyroiditis, there are no blood tests currently available that establish the diagnosis of idiopathic atrophy. Hence the diagnosis is one of exclusion; that is, if the tests for lymphocytic thyroiditis are negative, a diagnosis of idiopathic atrophy is made.

Neoplastic Destruction

Clinical signs of hypothyroidism may develop following destruction of more than 80% of the normal thyroid gland by an infiltrative tumor. Tumors may arise from the thyroid gland or

may metastasize to or invade the thyroid gland from adjacent tissues. Because most thyroid tumors are unilateral and do not destroy more than 80% of thyroid tissue, hypothyroidism due to thyroid gland destruction is only identified in approximately 10% of thyroid tumors. Interpretation of thyroid hormone concentrations in dogs with thyroid tumors is complicated by the effects of concurrent illness on serum thyroid hormone concentrations and because hypothyroidism may be a pre-existing condition in dogs with thyroid neoplasia (Benjamin et al, 1996). For more information on canine thyroid tumors, see Chapter 5.

Iodine Deficiency/Excess

The iodine requirement in the adult Beagle is estimated to be 140 µg/day. In one study, decreased concentrations of serum T_4 and serum T_3 did not occur until iodine intake was restricted to 20 to 50 µg/day, and even when thyroid hormone concentrations decreased, clinical signs of hypothyroidism did not develop (Belshaw et al, 1975). Free T_4 (fT_4) concentrations, determined by equilibrium dialysis, remained in the reference range regardless of the amount of dietary iodine restriction. Two histologic changes were observed in the thyroids of dogs with iodine deficiency. In one group, thyroid follicles were small and contained minimal amounts of colloid. Follicular cell hyperplasia was present, and increased uptake and rapid release of radioiodine occurred. In the second group, thyroid follicles were larger and contained more colloid. Increased uptake but slower release of radioiodine occurred. TSH-secreting cells of the pituitary were enlarged and sparsely granulated, suggesting increased activity and secretion of TSH. Iodine deficiency is a rare cause of hypothyroidism in dogs because commercial pet foods usually contain adequate amounts of iodine; however interest in bone and raw food diets has increased in recent years, and such diets may be deficient in iodine (Dillitzer et al, 2011). Clinical hypothyroidism due to iodine deficiency has been reported in working dogs fed all meat diets (Nuttall, 1986).

Excessive iodine intake inhibits iodide uptake and organification and thyroid hormone secretion by thyroid follicular cells, resulting in a small but significant compensatory increase in circulating TSH concentrations (Wolff-Chaikoff effect) (Roti and Vagenakis, 2013). Ingestion of diets containing an excessive amount of iodine caused impairment of thyroid function and hypothyroidism in puppies fed a high iodine diet for 45 days (Castillo et al, 2001). In humans, high iodine diets can result in transient or subclinical hypothyroidism (Roti and Vagenakis, 2013).

Miscellaneous Causes

Acquired primary hypothyroidism may rarely result from ingestion of goitrogens, administration of anti-thyroid medications (e.g., propylthiouracil and methimazole), and chronic use of high doses of potentiated sulfonamides. A palpable goiter may develop in dogs treated chronically with potentiated sulfonamides (Seelig et al, 2008; Taeymans and O'Marra, 2009). Surgical removal of the thyroid gland for treatment of thyroid neoplasia may also result in hypothyroidism, but because accessory thyroid tissue may be found from the base of the tongue to the base of the heart in dogs, hypothyroidism does not always occur after surgery. In a report of 15 dogs undergoing bilateral thyroidectomy for treatment of thyroid tumors, approximately 50% of dogs required long-term thyroid hormone supplementation (Tuohy et al, 2012). Use of high dose radioactive iodine (iodine-131 [^{131}I]) for treatment of thyroid neoplasia also results in hypothyroidism (Turrel et al, 2006). Other rare causes of primary hypothyroidism include leishmaniasis and congenital hypothyroidism (see Congenital Hypothyroidism).

case, secondary hypothyroidism may result from suppression of thyrotroph function and suppressed TSH secretion, rather than from destruction of thyrotrophs by the tumor.

Pituitary Thyrotroph Suppression

The most common cause of secondary hypothyroidism is believed to be suppression of TSH secretion due to concurrent illness, drugs, hormones, or malnutrition (see Factors Affecting Thyroid Gland Function Tests). Although endogenous and exogenous glucocorticoids are believed to suppress pituitary TSH secretion, in a study of 47 dogs with pituitary dependent hyperadrenocorticism, basal and TRH stimulated TSH concentrations did not differ from those of control dogs (Meij et al, 1997).

Miscellaneous Causes

In humans, secondary hypothyroidism may also develop following production of a defective TSH molecule or impaired interaction between TSH and the TSH receptor on follicular epithelial cells. These causes have not yet been reported in the dog. Secondary hypothyroidism can also result from radiation therapy or hypophysectomy for ACTH-secreting pituitary tumors (Lantz et al, 1988; Meij et al, 1998).

Tertiary Hypothyroidism

Tertiary hypothyroidism is defined as a deficiency in the secretion of TRH by peptidergic neurons in the supraoptic and paraventricular nuclei of the hypothalamus. Lack of TRH secretion causes deficiency of TSH secretion and follicular atrophy of the thyroid gland. In humans, impaired secretion of TRH by the hypothalamus may result from a congenital defect, acquired destruction secondary to a mass lesion or hemorrhage, a defective TRH molecule, or defective TRH-thyrotroph receptor interaction (Sunthornthepvarakul, 1994; Persani, 2013). Neurologic signs and additional pituitary dysfunction may be present, depending on the cause. Diagnosis of tertiary hypothyroidism is based on measurement of a low TSH concentration that increases after administration of TRH. Tertiary hypothyroidism is assumed to be rare in dogs. Unfortunately the poor sensitivity of the current canine TSH assay would make confirmation of this diagnosis difficult. Tertiary hypothyroidism was suspected in a 9-year-old Labrador Retriever with a highly infiltrative pituitary adenoma that invaded the hypothalamus (Shiel et al, 2007b).

Congenital Hypothyroidism

Congenital hypothyroidism is rare in dogs. Unfortunately, congenital hypothyroidism frequently results in early puppy death, and the cause of death is rarely documented. A defect anywhere in the hypothalamic-pituitary-thyroid axis or of the thyroid hormone receptor can result in congenital hypothyroidism (see Box 3-1). Congenital hypothyroidism with goiter (CHG) develops if the hypothalamic-pituitary-thyroid gland axis is intact. TSH binds appropriately with its receptor, but there is an intra-thyroidal defect in thyroid hormone synthesis (dyshormonogenesis). Increased serum TSH concentrations result in development of thyroid hyperplasia and a goiter. If the hypothalamic-pituitary-thyroid axis is not intact (e.g., as occurs with pituitary TSH deficiency), a goiter will not develop.

Documented causes of congenital primary hypothyroidism in the dog include dietary iodine deficiency, dyshormonogenesis (i.e. iodine organification defect), and thyroid dysgenesis (Chastain et al, 1983; Greco et al, 1985). CHG caused by a nonsense mutation in the TPO gene has been recognized in Toy Fox Terriers and Rat Terriers

Summary

Although there are several potential causes of canine hypothyroidism (see Box 3-1), lymphocytic thyroiditis and idiopathic atrophy account for most of the clinical cases of primary hypothyroidism diagnosed in dogs. Both cause progressive loss of thyroid function as a result of either immune-mediated destruction (lymphocytic thyroiditis) or degeneration (idiopathic atrophy) of the thyroid. The result is a deficiency in thyroid hormone synthesis and secretion and development of clinical signs of hypothyroidism.

Secondary Hypothyroidism

Secondary hypothyroidism results from failure of pituitary thyrotrophs to develop due to pituitary malformation or acquired dysfunction of the pituitary thyrotrophs causing impaired secretion of TSH. Deficiency of TSH leads to decreased thyroid hormone synthesis and secretion and thyroid gland hypoplasia. Histologically, the thyroid gland has small hypoplastic follicles that lack or contain only scant colloid and apical resorption follicles (Gal et al, 2012).

Potential causes of secondary hypothyroidism include congenital malformations of the pituitary gland, pituitary destruction, and pituitary suppression. In the dog, secondary hypothyroidism caused by naturally acquired defects in pituitary thyrotroph function or destruction of pituitary thyrotrophs (e.g., pituitary neoplasia) is uncommon. In contrast, suppression of pituitary thyrotroph function by hormones or drugs (e.g., glucocorticoids, spontaneous hyperadrenocorticism) is quite common. Serum TSH concentrations should be decreased or undetectable with secondary hypothyroidism. Unfortunately, current assays used to measure endogenous TSH in dogs are insensitive and unable to differentiate between decreased and normal concentrations (see Baseline Serum Thyrotropin Concentration), making confirmation of secondary hypothyroidism difficult; although one would expect the serum TSH concentration to be undetectable in a dog with secondary hypothyroidism, such a finding does not confirm the diagnosis.

Pituitary Malformation

Congenital abnormalities involving the pituitary gland have been recognized in many breeds but are reported most commonly in German Shepherd dogs. In German Shepherd dogs, pituitary dwarfism is caused by a simple autosomal recessive mutation of the LHX3 gene, which leads to combined pituitary hormone deficiency. Combined pituitary hormone deficiency is characterized by deficiency of growth hormone (GH), TSH, prolactin, and gonadotrophins. Because the various cell types of the adenohypophysis arise from the progenitor cells in a distinct order with corticotrophs differentiating first, secretion of adrenocorticotrophic hormone (ACTH) is unaffected. Pituitary cysts may be detected at a young age and gradually increase in size with time (Eigenmann, 1981; Hamann et al, 1999; Kooistra et al, 2000a). Because of the involvement of other anterior pituitary hormones—most notably GH, congenital defects affecting the anterior pituitary usually result in the development of proportionate dwarfism (see Chapter 2).

Pituitary Destruction

Although uncommon, pituitary tumors may cause secondary hypothyroidism, following destruction of thyrotrophs by an expanding, space-occupying mass. Other endocrinopathies, such as hypocortisolism (secondary adrenal insufficiency), diabetes insipidus, and reproductive dysfunction, may occur when pituitary dysfunction is due to neoplasia. The most common pituitary tumor affecting thyroid gland function in the dog is a functional corticotrophic tumor causing pituitary-dependent hyperadrenocorticism. In this

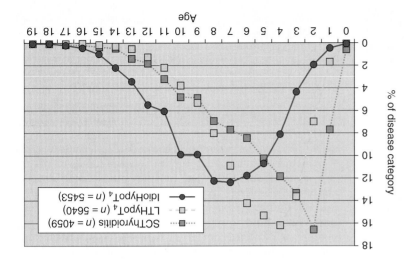

FIGURE 3-8 Age distribution profiles for different categories of thyroid disease and dysfunction based on findings in 143,800 samples submitted for the investigation of thyroid disease in which an age was provided. IdiolHypoT4, thyroglobulin autoantibody–negative hypothyroidism; LTHypoT4, thyroglobulin autoantibody–positive hypothyroidism; SC Thyroiditis, subclinical thyroglobulin autoantibody–positive thyroiditis. (From Graham PA, et al: Etiopathologic findings of canine hypothyroidism. *Vet Clin North Am Small Anim Pract* 37[4]: 620, 2007.)

breed popularity and geographic variation in breed distribution may influence the perception of which breeds are predisposed to the disease. Hypothyroidism is typically a disease of middle-aged to older dogs. Golden Retrievers and Doberman Pinschers are the breeds most commonly reported to be at increased risk for hypothyroidism, although many breeds are represented in published studies (Table 3-3). Based upon measurement of serum Tg and thyroid hormone autoantibodies, many breeds have been reported to have an increased incidence of lymphocytic thyroiditis (see Table 3-2), and this is likely due to a genetic predisposition to thyroiditis (Nachreiner et al, 2002; Kennedy et al, 2006a; 2006b). Thyroiditis is usually documented at an earlier age (2 to 4 years) than development of clinical signs (4 to 6 years), which fits with the hypothesis that thyroiditis may progress to complete thyroid failure over time. Of 143,800 serum samples from dogs with thyroid disease, the age distribution profile peaked at 2 years for dogs with subclinical hypothyroidism, 4 years for dogs with anti-Tg positive hypothyroidism, and 5 to 8 years for dogs with anti-Tg negative hypothyroidism (Graham et al, 2007; Fig. 3-8). Age of onset of symptomatic hypothyroidism may vary between breeds, presumably as a result of the underlying etiology and rate of progression of thyroid pathology. The majority of studies do not suggest a consistent association of hypothyroidism with sex or neuter status.

Clinical Signs

A deficiency in circulating thyroid hormone affects the metabolic function of almost all organ systems. Destruction of the thyroid gland is typically slowly progressive, and the onset of clinical signs may be gradual and initially subtle. Clinical signs are quite variable and may differ among breeds, different breeds have markedly different hair cycles and follicular morphology, which may influence the clinical and histologic features of the disease (Credille et al, 2001). Because of the slow progression of the disease, owners may fail to recognize the clinical signs until they become severe. Only after the dog returns to normal following initiation of thyroid hormone supplementation does the owner recognize that the problem existed for much longer than initially believed.

In the adult dog, the most consistent clinical signs of hypothyroidism are those due to decreased cellular metabolism and dermatologic manifestations (Box 3-2 and Table 3-4). Additional clinical signs may affect the cardiovascular system, neuromuscular system, gastrointestinal system, and reproductive system.

(Fyfe et al, 2003; Pettigrew et al, 2007). In a study of Rat Terrier puppies with congenital goiter and a mutation in the TPO gene, central nervous system (CNS) hypomyelination was demonstrated in affected puppies (Pettigrew et al, 2007). The hypomyelination was regionally distributed and most severe in the corpus callosum. Myelin reduction was paralleled by axon reduction, suggesting that hypomyelination was due to reduced axonal formation. Different mutations of the TPO gene cause CHG in Tenterfield Terriers and Spanish Water dogs (Dodgson et al, 2012; Fyfe 2013). Both defects are autosomal-recessive traits.

Secondary hypothyroidism resulting from an apparent deficiency of TSH was reported in a family of Giant Schnauzers (Greco et al, 1991) and a Boxer dog (Mooney and Anderson, 1993). Pedigree analysis suggested an autosomal recessive mode of inheritance in the family of Giant Schnauzers. Pituitary dwarfs with combined anterior pituitary hormone deficiencies usually lack TSH in addition to GH and prolactin (Hamann et al, 1999; Kooistra et al, 2000a; see Chapter 2). Lack of TSH may contribute to abnormal body maturation and growth in pituitary dwarfs.

CLINICAL FEATURES OF HYPOTHYROIDISM IN THE ADULT DOG

Signalment

Reports regarding breed incidence and genetics of canine hypothyroidism should always be examined critically, because confirming a definitive diagnosis of hypothyroidism is challenging, and

TABLE 3-3   BREED DISTRIBUTION OF 154 DOGS WITH PRIMARY HYPOTHYROIDISM*

BREED	NUMBER (%) OF DOGS
Golden Retriever	26 (17%)
Doberman Pinscher	21 (14%)
Labrador Retriever	7 (5%)
Mixed breed	24 (16%)
Other breeds	76 (49%)

*Based on four published and one unpublished study (Peterson et al, 1997; Scott-Moncrieff et al, 1998; Ramsey et al, 1997; Panciera, 1994).

General Metabolic Signs

Most adult dogs with acquired hypothyroidism have clinical signs that result from a generalized decrease in metabolic rate. Energy expenditure, as measured by indirect calorimetry, is approximately 15% lower in hypothyroid dogs, compared with healthy dogs, and energy expenditure returns to normal after initiating levothyroxine (L-thyroxine; L-T_4) sodium treatment (Greco et al, 1998). Clinical signs due to the decreased metabolic rate include mental dullness, lethargy, exercise intolerance or unwillingness to exercise, cold intolerance, and a propensity to gain weight without a corresponding increase in appetite or food intake. Obesity occurs in approximately 40% of hypothyroid dogs, but it is important to remember that the most common cause of obesity is overnutrition rather than hypothyroidism.

Metabolic signs are usually gradual in onset and initially very subtle but become more obvious with longer duration of hypothyroidism. Sometimes these clinical signs are missed on the history and physical examination and not recognized until the dog shows improvement in activity within 7 to 10 days of initiating thyroid hormone supplementation.

BOX 3-2	Clinical Manifestations of Hypothyroidism in the Adult Dog

Metabolic
Lethargy*
Mental dullness
Inactivity*
Weight gain*
Cold intolerance

Dermatologic
Endocrine alopecia*
Symmetric or asymmetrical
Areas of friction and pressure
"Rat tail"
Dry, brittle hair coat
Hyperpigmentation
Seborrhea
Pyoderma
Otitis externa
Myxedema

Reproductive
Prolonged parturition
Periparturient mortality
Low birth weight puppies
Female infertility
Inappropriate galactorrhea or gynecomastia

Neuromuscular
Polyneuropathy/myopathy
Vestibular signs (central or peripheral)
Facial/trigeminal nerve paralysis
Seizures
Disorientation/circling
Myxedema coma
Laryngeal paralysis (?)

Ocular
Corneal lipid deposits

Cardiovascular
Bradycardia
Cardiac arrhythmias

Gastrointestinal
Esophageal hypomotility (?)
Diarrhea
Constipation

Hematologic
Anemia*
Hyperlipidemia*

*Common.
?indicates that a causal relationship is not proven.

TABLE 3-4	INCIDENCE OF CLINICAL SIGNS IN 162 ADULT DOGS WITH HYPOTHYROIDISM
CLINICAL SIGN	**PERCENT OF DOGS**
Dermatologic	88
Obesity	49
Lethargy	48
Weakness	12
Neurologic	
Facial nerve paralysis	4
Peripheral vestibular	3
Polyneuropathy	2
Reproductive	<2
Cardiovascular (bradycardia)	10

Adapted from Panciera DL: Conditions associated with canine hypothyroidism, Vet Clin North Am 31:935, 2001.

Dermatologic Signs

Alterations in the skin and hair coat occur in 60% to 80% of hypothyroid dogs and are the most commonly observed abnormalities in dogs with hypothyroidism. Dermatologic changes can be quite varied and dependent on the breed of dog and severity and chronicity of the disease. The classic cutaneous sign of hypothyroidism is bilaterally symmetric, nonpruritic truncal alopecia. Thyroid hormone is necessary to initiate and maintain the anagen, or growing, phase of the hair cycle (Credille et al, 2001). With thyroid hormone deficiency, hair follicles prematurely enter the telogen phase of the hair cycle. Excessive shedding with lack of hair regrowth leads to alopecia. Decreased concentrations of cutaneous fatty acids and prostaglandin E_2 in canine hypothyroidism may lead to sebaceous gland atrophy, hyperkeratosis, scale formation, seborrhea sicca, and a dry and lusterless hair coat (Campbell and Davis, 1990). The hair coat may appear faded in color, and subtle changes in hair coat quality may initially be appreciated by the owner but not the veterinarian. In the early stages of hypothyroidism, hair loss is often asymmetric and develops over areas of excessive wear or pressure, such as the caudal thighs, ventral thorax, tail base, and tail (i.e., development of a "rat tail," Fig. 3-9). As hypothyroidism becomes more severe or chronic, alopecia becomes more symmetric and truncal, eventually developing into the classic cutaneous finding of bilaterally symmetric, nonpruritic truncal alopecia that tends to spare the head and distal extremities (Fig. 3-10). Although nonpruritic endocrine alopecia is not pathognomonic for hypothyroidism, when it is present in a dog with other signs of decreased metabolic rate and no polyuria or polydipsia, hypothyroidism is the most likely diagnosis.

There are breed variations in the dermatologic effects of hypothyroidism presumably because of differences in the hair cycle and follicular morphology. In some breeds, failure to shed leads to hypertrichosis, and in other breeds primary hairs are lost giving the hair coat a "wooly" appearance. In some dogs there is a loss of the undercoat, and the remaining primary hairs give the coat a coarse appearance. In some breeds the hair shafts within telogen follicles may be retained for long periods (months to years) without falling out. In a study evaluating the effect of induced hypothyroidism on the skin of Beagle dogs, none of the untreated hypothyroid dogs had a discernible alopecia after 10 months of observation despite the hypothyroid dogs having one-third fewer hair shafts than healthy Beagles (Credille et al, 2001). The most common finding was a failure of the hypothyroid dogs to regrow their hair after clipping. Retaining telogen hairs maintains the pelage, which explains why truncal alopecia does not usually develop in hypothyroid Beagle dogs.

Hyperpigmentation is common in hypothyroidism, especially in regions of alopecia and areas of wear such as the axilla and inguinal regions (Fig. 3-11). In severe cases of hypothyroidism, the

hygroscopic glycosaminoglycan, hyaluronic acid may accumulate in the dermis, bind water, and result in increased thickness and non-pitting edema of the skin, referred to as *myxedema*, or *cutaneous mucinosis* (Doliger et al., 1995). Myxedema predominantly affects the forehead, eyelids, and lips, and it contributes to the development of the classic "tragic facial expression" described in hypothyroid dogs (see Fig. 3-9). A rare complication of myxedema is cutaneous mucinous vesiculation (Miller and Buerger, 1990).

Thyroid hormone is believed to play a role in the normal immune response. Depletion of thyroid hormone suppresses humoral immune reactions, impairs T cell function, and reduces the number of circulating lymphocytes. Dogs with hypothyroidism may develop superficial bacterial infections (folliculitis, superficial spreading pyoderma, impetigo) characterized by papules, pustules, epidermal collarettes, and/or focal areas of alopecia. Bacterial infections are usually caused by *Staphylococcus spp* and are variably pruritic. Hypothyroidism may also predispose to adult onset demodicosis and chronic otitis externa (Duclos et al., 1994). The skin changes associated with hypothyroidism are generally nonpruritic; however secondary infection, seborrhea, or concurrent pruritic diseases (e.g., atopy or flea bite hypersensitivity) may cause pruritus. The presence of pruritic skin disease therefore does not rule out underlying hypothyroidism.

Neurologic Signs

Both the peripheral nervous system and CNS may be affected by hypothyroidism (Indrieri et al., 1987; Bichsel et al., 1988; Jaggy et al., 1994). Diffuse peripheral neuropathy characterized by exercise intolerance, weakness, ataxia, quadriparesis or paralysis, deficits of conscious proprioception, and decreased spinal reflexes has been reported to occur in dogs with hypothyroidism. Single or multifocal cranial nerve dysfunction with predisposition for the facial, vestibulocochlear, and trigeminal nerves has also been reported. Neurologic dysfunction may be multifocal, acute or chronic, and static or progressive. Other physical examination findings consistent with hypothyroidism may be absent. Hypothyroid dogs with vestibular deficits may have abnormal brainstem auditory evoked responses and electromyographic abnormalities identified in the appendicular muscles. Proposed mechanisms include nerve entrapment from accumulation of mucinous deposits, demyelination due to disrupted Schwann cell metabolism, vascular nerve damage due to alterations in the blood-nerve barrier, and disturbances in axonal cell transport. Although there are numerous reports of the association between hypothyroidism and periph- eral nerve dysfunction, the cause and effect relationship has been questioned, because in an experimental model of canine hypothy- roidism, it was not possible to reproduce a peripheral neuropathy (Rossmeisl, 2010). It has been proposed that other factors such as immune dysregulation may play a role in the pathogenesis of the peripheral neurologic abnormalities. Because immune-mediated thyroiditis is present in as many as 50% of hypothyroid dogs, it is conceivable that immune-mediated mechanisms contribute to the pathogenesis of the neuromuscular changes observed in hypo- thyroid dogs. Clinical signs of peripheral neuropathy resolve with L-T₄ sodium supplementation; however this finding must be interpreted carefully because peripheral vestibular disease, facial nerve paralysis, and polyradiculoneuritis of unknown etiology may also improve or resolve over time.

A subclinical myopathy has been well-documented in hypothy- roid dogs and also occurs in experimental models of canine hypo- thyroidism (Delauche, 1998; Rossmeisl et al., 2009). Hypothyroid myopathy is accompanied by increased plasma creatine kinase, aspartate aminotransferase, and lactate dehydrogenase activities.

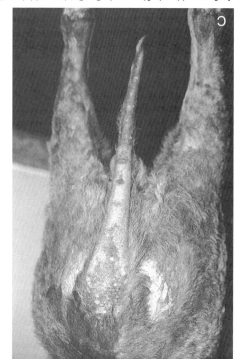

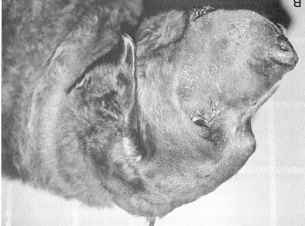

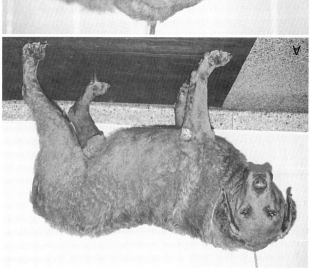

FIGURE 3-9 An 8-year-old male Chesapeake Bay Retriever with hypothyroidism. Note the poor hair coat, lethargic appearance, myxedema of the face with droop- ing of the eyelids (**A** and **B**), and "rat tail" (**C**).

Central vestibular dysfunction has also been reported in association with hypothyroidism. In 10 dogs with central vestibular dysfunction associated with hypothyroidism, lesions consistent with an infarct were identified in three dogs, but cranial imaging studies were normal in the other five dogs that were imaged (Higgins et al, 2006). Albuminocytologic dissociation was identified in five of six cerebrospinal fluid (CSF) analyses and most dogs had hypercholesterolemia or hypertriglyceridemia. Clinical signs completely resolved after 4 weeks of supplementation with L-thyroxine, apart

lethargy and exercise intolerance in canine hypothyroidism.

Histopathologic abnormalities include nemaline rod inclusions, predominance of type 1 myofibers, decrease in mean type II fiber area, subsarcolemmal accumulations of abnormal mitochondria, and myofiber degeneration (Delauche, 1998; Rossmeisl et al, 2009). Substantial depletion of skeletal muscle free carnitine has also been documented in affected dogs. Although an obvious clinical myopathy is not recognized associated with these changes, the abnormalities may contribute to nonspecific clinical signs, such as

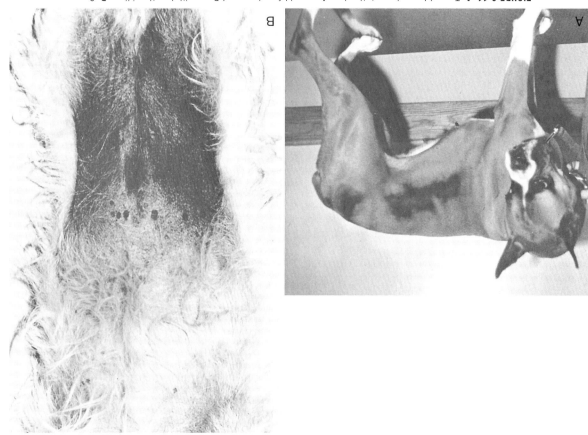

FIGURE 3-11 **A,** Truncal hyperpigmentation in a 4-year-old female spayed Boxer with hypothyroidism. **B,** Severe hyperpigmentation involving the inguinal region in a 6-year-old spayed mixed-breed dog with hypothyroidism.

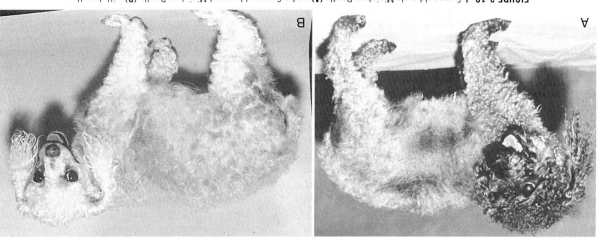

FIGURE 3-10 A 5-year-old male Miniature Poodle (**A**) and a 6-year-old spayed Miniature Poodle (**B**) with hypothyroidism. Note the truncal alopecia and hyperpigmentation, which have spared the head and extremities, in both dogs.

from residual head tilt in one dog. Cerebral dysfunction manifested by seizures, disorientation, and circling may also rarely occur in canine hypothyroidism, although there is little evidence to suggest that hypothyroidism is a common cause of seizure disorders in dogs. In a series of 113 dogs with seizure disorders, 38% of dogs with idiopathic epilepsy had thyroid hormone profiles consistent with nonthyroidal illness, but fewer than 3% of dogs were definitively diagnosed with hypothyroidism (von Klopmann et al, 2006). In a retrospective study of 96 dogs with metabolic and toxic causes of seizures, hypothyroidism was the suspected cause in only three dogs (Brauer et al, 2011). An incorrect diagnosis of hypothyroidism may be made in dogs already being treated for idiopathic epilepsy because anticonvulsant therapy may influence thyroid hormone testing (see Anticonvulsants). The reason for CNS dysfunction in canine hypothyroidism is poorly understood and is likely multifactorial. Atherosclerosis, hyperlipidemia, vascular encephalopathy, and functional metabolic derangements of neuronal or glial cell populations due to hypothyroidism may all play a role. Dogs with atherosclerosis, which is likely due to hypercholesterolemia, are over 50 times more likely to have hypothyroidism than dogs without atherosclerosis (Hess et al, 2003). Severe hyperlipidemia has been reported to cause neurologic dysfunction in hypothyroid dogs, and it has been proposed that Labrador Retrievers may be predisposed to this manifestation of hypothyroidism (Vitale et al, 2007). Dogs with experimentally induced hypothyroidism have disruption of the blood brain barrier as evidenced by albuminocytologic dissociation and increased CSF concentrations of plasma vascular endothelial growth factor (VEGF) (Pancotto et al, 2010). Two of nine dogs with induced hypothyroidism in this study developed CNS signs and evidence of cerebrovascular disease during the 18-month study. Myxedema coma or a pituitary tumor causing secondary hypothyroidism may also rarely cause CNS signs.

Other Neurologic Disorders

Laryngeal paralysis and megaesophagus may both occur in association with hypothyroidism; however, a causal relationship has not been established, and treatment of hypothyroidism does not consistently result in improvement of clinical signs of either disorder (MacPhail and Monnet, 2001; Gaynor et al, 1997). Myasthenia gravis has been identified in dogs with hypothyroidism (Dewey et al, 1995) and is a well-recognized cause of acquired megaesophagus in the dog. Concurrent hypothyroidism may exacerbate clinical signs of myasthenia gravis, such as muscle weakness and megaesophagus. In human beings, there is a link between autoimmune thyroiditis and acquired myasthenia gravis, and myasthenia gravis is a recognized component of polyglandular autoimmune syndrome type II. Presumably a common abnormality in immune function allows development of autoimmune attack on both the thyroid gland and acetylcholine receptors. Myasthenia gravis was documented in only 1 of 162 dogs with hypothyroidism reviewed by Panciera (2001), implying that hypothyroidism is rarely associated with myasthenia gravis. A causal relation between hypothyroidism and myasthenia gravis remains to be established.

Myxedema Coma

Myxedema coma is an extremely rare syndrome of severe hypothyroidism characterized by profound weakness, hypothermia, bradycardia, and a diminished level of consciousness, which can rapidly progress to stupor and then coma (Chastain et al, 1982; Kelly and Hill, 1984; Henik and Dixon, 2000; Atkinson and Aubert, 2004). Clinical signs in addition to the more typical clinical signs of hypothyroidism include mental dullness, depression, unresponsiveness, and weakness. Physical findings include profound weakness, hypothermia; non-pitting edema of the skin, face, and jowls (myxedema); bradycardia; hypotension; and hypoventilation. Myxedema results from the accumulation of acid and neutral mucopolysaccharides and hyaluronic acid in the dermis, which bind water and result in increased thickness of the skin. Laboratory findings may include hypoglycemia, hypercapnia, hypoxemia, and hypoglycemia in addition to the typical findings of hyperlipidemia, hypercholesterolemia, and nonregenerative anemia. Serum thyroid hormone concentrations are usually extremely low or undetectable; serum TSH concentration is variable but typically increased. There is commonly a precipitating event, such as hypothermia or infection. Mortality is high, likely because of late recognition and concurrent illness.

Alterations in Behavior

A relationship between thyroid function and behavioral changes is well established in humans. Neurologic and psychiatric symptoms (e.g., slowing of thought and speech, memory loss, poor concentration, anxiety, depression, and psychosis) may occur in hypothyroid adults (Schuff et al, 2013). These changes are proposed to result from alterations in expression of neurotransmitters, neuromodulators, and growth factors associated with thyroid dysfunction. The influence of thyroid dysfunction on serotonergic receptors has received particular attention because of the role of serotonin in depressive illness. It has been postulated that canine hypothyroidism may lead to aberrant behavior, including aggression, submissiveness, shyness, fearfulness, excitability, passivity, irritability, moodiness, and unstable temperament (Dodds, 1995). To date, most reports on alterations in behavior and hypothyroidism have been anecdotal and based on apparent improvement in behavior following initiation of thyroid hormone treatment. Proposed mechanisms for hypothyroidism associated aggression include a lowered threshold for aggression due to lethargy and irritability and disturbances in serotonergic or noradrenergic pathways. Two small prospective studies in dogs failed to demonstrate an association between hypothyroidism and behavioral problems, such as aggression (Carter et al, 2009; Radosta et al, 2012); however further larger prospective studies would be required to prove the absence of such a relationship. The benefits, if any, of using thyroid hormone to treat behavioral disorders remain to be clarified.

Reproductive Signs

Historically, hypothyroidism was believed to cause lack of libido, testicular atrophy, and oligospermia or azoospermia in male dogs. However, work by C. Johnson, et al. (1999) in Beagles failed to document any deleterious effect of experimentally induced hypothyroidism on any aspect of male reproductive function. Although other classic clinical signs and clinicopathologic abnormalities of hypothyroidism developed in the hypothyroid dogs studied, libido, testicular size, and the total sperm count per ejaculate remained normal. These findings suggest that hypothyroidism is an uncommon cause of reproductive dysfunction in male dogs; however, the duration of the study (2 years) may have been too short to allow reproductive abnormalities to develop, or the induced model used in the study may not have been representative of naturally occurring hypothyroidism, which commonly is due to lymphocytic thyroiditis. It is possible that lymphocytic thyroiditis and lymphocytic orchitis are comorbid conditions, which could account for the clinical observation of reproductive dysfunction in male hypothyroid dogs. Hypothyroidism appears to be an uncommon cause of infertility in male dogs. However, it should be considered when other causes for infertility cannot be identified, especially if decreased libido is part of the clinical picture.

Although thyroid hormone is believed to be necessary for normal follicle-stimulating hormone (FSH) and luteinizing hormone (LH) secretion, an association between hypothyroidism and infertility in the female dog has been poorly documented in the veterinary literature. Two prospective studies failed to identify an association between poor reproductive performance and hypothyroidism in pure bred dogs (Beale et al, 2009). In a prospective study of female dogs with experimentally induced hypothyroidism, short-term hypothyroidism (median 19 weeks) was associated with prolonged parturition and reduced periparturient puppy survival (Panciera et al, 2007). In the same study, dogs with more chronic hypothyroidism (56 weeks) had higher periparturient mortality and lower puppy birth weights than control dogs. Fertility was decreased in the hypothyroid dogs compared to control dogs, but the difference was not statistically significant, likely due to the small numbers of dogs in each group (Panciera et al, 2012). Hypothyroidism has also been implicated in causing prolonged interestrus intervals and failure to cycle in the female dog. However this was not documented in the studies by Panciera et al (2007, 2012). Additional reproductive abnormalities that have been reported in the veterinary literature include weak or silent estrus cycles, prolonged estrual bleeding, and inappropriate galactorrhea and gynecomastia. The latter is believed to develop following a thyroid hormone deficiency–induced increase in TRH secretion, which in turn stimulates prolactin secretion (Chastain and Schmidt, 1980; Cortese et al, 1997). Increased prolactin concentrations were documented in dogs with experimentally induced hypothyroidism 39 weeks after induction of hypothyroidism, but this was not associated with abnormalities in progesterone concentrations or ovulation (Kolster et al, 2010). Evaluation of thyroid gland function is recommended as part of the evaluation of female dogs for infertility, fetal resorption, or peripartum mortality, although it appears that hypothyroidism is an uncommon cause of reproductive failure.

Cardiovascular Signs

Clinical signs related to dysfunction of the cardiovascular system are uncommon in canine hypothyroidism. Abnormalities identified on physical examination may include bradycardia and a weak apex beat. Atrial fibrillation has been suggested to be associated with hypothyroidism in dogs (Gerritsen et al, 1996), but this appears to be rare based on findings in other studies (Panciera, 2001). More commonly, functional abnormalities are identified on electrocardiography or echocardiography in dogs exhibiting the more common clinical signs of hypothyroidism. Electrocardiographic abnormalities include sinus bradycardia, decreased amplitude of the P and R waves, inversion of the T waves, and first-degree and second-degree atrioventricular block (Panciera, 1994; 2001). Echocardiographic abnormalities include increased left ventricular end systolic diameter, prolonged preejection period, and decreases in left ventricular posterior wall thickness during systole, percentage change in left ventricular posterior wall thickness during systole to diastole, interventricular wall thickness during systole and diastole, aortic diameter, velocity of circumferential fiber shortening, and fractional shortening (Panciera, 1994; 2001). Many of the hemodynamic effects of hypothyroidism appear to be attributable to direct effects of hypothyroidism on the myocardium, which include decreased cardiac muscle myosin adenosine triphosphatase (ATPase) activity, decreased sarcoplasmic reticulum calcium-ATPase activity, decreased calcium channel activity, decreased sodium-potassium ATPase activity, and reduced β-adrenergic receptors in the myocardium (Bilezikian and Loeb, 1983; Haber and Loeb, 1988; Hawthorn et al, 1988; Dowell et al, 1994). Alterations in the circulatory system may also contribute to the decrease in cardiac output present in hypothyroidism, including

increased systemic vascular resistance, decreased vascular volume, and atherosclerosis (Klein, 1990; Hess et al, 2003). It is not known which of these alterations contribute to the myocardial abnormalities identified in dogs with hypothyroidism. Fortunately, the decrease in cardiac contractility in dogs with hypothyroidism is usually mild and asymptomatic, but it may become relevant during a surgical procedure requiring prolonged anesthesia and aggressive fluid therapy. Cardiac abnormalities are usually reversible with thyroid hormone supplementation although it may take months of supplementation to restore normal cardiovascular function (Panciera, 1994).

It is important to emphasize that although hypothyroidism can induce echocardiographic changes, thyroid hormone deficiency alone rarely causes heart failure. In most cases heart failure associated with primary hypothyroidism is considered to represent an exacerbation of intrinsic cardiac disease by the superimposed hemodynamic effects of thyroid hormone deficiency. Both cardiomyopathy and hypothyroidism are common problems in Doberman Pinschers, and Calvert, et al. speculated on a possible cause-and-effect relationship between these two disorders in 1982. However, subsequent studies failed to identify any relationship between hypothyroidism and cardiomyopathy in Doberman Pinschers (Lumsden et al, 1993; Calvert et al, 1998). Although low baseline serum thyroid hormone concentrations occur in dogs with idiopathic dilated cardiomyopathy and heart failure, the low thyroid hormone concentrations are due to nonthyroidal illness rather than hypothyroidism. One case report documented dramatic long-term improvement in cardiac function after treatment with T$_4$ in two Great Danes with concurrent dilated cardiomyopathy and hypothyroidism (Phillips, 2003). Pericardial disease has also been associated with canine hypothyroidism. Aortic thromboembolism and a cholesterol-based pericardial effusion that resolved after L-T$_4$ supplementation were reported in a 9-year-old mixed-breed dog with hypothyroidism (MacGregor, 2004).

Ocular Signs

Ocular signs are rare in hypothyroid dogs and most commonly are secondary to hyperlipidemia. Corneal lipid deposits (i.e, arcus lipoides corneae) have been described in a group of hypothyroid Alsatians with concomitant hyperlipidemia (Crispin, 1978). Corneal ulceration, uveitis, lipid effusion into the aqueous humor, secondary glaucoma, lipemia retinalis, retinal detachment, keratoconjunctivitis sicca (KCS), and Horner's syndrome have been reported in hypothyroid dogs, but the evidence for a causal association is weak (Kern and Riis, 1980; Gosselin et al, 1981b; Peruccio, 1982; Kern et al, 1989). Dogs with experimentally induced hypothyroidism did not develop ocular signs over a 6-month period (Miller, 1994). In another study decreased tear production was documented in hypothyroid dogs, compared to control dogs, but only 2 of 12 dogs evaluated had clinical signs of keratoconjunctivitis sicca (Williams et al, 2007).

Gastrointestinal Signs

Clinical signs related to the gastrointestinal system have been described but are not common in hypothyroid dogs. Constipation may occur, presumably as a result of alterations in electrical control activity and smooth muscle contractile responses in the gastrointestinal tract. Diarrhea has also been reported with hypothyroidism, although a cause-and-effect relationship has not been established, and some of these dogs may have had nonthyroidal illness rather than hypothyroidism.

Generalized megaesophagus has been identified in some dogs with hypothyroidism, and some investigators have theorized that megaesophagus is caused by hypothyroidism, presumably as a

result of hypothyroid-induced neuropathy or myopathy (Jaggy et al, 1994). Unfortunately, no published reports document a cause-and-effect relationship between hypothyroidism and megaesophagus, and one recent retrospective study failed to identify an association between hypothyroidism and acquired megaesophagus (Gaynor et al, 1997). As with cardiomyopathy, a low baseline thyroid hormone concentration in a dog with generalized megaesophagus more often represents nonthyroidal illness rather than hypothyroidism. The thyroid gland in most of these dogs is responsive to TSH, megaesophagus persists despite thyroid hormone supplementation, and treatment has minimal to no effect on clinical signs (Panciera, 1994; Jaggy et al, 1994).

CLINICAL FEATURES OF SECONDARY HYPOTHYROIDISM

The array of clinical signs is similar for primary and secondary hypothyroidism in the adult dog; however, other clinical signs may dominate depending on the underlying cause. If acquired secondary hypothyroidism is caused by a pituitary tumor, the clinical signs will depend on the degree of compression/destruction of surrounding structures. Clinical signs of hypoadrenocorticism or hyperadrenocorticism, diabetes insipidus, or hypothalamic/thalamic dysfunction (i.e., lethargy, stupor, anorexia, adipsia, loss of temperature regulation) may predominate. Subtle changes associated with hypothyroidism, GH deficiency, or reproductive dysfunction are less likely to be observed by an owner.

CLINICOPATHOLOGIC ABNORMALITIES OF HYPOTHYROIDISM

There are a number of laboratory abnormalities associated with hypothyroidism. Although most of the changes are nonspecific and observed in many other disorders, their presence adds support for a diagnosis of hypothyroidism in an animal with appropriate clinical signs.

Complete Blood Count

A normocytic, normochromic, nonregenerative anemia (packed cell volume [PCV], 28% to 36%) is identified in approximately 30% of dogs (Panciera, 2001). The cause is unknown but is believed to be due to decreased erythrocyte production. Decreased erythropoietin, decreased erythroid progenitor response to erythropoietin, and lack of a direct effect of thyroid hormone on early hemopoietic pluripotent stem cells may all contribute to the anemia. Erythrocyte

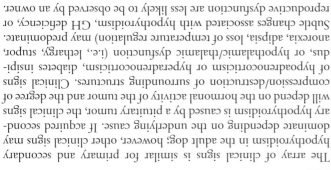

BOX 3-3 Clinical Signs Associated with Congenital Hypothyroidism

Dwarfism
Short, broad skull
Shortened mandible
Enlarged cranium
Shortened limbs
Kyphosis
Mental dullness
Constipation
Inappetence
Gait abnormalities
Delayed dental eruption
Alopecia
"Puppy" hair coat
Dry hair
Thick skin
Lethargy
Dyspnea
Goiter

CLINICAL FEATURES OF CONGENITAL HYPOTHYROIDISM

Normal physical and mental development depends on the presence of normal plasma thyroid hormone concentrations. Thyroid hormone is critical for normal neurologic development and bone growth. Thyroid hormone acts synergistically with GH and insulin-like growth factor-1 (IGF-1) to promote chondrogenesis. Retardation of growth and impaired mental development are the hallmarks of congenital hypothyroidism (cretinism) (Box 3-3). Clinical signs of hypothyroidism are not usually present at birth but develop postnatally. Abnormalities usually become obvious to owners between 2 and 12 weeks of age. Puppies with congenital hypothyroidism are typically of normal weight at birth, but fail to thrive and gain weight in the weeks after birth. They develop disproportionate dwarfism with a large, broad head, short thick neck, enlarged or protruding tongue, wide/square trunk, and short limbs (Fig. 3-12). This is in contrast to the proportionate dwarfism caused by GH deficiency (see Chapter 2). Delayed epiphyseal development and retarded epiphyseal growth with reduced long bone growth cause the disproportionate dwarfism of congenital hypothyroidism (Saunders and Jezyk, 1991).

Affected puppies are mentally dull and lethargic, may be unable to eat without assistance, and lack the typical playfulness seen in normal puppies. They often have stenotic ear canals and delayed opening of the eyelids. The soft, fluffy "puppy hair coat" persists, and diffuse truncal thinning of the hair with lack of guard hairs develops, which may progress to complete alopecia. Additional clinical signs may include inappetence, constipation, delayed dental eruption, and goiter (Fig. 3-13). The presence of goiter is variable and dependent on the underlying etiology (see Congenital Hypothyroidism).

Coagulopathy

In humans, hypothyroidism may cause several abnormalities in the coagulation system, including a reduction in concentration of factors VIII and IX, a reduction in factor VIII–related antigen (von Willebrand factor), reduced platelet adhesiveness, and increased capillary fragility (Hymes et al, 1981; Rogers et al, 1982; Dalton et al, 1987). These abnormalities account for the easy bruising observed in some humans with hypothyroidism. Numerous studies have evaluated the association between canine hypothyroidism and the concentration of factor VIII–related antigen both in euthyroid and hypothyroid dogs and found no evidence of an association (Avgeris et al, 1990; Heseltine, 2005; Panciera and Johnson, 1996). Evaluation of the coagulation cascade or factor VIII–related antigen is not recommended in dogs with untreated hypothyroidism unless concurrent bleeding problems are present. Thyroid hormone supplementation in euthyroid dogs with von Willebrand disease is not recommended.

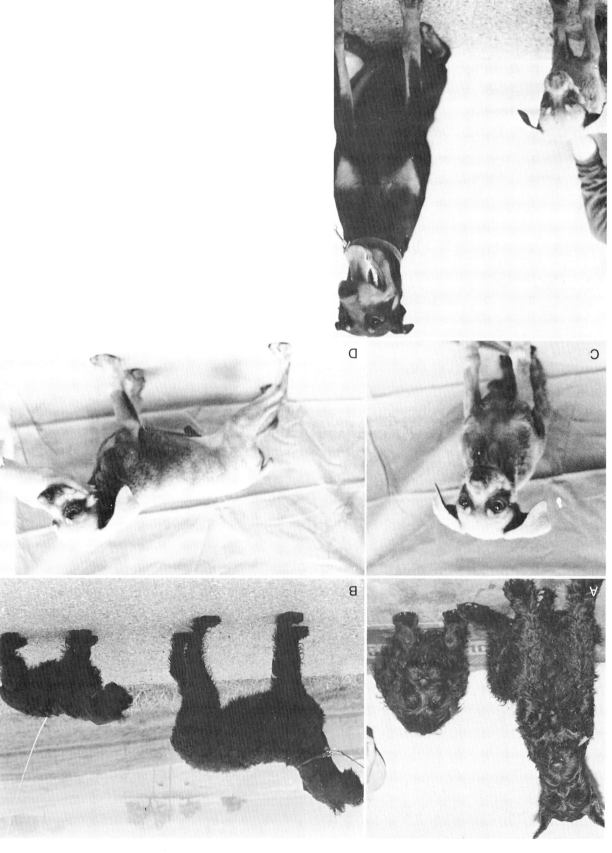

FIGURE 3-12 A and B, Eight-month-old female Giant Schnauzer littermates. The dog on the left is normal, whereas the smaller dog on the right has congenital hypothyroidism (cretinism). Note the small stature, disproportionate body size, large broad head, wide square trunk, and short limbs in the hypothyroid dog. **C and D,** A 3-year-old male Doberman Pinscher with congenital hypothyroidism. Note the small stature, juvenile appearance, and retention of a soft, fluffy puppy hair coat. **E,** Same dog as in **C** and **D,** shown next to his female littermate.

survival time is not affected by hypothyroidism. Evaluation of red blood cell morphology may reveal increased concentrations of leptocytes (target cells). These cells are believed to develop from increased erythrocyte membrane cholesterol loading, a direct result of the concomitant hypercholesterolemia associated with thyroid deficiency. Platelet counts are normal to increased, and platelet size is normal to decreased in dogs with hypothyroidism (Sullivan et al., 1993).

Serum Biochemistry Panel

The classic abnormality seen on a screening biochemistry panel is fasting hypercholesterolemia, which is present in approximately 75% of hypothyroid dogs. Fasting hypertriglyceridemia is also very common. Thyroid hormones stimulate virtually all aspects of lipid metabolism, including synthesis, mobilization, and degradation. Both the synthesis and degradation of lipids are depressed in hypothyroidism, with degradation affected more than synthesis. The net effect is an accumulation of plasma lipids in hypothyroidism and the potential for development of atherosclerosis (Hess et al., 2003). Lipoprotein electrophoretic evaluation of plasma from 26 hypothyroid dogs revealed three general groups of findings: (1) normal plasma lipid concentrations and lipoprotein electrophoresis; (2) hypercholesterolemia with increased intensity of the alpha$_2$-lipoprotein band; and (3) hypercholesterolemia and hypertriglyceridemia with prominent pre-beta, beta, and alpha$_2$-lipoprotein bands (Rogers et al., 1975). Hyperlipidemia and altered lipoprotein electrophoretic patterns normalized following supplementation with thyroid hormone. A more recent study used a combined ultracentrifugation and precipitation technique to quantify plasma lipoprotein concentrations in 10 dogs with hypothyroidism (Barrie et al., 1993). The plasma concentrations of cholesterol, very–low-density lipoprotein (VLDL) cholesterol, low-density lipoprotein (LDL) cholesterol, and high-density lipoprotein (HDL) cholesterol were significantly higher compared with healthy dogs. Thyroid hormone deficiency-induced decrease in hepatic LDL receptor activity and reduced activities of lipoprotein lipase and hepatic lipase were proposed as the underlying mechanisms responsible for the lipoprotein cholesterol abnormalities identified in hypothyroid dogs (Valdemarsson et al., 1983). Fasting hypercholesterolemia and hypertriglyceridemia can be associated with several other disorders (Box 3-4) and thus are not pathognomonic for hypothyroidism. However, their presence in a dog with appropriate clinical signs is strong supportive evidence for hypothyroidism.

BOX 3-4   Causes of Hyperlipidemia in the Dog and Cat

Postprandial hyperlipidemia
Secondary hyperlipidemia
  Hypothyroidism
  Hyperadrenocorticism
  Diabetes mellitus
  Pancreatitis
  Cholestasis
  Hepatic insufficiency
  Nephrotic syndrome
  Protein-losing enteropathy
Primary hyperlipidemia
  Idiopathic hyperlipoproteinemia (Miniature Schnauzer)
  Idiopathic hyperchylomicronemia (cat)
  Lipoprotein lipase deficiency (cat)
  Idiopathic hypercholesterolemia
  Drug-induced hyperlipidemia
    Glucocorticoids
    Megestrol acetate (cat)

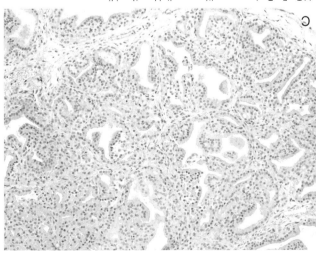
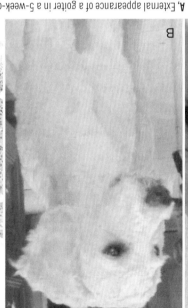
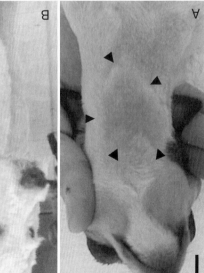

FIGURE 3-13 A, External appearance of a goiter in a 5-week-old Toy Fox Terrier puppy with congenital hypothyroidism. (Reprinted with permission from Fyfe JC, et al.: Congenital hypothyroidism with goiter in toy fox terriers, *J Vet Intern Med* 17:50, 2003.) **B,** A 16-month-old Spanish Water dog with congenital hypothyroidism and goiter. The dog was started on supplementation at 4- week-old and avoided all growth and morphologic abnormalities except the huge goiter. Histopathologic appearance of goiter from the Spanish Water dog shown above at 17-months-old. The gland measured 4.5 x 2.5 x 2 cm. There are typical dyshormonogenic features including diffuse follicular epithelial cell hyperplasia, with colloid spaces largely filled with cuboidal to columnar epithelial cells piled up as blunt papillae (Courtesy of Dr. John C. Fyfe, Associate Professor Microbiology and Molecular Genetics, Michigan State University.)

Mild hypercalcemia has been reported in some dogs with congenital hypothyroidism and has also been reported in an adult dog with hypothyroidism (Loberti, 2011). Hypercalcemia has been documented in hypothyroid children secondary to increased intestinal absorption and decreased urinary excretion of calcium (Henik and Dixon, 2000).

Hyponatremia occurs in dogs with myxedema coma (Atkinson and Aubert, 2004; Henik and Dixon, 2000).

Hypothyroid dogs may have a mild to moderate increase in serum lactate dehydrogenase (LDH), aspartate aminotransferase (AST), alanine aminotransferase (ALT), and alkaline phosphatase (AP) activities. These increases are believed to be associated with hypothyroid myopathy. In a study of nine dogs with experimentally induced hypothyroidism, a subclinical myopathy associated with increases in creatine kinase, AST, and lactate dehydrogenase was documented within 6 months of induction of hypothyroidism (Rossmeisl et al, 2009).

Urinalysis

Results of urinalysis are usually normal in dogs with hypothyroidism. In dogs with lymphocytic thyroiditis, concurrent immune-complex glomerulonephritis may result in proteinuria (Mansfeld and Mooney, 2006). Although an increased risk of glomerulonephritis would be expected in dogs with thyroiditis, there are few reports of dogs with both conditions in the published literature.

Other Hormone Concentrations

Hypothyroidism can affect the secretion of nonthyroidal hormones from other endocrine glands—most notably the pituitary gland. In dogs, chronic hypothyroidism induces hypersecretion of GH possibly due to transdifferentiation of somatotrophic pituitary cells to thyrosomatotropes (Diaz-Espiñeira 2008a; 2008b; 2009). Thyroid hormone deficiency–induced increase in TRH secretion can stimulate prolactin secretion, resulting in hyperprolactinemia and, in intact female dogs, inappropriate lactation (Chastain and Schmidt, 1980; Cortese et al, 1997, Diaz-Espiñeira, 2009).

DERMATOHISTOPATHOLOGIC FINDINGS IN HYPOTHYROIDISM

Histopathology of skin biopsies is sometimes recommended as part of the diagnostic evaluation for hypothyroidism. Unfortunately histopathology findings in the various disorders associated with noninflammatory alopecia are often nonspecific and do not discriminate between Alopecia X, hyperadrenocorticism, hyperestrogenism, recurrent flank alopecia, and hypothyroidism. Histopathologic findings common to all these disorders include increased kenogen (hairless) follicles, decreased anagen and catagen follicles, excessive trichilemmal keratinization, follicular atrophy, or follicular dystrophy. The only feature that distinguished hypothyroid biopsies from those of other noninflammatory causes of alopecia was a significantly thicker epidermis and dermis and fewer atrophic follicles (Münerer et al, 2012).

RADIOGRAPHY, ULTRASONOGRAPHY, AND NUCLEAR IMAGING

Conventional Radiography

Conventional radiography is not a routine procedure for evaluation of acquired canine hypothyroidism. Cervical radiography is ineffective in determining the status of the thyroid gland except when thyroid neoplasia is suspected (see Chapter 5). In congenital hypothyroidism, radiographic abnormalities include delayed epiphyseal ossification (Fig. 3-14): epiphyseal dysgenesis (i.e., irregularly formed, fragmented, or stippled epiphyseal centers), most common in the humeral, femoral, and proximal tibial condyles; short broad skulls; shortened vertebral bodies; and delayed maturation (Greco et al, 1991; Saunders and Jezyk, 1991; Mooney and Anderson, 1993). Ventral borders of vertebral bodies may be scalloped, suggesting lack of normal longitudinal growth (see Fig. 3-14). Overall length of the diaphyses of long bones is reduced, and carpal and tarsal bones appear to have retarded ossification. Valgus deformities are common. Accelerated epiphyseal ossification occurs during thyroid hormone supplementation, but degenerative joint changes with consequent osteoarthritis may develop despite thyroid hormone supplementation (Saunders and Jezyk, 1991).

Ultrasonography

The thyroid gland can be identified and its size, shape, and echogenicity determined using real-time ultrasonography in dogs. Ultrasonography is commonly employed for evaluation of suspected thyroid neoplasms, especially for guidance in performing needle biopsy (see Chapter 5). Ultrasound may also be helpful in differentiating between hypothyroidism and the euthyroid sick syndrome. The normal thyroid gland is homogenous and well delineated with a hyperechoic capsule. The parenchyma is hyperechoic to the surrounding muscles, and the size is correlated with the size (body surface area) of the dog (Bromel, 2006). The thyroid lobe in healthy dogs is fusiform in shape with a triangular to oval shape on the transverse view (Fig. 3-15). Differences in thyroid lobe size and echogenicity between hypothyroid and euthyroid dogs have been documented and are helpful in assessment of thyroid function (Bromel et al, 2005; Reese et al, 2005; Taeymans et al, 2007a; 2007b). In dogs with hypothyroidism, the thyroid lobes tend to be round or oval in shape on the transverse plane, are hypoechoic compared to surrounding musculature, and have a smaller volume and cross-sectional area relative to body size. One study reported a diagnostic specificity of 96% for diagnosis of hypothyroidism using relative thyroid volume and relative cross sectional area (Reese et al, 2005). Sensitivity was 98% for diagnosis of hypothyroidism when combining evaluation of relative thyroid volume and echogenicity relative to the sternothyroid muscle (Reese et al, 2005). Changes in the thyroid gland progress with time, and in early hypothyroidism the thyroid lobes may appear relatively normal on ultrasound examination. It is also important to recognize that there is relatively high interobserver variability for thyroid gland measurements, and sequential studies should ideally be performed by the same operator.

Nuclear Imaging

Thyroid scintigraphy is useful for evaluating the size, shape, and location of thyroid tissue (see Chapters 4 and 5). Either technetium-99m pertechnetate ($^{99m}TcO_4$) or iodine-123 (^{123}I) can be used for scintigraphy in dogs. $^{99m}TcO_4$ is concentrated but not organified by the thyroid gland and is the most commonly used isotope used for thyroid scintigraphy in veterinary medicine because of its low cost, short half-life, and safety (no beta emissions). On scintigraphy, normal canine thyroid lobes appear as two uniformly dense, symmetric ovals in the mid-cervical area (Fig. 3-16), although asymmetrical uptake has been reported in some euthyroid dogs, particularly Greyhounds (Pinilla et al, 2009). The thyroid lobes are slightly smaller than the parotid salivary glands, which also concentrate $^{99m}TcO_4$. A 1:1 thyroid-to-salivary ratio is considered normal in the dog, although there is some variability depending upon the time of the scan in relation to radioisotope administration (Adams 1997, Taeymans et al, 2007a). Percentage thyroidal uptake of radioisotope

can also be calculated with euthyroid dogs having a percentage uptake of approximately 1% of the administered dose. Scintigraphy is regarded as one of the gold standard methods for differentiating between hypothyroid and euthyroid dogs. Adult dogs with primary hypothyroidism typically have low or non-detectable accumulation of radioisotope by the thyroid gland, and the thyroid gland may also appear smaller than normal (see Fig. 3-16). Similar results are found in puppies with congenital hypothyroidism caused by thyroid dysgenesis and dogs with secondary hypothyroidism (Greco et al, 1991; Kintzer and Peterson, 1991). In contrast, puppies with congenital hypothyroidism caused by iodination defects have normal to enlarged thyroid lobes and normal to increased $^{99m}TcO_4$ uptake. Dogs with nonthyroidal illness should also have normal isotope uptake. In a study of 14 dogs with histologically confirmed hypothyroidism and 13 dogs with nonthyroidal illness, the percentage uptake of technetium at 60 minutes in the hypothyroid dogs ranged from 0.03% to 0.26% of the injected dose, whereas in the

dogs with nonthyroidal illness uptake ranged from 0.39% to 1.86% with no overlap between the groups (Diaz-Espiñeira et al, 2007; Fig. 3-17). In another study, however, some dogs had uptake in the equivocal range of 0.3% to 0.33% (Shiel et al, 2012). Thyroiditis may cause false positive results on scintigraphy (normal or increased uptake in a hypothyroid dog) and increased iodine intake may cause a false positive (low uptake in a euthyroid dog). Glucocorticoid administration may also cause suppression of thyroidal radioisotope uptake into the equivocal range (Shiel et al, 2012). Isotope uptake is typically normal or increased in dogs with hypothyroidism induced by potentiated sulfonamides (Hall et al, 1993; Gookin et al, 1999).

BLOOD TESTS OF THYROID GLAND FUNCTION

Function of the thyroid gland is typically initially assessed by measuring baseline serum thyroid hormone concentrations. Evaluating the responsiveness of the thyroid gland to provocative stimulation

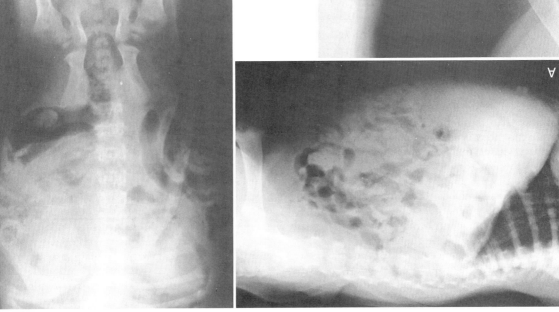
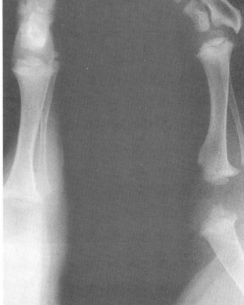

FIGURE 3-14 A and B, Lateral and ventrodorsal radiographs of the spine of a dog with congenital hypothyroidism. Note the shortened vertebral bodies with scalloped ventral borders and only partially calcified vertebral endplates. **C,** Lateral and anteroposterior radiograph of the tibia and fibula of a dog with congenital hypothyroidism, illustrating epiphyseal dysplasia and poor calcification of the bones.

(e.g., TSH stimulation test) is considered to be the gold standard for definitive diagnosis of thyroid dysfunction, but this is rarely performed in clinical practice because of the expense of recombinant TSH. Baseline tests to assess thyroid gland function include measurement of T_4, fT_4, 3,5,3'-T_3, free T_3 (fT_3), 3,3',5'-triiodothyronine (rT_3), and endogenous TSH concentration. T_4 accounts for the majority of the thyroid hormone secreted by the thyroid gland, with only small quantities of T_3 and minor amounts of rT_3 released. Once secreted into the circulation, more than 99% of T_4 is bound to plasma proteins. The unbound, or free, T_4 is biologically active, exerts negative feedback inhibition on pituitary TSH secretion (see Fig. 3-5), and is capable of entering cells throughout the body (Fig. 3-18). Protein-bound T_4 acts as a reservoir and buffer to maintain a steady concentration of free hormone in the plasma, despite rapid alterations in the delivery of thyroid hormone to tissues. Serum T_4 concentrations represent the sum of the

protein-bound and free levels circulating in the blood, whereas fT_4 concentration is a measure of the free hormone only.

Within the cell, fT_4 is de-iodinated to form either T_3 or rT_3, depending on the metabolic demands of the tissues at that particular time (see Fig. 3-18). T_3 is preferentially produced during normal metabolic states, whereas rT_3, which is biologically inactive, is produced during periods of illness, starvation, or excessive endogenous catabolism. Intracellular T_3 binds to nuclear receptors and exerts its physiologic effects by activation of target genes. T_3 is believed to be the primary hormone that induces physiologic effects, because of its greater biologic activity and volume of distribution compared with T_4, the preferential de-iodination of T_4 to T_3 within the cell, and the presence of specific intracellular receptors for T_3 (Yen and Brent, 2013).

All serum T_4, both protein-bound and free, comes from the thyroid gland. Therefore tests that measure the serum total and

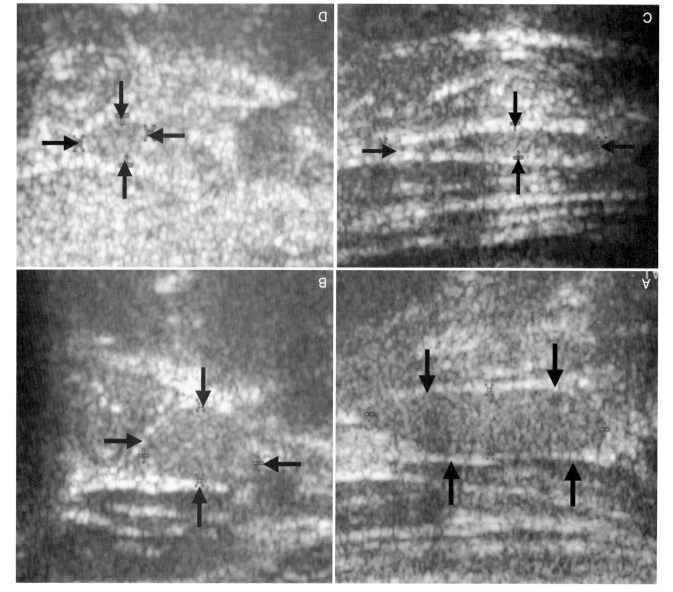

FIGURE 3-15 Longitudinal and transverse ultrasound images of the left thyroid lobe in a healthy Golden Retriever dog (**A and B**) and a Golden Retriever dog with hypothyroidism (**C and D**). Note the smaller size of the thyroid lobe in the dog with hypothyroidism compared with the healthy dog. The maximum length, width, and height of the thyroid lobe measured 24.8 mm, 7.9 mm, and 4.6 mm in the healthy dog and 20.2 mm, 4.1 mm, and 2.8 mm in the hypothyroid dog.

FT$_4$ concentrations, in conjunction with the serum TSH concentration, are currently recommended for the assessment of thyroid gland function in dogs suspected of having hypothyroidism. In contrast, most T$_3$ and rT$_3$ is formed through the deiodination of T$_4$ in extrathyroidal sites—most notably the liver, kidney, and muscle. Serum T$_3$ concentration is a poor gauge of thyroid gland function because of its predominant intracellular location and the minimal amount of T$_3$ secreted by the thyroid gland compared with T$_4$. Thus measurement of serum T$_3$, FT$_3$, or rT$_3$

concentration is not routinely recommended for the assessment of thyroid gland function in dogs.

Baseline Serum Total Thyroxine Concentration

Assay Technique

Baseline serum total T$_4$ concentration is the sum of both protein-bound and free hormone circulating in the blood. In the last few years, new methods for measurement of total T$_4$ have been

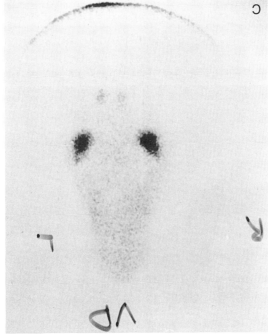

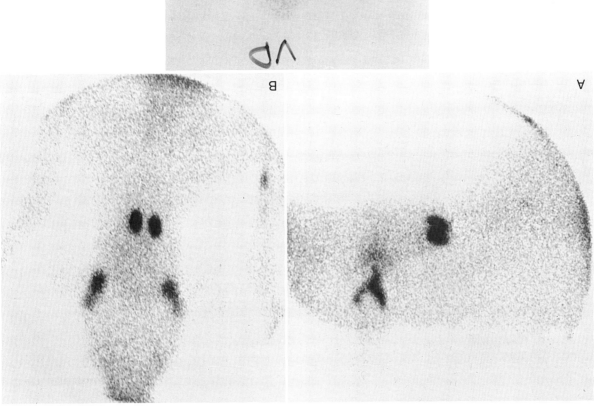

FIGURE 3-16 A and B, Lateral and ventrodorsal views of a sodium pertechnetate nuclear scan performed in a normal dog. The normal thyroid lobes appear as two uniformly dense symmetric spots in the cervical region. The parotid salivary glands are also visible. **C,** Ventrodorsal view of a sodium pertechnetate nuclear scan performed in a dog with primary hypothyroidism. Uptake of sodium pertechnetate is normal by the parotid salivary glands, which are readily visible, but is markedly reduced by the thyroid lobes, which are barely visible.

technique must be sensitive enough to detect T_4 concentrations less than 1.0 µg/dL to accurately differentiate hypothyroidism from euthyroidism in dogs. For most laboratories, the serum T_4 concentration in healthy dogs ranges between 1.0 and 3.5 µg/dL. The lower limit of the normal range varies between laboratories, depending on whether the laboratory wants greater specificity or sensitivity for the test (see Interpretation of Results later).

Chemiluminescent Immunoassays

Many reference laboratories now use chemiluminescent immunoassays for measurement of total T_4 in dogs, and studies suggest that these assays provide similar and consistent results compared to RIA (Kemppainen and Birchfield, 2006). In chemiluminescent assay systems, unlabeled hormone in the patient sample competes for antibody sites with a known amount of thyroid hormone labeled with an enzyme, such as alkaline phosphatase. The amount of the labelled hormone binding to the antibody in the tube is detected by addition of a chemiluminescent substrate rather than a radioactive label. Sample and reagents are automatically pipetted into the test unit, which is then incubated. Unbound material is removed by washing, and a chemiluminescent substrate is added to the test unit. Light emission is read with a sensitive photon counter. These assays have the advantage of speed, automation, and are much safer for laboratory personnel because radioactive isotopes are not utilized. Appropriate reference ranges provided by laboratories should be used to interpret the results.

Point-of-care enzyme-linked immunosorbent assays (ELISAs) for measuring serum T_4 in dogs and cats are also available for in clinic use. The advantage of an in-house test is that it is economical, quick, easy to perform, and it allows the clinician to make recommendations the same day the animal is evaluated. Evaluations of an in-house ELISA (Snap T_4 test kit and VetTest Snap Reader; IDEXX Laboratories Inc., Westbrooke, ME) for quantitative measurement of serum T_4 concentration in dogs and cats have been conflicting. In one study, substantial discrepancies between the in-house ELISA and RIA results for T_4 concentrations were detected (Lurye et al, 2002). In dogs, the in-house ELISA both overestimated and underestimated the serum T_4 concentration compared with a RIA assay. Interpretation of the ELISA results from 62% of 50 samples would have led to inappropriate clinical decisions. In cats, the in-house ELISA consistently overestimated the serum T_4 concentration obtained with RIA, and interpretation of the ELISA results from 50% of 50 samples would have led to inappropriate clinical decisions. In contrast, another study found good correlation between the in-house ELISA and both RIA and chemiluminescent assays for measurement of serum T_4 in feline and canine blood samples; in general total T_4 concentrations measured by RIA were lower than for the other two methods, emphasizing that laboratory-specific reference ranges should always be utilized (Kemppainen, 2006). Because a quality control system is an important part of maintaining assay consistency, accuracy of any point-of-care ELISA should always be documented in an ongoing quality control program by comparing ELISA and RIA results from the same blood samples.

Stability and Factors Interfering with Measurement

T_4 is a relatively stable hormone that is resistant to degradation by contact with cells in blood, long-term storage following centrifugation, hemolysis, or repeated thawing and freezing (Reimers et al, 1991). In addition, serum may be stored in plastic tubes for 8 days at room temperature and for 5 days at 37° C without affecting the concentration of T_4 (Behrend et al, 1998). This is also true for heparinized plasma and ethylenediaminetetraacetic acid

developed and are increasingly replacing the use of radioimmunoassays (RIAs), which have been considered the gold standard for measurement of serum T_4 concentration.

The reference range for serum T_4 concentration varies between laboratories because of differences in laboratory technique and the specific commercial kit utilized. There is excellent cross-reactivity for thyroid hormone between species. Most assays for measurement of serum thyroid hormones are manufactured for use in humans, although there are now some canine-specific commercial assays. Baseline serum T_4 concentrations are lower in healthy dogs than in humans (1.0 to 3.5 versus 4.0 to 10.0 µg/dL, respectively) because of weaker protein binding in dogs, hence the RIA

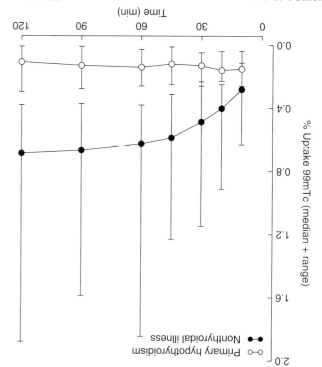

FIGURE 3-17 Median values and ranges for thyroidal uptake of $^{99m}TcO_4$- measured as percent uptake of injected dose, in 14 dogs with primary hypothyroidism and 13 dogs with nonthyroidal illness. (From Diaz-Espineira, Assessment of thyroid function in dogs with low plasma thyroxine concentration, *J Vet Intern Med* 21[1]:25-32, 2007.)

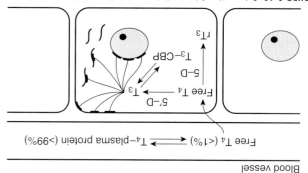

FIGURE 3-18 Schematic of intracellular metabolism of free T_4 (fT_4) to either triiodothyronine (T_3) or reverse T_3 (rT_3) by 5'- or 5-monodeiodinase, respectively. Intracellular T_3 formed from monodeiodination of fT_4 can interact with T_3 receptors on the cell membrane, mitochondria, or nucleus of the cell and stimulate the physiologic actions of thyroid hormone or bind to cytoplasmic binding proteins (*CBP*). The latter forms an intracellular storage pool for T_3.

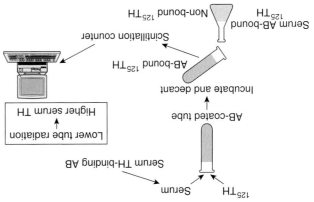

FIGURE 3-19 Schematic illustration of how anti-thyroid hormone antibodies may cause spuriously increased thyroid hormone values for a radioimmunoassay (RIA) using a single-step, antibody-coated tube separation system. Patient serum and radiolabeled thyroid hormone (which comes with the assay) are added to a test tube coated with anti-thyroid hormone antibody. Thyroid hormone in serum competes with radiolabeled thyroid hormone for antibody-binding sites in the tube. After incubation, the liquid in the tube is decanted, the radioactivity of the tube is measured in a scintillation counter, and the serum thyroid hormone concentration is determined based on the tube radioactivity. An inverse relationship exists between tube radioactivity and serum thyroid hormone concentration. If anti-thyroid hormone binding antibodies are present in the patient's serum, these antibodies compete with the antibodies attached to the tube for serum thyroid hormone and radiolabeled thyroid hormone. Because serum thyroid hormone and radiolabeled thyroid hormone are not attached to the tube, they are decanted along with any radiolabeled thyroid hormone that has bound to them. This causes a falsely low radioactivity of the tube and a correspondingly high serum thyroid hormone value. *AB,* Antibody; *TH,* thyroid hormone.

(EDTA) plasma samples; however, storage of serum or plasma at 37° C in glass can cause a significant increase in serum T_4 concentration, compared with storage at −20° C (Behrend et al., 1998). Because of potential for environmental extremes during shipping, whenever possible, blood samples should be centrifuged, serum should be decanted into plastic tubes, frozen, and sent to the laboratory on cold packs.

Many physiologic and pharmacologic factors influence the pituitary-thyroid axis and interfere with the accuracy of baseline serum T_4 concentration for differentiating hypothyroidism from euthyroidism (see Factors Affecting Thyroid Gland Function Tests). However, the only factor that directly interferes with the ability of an assay to measure T_4 is the presence of anti-T_4 antibodies in the serum sample. Anti-thyroid hormone antibodies occur in dogs with lymphocytic thyroiditis and are present in approximately 2% of dogs with clinical signs of hypothyroidism and 15% of hypothyroid dogs (Nachreiner et al., 2002; Graham et al., 2007). Anti-T_4 antibodies may cause spuriously increased or decreased serum T_4 values (Thacker et al., 1992). The effect of anti-thyroid hormone antibodies on the serum T_4 value depends on the type of assay being used by the laboratory, but in most currently utilized commercial assays, anti-T_4 antibodies cause a spurious increase in the measured T_4 concentration (Fig. 3-19). Although antibody interference can potentially lead to a falsely increased T_4 concentration, the probability of antibody interference resulting in a falsely normal T_4 concentration appears to be quite low (Piechotta et al., 2010). Hyperlipidemia and hemolysis do not affect measurement of T_4 in serum by RIA (Lee et al., 1991; Reimers et al., 1991); for other assay methods, the individual laboratory should be contacted for information about assay interference by hyperlipidemia and hemolysis.

Interpretation of Results

Measurement of the serum T_4 concentration can be used as the initial screening test for hypothyroidism or used in a thyroid panel, which typically includes T_4, FT_4, TSH, and an antibody test for lymphocytic thyroiditis (Fig. 3-20). Theoretically, the interpretation of baseline serum T_4 concentration should be straightforward: that is, dogs with hypothyroidism should have low values compared with healthy dogs. Unfortunately, the range of serum T_4 concentration overlaps between hypothyroid dogs and healthy dogs, and this overlap becomes more evident in euthyroid dogs with nonthyroidal illness (Fig. 3-21). In one study, the range of serum T_4 concentration in 62 healthy dogs was 1.0 to 3.3 μg/dL, and in 51 hypothyroid dogs it was from undetectable to 1.5 μg/dL (Nelson et al., 1991). The amount of residual thyroid gland function at the time the sample is obtained, the suppressive effects of extraneous factors especially concurrent nonthyroidal illness on serum thyroid hormone concentrations, and the presence of circulating anti-thyroid antibodies all affect the sensitivity and specificity of serum T_4 concentration in diagnosing hypothyroidism.

These overlap between euthyroidism and hypothyroidism creates a dilemma when a laboratory tries to establish its normal range for serum T_4 concentration. If the laboratory keeps the lower limit of the normal serum T_4 range high (e.g., 1.5 μg/dL), sensitivity of the test is sacrificed for specificity. That is, the number of hypothyroid dogs misdiagnosed as euthyroid is minimized, but the number of euthyroid dogs misdiagnosed as hypothyroid is increased, leading to inappropriate thyroid replacement treatment of euthyroid dogs. Alternatively, by decreasing the lower limit of the normal serum T_4 range (e.g., 0.8 μg/dL), specificity is sacrificed for sensitivity. The number of euthyroid dogs misdiagnosed as hypothyroid is minimized, but the number of hypothyroid dogs misdiagnosed as euthyroid increases.

The reference range for serum T_4 concentration also varies between breeds. The reference range is usually established based on the mean ± two standard deviations calculated from results of serum T_4 measured in a large population of dogs without regard for breed. The reference range for serum T_4 and FT_4 measured by modified equilibrium dialysis (MED) is now recognized to be lower in some breeds—most notably Sighthounds (Gaughan and Bruyette, 2001; Shiel et al., 2007a; Table 3-5). These findings suggest that breed-specific reference range values for thyroid hormone tests should be established and used when evaluating thyroid gland function. Until such information is established, interpretation of thyroid hormone test results in such breeds will continue to be challenging.

The use of an arbitrary serum T_4 value to separate euthyroidism from hypothyroidism is not recommended. Rather, the serum T_4 result should be evaluated in the context of the history, physical examination findings, and other clinicopathologic data (Tables 3-6 and 3-7; see Fig. 3-20). All of this information yields an index of suspicion for euthyroidism or hypothyroidism. For the clinician, it is difficult to judge the influence of extraneous factors, especially concurrent illness, on the serum T_4 concentration. Although nonthyroidal illness can suppress the baseline serum T_4 concentration to less than 0.5 μg/dL in a euthyroid dog, hypothyroid dogs rarely have serum T_4 concentrations greater than 1.5 μg/dL, so the baseline serum T_4 concentration is best used to rule out hypothyroidism. The higher the T_4 concentration, the more likely the dog is euthyroid. The one exception is the hypothyroid

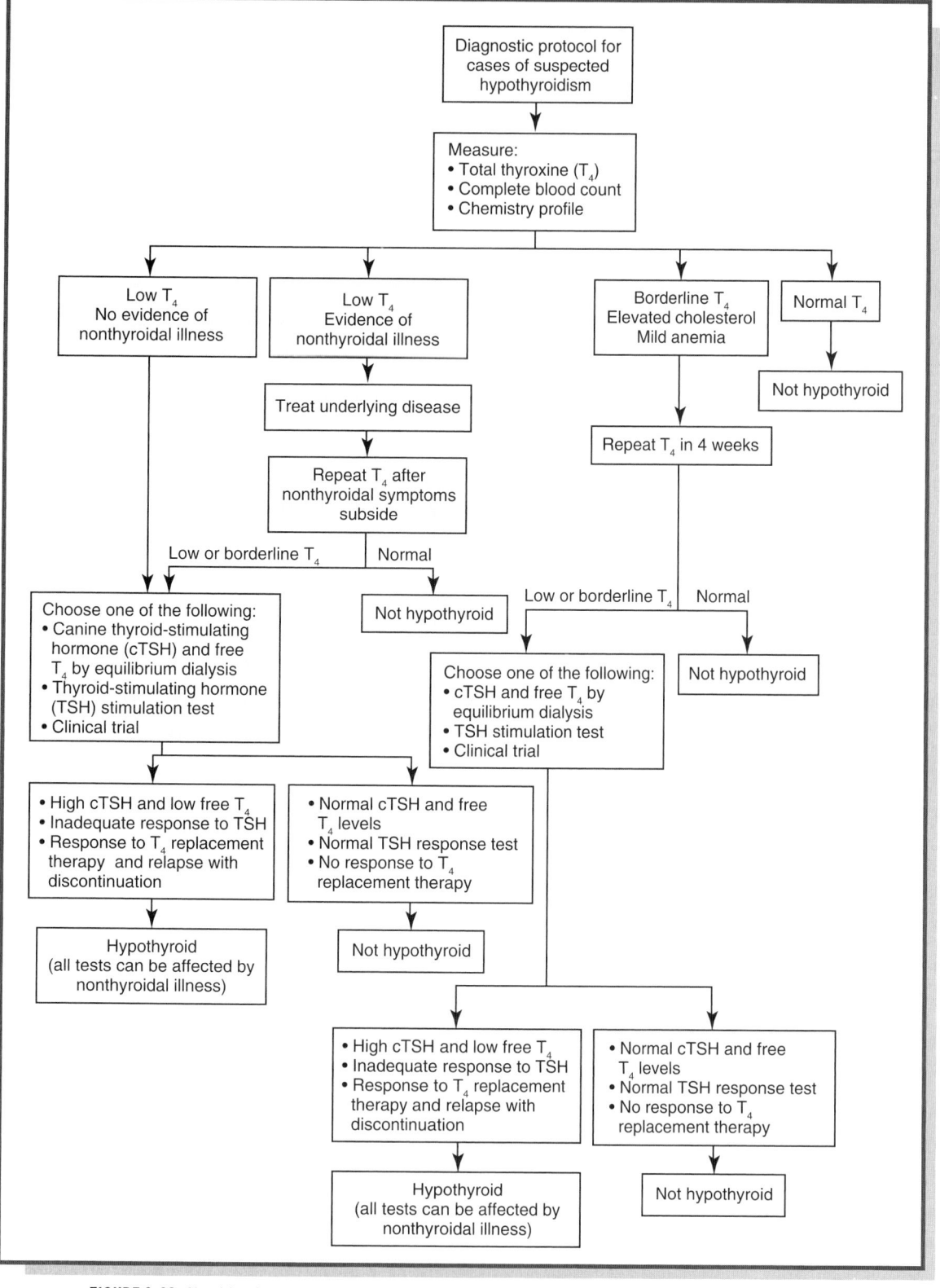

FIGURE 3-20 Algorithm for diagnosis of canine hypothyroidism. (From Ettinger SJ, Feldman EC, editors: *Textbook of veterinary internal medicine*, ed 7, St Louis, 2010, Elsevier, p. 1756.)

dog with circulating anti-thyroid hormone antibodies (see Fig. 3-19). Conversely, the lower the T_4 value, the more likely the dog has hypothyroidism, assuming the history, physical examination findings, and clinicopathologic data are also consistent with the disease and severe systemic illness is not present. If the clinician's index of suspicion is not high for hypothyroidism but the serum

T_4 concentration is low, other factors such as nonthyroidal illness should be strongly considered.

Interpretation: Concurrent Thyroid Hormone Supplementation

Occasionally, a clinician wants to determine whether a dog receiving thyroid supplementation is, in fact, hypothyroid. The

exogenous administration of thyroid hormone, either T_4 or T_3, will suppress pituitary TSH secretion and cause pituitary thyrotroph atrophy, and subsequently thyroid gland atrophy in a healthy euthyroid dog (Panciera et al, 1990). Immediately after withdrawal of exogenous supplementation, serum T_4, and fT_4, may be decreased or undetectable; the severity of the decrease is dependent on the severity of thyroid gland atrophy induced by the thyroid hormone supplement. Basal serum T_4 and response to TRH and TSH results may be suggestive of hypothyroidism, in a previously euthyroid dog, if the testing is performed within a month of discontinuing treatment (Panciera, 2002). Thyroid hormone supplementation must be discontinued, and the pituitary-thyroid axis must be allowed to recover function before meaningful results of baseline serum T_4, fT_4, and TSH concentrations can be obtained. The time interval between the discontinuation of thyroid hormone supplementation and the acquisition of meaningful results regarding thyroid gland function depends on the duration of treatment, the dosage and frequency of administration of the thyroid hormone supplement, and individual variability. As a

general rule, thyroid hormone supplements should be discontinued a minimum of 4 weeks and preferably 6 to 8 weeks before critically assessing thyroid gland function.

Baseline Serum Total Triiodothyronine Concentration

Assay Technique

Serum total T_3 concentrations are the sum of the protein-bound and free levels circulating in the blood. Almost all commercial laboratories currently use either RIA or chemiluminescent techniques for measuring T_3 concentrations in the blood. Most human RIAs for T_3 are suitable for use in the dog, because blood concentrations are similar for both species. Using the RIA technique, an approximate normal range for blood T_3 concentrations is 0.8 to 2.1 nmol/L—although the exact range varies from laboratory to laboratory because of differences in assays used and laboratory technique.

Stability and Factors Interfering with Measurement

Stability of serum T_3 and factors interfering with its measurement are as described for serum T_4. In dogs with suspected hypothyroidism, the incidence of anti-T_3 antibodies is greater than that of anti-T_4 antibodies (6% of dogs with suspected hypothyroidism) (Nachreiner et al, 2002).

Interpretation of Results

Measurement of baseline serum T_3 concentration is of minimal value in differentiating euthyroidism from hypothyroidism in the dog (Fig. 3-22). Essentially no difference exists in the mean or range of serum T_3 concentration between groups of healthy dogs, dogs with hypothyroidism, and dogs with concurrent illness (Nelson et al, 1991; Miller et al, 1992). The majority of circulating T_3 is produced from deiodination of T_4 at extra thyroidal sites, and thyroidal secretion of T_3 and peripheral tissue 5'-deiodination of T_4 to T_3 may increase with mild thyroid gland dysfunction (Ciger, 1980; Lum et al, 1984). In addition, the high proportion of anti-T_3 antibodies in hypothyroid dogs contributes to the poor diagnostic performance of T_3. When anti-T_3 positive dogs were excluded, the diagnostic performance of T_3 was similar to that of T_4 (Graham et al, 2007). Although serum T_3 is included as part of the canine thyroid panel run by some commercial diagnostic laboratories, it has limited diagnostic value. Measurement of T_3 may be justified in Greyhounds who tend to have low concentrations of T_4 and fT_4 but T_3 concentrations within the laboratory reference range (Shiel et al, 2007a; Pinilla et al, 2009; see Table 3-5).

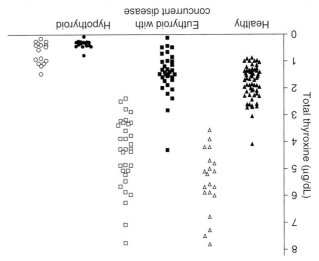

FIGURE 3-21 Serum total T_4 concentrations in healthy dogs, hypothyroid dogs, and euthyroid dogs with concurrent disease before and after administration of thyroid-stimulating hormone (TSH). (From Scott-Moncrieff J, Nelson RW. Change in serum thyroid-stimulating hormone concentration in response to administration of thyrotropin-releasing hormone to healthy dogs, hypothyroid dogs, and euthyroid dogs with concurrent disease. *J Am Vet Med Assoc* 213[10]:1435-1438, 1998.)

TABLE 3-5   CANINE BREEDS WITH UNIQUE THYROID HORMONE REFERENCE RANGES

BREED	TOTAL THYROXINE (↑ OR N)	FREE THYROXINE (↑ OR N)	TOTAL TRIIODOTHYRONINE (↑ OR N)	THYROTROPIN (↑ OR N)	THYROXINE RESPONSE TO TSH
Greyhound	↑	↑	Usually N	N	Decreased
Whippet	↑	N	—	N	
Saluki	↑	↑	↑	N or ↑	
Sloughi	↑	↑ or ↓ (ED)	—	↑	Normal to slightly decreased
Basenji	↑	—	—	N	—
Irish Wolfhound	↑	—	—	—	
Conditioned Alaskan sled dogs	↑	↑	↑		Variable

Baseline Serum Free Thyroxine Concentration

Although the gold standard technique for measurement of FT$_4$ is equilibrium dialysis, this technique is expensive and time consuming and is only performed in research laboratories. In commercial laboratories, canine serum FT$_4$ is measured by one of three methods: modified equilibrium dialysis (MED), analog RIA, or analog chemiluminescent assay. In MED assays, a short dialysis step is used to separate free from protein-bound T$_4$ followed by radioimmunoassay for FT$_4$. Analog methods measure FT$_4$ directly by RIA or chemiluminescence, but the reagents are optimized for human serum and depend upon the dominance of hormone binding by TBG (Ferguson, 2007). MED techniques are regarded as the most accurate commercially-available technique for determining serum FT$_4$ concentrations in dogs. In one study, the accuracy of one MED technique for FT$_4$ was 95% (Fig. 3-23) (Peterson et al, 1997). In

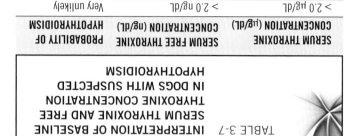

TABLE 3-6 INTERPRETATION OF BASAL THYROID HORMONE AND THYROTROPIN CONCENTRATIONS*

	NORMAL THYROXINE/FREE THYROXINE	DECREASED OR BORDER-LINE NORMAL THYROXINE/FREE THYROXINE
Normal dog	Hypothyroid, normal varia-tion, or concurrent illness	Consider further thyroid testing only if strong clinical suspi-cion of hypothyroidism
TSH Normal		Consider further diagnostic evaluation of thyroid function (e.g., thyroid au-toantibodies, provocative testing) or therapeutic trial
TSH Increased	Early subclinical hypothy-roidism or recovery from concurrent illness	Hypothyroid Consider revaluation of thyroid function in 1 to 3 months; if indicated, use therapeutic monitoring to adjust dose
		Lifelong therapy with L-T$_4$

*T$_4$, free T$_4$, TSH.

TABLE 3-7 INTERPRETATION OF BASELINE SERUM THYROXINE AND FREE THYROXINE CONCENTRATION IN DOGS WITH SUSPECTED HYPOTHYROIDISM

SERUM THYROXINE CONCENTRATION (µg/dL)	SERUM FREE THYROXINE CONCENTRATION (ng/dL)	PROBABILITY OF HYPOTHYROIDISM
> 2.0 µg/dL	> 2.0 ng/dL	Very unlikely
1.5 to 2.0 µg/dL	1.5 to 2.0 ng/dL	Unlikely
1.0 to 1.5 µg/dL	0.8 to 1.5 ng/dL	Unknown
0.5 to 1.0 µg/dL	0.5 to 0.8 ng/dL	Possible
< 0.5 µg/dL	< 0.5 ng/dL	Very likely*

*Assuming that a severe systemic illness is not present.

ATA, Anti-thyroglobulin antibody; L-T$_4$, levothyroxine, or L-thyroxine; T$_4$, thyroxine; TSH, thyroid-stimulating hormone, or thyrotropin.

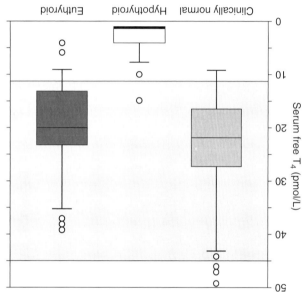

FIGURE 3-22 Baseline serum T$_3$ concentrations in 35 healthy dogs, 35 dogs with hypothyroidism, and 30 euthyroid dogs with concurrent dermatopathy. Note the overlap in serum T$_3$ results between the three groups of dogs.

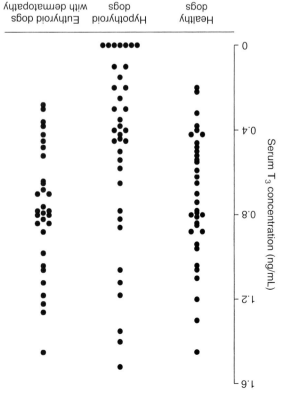

FIGURE 3-23 Box plots of serum free T$_4$ (fT$_4$) concentrations in 150 clinically normal dogs, 54 hypothyroid dogs, and 54 euthyroid dogs with nonthyroidal disease. The box represents the interquartile range (i.e., 25th to 75th percentile range, or the middle half of the data). The horizontal bar in the box represents the median value. For each box plot, the T bars represent the main body of data. Outlying data points are represented by open circles. The shaded area indicates the reference range for the serum free T$_4$ concentration. (From Peterson et al.: Measurement of serum total thyroxine, triiodothyronine, free thyroxine, and thyrotropin concentrations for diagnosis of hypothyroidism in dogs, *J Am Vet Med Assoc* 211[11]:1398, 1997.)

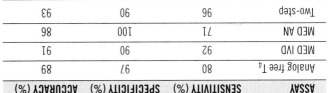

TABLE 3-8 | **SENSITIVITY, SPECIFICITY AND ACCURACY OF FOUR FREE THYROXINE ASSAYS IN DOGS***

ASSAY	SENSITIVITY (%)	SPECIFICITY (%)	ACCURACY (%)
Analog free T_4	80	97	89
MED IVD	92	90	91
MED AN	71	100	98
Two-step	96	90	93

T_4, Thyroxine.

*The dog population included 56 dogs with clinical signs of hypothyroidism (31 euthyroid, 25 hypothyroid). Assays included the IMMULITE 2000 Veterinary Free T_4 (*Analog free T_4*) (Siemens Health Care Diagnostics), Direct Free T_4 by Equilibrium Dialysis (*MED IVD*) (IVD technologies), free T_4 by equilibrium dialysis (*MED AN*) (Antech Diagnostics), and GammaCoat Free T_4 radioimmunoassay (RIA) (Diasorin Inc).

more recent studies, reported accuracy of different MED assays has ranged from 86% to 93%, compared with an accuracy of 75% to 85% for serum T_4 (Nelson et al, 1991; Scott-Moncrieff et al, 1994; 2011; Peterson et al, 1997). It is important to use a FT_4 assay that has been demonstrated to have adequate diagnostic performance in dogs, because some human analog assays for FT_4 have accuracy that is no better than measurement of total T_4 in dogs (Schachter, 2004), whereas others compare favorably to the MED methods (Table 3-8) (Scott-Moncrieff et al, 2011). Serum for measurement of FT_4 can be stored in plastic tubes and shipped without cooling if assayed within 5 days (Behrend et al, 1998); however, because of the potential for extremes of temperature during transportation, it is recommended that serum samples are frozen and shipped to the laboratory on ice packs. In general, serum FT_4 concentrations greater than 1.5 ng/ dL are consistent with euthyroidism, and values less than 0.8 ng/ dL (especially those less than 0.5 ng/dL) are suggestive of hypothyroidism, assuming that the history, physical examination, and clinicopathologic abnormalities are also consistent with the disorder and severe systemic illness is not present (see Table 3-7). Circulating anti-thyroid hormone antibodies do not affect the FT_4 results determined by the MED technique but may still influence FT_4 measured by analog methods. Serum FT_4 is less affected by the suppressive effects of nonthyroidal illness than is the serum T_4, although severe illness can cause FT_4 concentrations to decrease below 0.5 ng/dL; see Concurrent Illness (Nonthyroidal Illness Syndrome). The reference range for serum FT_4 concentration is also lower in some breeds, such as the Greyhound (see Table 3-5) (Shiel et al, 2007a).

Baseline Serum Free Triiodothyronine Concentration

Serum FT_3 is derived from intracellular 5'-deiodination of FT_4 in peripheral tissues and, to a lesser extent, in the thyroid gland. The theoretical principle behind measuring serum FT_3 is similar to that for FT_4. RIAs designed for measurement of serum FT_3 in humans have been used in the dog. A critical assessment of the sensitivity and specificity of these RIAs has not been reported in dogs, nor has the diagnostic usefulness of measuring serum FT_3 for evaluating thyroid gland function been demonstrated.

Baseline Serum Reverse Triiodothyronine Concentration

rT_3 is a relatively inactive product of T_4 5'-deiodination (see Fig. 3-4). The vast majority of rT_3 is produced intracellularly from T_4; very little is secreted by the thyroid gland. Serum rT_3 concentration

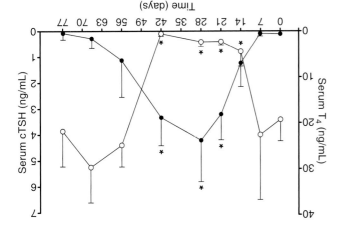

FIGURE 3-24 Mean serum thyroxine (T_4; ○) and canine thyroid-stimulating hormone (cTSH; •) concentrations after experimental induction of hypothyroidism (day 0) and treatment with levothyroxine (L-T_4 sodium, beginning on day 42). Bars represent SD. *Significantly (P < 0.05) different from day 0 values. (From Williams DA, et al.: Validation of an immunoassay for canine thyroid-stimulating hormone and changes in serum concentration following induction of hypothyroidism in dogs. *J Am Vet Med Assoc* 209[10]:1730, 1996.)

can be measured by specific RIAs that do not cross-react with T_4 or T_3. The clinical benefit of measuring rT_3 has not yet been demonstrated in dogs, and the assay has limited availability.

Baseline Serum Thyrotropin Concentration

TSH is a highly glycosylated molecule with an alpha and beta subunit. The alpha subunit is identical to that of the alpha subunit of the related glycoprotein hormones LH, FSH, and chorionic gonadotrophin, whereas the beta subunit is unique to TSH and confers the biologic properties of TSH. Assays for measurement of human TSH cannot be used to measure canine TSH. The first assay for canine TSH was validated in 1996 (Williams et al, 1996), and since that time there have been other commercial assays developed. Studies in dogs with ^{131}I-induced hypothyroidism have shown good assay performance with a 35-fold increase in the mean serum TSH concentration after induction of hypothyroidism and return of the mean serum TSH concentration to baseline after treatment with L-T_4 sodium (Fig. 3-24) (Williams et al, 1996). The assay used most commonly is the chemiluminescent TSH assay (Immulite Canine TSH), which has been demonstrated to have the highest precision compared to immunoradiometric and enzyme immunometric methods (Marca et al, 2001). Unfortunately all current commercial assays for canine TSH have poor sensitivity for diagnosis of spontaneous hypothyroidism. Twenty percent to 40% of dogs with hypothyroidism have TSH concentrations within the reference range, giving a test sensitivity of only 63% to 82% (Fig. 3-25). Although TSH as a stand-alone test has also poor specificity because of overlap in results between hypothyroid dogs and euthyroid dogs with concurrent illness (see Fig. 3-25), clinical studies have shown that a high serum TSH concentration has high specificity (90% or higher) for diagnosis of hypothyroidism in dogs when the baseline serum T_4 or FT_4 concentration is concurrently low (Dixon et al, 1996; Ramsey et al, 1997; Peterson et al, 1997; Scott-Moncrieff et al, 1998).

The reason for the low sensitivity of TSH for diagnosis of canine hypothyroidism has been the subject of investigation, because TSH is a highly sensitive diagnostic test in humans.

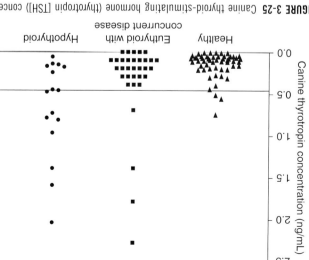

FIGURE 3-25 Canine thyroid-stimulating hormone (thyrotropin [TSH]) concentrations in healthy dogs, hypothyroid dogs, and euthyroid dogs with concurrent disease. (From Scott-Moncrieff JC, et al.: Comparison of serum concentrations of thyroid-stimulating hormone in healthy dogs, hypothyroid dogs, and euthyroid dogs with concurrent disease. *J Am Vet Med Assoc* 212[3]:389, 1998.)

Studies in dogs with ^{131}I-induced hypothyroidism demonstrated that over several months' time there was a loss of the TSH response to the low T_4 concentration, hypersecretion of GH, hyposecretion of prolactin, and pituitary enlargement (Fig. 3-26). The enlarged pituitary glands were characterized by thyrotroph hyperplasia, presence of large pale staining vacuolated "thyroid deficiency" cells similar to those observed in hypothyroid rats and humans, and double staining cells indicative of transdifferentiation of somatotrophs into thyrotrophs. The presence of mitoses in the thyrotrophs suggested that the division of pre-existing thyrotrophs or less differentiated stem cells contributed to the "thyroid deficiency" cells. It was hypothesized by the study authors that persistent stimulation of thyrotrophs via negative feedback led to TRH-receptor desensitization and gradual loss of TSH secretion (Diaz-Espiñeira, 2008b). Similar changes were demonstrated in dogs with spontaneous chronic hypothyroidism, and this is likely the reason for the poor sensitivity of the TSH assay in naturally occurring hypothyroidism (Diaz-Espiñeira, 2009). Other possible reasons that hypothyroid dogs might have serum TSH concentrations within the reference range include pulsatile TSH secretion, resulting in ultradian fluctuations (Fig. 3-27), secondary hypothyroidism, suppression of pituitary TSH secretion by concurrent disease or drug administration, and inability of the current TSH assay to detect all isoforms of circulating TSH (Kooistra et al, 2000b). Sample collection time does not appear to predictably influence serum TSH test results (Bruner et al, 1998; see Fig. 3-27). The lower limit of the reference range in dogs is currently below the sensitivity of the TSH assay, so it is not possible to differentiate low from normal serum TSH concentrations, which impairs the ability to identify secondary hypothyroidism, suppression of pituitary TSH secretion by concurrent drugs and diseases, and excess administration of L-T_4 sodium during treatment of hypothyroidism.

Because of the limitations discussed earlier, the serum TSH concentration should always be interpreted in conjunction with the serum T_4 or FT_4 concentration measured in the same blood sample and should never be used as the sole test for assessing thyroid gland function. A low serum T_4 or FT_4 concentration and a high TSH concentration in a blood sample obtained from a dog with appropriate history and physical examination findings supports

the diagnosis of primary hypothyroidism, whereas a finding of normal serum T_4, FT_4, and TSH concentrations rules out hypothyroidism. Any other combination of serum T_4, FT_4, and TSH results is difficult to interpret (see Table 3-6).

Thyrotropin Stimulation Test

The TSH stimulation test evaluates the thyroid gland's responsiveness to exogenous TSH administration and is a test of thyroid gland reserve. The TSH stimulation test is indicated in dogs with low basal thyroid hormone concentrations to differentiate hypothyroidism from nonthyroidal illness syndrome (NTIS). The biologic activity of the TSH molecule is not species-specific so human recombinant TSH can be used for the test; however, this product is extremely expensive and is only available in a vial containing 1.1 mg of lyophilized recombinant TSH synthesized in a genetically modified Chinese hamster ovary cell line. TSH (Thyrogen; Genzyme Corporation, Cambridge, ME) is reconstituted in 1.2 mL of sterile water for injection (final solution 0.9 mg/mL). This is sufficient TSH for 7 to 15 stimulation tests depending upon the dose used. Recombinant TSH can be reconstituted and stored at 4° C for 4 weeks or frozen at –20° C for up to 12 weeks (De Roover et al, 2007).

The protocol for the TSH stimulation test requires collection of a serum sample for measurement of T_4, followed by administration of 75 to 150 μg of TSH intravenous (IV). An additional blood sample for measurement of total T_4 is collected 6 hours later (Boretti et al, 2006a; 2006b; De Roover et al, 2006). The higher dose of TSH is recommended in dogs with concurrent disease and those receiving medication (e.g., glucocorticoids) that might suppress thyroid function (Boretti et al, 2009). Hypothyroidism is confirmed by a pre and post total T_4 concentration below the reference range for basal total T_4 concentration (< 1.5 μg/dL). Euthyroidism is confirmed by a post total T_4 concentration > 2.5 μg/dL and at least 1.5 times the basal T_4 concentration (see Fig. 3-21). Serum FT_4 concentrations increase in a manner similar to serum total T_4 concentrations but do not provide additional diagnostic information, and therefore are not routinely measured in the TSH stimulation test. Although the TSH stimulation is more accurate for assessment of thyroid function than measurement of basal thyroid hormone concentrations, false positive results can occur. In a study of 30 dogs in which the diagnosis of thyroid status was confirmed histopathologically, some euthyroid dogs failed to respond to bovine TSH administration, and nuclear imaging had higher discriminatory power for diagnosis of true thyroid status than TSH stimulation results (Diaz-Espiñeira et al, 2007). Stimulation results that fall in the intermediate range may also lead to interpretation difficulties especially in dogs with nonthyroidal illness. Interpretation of the results of the TSH stimulation test should take into consideration the clinical signs and severity of concurrent systemic disease, results of other thyroid testing (total T_4, FT_4, TSH, ATA concentration), and results of nuclear scintigraphy if available.

Thyrotropin-Releasing Hormone Stimulation Test

Indications

The TRH stimulation test evaluates the pituitary gland's responsiveness to TRH and the thyroid gland's responsiveness to TSH secreted in response to TRH administration. In humans, the TRH stimulation test is used to differentiate secondary and tertiary hypothyroidism. TRH response tests are not routinely performed for evaluation of humans with suspected primary hypothyroidism; however, there is a greater and more prolonged increase in TSH

concentration after TRH administration in humans with primary hypothyroidism than in healthy humans. In contrast, dogs with primary hypothyroidism have a lower change in TSH concentration after TRH administration than do healthy dogs (Scott-Moncrieff et al, 1998). This finding has been attributed to TRH receptor desensitization due to persistent stimulation of the pituitary thyrotrophs by the negative feedback loop (Diaz-Espineira, 2008b). In dogs, the TRH stimulation test has been used to differentiate between hypothyroidism and the NTIS in dogs with low basal thyroid hormone concentrations; however the test can be difficult to interpret because of the relatively small increase in serum T_4 concentration after TRH administration, and the test has little advantage for diagnosis of hypothyroidism over measurement of baseline TSH and total or free T_4 concentration. The primary current use of the TRH stimulation test is to assess anterior pituitary function as part of a combined pituitary function test.

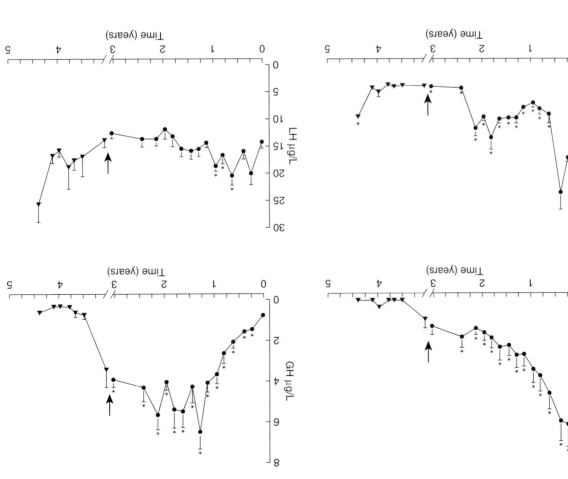

FIGURE 3-26 Mean basal plasma concentrations of thyrotropin *(TSH)*, growth hormone *(GH)*, prolactin *(PRL)*, luteinizing hormone *(LH)*, and adrenocorticotropic hormone *(ACTH)* measured at monthly intervals in seven Beagle dogs with hypothyroidism induced at time 0. Three of these dogs were followed up for another 1½ years while on levothyroxine (L-thyroxine; L-T_4) sodium supplementation *(arrow)*. (From Diaz-Espineira MM, et al.: Functional and morphological changes in the adenohypophysis of dogs with induced primary hypothyroidism: loss of TSH hypersecretion, hypersomatotropism, hypoprolactinemia, and pituitary enlargement with transdifferentiation. *Domest Anim Endocrinol* 35[1]:98-111, 2008.)

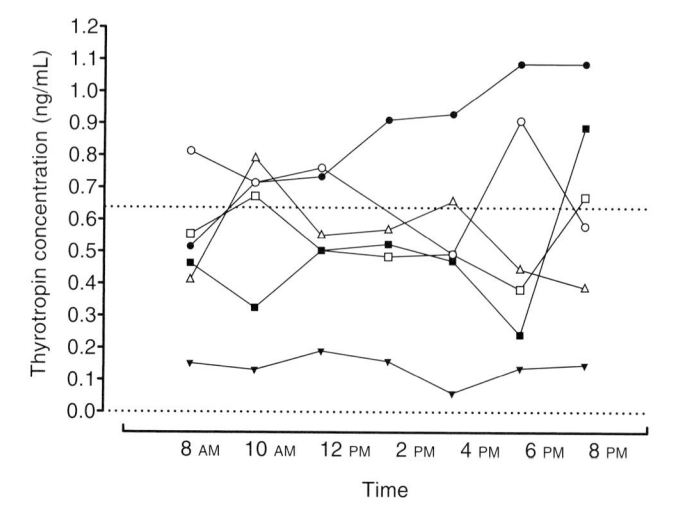

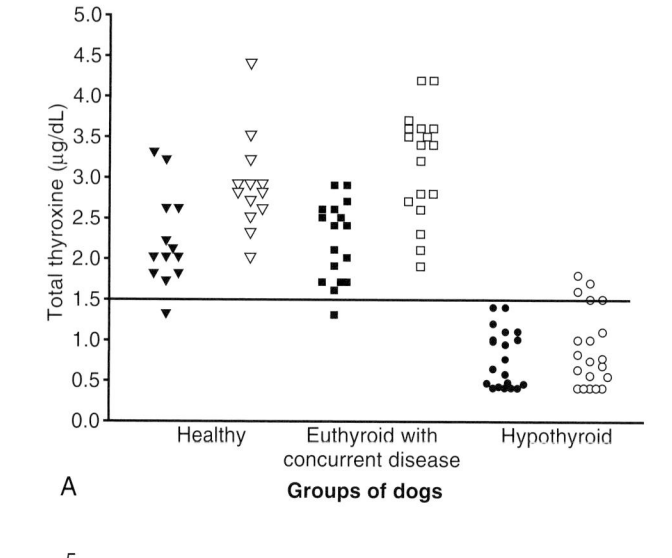

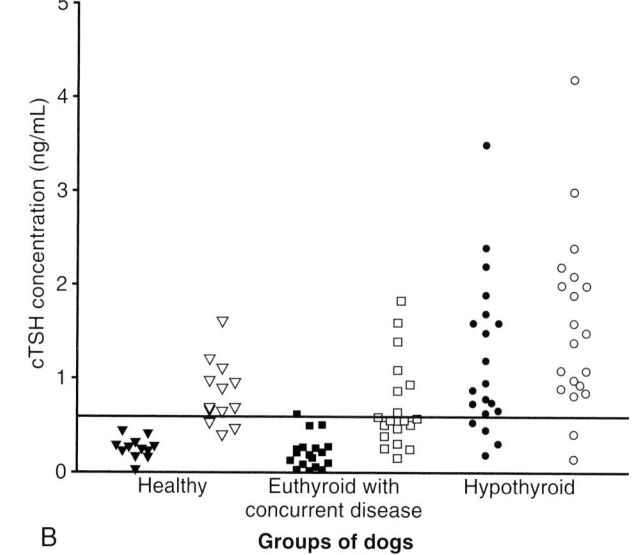

FIGURE 3-27 Serum thyrotropin (TSH) concentrations measured at 2-hour intervals from 8 AM to 8 PM in six dogs with naturally developing hypothyroidism. Reference range is between the *horizontal dotted lines.* Each symbol represents values obtained for one hypothyroid dog. (From Bruner JM, et al.: Effect of time of sample collection on serum thyroid-stimulating hormone concentrations in euthyroid and hypothyroid dogs, *J Am Vet Med Assoc* 212[10]:1572, 1998.)

Protocol

TRH is administered at a dose of 10 μg/kg or 200 μg/dog IV; blood for serum total T4 determination is obtained before and 4 hours after TRH administration, and blood for serum TSH determination is obtained before and 30 minutes after TRH administration (Scott-Moncrieff and Nelson, 1998). Measurement of serum TSH concentration after TRH administration is used to assess pituitary responsiveness to TRH, whereas measurement of serum T_4 concentration is used to assess the thyroid gland's responsiveness to the TRH-induced increase in pituitary TSH secretion. Serum fT_4 concentrations increase in a manner similar to serum T_4, do not provide additional diagnostic information, and therefore are not routinely measured.

Interpretation

The increase in serum total T_4 concentration is less dramatic with TRH than with TSH (Frank, 1996). Euthyroid dogs should have a post-TRH serum T_4 concentration greater than 1.5 to 2.0 μg/dL (Scott-Moncrieff et al, 1998). In contrast, dogs with primary hypothyroidism have a post-TRH serum T_4 concentration below the normal baseline serum T_4 range (i.e., < 1.5 μg/dL) (Fig. 3-28), but there is substantial overlap between the groups, and some euthyroid dogs fail to have any increase in T_4 after TRH administration. Because of these findings, there is currently little indication for the use of the TRH stimulation test in the evaluation of dogs with suspected hypothyroidism. TRH is not currently commercially available in the United States.

![] TESTS FOR LYMPHOCYTIC THYROIDITIS

During the inflammatory phase of lymphocytic thyroiditis, antibodies are released into the circulation. In dogs, the predominant antibody that arises is directed against Tg. Tg is a large complex protein molecule with several epitopes and antibodies formed against it are heterogenous. The thyroid hormones T_3 and T_4 are haptens and do not elicit an antibody response unless attached to a larger protein molecule (Gaschen et al, 1993). When an epitope contains a hormonogenic site, antibodies that cross-react with either T_3 or T_4 may develop. These antibodies are a subset of total

FIGURE 3-28 Thyroxine (T_4) concentration (**A**) and thyrotropin (TSH) concentration (**B**) before *(solid symbol)* and 30 minutes (for TSH) and 4 hours (for T_4) after *(open symbols)* administration of TRH to healthy dogs, hypothyroid dogs, and euthyroid dogs with concurrent diseases. The *horizontal line* represents the upper limit of the reference range for T_4 (**A**) and TSH (**B**). (From Scott-Moncrieff JC, Nelson RW: Change in serum thyroid-stimulating hormone concentration in response to administration of thyrotropin-releasing hormone to healthy dogs, hypothyroid dogs, and euthyroid dogs with concurrent disease, *J Am Vet Med Assoc* 213[10]:1435, 1998.)

ATAs and therefore dogs with thyroid hormone autoantibodies also have autoantibodies against Tg, whereas the converse is not true (Graham et al, 2007). Thus the Tg autoantibody test is a more sensitive test for lymphocytic thyroiditis than is measurement of anti-T_3 and anti-T_4 antibodies. Anti-TPO antibodies are the most common antibodies detected in human thyroiditis, but they are only detected in 17% of dogs with thyroiditis and are not detected in dogs that lack ATAs (Skopek et al, 2006). Assays for anti-TPO antibodies, therefore, have little clinical utility and are not currently commercially available.

Serum Thyroglobulin Autoantibodies

Circulating Tg autoantibodies are detected in approximately 50% of hypothyroid dogs (Nachreiner et al, 1998; Graham et al, 2007).

A commercially available ELISA (Oxford Biomedical Research Inc., Oxford, MI) for detection of T$_g$ autoantibodies has been shown to be sensitive and specific for identification of T$_g$ autoantibodies (Nachreiner et al, 1998). This ELISA is currently the most common T$_g$ autoantibody assay used by commercial laboratories and results are expressed as a percentage of a standardized positive control. Non-specific binding ELISA plates that do not contain T$_g$ are included to reduce the effect of nonspecific immunoglobulin G (IgG). Some of the initial concern about borderline positive results after vaccination may have been related to nonspecific antibody binding.

Presence of serum T$_g$ autoantibodies implies the presence of thyroiditis within the thyroid gland but provides no information on the severity or progressive nature of the inflammatory response or the function of the thyroid gland. Detection of T$_g$ autoantibodies should not be used as the sole criteria to establish the diagnosis of hypothyroidism but can increase the index of suspicion for

hypothyroidism in dogs with consistent clinical findings and equivocal basal thyroid hormone concentrations. Dogs with confirmed hypothyroidism can have negative T$_g$ autoantibody concentrations, and euthyroid dogs can be positive for T$_g$ autoantibodies. The value of serum T$_g$ autoantibodies as a marker for eventual development of hypothyroidism remains to be clarified. A 1 year longitudinal study of 171 dogs with positive T$_g$ autoantibody and normal serum FT$_4$ and TSH test results, found that approximately 20% of dogs developed decreased FT$_4$ and/or increased TSH concentrations consistent with hypothyroidism during the 1 year of follow-up. Fifteen percent of dogs reverted to negative T$_g$ autoantibody status with no change in FT$_4$ and TSH concentrations, and 65% remained T$_g$ autoantibody positive or had an inconclusive result with no change in FT$_4$ and TSH test results (Graham et al, 2001).

The prevalence of T$_g$ autoantibodies varies with the breed (Table 3-2). Measurement of T$_g$ autoantibodies has been advocated for

TABLE 3-9 ODDS OF HAVING SERUM THYROID HORMONE AUTOANTIBODIES (THAA) AMONG BREEDS WITH AN INCREASED RISK OF THAA COMPARED WITH DOGS OF ALL OTHER BREEDS

| BREED | NUMBER OF DOGS | Percentage with Autoantibodies | | | | ODDS RATIO | PVALUE |
		TRIIODOTHYRONINE AUTOANTIBODIES	THYROXINE AUTOANTIBODIES	BOTH	TOTAL		
Pointer	118	11.86	0.85	6.78	19.49	3.61	0.001
English Setter	1,246	13.88	1.2	3.53	18.61	3.44	0.001
English Pointer	66	14.14	2.02	2.02	18.18	3.31	0.001
Skye Terrier	53	13.21	1.89	1.89	16.99	3.04	0.001
German Wirehaired Pointer	324	11.42	1.54	2.47	15.43	2.72	0.001
Old English Sheepdog	1,031	10.96	0.87	3.20	15.03	2.65	0.001
Boxer	5,239	9.14	0.88	3.47	13.49	2.37	0.001
Maltese	962	9.56	0.94	2.60	13.10	2.25	0.001
Kuvasz	180	10.56	2.22	0.00	12.78	2.18	0.001
Petit Basset Griffon Vendeen	63	6.35	3.17	3.17	12.69	2.16	0.036
American Staffordshire Terrier	246	8.54	1.22	1.22	10.98	1.84	0.003
Beagle	3,988	7.70	0.80	2.16	10.66	1.79	0.001
American Pit Bull Terrier	676	9.02	0.44	1.18	10.64	1.78	0.001
Dalmatian	2,332	6.82	1.07	2.53	10.42	1.74	0.001
Giant Schnauzer	406	8.37	0.74	1.23	10.34	1.72	0.001
Rhodesian Ridgeback	1,025	8.39	0.39	1.56	10.34	1.72	0.001
Golden Retriever	36,016	7.19	0.77	2.37	10.33	1.90	0.001
Shetland Sheepdog	11,423	7.84	0.61	1.51	9.96	1.69	0.001
Chesapeake Bay Retriever	1,005	7.26	0.70	1.49	9.45	1.56	0.001
Siberian Husky	1,153	6.94	0.69	1.21	8.84	1.45	0.001
Brittany	1,257	6.76	0.72	1.19	8.67	1.42	0.001
Borzoi	527	7.21	0.19	1.14	8.54	1.39	0.034
Australian Shepherd	1,328	5.72	0.60	1.58	7.90	1.28	0.016
Doberman Pinscher	11,084	6.21	0.64	0.77	7.62	1.24	0.001
Malamute	1,449	6.21	0.48	0.90	7.59	1.22	0.042
Cocker Spaniel	18,976	5.83	0.63	0.76	7.22	1.17	0.001
Mixed	42,647	4.92	0.66	0.99	6.57	1.05	0.012
Total all breeds	**287,948**	4.64	0.63	1.03	6.30	NA	NA

From Nachreiner RF, et al.: Prevalence of serum thyroid hormone autoantibodies in dogs with clinical signs of hypothyroidism. J Am Vet Med Assoc 220:468, 2002.

NA, Not applicable.

hypothyroidism caused by lymphocytic thyroiditis if the dog has clinical signs, physical findings, and thyroid hormone test results consistent with the disorder.

FACTORS AFFECTING THYROID GLAND FUNCTION TESTS

Correct interpretation of tests of thyroid gland function is one of the primary diagnostic challenges in canine clinical endocrinology. There are many factors that influence baseline thyroid hormone and endogenous TSH concentrations, including age, breed, body size, diurnal or random fluctuations, athletic training, gender, reproductive status, concurrent illness, and drug therapy. Because many of these factors decrease baseline thyroid hormone concentrations and some can concomitantly increase endogenous TSH in euthyroid dogs, misdiagnosis of hypothyroidism may occur if the clinician accepts the results out of context. In our experience, the most common factors that result in lower baseline thyroid hormone concentrations in euthyroid dogs are concurrent illness (i.e., NTIS), use of drugs (especially glucocorticoids), and random fluctuations in thyroid hormone concentrations. In any given dog, other factors may also influence baseline thyroid hormone concentrations. It is important to recognize the potential influence of these factors when interpreting thyroid hormone test results.

Age

In dogs there is a progressive decline in T_4 concentration with age; serum T_4 concentration is highest in puppies, and the T_4 concentration progressively declines during adulthood. In a study of 27 female Beagles of different ages, mean serum T_4 concentrations in old dogs were 40% lower than those of young adult dogs (Gonzalez and Quadri, 1988). In a larger study of serum collected from 1074 healthy dogs of differing ages, the mean total T_4 concentration was 21% lower in dogs older than 6 years of age compared to young adult dogs; similar trends with age were not identified for serum T_3 concentration (Reimers et al, 1990; Fig. 3-29). In a longitudinal study of 48 Labrador Retrievers studied for 12 years, the mean total T_4 decreased by 29% from the age of 6 to 12 years of age (Lawler et al, 2007). Similar trends occur for FT_4 and serum total T_3 concentrations, although this was not true in a study of healthy Salukis (Reimers et al, 1990; Lawler et al, 2007; Shiel et al, 2010). Older dogs have a higher mean TSH concentration than younger dogs (Bhatti et al, 2006) and middle-aged and older dogs also have a blunted T_4 response to TSH compared to young animals (Gonzalez and Quadri, 1988). Changes in other parameters of thyroid function have been less studied, but increases in anti-T_4 antibody in older dogs have been reported (Lawler et al, 2007). Although older dogs as a group have lower total T_4 concentrations than younger animals, the mean and median total T_4 concentration still falls within the lower end of most reference ranges (Table 3-10). None of the studies cited earlier reported a range for total T_4 in healthy geriatric dogs; it is likely that for many geriatric dogs a total T_4 below the reference range is a normal age related change. Reasons for the decline in thyroid hormone concentrations with age in dogs are not fully understood; proposed reasons include effect of concurrent illness, change in responsiveness of the thyroid gland to TSH, subclinical thyroid pathology (fibrosis, atrophy, degenerative changes), and decreased biologic activity of TSH with age.

screening breeding stock with the aim of ultimately eliminating heritable forms of thyroiditis. The Orthopedic Foundation for Animals (OFA) maintains a thyroid registry and issues a breed-database number to all dogs found to have normal thyroid function at 12 months of age (based on measurement of FT_4, TSH, and T_3 autoantibodies by an OFA-approved laboratory). Each dog also must be examined by a veterinarian. Because hypothyroidism usually develops after 1 year of age, it is recommended that reexamination and retesting occur at 2, 3, 4, 6, and 8 years of age.

Serum Thyroid Hormone Autoantibodies

Thyroid hormone autoantibodies are also considered an indicator of lymphocytic thyroiditis and may be a better predictor of the potential for development of hypothyroidism in dogs. In a recent study, thyroid hormone autoantibodies were detected in 6.3% of 287,948 serum samples from dogs with clinical signs consistent with hypothyroidism (Nachreiner et al, 2002; Table 3-9). T_3 autoantibodies alone were detected in 4.64%, T_4 autoantibodies alone were detected in 0.63%, and both T_3 and T_4 antibodies were detected in 1.03% of the serum samples. An inverse correlation existed between prevalence of thyroid hormone autoantibodies and age of the dogs; females had a significantly higher chance of being positive for thyroid hormone autoantibodies than did males, and neutered males and females had a significantly higher prevalence of thyroid hormone autoantibodies than did sexually intact dogs. Breeds at increased risk for having thyroid hormone autoantibodies were also identified (Table 3-9).

Measurement of serum T_4 and T_3 autoantibodies is offered by some commercial endocrine laboratories as part of an extensive thyroid panel. Testing for serum T_3 and T_4 autoantibodies is indicated in dogs with unexpected or unusual serum T_3 or T_4 test results. T_3 and T_4 autoantibodies may interfere with the RIAs used to measure serum T_3 or T_4 concentrations, causing unexpected and often confusing test results (Graham et al, 2007; see Fig. 3-19). The type of interference depends on the separation system employed in the RIA. Falsely low results are obtained if nonspecific separation methods are used (e.g., ammonium sulfate, activated charcoal); falsely increased values are obtained if single-step separation systems utilizing antibody-coated tubes are used. For most commercially available T_4 assays, T_4 autoantibodies will falsely increase the measured T_4 concentration. The false increase may be enough to raise a hypothyroid dog's result into the reference or hyperthyroid range. The same false increase occurs with non-dialysis (direct) RIAs used for measuring serum FT_4 concentrations (Kemppainen et al, 1996). False elevations in serum FT_4 concentration do not occur if FT_4 is measured using an assay that includes a dialysis step (MED assays), because autoantibodies cannot pass through the dialysis membrane and interfere with the assay. Thus evaluation of serum FT_4 concentration measured by MED should be performed in lieu of measurement of serum T_4 in dogs suspected of having T_4 autoantibodies. Fortunately spurious T_4 values resulting from clinically relevant concentrations of T_4 autoantibody are uncommon (Nachreiner et al, 2002; Piechotta et al, 2010).

Positive serum thyroid hormone autoantibody test results imply pathology in the thyroid gland but provide no information on the severity or progressive nature of the inflammatory response or the extent of thyroid gland involvement, nor are these tests an indicator of thyroid gland function. Dogs with confirmed hypothyroidism should not be used as the sole criteria for establishing the diagnosis of hypothyroidism. T_3 and T_4 autoantibodies can be negative and euthyroid dogs can be positive for thyroid hormone autoantibodies. Identification of T_3 or T_4 autoantibodies support

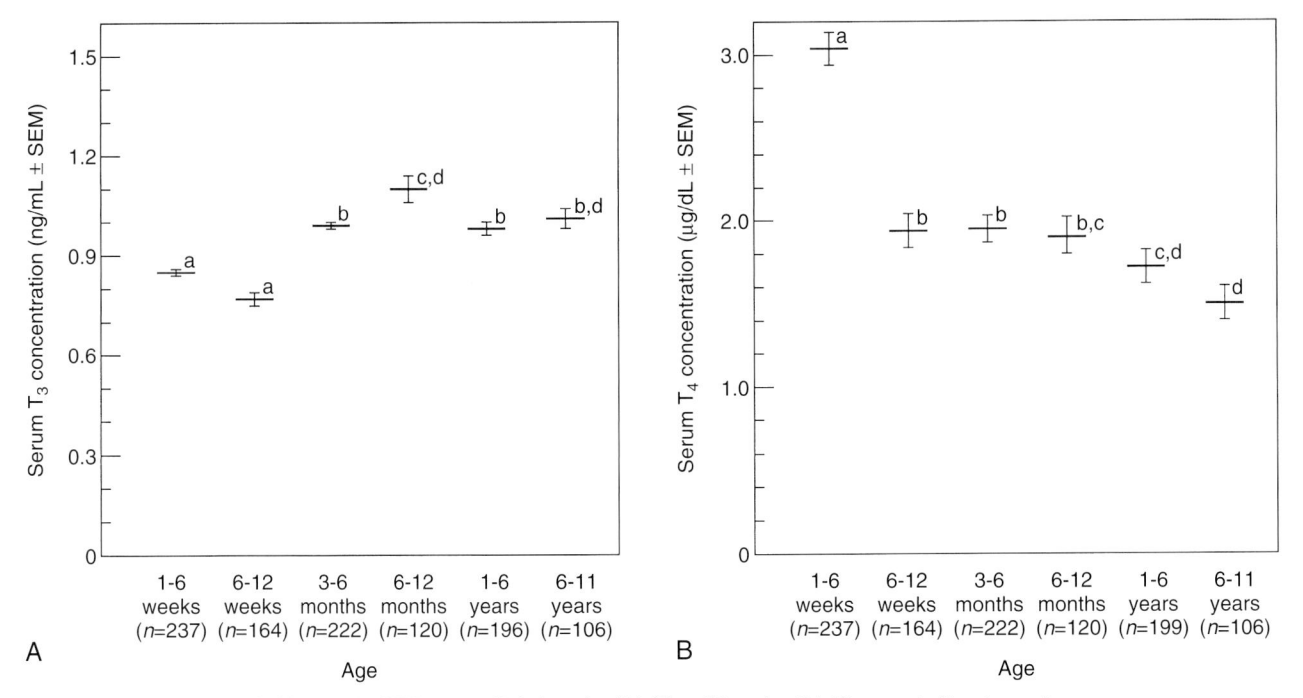

FIGURE 3-29 Mean (± SEM) serum triiodothyronine (T_3) **(A)** and thyroxine (T_4) **(B)** concentrations in nursing puppies (1 to 6 weeks), weanling puppies (6 to 12 weeks), juvenile dogs (3 to 6 months), young adults (6 to 12 months), middle-aged adults (1 to 6 years), and old dogs (6 to 11 years). Means having different superscripts are significantly ($P < 0.05$) different. (Adapted from Reimers TJ, et al.: Effects of age, sex, and body size on serum concentrations of thyroid and adrenocortical hormones in dogs, *Am J Vet Res* 51[3]:454, 1990.)

	TABLE 3-10	**MEAN AND MEDIAN SERUM TOTAL THYROXINE CONCENTRATION OF SAMPLES SUBMITTED TO A REFERENCE LABORATORY FOR DOGS OF DIFFERENT AGES***		
AGE, y	**MEAN THYROXINE, μg/dL**	**MEDIAN THYROXINE, μg/dL**	**NUMBER OF PATIENTS**	
0 to 2	1.94	1.9	1043	
3 to 5	1.91	1.8	2773	
6 to 8	1.83	1.6	6975	
9 to 11	1.75	1.5	5064	
12 to 14	1.67	1.4	4016	
> 14	1.46	1.2	736	
All ages	1.78	1.5	20,607	
Total T_4 reference range	1.0-4.0			

Data was provided by IDEXX Laboratories, Inc., Westbrook, ME.
Modified from Scott-Moncrieff CJ: Thyroid disorders in the geriatric veterinary patient, *Vet Clin North Am Small Anim Pract* 42(4):709, 2012.
*Patients with an age listed as 0 were excluded.

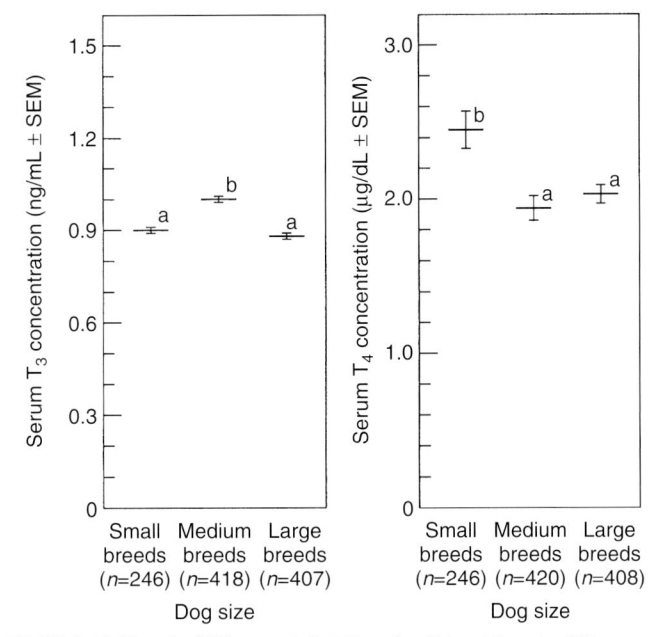

FIGURE 3-30 Mean (± SEM) serum triiodothyronine (T_3) and thyroxine (T_4) concentration in small breed dogs (mean body weight, 7.1 kg), medium breed dogs (mean body weight, 23.3 kg), and large breed dogs (mean body weight, 30.6 kg). Means having different superscripts are significantly ($P < 0.05$) different. (Adapted from Reimers TJ, et al.: Effects of age, sex, and body size on serum concentrations of thyroid and adrenocortical hormones in dogs, *Am J Vet Res* 51[3]:454, 1990.)

Body Size

Comparison of normal thyroid hormone values between groups of dogs based on body size has identified differences in mean serum T_4 and T_3 concentrations (Reimers et al, 1990; Fig. 3-30). Dogs were divided into three groups based on body size. Small dogs had

a mean middle-aged body weight of 7.1 kg and included Poodles, Beagles, and Miniature Schnauzers; medium-sized dogs had a mean middle-aged body weight of 23.3 kg and included English Pointers, English Setters, and Siberian Huskies; large dogs had a mean middle-aged body weight of 30.6 kg and included Black

Breed

Most laboratories report reference ranges based on measurement of thyroid hormone concentrations in large groups of dogs of various breeds and ages; however there are significant differences between breeds in regard to thyroid hormone concentration, particularly for Sighthounds. In a study of 46 young healthy Greyhounds, 91% of the dogs had total T_4 concentration below the non-breed specific reference range, and 16% had total T_4 concentrations that were either at or below the limit of detection of the assay (Shiel et al, 2007a). Free T_4 was lower than the non-breed specific reference range in 21% of dogs and at or below the limit of detection in 13% of dogs. In the same study, T_3 concentrations were all within the non-breed specific reference range. Differences in reference ranges have also been reported for Whippets, Salukis, Sloughis, Basenjis, Borzois, Scottish Deerhounds, Irish Wolfhounds, and conditioned Alaskan sled dogs (van Geffen, 2006; Panacova, 2008; Seavers, 2008; see Table 3-5). The reason for the difference in thyroid hormone concentrations between Greyhounds and other breeds has not yet been elucidated, but studies suggest that it is not due to changes in concentration or function of thyroid binding globulin (Shiel et al, 2011). These findings suggest that breed-specific reference ranges for thyroid hormone tests need to be established and used when evaluating thyroid gland function especially in Sighthounds. For breeds in which total T_4 and fT_4 concentrations are close to the limit of detection in many healthy dogs, diagnosis of hypothyroidism should rely on history, physical examination, results of the complete blood count (CBC) and serum biochemistry panel and multiple tests of thyroid gland function. Measurement of total T_3 may be more useful in Greyhounds than in other breeds, because it is the only measurement that typically falls within the non-breed specific reference range, and because there is a low prevalence of thyroiditis in this breed (Nachreiner et al, 2002).

Athletic Training

Most studies on the effect of athletic training on thyroid function have focused on Alaskan sled dogs and Greyhounds. After sprint racing, total T_4 but not fT_4 concentration decreased after adjustment for hemoconcentration (Hill et al, 2001). Concentrations of T_4, T_3, and fT_4 are below the non-breed specific reference range in conditioned Alaskan sled dogs, and these concentrations decrease further during prolonged endurance racing (Panciera et al, 2003; Lee et al, 2004; Evason et al, 2004). The reported effect of conditioning and racing on serum TSH is variable. Reasons for the change in thyroid hormone concentrations after endurance exercise are poorly defined but likely include nutritional changes, effect of ambient temperature, or an appropriate physiologic response to increased metabolic rate associated with racing.

Gender and Reproductive Stage of the Female

When the specific stage of the female reproductive cycle is not considered and dogs are merely classified as male or female, gender has no apparent effect on serum thyroid hormone concentrations (Reimers et al, 1990). The mean (± SE) serum T_4 and T_3 concentrations in approximately 550 female versus 515 male dogs were 2.11 ± 0.04 versus 2.08 ± 0.04 µg/dL and 0.94 ± 0.01 versus 0.92 ± 0.01 ng/mL, respectively.

Testosterone decreases thyroid-binding protein and can decrease serum T_4 while having little effect on serum fT_4 concentrations (Wenzel, 1981). The effect of testosterone on thyroid hormone test results in dogs is unclear. In one study, serum T_4 concentration increased significantly after male Greyhound dogs were castrated and when not in training (Hill et al, 2001). There was no effect of castration on serum fT_4 or TSH concentration. However, in another study, serum T_4, fT_4, and TSH concentrations were not different between testosterone-treated and untreated female Greyhound dogs, suggesting that exogenous testosterone administration may not affect thyroid hormone test results (Gaughan and Bruyette, 2001).

In the female dog, progesterone (but not estrogen) affects serum T_4 and T_3 concentrations. In one study, serum T_4 and T_3 concentrations were greater in diestrus females, than in females in anestrus, proestrus, lactating females, or male dogs (Reimers et al, 1984). Medroxyprogesterone treatment of five euthyroid bitches once a month for 11 months did not change basal plasma TSH concentration or TRH stimulated TSH concentration (Beierink et al, 2007). In another study, dogs with hyperestrogenism did not have changes in baseline serum T_4 or T_3 concentrations, although the T_4 response to TSH administration was mildly depressed (Gosselin et al, 1980). It has been postulated that progesterone (elevated during pregnancy with or without pregnancy) may enhance the binding affinity of plasma proteins for thyroid hormones, resulting in an increase in serum concentrations of total T_4 and T_3 (Wenzel, 1981).

TABLE 3-11 THYROID FUNCTION TEST RESULTS IN HEALTHY AKITAS, GOLDEN RETRIEVERS, BEAGLES, AND MINIATURE AND TOY POODLES*

VARIABLE	AKITA (N = 12)	GOLDEN RETRIEVER (36)	BEAGLE (12)	TOY AND MINIATURE POODLES (12)	REFERENCE RANGE
Serum T_4 (µg/dL)	2.4 ± 0.9	2.0 ± 0.5	1.9 ± 0.6	1.9 ± 0.5	1.0-3.6
Serum fT_4 (ng/dL)	1.1 ± 0.3	1.1 ± 0.4	1.3 ± 0.5	1.3 ± 0.5	0.8-3.5
Serum cTSH (ng/mL)	0.1 ± 0.1	0.1 ± 0.1	0.2 ± 0.1	0.2 ± 0.1	0.0-0.6
Thyroglobulin autoantibody positive sera	None	None	None	None	NA

From Brömel C, et al.: Compari of ultrasonographic characteristics of the thyroid gland in healthy small-, medium-, and large-breed dogs, *Am J Vet Res* 67(1):72, 2006.

*Data for serum hormone concentrations are presented as mean ± SD.

Diurnal Rhythm

In a study of 11 healthy mixed breed dogs in which blood samples were collected every 3 hours between 8 AM and 8 PM, total T_4 concentration was higher between 11 AM and 8 PM compared to 8 AM (Hoh et al, 2006). For FT_4, the concentrations at 11 AM and 2 PM were higher than those at 8 AM. This suggests the possibility of a diurnal rhythm with a peak in serum thyroid hormone concentration at mid-day in the dog. Further studies are needed to confirm this finding. A diurnal rhythm in TSH secretion was not identified in healthy euthyroid dogs (Bruner et al, 1998; see Fig. 3-27).

Random Fluctuations

Random or pulsatile fluctuations in baseline serum T_3, and T_4, occur in healthy dogs, euthyroid dogs with concurrent illness, and hypothyroid dogs (Fig. 3-31; Kemppainen and Sarin, 1984; Miller et al, 1992). Although there was little fluctuation in TSH concentration during the day in euthyroid dogs, sporadic and pulsatile fluctuations in TSH concentrations during the day were documented in hypothyroid dogs (Bruner et al, 1998; Kooistra et al, 2000a; see Fig. 3-27).

Concurrent Illness (Nonthyroidal Illness Syndrome)

The nonthyroidal illness syndrome (NTIS; euthyroid sick syndrome) refers to suppression of serum thyroid hormone concentrations that occur in euthyroid patients due to concurrent illness. Causes of NTIS include almost any systemic illness, surgery, and trauma, as well as inadequate caloric intake. Disorders such as dermatologic diseases and osteoarthritis are unlikely to cause NTIS (Paradis et al, 2003). Although drugs may also affect thyroid function, thyroid suppression induced by drugs is not

generally included within the definition of NTIS. Mechanisms that are believed to contribute to NTIS include decreased TSH secretion, decreased synthesis of T_4, decreased concentration or binding affinity of circulating binding proteins, presence of serum protein binding inhibitors, inhibition of the de-iodination of T_4 to T_3, or any combination of these factors (Wiesinga and Van den Berghe, 2013). Decreased serum thyroid hormone concentrations are believed to be a physiologic adaptation that decreases cellular metabolism during illness. Generally, the magnitude of the change in serum thyroid hormone concentrations is not related to the specific disorder but rather reflects the severity of the illness, with more severe systemic illness resulting in more severe suppression of serum thyroid hormone concentrations (Kaptein, 1988; Kantrowitz et al, 2001; Mooney et al, 2008; Fig. 3-32). In a study of dogs with idiopathic epilepsy, there was a significant correlation between seizure frequency and thyroid hormone concentrations; the longer the interval between seizures the higher the thyroid hormone concentration (von Klopmann et al, 2006). There was no correlation with the time span between the most recent seizure episode and blood collection, suggesting that it was the severity of illness rather than the seizure itself that suppresses thyroid hormone concentrations. Disorders that are frequently associated with NTIS in dogs include neoplasia, renal disease, hepatic disease, cardiac failure, neurologic disease, inflammatory disorders, and diabetic ketoacidosis. It may be difficult or impossible to establish a diagnosis of concurrent hypothyroidism in dogs with NTIS, especially when relying on results of a single test of thyroid gland function. Normal test results are indicative of euthyroidism, but abnormal test results do not confirm a diagnosis of hypothyroidism because dogs with NTIS often have serum T_4 concentrations that are indistinguishable from true hypothyroidism.

In humans the pattern of thyroid hormone suppression is quite predictable, and T_3 is more commonly suppressed than total T_4 or fT_4 (low T_3 syndrome). In dogs, however, most studies have

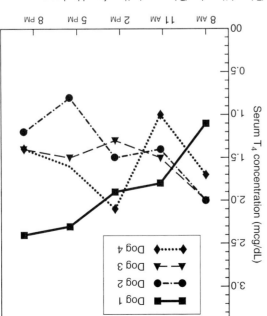
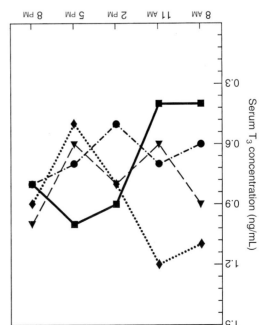

FIGURE 3-31 Sequential baseline serum triiodothyronine (T_3) and thyroxine (T_4) concentrations from blood samples obtained at 8 AM, 11 AM, 2 PM, 5 PM, and 8 PM in four healthy dogs. Note the random fluctuation in serum T_3 and T_4 concentrations throughout the day and the occasional low value, which could result in a misdiagnosis of hypothyroidism.

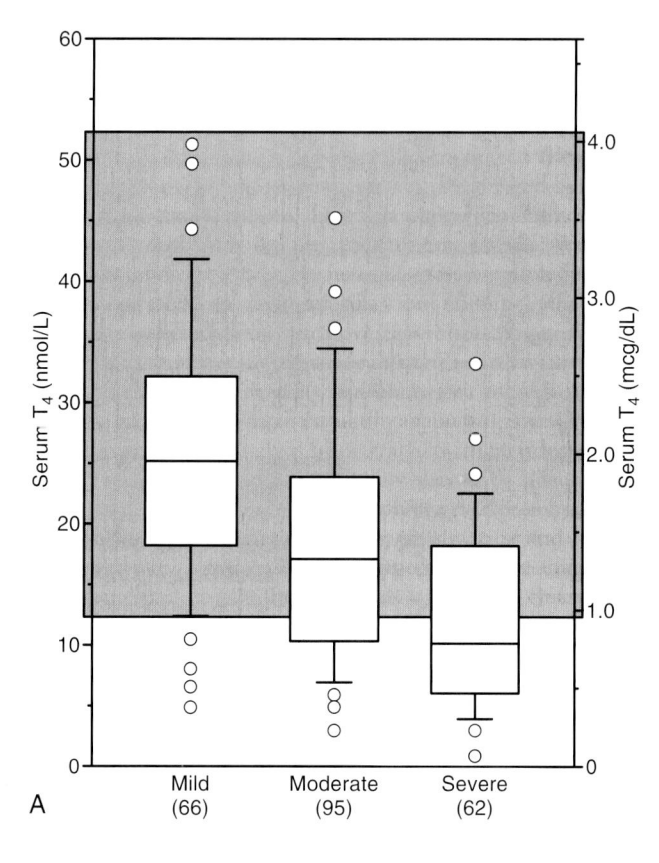

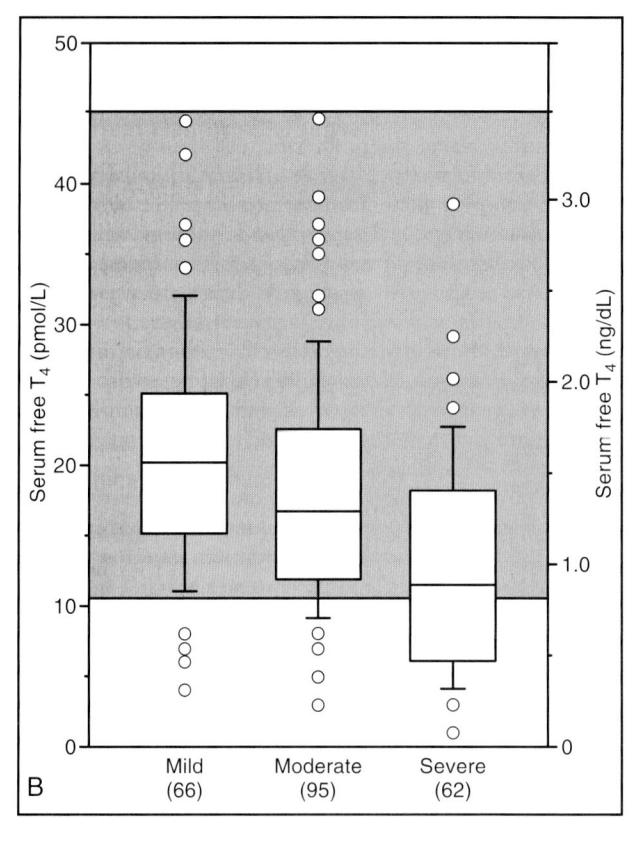

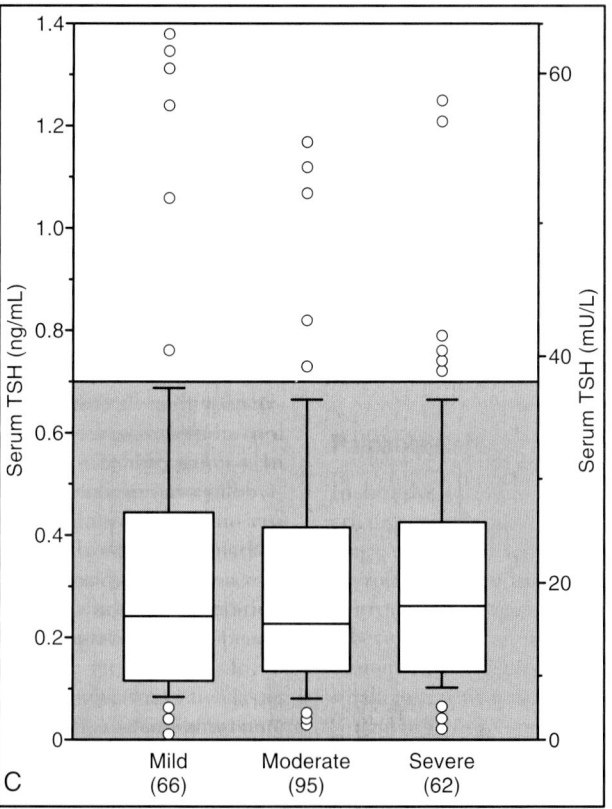

FIGURE 3-32 Box plots of serum concentrations of total thyroxine (T$_4$) **(A),** free T$_4$ (fT$_4$) **(B),** and thyrotropin (TSH) **(C)** in 223 dogs with nonthyroidal disease stratified according to severity of disease. For each box plot, T-bars represent the main body of data, which in most instances is equal to the range. Each box represents interquartile range (25th to 75th percentile). The *horizontal bar* in each box is the median. *Open circles* represent outlying data points. *Numbers in parentheses* indicate the numbers of dogs in each group. Reference range is indicated by the *shaded area.* (From Kantrowitz LB, et al.: Serum total thyroxine, total triiodothyronine, free thyroxine, and thyrotropin concentrations in dogs with nonthyroidal disease, *J Am Vet Med Assoc* 219[6]:765, 2001.)

reported that the most common finding in systemically ill dogs is a decreased total T_3. FT_4, and TSH are more variable and may depend in part on the pathophysiologic mechanisms involved in the illness. Although serum FT_4 concentrations are decreased to a lesser extent than total T_4 concentrations (Peterson et al., 1997; Kantrowitz et al., 2001), in the presence of severe systemic illness, FT_4 concentrations can also be suppressed and suggestive of true hypothyroidism. Serum TSH concentrations are usually normal but may be increased in a small percentage of patients especially during recovery from NTIS. In one study of 223 dogs with NTIS, approximately 31% of dogs had low total T_4 concentrations and 22% had low FT_4, whereas only 8% had high serum TSH concentrations (Kantrowitz et al., 2001). In a more recent study of 196 dogs with NTIS, total T_3, total T_4, and FT_4 were decreased in 76%, 35%, and 5% of dogs respectively, whereas canine TSH was increased in only 3% of dogs (Mooney et al., 2008). In this study, decreased total T_3 concentrations were relatively common, and total T_3 was significantly lower in dogs that were euthanized compared to those that survived. The high percentage of dogs in this study with a low total T_3 is more similar to what is typically reported in humans with NTIS. Multiple studies in dogs, cats, and humans with NTIS have confirmed that the severity of suppression of serum thyroid hormone concentrations can be used as a prognostic indicator. Lower serum thyroid hormone concentrations are associated with a higher mortality rate (Peterson and Gamble, 1990; Elliott et al., 1995; Mooney et al., 2008; Schoeman et al., 2007). In a study of 63 critically ill puppies with parvoviral enteritis, serum T_4 and FT_4 were significantly lower in non-survivors than survivors (Schoeman et al., 2007). Similar findings have been documented in dogs with other severe systemic illness.

The existence of NTIS makes it very difficult to confirm a diagnosis of concurrent hypothyroidism in systemically ill dogs. If possible, evaluation of thyroid function should be postponed until resolution of the underlying illness. In some circumstances, however, treatment of concurrent hypothyroidism could improve outcome if hypothyroidism is contributing to the pathogenesis of the disorder. Examples of clinical situations in which this might occur are dogs with laryngeal paralysis and megaesophagus in which hypothyroidism may contribute to decreased neurologic function. In this situation multiple thyroid parameters should be evaluated in the context of history, physical examination findings, and other laboratory data. The simultaneous occurrence of low T_4, FT_4, and high TSH concentration is uncommon in NTIS, occurring in only 1.8% of 223 dogs with nonthyroidal illness in one study and in none of 66 dogs in another study (Kantrowitz et al., 2001; Torres, 2003). Therefore if this combination of findings is identified in a dog with supportive clinical findings, a diagnosis of true hypothyroidism is more likely. A TSH stimulation test, thyroid scintigraphy, or a therapeutic trial may all be appropriate options in such a scenario.

Treatment of NTIS should be directed at resolution of the concurrent illness. Serum thyroid hormone concentrations return to normal once the concurrent illness is corrected. Because NTIS is believed to be a physiologic protective mechanism, it is not recommended to treat affected patients with thyroid supplementation, and there are no studies that document a benefit of such treatment. In a study of euthyroid dogs with congestive heart failure, supplementation with thyroid hormone did not improve survival (Tidholm et al., 2003). Although many dogs with euthyroid sick syndrome are inadvertently treated with L-T_4 sodium

without obvious deleterious consequences, it is not recommended—especially if the concurrent illness is severe and there is nothing in the history, physical examination, or blood work to support a diagnosis of concurrent hypothyroidism.

Dermatologic Disorders

Hypothyroidism is frequently included in the differential diagnosis of many dermatologic disorders in the dog. Studies suggest that common dermatologic disorders (e.g., pyoderma, flea hypersensitivity, allergic dermatitis) do not typically cause serum thyroid hormone concentrations to decrease into the hypothyroid range in euthyroid dogs (Slade et al., 1984; Nelson et al., 1991; Beale et al., 1992a; Daminet et al., 2000). Borderline serum T_4 and FT_4 concentrations however may occur in individual euthyroid dogs with skin disease.

Diabetes Mellitus

Thyroid hormones play an important role in glucose homeostasis, and hypothyroidism and diabetes mellitus can occur together (Hess et al., 2003; Dixon et al., 1999). Concurrent hypothyroidism in diabetic dogs may cause insulin resistance (Ford et al., 1993), although in most hypothyroid dogs increased secretion of insulin results in maintenance of normal blood glucose concentration. Increased concentrations of IGF-1 and GH have been documented in hypothyroid dogs and likely contribute to insulin resistance (Diaz-Espiñeira, 2009; Hofer-Inteeworn, 2012). Hypothyroid dogs have increased fructosamine concentrations due to decreased metabolic rate and resultant decreased protein turnover, which may complicate the assessment of glycemic control in hypothyroid diabetic dogs (Reusch, 2002). Recognition of hypothyroidism may be difficult in dogs with poorly controlled diabetes mellitus, because clinical signs (e.g., lethargy and weakness) and abnormalities in clinical pathologic values (e.g., lipemia and hypercholesterolemia) may be present in both disorders. Reliance on baseline serum thyroid hormone concentrations can be misleading because of NTIS. Evaluation of baseline thyroid hormone and TSH concentrations in the diabetic dog should not be undertaken until after treatment for diabetes mellitus has improved the initial systemic signs of illness. Interpretation of test results should take into consideration the degree of success achieved in controlling hyperglycemia and the impact that poorly controlled diabetes mellitus may have on serum T_4, FT_4, and TSH concentrations. If hypothyroidism is diagnosed and treated in a diabetic patient, the blood glucose should be carefully monitored when thyroid supplementation is initiated because establishment of euthyroidism results in increased insulin sensitivity and a decreased need for insulin.

Hyperadrenocorticism

Endogenously produced and exogenously administered glucocorticoids lower baseline serum T_3, T_4, and FT_4 concentrations in the dog (Peterson et al., 1984; Nelson et al., 1991; Ferguson and Peterson, 1992). Most studies suggest that 40% to 50% of dogs with spontaneous hyperadrenocorticism have decreased total T_4 and T_3 concentrations, whereas FT_4 is usually maintained within the reference range (Peterson et al., 1984; Ferguson and Peterson, 1992). There are several proposed mechanisms for the alterations in serum thyroid hormone concentrations in dogs with hyperadrenocorticism (Box 3-5), including inhibition of TSH secretion, reduced serum protein binding of T_4, reduced T_3 production and degradation, and possibly inhibition of peripheral 5'-deiodination of T_4 (Kemppainen et al., 1983; Ferguson and Peterson, 1992). Although glucocorticoids are believed to suppress pituitary TSH secretion, in a study of 47

dogs with pituitary dependent hyperadrenocorticism, basal and TRH stimulated TSH concentrations did not differ from those of control dogs (Meij et al, 1997).

In some cases it can be difficult to clinically differentiate hyperadrenocorticism from hypothyroidism in dogs with endocrine alopecia, although usually the history (e.g., polydipsia, polyuria, polyphagia in hyperadrenocorticism but not hypothyroidism), the presence of additional physical abnormalities, and the presence of abnormalities on a CBC, urinalysis, and serum biochemical panel (e.g., increased alkaline phosphatase activity) are helpful. If hyperadrenocorticism is considered possible, a screening test, such as the urine cortisol/creatinine ratio or low dose dexamethasone suppression test, should be considered in addition to tests of thyroid gland function to avoid a misdiagnosis of hypothyroidism in a dog with hyperadrenocorticism. If a dog with hyperadrenocorticism is inadvertently treated with L-T_4, a poor response to treatment or development of additional clinical manifestations of hyperadrenocorticism (e.g., polyuria and polydipsia) will eventually lead the clinician back toward the diagnosis of hyperadrenocorticism.

Environmental and Body Temperature

Seasonal influence on thyroid hormone concentrations was evaluated in healthy outdoor dogs in Hokkaido, Japan (Ohashi et al, 2001). Serum T_4 concentration decreased in January and increased in August and September; FT_4 concentration increased in January and November, and there was no significant seasonal variation in serum TSH concentration. It is not known whether a similar seasonal variation occurs in dogs housed indoors or whether temperature variation, photoperiod, or region of the world may impact the results. Acute cold exposure may increase serum concentrations of TSH and thyroid hormones in the rat and possibly in humans, and acute exposure to heat may decrease serum TSH, T_4, and T_3 and increase serum rT_3 (Wartofsky and Burman, 1982). Hypothermia and hyperpyrexia may also alter serum T_4, T_3, rT_3, and TSH. It is not known, however, whether these alterations are a result of temperature fluctuations or other factors associated with NTIS.

Obesity, Fasting, and Cachexia

An increase in serum T_3 and T_4 concentrations has been reported in obese euthyroid dogs (Gosselin et al, 1980; Daminet et al, 2003a). It is believed that increased serum thyroid hormone levels are the result of increased caloric intake rather than obesity itself. The changes reported are small and unlikely to influence clinical interpretation of thyroid hormone concentrations.

In humans, fasting causes a significant rapid decrease in serum concentrations of T_3 and an increase in serum rT_3 without affecting serum T_4 or TSH concentrations (Wartofsky and Burman, 1982). Re-feeding with either a mixed-nutrient or carbohydrate-rich diet causes the fasting-induced changes to reverse quickly. Impaired conversion of T_4 to T_3 from inhibition of peripheral 5'-deiodinase has been proposed to account for these abnormalities (Borst et al, 1983), although studies in rats have also shown decreased thyroidal secretion of T_4. Fasting for up to 36 hours did not affect baseline serum T_4 or T_3 concentrations in euthyroid Beagles (Reimers et al, 1986). However, fasting in excess of 48 hours did decrease T_3 concentrations in dogs (de Bruijne et al, 1981). In Labrador Retrievers subjected to life-time caloric restriction, only T_3 concentrations were consistently lower in dogs subjected to dietary restriction (Lawler et al, 2007). Serum T_4 and T_3 but not FT_4 concentrations were significantly lower in dogs with chronic weight loss causing cachexia, compared with dogs that had not undergone weight loss (Vail et al, 1994). The decrease in serum T_4 and T_3 concentration was proportional to the degree of weight loss associated with their disease. The decline in serum T_4 and T_3 was believed to be related to the severity of the illness or an abnormal nutritional state.

Drugs

Our knowledge of the effect, if any, of various drugs and hormones on serum thyroid hormone and TSH concentrations in dogs is gradually expanding as investigators continue to examine the interplay between medications and thyroid hormone test results (Tables 3-12 and 3-13). Undoubtedly, many more as yet unrecognized drugs also affect serum thyroid hormone and TSH concentrations in dogs. Until proved otherwise, any drug should be suspected of influencing thyroid hormone test results, especially if the drug has been shown to alter serum thyroid hormone concentrations in humans (see Table 3-13; Box 3-6).

Glucocorticoids

Glucocorticoids are the most commonly used drugs that influence serum thyroid hormone concentrations. The effect of exogenously administered glucocorticoids on serum thyroid hormone concentrations is similar to that seen with naturally occurring hyperadrenocorticism (see Chapter 10). Serum T_4, FT_4, and T_3 concentrations are decreased, often into the hypothyroid range. Proposed mechanisms for this decrease include decreased binding of T_4 to carrier proteins, alterations in clearance and metabolism of thyroid hormones, decreased conversion of T_4 to T_3 at peripheral sites, and suppressed pituitary TSH secretion (Woltz et al,

---

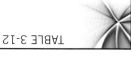

BOX 3-5 Proposed Alterations in Thyroid Hormone Physiology Caused by Glucocorticoids

Decreased 5'-monodeiodination enzyme activity
Decreased binding affinity of plasma proteins for T_4, T_3
Decreased cellular binding of T_4, T_3
Increased metabolic clearance rate of T_4
Decreased metabolic clearance rate of T_3, rT_3
Inhibition of TSH secretion (secondary hypothyroidism)
Inhibition of TRH secretion

T_3, Triiodothyronine; T_4, thyroxine; TRH, thyrotropin-releasing hormone; TSH, thyroid-stimulating hormone (also known as thyrotropin).

TABLE 3-12 MECHANISMS BY WHICH DRUGS INFLUENCE THYROID FUNCTION IN HUMANS

MECHANISM	EXAMPLE
Decrease TSH secretion	Glucocorticoids
Change thyroid hormone secretion	Amiodarone
Decrease gastrointestinal absorption	Sucralfate
Alter serum binding	Phenylbutazone
Change hepatic metabolism	Phenobarbital
Inhibit TPO	Sulfonamides

TPO, Thyroid peroxidase; TSH, thyroid-stimulating hormone (also known as thyrotropin).

1984; Kaptein et al., 1992; Moore et al., 1993). Because serum TSH concentrations are not increased in dogs with hyperadrenocorticism, measurement of TSH can be helpful in distinguishing hyperadrenocorticism and hypothyroidism. An increased TSH concentration is consistent with hypothyroidism rather than hyperadrenocorticism, although it is important to recognize that the two disorders can occur together. The magnitude and duration of suppression of serum thyroid hormone concentrations depend on the type of glucocorticoid, dosage, route of administration, and duration of glucocorticoid administration. The higher the dosage, the longer the administration, and the more potent the glucocorticoid administration, the more severe the suppression of serum thyroid hormone concentrations. Topical glucocorticoids can have a similar effect as parenterally-administered glucocorticoids (Gottschalk, 2011). Administration of exogenous glucocorticoids does not typically result in clinical signs of hypothyroidism, although clinical signs of iatrogenic hyperadrenocorticism may mimic clinical signs of hypothyroidism particularly in regard to dermatologic signs. Because of the overlap in clinical signs between iatrogenic hyperadrenocorticism and the effects of glucocorticoids on laboratory evaluation of the thyroid axis, in some situations it can be difficult or impossible to determine whether glucocorticoid induced hypothyroidism is contributing to a dog's clinical signs and on rare occasions a therapeutic trial may be appropriate.

Because of the common use of glucocorticoid therapy in the management of various medical and dermatologic disorders, a thorough history regarding prior glucocorticoid therapy is extremely important before evaluating thyroid gland function, because failure to identify prior glucocorticoid administration can result in a misdiagnosis of hypothyroidism. If glucocorticoids have been administered in the recent past, measurement of baseline serum thyroid hormone concentrations should be delayed or interpreted carefully. Normal serum T_4, FT_4, and TSH concentrations in these dogs confirm normal thyroid function, whereas low serum T_4 and FT_4 concentrations in conjunction with high TSH concentrations suggest hypothyroidism if clinical signs and

physical examination findings are consistent with the disease. Any other combination of test results is difficult to interpret, and the ideal approach is to discontinue glucocorticoid treatment and reassess serum thyroid hormone and TSH concentrations 4 to 8 weeks later. In hypothyroid dogs already being treated with thyroid hormone supplementation, prednisone at a dose of 1.0 mg/kg for 7 days decreased total T_4 but not FT_4 or TSH. Every other day treatment at the same dose did not alter any thyroid parameter over a 28-day period (O'Neill and Reynolds, 2011).

Anticonvulsants

In dogs, phenobarbital treatment at therapeutic dosages decreases serum T_4 and FT_4 concentrations into the range consistent with hypothyroidism (Gaskill et al., 1999; Kantrowitz et al., 1999; Gieger et al., 2000; Muller et al., 2000). Although the mechanism remains unproven in dogs, increased metabolism and excretion of T_4 secondary to hepatic microsomal enzyme induction is believed to be the primary cause, although other mechanisms such as displacement of T_4 from plasma protein binding sites may also play a role. A delayed increase in serum TSH concentration occurs as serum T_4 and FT_4 concentrations decline, although TSH concentrations do not usually exceed the upper limit of the reference range (Muller et al., 2000). Increased serum TSH concentrations quickly return to the reference range following discontinuation of phenobarbital treatment, whereas serum T_4 and FT_4 concentrations may take up to 4 weeks to return to pretreatment values (Gieger et al., 2000). Although in most cases clinical signs of hypothyroidism do not develop in phenobarbital-treated dogs, rarely we have seen dogs with clinical signs suggestive of hypothyroidism in dogs treated chronically with phenobarbital.

Bromide, a halide similar to iodide, could potentially affect the thyroid axis by interfering with iodide uptake or iodide organification by the thyroid gland. Potassium bromide treatment did not have a significant effect on serum T_4, T_3, FT_4, and TSH concentrations in five healthy dogs or in eight dogs with a seizure disorder (Kantrowitz et al., 1999; Paull et al., 2003).

TABLE 3-13   DRUGS THAT HAVE BEEN DEMONSTRATED TO INFLUENCE THYROID FUNCTION IN DOGS

DRUG	TOTAL THYROXINE (↓ OR N)	FREE THYROXINE (↓ OR N)	THYROTROPIN (↑ OR N)	CLINICAL SIGNS OF HYPOTHYROIDISM? (Y/N)	NOTES
Glucocorticoids	↓	↓ (↓ or N)	N	N	Effect dose and duration dependent
Phenobarbital	↓	↓	Slight ↑	N	TSH not increased outside reference range
Trimethoprim/sulfonamides	↓	↓	↑	Y	Effect dose and duration dependent
Nonsteroidal anti-inflammatory drugs					Effect varies depending on specific drug used
Aspirin	↓	N or ↓	N	N	
Deracoxib	N	N	N	N	
Ketoprofen	N	N	N	N	
Meloxicam	N	N	N	N	
Carprofen	N	N	N	N	
Etodolac	N or ↓	N	N or ↓	N	
Clomipramine	↓	↓	N	N	

TSH, Thyroid-stimulating hormone (also known as thyrotropin).

BOX 3-6 Some Drugs and Diagnostic Agents that can Alter Basal Serum Thyroid Hormone Concentrations in Humans and Possibly Dogs

Decrease T_4 and/or T_3
Amiodarone (T_3)
Androgens
Cholecystographic agents
Diazepam
Dopamine
Flunixin
Furosemide
Glucocorticoids
Heparin
Imidazole
Iodide
Methimazole
Mitotane
Nitroprusside
Penicillin
Phenobarbital
Phenothiazines
Phenylbutazone
Phenytoin
Primidone
Propranolol
Propylthiouracil
Radiopaque dyes (ipodate) (T_3)
Salicylates
Sulfonamides (sulfamethoxazole)
Sulfonylureas

Increase T_4 and/or T_3
Amiodarone (T_4)
Estrogens
5-Fluorouracil
Halothane
Insulin
Narcotic analgesics
Radiopaque dyes (e.g., ipodate) (T_4)
Thiazides

T_3, triiodothyronine; T_4, thyroxine.

Sulfonamide Antibiotics

Sulfonamides interfere with thyroid hormone synthesis by means of dosage- and duration-dependent inhibition of TPO activity (Doerge and Decker, 1994). TPO is responsible for oxidation of iodide, iodination of tyrosine residues on Tg, and coupling of tyrosine residues prior to thyroid hormone secretion. Decreases in serum T_4, fT_4, and T_3 and an increase in TSH concentrations have been documented in dogs treated with potentiated sulfonamides (e.g., trimethoprim-sulfamethoxazole, trimethoprim-sulfadiazine; Hall et al, 1993; Torres et al, 1996; Gookin et al, 1999). Serum T_4 concentrations can decrease into the hypothyroid range within 1 to 2 weeks, and serum TSH concentrations can increase above the reference range within 2 to 3 weeks after initiating sulfonamide therapy at doses of 15 mg/kg every 12 hours or higher (Hall et al, 1993; Williamson et al, 2002; Frank et al, 2005). Clinical signs of hypothyroidism may develop with sulfonamide administration and chronic treatment may result in a palpable goiter due

to persistent TSH stimulation (Torres et al, 1996; Seelig et al, 2008). Thyroid gland function tests return to normal within 1 to 12 weeks after cessation of the antibiotic depending upon the dose and chronicity of treatment (Hall et al, 1993; Williamson et al, 2002; Frank et al, 2005). Administration of sulfadiazine in combination with trimethoprim during the last 4 weeks of pregnancy in female dogs did not affect the thyroid gland in the neonates (Post et al, 1993).

Nonsteroidal Anti-Inflammatory Drugs

Nonsteroidal anti-inflammatory drugs (NSAIDs) may decrease serum T_4, fT_4, T_3, and TSH concentrations in humans and other species (Bishnoi et al, 1994). Proposed mechanisms include displacement of thyroid hormone binding to plasma proteins, decreased thyroid hormone de-iodination and inhibition of binding of thyroid hormone to receptors in the plasma membrane, cytoplasm, and nucleus. The effect of NSAIDs on thyroid function tests varies depending on the drug. In dogs, administration of aspirin causes a decrease in total T_4 and fT_4 concentration but no change in TSH concentration. Etodolac, deracoxib, ketoprofen, meloxicam, and carprofen do not result in significant alterations in thyroid hormone concentrations in dogs (Ferguson, 1999; Panciera and Johnston, 2002; Daminet, 2003b; Ness, 2003; Sauve, 2003; Panciera, 2006; see Table 3-13).

Tricyclic Antidepressants

Clomipramine is a tricyclic antidepressant commonly used in dogs with behavioral problems. Clomipramine inhibits thyroid hormone synthesis by altering thyroid follicular cell uptake of iodide and inhibition of TPO. Clomipramine at a dose of 3 mg/kg every 12 hours decreased total T_4 and fT_4 in dogs after 28 days of treatment but did not change TSH concentrations during the 112 days of the study (Gulickers and Panciera, 2003). Because hypothyroidism has been implicated in causing behavioral changes in dogs, it is important that thyroid function is not evaluated while dogs are being treated with clomipramine.

THYROID BIOPSY

The gold standard method for identifying pathology of the thyroid gland is histologic evaluation of a thyroid biopsy specimen. Severe lymphocytic thyroiditis or thyroid atrophy are readily identified histologically (see Figs. 3-6 and 3-7), and in the dog with appropriate clinical signs and diagnostic test results, these findings confirm the diagnosis of primary hypothyroidism (Diaz-Espiñeira et al, 2007). Unfortunately, histologic evaluation of a thyroid biopsy does not always clarify the status of thyroid gland function, especially when clinical signs or diagnostic test results are vague and changes in thyroid pathology are less severe. Thyroiditis can be present in the thyroid gland without causing overt clinical thyroid failure and does not always progress to cause clinical hypothyroidism. Approximately 80% of both thyroid lobes must be destroyed before clinical thyroid gland failure is evident. Variants of normal can be also difficult to differentiate from secondary hypothyroidism, primary atrophy, and follicular cell hyperplasia, especially when the last two conditions are in the early stages of development. The influence of concurrent illness on thyroid gland morphology may also affect biopsy results. Biopsies of the thyroid gland must be obtained surgically and are rarely performed because of the invasiveness of the procedure, cost to the client, and lack of guarantee that diagnostically useful information will be obtained. The only clinical indication for thyroid biopsy in dogs is identification of an enlarged thyroid gland when thyroid neoplasia is suspected.

ESTABLISHING THE DIAGNOSIS

Recommendations regarding the approach to the diagnosis of hypothyroidism are shown in Fig. 3-20. The presence of appropriate clinical signs is imperative, especially when relying on baseline thyroid hormone concentrations for a diagnosis. Identification of a mild nonregenerative anemia on the CBC and especially an increased serum cholesterol concentration on a serum biochemistry panel adds further support for hypothyroidism. Baseline serum T_4 concentration is often used as the initial screening test for thyroid gland function, in part because it is widely available at low cost and can be measured in-house. It is important to remember that serum T_4 concentrations can be suppressed by a variety of factors, most notably NTIS. Thus measurement of the serum T_4 concentration should be used to confirm a euthyroid state. A normal serum T_4 concentration establishes euthyroidism in the vast majority of dogs. The exceptions are a very small number of hypothyroid dogs with lymphocytic thyroiditis and serum T_4 autoantibodies that interfere with the RIA used to measure T_4 (see Fig. 3-19). A low serum T_4 concentration (i.e., less than 0.5 μg/dL) in conjunction with hypercholesterolemia and clinical signs strongly suggestive of the disease, supports the diagnosis of hypothyroidism, especially if systemic illness is not present.

Although measurement of serum T_4 concentration can be used as an initial screening test, measuring a combination of thyroid gland tests is preferred to confirm the diagnosis. Many diagnostic laboratories offer a variety of thyroid panels that incorporate two or more of the following: serum T_4, fT_4 by RIA or MED, T_3, fT_3, rT_3, TSH, and antibody tests for lymphocytic thyroiditis. A normal serum T_4, fT_4, and TSH concentration rules out hypothyroidism. Low serum T_4 and fT_4 and increased serum TSH concentrations in a dog with appropriate clinical signs and clinicopathologic abnormalities strongly support the diagnosis of hypothyroidism, especially if systemic illness is not present and drugs known to affect thyroid test results have not been recently administered. Concurrent presence of Tg autoantibodies suggests lymphocytic thyroiditis as the underlying etiology.

Unfortunately, discordant test results are common. In this situation, reliance on presence of clinical signs, clinicopathologic abnormalities, and clinician index of suspicion become the most important parameters in deciding whether to treat the dog with L-T_4 sodium (see Table 3-6). Serum fT_4 concentration measured by MED is the single most accurate test of thyroid gland function. The combination of a high TSH concentration and a low fT_4 or total T_4 has high specificity for a diagnosis of hypothyroidism. Positive anti-thyroid antibodies alone do not equate with a diagnosis of hypothyroidism but increase the likelihood of the disease in the presence of borderline or discordant thyroid hormone concentrations. Ultimately when discordant test results occur, the clinician must decide whether to initiate trial therapy with L-T_4 sodium or to repeat the testing in 3 to 6 months. In general the most important factor influencing this decision is the severity of clinical signs consistent with hypothyroidism.

Trial therapy should be considered only when thyroid hormone supplementation does not pose a risk to the patient. Response to trial therapy with L-T_4 sodium is nonspecific. Because of the general increase in the metabolic rate that can result from pharmacologic doses of thyroid hormone, thyroid hormone supplementation can temporarily improve clinical signs in a dog without thyroid dysfunction. The effect on the quality of the hair coat is most notable. Thyroid hormone supplementation stimulates telogen hair follicles to become anagen follicles and improves the hair coat, presumably even in euthyroid dogs (Gunaratnam, 1986;

Credille et al, 2001). For this reason, a dog that has a positive response to therapy either has hypothyroidism or has "thyroid-responsive disease." Therefore, if a positive response to trial therapy is observed, thyroid supplementation should be discontinued once clinical signs have resolved. If clinical signs recur, hypothyroidism is confirmed, and the supplement should be reinitiated. If clinical signs do not recur, a "thyroid-responsive disorder" or a beneficial response to concurrent therapy (e.g., antibiotics, flea control) should be suspected.

Diagnosis in a Previously Treated Dog

Occasionally, a clinician wants to determine whether a dog receiving thyroid hormone supplementation is, in fact, hypothyroid. The exogenous administration of thyroid hormone, either T_4 or T_3, to a healthy euthyroid dog, suppresses pituitary TSH secretion and causes pituitary thyrotroph atrophy and, subsequently, thyroid gland atrophy. Once the supplement is withdrawn, serum T_4, and T_3 concentrations may be suggestive of hypothyroidism, even in a previously euthyroid dog, if testing is performed within a month of discontinuing treatment (Panciera et al, 1989). Thyroid hormone supplementation must be discontinued and the pituitary-thyroid axis allowed to regain function before meaningful baseline serum T_4 concentrations can be obtained. The time between the discontinuation of thyroid hormone supplementation and the acquisition of meaningful results regarding thyroid gland function depends on the duration of treatment, the dose and frequency of administration of the thyroid hormone supplement, and individual variability. As a general rule, thyroid hormone supplements should be discontinued for a minimum of 4 weeks, but preferably 6 to 8 weeks, before thyroid gland function is critically assessed.

Diagnosis in Puppies

An approach similar to the one described earlier is used to diagnose congenital hypothyroidism. In general, the clinical signs are more obvious in dogs with congenital hypothyroidism; and if the hypothalamic-pituitary-thyroid gland axis is intact, a goiter will be present (see Fig. 3-13). Serum TSH concentrations in dogs with congenital hypothyroidism are also dependent on the etiology of hypothyroidism. Serum TSH concentrations will be increased in dogs with primary dysfunction of the thyroid gland (e.g., iodine organification defect) and an intact hypothalamic-pituitary-thyroid gland axis. However, serum TSH concentrations will not be increased in dogs with congenital hypothyroidism in which pituitary or hypothalamic dysfunction is the cause of the hypothyroidism.

TREATMENT

The initial treatment of choice, regardless of the underlying cause of hypothyroidism, is synthetic L-T_4 sodium (Fig. 3-33; Box 3-7). The same treatment protocol is used for both a therapeutic trial and definitive therapy. Treatment with L-T_4 sodium preserves normal regulation of T_4 to T_3 de-iodination, which allows physiologic regulation of individual tissue T_3 concentrations and decreases the risk of iatrogenic hyperthyroidism. The plasma half-life of L-T_4 sodium in dogs ranges from 9 to 14 hours and depends, in part, on the dosage and frequency of administration, with higher dosages and more frequent administration associated with a shorter half-life of L-T_4 sodium (Nachreiner et al, 1993; Le Traon, 2007). In one study, the mean (± SD) serum half-life of L-T_4 sodium was 9.0 ± 5.9 and 14.6 ± 6.3 hours when L-T_4 sodium was administered at 22 μg/kg once a day or divided twice a day, respectively (Nachreiner et al, 1993). At this dosage, mean time to peak serum T_4 concentration was 3.8

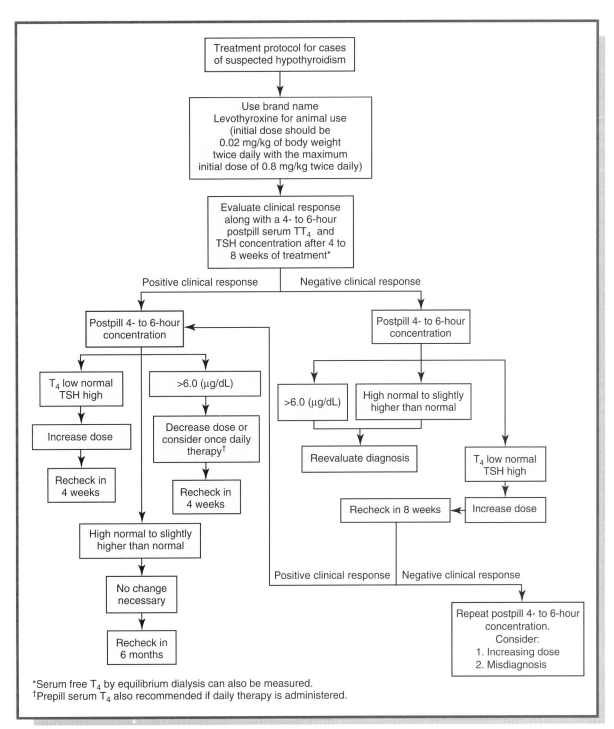

FIGURE 3-33 Algorithm for treatment of canine hypothyroidism. *TSH,* thyroid-stimulating hormone, also known as thyrotropin; *TT₄,* total thyroxine. (Modified from Ettinger SJ, Feldman EC, editors: *Textbook of veterinary internal medicine,* ed 7, St Louis, 2010, Elsevier, p. 1760.)

± 2.0 hours after L-T$_4$ sodium administration. Maximal and minimal serum T$_4$ concentrations were higher and lower, respectively with once daily L-T$_4$ sodium administration, than with twice-daily administration. As a result, serum T$_4$ concentrations were above the physiologic range for a number of hours with single L-T$_4$ sodium administration, whereas concentrations closer to physiologic ranges were achieved by use of divided doses. The ideal dose and frequency of L-T$_4$ sodium supplementation varies among dogs because of variability in T$_4$ absorption and serum half-life between individual dogs. A dose of 0.02 mg/kg every 24 hours normalizes TSH concentration in most dogs; higher doses (0.04 mg/kg every 12 hours) are required

to consistently normalize T$_3$ concentration, but there is no evidence that normalization of T$_3$ is necessary for a good clinical response. The recommended initial dose for otherwise healthy hypothyroid dogs is 0.02 mg/kg by mouth every 12 hours (0.1 mg/10 lb; maximum starting dose, 0.8 mg). This dosage is similar to the average calculated oral replacement dosage (0.018 mg/kg) determined in a study evaluating replacement T$_4$ requirements in thyroidectomized dogs (Ferguson and Hoenig, 1997). The dose for treatment of hypothyroid dogs is 10 times higher than the dose used in hypothyroid humans because of poorer gastrointestinal absorption and a shorter serum half-life of T$_4$ in dogs compared to humans. Some

---

BOX 3-7   Recommendations for the Initial Treatment and Monitoring of Hypothyroidism in Dogs

Initial Treatment

Use a name brand synthetic L-T$_4$ sodium product approved for animal use.
The initial dosage per administration should be 0.02 mg/kg of body weight (0.1 mg/10 pounds) with a maximum initial dose of 0.8 mg.
The initial frequency of administration is every 12 hours.

Initial Monitoring

Response to treatment should be critically evaluated 6 to 8 weeks after initiating treatment.
Serum T$_4$ or fT$_4$ (measured by equilibrium dialysis) and TSH concentration should be measured 4 to 6 hours after administration of thyroid hormone.
  Serum T$_4$ or fT$_4$ concentration should be in the normal range or increased.
  Serum TSH concentration should be in the normal range.
Measuring serum T$_4$ or fT$_4$ (measured by equilibrium dialysis) concentration immediately prior to thyroid hormone administration (i.e., trough level) is optional but is recommended if thyroid hormone is being given once a day.
  Serum T$_4$ or fT$_4$ concentration should be in the normal range at this time.

Adapted from consensus recommendations reached at an international symposium on canine hypothyroidism held in August 1996 (*Canine Practice*, vol 77, 1997).
fT$_4$, Free thyroxine; *L-T$_4$*, levothyroxine (also known as L-thyroxine), *T$_4$*, thyroxine; *TSH*, thyroid-stimulating hormone (also known as thyrotropin).

---

investigators believe that the dose of L-T$_4$ sodium may correlate better with body surface area than with body weight (Chastain, 1982). The recommended dosage of L-T$_4$ sodium based on body surface area is 0.5 mg/m^2, however the authors prefer to dose L-T$_4$ sodium based on body weight rather than body surface area. Most studies have shown that the majority of dogs have a good clinical response to treatment with once daily L-T$_4$ sodium; however dose adjustments are required in 20% to 50% of dogs started on once a day therapy (Le Traon et al, 2009; Dixon et al, 2002). Twice daily administration of T$_4$ is recommended initially to improve the likelihood of a positive response to treatment, which is especially important when performing a therapeutic trial. If clinical signs resolve and T$_4$ concentrations are within the therapeutic range, the frequency of T$_4$ administration can be decreased to once daily. The final L-T$_4$ sodium dose should be adjusted based on the measured serum T$_4$ concentration and TSH concentration (see Fig. 3-33). In humans the TSH concentration is used to titrate the dose, but this is problematic in dogs because of the lower sensitivity of the TSH assay.

Most L-T$_4$ sodium products are formulated as a tablet ranging in strength from 0.1 to 0.8 mg; chewable L-T$_4$ sodium formulations and an L-T$_4$ sodium solution (Leventa Merck Animal Health) solution are also available. There are differences in potency and bioavailability between different brands and formulations of L-T$_4$ sodium supplements. Unfortunately, even in human patients, not all available products have been directly compared for bioequivalence, and even when products have been documented to be bioequivalent, the biologic response can vary between products in individual patients. The methods used to establish bioequivalence in humans also have some limitations. One concern is that the methods rely on administration of a supra-physiologic dose of L-T$_4$ sodium to euthyroid volunteers. The outcome measures are area under the curve, maximum concentration, and time to maximum concentration, rather than measurement of TSH concentration and adjustment for endogenous T$_4$ secretion is not required (Di Girolamo et al, 2008). The Food and Drug Administration

(FDA) allows variability in potency of 80% to 125%, which for a drug such as L-T$_4$ sodium with a relatively narrow therapeutic window could have clinical consequences. In dogs the relative bioavailability of a liquid L-T$_4$ sodium solution was demonstrated to be 50% higher than that of a tablet formulation in euthyroid dogs; however, the dose required for establishment of euthyroidism in hypothyroid dogs (0.02 mg/kg every 24 hours) was similar to that required for an oral tablet formulation (Soloxine, Daniels Pharmaceuticals) (Le Traon et al, 2007; 2009; Dixon et al, 2002). Because of the limitations of bioequivalence studies, it is recommended that clinicians use one formulation of L-T$_4$ sodium consistently; and if a change in formulation needs to be made, therapeutic monitoring should be used to confirm that the dose of the new product is appropriate. Many other factors, including concurrent drug administration, nutritional supplements, food type, timing of meals, concurrent illness, and physiologic conditions such as age and obesity influence L-T$_4$ sodium absorption from the gastrointestinal tract. For example in people, consumption of a meal at the time of L-T$_4$ sodium administration decreases absorption. Administration of L-T$_4$ sodium with food has been shown to decrease bioavailability of liquid L-T$_4$ sodium formulations in dogs (Le Traon et al, 2007). If possible, it is recommended to avoid giving L-T$_4$ sodium supplements at the time of a meal. When therapeutic monitoring is performed, it is important not to change any of the aforementioned variables. For example, if the medication is given at the time of a meal, the same protocol should be followed on the day of testing.

Response to Levothyroxine Sodium Therapy

Thyroid hormone supplementation should be continued for a minimum of 6 to 8 weeks before critically evaluating the effectiveness of treatment. With appropriate therapy, all of the clinical signs and clinicopathologic abnormalities associated with hypothyroidism should resolve (Fig. 3-34). An increase in mental alertness and activity usually occurs within the first week of treatment (Table 3-14); this is an important early indicator that the diagnosis of hypothyroidism was correct. Although some hair regrowth may be observed during the first month in dogs with endocrine alopecia, it may take several months for complete regrowth and a marked reduction in hyperpigmentation of the skin to occur. Initially, the hair coat may appear to worsen as hairs in the telogen stage of the hair cycle are shed (Credille et al, 2001). If obesity is caused by hypothyroidism, it should also begin to improve within 2 months after initiating L-T$_4$ sodium therapy along with adjustments in diet and exercise (Fig. 3-35). Improvement in myocardial function is usually evident within 1 to 2 months, but it may be delayed for as long as 12 months. Neurologic deficits improve rapidly after treatment, but complete resolution may take 2 to 3 months (Jaggy et al, 1994).

Therapeutic Monitoring

Therapeutic monitoring includes evaluation of the clinical response to thyroid hormone supplementation and measurement of serum T$_4$ and TSH concentrations before or after L-T$_4$ sodium administration, or both. Therapeutic monitoring allows treatment to be individualized to the patient based on clinical response, thyroid hormone concentrations, and presence or absence of concurrent illness. Serum T$_4$ and TSH should be measured 6 to 8 weeks after initiating therapy, whenever signs of thyrotoxicosis develop, or when there is a poor response to therapy. T$_4$ concentration and TSH should also be measured 2 to 4 weeks after any adjustment in L-T$_4$ sodium therapy.

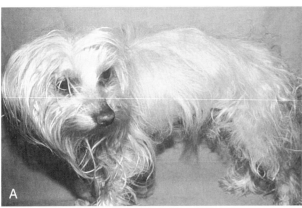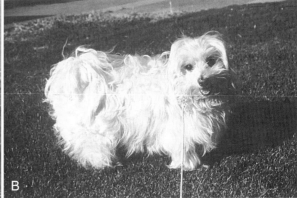

FIGURE 3-34 A, A 7-year-old male Maltese with hypothyroidism and diabetes mellitus. **B,** Same dog as in **A** after 3 months of levothyroxine (L-T₄) sodium treatment. Note the marked improvement in appearance and hair coat.

TABLE 3-14	ANTICIPATED TIME OF CLINICAL RESPONSE TO SODIUM LEVOTHYROXINE TREATMENT IN DOGS WITH HYPOTHYROIDISM

AREA OF IMPROVEMENT	TIME TO IMPROVEMENT
Mentation and activity	2 to 7 days
Lipemia and clinical pathology	2 to 4 weeks
Dermatologic abnormalities	2 to 4 months
Neurologic abnormalities	1 to 3 months
Cardiac abnormalities	1 to 2 months
Reproductive abnormalities	3 to 10 months

Serum T_4 and TSH concentrations are typically evaluated 4 to 6 hours after the administration of L-T_4 sodium in dogs receiving the medication twice daily and just before and 4 to 6 hours after administration in dogs receiving it once a day (Nachreiner and Refsal, 1992). This information allows the clinician to evaluate the dose, frequency of administration, and adequacy of intestinal absorption of L-T_4 sodium. Measurement of serum fT_4 by the MED technique can be done in lieu of T_4 but is more expensive and usually does not have benefit except in dogs with serum T_4 autoantibodies. Although the presence of thyroid hormone auto-antibodies does not interfere with the physiologic actions of thyroid hormone supplements, they will interfere with measurement of total T_4 concentration (see Fig. 3-19). Results of serum fT_4 measured by assays that use a dialysis step (e.g., MED technique) are not affected by thyroid hormone autoantibodies. Measurement of serum TSH is only useful in dogs in which the TSH concentration was above the reference range at the time of diagnosis.

Post dosing serum T_4 and TSH results and recommendations for changes in therapy are given in Fig. 3-33. If the dose of the thyroid hormone supplement and the dosing schedule are appropriate, the serum T_4 concentration should be in the upper half of or a little above the reference baseline range (i.e., 3.0 to 6.0 µg/dL) when measured 4 to 6 hours after thyroid hormone administration, and the serum TSH concentration should be in the reference range (i.e., less than 0.6 ng/mL) in all blood samples evaluated. If the clinical signs do not resolve and the post-pill T_4 is below or within the lower half of the reference range (< 2.0 µg/dL), the dose of L-T_4 sodium should be increased. If the clinical signs

have resolved but the post-pill concentration is in lower half of the reference range, a serum TSH should be measured. If this is within the reference range indicating good biological response to supplementation, the dose does not need to be adjusted. Post dosing serum T_4 concentrations measured at times other than 4 to 6 hours after L-T_4 sodium administration should be interpreted with the realization that serum T_4 may not be at peak concentrations. Ideally, all post-pill serum T_4 concentrations should be greater than 1.5 µg/dL, regardless of the time interval between L-T_4 sodium administration and post-pill blood sampling. The post-dosing serum T_4 concentration may also be affected by the pharmaceutical preparation administered, concurrent drugs such as glucocorticoids, and possibly diet. Post-dosing serum T_4 concentrations are frequently above the reference range. The finding of an increased post-dosing serum T_4 concentration is not an absolute indication to reduce the dose of L-T_4 sodium, especially if there are no clinical signs of thyrotoxicosis. However, we recommend a reduction in the dose whenever serum T_4 concentrations exceed 6.0 µg/dL. Dogs are relatively resistant to development of iatrogenic hyperthyroidism because of the short half-life of T_4 in this species; however, the risk of long-term over-supplementation of thyroid hormone in dogs has not been investigated. Current assays for TSH are not sensitive enough to distinguish a normal from a low TSH concentration and thus cannot distinguish between those dogs that are adequately supplemented and those that are over-supplemented. If the clinical response is poor to thyroid hormone supplementation, post dosing serum T_4 concentrations are within or above the reference range, and serum TSH concentrations are less than 0.6 ng/mL, other causes of the clinical signs of concern should be investigated. Although trial therapy with liothyronine sodium may be attempted, it is usually ineffective in producing a beneficial response in a dog that has failed to respond to L-T_4 sodium and whose serum T_4 concentrations are in the normal range during treatment.

Treatment of Dogs with Concurrent Nonthyroidal Illness
Cardiomyopathy
Because euthyroid dogs with cardiac disease may have decreased thyroid hormone concentrations, accurate diagnosis of hypothyroidism may be challenging. It is important to be confident of the diagnosis in such dogs to avoid inappropriate treatment. In hypothyroid dogs with cardiac disorders, thyroid hormone supplementation increases myocardial oxygen demand, increases heart rate, and may reduce ventricular filling time. Decompensation of the

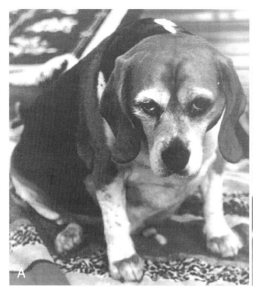
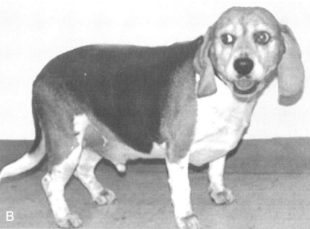

FIGURE 3-35 A, An 8-year-old male castrated Beagle with hypothyroidism. The primary owner complaints were obesity, lethargy, and weakness. The dog weighed 31 kg. **B,** Same dog as in **A** after 6 months of levothyroxine (L-T$_4$) sodium treatment and adjustments in caloric intake and type of diet to promote weight loss. The owner reported marked improvement in the dog's alertness and activity, and its body weight had decreased to 19 kg.

cardiac disease can therefore occur with initiation of thyroid hormone supplementation. Because of these concerns the initial dose of thyroid hormone replacement in dogs with cardiac diseases such as cardiomyopathy should be 25% to 50% of the usual starting dose. The dose may then be increased incrementally based on the results of therapeutic monitoring and reevaluation of cardiac function.

Hypoadrenocorticism

In dogs with concurrent hypoadrenocorticism and hypothyroidism, replacement of mineralocorticoid and glucocorticoid deficiency should be initiated before treatment with L-T$_4$ sodium, because the increased basal metabolic rate resulting from thyroid hormone supplementation may exacerbate electrolyte disturbances and cause decompensation of hypoadrenocorticism.

Diabetes Mellitus

In dogs with concurrent hypothyroidism and diabetes mellitus, hypothyroidism can cause insulin resistance that resolves with treatment of hypothyroidism (Ford et al, 1993). When hypothyroidism is diagnosed and treated in a diabetic patient, the blood glucose should be carefully monitored for hypoglycemia during the 1 to 2 weeks after initiation of thyroid supplementation. Once euthyroidism is reestablished, increased insulin sensitivity and a decreased need for insulin may lead to hypoglycemia.

Other Concurrent Illness

The appropriate therapeutic range for hypothyroid dogs with concurrent nonthyroidal illness, for geriatric dogs, and for dogs being treated with drugs, such as phenobarbital and glucocorticoids, that influence serum total T$_4$, is unknown. The target serum total T$_4$ concentration should be lower in dogs with concurrent illness and those being treated with drugs known to lower thyroid hormone concentrations. In such cases, the decision whether to adjust the dose of thyroid supplementation should be based primarily on response to therapy. If a positive response to therapy occurs but the post-pill T$_4$ concentration is low, no further dosage increase should be recommended.

BOX 3-8   Potential Reasons for Poor Clinical Response to Treatment with Levothyroxine Sodium (Synthetic Thyroxine)

Owner compliance problems
Use of inactivated or outdated product
Use of some generic levothyroxine (L-T$_4$) sodium preparations
Inappropriate L-T$_4$ sodium dose
Inappropriate frequency of administration
Use of thyroid extracts or combination thyroxine/triiodothyronine products
Poor bioavailability (e.g., poor gastrointestinal absorption)
Inadequate time for clinical response to occur
Incorrect diagnosis of hypothyroidism
Concurrent disease causing clinical signs (e.g., allergic dermatitis)

Treatment Failure

There are several possible reasons for a poor response to T$_4$ supplementation (Box 3-8). An inappropriate diagnosis of hypothyroidism is the most common cause. Hyperadrenocorticism can be mistaken for hypothyroidism especially if other clinical signs, such as polyuria and polydipsia, characteristic of hyperadrenocorticism are not present. This confusion results because of the suppressive effects of cortisol on serum thyroid hormone concentrations. Other causes of skin disorders (e.g., atopy and flea allergic dermatitis) may also be confused with hypothyroidism. Failure to recognize the impact of concurrent illness on thyroid hormone test results is another common cause for misdiagnosing hypothyroidism. When a dog shows a poor response to L-T$_4$ sodium therapy, the history, physical examination findings, and diagnostic test results that prompted the initiation of L-T$_4$ sodium therapy should be critically reevaluated and a thorough evaluation for concurrent disease undertaken. In addition, problems with the treatment regimen should be investigated, including poor owner compliance in administering the hormone, the use of outdated preparations, an inappropriate dose or frequency of administration of L-T$_4$ sodium, the use of some generic L-T$_4$ sodium products, the use of thyroid extracts or combination thyroxine/triiodthyronine products, or poor intestinal absorption of L-T$_4$ sodium due to concurrent gastrointestinal disorders or administration of thyroid supplements with food. If poor gastrointestinal absorption is suspected, T$_3$ may be substituted for T$_4$.

Treatment with Liothyronine Sodium (Synthetic Triiodothyronine)

Liothyronine sodium is not the initial thyroid hormone supplement of choice for the treatment of hypothyroidism. Liothyronine sodium supplementation results in normal serum T$_3$ but low to non-detectable serum T$_4$ concentrations. In contrast, L-T$_4$ sodium therapy results in normal serum concentrations of both T$_3$ and T$_4$ because L-T$_4$ sodium is converted to T$_3$. Treatment with L-T$_4$ sodium preserves normal regulation of T$_4$ to T$_3$ conversion, which allows physiologic regulation of tissue T$_3$ concentrations and decreases the risk of iatrogenic hyperthyroidism (Siegmund et al, 2004).

Liothyronine therapy is indicated when L-T$_4$ sodium therapy has failed to achieve a response in a dog with confirmed hypothyroidism, when gastrointestinal malabsorption is the suspected cause for failure to respond to the L-T$_4$ supplement. Impaired absorption of L-T$_4$ sodium should be suspected when baseline serum T$_4$ concentrations are low, serum TSH is high, and no increase in serum T$_4$ concentration occurs following oral L-T$_4$ sodium administration. Thyroid hormone autoantibodies that interfere with the RIA technique should also be considered in this scenario. Gastrointestinal absorption of ingested T$_3$ approaches 100%, whereas absorption of L-T$_4$ sodium is only 10% to 50% of the administered dose. This more complete absorption of T$_3$ reflects less binding affinity of intestinal contents for T$_3$, especially plasma proteins secreted in the bowel lumen.

Historically, liothyronine sodium has been used for treatment of hypothyroidism in dogs with normal serum T$_4$ but low serum T$_3$ concentration. These dogs were often suspected of having a defect in the conversion of T$_4$ to T$_3$. It is now recognized that most of these dogs are either normal, have NTIS, or have T$_3$ autoantibodies that cause a false lowering of the serum T$_3$ concentration. T$_4$ to T$_3$ conversion abnormalities have not been documented in any species, including dogs. Conceptually, conversion defects are most likely to be congenital, and thus, affected puppies should either die shortly after birth or develop cretinism. If the decision is made to treat the dog with normal serum T$_4$ and low serum T$_3$ concentration, L-T$_4$ sodium should be used initially.

The initial dosage of liothyronine is 4 to 6 µg/kg body weight every 8 hours. As with L-T$_4$ sodium, the plasma half-life and time of peak plasma concentration after administration of liothyronine are variable among dogs. In most dogs, the plasma half-life of liothyronine is approximately 5 to 6 hours, with peak plasma concentrations occurring 2 to 5 hours after administration. Once clinical improvement is observed, the frequency of administration may be reduced to twice a day. If clinical signs recur, three daily doses should be reinstituted.

Blood for therapeutic monitoring should be obtained just before and 2 to 4 hours after administration of liothyronine sodium. Evaluation of serum T$_3$ is mandatory with this supplement because the risk of thyrotoxicosis is much higher. Serum T$_4$ concentrations are low to non-detectable with adequate T$_3$ supplementation because of the negative feedback suppression of TSH and the inability of T$_3$ to be converted to T$_4$. Guidelines for adjustments in T$_3$ therapy are similar to those for T$_4$ supplements. Serum T$_3$ concentrations before and following T$_3$ administration should be within the normal range in a dog receiving an adequate dosage of a T$_3$ supplement.

Combination Thyroxine/Triiodothyronine Products

Synthetic preparations are available that contain both L-T$_4$ sodium and liothyronine (Liotrix, Thyrolar). The T$_4$-to-T$_3$ ratio is generally 4 to 1 and the unphysiologic proportion of T$_3$ can make it difficult to maintain euthyroidism (Siegmund et al, 2004). Whether there are benefits to using such products for treatment of hypothyroid human patients is controversial. Although most controlled studies have not provided evidence that treatment with combination products improves patient outcome (Siegmund et al, 2004), anecdotally some patients report improved quality of life when treated with combination products. Combination T$_4$/T$_3$ products are not recommended in dogs for the following reasons: (1) the rate of metabolism and thus the frequency of administration differ between L-T$_4$ sodium and liothyronine; (2) L-T$_4$ sodium therapy provides adequate serum concentrations of both T$_4$ and T$_3$; and (3) the use of synthetic combinations may result in serum concentrations of T$_3$ that could cause thyrotoxicosis. In addition, synthetic combination products tend to be more expensive than either synthetic L-T$_4$ sodium or liothyronine alone.

Thyroid Extracts

Animal-origin preparations are desiccated thyroid that is derived from cleaned, dried, and powdered thyroid glands of slaughterhouse origin. The porcine product is the most commonly available (Armour Thyroid). The United States Pharmacopeia requires thyroid extracts to contain approximately 38 µg of T$_4$ and 9 µg of T$_3$ for each 60 to 65 mg tablet giving a T$_4$-to-T$_3$ ratio of approximately 4:1, which is similar to combination products. Potential problems with such products include the potential for allergy or sensitivity, batch to batch variability, variable shelf life, and the difficulties outlined earlier in maintaining euthyroidism with the unphysiologic ratio of T$_4$ to T$_3$. For these reasons crude animal-origin thyroid preparations are not recommended for the treatment of hypothyroidism in dogs.

Treatment of Myxedema Coma

Early recognition and aggressive therapy are critical to survival of myxedema coma. Consequently, the diagnosis should be made clinically, and therapy should be initiated without waiting for results of serum thyroid hormone concentrations if this disorder is suspected. Treatment consists of thyroid hormone administration and correction of the associated physiologic disturbances, such as hypothermia, hypovolemia, electrolyte disturbances, and hypoventilation. Because concurrent nonthyroidal disorders commonly precipitate myxedema coma, diagnosis and treatment of these disorders is critical. Because of the sluggish circulation and severe hypometabolism of profound hypothyroidism, absorption of therapeutic agents from the gut or from subcutaneous or intramuscular sites is unpredictable, and if possible, thyroid hormone should be administered intravenously. The recommended initial dosage for injectable L-T$_4$ sodium is 4 to 5 µg/kg every 12 hours (Pullen and Hess, 2006). A 50% to 75% reduction in the dosage should be considered if there is pre-existing cardiac disease or failure (Henik and Dixon, 2000). Oral administration of L-T$_4$ sodium can also be administered every 12 hours to provide sustained delivery of T$_4$. Appropriate supportive care should also be initiated, including IV sodium-containing fluids with dextrose supplementation; slow, passive rewarming with blankets; and assisted ventilation, if needed. Clinical improvement is usually seen within 24 hours, although death due to concurrent illness is common. Once the dog has stabilized, oral thyroid hormone treatment can be started.

Thyrotoxicosis

It is unusual for thyrotoxicosis to develop as a result of excessive administration of L-T$_4$ sodium in the dog, because of the short half-life of L-T$_4$ sodium in the dog as well as physiologic adaptations that impair gastrointestinal tract absorption and enhance clearance of thyroid hormone by the liver and kidneys (Nachreiner and Refsal, 1992). Nevertheless, thyrotoxicosis may develop in dogs receiving excessive amounts of L-T$_4$ sodium (especially in dogs receiving L-T$_4$ sodium twice daily) and in dogs with impaired metabolism of L-T$_4$ sodium (e.g., concurrent renal or hepatic insufficiency).

Clinical signs of thyrotoxicosis include panting, nervousness, anxiety, tachycardia, aggressive behavior, polyuria, polydipsia, polyphagia, and weight loss. Sinus tachycardia, atrial flutter, and syncope have been reported in dogs with iatrogenic hyperthyroidism and concurrent cardiac disease (Fine et al, 2010). Documentation of mild to marked increased serum thyroid hormone concentrations supports the diagnosis; however, these concentrations can occasionally be within the upper end of the reference normal range in a dog with signs of thyrotoxicosis, and conversely some dogs with increased thyroid hormone concentrations have no clinical signs of thyrotoxicosis. A cardiac evaluation should be performed in dogs with arrhythmias due to suspected thyrotoxicosis. Adjustments in the dose or frequency of administration of thyroid hormone medication are indicated if clinical signs of thyrotoxicosis develop in a dog receiving thyroid hormone supplements. Supplementation may have to be discontinued for a few days in such animals if the clinical signs are severe. Signs of thyrotoxicosis should resolve within 1 to 3 days if they are due to the thyroid medication and the adjustment in treatment has been appropriate, although the presence of underlying heart disease may lead to persistence of cardiac arrhythmias. It is recommended that therapeutic monitoring should be repeated 2 to 4 weeks after the dose of L-T$_4$ sodium has been decreased. It is also important to review the criteria used for diagnosis in order to determine whether T$_4$ supplementation was appropriate in the first place.

PROGNOSIS

The prognosis for dogs with hypothyroidism depends on the underlying cause. The life expectancy of an adult dog with primary hypothyroidism that is receiving appropriate therapy should be normal. All the clinical manifestations should resolve in response to thyroid hormone supplementation. Prognosis in myxedema coma is dependent on early recognition and treatment. The prognosis for puppies with hypothyroidism (i.e., cretinism) is guarded and depends on the severity of skeletal and joint abnormalities at the time treatment is initiated. Although many of the clinical signs resolve with therapy, musculoskeletal problems, especially degenerative osteoarthritis, may develop as a result of abnormal bone and joint development (Greco et al, 1991; Saunders and Jezyk, 1991). Degenerative osteoarthritis is more prevalent in joints with adjacent epiphyseal dysgenesis. Epiphyseal dysgenesis may result in increased susceptibility to trauma, articular cartilage damage, osteochondrosis-type lesions, and degenerative joint changes. Contributing to these changes

are the biomechanical abnormalities caused by radial bowing with subsequent humeroradial joint widening and humeroulnar joint subluxation, which is seen in some dogs with congenital hypothyroidism. In puppies with CHG due to TPO deficiency, the goiter persists and TSH concentrations remain high despite normalization of total T$_4$ concentrations with twice daily L-T$_4$ sodium at appropriate doses (Fyfe, 2003; Pettigrew et al, 2007). Whether further adjustment of thyroid hormone supplementation by therapeutic monitoring would result in resolution of the goiter is unknown.

The prognosis for dogs with secondary hypothyroidism caused by malformation or destruction of the pituitary gland is guarded to poor. The life expectancy is shortened in dogs with congenital malformation of the pituitary gland (i.e., pituitary dwarfism), primarily because of the multiple problems that develop in early life (see Chapter 2). Acquired secondary hypothyroidism is usually caused by destruction of the pituitary by a space-occupying mass, which has the potential to expand into the brainstem.

FELINE HYPOTHYROIDISM

Naturally acquired hypothyroidism is a rare clinical entity in the cat, and most clinical descriptions of feline hypothyroidism in the veterinary literature have been case reports of either primary congenital or adult onset hypothyroidism (Arnold et al, 1984; Sjollema et al, 1991; Jones et al, 1992, Rand et al, 1993; Mellanby et al, 2005; Traas et al, 2008; Blois et al, 2010; Quante et al, 2010). In contrast, iatrogenic hypothyroidism following any of the three common treatments for hyperthyroidism is well recognized (Nykamp et al, 2005; Williams et al, 2010).

Low serum T$_4$ concentrations in cats are frequently documented by veterinarians because of inclusion of serum T$_4$ concentration in the typical "feline geriatric panel" offered by many commercial laboratories. Unfortunately, the blood sample is usually submitted for evaluation of another problem (e.g., systemic illness) and the low T$_4$ concentration is almost always the result of the suppressive effects of nonthyroidal illness on serum T$_4$ concentration (i.e., NTIS) and not hypothyroidism.

ETIOLOGY

Iatrogenic Hypothyroidism

Iatrogenically induced hypothyroidism is usually the result of treatment of hyperthyroidism and is far more common than naturally acquired hypothyroidism in cats. Iatrogenic hypothyroidism can result from bilateral thyroidectomy, radioactive iodine treatment, or treatment with anti-thyroid drugs. Depending on the treatment used for hyperthyroidism, plasma thyroid hormone concentrations can decline to subnormal concentrations within hours (surgery), days (anti-thyroid drugs), or weeks to months (radioactive iodine) after treatment. In a study of 165 cats treated with radioactive iodine, 30% developed hypothyroidism defined by a total T$_4$ concentration less than the lower reference limit 3 months after treatment (Nykamp et al, 2005). Cats that had evidence of bilateral thyroid disease were more likely to become hypothyroid than those with unilateral dysfunction. In another study of 80 non-azotemic hyperthyroid cats treated with anti-thyroid drugs, 35% became hypothyroid (as defined by a total T$_4$ concentration below the reference range and a serum TSH concentration above the reference range) 6 months after initiating treatment (Williams et al, 2010). Hypothyroid cats were more likely to become azotemic after treatment than euthyroid cats, and cats that were both hypothyroid and azotemic had shorter survival times than those that were azotemic but not hypothyroid. Azotemia was presumed to be due to a decrease in glomerular filtration rate in cats with underlying chronic kidney disease and concurrent hypothyroidism. Prolonged iatrogenic hypothyroidism should therefore be avoided especially in cats with known concurrent chronic kidney disease. In cats with iatrogenic hypothyroidism, the clinical signs are usually mild with decreased activity and weight gain typically observed. These clinical signs are usually not worrying to the owner of a previously hyperthyroid cat; however, because of the risk of progressive azotemia, thyroid hormone supplementation should be instituted in hypothyroid azotemic cats, in cats with clinical signs of hypothyroidism, and in cats with hypothyroidism that persists 3 to 6 months beyond definitive treatment with radioactive iodine or thyroidectomy. In cats treated with oral anti-thyroid drugs that become hypothyroid, a decreased drug dose should be implemented.

Adult-Onset Hypothyroidism

Naturally acquired adult-onset primary hypothyroidism is rarely documented in the cat. Two well documented cases have been published. One cat had lymphocytic thyroiditis, whereas in another cat the thyroid gland could not be identified at necropsy (Rand et al, 1993; Blois et al, 2010). Secondary hypothyroidism due to head trauma was reported in an 18-month-old cat with stunted growth and a history of head trauma at 8 weeks of age (Mellanby et al, 2005). The diagnosis was made by documentation of low total T_4 and TSH and no increase in T_4 or TSH after administration of TRH. A magnetic resonance imaging (MRI) scan of the brain revealed an almost empty sella turcica and a very small pituitary gland.

Congenital Hypothyroidism

Congenital primary hypothyroidism causing disproportionate dwarfism is recognized more frequently than adult-onset hypothyroidism in the cat. Reported causes of congenital hypothyroidism include thyroid dyshormonogenesis (Sjollema et al, 1991; Jones et al, 1992), thyroid dysmorphogenesis (Traas et al, 2008), and TSH resistance. Goiter is expected in congenital hypothyroidism due to dyshormonogenesis. An inherited defect in iodine organification was documented in a family of Abyssinian cats with congenital hypothyroidism and goiter (Jones et al, 1992); an autosomal recessive mode of inheritance was suspected. CHG due to TPO deficiency was reported in a family of Domestic Short-Hair cats and was also thought to be inherited as an autosomal recessive trait (Mazrier et al, 2003). A colony of cats with hypothyroidism and thyroiditis with severe signs of hypothyroidism developing 40 to 60 days after birth has also been reported (Schumm-Draeger et al, 1996). The severity of thyroiditis was decreased by early treatment with thyroid hormone. TSH resistance was proposed to be the cause of inherited primary hypothyroidism in a colony of Japanese cats (Tanase et al, 1991). The cats in this colony of hypothyroid cats did not develop a goiter, and the defect was inherited as an autosomal recessive trait. Although rare, iodine deficiency has been reported to cause hypothyroidism in kittens fed a strict all-meat diet.

 CLINICAL SIGNS

Adult-Onset Hypothyroidism

The clinical signs that have been associated with feline hypothyroidism are listed in Box 3-9. Of these, the most commonly seen

BOX 3-9 Clinical Manifestations of Feline Hypothyroidism

Adult-Onset Hypothyroidism
Lethargy
Inappetence
Obesity
Dermatologic
Seborrhea sicca
Dry, lusterless hair coat
Easily epilated hair
Poor regrowth of hair
Endocrine alopecia
Alopecia of pinnae
Thickened skin
Myxedema of the face
Bradycardia
Mild hypothermia

Congenital Hypothyroidism
Disproportionate dwarfism
    Failure to grow
    Large head
    Short, broad neck
    Short limbs
Lethargy
Mental dullness
Constipation
Hypothermia
Bradycardia
Retention of kitten hair coat
Retention of deciduous teeth

are lethargy, inappetence, dermatologic abnormalities, and obesity (Fig. 3-36). Lethargy and inappetence may become severe. Dermatologic signs are quite variable and often develop secondary to a decrease in grooming behavior by the cat. Affected cats develop a dull, dry, unkempt hair coat with matting and seborrhea. Easily epilated and poor regrowth of hair may lead to alopecia affecting the pinnae, pressure points, and the dorsal and lateral tail base region (Peterson, 1989; Rand et al, 1993; Blois et al, 2010). Asymmetric or bilaterally symmetric alopecia involving the lateral neck, thorax, and abdomen may also develop. Myxedema of the face, causing a "puffy" appearance, was reported in one cat with naturally acquired adult-onset hypothyroidism (Rand et al, 1993). Bradycardia and mild hypothermia may be additional findings on physical examination.

Congenital Hypothyroidism

The clinical signs of congenital hypothyroidism are similar to those in dogs. Affected kittens typically appear normal at birth, but a decrease in growth rate usually becomes evident by 6 to 8 weeks of age. Disproportionate dwarfism develops over the ensuing months with affected kittens developing large heads, short broad necks, and short limbs. Additional findings include lethargy, mental dullness, constipation, hypothermia, bradycardia, and prolonged retention of deciduous teeth (Arnold et al, 1984; Peterson, 1989; Sjollema et al, 1991; Jones et al, 1992; Traas et al, 2008; Fig. 3-37). The hair coat consists mainly of the undercoat with primary guard hair scattered thinly throughout. Radiographic abnormalities are similar to those described for the dog. Two littermate kittens with hypothyroidism had a concurrent

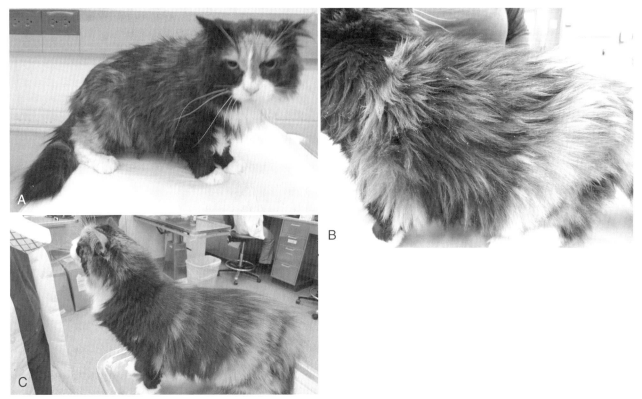

FIGURE 3-36 A, A 12-year-old spayed female cat with spontaneous adult onset hypothyroidism. The cat presented for evaluation of obesity, lethargy, and a dull dry hair coat. **B,** Close up of the hair coat showing dry dull coat with dry flaky skin. **C,** Same cat after 3 months of thyroid supplementation. Clinical signs had all resolved.

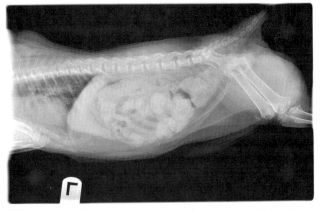

FIGURE 3-37 Lateral abdominal radiograph of a young cat with constipation due to hypothyroidism.

seizure disorder but whether the seizures were related to hypothyroidism was unclear (Traas et al, 2008).

 TESTS OF THYROID GLAND FUNCTION

Hormone measurements that have been used for documentation of feline hypothyroidism include total T_4, fT_4, total T_3, and TSH concentration. For a detailed discussion of thyroid hormone assays in cats see Chapter 4.

Baseline Serum Thyroxine Concentration

Measurement of baseline serum T_4 concentration is the best initial screening test for hypothyroidism in a cat with appropriate clinical signs. Cats with hypothyroidism typically have baseline serum T_4 concentrations below the lower limit of the reference range, and sometimes T_4 is undetectable. A total T_4 within the reference range is useful to exclude a diagnosis of hypothyroidism, but because nonthyroidal illness and administration of drugs (e.g., glucocorticoids) can lower serum T_4 concentration into the hypothyroid range (Fig. 3-38), a low serum T_4 concentration does not, by itself, confirm hypothyroidism. As in the dog, the total T_4 should be interpreted in the context of the clinical signs and presence or absence of other concurrent illness and concurrent drug therapy. If the history and physical findings are consistent with the disease, the lower the T_4 value, the more likely it is that the cat truly has hypothyroidism. If the clinician's index of suspicion is not high for hypothyroidism but the serum T_4 concentration is low, then other factors such as nonthyroidal illness are much more likely.

Baseline Serum Triiodothyronine Concentration

Measurement of baseline serum T_3 concentration is not routinely performed in cats, and reported total T_3 concentrations have been variable in those cases of feline hypothyroidism in which it has been measured. Presumably, the problems encountered with serum T_3 measurements in differentiating euthyroidism from hypothyroidism in the dog also exist in the cat. Ideally, baseline serum T_3 concentration should be less than the lower limit of normal for the laboratory used in the cat with

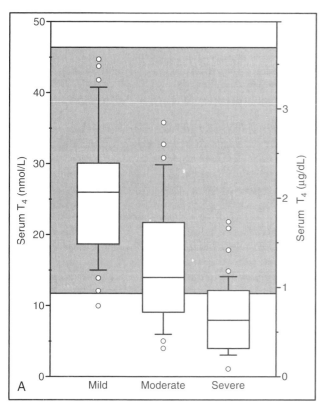 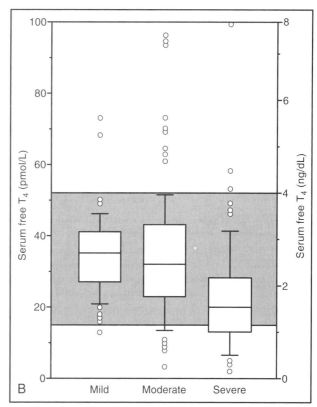

FIGURE 3-38 Box plots of serum total thyroxine (T_4) **(A)** and free T_4 (fT_4) **(B)** concentrations in 221 cats with nonthyroidal disease stratified according to severity of disease. Of the 221 cats, 65 had mild disease, 83 had moderate disease, and 73 had severe disease. For each box plot, T-bars represent the main body of data, which in most instances is equal to the range. Each box represents the interquartile range (25th to 75th percentile). The *horizontal bar* in each box is the median. *Open circles* represent outlying data points. The *shaded area* indicates the reference range. (From Peterson ME, et al.: Measurement of serum concentrations of free thyroxine, total thyroxine, and total triiodothyronine in cats with hyperthyroidism and cats with nonthyroidal disease, *J Am Vet Med Assoc* 218[4]:529, 2001.)

hypothyroidism. However, a normal serum T_3 concentration in a cat with appropriate history, physical examination findings, and low serum T_4 concentration does not rule out hypothyroidism. Similarly, a low serum T_3 concentration in a cat with normal serum T_4 concentration is not consistent with hypothyroidism, especially if the remainder of the clinical picture does not support the diagnosis.

Baseline Serum Free Thyroxine Concentration

Cats with hypothyroidism should have baseline serum fT_4 concentrations below the lower limit of normal for the laboratory used. As with serum T_4, a low serum fT_4 concentration does not, by itself, confirm hypothyroidism. Nonthyroidal factors, most notably concurrent illness and administration of drugs (e.g., glucocorticoids), can falsely lower the serum fT_4 concentration into the hypothyroid range (see Fig. 3-38). Serum fT_4 is believed to be less influenced by factors such as nonthyroidal illness and administration of drugs than serum T_4, but serum fT_4 concentrations have been reported to increase rather than decrease in some euthyroid cats with nonthyroidal illness (Mooney et al, 1996a; Peterson et al, 2001). The comparative sensitivity and specificity of serum fT_4 versus serum T_4 for evaluation of thyroid gland function in cats with suspected hypothyroidism is unknown.

Baseline Serum Thyroid-Stimulating Hormone Concentration

A canine TSH assay (Immulite canine TSH assay, Diagnostic Products Corporation). has been validated for use in cats (Wakeling et al, 2008; 2011). Although the sensitivity of the assay is suboptimal, a high TSH concentration in a cat with a concurrent decrease in total T_4 is highly specific for a diagnosis of hypothyroidism. Increased TSH has been documented in cats with congenital hypothyroidism, spontaneous adult unset hypothyroidism, and iatrogenic hypothyroidism.

Tests for Lymphocytic Thyroiditis

Tests for the presence of circulating Tg and microsomal antibodies were reported to be positive in a colony of cats with early onset thyroiditis; however commercial assays for these antibodies are not currently available in the cat (Schumm-Draeger et al, 1996).

Factors Affecting Baseline Thyroid Hormone Concentrations

Many of the nonthyroidal factors known to influence serum thyroid hormone concentrations in dogs have yet to be evaluated in cats. The effects of age, gender, and breed on serum T_4 and T_3 concentrations in cats are controversial. In one study, serum T_4 and, to a lesser extent, serum T_3 concentrations in both genders tended to decrease until approximately 5 years of age and then increase again; females (intact and neutered) had significantly higher serum T_4 but not T_3 concentrations than males (intact or neutered); and serum T_3 but not T_4 concentration was significantly higher in pedigree cats than in Domestic Short- and Long-Haired cats (Thoday et al, 1984). Serum thyroid hormone concentrations remained within the reference range in these cats regardless of any influence of age, gender, or breed on blood thyroid hormone levels. In another study, Zerbe, et al. (1998) identified values for serum T_4 and fT_4 concentrations within reference range for adult cats in kittens from birth to 12 weeks of age, whereas serum T_3 concentrations were low until kittens were 5 weeks of age. Other investigators have not identified an effect of age, gender, and/or breed on serum thyroid hormone concentrations. A diurnal variation in blood thyroid hormone concentrations apparently does not occur in the cat (Hoenig and Ferguson, 1983), so the time of day that the blood is sampled should not affect the results.

Nonthyroidal illness causing NTIS has been documented in the cat (Peterson and Gamble, 1990; Mooney et al, 1996a; Peterson et al, 2001; see Fig. 3-38). As with the dog, serum T_4 and T_3 concentrations are more likely to be decreased with nonthyroidal illness than serum fT_4 concentrations, and there is a direct correlation between the severity of illness and the magnitude of the decrease in serum thyroid hormone concentrations (see Fig. 3-38). The more severe the nonthyroidal illness, the more likely serum thyroid hormone concentrations will decrease into the hypothyroid range. Serum T_4 values less than 0.5 μg/dL and fT_4 values less than 0.5 ng/dL may occur with severe systemic illness in a euthyroid cat. It is interesting to note that some euthyroid cats with nonthyroidal disease will have decreased serum T_4 concentrations but increased serum fT_4 concentrations when an equilibrium dialysis technique is used to measure fT_4. Increased serum fT_4 concentrations were found in 12% of 98 euthyroid cats with nonthyroidal illness in one study (Mooney et al, 1996a) and 6.3% of 221 euthyroid cats with nonthyroidal illness in another study (Peterson et al, 2001). Nonthyroidal illnesses in these cats included diabetes mellitus, gastrointestinal tract disease, hepatic disease, renal insufficiency, and neoplasia. The reason for increased serum fT_4 concentrations in some cats with nonthyroidal illness is not known but may be related to decreased protein binding of circulating T_4 and/or impaired clearance of T_4 from the circulation.

The effects of drugs on serum thyroid hormone concentrations have not been extensively evaluated in the cat. Two classes of drugs that can decrease serum thyroid hormone concentrations into the hypothyroid range are glucocorticoids and anti-thyroid hormone drugs (i.e., methimazole, propylthiouracil). Undoubtedly, many more drugs also affect serum thyroid hormone concentrations in cats. Until proven otherwise, any drug should be suspected of affecting thyroid hormone test results, especially if the drug has been shown to alter serum thyroid hormone concentrations in humans and dogs (see Table 3-13 and Box 3-6) and the history and clinical signs of the patient do not support a diagnosis of hypothyroidism.

Thyroid-Stimulating Hormone Stimulation Test

The indications, protocol, and interpretation of the TSH stimulation test are similar for the cat and dog except that a lower dose of recombinant human thyrotropin (rhTSH) (25 micrograms IV) is used in the cat (Stegeman et al, 2003; van Hoek et al, 2010). In euthyroid cats, there is a two- to threefold increase in total T_4 6 to 8 hours after TSH administration. Although responses of healthy euthyroid cats to TSH have been studied, there are few studies reporting changes in total T_4 after TSH administration in cats with nonthyroidal illness or hypothyroidism. In one small study, the percent increase after TSH administration in healthy cats

ranged from 111% to 300%, and in cats with nonthyroidal illness total T_4 increased by 146% to 414% (van Hoek et al, 2010). Cats with iatrogenic hypothyroidism after radioactive iodine treatment had a percent increase in total T_4 of 11% or less. These results suggest that the TSH stimulation test is useful for diagnosis of hypothyroidism in cats; however, the TSH stimulation test is rarely used clinically because of the expense of rhTSH.

Thyrotropin-Releasing Hormone Stimulation Test

The TRH stimulation test has been recommended for diagnosis of hyperthyroidism in cats (see Chapter 4) but is currently rarely used for this purpose and it has not been evaluated for diagnosis of hypothyroidism in cats. Theoretically in a cat with a functionally intact pituitary-thyroid axis, the serum T_4 concentration should increase 1 to 2 μg/dL or greater than 50% above baseline serum T_4 concentration, after administration of TRH. Failure of serum T_4 concentration to increase after TRH administration suggests dysfunction of either the pituitary or the thyroid gland or suppression of the pituitary-thyroid axis by nonthyroidal factors. If results of a previous TSH stimulation test were normal, an abnormal TRH stimulation test implies pituitary dysfunction.

 ## ESTABLISHING THE DIAGNOSIS

The diagnosis of hypothyroidism in the cat should be based on a combination of history, clinical signs, physical examination findings, low serum thyroid hormone concentrations and increased serum TSH concentration. A minimum data base of CBC, serum chemistry profile, and urinalysis should be performed to identify changes supportive of hypothyroidism and assess for the presence of nonthyroidal illness. The most consistent findings in hypothyroid cats include hypercholesterolemia; normocytic, normochromic non-regenerative anemia; and an increase in creatine kinase. A low serum T_4 concentration in conjunction with an increased TSH concentration supports the diagnosis of primary hypothyroidism. Hypothyroidism is much more likely in a cat that has undergone thyroidectomy or radioactive iodine treatment or a kitten with disproportionate dwarfism; spontaneous adult onset hypothyroidism is so rare that nonthyroidal illness should be carefully considered prior to making a diagnosis of hypothyroidism. Further diagnostic testing that should be considered to confirm the diagnosis and localize the location of the defect includes scintigraphy and a TSH stimulation test. Response to trial therapy with L-T_4 sodium also supports the diagnosis.

Because naturally acquired primary hypothyroidism is rare and a low serum T_4 concentration in an adult cat is almost always caused by nonthyroidal illness, it is important to avoid making a diagnosis of hypothyroidism based solely on serum T_4 concentration in an adult cat that has not been previously treated for hyperthyroidism (see Chapter 4). A serum fT_4 concentration and TSH concentration should be measured prior to confirming the diagnosis. It is important to remember that response to trial therapy with L-T_4 sodium is nonspecific and does not, by itself, prove the diagnosis.

 ## TREATMENT AND PROGNOSIS

For cats with iatrogenic hypothyroidism due to thyroidectomy or radioactive iodine treatment, transient hypothyroidism is expected after treatment, but cats should become euthyroid after 2 to 3 months. Treatment with L-T_4 sodium is indicated if clinical signs of hypothyroidism are present, if the cat is azotemic, or if hypothyroidism does not resolve by 3 to 6 months after treatment.

Treatment of hypothyroidism is similar for the cat and dog. L-T_4 sodium is the recommended thyroid hormone supplement. The initial dosage for cats is 0.05 to 0.1 mg once daily. A minimum of 6 to 8 weeks should elapse before critically assessing the cat's clinical response to treatment. Subsequent reevaluations should include history, physical examination, and measurement of serum thyroid hormone concentrations and serum TSH (see Therapeutic Monitoring). The goal of therapy is to resolve the clinical signs of hypothyroidism while avoiding signs of hyperthyroidism. This can usually be accomplished by maintaining serum T_4 concentration between 1.0 and 3.0 μg/dL. The dosage and frequency of L-T_4 sodium administration may need modification to achieve these goals. If serum thyroid hormone concentrations are normal after 6 to 8 weeks of treatment but there is no clinical response, the clinician should reassess the diagnosis.

The prognosis for feline hypothyroidism depends on the underlying cause and the age of the cat at the time clinical signs develop. With appropriate therapy, the clinical manifestations should resolve following thyroid hormone supplementation and the life expectancy of an adult cat with primary hypothyroidism should be normal. The prognosis for kittens with congenital hypothyroidism is guarded and depends on the severity of skeletal changes at the time treatment is initiated and neurologic status. Although many of the clinical signs resolve with therapy, musculoskeletal and neurologic problems may persist.

REFERENCES

Canine Hypothyroidism

Adams WH, et al.: Quantitative 99 m Tc-pertechnetate thyroid scintigraphy in normal beagles, *Vet Radiol Ultrasound* 38(4):323, 1997.

Atkinson K, Aubert I: Myxedema coma leading to respiratory depression in a dog, *Can Vet J* 45(4):318, 2004.

Avgeris S, et al.: Plasma von Willebrand factor concentration and thyroid function in dogs, *J Am Vet Med Assoc* 196:921, 1990.

Barrie J, et al.: Plasma cholesterol and lipoprotein concentrations in the dog: the effects of age, breed, gender and endocrine disease, *J Small Anim Pract* 34:507, 1993.

Beale KM, et al.: Serum thyroid hormone concentrations and thyrotropin responsiveness in dogs with generalized dermatologic disease, *J Am Vet Med Assoc* 201:1715, 1992a.

Beale K, et al.: Correlation of racing and reproductive performance in Greyhounds with response to thyroid function testing, *J Am Anim Hosp Assoc* 28:263, 1992b.

Behrend EN, et al.: Effect of storage conditions on cortisol, total thyroxine, and free thyroxine concentrations in serum and plasma of dogs, *J Am Vet Med Assoc* 212:1564, 1998.

Beijerink NJ, et al.: Adenohypophyseal function in bitches treated with medroxyprogesterone acetate, *Domest Anim Endocrinol* 32:63, 2007.

Belshaw BE, et al.: The iodine requirement and influence of iodine intake on iodine metabolism and thyroid function in the adult beagle, *Endocrinology* 96:1280, 1975.

Benjamin SA, et al.: Associations between lymphocytic thyroiditis, hypothyroidism, and thyroid neoplasia in beagles, *Vet Pathol* 33:486, 1996.

Bhatti SFM, et al.: Effects of growth hormone secretagogues on the release of adenohypophyseal hormones in young and old healthy dogs, *Vet J* 172:515, 2006.

Bianco AC, Kim BW: Intracellular pathways of iodothyronine metabolism: implications of deiodination for thyroid hormone action. In Braverman LE, Cooper DS, editors: *The thyroid: a fundamental and clinical text*, ed 10, Philadelphia, 2013, WB Saunders, p 103.

Bichsel P, et al.: Neurologic manifestations associated with hypothyroidism in four dogs, *J Am Vet Med Assoc* 192:1745, 1988.

Bilezikian JP, Loeb JN: Increased myocardial beta-receptor and adrenergic responsiveness, *Endocr Rev* 4:3378, 1983.

Bishnoi A, et al.: Effects of commonly prescribed nonsteroidal anti-inflammatory drugs on thyroid hormone measurements, *Am J Med* 96:235, 1994.

Blois SL, et al.: Multiple endocrine diseases in dogs: 35 cases (1996-2009), *J Am Vet Med Assoc* 238:1616, 2011.

Boretti FS, et al.: Evaluation of recombinant human thyroid-stimulating hormone to test thyroid function in dogs suspected of having hypothyroidism, *Am J Vet Res* 67(12):2012, 2006a.

Boretti FS, et al.: Comparison of the biological activity of recombinant human thyroid-stimulating hormone with bovine thyroid-stimulating hormone and evaluation of recombinant human thyroid-stimulating hormone in healthy dogs of different breeds, *Am J Vet Res* 67(7):1169, 2006b.

Boretti FS, et al.: Comparison of 2 doses of recombinant human thyrotropin for thyroid function testing in healthy and suspected hypothyroid dogs, *J Vet Intern Med* 23(4):856, 2009.

Borst GC, et al.: Fasting decreases thyrotropin responsiveness to thyrotropin-releasing hormone: a potential cause of misinterpretation of thyroid function tests in the critically ill, *J Clin Endocrinol Metab* 57:380, 1983.

Bowen D, et al.: Autoimmune polyglandular syndrome in a dog: a case report, *J Am Anim Hosp Assoc* 22:649, 1986.

Brauer C, et al.: Metabolic and toxic causes of canine seizure disorders: a retrospective study of 96 cases, *Vet J* 187:272, 2011.

Braund KG, et al.: Hypothyroid myopathy in two dogs, *Vet Pathol* 18:589, 1981.

Brömel C, et al.: Ultrasonographic evaluation of the thyroid gland in healthy, hypothyroid, and euthyroid Golden Retrievers with nonthyroidal illness, *J Vet Intern Med* 19(4):499, 2005.

Brömel C, et al.: Comparison of ultrasonographic characteristics of the thyroid gland in healthy small-, medium-, and large-breed dogs, *Am J Vet Res* 67(1):70, 2006.

Bruner JM, et al.: Effect of time of sample collection on serum thyroid-stimulating hormone concentrations in euthyroid and hypothyroid dogs, *J Am Vet Med Assoc* 212:1572, 1998.

Calvert CA, et al.: Congestive cardiomyopathy in Doberman Pinscher dogs, *J Am Vet Med Assoc* 181:598, 1982.

Calvert CA, et al.: Thyroid-stimulating hormone stimulation tests in cardiomyopathic Doberman Pinschers: a retrospective study, *J Vet Intern Med* 12:343, 1998.

Campbell KL, Davis CA: Effects of thyroid hormones on serum and cutaneous fatty acid concentrations in dogs, *Am J Vet Res* 51:752, 1990.

Carter GR, et al.: Serum total thyroxine and thyroid stimulating hormone concentrations in dogs with behavior problems, *J Vet Behavior* 4:230, 2009.

Castillo VA, et al.: Nutrition: commercial diet induced hypothyroidism due to high iodine. A histological and radiological analysis, *Vet Quarterly* 23:218, 2001.

Chastain CB: Canine hypothyroidism, *J Am Vet Med Assoc* 181:349, 1982.

Chastain CB, Schmidt B: Galactorrhea associated with hypothyroidism in intact bitches, *J Am Anim Hosp Assoc* 16:851, 1980.

Chastain CB, et al.: Myxedema coma in two dogs, *Canine Pract* 9:20, 1982.

Chastain CB, et al.: Congenital hypothyroidism in a dog due to an iodide organification defect, *Am J Vet Res* 44:1257, 1983.

Conaway DH, et al.: The familial occurrence of lymphocytic thyroiditis in Borzoi dogs, *Am J Med Genet* 22:409, 1985a.

Conaway DH, et al.: Clinical and histological features of primary progressive, familial thyroiditis in a colony of Borzoi dogs, *Vet Pathol* 22:439, 1985b.

Cortese L, et al.: Hyperprolactinaemia and galactorrhoea associated with primary hypothyroidism in a bitch, *J Small Anim Pract* 38:572, 1997.

Credille KM, et al.: The effects of thyroid hormones on the skin of Beagle dogs, *J Vet Intern Med* 15:539, 2001.

Crispin SM, Barnett KC: Arcus lipoides corneae secondary to hypothyroidism in the Alsatian, *J Small Anim Pract* 19:127, 1978.

Dalton RG, et al.: Hypothyroidism as a cause of acquired von Willebrand's disease, *Lancet* 1:1007, 1987.

Daminet S, Paradis M: Evaluation of thyroid function in dogs suffering from recurrent flank alopecia, *Can Vet J* 41:699, 2000.

Daminet S, et al.: Evaluation of thyroid function in obese dogs and in dogs undergoing a weight loss protocol, *J Vet Med A Physiol Pathol Clin Med* 50(4):213, 2003a.

Daminet S, et al.: Influence of acetylsalicylic acid and ketoprofen on canine thyroid function tests, *Vet J* 166(3):224, 2003b.

Daminet S, et al.: Use of recombinant human thyroid-stimulating hormone for thyrotropin stimulation test in healthy hypothyroid and euthyroid sick dogs, *Can Vet J* 48:1273, 2007.

de Bruijne J, et al.: Fat mobilization and plasma hormone levels in fasted dogs, *Metabolism* 30:190, 1981.

Delauche AJ, et al.: Nemaline rods in canine myopathies: 4 case reports and literature review, *J Vet Intern Med* 12:424, 1998.

Dewey CW, et al.: Neuromuscular dysfunction in five dogs with acquired myasthenia gravis and presumptive hypothyroidism, *Prog Vet Neurol* 6:117, 1995.

De Roover K, et al.: Effect of storage of reconstituted recombinant human thyroid-stimulating hormone (rhTSH) on thyroid-stimulating hormone (TSH) response testing in euthyroid dogs, *J Vet Intern Med* 20:812, 2006.

Diaz-Espiñeira MM, et al.: Assessment of thyroid function in dogs with low plasma thyroxine concentrations, *J Vet Intern Med* 21:25, 2007.

Diaz-Espiñeira MM, et al.: Thyrotropin releasing hormone-induced growth hormone secretion in dogs with primary hypothyroidism, *Domestic Anim Endocrinol* 34(2):176, 2008a.

Diaz-Espiñeira MM, et al.: Functional and morphological changes in the adenohypophysis of dogs with induced primary hypothyroidism: loss of TSH hypersecretion, hypersomatotropism, hypoprolactinemia, and pituitary enlargement with transdifferentiation, *Domestic Anim Endocrinol* 35(1):98, 2008b.

Diaz-Espiñeira MM, et al.: Adenohypophyseal function in dogs with primary hypothyroidism and nonthyroidal illness, *J Vet Intern Med* 23:100, 2009.

Di Girolamo G, et al.: Bioequivalence of two levothyroxine tablet formulations without and with mathematical adjustment for basal thyroxine levels in healthy Argentinian volunteers: a single dose, randomized, open-label, crossover study, *Clin Ther* 30(11):2015, 2008.

Dillitzer N, et al.: Intake of minerals, trace elements and vitamins in bone and raw food rations in adult dogs, *Br J Nutr* 106:S53, 2011.

Dixon RM, et al.: Serum thyrotropin concentrations: a new diagnostic test for canine hypothyroidism, *Vet Rec* 138:594, 1996.

Dixon RM, et al.: Epideiological, clinical, haematological and biochemical characteristics of canine hypothyroidism, *Vet Rec* 145:481, 1999.

Dixon RM, et al.: Treatment and therapeutic monitoring of canine hypothyroidism, *J Small Anim Pract* 43:334, 2002.

Dodds WJ: Estimating disease prevalence with health surveys and genetic screening, *Adv Vet Sci Comp Med* 39:29, 1995.

Dodgson SE, et al.: Congenital hypothyroidism with goiter in Tenterfield Terriers, *J Vet Intern Med* 26:1350, 2012.

Doerge DR, Decker CJ: Inhibition of peroxidase-catalyzed reactions by arylamines: mechanism for the anti-thyroid action of sulfamethazine, *Chem Res Toxicol* 7:164, 1994.

Doliger S, et al.: Histochemical study of cutaneous mucins in hypothyroid dogs, *Vet Pathol* 32:628, 1995.

Dowell RT, et al.: Beta-adrenergic receptors, adenylate cyclase activation, and myofibril enzyme activity in hypothyroid rats, *Am J Physiol* 266:H2527, 1994.

Duclos DD, et al.: Prognosis for treatment of adult onset demodicosis in dogs: 34 cases, *J Am Vet Med Assoc* 204:616, 1994.

Eigenmann JE: Diagnosis and treatment of dwarfism in a German Shepherd dog, *J Am Anim Hosp Assoc* 17:798, 1981.

Eisenbarth GS, et al.: Autoimmune polyendocrine syndromes, *N Engl J Med* 350:20, 2004.

Elliott DA, et al.: Thyroid hormone concentrations in critically ill canine intensive care patients, *J Vet Emerg Crit Care* 5:17, 1995.

Evason MD, et al.: Alterations in thyroid hormone concentrations in healthy sled dogs before and after athletic conditioning, *Am J Vet Res* 65(3):333, 2004.

Ferguson DC: Testing for hypothyroidism in dogs, *Vet Clin Small Anim* 37:647, 2007.

Ferguson DC, Hoenig M: Re-examination of dosage regimens for l-thyroxine (T$_4$) in the dog: bioavailability and persistence of TSH suppression (abstract), *J Vet Intern Med* 11:120, 1997.

Ferguson DC, Peterson ME: Serum free and total iodothyroinine concentrations in dogs with hyperadrenocorticism, *Am J Vet Res* 53:1636, 1992.

Ferguson DC, et al.: Carprofen lowers total T$_4$ and TSH, but not free T$_4$ concentrations in dogs (abstract), *J Vet Intern Med* 13:243, 1999.

Ferm K, et al.: Prevalence of diagnostic characteristics indicating canine autoimmune lymphocytic thyroiditis in giant schnauzer and hovawart dogs, *J Small Anim Pract* 50:176, 2009.

Fine DM, et al.: Cardiovascular manifestations of iatrogenic hyperthyroidism in two dogs, *J Vet Cardiology* 12:141, 2010.

Ford SL, et al.: Insulin resistance in three dogs with hypothyroidism and diabetes mellitus, *J Am Vet Med Assoc* 202:1478, 1993.

Frank LA: Comparison of thyrotropin-releasing hormone (TRH) to thyrotropin (TSH) stimulation for evaluating thyroid function in dogs, *J Am Anim Hosp Assoc* 32:481, 1996.

Frank LA, et al.: Effects of sulfamethoxazole-trimethoprim on thyroid function in dogs, *Am J Vet Res* 66(2):256, 2005.

Fritz TE, et al.: Pathology and familial incidence of orchitis and its relation to thyroiditis in a closed beagle colony, *Exp Mol Pathol* 24:142, 1976.

Fyfe JC, et al.: Congenital hypothyroidism with goiter in toy fox terriers, *J Vet Intern Med* 17:50, 2003.

Fyfe JC, et al.: A thyroid peroxidase (TPO) mutation in dogs reveals a canid-specific gene structure, *Mamm Genome* 24:127, 2013.

Gal A, et al.: Congenital adenohypophyseal hypoplasia associated with secondary hypothyroidism in a 2 week old Portuguese water dog, *Can Vet J* 53:659, 2012.

Gaschen F, et al.: Recognition of triiodothyronine-containing epitopes in canine thyroglobulin by circulating thyroglobulin autoantibodies, *Am J Vet Res* 54:244, 1993.

Gaskill CL, et al.: Effects of phenobarbital treatment on serum thyroxine and thyroid-stimulating hormone concentrations in epileptic dogs, *J Am Vet Med Assoc* 215:489, 1999.

Gaughan KR, Bruyette DS: Thyroid function testing in Greyhounds, *Am J Vet Res* 62:1130, 2001.

Gaynor AR, et al.: Risk factors for acquired megaesophagus in dogs, *J Am Vet Med Assoc* 211:1406, 1997.

Gerritsen RJ, et al.: Relationship between atrial fibrillation and primary hypothyroidism in the dog, *Vet Quart* 18:49, 1996.

Gieger TL, et al.: Thyroid function and serum hepatic enzyme activity in dogs after phenobarbital administration, *J Vet Intern Med* 14:277, 2000.

Gonzalez E, Quadri SK: Effects of aging on the pituitary-thyroid axis in the dog, *Exp Gerontology* 23:151, 1988.

Gookin JL, et al.: Clinical hypothyroidism associated with trimethoprim-sulfadiazine administration in a dog, *J Am Vet Med Assoc* 214:1028, 1999.

Gosselin SJ, et al.: Biochemical and immunological investigation on hypothyroidism in dogs, *Can J Comp Med* 44:158, 1980.

Gosselin SJ, et al.: Lymphocytic thyroiditis in dogs: induction with a local graft-versus-host reaction, *Am J Vet Res* 42:1856, 1981a.

Gosselin SJ, et al.: Histopathologic and ultrastructural evaluation of thyroid lesions associated with hypothyroidism in dogs, *Vet Pathol* 18:299, 1981b.

Gosselin SJ, et al.: Induced lymphocytic thyroiditis in dogs: effect of intrathyroidal injection of thyroid autoantibodies, *Am J Vet Res* 42:1565, 1981c.

Gottschalk J, et al.: Influence of topical dexamethasone applications on insulin, glucose, thyroid hormone and cortisol levels in dogs, *Res Vet Sci* 90:491, 2011.

Graham PA, et al.: Lymphocytic thyroiditis, *Vet Clin North Am* 31:915, 2001.

Graham PA, et al.: Etiopathologic findings of canine hypothyroidism, *Vet Clin Small Anim* 37:617, 2007.

Greco DS: Polyendocrine gland failure in dogs, *Vet Med* 95:477, 2000.

Greco DS, et al.: Juvenile-onset hypothyroidism in a dog, *J Am Vet Med Assoc* 187:948, 1985.

Greco DS, et al.: Congenital hypothyroid dwarfism in a family of Giant Schnauzers, *J Vet Intern Med* 5:57, 1991.

Greco DS, et al.: The effect of levothyroxine treatment on resting energy expenditure of hypothyroid dogs, *J Vet Intern Med* 12:7, 1998.

Greenspan FS: The thyroid gland. In Greenspan FS, Gardner, editors: *Basic and clinical endocrinology*, ed 6, New York, 2001, Lange Medical Books/ McGraw Hill, p 201.

Gulickers KP, Panciera DL: Evaluation of the effects of clomipramine on canine thyroid function tests, *J Vet Intern Med* 17:44, 2003.

Gunaratnam P: The effects of thyroxine on hair growth in the dog, *J Small Anim Pract* 27:17, 1986.

Haber RS, Loeb JN: Selective induction of high-ouabain-affinity isoform of Na+-K+-ATPase by thyroid hormone, *Am J Physiol* 255:E912, 1988.

Haines DM, Penhale WJ: Antibodies to pancreatic islet cells in canine diabetes mellitus, *Vet Immunol Immunopathol* 8:149, 1985.

Hall IA, et al.: Effect of trimethoprim/sulfamethoxazole on thyroid function in dogs with pyoderma, *J Am Vet Med Assoc* 202:1959, 1993.

Hamann F, et al.: Pituitary function and morphology in two German Shepherd dogs with congenital dwarfism, *Vet Rec* 144:644, 1999.

Hargis AM, et al.: Relationship of hypothyroidism to diabetes mellitus, renal amyloidosis, and thrombosis in pure-bred Beagles, *Am J Vet Res* 42:1077, 1981.

Hawthorn MH, et al.: Effect of thyroid status on beta-adrenoreceptors and calcium channels in rat cardiac and vascular tissue, *Naunyn Schmiedebergs Arch Pharmacol* 337:539, 1988.

Henik RA, Dixon RM: Intravenous administration of levothyroxine for treatment of suspected myxedema coma complicated by severe hypothermia in a dog, *J Am Vet Med Assoc* 216:713, 2000.

Heseltine JC, et al.: Effect of levothyroxine administration on hemostatic analytes in Doberman Pinschers with von Willebrand disease, *J Vet Intern Med* 19:523, 2005.

Hess RS, et al.: Association between diabetes mellitus, hypothyroidism or hyperadrenocorticism and atherosclerosis in dogs, *J Vet Intern Med* 17:489, 2003.

Higgins MA, et al.: Hypothyroid associated central vestibular disease in 10 dogs: 1999-2005, *J Vet Intern Med* 20:1363, 2006.

Hill RC, et al.: Effects of racing and training on serum thyroid hormone concentrations in racing Greyhounds, *Am J Vet Res* 62:1969, 2001.

Hofer-Inteeworn N, et al.: Effect of hypothyroidism on insulin sensitivity and glucose tolerance in dogs, *Am J Vet Res* 73:529, 2012.

Hoh WP, et al.: Circadian variations of serum thyroxine, free thyroxine, and 3,5,3′triiodothyronine concentrations in healthy dogs, *J Vet Sci* 7:25, 2006.

Hymes K, et al.: Easy bruising, thrombocytopenia, and elevated platelet immunoglobulin G in Graves' disease and Hashimoto's thyroiditis, *Ann Intern Med* 94:27, 1981.

Indrieri RJ, et al.: Neuromuscular abnormalities associated with hypothyroidism and lymphocytic thyroiditis in three dogs, *J Am Vet Med Assoc* 190:544, 1987.

Jaggy A, et al.: Neurological manifestations of hypothyroidism: a retrospective study of 29 dogs, *J Vet Intern Med* 8:328, 1994.

Johnson C, et al.: Effect of ^{131}I-induced hypothyroidism on indices of reproductive function in adult male dogs, *J Vet Intern Med* 13:104, 1999.

Kantrowitz LB, et al.: Serum total thyroxine, total triiodothyronine, free thyroxine, and thyrotropin concentrations in epileptic dogs treated with anticonvulsants, *J Am Vet Med Assoc* 214:1804, 1999.

Kantrowitz LB, et al.: Serum total thyroxine, total triiodothyronine, free thyroxine, and thyrotropin concentrations in dogs with nonthyroidal illness, *J Am Vet Med Assoc* 219:765, 2001.

Kaptein EM, et al.: Effects of prednisone on thyroxine and 3,5,3′-triiodothyronine metabolism in normal dogs, *Endocrinology* 130:1669, 1992.

Kelly MJ, Hill JR: Canine myxedema stupor and coma, *Comp Cont Ed Pract Vet* 6:1049, 1984.

Kemppainen RJ, Birchfield JR: Measurement of total thyroxine concentration in serum from dogs and cats by use of various methods, *Am J Vet Res* 67:259, 2006.

Kemppainen RJ, Sartin JL: Evidence for episodic but not circadian activity in plasma concentrations of adrenocorticotrophin, cortisol, and thyroxine in dogs, *J Endocrinol* 103:219, 1984.

Kemppainen RJ, et al.: Effects of prednisone on thyroid and gonadal endocrine function in dogs, *J Endocrinol* 96:293, 1983.

Kemppainen RJ, et al.: Autoantibodies to triiodothyronine and thyroxine in a Golden Retriever, *J Am Anim Hosp Assoc* 32:195, 1996.

Kennedy LJ, et al.: Association of hypothyroid disease in Doberman Pinscher with a rare major histocompatibility complex DLA class II haplotype, *Tissue Antigens* 67:53, 2006a.

Kennedy LJ, et al.: Association of canine hypothyroidism with a common major histocompatibility complex DLA class II allele, *Tissue Antigens* 68:82, 2006b.

Kern TJ, Riis RC: Ocular manifestations of secondary hyperlipidemia associated with hypothyroidism and uveitis in a dog, *J Am Anim Hosp Assoc* 16:907, 1980.

Kern TJ, et al.: Horner's syndrome in dogs and cats: 100 cases (1975-1985), *J Am Vet Med Assoc* 195:369, 1989.

Kintzer PP, Peterson ME: Thyroid scintigraphy in small animals, *Semin Vet Med Surg Small Anim* 6:131, 1991.

Klein I: Thyroid hormone and the cardiovascular system, *Am J Med* 88:631, 1990.

Kolster KA, et al.: Control of prolactin secretion in canine hypothyroidism, *Clin Theriogenol* 2:185, 2010.

Kooistra HS, et al.: Polyglandular deficiency syndrome in a Boxer dog: thyroid hormone and glucocorticoid deficiency, *Vet Quart* 17:59, 1995.

Kooistra HS, et al.: Combined pituitary hormone deficiency in German Shepherd dogs with dwarfism, *Domest Anim Endocrinol* 19:177, 2000a.

Kooistra HS, et al.: Secretion pattern of thyroid-stimulating hormone in dogs during euthyroidism and hypothyroidism, *Domest Anim Endocrinol* 18:19, 2000b.

Lantz GC, et al.: Transsphenoidal hypophysectomy in the clinically normal dog, *Am J Vet Res* 49:1134, 1988.

Lawler DF, et al.: Influence of lifetime food restriction on physiologic variables in Labrador retriever dogs, *Exp Gerontology* 42:204, 2007.

Lee DE, et al.: Effects of hyperlipemia on radioimmunoassays for progesterone, testosterone, thyroxine, and cortisol in serum and plasma samples from dogs, *Am J Vet Res* 52:1489, 1991.

Lee JA, et al.: Effects of racing and nontraining on plasma thyroid hormone concentrations in sled dogs, *J Am Vet Med Assoc* 224:226, 2004.

Le Traon G, et al.: Pharmacokinetics of total thyroxine in dogs after administration of an oral solution of levothyroxine sodium, *Vet Pharmacol Therap* 31:95, 2007.

Le Traon G, et al.: Clinical evaluation of a novel liquid formulation of L-thyroxine for once daily treatment of dogs with hypothyroidism, *J Vet Intern Med* 23(1):43, 2009.

Lobetti RG: Hypercalcemia in a dog with primary hypothyroidism, *J S Afr Vet Assoc* 82:242, 2011.

Lum SMC, et al.: Peripheral tissue mechanism for maintenance of serum triiodothyronine values in a thyroxine-deficient state in man, *J Clin Invest* 73:570, 1984.

Lumsden JH, et al.: Prevalence of hypothyroidism and von Willebrand's disease in Doberman Pinschers and the observed relationship between thyroid, von Willebrand, and cardiac status, *J Vet Intern Med* 7:115, 1993 (abstract).

Lurye JC, et al.: Evaluation of an in-house enzyme-linked immunosorbent assay for quantitative measurement of serum total thyroxine concentration in dogs and cats, *J Am Vet Med Assoc* 221:243, 2002.

MacGregor JM, et al.: Cholesterol based pericardial effusion and aortic thromboembolism in a 9-year-old mixed-breed dog with hypothyroidism, *J Vet Intern Med* 18:354, 2004.

MacPhail CM, Monnet E: Outcome of and postoperative complications in dogs undergoing surgical treatment of laryngeal paralysis: 140 cases (1985-1998), *J Am Vet Med Assoc* 218:1949, 2001.

Mansfield CS, Mooney CT: Lymphocytic-plasmacytic thyroiditis and glomerulonephritis in a boxer, *J Small Anim Pract* 47(7):396, 2006.

Marca MC, et al.: Evaluation of canine serum thyrotropin (TSH) concentration: comparison of three analytical procedures, *J Vet Diag Invest* 13:106, 2001.

Meij BP, et al.: Alterations in anterior pituitary function of dogs with pituitary dependent hyperadrenocorticism, *J Endocrinol* 154:505, 1997.

Meij BP, et al.: Results of transsphenoidal hypophysectomy in 52 dogs with pituitary-dependent hyperadrenocorticism, *Vet Surg* 27:246, 1998.

Miller AB, et al.: Serial thyroid hormone concentrations in healthy euthyroid dogs, dogs with hypothyroidism, and euthyroid dogs with atopic dermatitis, *Br Vet J* 148:451, 1992.

Miller PE, Panciera DL: Effects of experimentally induced hypothyroidism on the eye and ocular adnexa in dogs. *AJVR* 55:692, 1994.

Miller WH, Buerger RG: Cutaneous mucinous vesiculation in a dog with hypothyroidism, *J Am Vet Med Assoc* 196:757, 1990.

Mooney CT, et al.: Thyroid hormone abnormalities and outcome in dogs with non-thyroidal illness, *J Small Anim Pract* 49:11, 2008.

Mooney CT, Anderson TJ: Congenital hypothyroidism in a Boxer dog, *J Small Anim Pract* 34:31, 1993.

Moore GE, et al.: Effects of oral administration of anti-inflammatory doses of prednisone on thyroid hormone response to thyrotropin-releasing hormone and thyrotropin in clinically normal dogs, *Am J Vet Res* 54:130, 1993.

Muller PB, et al.: Effects of long-term phenobarbital treatment on the thyroid and adrenal axis and adrenal function tests in dogs, *J Vet Intern Med* 14:157, 2000.

Müntener T, et al.: Canine noninflammatory alopecia: a comprehensive evaluation of common and distinguishing histological characteristics, *Vet Derm* 23:206, 2012.

Nachreiner RF, Refsal KR: Radioimmunoassay monitoring of thyroid hormone concentrations in dogs on thyroid replacement therapy: 2,674 cases (1985-1987), *J Am Vet Med Assoc* 201:623, 1992.

Nachreiner RF, et al.: Pharmacokinetics of l-thyroxine after its oral administration in dogs, *Am J Vet Res* 54:2091, 1993.

Nachreiner RF, et al.: Prevalence of autoantibodies to thyroglobulin in dogs with nonthyroidal illness, *Am J Vet Res* 59:951, 1998.

Nachreiner RF, et al.: Prevalence of serum thyroid hormone autoantibodies in dogs with clinical signs of hypothyroidism, *J Am Vet Med Assoc* 220:466, 2002.

Nelson RW, et al.: Serum free thyroxine concentration in healthy dogs, dogs with hypothyroidism, and euthyroid dogs with concurrent illness, *J Am Vet Med Assoc* 198:1401, 1991.

Ness TA, et al.: Effect of dosing and sampling time on serum thyroxine, free thyroxine, and thyrotropin concetrations in dogs following multidose etodolac administration, *Vet Ther* 4:340, 2003.

Nuttall WO: Iodine deficiency in working dogs, *N Z Vet J* 34:72, 1986.

O'Neill SH, Reynolds LM: Effect of an anti-inflammatory dose of prednisone on thyroid hormone monitoring in hypothyroid dogs, *Vet Dermatol* 22:202, 2011.

Oohashi E, et al.: Seasonal changes in serum total thyroxine, free thyroxine, and canine thyroid-stimulating hormone in clinically healthy Beagles in Hokkaido, *J Vet Med Sci* 63:1241, 2001.

Panacova L, et al.: Thyroid testing in Sloughis, *J Vet Intern Med* 22:1144, 2008.

Panciera DL: An echocardiographic and electrocardiographic study of cardiovascular function in hypothyroid dogs, *J Am Vet Med Assoc* 205:996, 1994.

Panciera DL: Conditions associated with canine hypothyroidism, *Vet Clin North Am* 31:935, 2001.

Panciera DL, Johnson GS: Plasma von Willebrand factor antigen concentration in dogs with hypothyroidism, *J Am Vet Med Assoc* 205:1550, 1994.

Panciera DL, Johnson GS: Plasma von Willebrand factor antigen concentration and buccal mucosal bleeding time in dogs with experimental hypothyroidism, *J Vet Intern Med* 10:60, 1996.

Panciera DL, Johnston SA: Results of thyroid function tests and concentrations of plasma proteins in dogs administered etodolac, *Am J Vet Res* 63:1492, 2002.

Panciera DL, et al.: Thyroid function tests in euthyroid dogs treated with l-thyroxine, *Am J Vet Res* 51:22, 1989.

Panciera DL, et al.: Quantitative morphologic study of the pituitary and thyroid glands of dogs administered l-thyroxine, *Am J Vet Res* 51:27, 1990.

Panciera DL, et al.: Plasma thyroid hormone concentrations in dogs competing in a long-distance sled dog race, *J Vet Intern Med* 17:593, 2003.

Panciera DL, et al.: Effects of deracoxib and aspirin on serum concentrations of thyroxine, 3,5,3'-triiodothyronine, free thyroxine, and thyroid stimulating hormone in dogs, *Am J Vet Res* 67:599, 2006.

Panciera DL, et al.: Effect of short-term hypothyroidism on reproduction in the bitch, *Theriogenology* 68:316, 2007.

Panciera DL, et al.: Reproductive effects of prolonged experimentally induced hypothyroidism in bitches, *J Vet Intern Med* 26:326, 2012.

Pancotto T, et al.: Blood-brain-barrier disruption in chronic canine hypothyroidism, *Vet Clin Path* 39:485, 2010.

Paradis M, et al.: Effects of moderate to severe osteoarthritis in canine thyroid function, *Can Vet J* 44:407, 2003.

Paull LC, et al.: Effect of anticonvulsant dosages of potassium bromide on thyroid function and morphology in dogs, *J Am Anim Hosp Assoc* 39:193, 2003.

Persani L, Beck-Peccoz P: Central hypothyroidism. In Braverman LE, et al, editors: *Werner and Ingbar's the thyroid*, ed 10, Philadelphia, 2013, Lippincott Williams &Wilkins.

Peruccio C: *Incidence of hypothyroidism in dogs affected by keratoconjunctivitis sicca*, Las Vegas, 1982, Proceedings of the American Society of Veterinary Ophthalmology. p 47.

Peterson ME, Ferguson DC: Thyroid diseases. In Ettinger SJ, editor: *Textbook of veterinary internal medicine*, ed 3, Philadelphia, 1989, WB Saunders, p 1632.

Peterson ME, Gamble DA: Effect of nonthyroidal illness on serum thyroxine concentrations in cats: 494 cases (1988), *J Am Vet Med Assoc* 197:1203, 1990.

Peterson ME, et al.: Effects of spontaneous hyperadrenocorticism on serum thyroid hormone concentrations in the dog, *Am J Vet Res* 45:2034, 1984.

Peterson ME, et al.: Pretreatment clinical and laboratory findings in dogs with hypoadrenocorticism: 225 cases (1979-1993), *J Am Vet Med Assoc* 208:85, 1996.

Peterson ME, et al.: Measurement of serum total thyroxine, triiodothyronine, free thyroxine, and thyrotropin concentrations for diagnosis of hypothyroidism in dogs, *J Am Vet Med Assoc* 211:1396, 1997.

Pettigrew R, et al.: CNS hypomyelination in rat terrier dogs with congenital goiter and a mutation in the thyroid peroxidase gene, *Vet Pathol* 44:50, 2007.

Phillips DE, Harkin KR: Hypothyroidism and myocardial failure in two Great Danes, *J Am Vet Med Assoc* 39:133, 2003.

Piechotta M, et al.: Autoantibodies against thyroid hormones and their influence on thyroxine determination with chemiluminescent immunoassay in dogs, *J Vet Sci* 11:191, 2010.

Pinilla M, et al.: Quantitative thyroid scintigraphy in greyhounds suspected of primary hypothyroidism, *Vet Radiol Ultrasound* 50(2):224, 2009.

Post K, et al.: Lack of effect of trimethoprim and sulfadiazine in combination in mid- to late gestation on thyroid function in neonatal dogs, *J Reprod Fertil* 47(Suppl):477, 1993.

Pullen WH, Hess RS: Hypothyroid dogs treated with intravenous levothyroxine, *J Vet Intern Med* 20:32, 2006.

Radosta LA, et al.: Comparison of thyroid analytes in dogs aggressive to familiar people and in non-aggressive dogs, *Vet J* 192:472, 2012.

Ramsey IK, et al.: Thyroid-stimulating hormone and total thyroxine concentrations in euthyroid, sick euthyroid and hypothyroid dogs, *J Small Anim Pract* 38:540, 1997.

Reese S, et al.: Thyroid sonography as an effective tool to discriminate between euthyroid sick and hypothyroid dogs, *J Vet Intern Med* 19:491, 2005.

Reimers TJ, et al.: Effects of reproductive state on concentrations of thyroxine, 3,5,3'-triiodothyronine, and cortisol in serum of dogs, *Biol Reprod* 31:148, 1984.

Reimers TJ, et al.: Effect of fasting on thyroxine, 3,5,3'-triiodothyronine, and cortisol concentrations in serum of dogs, *Am J Vet Res* 47:2485, 1986.

Reimers TJ, et al.: Effects of age, sex, and body size on serum concentrations of thyroid and adrenocortical hormones in dogs, *Am J Vet Res* 51:454, 1990.

Reimers TJ, et al.: Effects of hemolysis, and storage on quantification of hormones in blood samples from dogs, cattle, and horses, *Am J Vet Res* 52:1075, 1991.

Reusch CE, et al.: Serum fructosamine concentrations in dogs with hypothyroidism, *Vet Res Commun* 26:531, 2002.

Rogers JS, et al.: Factor VIII activity and thyroid function, *Ann Intern Med* 97:713, 1982.

Rogers WA, et al.: Lipids and lipoproteins in normal dogs and in dogs with secondary hyperlipoproteinemia, *J Am Vet Med Assoc* 166:1092, 1975.

Rossmeisl JH: Resistance of the peripheral nervous system to the effects of chronic canine hypothyroidism, *J Vet Intern Med* 24:875, 2010.

Rossmeisl JH, et al.: Longitudinal study of the effects of chronic hypothyroidism on skeletal muscle in dogs, *Am J Vet Res* 70:879, 2009.

Roti E, Vagenakis AG: Effect of excess iodide: clinical aspects. In Braverman LE, Cooper DS, editors: *The thyroid: a fundamental and clinical text*, ed 10, Philadelphia, 2013, WB Saunders, p 242.

Salvatore D, et al, editors: Thyroid physiology and diagnostic evaluation of patients with thyroid disorders. In Melmed S, et al.: *Williams textbook of endocrinology*, ed 12, Philadelphia, 2011, Elsevier/Saunders.

Saunders HM, Jezyk PK: The radiographic appearance of canine congenital hypothyroidism: skeletal changes with delayed treatment, *Vet Radiol* 32:171, 1991.

Sauvé F, et al.: Effects of oral administration of meloxicam, carprofen, and a nutraceutical on thyroid function in dogs with osteoarthritis, *Can Vet J* 44:474, 2003.

Schachter S, et al.: Compariosn of serum-free thyroxine concentrations determined by standard equilibrium dialysis, modified equilibrium dialysis, and five radioimmunoassays in dogs, *J Vet Intern Med* 18:259, 2004.

Schoeman JP, et al.: Serum cortisol and thyroxine concentrations as predictors of death in critically ill puppies with parvoviral diarrhea, *J Am Vet Med Assoc* 231:1534, 2007.

Schuff KG, et al.: Psychiatric and cognitive effects of hypothyroidism, In Braverman LE, Cooper DS, editors: *The thyroid, a fundamental and clinical text*, ed 10, Philadelphia, 2013, WB Saunders, p 596.

Scott-Moncrieff JCR, Nelson RW: Change in serum thyroid-stimulating hormone concentration in response to administration of thyrotropin-releasing hormone to healthy dogs, hypothyroid dogs, and euthyroid dogs with concurrent disease, *J Am Vet Med Assoc* 213:1435, 1998.

Scott-Moncrieff JCR, et al.: Measurement of serum free thyroxine by modified equilibrium dialysis in dogs (abstract), *J Vet Intern Med* 8:159, 1994.

Scott-Moncrieff JCR, et al.: Comparison of serum concentrations of thyroid-stimulating hormone in healthy dogs, hypothyroid dogs, and euthyroid dogs with concurrent disease, *J Am Vet Med Assoc* 212:387, 1998.

Scott-Moncrieff JCR, et al.: Evaluation of antithyroglobulin antibodies after routine vaccination in pet and research dogs, *J Am Vet Med Assoc* 221:515, 2002.

Scott-Moncrieff JCR, et al.: Lack of association between repeated vaccination and thyroiditis in laboratory beagles, *J Vet Intern Med* 20:818, 2006.

Scott-Moncrieff JCR, et al.: Accuracy of serum free thyroxine concentrations determined by a new veterinary chemiluminescent immunoassay in euthyoid and hypothyroid dogs (abstract), *J Vet Intern Med* 25:1493, 2011.

Seavers A, et al.: Evaluation of the thyroid status of Basenji dogs in Australia, *Australian Vet J* 86:429, 2008.

Seelig DM, et al.: Goitrous hypothyroidism associated with treatment with trimethoprim-sulfamethoxazole in a young dog, *J Am Vet Med Assoc* 232:1181, 2008.

Segalini V, et al.: Thyroid function and infertility in the dog: a survey of five breeds, *Reprod Dom Anim* 44:211, 2009.

Shiel RE, et al.: Thyroid hormone concentrations in young healthy pretraining greyhounds, *Vet Rec* 161:616, 2007a.

Shiel RE, et al.: Tertiary hypothyroidism in a dog, *Irish Vet J* 60:88, 2007b.

Shiel RE, et al.: Assessment of criteria used by veterinary practitioners to diagnose hypothyroidism in sighthounds and investigation of serum thyroid hormone concentrations in healthy Salukis, *J Am Vet Med Assoc* 236:302, 2010.

Shiel E, et al.: Qualitative and semiquantitative assessment of thyroxine binding globulin in the greyhound and other dog breeds (abstract), *J Vet Intern Med* 25:1494, 2011.

Shiel RE, et al.: Assessment of the value of quantitative thyroid scintigraphy for determination of thyroid function in dogs, *J Small Anim Pract* 53:278, 2012.

Siegmund W, et al.: Replacement therapy with levothyroxine plus triiododthyronine (bioavailable molar ratio 14:1) is not superior to thyroxine alone to improve well-being and cognitive performance in hypothyroidism, *Clinical Endocrinol* 60:750, 2004.

Skopek E, et al.: Detection of autoantibodies against thyroid peroxidase in serum samples of hypothyroid dogs, *Am J Vet Res* 67:809, 2006.

Slade E, et al.: Serum thyroxine and triiodothyronine concentrations in canine pyoderma, *J Am Vet Med Assoc* 185:216, 1984.

Sullivan P, et al.: Altered platelet indices in dogs with hypothyroidism and cats with hyperthyroidism, *Am J Vet Res* 54:2004, 1993.

Sunthornthepvarakui T, et al.: Brief report: Resistance to thyrotropin caused by mutations in the thyrotropin-receptor gene, *N Engl J Med* 332:155, 1994.

Taeymans O, O'Marra SK: Imaging diagnosis: acquired goitrous hypothyroidism following treatment with trimethoprim sulfamethoxazole, *Vet Radiol Ultrasound* 50:443, 2009.

Taeymans O, et al.: Thyroid imaging in the dog: current status and future directions, *J Vet Intern Med* 21:673, 2007a.

Taeymans O, et al.: Pre- and post-treatment ultrasonography in hypothyroid dogs, *Vet Rad and Ultrasound* 48:262, 2007b.

Tani H, et al.: Proliferative responses to canine thyroglobulin of peripheral blood mononuclear cells from hypothyroid dogs, *J Vet Med Sci* 67:363, 2005.

Thacker EL, et al.: Prevalence of autoantibodies to thyroglobulin, thyroxine, or triiodothyronine and relationship of autoantibodies and serum concentrations of iodothyronines in dogs, *Am J Vet Res* 53:449, 1992.

Tidholm A, et al.: Effect of thyroid hormone supplementation on survival of euthyroid dogs with congestive heart failure due to systolic myocardial dysfunction: a double blind placebo-controlled trial, *Res Vet Sci* 75:195, 2003.

Torres SM, et al.: Comparison of colloid, thyroid follicular epithelium, and thyroid hormone concentrations in healthy and severely sick dogs, *J Am Vet Med Assoc* 222:1079, 2003.

Torres SMF, et al.: Hypothyroidism in a dog associated with trimethoprim-sulfadiazine therapy, *Vet Derm* 7:105, 1996.

Tuohy JL, et al.: Outcome following simultaneous bilateral thyroid lobectomy for treatment of thyroid gland carcinoma in dogs: 15 cases (1994-2010), *J Am Vet Med Assoc* 241:95, 2012.

Turrel JM, et al.: Sodium iodide I 131 treatment of dogs with nonresectable thyroid tumors: 39 cases (1990-2003), *J Am Vet Med Assoc* 229:542, 2006.

Utiger RD: Decreased extrathyroidal triiodothyronine production in nonthyroidal illness: benefit or harm? *Am J Med* 69:807, 1980.

Vail DM, et al.: Thyroid hormone concentrations in dogs with chronic weight loss with special reference to cancer cachexia, *J Vet Intern Med* 8:122, 1994.

Valdermarsson S, et al.: Relations between thyroid function, hepatic and lipoprotein lipase activities and plasma lipoprotein concentrations, *Acta Endocrinologica* 104:50, 1983.

van Geffen C, et al.: Serum thyroid hormone concentrations and thyroglobulin autoantibodies in trained and non-trained healthy whippets, *Vet J* 172:135, 2006.

Vitale CL, et al.: Neurologic dysfunction in hypothyroid hyperlipidemic labrador retrievers, *J Vet Intern Med* 21:1316, 2007.

von Klopmann T, et al.: Euthyroid sick syndrome in dogs with idiopathic epilepsy before treatment with anticonvulsant drugs, *J Vet Intern Med* 20(3):516, 2006.

Wartofsky L, Burman KD: Alterations in thyroid function in patients with systemic illness: the euthyroid sick syndrome, *Endocrinol Rev* 3:164, 1982.

Wenzel KW: Pharmacological interference with in vitro tests of thyroid function, *Metabolism* 30:717, 1981.

Wiesinga WM, Van den Berghe G: Nonthyroidal illness syndrome. In Braverman LE, Cooper DS, editors: *The thyroid: a fundamental and clinical text*, ed 10, Philadelphia, 2013, WB Saunders, p 596.

Wilbe M, et al.: Increased genetic risk or protection for canine autoimmune lymphocytic thyroiditis in Giant Schnauzers depends on DLA class II genotype, *Tissue Antigens* 75:712, 2010.

Williams DA, et al.: Validation of an immunoassay for canine thyroid-stimulating hormone and changes in serum concentration following induction of hypothyroidism in dogs, *J Am Vet Med Assoc* 209:1730, 1996.

Williams DL, et al.: Reduced tear production in three canine endocrinopathies, *J Small Anim Pract* 48:252, 2007.

Williamson NL, et al.: Effects of short-term trimethoprim-sulfamethoxazole administration on thyroid function in dogs, *J Am Vet Med Assoc* 221:802, 2002.

Woltz HH, et al.: Effect of prednisone on thyroid gland morphology on plasma thyroxine and triiodothyronine concentrations in the dog, *Am J Vet Res* 44:2000, 1984.

Yen PM, Brent GA: Genomic and non-genomic actions of thyroid hormones. In Braverman LE, Cooper DS, editors: *The thyroid: a fundamental and clinical text*, ed 10, Philadelphia, 2013, WB Saunders, p 127.

Feline Hypothyroidism

Arnold U, et al.: Goitrous hypothyroidism and dwarfism in a kitten, *J Am Anim Hosp Assoc* 20:753, 1984.

Blois SL, et al.: Use of thyroid scintigraphy and pituitary immunohistochemistry in the diagnosis of spontaneous hypothyroidism in a mature cat, *J Feline Med Surg* 12:156, 2010.

Hoenig M, Ferguson DC: Assessment of thyroid functional reserve in the cat by the thyrotropin-stimulation test, *Am J Vet Res* 44:1229, 1983.

Jones BR, et al.: Preliminary studies on congenital hypothyroidism in a family of Abyssinian cats, *Vet Rec* 131:145, 1992.

Mazrier H, et al.: Goiterous congenital hypothyroidism caused by thyroid peroxidase deficiency in a family of domestic shorthair cats, *J Vet Intern Med* 17:395, 2003.

Mellanby RJ, et al.: Secondary hypothyroidism following head trauma in a cat, *J Feline Med Surg* 7:135, 2005.

Miller PE, Panciera DL: Effects of experimentally induced hypothyroidism on the eye and ocular adnexa in dogs, *Am J Vet Res* 55:692, 1994.

Mooney CT, et al.: Effect of illness not associated with the thyroid gland on serum total and free thyroxine concentrations in cats, *J Am Vet Med Assoc* 208:2004, 1996a.

Nykamp SG, et al.: Association of the risk of development of hypothyroidism after iodine 131 treatment with the pretreatment pattern of sodium pertechnetate Tc 99m uptake in the thyroid gland in cats with hyperthyroidism. 165 cases (1990-2002), *J Am Vet Med Assoc* 226:1671, 2005.

Peterson ME, Gamble DA: Effect of nonthyroidal illness on serum thyroxine concentrations in cats: 494 cases (1988), *J Vet Intern Med* 197:1203, 1990.

Peterson ME, et al.: Measurement of serum concentrations of free thyroxine, total thyroxine, and total triiodothyronine in cat with hyperthyroidism and cats with nonthyroidal illness, *J Am Vet Med Assoc* 218:529, 2001.

Quante S, et al.: Congenital hypothyroidism in a kitten resulting in decreased IGF-1 concentration and abnormal liver function tests, *J Feline Med Surg* 12:487, 2010.

Rand JS, et al.: Spontaneous adult-onset hypothyroidism in a cat, *J Vet Intern Med* 7:272, 1993.

Schumm-Draeger PM, et al.: Spontaneous Hashimoto-like thyroiditis in cats, *Verh Dtsch Ges Path* 80:297, 1996.

Sjollema BE, et al.: Congenital hypothyroidism in two cats due to defective organification: Data suggesting loosely anchored thyroperoxidase, *Acta Endocrinol* 125:435, 1991.

Stegeman JR, et al.: Use of recombinant human thyroid-stimulating hormone for thyrotropin-stimulation testing of euthyroid cats, *Am J Vet Res* 64:149, 2003.

Tanase H, et al.: Inherited primary hypothyroidism with thyrotrophin resistance in Japanese cats, *J Endocrinology* 129:245, 1991.

Thoday KL, et al.: Radioimmunoassay of serum total thyroxine and triiodothyronine in healthy cats: Assay methodology and effects of age, sex, breed, heredity and environment, *J Small Anim Pract* 25:457, 1984.

Traas AM, et al.: Congenital thyroid hypoplasia and seizures in 2 littermate kittens, *J Vet Intern Med* 22:1427, 2008.

Van Hoek IM, et al.: Effect of recombinant human thyroid stimulating hormone on serum thyroxin and thyroid scintigraphy in euthyroid cats, *J Feline Med Surg* 11:309, 2009.

Van Hoek IM, et al.: Thyroid stimulation with recombinant human thyrotropin in healthy cats, cats with non-thyroidal illness, and in cats with low serum thyroxin and azotaemia after treatment of hyperthyroidism, *J Feline Med Surg* 12:117, 2010.

Wakeling J, et al.: Diagnosis of hyperthyroidism in cats with mild kidney disease, *J Small Anim Pract* 49:287, 2008.

Wakeling J, et al.: Evaluation of predictors for the diagnosis of hyperthyroidism in cats, *J Vet Intern Med* 25:1057, 2011.

Williams TL, et al.: Association of iatrogenic hypothyroidism with azotemia and reduced survival time in cats treated for hyperthyroidism, *J Vet Intern Med* 24:1086, 2010.

Zerbe CA, et al.: Thyroid profiles in healthy kittens from birth to 12 weeks of age, *Proc Annu Meet American College of Veterinary Internal Medicine* 16:702, 1998.

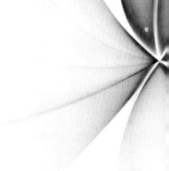

CHAPTER 4 | **Feline Hyperthyroidism**

J. Catharine Scott-Moncrieff

Hyperthyroidism, caused by autonomous growth and function of the thyroid follicular cells, was initially described in humans by Henry Plummer in 1913. Clinical observations led him to characterize two types of hyperthyroidism: exophthalmic goiter (Graves' disease) and toxic adenomatous goiter. In Graves' disease, the hyperthyroidism was associated with diffuse hyperplasia of the thyroid glands. Toxic adenomatous goiter was associated with either single or multiple nodules and variable histologic patterns. The latter disease involved the slow growth of autonomous functioning follicles. Toxic adenomatous goiter is very similar to the disorder seen in hyperthyroid cats, initially described as a clinical entity in 1979 by Peterson and colleagues and in 1980 by Holzworth and colleagues. For detailed information on the anatomy and physiology of the normal thyroid gland, see Chapter 3.

DEFINITION

Naturally occurring hyperthyroidism (thyrotoxicosis) is a clinical condition that results from excessive production and secretion of thyroxine (T_4) and triiodothyronine (T_3) by the thyroid gland. Hyperthyroidism in cats is almost always the result of a primary autonomous condition of the thyroid gland itself, most commonly due to adenomatous hyperplasia or a benign adenoma. Adenomatous hyperplasia is the most common pathologic change. Feline hyperthyroidism may also be caused by functional thyroid carcinoma. Thyroid-stimulating hormone (also known as thyrotropin; TSH) secreting pituitary adenoma is a rare cause of hyperthyroidism in people (Beck-Peccoz et al, 2009), but has yet to be described in cats. Other causes of hyperthyroidism, such as ingestion of excessive quantities of exogenous thyroid hormone (Köhler et al, 2012) or acute destruction of thyroid tissue causing excessive release of thyroid hormone, have also not been reported in cats.

HISTORY OF HYPERTHYROIDISM

Veterinary clinicians were not aware of the clinical syndrome of feline hyperthyroidism until the publication of three clinical reports by Peterson, et al., in 1979, Holzworth, et al., 1980, and Jones and Johnstone, 1981. After these publications, practitioners increasingly started to recognize cats with signs suggestive of hyperthyroidism (thyrotoxicosis). From 1980 to 1985, 125 hyperthyroid cats were identified at the University of California. During a similar period, hyperthyroid cats were being recognized at a rate of three per month at the Animal Medical Center in New York City (Peterson et al, 1983). By 1993, hyperthyroidism was a common disease in both the United States and the United Kingdom (Thoday and Mooney, 1992; Broussard et al, 1995). By 2004, a retrospective study suggested that the prevalence of feline hyperthyroidism in the United States was 3% of hospital visits (Edinboro et al, 2004). Feline hyperthyroidism is now recognized as a common clinical problem of cats in many countries in the world including Europe, Australia, New Zealand, Japan, and Hong Kong. Interestingly prevalence rates appear to vary

substantially by geographic region. For example, the prevalence of hyperthyroidism in an urban area of Germany was estimated to be 11.4% (Sassnau, 2006), whereas the prevalence rate in Hong Kong was estimated to be 3.9% (De Wet et al, 2009). It has been proposed that the emergence of clinical hyperthyroidism is related to the gradual introduction of commercially-prepared cat foods by different cultures around the world. It is interesting that commercial cat foods were first test-marketed on both coasts of the United States in the mid-1960s. This means that the first generation of cats raised and maintained almost entirely on commercial foods was reaching middle and old age in the late 1970s and early 1980s, which coincides with the recognition of feline hyperthyroidism in Boston, New York, Philadelphia, Los Angeles, and San Francisco.

Factors that have contributed to the increased recognition of feline hyperthyroidism since the 1980s include increased awareness by owners and veterinarians, inclusion of total T_4 measurement on routine biochemical profiles for geriatric cats, improved feline health care, and increased feline life spans; however, there is little doubt that the true prevalence of the disease has also increased from the time the first reports in 1979 and 1980 were published until today. Unfortunately although there have been a number of epidemiological studies investigating the risk factors for feline hyperthyroidism, no single risk factor has been identified and it is thus believed that the cause is likely multifactorial.

PATHOLOGY

Background

A thorough review of feline thyroid pathology has not been published in the 20 to 25 years since clinical feline hyperthyroidism became common. However, reviews of surgically removed tissue and necropsy specimens have confirmed that multinodular adenomatous goiter is the most common pathologic abnormality. Benign tumors are much more common than malignant tumors.

Benign Thyroid Tumors

Multinodular Adenomatous Goiter

Follicular cell adenoma and multinodular adenomatous hyperplasia are the most common thyroidal histological abnormalities described in the thyroid glands from hyperthyroid cats. Both histopathologic abnormalities are benign changes, and both may occur together within the same thyroid gland. In both thyroid adenoma and adenomatous hyperplasia, the follicular cells are uniform and cuboidal to columnar in shape with occasional papillary infoldings that form follicles containing variable amounts of colloid (Maxie, 2007). Thyroid adenomas are grossly visible, have a thin fibrous capsule, and may compress the surrounding normal thyroid tissue. In thyroid adenomatous hyperplasia, one or more nodules of hyperplastic follicular cells are present within the thyroid gland. The nodules of hyperplastic tissue range in size from less than 1 mm to greater than 3 cm in diameter (Fig. 4-1). There is no clinically relevant difference between an adenoma

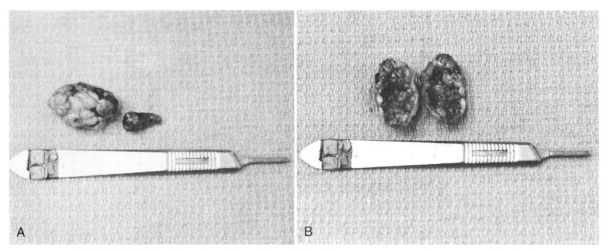

FIGURE 4-1 A, Multinodular adenomatous goiter, which has the gross appearance of a compressed cluster of grapes. This is an example of bilaterally asymmetric thyroid enlargement. **B,** After the larger mass is cut in half, cystic changes are revealed.

and adenomatous hyperplasia, and the two can coexist within the same thyroid gland. Adenomatous hyperplasia and adenomas are bilateral in approximately 70% of cats and unilateral in the remaining 30% of cats. Focal areas of necrosis, mineralization, and cystic degeneration are often present in larger adenomas and rarely may form large fluid filled cystadenomas. Normal follicular cells surrounding adenomas and hyperplastic nodules are low cuboidal or atrophied with little evidence of endocytotic activity (Maxie, 2007).

Malignant Thyroid Tumors

Thyroid Carcinoma

Malignant neoplasia is recognized to be the cause of hyperthyroidism in approximately 1% to 3% of hyperthyroid cats and may involve one or both thyroid lobes. There are a variety of clinical presentations ranging from tumors that are well encapsulated, freely moveable, and clinically indistinguishable from benign thyroid neoplasia, to thyroid masses that are very large, locally invasive, attached to overlying and underlying tissues, and metastatic to local lymph nodes. There may be multiple masses throughout the cervical region and may also be distant metastases. In cats, thyroid carcinomas are usually well differentiated adenocarcinomas that are composed of a uniform pattern of small follicles containing variable amounts of colloid (Maxie, 2007). Mixed compact and follicular morphologic patterns are most common although primary follicular and papillary patterns have also been reported (Turrel et al, 1988). There may be neoplastic invasion of blood vessels and the connective tissue capsule. The neoplastic cells may be subdivided into small lobules by strands of connective tissue with an abundant capillary network. Nonfunctional thyroid tumors in cats are rare (Turrel et al, 1988; Guptill et al, 1995). In one case series, the nonfunctional thyroid tumor was of the papillary type (Turrel et al, 1988).

Distinguishing between well-differentiated thyroid follicular carcinoma and benign proliferation of thyroid follicular epithelium on the basis of histologic features alone is not always possible (Guptill et al, 1995). Criteria used to diagnose follicular carcinoma include evidence of capsular and vascular invasion, cellular pleomorphism, extracapsular extension or distant metastasis. Clinical behavior of the tumor must be taken into consideration when interpreting the histopathology findings.

ETIOLOGY

Evidence for Primary Thyroid Dysfunction

Early studies of hyperthyroid cats in the 1980s suggested feline hyperthyroidism was due to a primary abnormality of the thyroid gland rather than the result of thyroid stimulation by a circulating hormone, such as TSH, thyrotropin-releasing hormone (TRH), or thyroid stimulating immunoglobulins. Thyroid tissue from hyperthyroid cats was transplanted subcutaneously into nude mice that had endogenous TSH secretion suppressed by administration of levothyroxine (also known as L-thyroxine; L-T$_4$). It was demonstrated that the thyroid cells retained their cuboidal shape, high growth potential, and functional autonomy in the nude mice (Peter et al, 1987). Furthermore administration of serum from hyperthyroid cats failed to stimulate iodine uptake in either normal or hyperplastic thyroid tissue. Similar findings have more recently been demonstrated in cells transfected with the feline TSH receptor (Nguyen et al, 2002).

Genetic Cause of Thyroid Autonomy

Stimulation of thyroid follicular cells by TSH results in thyroid follicular cell growth as well as synthesis and secretion of thyroid hormone via the receptor G protein–cyclic adenosine monophosphate (cAMP) signal transduction system. The normal feline thyroid gland contains subpopulations of follicular cells with high growth potential and TSH receptors that have detectable basal constitutive activity (Nguyen et al, 2002). In the thyroid gland of a cat that is destined to become hyperthyroid, subpopulations of follicular cells begin replicating autonomously. Once these subpopulations are present in sufficient numbers, growth and thyroid hormone synthesis becomes autonomous (Peter et al, 1991). It has been hypothesized that chronic stimulation of cells with a high growth potential ultimately causes them to become autonomous due to development of follicular cell mutations (Ward et al, 2005a). In humans, gain-of-function mutations of the TSH receptor or the alpha subunit of stimulatory G proteins have been described. Altered expression of the alpha subunits of the stimulatory and inhibitory G proteins has also been reported. Eleven TSH receptor mutations were detected in 134 hyperplastic nodules from 50 hyperthyroid cats (Watson et al, 2005). Five of

| | TABLE 4-1 | RISK FACTORS FOR FELINE HYPERTHYROIDISM IDENTIFIED IN CASE CONTROL STUDIES |

STUDY LOCATION	NUMBERS OF CASES (CONTROLS)	STUDY DATES	DIET STUDIED	REPORTED RISK FACTORS
New York State College of Veterinary Medicine, USA	56 (117)	1982-1985	Diet for past 5 years	• Non-Siamese breeds • More than 50% canned food • Partial or complete indoor housing • Exposure to lawn or flea control products
University of California, Davis, and Animal Medical Center, New York, USA	379 (351)	1986	Current and one previous diet	• Non-Siamese or Himalayan breeds • More than 50% canned food • Exposure to cat litter
Seattle, WA, USA	100 (163)	1996-1997	Diet for past 5 years	• Increasing age • Preference for certain canned food flavors
New Zealand	125 (250)	1996-1998	Current diet*	• Increasing age • Female sex • Domestic Short-Hair • Canned food of multiple flavors • Sleeping on the floor • Contact with flea and fly control products • Drinking puddle water and exposure to organic fertilizers
Purdue University, IN, USA	109 (173)	1998-2000	Lifetime diet until 1 year before presentation	• Increasing age • Female sex • More than 50% canned food • Food from pop-top cans • Baby food in regular kitten diet or as treat • Lack of iodine supplement in label ingredients • Increasing frequency of carpet cleaning • Increasing years of exposure to well water • Increasing years to exposure of gas fireplaces
Hong Kong	12 (293)	2006-2007	Not stated	• Increasing age • Non-domestic Short-Hair breed
United Kingdom	109 (196)	2006-2007	Diet for past 5 years	• Increasing age • Non-purebred • Litter box use • More than 50% wet (canned/pouched) food • Canned foods • Fish in diet • Lack of deworming medication

From Edinboro CH, et al.: Feline hyperthyroidism: potential relationship with iodine supplement requirements of commercial cat foods, *J Feline Med Surg* 12(9):672-679, 2010.
*This was not explicitly reported but apparent from the context.

the mutations that were identified have also been associated with human hyperthyroidism. Interestingly of the 41 cats for which more than one nodule was available, 14 had nodules with different mutations. In an in vitro study of thyroid adenomas obtained from hyperthyroid cats, a decreased amount of an inhibitory G protein was identified (Hammer et al, 2000). Decreased expression of this G protein in thyroid follicular cells could reduce the inhibitory effect on the cAMP cascade, leading to autonomous growth and hypersecretion of thyroxine (Ward et al, 2005b). A further study suggested that decreased expression of certain subsets of inhibitory G proteins, rather than a change in TSH-stimulated G protein activity, contributes to the molecular pathogenesis of feline hyperthyroidism (Ward et al, 2010). In another study, overexpression of the product of the oncogene c-Ras was detected in areas of nodular hyperplasia/adenoma in thyroid tissue from 18 hyperthyroid cats (Merryman et al, 1999). Taken together

these studies suggest that multiple mutations in thyroid follicular cells may ultimately result in thyroid cell autonomy. What is still unclear is the underlying cause of these mutations and why clinical feline hyperthyroidism has become more common in the last 30 years.

Epidemiological Studies

Risk Factors

Numerous epidemiological studies have been performed in the last 25 years in an attempt to elucidate the cause of feline hyperthyroidism (Table 4-1). The first study published in 1988 suggested that feeding of canned cat foods, living strictly indoors, being a non-Siamese breed, and having reported exposure to flea sprays, fertilizers, insecticides, and herbicides increased the risk of developing hyperthyroidism (Scarlett et al, 1988). In another study, two genetically related cat breeds (Siamese and Himalayan) were found to have a diminished risk of developing hyperthyroidism. In addition, there was a twofold to threefold increase in risk of developing hyperthyroidism among cats fed mostly canned cat food. There was also a threefold increase in risk among cats using cat litter (Kass et al, 1999). In a more recent study, there was no breed association with risk for developing hyperthyroidism. Exposure to fertilizers, herbicides, plant pesticides, or flea control products or the presence of a smoker in the home was not significantly associated with an increased risk for developing hyperthyroidism. Cats that preferred fish-flavored or liver and giblets–flavored canned cat food had an increased risk of hyperthyroidism (Martin et al, 2000). Finally in a study published in 2004, Edinboro et al. identified consumption of canned cat food (especially food consumed from pop top cans) as a risk factor for developing hyperthyroidism. In this study, female cats were at increased risk of developing hyperthyroidism. Other identified risk factors were consumption of baby food, lack of iodine supplement in label ingredients, and increasing frequency of carpet cleaning; increasing years of exposure to well water and increasing years of exposure to gas fireplaces were also identified as risk factors (Edinboro et al, 2010). Similar risk factors have been identified in widely diverse geographic locations, such as the United Kingdom, Germany, New Zealand, and Hong Kong (Wakeling et al, 2009b) (Table 4-1). These studies collectively suggest that the cause of feline hyperthyroidism is probably multifactorial; however the consistent identification of canned cat food as a risk factor suggests that diet likely plays a major role. Candidate dietary candidate risk factors fall into two categories; nutritional deficiencies or excesses and consumption of goitrogens (Peterson, 2012).

Nutritional Deficiencies or Excesses

Iodine

Iodine deficiency causes hypothyroidism and goiter in humans and other species. Low thyroid hormone concentrations cause increased TSH concentrations, which lead to thyroid hyperplasia and goiter. Mild or moderate iodine deficiency increases the risk of toxic nodular goiter in elderly humans (Laurberg et al, 1991; Pedersen et al, 2002). In some individuals, correction of iodine deficiency or administration of excess iodine can lead to thyrotoxicosis, which may be transient or persistent. Causes of iodine-induced thyrotoxicosis in humans include iodine supplementation for endemic iodine deficiency goiter, iodine administration to patients with euthyroid Graves' disease or underlying nodular or diffuse goiter, and administration of radiographic contrast material to patients with underlying thyroid disease. In areas of mild to moderate iodine deficiency, iodide administration can cause thyrotoxicosis in patients with no underlying thyroid disease (Roti and Vagenakis, 2013). It is therefore possible that iodine excess or deficiency could contribute to the pathogenesis of feline hyperthyroidism. Although acute changes in iodine intake result in inverse changes in thyroid hormone concentrations in cats, longer-term studies suggest that cats are able to auto regulate thyroid hormone synthesis and maintain thyroid hormone concentrations within reference range despite variable iodide intake (Mumma et al, 1986; Johnson et al, 1992; Edinboro et al, 2013). Longer-term effects of variation in iodide intake however are unknown. In a case control study of cats with hyperthyroidism, cats consuming diets that did not have iodine supplementation identified as a labeled ingredient were four times more likely to be hyperthyroid than those that did; however it should be recognized that iodine

in the diet can result from overt supplementation, or be naturally present in the diet from both plant and animal sources—especially ocean fish. Thus the lack of explicit iodine supplementation in a diet does not necessarily equate with iodine deficiency. Studies have documented that the iodine content of commercial diets, especially canned diets, is extremely variable with some commercial diets being deficient in iodine while others contain iodine in excess (Johnson et al, 1992; Edinboro et al, 2013). There has been a recent trend toward less iodine supplementation of commercial cat foods, because recommended dietary requirements of iodine for cats have decreased over the last 30 years (Edinboro et al, 2010). In a study of urinary iodide concentrations in hyperthyroid cats, before and after treatment with radioactive iodine, it was demonstrated that iodine concentrations were lower in hyperthyroid cats compared to euthyroid cats (Wakeling et al, 2009a). Although it is possible that these findings indicate decreased iodine intake during development of hyperthyroidism, there are many complex influences on iodine metabolism in cats and further studies are necessary to establish a cause and effect relationship. Although it is unlikely that iodine deficiency is the sole cause of feline hyperthyroidism, it is possible that dramatic fluctuations in iodine intake or chronic iodine deficiency may contribute to the current increase in feline thyrotoxicosis.

Soy Isoflavones

Dietary soy is a potential dietary goitrogen that is commonly used as a source of high-quality vegetable protein in commercial cat food. In one study, soy isoflavones were identified in in 24 of 42 commercial cat foods with concentrations ranging from 1 to 163 µg/g of food; these amounts are predicted to have a biologic effect (Court and Freeman, 2002). Although soy is more commonly used as an ingredient in dry food, it is also present in some canned diets. The soy isoflavones genistein and daidzein are known to inhibit thyroid peroxidase, which is an enzyme essential to thyroid hormone synthesis (Doerge and Sheehan 2002), and also inhibit 5′-deiodinase activity, resulting in decreased conversion of T_4 to T_3. These compounds may also induce hepatic enzymes that are responsible for hepatic clearance of T_3 and T_4 (White et al, 2004). In a study of normal cats fed either soy or soy-free diets for 3 months, soy fed cats had a measurable increase in total T_4 and free T_4 (fT_4) concentrations with no change in total T_3 concentrations (White et al, 2004). These changes were hypothesized to be due to deiodinase inhibition and resulted in some cats having a fT_4 concentration above the reference range. These finding are consistent with the hypothesis that decreased total T_3 concentrations cause increased TSH, which stimulates the thyroid gland to increase thyroid hormone synthesis and normalize total T_3 concentrations. These compounds, therefore, could potentially cause chronic thyroid gland hyperplasia and play an etiologic role in feline thyrotoxicosis. Although compelling, this theory does not explain the increased risk of hyperthyroidism in cats fed canned food, because soy is less commonly found in canned diets. Interestingly the effects of soy on thyroid function are exacerbated in the presence of iodine deficiency (Doerge and Sheehan, 2002). It is conceivable that soy diets contribute to the pathogenesis of feline hyperthyroidism by interacting with other factors that impact the thyroid gland such as iodine deficiency. Further studies are necessary to confirm this hypothesis.

Selenium

The thyroid gland contains more selenium per gram than any other tissue, which suggests an important role for this trace element in thyroid homeostasis. Selenium modifies thyroid hormone metabolism through the activity of selenoproteins, such as glutathione peroxidases and thioredoxin reductase, which protect thyrocytes from oxidative damage. In cats, the type I deiodinase is a selenium dependent enzyme, and selenium deficiency may impair thyroid function. In kittens fed a low selenium diet, total T_4 increased and total T_3 decreased (Yu et al, 2002). There was no difference in plasma selenium concentrations of either euthyroid or hyperthyroid cats from two geographic areas with an allegedly high incidence of hyperthyroidism (UK, Eastern Australia) and two regions with a lower incidence (Denmark, Western Australia); however, cats had higher concentrations of selenium in their plasma than do other species such as rats and humans (Foster et al, 2001). In another study, selenium concentrations were not different between hyperthyroid cats and control cats (Sabatino et al, 2013). The role, if any, of selenium in the pathogenesis of feline hyperthyroidism remains to be determined.

Goitrogens (Thyroid Disrupters)

A large number of environmental chemicals are known to disrupt thyroid function in various species, including humans (Boas et al, 2012). Known endocrine disrupting chemicals include polychlorinated biphenyls, dioxins, polybrominated diphenyl ether (PBDE) flame retardants, perfluorinated chemicals, phthalates, bisphenol A (BPA), and perchlorate. Many of these compounds have a high degree of structural similarity to T_4 (Fig. 4-2) and most are metabolized via glucuronidation, a process that is unusually slow in cats (Court and Greenblatt, 2000). The mechanisms by which goitrogens disrupt thyroid function are many and complex and include binding to the TSH receptor, stimulation or inhibition of the sodium iodide symporter, inhibition of thyroid peroxidase, binding to thyroid hormone plasma binding proteins, interference with other receptors on the thyrocyte, interference with membrane thyroid hormone transporters, changes in thyroid receptor (TR) expression or binding, and stimulation of hepatic enzymes responsible for thyroid hormone clearance. Although there are a large number of chemicals that have the potential to disrupt thyroid function in cats, recently most attention has focused on BPA and the PBDE flame retardants.

Bisphenol A

BPA is a chemical used to make epoxy resins and polycarbonate plastics. It has estrogenic activity and has been demonstrated to disrupt thyroid function both by inhibiting thyroid peroxidase and by binding to the thyroid hormone receptor, inhibiting TR mediated transcription. Epoxy resins are widely used for lining the interior of metal cans to prevent corrosion and maintain flavor and shelf life. BPA has been demonstrated to migrate from food can linings into human and pet food products during the cooking process (Kang and Kondo, 2002). It is hypothesized that BPA migration into canned cat food could explain the increased risk of hyperthyroidism in cats fed canned food (Edinboro et al, 2004). Further studies are needed to establish the relationship between BPA and hyperthyroidism in cats.

Polybrominated Diphenyl Ether Flame Retardants

PBDEs are a group of synthetic brominated compounds that are widely used as flame retardants in many consumer products. These chemicals interfere with thyroid function at multiple levels including binding with the TR, interacting with thyroid hormone binding proteins, inhibition of deiodinases, and increasing hepatic clearance of thyroid hormone. Studies have demonstrated that house cats have high plasma concentrations of a variety of PBDEs, although concentrations do not differ between euthyroid and hyperthyroid cats. In a recent study, although the serum concentrations of PBDEs did not differ between euthyroid and hyperthyroid cats, there were higher concentrations of PBDEs in dust collected from the households of hyperthyroid cats than from the households of euthyroid cats (Mensching et al, 2012). Clearly domestic cats have a significant burden of PBDEs presumably due to ingestion of household dust during grooming; however a causal association between PBDEs and feline hyperthyroidism has yet to be proven.

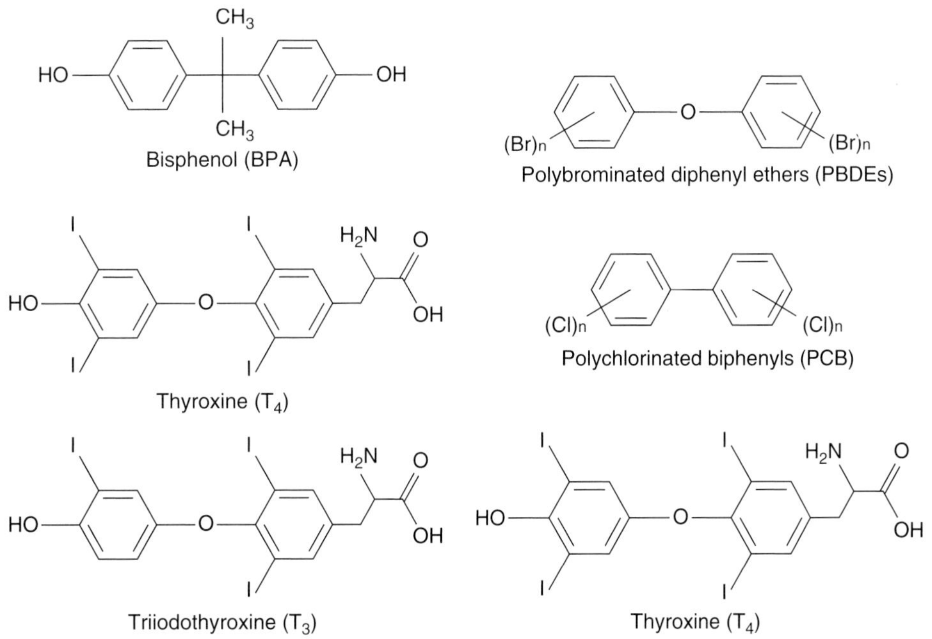

FIGURE 4-2 Chemical structure of bisphenol A (BPA), polybrominated diphenyl ethers (PBDEs), polychlorinated biphenyls (PCB), thyroxine (T_4), and triiodothyronine (T_3). (From Peterson ME: Hyperthyroidism in cats: what's causing this epidemic of thyroid disease and can we prevent it? *J Feline Med Surg* 14[11]:804-818, 2012.)

CLINICAL FEATURES OF FELINE HYPERTHYROIDISM

Signalment

Hyperthyroidism is the most common endocrinopathy affecting cats (Edinboro et al, 2004). The reported age range is 4 to 22 years with a mean of 13 years. Interestingly the mean age of onset has not changed over the time period of 1983 to 2004 (Peterson et al, 1983; Broussard et al, 1995; Edinboro et al, 2004). A small number of cats younger than 4 years has been diagnosed with hyperthyroidism, although the disorder remains rare in this age group (Gordon et al, 2003). Fewer than 5% of cats diagnosed with hyperthyroidism are younger than 8 years of age. Pure bred cats, particularly Siamese and Himalayan cats, have a decreased risk of developing hyperthyroidism (Scarlett et al, 1988; Kass et al, 1999; Olczak et al, 2005).

Clinical Signs and Pathophysiology

Overview

Most hyperthyroid cats have a range of clinical signs that reflect the effects of thyroid hormone on almost every organ in the body. Feline hyperthyroidism is a chronically progressive and insidious disease, and the clinical effects can vary from mild to severe. Early in the disease process, the clinical signs are subtle enough to be missed by both the owner and the veterinarian and the diagnosis may only be made when routine thyroid hormone testing is performed. Even if the diagnosis is made by routine testing, clinical signs (e.g., weight loss) can often be identified retrospectively. In some cases, weight loss is ignored because it occurs after intentional calorie restriction to manage obesity, but the weight loss continues even after calorie restriction is discontinued. In other cases, subtle clinical changes (e.g., tachycardia and increased activity) are blamed on stress during the office visit. Clinical signs may be present for months to 1 to 2 years prior to the diagnosis being made (Thoday and Mooney, 1992). Because hyperthyroid cats usually have a good to ravenous appetite and are active or even overactive, the owners often perceive that an elderly cat has a new lease on life and do not initially worry about the clinical signs. Only when the signs worsen or other more serious clinical signs appear do owners seek veterinary help. The most common reasons for owners to seek veterinary care are weight loss, polyphagia, polydipsia/polyuria, vomiting, and/or diarrhea. The spectrum of clinical signs reported in the first large case series reported in the veterinary literature is shown in Table 4-2.

Because owner and veterinary awareness of the clinical syndrome of feline hyperthyroidism is now very high and measurement of serum thyroxine concentration is a routine component of geriatric feline serum biochemistry profiles, cats with hyperthyroidism are being diagnosed earlier in the course of the disease. This means that the clinical signs observed by owners and veterinarians are less severe than those which were described when the disease was first recognized in the 1980s; thus diagnosis of feline hyperthyroidism has become more challenging particularly in cats with other concurrent illness (Broussard et al, 1995; Bucknell, 2000). There was a dramatic decrease in the frequency and severity of clinical findings in cats diagnosed with hyperthyroidism from 1983 to 1993 (Broussard et al, 1995; Fig. 4-3). Unfortunately studies evaluating the frequency of clinical signs in hyperthyroid cats have not been published in the peer reviewed literature since 2000, but subjectively the trend for decreasing severity of clinical signs at the time of diagnosis has continued. A significant percentage of cats presented for radioactive

iodine treatment at our institution did not have clinical signs recognized by the owner prior to diagnosis of hyperthyroidism.

Weight Loss

Weight loss is the most common clinical sign observed in cats with hyperthyroidism. Approximately 90% of hyperthyroid cats have evidence of mild to severe weight loss documented at the time of diagnosis. Some hyperthyroid cats become severely cachectic (Fig. 4-4), but this is less common now than previously because of the increased awareness of the disease and resultant earlier diagnosis. The weight loss typically occurs gradually over a period of months to years. Owners may comment that the weight loss was not recognized until someone who had not seen the cat for several months noticed the change.

Polyphagia

Polyphagia and weight loss are quite common in feline hyperthyroidism. This is an extremely important historical finding, because the combination of polyphagia and weight loss has fewer differential diagnoses than anorexia and weight loss (Box 4-1). Cats previously thought to be finicky eaters may develop excellent appetites, which is a change that may not initially be perceived as a problem by the owner. In severe cases of polyphagia, cats can become aggressive in obtaining food.

Polyphagia and weight loss occur due to the increased metabolic rate and increased energy expenditure of the hyperthyroid state, which results in reduced efficiency of physiologic functions.

TABLE 4-2	**HISTORICAL AND PHYSICAL EXAMINATION FINDINGS FROM THE FIRST LARGE CASE SERIES OF 131 CATS WITH HYPERTHYROIDISM**

SIGN	PERCENT OF CATS
Weight loss	98
Polyphagia	81
Increased activity/restless	76
Tachycardia	66
Polydipsia/polyuria	60
Vomiting	55
Cardiac murmur	53
Diarrhea	33
Increased fecal volume	31
Anorexia	26
Polypnea	25
Muscle weakness	25
Muscle tremor	18
Congestive heart failure	12
Increased nail growth	12
Dyspnea	11
Alopecia	7
Ventroflexion of neck	3

Modified from Peterson ME, et al.: Feline hyperthyroidism: pretreatment clinical and laboratory evaluation of 131 cases, *J Am Vet Med Assoc* 183(1):103-110, 1983.

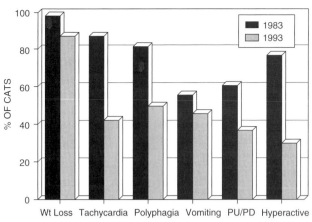
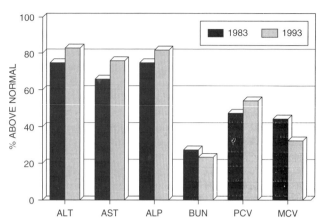

FIGURE 4-3 Percentage of cats with common clinical findings in 1983 (n = 131) compared to 1993 (n = 202). (From Broussard JD, et al.: Changes in clinical and laboratory findings in cats with hyperthyroidism from 1983 to 1993, *J Am Vet Med Assoc* 206[3]:302-305, 1995.) *ALP,* alkaline phosphatase; *ALT,* alanine aminotransferase; *AST,* aspartate aminotransferase; *BUN,* blood urea nitrogen; *MCV,* mean corpuscular volume; *PCV,* packed cell volume; *PD,* polydipsia; *PU,* polyuria.

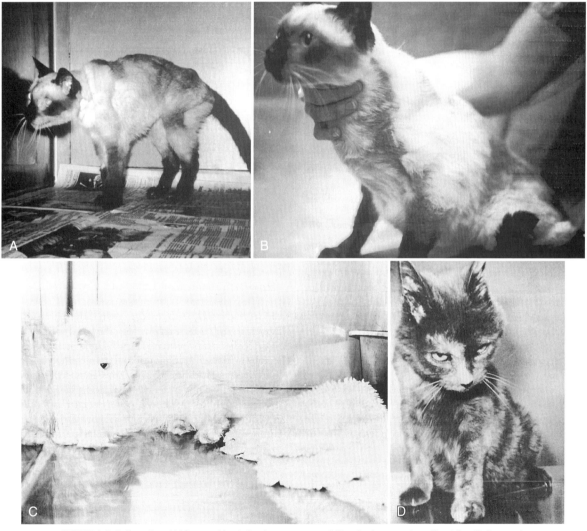

FIGURE 4-4 A, Hyperthyroid 13-year-old cat showing severe emaciation due to severe hyperthyroidism **B,** Same cat as in **A** 2 months after return to a euthyroid condition. **C,** Hyperthyroid cat choosing the cool cage floor rather than a warm fleece pad. **D,** Hyperthyroid cat with marked ventroflexion of the head, a finding suggestive of concomitant thiamine or potassium deficiency. (**D,** Courtesy of Dr. Jane Turrel, Pacifica, CA.)

> **BOX 4-1   Differential Diagnosis for Cats with Polyphagia and Weight Loss**
>
> Hyperthyroidism
> Diabetes mellitus
> Poor quality or insufficient diet
> Gastrointestinal disease
>   Malabsorption (inflammatory bowel disease, gastrointestinal lymphoma, gastrointestinal parasitism)
>   Maldigestion (exocrine pancreatic insufficiency)
> Hyperadrenocorticism

TABLE 4-3 PHYSICAL EXAMINATION FINDINGS ASSOCIATED WITH HYPERTHYROIDISM IN CATS	
FINDING	**PERCENT OF CATS**
Palpable thyroid	91
Thin	71
Tachycardia (more than 240 beats/min)	48
Hyperactive/difficult to examine	48
Heart murmur	41
Skin changes (patchy alopecia, matting, dry coat, greasy seborrhea, thin skin)	36
Small kidneys	26
Increased rectal temperature	14
Gallop cardiac rhythm	12
Easily stressed	12
Dehydrated/cachectic appearance	11
Aggressive behavior	8
Premature cardiac beats	8
Increase nail growth	2
Depressed/weak	2
Ventroflexion of the neck	< 1

Increased food intake and utilization of stored energy can initially compensate for the increased energy expenditure; however, ultimately chronic caloric and nutritional deficiency occurs. Although both synthesis and degradation of proteins are increased, the net effect is protein catabolism. In addition to weight loss, negative nitrogen balance is evidenced by muscle wasting and weakness. The exact mechanism for the increase in appetite associated with hyperthyroidism is poorly understood but studies suggest that suppression of leptin, increased hypothalamic neuropeptide Y, and enhanced phosphorylation of adenosine monophosphate (AMP)-activated protein kinase may play a role (Pétervári et al, 2005; Ishii et al, 2008). Although polyphagia is one of the most common clinical signs of hyperthyroidism, a small percentage of hyperthyroid cats exhibit periods of decreased appetite (see Decreased Appetite).

Nervousness, Hyperactivity, Aggressive Behavior

Approximately 50% of humans with thyrotoxicosis exhibit trembling, nervousness, emotional lability, and depression and anxiety, which are presumably due to a direct effect of thyroid hormone concentrations on the nervous system (Burch, 2013). In cats, these signs are characterized by restlessness, irritability, and/or aggressive behavior (see Table 4-2; Table 4-3). Many hyperthyroid cats appear to have an intense desire to move about constantly. Owners may note that their cats wander, pace, sleep for only brief periods, and waken easily. Many hyperthyroid cats appear "anxious" and cannot be held for the short time required to complete a physical examination. Some become aggressive if an attempt is made to further restrain them. The cause of these clinical signs is multifactorial; however some of the signs are due to increased adrenergic activity, because a degree of improvement occurs during treatment with adrenergic antagonists.

Polydipsia and Polyuria

Polyuria and polydipsia are commonly reported in feline hyperthyroidism. Although the two clinical signs invariably occur together, it is common for owners to report polydipsia in the absence of polyuria, or vice versa. Polyuria and polydipsia occur in 30% to 40% of hyperthyroid cats, and changes in the amount of water consumed and urine excreted are highly variable. There are a number of mechanisms involved in the pathogenesis of polydipsia and polyuria in hyperthyroidism. Primary (psychogenic) polydipsia increases water and solute intake, and down regulation of Aquaporin 1 and Aquaporin 2 channels may contribute to the polyuria (Wang et al, 2007). Occult renal disease may also play a role. Polyuria and polydipsia may be present in hyperthyroid cats without evidence of renal disease, but because hyperthyroidism increases glomerular filtration rate (GFR) and decreases urine

specific gravity (USG), it is difficult to assess true renal function in hyperthyroid cats. After resolution of hyperthyroidism (regardless of the treatment method), renal perfusion typically decreases, which in some cats may unmask occult renal failure (see Treatment of Hyperthyroidism and Renal Function).

Gastrointestinal Dysfunction

The most common clinical signs of hyperthyroidism referable to the gastrointestinal tract are polyphagia and weight loss (see earlier). Other signs of gastrointestinal dysfunction include anorexia, vomiting, diarrhea, increased fecal volume, increased frequency of defecation, and foul smelling feces. Vomiting is relatively common, occurring in approximately 50% of hyperthyroid cats. Anorexia and watery diarrhea are less common but when present are usually seen in cats with severe hyperthyroidism or in those with coexistent primary intestinal problems. Reasons for diarrhea and increased frequency of defecation in hyperthyroidism include hypermotility of the gastrointestinal tract, leading to rapid gastric emptying, and shortened intestinal transit times (Papasouliotis et al, 1993; Schlesinger et al, 1993). Rapid eating or overeating leading to gastric distension and direct action of thyroid hormone on the chemoreceptor trigger zone are potential causes of vomiting. Steatorrhea is also reported in cats with severe hyperthyroidism; however, fat malabsorption may be due to other concurrent illness, such as exocrine pancreatic insufficiency.

Hair Loss/Unkempt Coat

Nonspecific hair coat changes (e.g., unkempt hair, matted hair, and a lusterless coat) occur commonly in hyperthyroid cats. Less commonly, patchy alopecia may occur due to excessive grooming activity. Some cats may pull hair out in clumps. Heat intolerance is a classic sign of thyrotoxicosis in humans, and hair pulling may also be a result of heat intolerance in cats.

Panting and Respiratory Distress

Open-mouth breathing (panting) is rare in cats and is usually associated with heart or respiratory disease. Some hyperthyroid cats exhibit panting, dyspnea, or hyperventilation at rest; these signs are most common in hyperthyroid cats that are stressed by physical restraint or transportation. Dyspnea on exertion is common in thyrotoxic people and is due to respiratory muscle weakness, enhanced ventilatory drive, decreased pulmonary compliance, and concurrent cardiovascular complications (Burch, 2013). Thyrotoxicosis is associated with shallow rapid breathing, enhanced oxygen utilization and carbon dioxide output, and a low anaerobic threshold (Burch, 2013).

Decreased Appetite

Although most hyperthyroid cats are polyphagic, some hyperthyroid cats exhibit inappetence, anorexia, or a waxing and waning appetite. Potential causes of a poor appetite include congestive heart failure, severe debilitation and muscle weakness, thiamine or cobalamine deficiency, hypokalemia, or other concurrent nonthyroidal illness (e.g., inflammatory bowel disease, pancreatitis, renal disease, and neoplasia) (Cook et al, 2011).

Weakness and Lethargy

Decreased activity, weakness, fatigability, and lethargy occur in some cats with severe hyperthyroidism. Some cats progress from over-activity and restlessness to listlessness and weakness. Weakness and fatigability are also frequent complaints in humans with thyrotoxicosis. In one study, 67% of hyperthyroid people had complaints of muscle weakness, mainly in the proximal muscles of the legs, and 19% had symmetrical distal sensory abnormalities and depressed distal tendon reflexes (Duyff et al, 2000). The biochemical basis of the muscular weakness is uncertain; it may simply be caused by weight loss and the catabolic state. Hypokalemia, cobalamine deficiency, and thiamine deficiency may also contribute to muscle weakness and weight loss (Ruaux et al, 2005).

Heat and Stress Intolerance

Heat intolerance is a subtle sign that may be observed by cat owners. Most normal cats seek warm, sunny places to sleep. Hyperthyroid cats may reverse this heat-seeking behavior and sleep in cool places, such as the bath tub or a cool tile floor (see Fig. 4-4, *C*). In addition to heat intolerance, some hyperthyroid cats have an obvious impaired tolerance for stress. Brief car rides, bathing, and visits to boarding kennels or veterinary hospitals may cause marked clinical deterioration, respiratory distress, weakness, or even cardiac arrest. The clinician should always take into consideration this inability to cope with stress when diagnostic or therapeutic procedures are being planned.

Heat intolerance and an inability to cope with stress are classic clinical signs of human thyrotoxicosis. Many of these effects are similar to those induced by epinephrine, including heat intolerance, excessive sweating (in humans), tremor, and tachycardia. Because these signs are partly alleviated by adrenergic antagonists, it has been hypothesized that a state of increased adrenergic activity exists in thyrotoxicosis; however investigators have been unable to demonstrate increased catecholamine production, increased concentrations of serum catecholamine concentrations, or excretion of urinary catecholamine metabolites. Furthermore, although increased numbers of adrenergic receptors have been demonstrated in thyrotoxicosis, evidence of increased sensitivity to catecholamines in thyrotoxicosis is lacking (Liggert et al, 1989).

Concurrent Nonthyroidal Illness

Because feline hyperthyroidism is a geriatric disease, concurrent nonthyroidal illness is common and often complicates the clinical picture. Because the clinical signs of hyperthyroidism are so variable and overlap with those of many other concurrent illnesses, the presence or absence of any one clinical sign cannot be used to diagnose or exclude hyperthyroidism. In some cases, the only way to determine whether all the clinical signs exhibited by a particular patient can be explained by hyperthyroidism is to treat the hyperthyroidism and determine if the clinical signs resolve.

Subclinical Hyperthyroidism

Subclinical hyperthyroidism is defined in humans as the presence of hormone test results indicating hyperthyroidism (usually decreased TSH) in a person without clinical signs of hyperthyroidism (Biondi et al, 2005). It is likely that a similar condition exists in cats; however, documentation of this condition is hampered by the lack of a sensitive assay for TSH in cats. In one study of 104 geriatric cats with normal thyroid hormone concentrations, 7.5% of cats became hyperthyroid during 12 months of follow up (Wakeling et al, 2011). Cats with undetectable TSH at baseline were more likely to become hyperthyroid, but not all cats with a suppressed TSH became hyperthyroid. Furthermore, geriatric cats with a low TSH are more likely to have histologic evidence of nodular thyroid disease (Wakeling et al, 2007).

 PHYSICAL EXAMINATION

General

Although many cats with mild hyperthyroidism appear asymptomatic to the owner, in the vast majority of cases abnormalities consistent with a diagnosis of hyperthyroidism can be detected by a careful physical examination. Weight loss and tachycardia are usually present and support a diagnosis of hyperthyroidism. Most importantly, a palpable cervical mass is detected in over 90% of hyperthyroid cats at the time of diagnosis.

Palpable Cervical Mass (Goiter)

In healthy cats, the thyroid lobes are positioned just below the cricoid cartilage and extend ventrally over the first few tracheal rings; they lie dorsolateral to and on either side of the trachea. The thyroid lobes are not palpable in normal cats. Hyperthyroidism is invariably associated with enlargement of one or both thyroid lobes (goiter)—an enlargement that is palpable in more than 90% of hyperthyroid cats. Careful palpation is required to identify small goiters, which can be challenging in a stressed cat.

Palpation of a cervical mass is not pathognomonic for hyperthyroidism; some cats with palpable thyroid glands are clinically normal, and some cervical masses arise from structures other than the thyroid gland. In one study of euthyroid geriatric cats (more than 9 years of age) a palpable goiter was present in 27 of 104 (26%) of cats. Sixteen percent of these cats ultimately became hyperthyroid over 4½ years of follow up (Wakeling et al, 2011). Causes of thyroid gland enlargement, other than adenomatous hyperplasia or adenoma, include thyroiditis, and thyroid cystadenoma (Norsworthy et al, 2002). Other causes of palpable cervical masses

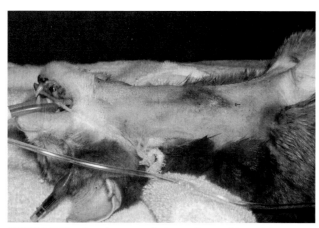

FIGURE 4-5 The clipped ventrocervical area of a cat with an obvious goiter.

include salivary mucoceles, parathyroid gland masses or cysts, thyroglossal cysts, dermoid cysts, and pharyngeal (branchial) cysts (Norsworthy et al, 2002; Phillips et al, 2003; Lynn et al, 2009; Tolbert et al, 2009; Nelson et al, 2012).

Because the thyroid lobes are only loosely attached to the trachea, the increased weight associated with thyroid enlargement causes migration of the lobes ventrally in the neck. Sometimes the abnormal lobe (or lobes) descends through the thoracic inlet and into the anterior mediastinum. This may be one explanation for being unable to palpate a goiter in a hyperthyroid cat. In cats with thyroid carcinoma, thyroid gland palpation may be similar to that of a hyperthyroid cat with benign disease; however, in other cases the masses associated with thyroid carcinoma are large, fixed rather than freely moveable and attached to underlying or overlying tissues.

Palpation Technique

Evaluation of the thyroid area should be part of the physical examination of every cat seen by a veterinarian. This allows the clinician to develop expertise and confidence when palpating a cat suspected of having hyperthyroidism, and it occasionally allows identification of a mass that would otherwise go undetected.

For the evaluation, the cat's head should be gently extended. The thumb and index finger of one hand are gently placed on either side of the trachea in the jugular furrows at the level of the larynx. The area is gently compressed, and the fingers are smoothly slid down to the thoracic inlet and back up again to the larynx. The fingertips should remain within the jugular furrows. Thyroid enlargement is usually felt as a somewhat movable, subcutaneous (SC) nodule that may vary between the size of a lentil and the size of a lima bean. Success in this maneuver depends on not squeezing too hard; the pressure exerted must be gentle enough to allow the abnormal nodule to slide under the fingertips but firm enough to detect the mass. Sometimes it is possible for owners to visualize a goiter by moistening the neck with alcohol; the enlarged thyroid glands can often be visualized as the fingers palpating the neck slide toward the thoracic inlet. Occasionally a large cervical mass can be directly direct visualized if the ventrocervical area is clipped free of hair (Fig. 4-5). If thyroid enlargement is not palpated after two or three attempts in a cat with compatible clinical signs, the cats head and neck should be extended further and the palpation repeated. This maneuver will sometimes result in an intrathoracic nodule moving back out into the neck where it can be palpated. Alternatively gradual pressure applied just below the thoracic inlet may move a thyroid mass located just inside the thoracic inlet back into the neck.

Alternative Palpation Technique

An alternative semi-quantitative palpation technique has been described in which the clinician stands behind the cat and elevates the head at a 45-degree angle while turning the head to the right and left (Norsworthy et al, 2002). The size of the thyroid gland is scored from 0 to 6 with 0 being a non-palpable thyroid gland, 1 being a barely palpable thyroid gland and 6 being a lobe measuring 2.5 cm or greater in length. Using this technique, an enlarged thyroid gland was detected in 96% of hyperthyroid cats and 59% of euthyroid cats (Norsworthy et al, 2002); however, the technique was not compared to the standard palpation technique. None of the enlarged thyroid glands detected in euthyroid cats had a score of 3 or more, whereas 18 of the 23 hyperthyroid cats had a score of 4 or greater.

Cardiac Disturbances

Tachycardia, Murmurs, Premature Beats, and Gallop Rhythm

The heart is very sensitive to the effects of thyroid hormone, and many hyperthyroid cats have clinical evidence of heart disease. Common cardiovascular abnormalities include tachyarrhythmias, heart murmurs, and gallop rhythms. Less commonly, clinical signs of congestive heart failure (e.g., dyspnea, muffled heart sounds, and ascites) may be present. In a study of approximately 200 hyperthyroid cats evaluated from 1992 to 1993, 8% of cats had evidence of congestive heart failure compared to 20% of cats evaluated between 1979 and 1982 (Fox et al, 1999). Congestive heart failure due to feline hyperthyroidism is even less common now that it was in the 1990s (Connolly et al, 2005).

Tachycardia is the most common cardiovascular abnormality present in hyperthyroid cats, but it is sometimes difficult to distinguish tachycardia due to thyrotoxicosis from other causes of tachycardia, such as stress, hypovolemia, and primary cardiac disease. Sinus tachycardia is the most common cause of tachycardia and is reported in about 30% of hyperthyroid cats. Other less common arrhythmias include atrial extrasystoles, atrial tachycardia, ventricular extrasystoles, first degree atrioventricular block, left anterior fascicular block, right bundle branch block, and left bundle branch block.

The tachycardia present in the majority of hyperthyroid cats is due to both an increase in sympathetic tone and a decrease in parasympathetic tone (Fig. 4-6; Klein and Ojamaa, 2001). Cardiac output is increased due to tachycardia, increased ejection fraction, increased blood volume, and decreased vascular resistance (Klein and Ojamaa, 2001). The direct vasodilatory effect of T_3 on smooth muscle results in decreased peripheral resistance that leads to activation of the renin-angiotensin-aldosterone system (RAAS) and increased blood volume. Thyroid hormones also directly activate genes that encode structural and regulatory cardiac proteins (Box 4-2), which ultimately results in an increase in contractile function (Connolly et al, 2005; Klein and Ojamaa, 2001). The increased metabolic rate of the hyperthyroid state increases peripheral oxygen demand and also contributes to the high-output state. The normal heart compensates for these changes by cardiac dilation and hypertrophy. Although the increased heart rate and increased cardiac output of the hyperthyroid state resemble a state of increased adrenergic activity and various components of the adrenergic receptor complex in the plasma membrane are altered by changes in thyroid hormone concentrations, there is no net effect on the sensitivity of the heart to adrenergic stimulation (Klein and Ojamaa, 2001).

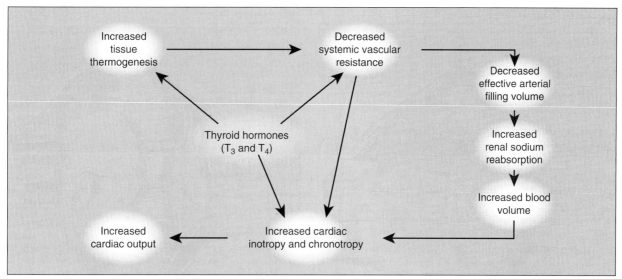

FIGURE 4-6 Effects of thyroid hormone on cardiovascular dynamics. The diagram shows the way that thyroid hormones increase cardiac output by affecting tissue oxygen consumption, vascular resistance, blood volume, cardiac contractility, and heart rate. T_3, Triiodothyronine; T_4, thyroxine. (Adapted from Klein I, Ojamaa K: Thyroid hormone and the cardiovascular system, *N Engl J Med* 344[7]:501-509, 2001.)

BOX 4-2 Regulation of Genes Coding for Cardiac Proteins by Thyroid Hormone

Positive Regulation
α-Myosin heavy chain
Sarcoplasmic reticulum Ca^{2+}-ATPase
β_1-Adrenergic receptors
Guanine-nucleotide-regulatory proteins
Na^+/K^+-ATPase
Voltage-gated potassium channels (Kv1.5, Kv4.2, Kv4.3)

Negative Regulation
β-Myosin heavy chain
Phospholamban
Adenylyl cyclase types V and VI
Triiodothyronine (T_3) nuclear receptor $\alpha1$
Na^+/Ca^{2+} exchanger

From Klein I, Ojamaa K: Thyroid hormone and the cardiovascular system, *N Eng J Med* 344(7):504, 2001.
ATPase, Adenosine triphosphatase.

Some cats with hyperthyroidism develop secondary hypertrophic cardiomyopathy, which may result in heart failure. In a study of 103 hyperthyroid cats, the most common echocardiographic findings were ventricular or interventricular hypertrophy; only four cats had subnormal cardiac performance and ventricular dilatation, and all of these cats had clinical and radiographic evidence of congestive heart failure (Bond et al, 1988). Severe heart failure appears to be more common among hyperthyroid cats with the dilated form of cardiomyopathy (Jacobs et al, 1986; Jacobs and Panciera, 1992). Dilated cardiomyopathy in hyperthyroid cats may be due to concurrent primary heart disease rather than secondary to hyperthyroidism. Approximately 50% of hyperthyroid cats have detectable concentrations of serum troponin I, which is a sensitive and specific marker of myocardial cellular damage (Connolly et al, 2005); this would be expected in a systemic disease that increases myocardial oxygen demand and predisposes

the myocardium to cellular hypoxia. The serum troponin concentrations normalize in most cats after effective treatment of hyperthyroidism.

Ventroflexion of the Head

Early reports of hyperthyroid cats included occasional cats exhibiting pronounced ventroflexion of the head (see Fig. 4-4, *D*). The head of an affected cat could be lifted without difficulty, but the cat immediately resumed the abnormal posture when released. Clinical signs usually seen in association with cervical ventroflexion were anorexia, mild ataxia, and mydriasis. There have been no published reports of this syndrome since 1994 (Nemzek et al, 1994). It has been hypothesized that either thiamine deficiency or hypokalemia could be the cause of cervical ventroflexion; but because it is now so rare, there have been no further investigations of the pathogenesis. Potassium depletion may occur in hyperthyroidism secondary to vomiting, diarrhea, anorexia, or excess urine loss. Vitamin deficiencies (e.g., thiamine and cobalamine deficiency) occur in hyperthyroidism secondary to polyuria, malabsorption, diarrhea, vomiting, and anorexia.

Ocular Lesions

Systolic hypertension is documented in approximately 10% to 15% of hyperthyroid cats at the time of diagnosis (Williams et al, 2010). Despite this, retinopathy secondary to hypertension is uncommonly detected in feline hyperthyroidism. In a study of 100 hyperthyroid cats and 30 control cats, there were no ophthalmologic abnormalities that were more commonly identified in hyperthyroid cats than in euthyroid cats (van der Woerdt and Peterson, 2000). Two hyperthyroid cats had retinal changes consistent with hypertensive retinopathy, including retinal hemorrhage and focal retinal detachment with subretinal effusion. The authors concluded that ocular abnormalities are uncommon in hyperthyroid cats (see also Blood Pressure and Hypertension).

Thyroid Storm

Thyroid storm is the term used in humans to describe an acute exacerbation of clinical signs of thyrotoxicosis in conjunction with varying degrees of organ decompensation. The cause is believed to be an increased cellular response to thyroid hormone in conjunction with increased or abrupt availability of free thyroid hormones. Thyroid storm is usually precipitated by a superimposed insult, such as infection, thyroid surgery, other nonthyroidal illness, or withdrawal of anti-thyroid drugs (Chiha et al, 2013). The diagnosis is based on documentation of four major clinical signs: fever, central nervous system (CNS) manifestations, gastrointestinal or hepatic dysfunction, and cardiovascular effects, such as tachycardia, atrial fibrillation, and congestive heart failure. Although cats with hyperthyroidism may have an acute exacerbation of clinical signs either due to complications of thyrotoxicosis (e.g., congestive heart failure, hypertension) or presence of concurrent nonthyroidal illness, thyroid storm as defined in humans has yet to be described (Ward, 2007; Tolbert, 2010).

IN-HOSPITAL DIAGNOSTIC EVALUATION

Background

Cats with hyperthyroidism are usually geriatric, and therefore abnormalities identified on the diagnostic evaluation may be due either to thyrotoxicosis or other underlying concurrent disease. It can sometimes be difficult to distinguish which abnormalities are due to hyperthyroidism and which are due to other concurrent illness. In addition, hyperthyroidism increases the metabolic rate and GFR and can mask underlying chronic kidney disease (CKD). The goals of the diagnostic evaluation in a cat with suspected hyperthyroidism are to confirm the diagnosis, identify complications of hyperthyroidism (e.g., hypertension and heart failure that require either further evaluation or specific treatment), and evaluate for the presence of other disorders that require treatment or whose presence may influence the choice of treatment for hyperthyroidism. Minimum diagnostic testing should include a complete blood count (CBC), serum biochemistry profile, urinalysis, serum T_4 concentration, thoracic radiography, and measurement of indirect blood pressure. Electrocardiography and echocardiography are indicated if clinically significant heart disease is suspected. Further diagnostic testing may be necessary in cats in which the diagnosis of hyperthyroidism cannot be confirmed by measurement of serum T_4 concentration alone, and in those cats in which the initial evaluation reveals abnormalities that cannot be explained by hyperthyroidism alone.

Complete Blood Count

Erythron

Approximately 40% to 50% of hyperthyroid cats have a mild elevation in the packed cell volume (PCV) (Broussard et al, 1995). The increase in the red blood cell count may be directly related to thyrotoxicosis, because thyroid hormone stimulates secretion of erythropoietin (Klein and Ojamaa, 2001). Additionally, 20% of hyperthyroid cats have macrocytosis (Broussard et al, 1995). Heinz bodies are a more common finding on evaluation of the blood film in hyperthyroid cats than in control cats. Although cats with Heinz bodies tend to have a lower hematocrit than those without Heinz bodies, anemia is a rare finding in hyperthyroid cats (Christopher, 1989). Depletion of antioxidants and excessive fat and protein catabolism has been proposed as the reason for

Heinz body formation in hyperthyroid cats (Christopher, 1989; Branter et al, 2012).

Leukon

Hyperthyroid cats usually have a normal leukogram or may have nonspecific changes, such as a stress response characterized by leukocytosis, neutrophilia, lymphopenia, and eosinopenia.

Platelets

Hyperthyroid cats have been demonstrated to have larger platelets than normal control cats, but platelet counts were similar (Sullivan et al, 1993).

Serum Chemistry Profile

Liver Enzyme Activities

Increased liver enzymes are among the most frequently observed screening test alterations seen in hyperthyroid cats (Table 4-4). More than 75% of hyperthyroid cats have abnormalities in both serum alanine aminotransferase (ALT) and serum alkaline phosphatase (ALP) activities, and more than 90% show increases of at least one of these enzymes. The increases are usually only mild to moderate (less than 500 IU/L), although higher values are noted occasionally. The influence of underlying concurrent hepatic disease should be considered in hyperthyroid cats with more markedly increased liver enzyme activities (more than 500 IU/L), although not all hyperthyroid cats with higher increases in ALT have concurrent hepatic dysfunction. Hepatic hypoxia is thought to be the major cause of abnormalities in

TABLE 4-4	LABORATORY ABNORMALITIES ON ROUTINE TESTING OF HYPERTHYROID CATS
TEST	**PERCENTAGE OF CATS**
Complete Blood Count	
Erythrocytosis	39
Increase in MCV	27
Lymphopenia	22
Leukocytosis	19
Eosinopenia	13
Serum Chemistry Profile	
Increased ALT	85
Increased serum ALP	62
Azotemia (increased BUN)	26
Increased creatinine	23
Hyperphosphatemia	18
Electrolyte abnormalities	11
Hyperglycemia	5
Hyperbilirubinemia	3
Urinalysis	
Specific gravity > 1.035	63
Specific gravity < 1.015	4
Glucosuria	4
Inflammation/infection	2

ALP, Alkaline phosphatase; *ALT*, alanine aminotransferase; *BUN*, blood urea nitrogen; *MCV*, mean cell volume.

ALT but increased hepatic enzyme activity may also be due in part to malnutrition, congestive heart failure, infection, and direct toxic effects of thyroid hormones on the liver. Separation of the different isoenzymes of serum ALP has demonstrated that 50% to 80% of the increased serum ALP in hyperthyroid cats is the bone isoenzyme of serum ALP, presumably because of increased bone turnover (Archer and Taylor, 1996; Foster and Thoday, 2000). Increased AST and creatine kinase (CK) have also been reported in some hyperthyroid cats (Archer and Taylor, 1996). Increases in gamma glutamyl transferase (GGT) have not been reported in hyperthyroid cats (Archer and Taylor, 1996; Berent et al, 2007).

Liver Dysfunction

In addition to increased hepatic enzymes, cats with hyperthyroidism have significantly higher fasting serum ammonia concentrations than euthyroid cats; these values return to normal with effective treatment of the hyperthyroidism (Berent et al, 2007). The reason for increased ammonia concentrations is unknown, but it may be secondary to accelerated protein catabolism and deamination due to the increased metabolic rate. Pre and post prandial bile acid concentrations and results of hepatic ultrasonography were normal in all hyperthyroid cats with increased ammonia concentrations. Four of the 19 hyperthyroid cats evaluated had ALT concentrations greater than 500 I/L; however, the ALT returned to normal in all cats after treatment. This implies that there were no functional or clinically relevant hepatic changes in these hyperthyroid cats and that a high ALT with no other indication of hepatic dysfunction should not necessarily prompt further hepatic evaluation in a cat whose clinical signs are consistent with hyperthyroidism. Other indicators of hepatic dysfunction may include hypoglycemia, hypocholesterolemia, hypoalbuminemia, and decreased blood urea nitrogen (BUN). In the cats studied by Berent et al., (2007), none of the hyperthyroid cats were hypoglycemic or hypocholesterolemic, although the hyperthyroid cats had lower concentrations of glucose and cholesterol than age matched control cats. These changes also normalized after treatment of the hyperthyroidism. Serum albumin and BUN concentrations did not differ between hyperthyroid cats and age matched control cats and did not change after treatment. The differences likely relate to the increased metabolic rate of hyperthyroid cats, but the changes do not appear to be clinically relevant or supportive of hepatic dysfunction. There have been no published studies evaluating hepatic histopathology in cats with hyperthyroidism. One author reported that liver biopsies typically reveal increased pigment within hepatocytes, aggregates of mixed inflammatory cells in the portal regions, and focal areas of fatty degeneration; and some cats have mild hepatic necrosis (Feldman and Nelson, 2004). In severe cases of thyrotoxicosis, it was reported that centrilobular fatty infiltration may occur together with patchy portal fibrosis, lymphocytic infiltration, and proliferation of bile ducts (Feldman and Nelson, 2004). Liver enzyme activities, regardless of their origin, usually return to normal with successful management of the hyperthyroidism (Berent et al, 2007).

Altered Bone Metabolism

People with hyperthyroidism have decreased bone mineral density and increased concentrations of bone resorption markers and bone formation markers such as ALP and osteocalcin (Williams, 2013). There is believed to be an increased risk of fracture in people with either overt or subclinical hyperthyroidism, but studies are confounded by multiple other factors that influence fracture risk, such as age, sex, use of hormone therapy, and other factors. Increased bone metabolism is attributed to the direct effects of thyroid hormones on osteoclasts and osteoblasts.

Hyperthyroid cats also have evidence of increased bone turnover as evidenced by increased activity of the bone isoenzyme of serum ALP and osteocalcin concentrations (Archer and Taylor, 1996; Foster and Thoday, 2000). In a study of 36 hyperthyroid cats, 44% of cats had increased osteocalcin concentrations. There were no correlations between magnitude of serum ALP bone isoenzyme, osteocalcin, and serum thyroxine concentrations (Archer and Taylor, 1996). Derangements in calcium homeostasis also occur in hyperthyroid cats. Hyperthyroid cats have been reported to have increased serum phosphate concentrations and decreased ionized calcium concentrations (Archer and Taylor, 1996; Williams et al, 2012; Barber and Elliott, 1996). The mechanism for ionized hypocalcemia in hyperthyroid cats is unknown but does not appear to be due to concurrent CKD or reduced plasma calcitriol concentrations (Williams et al, 2013). In a study of 30 cats with untreated hyperthyroidism, hyperthyroid cats had lower blood ionized calcium concentrations and higher phosphate concentrations than a group of age matched controls; 43% of the cats were hyperphosphatemic, and 27% of the cats had an ionized calcium concentration below the reference range (Barber and Elliott, 1996). Hyperparathyroidism was documented in 77% of the cats with parathyroid hormone (PTH) concentrations reaching up to 19 times the upper limit of the reference range. Other studies also suggest that 60% to 80% of hyperthyroid cats have increased serum concentrations of PTH (Williams et al, 2012; Barber and Elliott, 1996). This finding is very different from thyrotoxic human patients that typically have hypoparathyroidism. The changes usually normalize after treatment of hyperthyroidism (Williams et al, 2012), although some cats with underlying CKD have persistent increases in PTH presumably due to secondary renal hyperparathyroidism. Although indications of increased bone turnover have been documented in hyperthyroid cats, clinical consequences (e.g., increased fracture risk) are very rare.

Blood Glucose

Cats have a remarkable ability to increase their blood glucose concentrations in response to acute stress. Acutely stressed cats can have blood glucose concentrations as high as 300 mg/dL (17 mmol/l) (Rand et al, 2002). This hyperglycemia is believed to result from an acute release of epinephrine. Blood glucose concentrations may become even higher (400 to 500 mg/dL, 22-28 mmol/L) due to the stress of chronic illness, although it is difficult to assess the contribution of concurrent beta cell dysfunction in clinically ill cats. Surprisingly the majority of hyperthyroid cats have normal blood glucose concentrations, and as a group, hyperthyroid cats have lower blood glucose concentrations than age matched controls.

In humans, the increased energy expenditure of thyrotoxicosis is compounded by the inefficient maintenance of basic physiologic functions. To compensate for increased energy expenditure, increases in food consumption, utilization of stored energy, and enhanced oxygen expenditure alter the metabolism of carbohydrate, lipid, and protein. Intestinal absorption of glucose and the rate of glucose production from glycogen, lactate, glycerol, and amino acids are increased. Hepatic glycogen stores are decreased, owing to increased glucose utilization by muscle and adipose tissue. It is likely that multiple factors influence the blood glucose concentration in hyperthyroid cats with factors such as depletion of hepatic glycogen stores tending to decrease the blood sugar, whereas stress and peripheral insulin resistance tend to increase the blood glucose. Diabetes mellitus and hyperthyroidism are both common diseases of the geriatric cat and occasionally can occur together. This scenario should be considered in hyperthyroid cats with persistent mild hyperglycemia (more than 200 mg/dL; 11 mmol/l) (Hoenig and Ferguson, 1989).

Cholesterol

Serum cholesterol concentration is usually within the reference range in hyperthyroid cats. The synthesis and especially clearance of cholesterol and triglycerides are increased in hyperthyroidism, resulting in modest reductions in both the serum cholesterol and triglyceride concentrations, although the cholesterol concentrations do not typically decrease below the reference range. Lipolysis is also accelerated, resulting in increased plasma free fatty acid concentrations.

Blood Urea Nitrogen and Creatinine

CKD is estimated to be present in 15% of cats older than 15 years of age and is therefore a common concurrent disorder in hyperthyroid cats. Recent studies suggest that approximately 10% of hyperthyroid cats are azotemic at the time of diagnosis of hyperthyroidism based on measurement of a serum creatinine above the laboratory reference range (Williams et al, 2010). Increased serum BUN is found in a slightly larger number (10% to 20%) of hyperthyroid cats. It is important to recognize, however, that merely including the proportion of cats with azotemia underestimates the prevalence of CKD in hyperthyroid cats because of physiologic changes in hyperthyroidism that lead to an increased GFR. Untreated hyperthyroid cats have a higher GFR, as measured by iohexol clearance or scintigraphy, than the same cats after reestablishment of the euthyroid state (Adams et al, 1997; Graves et al, 1994; DiBartola et al, 1996; van Hoek et al, 2008a). Hyperthyroidism increases renal blood flow due to increased cardiac output and intra-renal vasodilation. Changes in afferent and efferent arteriolar resistance increases the glomerular transcapillary hydraulic pressure, which increases GFR. Activation of the RAAS possibly via changes in β-adrenergic activity has been implicated as a mechanism for this alteration in renal hemodynamics. Despite the increase in renal perfusion pressure in hyperthyroidism, resorption of sodium and chloride from the proximal tubule and loop of Henle is increased rather than decreased due to impairment of the pressure-diuresis-natriuresis response (Syme, 2007), which may explain how plasma volume can increase and sodium excretion can decrease. In addition to the renal hemodynamic changes in hyperthyroidism, weight loss and muscle atrophy further decrease serum creatinine concentrations in hyperthyroid cats. For these reasons, it may be difficult or impossible to diagnose CKD in cats with concurrent hyperthyroidism.

The increased GFR normalizes after treatment of hyperthyroidism, so from 15% to 49% of cats that are non-azotemic at the time of diagnosis of hyperthyroidism become azotemic after treatment. The variability in the percentage of cats becoming azotemic likely reflects variability in adequacy of control of hyperthyroidism (Williams et al, 2010b). Numerous studies have failed to identify pretreatment parameters other than measurement of GFR that allow prediction of which cats will have clinically significant worsening of azotemia after treatment. The fact that cats with hyperthyroidism and CKD may have similar clinical signs (e.g., polyuria, polydipsia, and weight loss) and that the two diseases commonly occur together compounds the problem of establishing the severity of CKD in hyperthyroid cats. Whether the long-term effects of hyperthyroidism actually contribute to progression of renal disease in cats is still unclear. Glomerular hypertension, proteinuria, and hyperparathyroidism have all been proposed as mechanisms for

intrinsic progression of CKD in the cat. Further epidemiological studies are required to determine whether CKD is more common in hyperthyroid cats than in the population at large.

Urinalysis

Urine abnormalities that may be present in hyperthyroid cats include a decreased USG, proteinuria, evidence of urinary tract infection, and ketonuria. As discussed earlier, concurrent CKD is common in hyperthyroid cats and may result in a decreased USG. Polyuria and polydipsia may also occur in hyperthyroid cats without CKD by mechanisms that are poorly understood. Mechanisms that have been proposed include disturbances in the vasopressin axis and primary polydipsia possibly due to heat intolerance (Feldman and Nelson, 2004). In one study of 21 hyperthyroid cats treated with radioactive iodine, USG did not change after treatment in most cats (van Hoek et al, 2009a) suggesting that CKD was the most common reason for a low USG. Proteinuria is detected in 75% to 80% of hyperthyroid cats and usually resolves following treatment (Berent et al, 2007; van Hoek et al, 2009a; Williams et al, 2010b). Studies suggest that the proteinuria associated with hyperthyroidism is primarily due to increased excretion of proteins other than albumin (Williams et al, 2010b). Reasons for proteinuria in hyperthyroid cats could include glomerular hypertension and hyperfiltration, changes in tubular protein handling, and changes in the structure of the glomerular barrier (van Hoek et al, 2009a). Although proteinuria usually resolves after treatment of hyperthyroidism, its presence prior to treatment is correlated with reduced survival but not development of azotemia (Williams et al, 2010b). Urinary tract infection is relatively common in cats with hyperthyroidism. In one study urine culture was positive in 11 of 90 (12%) of hyperthyroid cats, and 17 of 77 (22%) cats with CKD. Only two of the hyperthyroid cats had clinical signs of lower urinary tract disease (Mayer-Roenne et al, 2007). Interestingly in one study, trace ketonuria was detected in 9 of 19 hyperthyroid cats (Berent et al, 2007). This had not been previously reported in hyperthyroid cats but has been described in humans with hyperthyroidism. Potential reasons for ketonuria in hyperthyroidism include β-adrenergic induced lipolysis, which results in increased fatty acid delivery to the liver, or increased hepatic ketogenesis due to carnitine deficiency (Wood and Kinlaw, 2004). A number of recent studies have investigated urinary markers of renal tubular injury such as urinary retinol binding protein and N-acetyl-β–D-glucosaminidase that might be useful in prediction of azotemia after treatment of hyperthyroid cats. Although these markers are present in the urine of hyperthyroid cats, they have not proved useful in predicting which cats are likely to become azotemic after treatment (Lapointe et al, 2008; van Hoek et al, 2009b).

Plasma Cortisol/Urine Cortisol:Creatinine Ratio

Adrenocortical hyperplasia is an uncommon finding in cats, but it was found in one-third of hyperthyroid cats in one study (Liu et al, 1984). Increased cortisol secretion due to increased pituitary secretion of adrenocorticotropic hormone (ACTH) also occurs in hyperthyroid humans, although it does not result in hypercortisolemia, because hyperthyroidism in humans is also associated with increased metabolic clearance of cortisol. In a study of 17 hyperthyroid cats, 18 healthy geriatric cats, and 18 cats with concurrent nonthyroidal illness, basal and ACTH stimulated cortisol concentrations were higher in hyperthyroid cats than in control cats, but the urinary cortisol creatinine ratio (UCCR) and adrenal size as measured by ultrasound were not different between the groups (Ramspott et al, 2012).

Other studies have documented mild adrenomegaly in hyperthyroid cats compared with healthy euthyroid cats, and higher UCCR in hyperthyroid cats compared to healthy cats (de Lange et al, 2004; Combes et al, 2012). Taken together, these studies suggest that there is some degree of hypercortisolemia and adrenal gland hyperplasia in hyperthyroid cats. These findings are important because although hyperadrenocorticism is rare in cats, there are some similarities between the clinical signs of the two diseases.

Serum Fructosamine

Fructosamine is produced by an irreversible reaction between glucose and plasma proteins. Serum fructosamine concentrations in cats are thought to reflect the mean blood glucose concentration during the preceding 1 to 2 weeks (Link and Rand, 2008). However, fructosamine concentrations are also affected by the concentration and metabolism of serum proteins, and hyperthyroidism increases protein metabolism. Serum fructosamine concentrations in hyperthyroid cats have been documented to be significantly lower than in healthy control cats (Reusch and Tomsa, 1999). Fifty percent of hyperthyroid cats had serum fructosamine concentrations less than the reference range. Serum fructosamine concentrations in hyperthyroid, normoproteinemic cats did not differ from values in hypoproteinemic cats. During treatment for hyperthyroidism, an increase in serum fructosamine concentration was documented. It was concluded that the concentration of serum fructosamine in hyperthyroid cats may be low because of accelerated protein turnover—independent of blood glucose concentration. For these reasons, the serum fructosamine concentration should not be considered a reliable monitoring tool in hyperthyroid cats with concurrent diabetes mellitus. Additionally, serum fructosamine concentrations should not be considered reliable for differentiating between diabetes mellitus and stress-related hyperglycemia in hyperthyroid cats (Reusch and Tomsa, 1999).

Blood Pressure and Hypertension

Although in earlier studies systolic hypertension was reported to be common in hyperthyroid cats (Kobayashi et al, 1990), more recent studies suggest that only 10% to 20% of hyperthyroid cats have hypertension diagnosed at the time of diagnosis of hyperthyroidism; end-organ damage due to hypertension (e.g., retinal detachment) appears to be extremely uncommon (van der Woerdt and Peterson, 2000; Syme, 2007; Williams et al, 2010). Reasons for the lower prevalence of hypertension in more recent studies include earlier diagnosis of feline hyperthyroidism, more conservative cut-offs for diagnosis of hypertension (blood pressure of more than170 mm Hg on a least two occasions, or more than170 mmHg and evidence of hypertensive retinopathy), and increased recognition of the white coat effect (Belew et al, 1999; see also Ocular Lesions). The low prevalence of hypertension is similar to findings in humans and is likely because the decrease in systemic vascular resistance results in a decrease in diastolic resistance, and the increase in cardiac output results in only modest increases in systolic blood pressure (Syme, 2007). Interestingly a recent report found that approximately 20% to 25% of cats that were normotensive prior to treatment of hyperthyroidism became hypertensive several months (median 5 months) after treatment of hyperthyroidism (Syme and Elliott, 2003). Whether this is due to a decline in renal function after treatment or other undetermined mechanism is unclear. Posttreatment hypertension was not limited to cats that became azotemic after therapy, and no differences were detected between cats that developed hypertension and those that did not in regard to RAAS activation (Syme, 2007).

Radiography

Thoracic radiographs should ideally be performed as part of the diagnostic evaluation of all hyperthyroid cats to assess for evidence of heart disease or concurrent illness. Even if there are no clinical signs of heart disease, thoracic radiographs allow detection of occult concurrent illness, such as pulmonary or cranial thoracic neoplasia. Abnormalities on physical examination that increase the importance of obtaining thoracic radiographs include respiratory distress, tachypnea or panting, muffled heart sounds, tachycardia, arrhythmias, or a heart murmur. The most common findings on thoracic radiographs include mild cardiomegaly. Signs of congestive heart failure such as pulmonary edema, enlarged pulmonary vessels, and pleural effusion are uncommon in hyperthyroid cats (Jacobs et al, 1986). In a study reporting radiographic abnormalities in hyperthyroid cats diagnosed from 1992 to 1993, 8% of cats had radiographic evidence of congestive heart failure compared to 20% in cats evaluated from 1979 to 1982 (Fox et al, 1999). The prevalence of congestive heart failure in hyperthyroid cats is now likely even lower than it was in the 1990s.

Electrocardiography

Electrocardiographic changes are common in hyperthyroid cats but rarely require specific treatment. The electrocardiographic changes seen in cats with thyrotoxicosis are listed in Table 4-5 and are illustrated in Figs. 4-7 to 4-9. Tachycardia (heart rate above 240/min) and an increased R-wave amplitude in lead II (greater than 1.0 mv) are the abnormalities most frequently seen, although each is now detected less commonly than in the 1980s (Broussard et al, 1995). Other less common arrhythmias include atrial extrasystoles, atrial tachycardia, ventricular extrasystoles, first degree atrioventricular block, left anterior fascicular block, right bundle branch block, and left bundle branch block. In a study of hyperthyroid cats evaluated in 1993, evidence of right or left atrial enlargement was present on the electrocardiogram (ECG) in 42% of cats (Fox et al, 1999). Most electrocardiographic abnormalities resolve with successful management of the thyrotoxicosis.

TABLE 4-5	**PRETREATMENT ELECTROCARDIOGRAM FINDINGS IN 131 CATS WITH HYPERTHYROIDISM PRESENTING IN 1992-1993**
FINDING	**PERCENTAGE OF CATS**
Sinus tachycardia	66
Increased R-wave amplitude (lead II)	29
Left anterior fascicular block	8
Atrial asystoles	7
Ventricular asystoles	2
First degree atrioventricular block	2
Right bundle branch block	2
Atrial tachycardia	1

Data modified from Fox PR, et al.: Electrocardiographic and radiographic changes in cats with hyperthyroidism: comparison of populations evaluated during 1992-1993 vs. 1979-1982, *J Am Anim Hosp Assoc* 35(1):27-31, 1999.

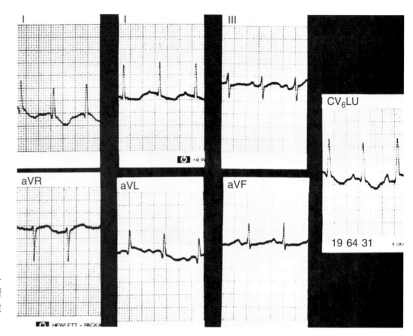

FIGURE 4-7 Electrocardiogram (ECG) from a thyrotoxic cat showing R waves of increased amplitude in all leads and deviation of the mean electrical axis to 30 degrees, suggestive of left heart enlargement.

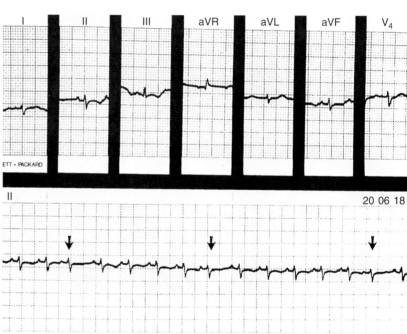

FIGURE 4-8 Electrocardiogram (ECG) from a thyrotoxic cat showing normal P-QRS-T complex amplitudes. However, three atrial premature contractions can be seen in the rhythm strip *(arrows)*, and an abnormal heart rate of 300 beats per minute is present.

Echocardiography

Echocardiographic abnormalities frequently identified in hyperthyroid cats include left ventricular caudal wall hypertrophy and hypertrophy of the interventricular septum; these changes are largely reversible after treatment of the hyperthyroidism state (Bond et al, 1988). Hyperthyroid cats also may have increased left atrial diameter, aortic end-diastolic diameter, and left atrial to aortic root ratio. Myocardial hypercontractility is also common as evidenced by increased percentage of shortening of the minor axis and velocity of circumferential shortening (Bond et al, 1988). Less commonly, a dilated form of cardiomyopathy is observed. Echocardiographic abnormalities in these cats include subnormal myocardial contractility and marked ventricular dilation. These cats usually have radiographic evidence of congestive heart failure (Jacobs et al, 1986; Bond et al, 1988).

The radiographic, electrocardiographic, and echocardiographic changes observed in feline hyperthyroidism occur due to the marked cardiovascular effects of thyroid hormone on the heart. Increased cardiac output, decreased systemic vascular resistance, direct positive chronotropic and inotropic stimulation, β-adrenergic stimulation, and underlying cardiomyopathy all may contribute to the abnormalities detected. In a study of 91 cats that were studied before and 2 to 3 months after treatment with radioiodine, 37% of cats had one or more echocardiographic variables outside the reference range prior to treatment. The most common findings were primarily increases in interventricular septal and left ventricular wall thickness; the findings were considered clinically relevant in less than 10% of cats (Table 4-6) (Weichselbaum et al, 2005). Interestingly 32% of the cats studied had one or more echocardiographic abnormalities present following treatment; almost half of these cats had been normal before

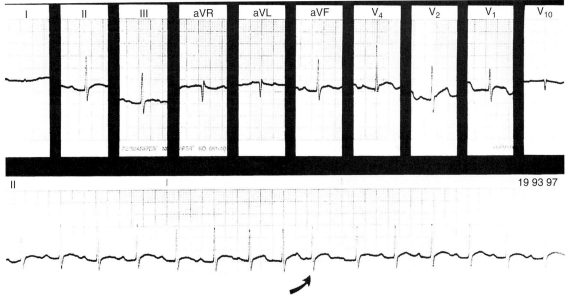

FIGURE 4-9 Electrocardiogram (ECG) from a thyrotoxic cat showing both increased amplitude in the R waves and an atrial premature contraction *(arrow)*.

TABLE 4-6 NORMAL FELINE REFERENCE, PRE-RADIOIODINE, AND POST-RADIOIODINE M-MODE ECHOCARDIOGRAPHIC VALUES FOR 91 HYPERTHYROID CATS

	Feline Normal Reference Values (2.7 to 8.2 kg*)			Feline Pre- and Post-Radioiodine Treatment Values (2.2 to 8.9 kg*)					
	Observed Range				Observed Range			Observed Range	
ECHOCARDIOGRAPH VARIABLE (UNIT)	MEAN ± SD	MINIMUM	MAXIMUM	PRERADIOIODINE MEAN ± SD	MINIMUM	MAXIMUM	POSTRADIOIODINE MEAN ± SD	MINIMUM	MAXIMUM
Number of cats	76-79			91			91		
IVSED (cm)	0.42 ± 0.07	0.30	0.60	0.44 ± 0.07	0.27	0.72	0.43 ± 0.13	0.27	0.55
IVSES (cm)	0.67 ± 0.12	0.40	0.90	0.78 ± 0.12	0.41	1.14	0.72 ± 0.11	0.34	1.08
LVEDD (cm)	1.50 ± 0.20	1.08	2.14	1.63 ± 0.22	0.64	2.09	1.64 ± 0.22	1.17	2.22
LVESD (cm)	0.72 ± 0.15	0.40	1.12	0.80 ± 0.15	0.42	1.13	0.87 ± 0.19	0.55	1.73
LVWED (cm)	0.41 ± 0.07	0.25	0.60	0.47 ± 0.10	0.28	0.89	0.42 ± 0.56	0.29	0.59
LVWES (cm)	0.68 ± 0.11	0.43	0.98	0.78 ± 0.10	0.49	1.02	0.69 ± 0.80	0.53	0.90
A_0 (cm)	0.95 ± 0.14	0.60	1.21	0.99 ± 0.11	0.72	1.21	1.02 ± 0.13	0.72	1.36
LA (cm)	1.17 ± 0.17	0.70	1.70						
LA Max (cm)				1.34 ± 0.15	0.99	1.82	1.32 ± 0.18	0.99	2.14
FS (%)	52.1 ± 7.11	40.00	66.70	50.60 ± 7.29	34.00	66.00	46.60 ± 7.24	21.00	62.90

From Weichselbaum RC, et al.: Relationship between selected echocardiographic variables before and after radioiodine treatment in 91 hyperthyroid cats, *Vet Radiol Ultrasound* 46(6):506-513, 2005.

A_0, Aortic root maximum dimension (from M-mode); *FS*, LV fractional shortening, i.e.,¼((LVEDDLVESD)/LVEDD) 100); *IVSED*, interventricular septum at end-diastole (from M-mode); *IVSES*, interventricular septum at end-systole (from M-mode); *LA*, left atrium dimension (from M-mode); *LA Max*, left atrium maximum dimension (from two-dimensional long-axis); *LVEDD*, left ventricular end-diastolic dimension (from M-mode); *LVESD*, left ventricular end-systolic dimension (from M-mode); *LVWED*, left ventricular posterior wall thickness at end-diastole (from M-mode); *LVWES*, left ventricular posterior wall thickness at end-systole (from M-mode).
*Body weight range.

treatment. The conclusions of the authors were that changes in echocardiographic variables in hyperthyroid cats are less common than previously reported, presumably due to earlier diagnosis. The emergence of new abnormalities after treatment of hyperthyroidism may reflect underlying cardiac disease unrelated to hyperthyroidism, permanent hyperthyroidism related damage, or incomplete recovery from the effects of hyperthyroidism or possibly the effects of iatrogenic hypothyroidism. These findings underscore the complexity of the interactions between hyperthyroidism and the heart. There was no correlation between the total T_4 concentration and the presence of clinically relevant echocardiographic changes. The heart rate of hyperthyroid cats rather than presence of echocardiographic changes may be a more useful parameter for determining which cats require medical management with cardiac drugs during and after treatment of hyperthyroidism (Weichselbaum et al, 2005).

 ## DIFFERENTIAL DIAGNOSIS

Because hyperthyroidism is a disease of geriatric cats and because the clinical signs of hyperthyroidism often mimic those of other disorders, the differential diagnosis for hyperthyroidism is extensive (Table 4-7). The most common disorders that should be considered in the differential diagnosis include CKD, gastrointestinal disorders, heart disease, and diabetes mellitus.

 ## SERUM THYROID HORMONE CONCENTRATIONS

For an overview of thyroid hormone physiology and the assays used for diagnosis of thyroid disorders in dogs and cats, see Chapter 3. Thyroid hormone measurements commonly used to confirm the diagnosis of feline hyperthyroidism include the serum total T_4 and fT_4 concentrations. Measurement of serum T_3 concentration is rarely useful for diagnosis of feline hyperthyroidism, and serum TSH concentrations have limited utility because of poor sensitivity of the current commercial assays for measurement of feline TSH.

Basal Total Serum Thyroxine Concentration

The initial screening test of choice for diagnosis of feline hyperthyroidism is the basal serum T_4 concentration. Reference range for

total T_4 is typically 1 to 4.5 µg/dL for healthy cats, although the reference ranges of individual laboratories vary. The total T_4 concentration has both high sensitivity and specificity for diagnosis of feline hyperthyroidism. In a study of 917 untreated hyperthyroid cats, 221 cats with nonthyroidal illness, and 172 normal cats, 91% of the hyperthyroid cats had high serum total T_4 concentrations, whereas none of the cats with nonthyroidal illness had high total T_4 concentrations, giving an assay sensitivity of 91% and assay specificity of 100% (Peterson et al, 2001; Fig. 4-10). Similar findings have been reported in other smaller studies. Commercial veterinary laboratories now include serum total T_4 concentrations as a component of most geriatric feline chemistry profiles, which has resulted in the diagnosis of feline hyperthyroidism being made much earlier in the disease process. This approach to screening is appropriate for diagnosis of feline hyperthyroidism because of the high specificity of total T_4 for diagnosis of hyperthyroidism; however the cautions that apply to evaluation of a low total T_4 concentration in the dog also apply to the cat because of the influence of nonthyroidal illness on the measured total T_4 concentration. Despite the high specificity of total T_4 concentration for diagnosis of feline hyperthyroidism, if the total T_4 is increased in a cat with no reported clinical signs of hyperthyroidism, it is important to rule out laboratory and other sample handling errors before confirming the clinical diagnosis; in most cats with

TABLE 4-7	DIFFERENTIAL DIAGNOSIS FOR HYPERTHYROIDISM IN CATS
DIFFERENTIAL DIAGNOSIS	**MAJOR CLINICAL AREAS OF OVERLAP WITH HYPERTHYROIDISM**
Nonthyroid endocrine disease	
Diabetes mellitus	PD, PU, polyphagia, weight loss
Hyperadrenocorticism (rare)	PD, PU, polyphagia, weight loss
Diabetes insipidus (rare)	PD, PU, mild weight loss
Acromegaly (uncommon)	PD, PU, polyphagia
Renal disease	PD, PU, anorexia, weight loss, elevated BUN
Heart disease and failure	
Hypertrophic cardiomyopathy	Respiratory distress, weight loss,
Congestive cardiomyopathy	tachycardia, murmur, arrhythmia:
Idiopathic arrhythmia	radiography, ECG, echocardiogram abnormalities are not specific for hyperthyroidism
Gastrointestinal disease	
Pancreatic exocrine insufficiency	Bulky, foul-smelling stool, weight loss, polyphagia
Diffuse gastrointestinal disorders	
Inflammatory	Diarrhea, vomiting, anorexia, chronic weight loss
Cancer (including lymphosarcoma)	
Hepatopathy	Elevated liver enzymes
Inflammatory	
Cancer	
Pulmonary disease	Respiratory distress, panting

BUN, Blood urea nitrogen; *ECG*, electrocardiogram; *PD*, polydipsia; *PU*, polyuria.

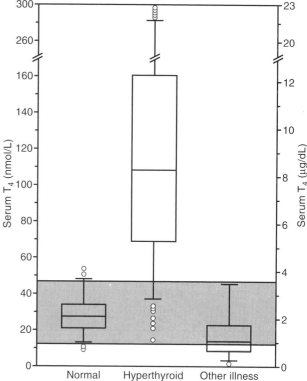

FIGURE 4-10 Box plots of serum total thyroxine (T_4) concentrations in 172 clinically normal cats, 917 cats with untreated hyperthyroidism, and 221 cats with nonthyroidal disease. The box represents the interquartile range (i.e., 25th to 75th percentile range, or the middle half of the data). The horizontal bar in the box represents the median value. For each box plot, the *T bars* represent the main body of data, which in most instances is equal to the range. Outlying data points are represented by *open circles*. The *shaded area* indicates the reference range for the serum T_4 concentration. (From Peterson ME, et al.: Measurement of serum concentrations of free thyroxine, total thyroxine, and total triiodothyronine in cats with hyperthyroidism and cats with nonthyroidal disease, *J Am Vet Med Assoc* 218[4]:529-536, 2001).

apparent asymptomatic hyperthyroidism, there are usually some subtle clinical signs detected once a more detailed history is collected and a physical examination is performed.

Although the total T_4 concentration is a relatively sensitive assay, in some cats with early hyperthyroidism and those with concurrent nonthyroidal illness, the initial measured total T_4 concentration may be within the reference range (usually within the upper 50% of the reference range).

Fluctuations in Serum Thyroxine Concentrations

In a study in which blood samples were collected from hyperthyroid cats hourly during the day and daily over a 15 day period, there were hourly and daily fluctuations in the measured serum total T_4 concentration that sometimes exceeded the expected coefficient of variation of the assay (Peterson et al, 1987), although another study showed less variability (Broome et al, 1988a). Despite fluctuations in total T_4, the measured total T_4 concentration in most hyperthyroid cats is usually persistently above the reference range (Fig. 4-11); however, in cats with only mild increases in the total T_4 concentration, the serum T_4 concentration may fluctuate in and out of the reference range. For this reason, in a cat that has appropriate clinical signs and physical examination findings, a diagnosis of hyperthyroidism should not be excluded on the basis of one "normal" total T_4 measurement (especially if there is a palpable thyroid gland).

Effect of Nonthyroidal Illness on Serum Total Thyroxine Concentrations

As in dogs, the presence of concurrent illness can influence the measured total T_4 concentration. In a study of 98 euthyroid cats with concurrent illness, 76 cats had values within the reference range, 21 cats had values below the reference range, and one cat had a very mild increase in serum total T_4 concentration (less than 3 SD from the reference mean) (Mooney et al, 1996a). In another study that included 221 euthyroid ill cats, none had an abnormally increased serum total T_4 concentration, whereas 38% of the cats had a low concentration (Peterson et al, 2001; see Fig. 4-10). These studies demonstrate that illness can lower serum T_4 concentrations in euthyroid cats with the severity of the decrease correlated with the severity of the disease (Fig. 4-12). In fact the total T_4 concentration is a good prognostic indicator in cats with nonthyroidal illness syndrome (NTIS); mortality increases as the

measured total T_4 decreases (Mooney et al, 1996a; Peterson et al, 2001). Diseases that are commonly associated with a decreased total T_4 concentration include diabetes mellitus, hepatopathy, CKD, gastrointestinal disease, and systemic neoplasia; however, severity of disease has more significant effect than does disease category (Peterson et al, 1990b; 2001). The presence of concurrent

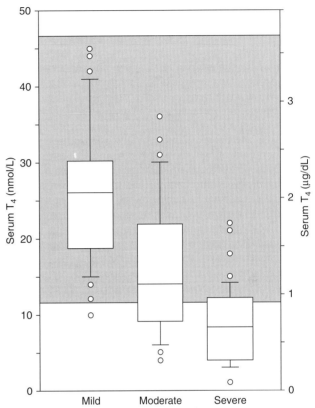

FIGURE 4-12 Box plots of serum total T_4 concentration in 221 cats with nonthyroidal illness grouped according to severity of illness. Of the 221 cats, 65 had mild disease, 83 had moderate disease, and 73 had severe disease (see Fig. 4-10 for key). (Peterson ME, et al.: Measurement of serum concentrations of free thyroxine, total thyroxine, and total triiodothyronine in cats with hyperthyroidism and cats with nonthyroidal disease, *J Am Vet Med Assoc* 218[4]:529-536, 2001.)

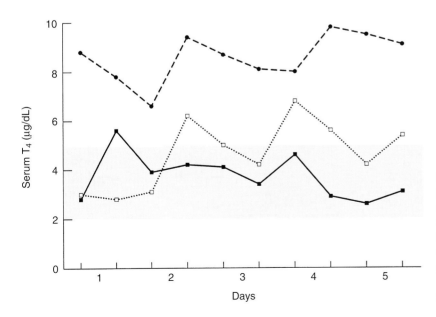

FIGURE 4-11 Serum thyroxine (T_4) concentrations fluctuate in normal and hyperthyroid cats. This figure demonstrates the amount of fluctuation typical of cats with hyperthyroidism. Cats with significantly increased serum T_4 concentrations usually have persistently abnormal results *(dashed line)*, whereas cats with "borderline" values have serum T_4 concentrations that can be "non-diagnostic" and occasionally abnormally increased *(dotted line)* or *(solid line)*. *Light gray area* is the reference range. T_4 laboratory reference range: 2.4 to 4.6 µg/dL.

illness also decreases the measured total T_4 in cats with hyperthyroidism. In one study of 110 cats with hyperthyroidism, systemic disease was diagnosed in 36% of the cats, and the serum total T_4 was significantly lower in the cats with nonthyroidal illness than in those without (McLoughlin et al, 1993). Fourteen of the hyperthyroid cats in this study had serum T_4 concentrations within or below the reference range with total T_4 concentrations ranging from 1.3 to 4.0 µg/dL. Ten of these 14 cats had evidence of nonthyroidal illness. For this reason, the history and physical examination findings are critical in determining whether the diagnosis of hyperthyroidism should be pursued further in a cat with a normal or subnormal total T_4 concentration. Although in most hyperthyroid cats with NTIS, the total T_4 is in the upper half of the reference range, as in the study discussed above with severe concurrent illness the T_4 can occasionally be below the reference range in a cat with confirmed hyperthyroidism (Tomsa et al, 2001). The effect of nonthyroidal illness on the total serum T_4 concentration in hyperthyroid cats was further evaluated in a study of cats with hyperthyroidism and concurrent CKD. In 16 cats with a normal serum total T_4 that were later confirmed to be hyperthyroid, the total T_4 ranged from 1.8 to 3.6 µg/dL whereas the total T_4 in cats with CKD alone ranged from 0.4 to 2.3 µg/dL. Most of the hyperthyroid cats with CKD had a total T_4 greater than 2.3 µg/dL, whereas all the cats with CKD alone had a total T_4 less than 2.3 µg/dL (Wakeling et al, 2008).

Other Factors Affecting Serum Total Thyroxine Concentrations

Factors other than NTIS that are believed to influence serum total T_4 concentrations in cats include age and concurrent medication administration. There is little published information on how thyroid hormone concentrations change with age in cats. In a group of more than 13,000 cats of varying ages that had total T_4 concentrations either within or below the reference range, there was no decline in total T_4 with age (Table 4-8). There is also limited information on the effect of drugs on the thyroid axis in cats. It is presumed that most of the medications that influence thyroid hormone concentrations in dogs have similar effects in cats, but the data is lacking to confirm this. Drugs that are known to influence thyroid hormone concentrations in cats include thioureylene drugs, iodinated contrast agents, and glucocorticoids.

APPROACH TO CATS WITH SUSPECTED HYPERTHYROIDISM THAT HAVE A THYROXINE CONCENTRATION WITHIN THE REFERENCE RANGE

If hyperthyroidism is suspected in a cat based on the history and physical examination, but the total T_4 concentration is within the upper half of the reference range, it is possible that the cat either has mild disease in which the total T_4 is fluctuating in and out of the reference range, or that the cat has hyperthyroidism and concurrent nonthyroidal illness (Fig. 4-13). The clinical approach to diagnosis depends upon the severity of clinical signs. If the signs are mild and early hyperthyroidism is considered likely, the most appropriate approach is to repeat the total T_4 at later date. Because thyroid hormone concentrations vary more over a period of days than over a period of several hours, repeat measurement of the serum T_4 concentration should be performed days to weeks after the initial result was obtained (Peterson et al, 1987). This also allows for disease progression such that there is less likely to be fluctuation into the reference range. If the cat has more severe clinical signs and it is therefore important that a diagnosis be made in a more timely fashion, further diagnostic testing such as measurement of serum fT_4 concentration, a T_3 suppression test, or thyroid scintigraphy should be considered. TRH stimulation tests have also been recommended in this situation; however, they are rarely performed because they are expensive and do not perform well in the presence of concurrent nonthyroidal illness (Tomsa et al, 2001). Administration of TRH also causes adverse clinical signs in cats. If concurrent NTIS is diagnosed and the disease is amenable to treatment, the most appropriate course of action is to reassess thyroid function after resolution of any nonthyroidal illness if immediate treatment of hyperthyroidism is not required.

76.61 PT	TABLE 4-8	**MEAN AND MEDIAN SERUM TOTAL THYROXINE CONCENTRATION OF SAMPLES SUBMITTED TO A REFERENCE LABORATORY FOR CATS OF DIFFERENT AGES**	
76.61 PT	**MEAN THYROXINE, µG/DL**	**MEDIAN THYROXINE, µG/DL**	**NUMBER OF PATIENTS**
0-2	1.93	2.0	414
3-5	2.01	2.1	733
6-8	2.02	2.1	2183
9-11	2.08	2.1	2480
12-14	2.12	2.1	3644
> 14	2.13	2.1	4477
All ages	2.08	2.1	13,931
Total T_4 reference range	0.8-4.7		

Data provided by IDEXX Laboratories, Inc.; From Scott-Moncrieff JC: Thyroid disorders in the geriatric veterinary patient, *Vet Clin North Am Small Anim Pract* 42(4):707-725, 2012. Patients with an age listed as 0 were excluded. Samples from cats in which the thyroxine (T_4) concentration was greater than 4.7 µg/dL were excluded from the analysis.

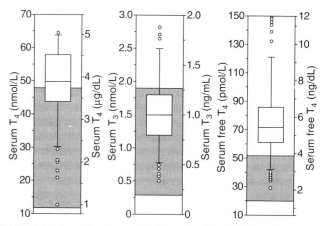

FIGURE 4-13 Box plots of serum total thyroxine (T_4), triiodothyronine (T_3), and free T_4 (fT_4) concentrations in 205 cats with mild hyperthyroidism (defined as total T_4 concentration less than 66 nmol/L; see Fig. 4-10 for key.) (From Peterson ME, et al.: Measurement of serum concentrations of free thyroxine, total thyroxine, and total triiodothyronine in cats with hyperthyroidism and cats with nonthyroidal disease, *J Am Vet Med Assoc* 218[4]:529-536, 2001.)

Basal Total Serum Triiodothyronine Concentrations

T_3 is the most biologically active thyroid hormone; however, the primary hormone secreted from the canine and feline thyroid gland is T_4, which is metabolized to T_3. Studies suggest that as many as 25% to 33% of cats with confirmed hyperthyroidism have serum T_3 concentrations within the reference range (Broussard et al, 1995; Peterson et al, 2001; Fig. 4-14). For this reason routine measurement of T_3 concentration for diagnosis of feline hyperthyroidism is not recommended and is rarely performed. A small percentage (< 5%) of human patients with hyperthyroidism have a normal total and fT_4 but an increased T_3 concentration (so-called T_3 thyrotoxicosis; Ladenson 2013). This syndrome has not been reported in cats, although as noted earlier T_4 thyrotoxicosis (high total T_4 and normal T_3) is relatively common in cats (Peterson et al, 2001).

Basal Free Thyroxine Concentration

The total T_4 concentration includes both the protein-bound fraction (more than 99% of the total) and the free, unbound fraction of thyroid hormone (< 1% of the total). Only the free fraction of thyroid hormone is available for entry into cells and is biologically active. Measured serum thyroid hormone concentrations can be altered by many illnesses that do not directly affect the thyroid gland (NTIS; see Effect of Nonthyroidal Illness on Serum Total Thyroxine Concentrations and also Chapter 3). Total T_4 concentrations can also be affected by alterations in metabolism, hormone binding to plasma carrier proteins, transport into cells, and

intracellular binding. For these reasons, measurement of serum free thyroid hormone concentrations (fT_4) should provide a more consistent assessment of thyroid gland function than measurement of the total thyroid hormone concentration.

Although the gold standard technique for measurement of fT_4 is equilibrium dialysis, this technique is expensive and time consuming and is usually only performed in research laboratories. In commercial laboratories feline serum fT_4 is measured by one of three methods: modified equilibrium dialysis (MED), analog radioimmunoassay (RIA), or analog chemiluminescent assay. In MED assays, a short dialysis step is used to separate free from protein-bound T_4 followed by radioimmunoassay for fT_4. MED techniques have been regarded as the gold standard technique for determining serum fT_4 concentrations in cats. In one study, the sensitivity and specificity of fT_4 concentration for diagnosis of hyperthyroidism in cats measured using the MED technique was 98.5% and 93%, respectively (Peterson et al, 2001; Fig. 4-15). It is important to note that in this study, although the sensitivity of fT_4 measurement was higher than measurement of total T_4, specificity was lower, because some euthyroid cats with nonthyroidal illness had a fT_4 that was above the reference range. Other studies have confirmed that approximately 6% to 12% of euthyroid cats with nonthyroidal illness may have fT_4 concentrations above the reference range using the MED assay. Other commercial assays have now been validated for measurement of fT_4 in cats (Table 4-9). Although the specificity and sensitivity of the assays vary, overall diagnostic accuracy is remarkably similar and all of the assays listed in the table appear to have acceptable performance for the

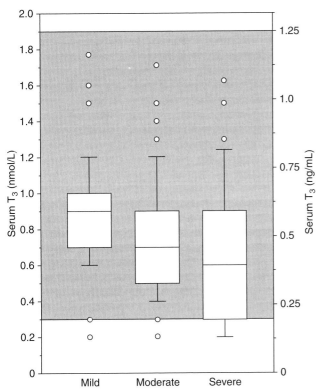

FIGURE 4-14 Box plots of serum T_3 concentrations in 221 cats with nonthyroidal illness grouped according to severity of illness. Of the 221 cats, 65 cats had mild disease, 83 had moderate disease, and 73 had severe disease. (From Peterson ME, et al.: Measurement of serum concentrations of free thyroxine, total thyroxine, and total triiodothyronine in cats with hyperthyroidism and cats with nonthyroidal disease, *J Am Vet Med Assoc* 218[4]:529-536, 2001.)

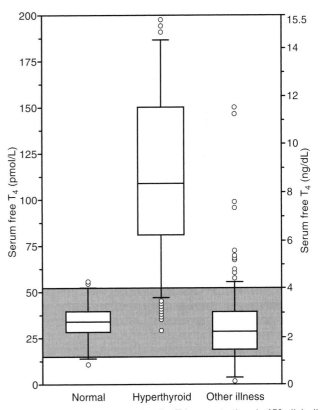

FIGURE 4-15 Box plots of serum free T_4 (fT_4) concentrations in 172 clinically normal cats, 917 cats with untreated hyperthyroidism, and 221 cats with nonthyroidal disease (see Fig. 4-10 for key). (From Peterson ME, et al.: Measurement of serum concentrations of free thyroxine, total thyroxine, and total triiodothyronine in cats with hyperthyroidism and cats with nonthyroidal disease, *J Am Vet Med Assoc* 218[4]:529-536, 2001.)

TABLE 4-9	PERFORMANCE OF FREE THYROXINE ASSAY IN DIAGNOSIS OF FELINE HYPERTHYROIDISM		
ASSAY	**SENSITIVITY (%)**	**SPECIFICITY (%)**	**ACCURACY (%)**
Analog free T_4 (fT_4)	87	100	89
MED IVD	87	100	89
MED AN	92	67	89
Two step Diasorin	89	100	91

From Peterson ME, et al.: Accuracy of serum free thyroxine concentrations determined by a new veterinary chemiluminescent immunoassay in euthyroid and hyperthyroid cats [abstract]. Proceedings of the 21st ECVIM-CA Congress. Seville (Spain), September 8-10, 2011.

Sensitivity, sensitivity, and accuracy of four assays for fT_4 in cats. The cat population included 53 clinically healthy cats and 45 cats with clinical signs of hyperthyroidism (6 euthyroid, 39 hyperthyroid). Assays included the Immulite 2000 Veterinary fT_4 (analog fT_4), Direct fT_4 by dialysis (IVD technologies; MED IVD), fT_4 by equilibrium dialysis (Antech Diagnostics; MED AN), and the Gammacoat fT_4 (two step) Radioimmunoassay (Diasorin).

diagnosis of hyperthyroidism in cats (Peterson et al, 2011). It should be noted however that none of the assays evaluated in this study, including the MED assays, had as good sensitivity as was originally reported in the first study evaluating performance of the MED assay by Peterson and colleagues in 2001. Because of the problem of specificity of the fT_4 measurement, an increased fT_4 concentration must never be used alone for diagnosis of feline hyperthyroidism; rather it should be interpreted in conjunction with the history, physical examination, and total T_4 concentration. Measurement of fT_4 concentration is most useful for evaluation of cats with suspected hyperthyroidism that have a total T_4 concentration in the upper half of the normal reference range. In cats with a high fT_4 and a low normal or low total T_4 concentration, other diagnostic testing (e.g., scintigraphy) should be utilized for confirmation of the diagnosis if hyperthyroidism is suspected clinically.

Baseline Serum Thyrotropin Concentration

TSH is a highly glycosylated glycoprotein hormone that has an alpha and beta subunit. The alpha subunit is identical to that of the alpha subunit of the related glycoprotein hormones luteinizing hormone (LH), follicle-stimulating hormone (FSH), and chorionic gonadotrophin, whereas the beta chain is unique and confers the unique biologic properties of TSH. Human TSH assays cannot be used to measure TSH in other species. The first assay for canine TSH was validated in 1996, and since that time there have been a number of commercial assays developed. A canine TSH assay (Immulite canine TSH assay, DPC) has been validated for use in cats (Wakeling et al, 2008; 2011). Although the sensitivity of the assay is suboptimal, a high TSH concentration in a cat with a low total T_4 concentration is highly specific for a diagnosis of hypothyroidism. Because of the extremely poor sensitivity of this TSH assay in cats, measurement of TSH has a limited role in diagnosis of feline hyperthyroidism; however in one study of 104 geriatric cats evaluated for a routine health evaluation, cats with an undetectable TSH at baseline were significantly more likely to be diagnosed with hyperthyroidism

in the follow-up time period of up to 54 months (Wakeling et al, 2011). It should be noted however that not all cats with an undetectable TSH became hyperthyroid during the study period.

Triiodothyronine Suppression Test

Traditionally, humans suspected of having hormonal deficiencies are tested with provocative (stimulation) tests, and those suspected of having hormonal excesses are tested with suppression tests. Administration of thyroid hormone to an individual with a normal pituitary-thyroid axis should suppress pituitary TSH secretion and in turn suppress endogenous thyroid hormone secretion. Administration of T_3 to normal cats should suppress pituitary TSH secretion, causing a subsequent decrease in the serum T_4 concentration. Measurement of serum T_4 is a valid marker of thyroid gland function, because exogenous T_3 cannot be converted to T_4.

Cats with hyperthyroidism have autonomous secretion of thyroid hormone (i.e., hormone secretion is independent of pituitary control). Thus administration of T_3 to hyperthyroid cats has no effect on the serum T_4 concentration, because pituitary TSH secretion has already been chronically suppressed and T_3 administration has no further suppressive effect. The T_3 suppression test should therefore allow discrimination between cats with a normal pituitary-thyroid axis from those with autonomous thyroid secretion resulting in hyperthyroidism. The protocol for T_3 suppression testing in cats involves measurement of serum T_3 and T_4 concentration and takes advantage of the relatively short (6 to 8 hours) serum half-life of T_3 in cats (Broome et al, 1987; Hays et al, 1988; Peterson et al, 1990a; Refsal et al, 1991).

Protocol

Initially, serum is obtained for determination of both serum T_3 and T_4 concentrations. Owners are then instructed to administer T_3 (liothyronine [Cytomel]; King Pharmaceuticals) beginning the next morning at a dosage of 25 µg given orally three times daily for 2 days. On the morning of day 3, a seventh 25 µg dose should be administered and the cat returned to the hospital so that a second blood sample can be obtained. This blood sample, for measurement of both serum T_3 and T_4 concentrations, should be obtained 2 to 4 hours after administration of the seventh dose of liothyronine (Peterson et al, 1990a; Table 4-10). The pretreatment and posttreatment serum samples should be submitted to the laboratory together to eliminate any concern about a possible effect of interassay variation on the results.

Change in Serum Thyroxine

Normal cats demonstrate a marked reduction in the serum T_4 concentration after seven doses of synthetic T_3. Cats with hyperthyroidism, however, demonstrate minimal or no decrease in serum T_4 concentrations (Fig. 4-16). This is true even for cats with mild hyperthyroidism and high-normal or marginally increased resting T_4 concentrations. Normal cats consistently have post-pill serum T_4 concentrations of less than 1.5 µg/dL (20 nmol/l). Hyperthyroid cats have post-pill T_4 concentrations greater than 1.5 µg/dL. Values close to the cut-off of 1.5 µg/dL should be considered nondiagnostic. The percentage of decrease in the serum T_4 concentration is not as reliable a criterion as the absolute value, although suppression of greater than 50% below the baseline value was observed only in euthyroid

TABLE 4-10	COMMONLY USED PROTOCOLS FOR DYNAMIC THYROID FUNCTION TESTS IN CATS*		
	TRIIODOTHYRONINE SUPPRESSION	**THYROID-STIMULATING HORMONE STIMULATION**	**THYROTROPIN-RELEASING HORMONE STIMULATION**
Drug	Liothyronine (Cytomel)	Human recombinant TSH	TRH
Dose	25 µg every 8 hours × 7 doses	0.025 to 0.2 mg	0.1 mg/kg
Route	Oral	IV	IV
Sampling times	Before and 2 to 4 hours after last dose	0 and 6 to 8 hours	0 and 4 hours
Assays	Total T_3 and T_4	Total T_4	Total T_4
Interpretation			
a) Euthyroid	< 1.5 µg/dL (20 nmol/L) with > 50% suppression	> 100%	> 60%
b) Hyperthyroid	> 1.5 µg/dL (20 nmol/L) ± < 50% suppression	Minimal or no increase from baseline	< 50%
Reference	Peterson et al, 1990a	Mooney et al, 1996b	Peterson et al, 1994

IV, Intravenous; T_3, triiodothyronine; T_4, thyroxine; *TRH*, thyrotropin-releasing hormone; *TSH*, thyroid-stimulating hormone.
*Values quoted are guidelines only. Each laboratory should furnish its own reference ranges.

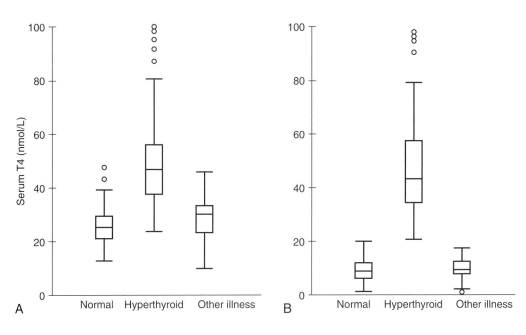

FIGURE 4-16 Box plots of the serum thyroxine (T_4) concentrations before (**A**) and after (**B**) administration of liothyronine to 44 clinically normal cats, 77 cats with hyperthyroidism, and 22 cats with nonthyroidal disease. Data plotted as described in Fig. 4-10. (From Peterson ME, et al.: Triiodothyronine [T_3] suppression test: an aid in the diagnosis of mild hyperthyroidism in cats, *J Vet Intern Med* 4[5]:233-238, 1990.)

cats (Peterson et al, 1990a; Refsal et al, 1991). As for any endocrine test, it is important for laboratory to establish laboratory specific reference ranges.

Change in Serum Triiodothyronine

Assay results for the serum T_3 concentration are not used to evaluate the status of the pituitary-thyroid axis. Rather, serum T_3 results are used to determine whether the owner successfully administered the T_3. The serum T_3 concentration should increase in all cats that are successfully medicated, regardless of the status of thyroid gland function (Fig. 4-17). If the serum T_4 concentration fails to decline in a cat that does not demonstrate an increase in the serum T_3 concentration, problems with owner compliance could explain these results, and the test results should not be trusted.

The T_3 suppression test is particularly useful in distinguishing euthyroid from mildly hyperthyroid cats with borderline resting serum T_4 concentrations. The disadvantages of the test are the 3 days required to complete the regimen and the need to rely on

owners to administer the drug seven times (Peterson et al, 1990a; Refsal et al, 1991).

Thyroid-Stimulating Hormone Response Test

The TSH response test is the gold standard for diagnosis of canine hypothyroidism and may have value for evaluating cats suspected of having hypothyroidism (see Chapter 3). The TSH stimulation test has also been evaluated for diagnosis of hyperthyroidism in cats (see Table 4-10). The test involves obtaining serum for determination of the T_4 level before and after TSH administration. The most recently reported protocol evaluated in healthy cats used intravenous (IV) administration of 0.025 to 0.2 mg recombinant human thyrotropin (rhTSH) with total T_4 concentration measured prior to injection and 6 to 8 hours later (Stegeman et al, 2003).

Interpretation

Euthyroid cats have greater responsiveness to TSH than hyperthyroid cats; however, hyperthyroid cats with a normal or

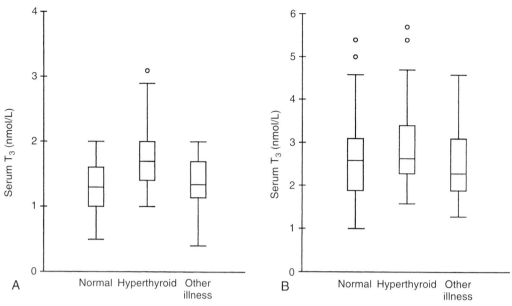

FIGURE 4-17 Box plots of the serum triiodothyronine (T_3) concentrations before **(A)** and after **(B)** administration of liothyronine to 44 clinically normal cats, 77 cats with hyperthyroidism, and 22 cats with nonthyroidal disease. Data plotted as described in Fig. 4-10. (From Peterson ME, et al.: Triiodothyronine [T_3] suppression test: an aid in the diagnosis of mild hyperthyroidism in cats, *J Vet Intern Med* 4[5]:233-238, 1990.)

borderline T_4 concentration are indistinguishable from euthyroid cats. Therefore the TSH stimulation test is not recommended for diagnosing feline hyperthyroidism (Mooney et al, 1996b).

Thyrotropin-Releasing Hormone Stimulation Test

Protocol

In cats, the TRH stimulation test (see Table 4-10) is performed by evaluating changes in the serum T_4 concentration in response to TRH (Peterson et al, 1994). Blood is collected for serum T_4 determination before and 4 hours after IV administration of TRH at a dosage of 0.1 mg/kg body weight. Adverse reactions (e.g., salivation, vomiting, tachypnea, defecation) are common with IV administration of TRH. Side effects usually begin immediately after TRH administration and may continue as long as 4 hours. Side effects are reported to be the result of activating central cholinergic and catecholaminergic mechanisms and direct neurotransmitter effects of TRH on specific binding sites (Holtman et al, 1986; Beleslin et al, 1987a; 1987b).

Interpretation

Healthy cats and those with nonthyroidal illness usually have a twofold increase in the serum T_4 concentration 4 hours after IV administration of TRH. Cats with mild hyperthyroidism have little or no increase in the serum T_4 concentration (see Fig. 4-18; Fig. 4-19). Serum T_3 assessments have been less consistent and are not recommended. A percentage increase in the post-TRH serum T_4 concentration of less than 50% above basal values was also consistent with the diagnosis of hyperthyroidism. Post-TRH T_4 values greater than 60% above basal concentrations were observed only in normal cats and in those with nonthyroidal illness. Increases of 50% to 60% should be considered nondiagnostic (Peterson et al, 1994; Tomsa et al, 2001).

The TRH stimulation test has been reported to be as reliable as the T_3 suppression test for diagnosis of hyperthyroidism in cats and has the advantage of being less time-consuming and less dependent on owner compliance (Sparkes et al, 1991; Peterson and Becker, 1995). However, in the most recent study investigating this test, the TRH stimulation test did not reliably distinguish between sick euthyroid and sick hyperthyroid cats (Tomsa et al, 2001). Because this is the population of cats that is most likely to need additional testing beyond measurement of the total T_4 and the fT_4, the TSH stimulation test currently has little place in diagnostic evaluation for hyperthyroidism.

Summary of Diagnostic Testing for Hyperthyroidism

The clinician should gain a suspicion of hyperthyroidism based on careful review of the history and physical examination findings. Careful palpation of the cat's neck, especially in the area of the thoracic inlet, is very important. Most cats with hyperthyroidism have a palpable thyroid mass. If a thyroid mass is not palpable, the clinician should consider that the abnormal thyroid tissue might be in the mediastinum, but other possible causes of the clinical signs observed by the owners should be considered (see Table 4-7).

The diagnosis of hyperthyroidism can usually be confirmed by evaluating a single, random, serum total T_4 concentration (Fig. 4-20). If a cat that appears to be hyperthyroid does not have a diagnostic baseline serum total T_4 concentration and no other cause for the clinical signs is identified, the test should be repeated days to weeks later, together with a serum fT_4 concentration. If the serum T_4 concentrations (total and free) fail to confirm hyperthyroidism at the time of the second evaluation, the T_3 suppression test or a radionuclide imaging (scintigraphy) should be considered. Trial therapy with methimazole as a means to confirm the diagnosis is not recommended.

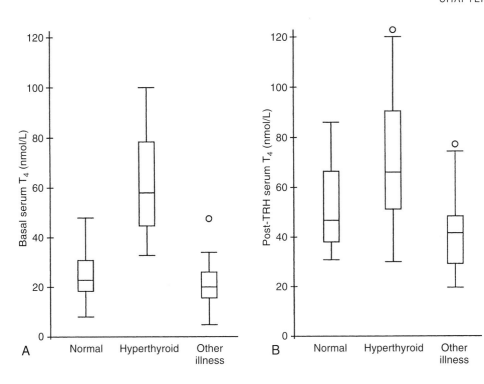

FIGURE 4-18 Box plots of the serum thyroxine (T$_4$) concentrations before **(A)** and after **(B)** thyrotropin-releasing hormone (TRH) stimulation in 31 clinically normal cats, 35 cats with hyperthyroidism, and 15 cats with nonthyroidal illness. Data plotted as described in Fig. 4-10. (From Peterson ME, et al.: Use of the thyrotropin releasing hormone stimulation test to diagnose mild hyperthyroidism in cats, *J Vet Intern Med* 8[4]:279-286, 1994.)

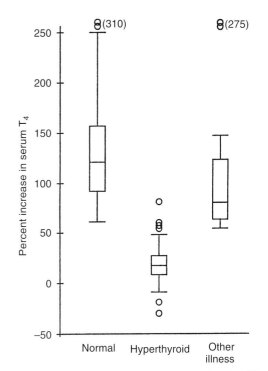

FIGURE 4-19 Box plots of the relative change in serum thyroxine (T$_4$) concentrations after thyrotropin-releasing hormone (TRH) administration (percent increase) in 31 clinically normal cats, 35 cats with hyperthyroidism, and 15 cats with nonthyroidal disease. Data plotted as described in Fig. 4-10. (From Peterson ME, et al.: Use of the thyrotropin releasing hormone stimulation test to diagnose mild hyperthyroidism in cats, *J Vet Intern Med* 8[4]:279-286, 1994.)

RADIONUCLIDE IMAGING: THYROID SCINTIGRAPHY

Thyroid scintigraphy provides both anatomic and functional information about the thyroid gland. Scintigraphy is useful for

determining the functional status of the thyroid gland, establishing whether thyroid disease is unilateral or bilateral, identifying ectopic tissue or metastatic thyroid tissue and may give insight into differentiation of malignant from benign thyroid disease. Thyroid scintigraphy can also be used to determine the dose of radioactive iodine for treatment of a hyperthyroid cat (see Dose Determination). Several radionuclides are available for thyroid scintigraphy in cats. The iodine isotopes (iodine-131 [^{131}I] and iodine-123 [^{123}I]) are both trapped and concentrated within thyroid follicular cells in a similar manner to stable iodine and are incorporated into the tyrosine groups of thyroglobulin and then into T$_3$ and T$_4$. Radioactive technetium-99m pertechnetate (^{99m}TcO$_4$) is referred to as a *pseudohalogen* because it mimics the biologic behavior of iodine and chloride. It is therefore trapped and concentrated within thyroid follicular cells, although it is not incorporated into thyroid hormone and therefore is not retained in the thyroid gland. Some other epithelial structures (salivary glands, gastric mucosa) also concentrate iodine and pertechnetate without organic binding or storage within the tissue (Nap et al, 1994). Both iodine and pertechnetate are primarily excreted in the urine, so the bladder is also visible on whole body scintigraphy.

Choice of Radionuclide

All three radionuclides (^{131}I, ^{123}I, and pertechnetate) provide excellent thyroid images, but pertechnetate, for several reasons, is the most commonly used radionuclide for thyroid scintigraphy (Table 4-11). ^{131}I is inexpensive and readily available, but it has a long physical half-life (8 days) and emits a high-energy γ-photon (364 keV) that is inefficiently collimated by the camera. ^{131}I also emits beta-particles that are not detected by the camera but that increase total body and thyroid radiation exposure. The increased risk to technicians administering ^{131}I makes this material less suitable for routine use (Beck et al, 1985). In contrast to ^{131}I, ^{123}I has a short physical half-life (13.3 hours), emits low-energy γ-rays (159 keV) that are well

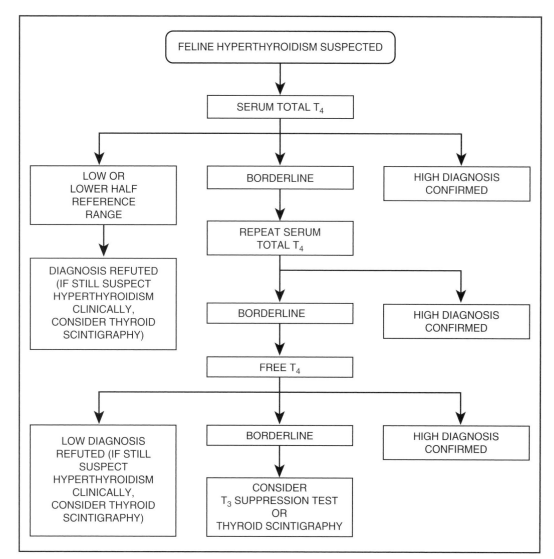

FIGURE 4-20 Algorithm for the diagnosis of hyperthyroidism in cats.

suited for scanning, and has no β-emission. The imaging procedure can begin as soon as 4 hours after administration. For these reasons, ^{123}I is a good agent for thyroid scanning; until recently the high cost of ^{123}I limited its use, but it has recently become more affordable.

Pertechnetate, a widely available and relatively inexpensive radionuclide, is considered by most investigators to be the best choice for routine imaging of thyroid glands in humans and cats (Broome et al, 2006). Pertechnetate has a short physical half-life (6 hours), and imaging procedures can begin as soon as 20 minutes after administration because of its rapid uptake by the thyroid. Pertechnetate emits low-energy γ-particles (140 keV), has no β-emission, and gives the lowest radiation dose to the thyroid of all available scanning agents.

Protocol for Technetium-99m Pertechnetate

Thyroid scanning using pertechnetate is accomplished after IV administration of radiolabeled pertechnetate (37 to 185 MBq [1 to 5 mCi]). One report described successful thyroid scintigraphy in cats after SC administration of the isotope; however, a direct comparison between IV and SC administration was not made (Page et al, 2006). The image is typically acquired 60 minutes after isotope administration; however, good quality scans can

be acquired any time from 20 minutes to 2 hours after isotope administration (Broome et al, 2006). At the time of scanning, the cat is placed over a gamma scintillation camera, using a low energy all purpose (LEAP) collimator that interfaces with a dedicated nuclear imaging computer. Ventral, dorsal, and right and left lateral images are acquired of the cervical region and ventral and right and left lateral views of the thorax (after shielding the activity arising from the stomach and thyroid area to increase the count density within the thoracic region). Some protocols also use a pin-hole collimator that acquires a magnified image to acquire a more detailed image of the thyroid gland(s). Although many facilities perform scintigraphy without sedation or anesthesia, sedation is required when using a pinhole collimator, because the effect of patient motion is exacerbated when using a pin-hole collimator. In one of our hospitals all scintigraphy in small animal patients is done under general anesthesia to minimize exposure of personnel to radiation; in other hospitals anesthesia is not used.

Protocol for Iodine-123

Thyroid scanning using ^{123}I is accomplished after oral or IV administration of 200 to 400 μCi [123]I. The image is typically acquired 8 and 24 hours after isotope administration (Nieckarz and Daniel, 2001; van Hoek et al, 2008b).

		PRINCIPAL GAMMA ENERGY (KEV)	TIME FROM INJECTION TO SCANNING PROCEDURE	PHYSICAL HALF-LIFE	RISK TO TECHNICIANS
ISOTOPE	**EXPENSE/AVAILABILITY**				
Iodine-131	Inexpensive/available	364	24 hours	8.1 days	Yes
Iodine-123	More expensive/less available	159	8, 24 hours	13.3 hours	Low
$^{99m}TcO_4$ (pertechnetate)	Inexpensive/available	140	20 minutes	6.0 hours	Low

TABLE 4-11   RADIONUCLIDES USED IN THYROID IMAGING STUDIES

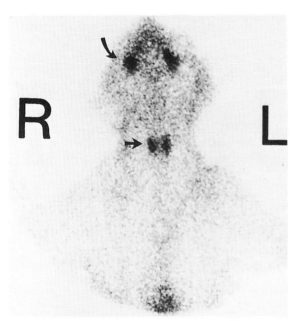

FIGURE 4-21 Thyroid scan (radioactive technetium-99m [^{99m}Tc]) of a normal cat. Note the similar size and density of the thyroid lobes *(straight arrow)* and the salivary glands *(curved arrow)*.

Tissue Identified

Scintigraphy identifies all functional thyroid tissue in the body and allows determination of whether the abnormal thyroid tissue is unilateral, bilateral, or ectopic. In a study of 120 hyperthyroid cats, 12% had ectopic thyroid tissue identified on scintigraphy (Harvey et al, 2009). Pertechnetate also concentrates in the gastric mucosa, the salivary glands, and the bladder; the relative uptake of technetium by the thyroid glands and the salivary glands is used to subjectively assess thyroid gland function. A euthyroid cat should have close to a 1:1 ratio of salivary gland to thyroid lobe uptake (Fig. 4-21). In most hyperthyroid cats, the thyroid lobe(s) have much more intense uptake than the salivary glands, and this is usually easily determined by subjective visual inspection of the images (Figs. 4-22 to 4-25) (Broome et al, 2006; Harvey et al, 2009). The relative uptake of the thyroid lobe(s) and the salivary tissue can be also be quantified by drawing regions of interest around the thyroid lobe(s) and the ipsilateral zygomatic/molar salivary gland. The percentage uptake of radioisotope by the thyroid gland, the thyroid-to-salivary (T:S) ratio, and rate of isotope uptake by the thyroid gland are all significantly correlated with the T_4 concentration, indicating that scintigraphy is a good indicator of the metabolic activity of the thyroid gland (Daniel et al, 2002). The best correlation is obtained by using the 20 minute T:S ratio using only the most intense of the thyroid lobes (Daniel et al, 2002). It is important to remember that in

certain circumstances other tissues can concentrate pertechnetate. In one study, in addition to concentrating in the tissues previously described, the imaging radionuclides accumulated in bronchogenic carcinomas in two cats (Cook et al, 1993).

Clinical Indications for Scintigraphy

Clinical indications for performing thyroid scintigraphy in cats are shown in Box 4-3.

Determine Whether Thyroid Autonomy Is Unilateral or Bilateral

Approximately 30% of hyperthyroid cats have unilateral hyperthyroidism, whereas in 70% of cats there is autonomous tissue present within both thyroid lobes. In either case, the normal thyroid tissue is atrophic due to lack of stimulation by TSH. In cats with unilateral disease, surgical thyroidectomy is a straightforward and simple procedure, whereas in cats with bilateral disease it may be complicated by postoperative hypothyroidism and/or hypoparathyroidism—so other modes of therapy may be more appropriate. Unfortunately it is not always possible to determine the functional activity of the thyroid glands by palpation or by visual inspection at surgery. In some cases, both glands are grossly enlarged and both are clearly abnormal, but in other cases, a small lobe may contain small numbers of adenomatous cells but be grossly indistinguishable from an atrophic normal thyroid gland. Scintigraphy allows determination of the functional status of both thyroid glands prior to thyroidectomy so that treatment planning can be optimized (see General Concepts in Treatment for more information on treatment choice for hyperthyroid cats). In cats with unilateral disease, only one thyroid lobe is detected on the scan, because there is no uptake of isotope into the contralateral atrophic thyroid gland (see Fig. 4-22). If any isotope uptake is visualized in the contralateral thyroid gland, bilateral disease should be assumed to be present (see Figs. 4-23 to 4-25). It is important to review all the cervical views of the scintigram in order to determine whether the disease is unilateral or bilateral, because particularly on the lateral views, one thyroid gland may overlie the other, leading to the appearance of unilateral disease when actually both thyroid glands are abnormal.

Determine Presence of Mediastinal or Ectopic Thyroid Tissue

In some hyperthyroid cats, an enlarged thyroid lobe may descend into the thoracic cavity where it is not palpable. In addition, additional ectopic thyroid tissue may be present anywhere from the base of the tongue to within the thoracic cavity (Knowles et al, 2010; Reed et al, 2011). A study of 120 hyperthyroid cats undergoing scintigraphy documented that 12% of hyperthyroid cats had more than two areas of increased radionuclide uptake (IRU) with the number of areas of IRU ranging from 1 to 5 (Harvey et al, 2009). Areas of IRU were located in the neck in 61% of cats, the thoracic inlet in in 53% of cats, and the thorax in in 22% of cats. Most of the cats with more than two areas of IRU had IRU

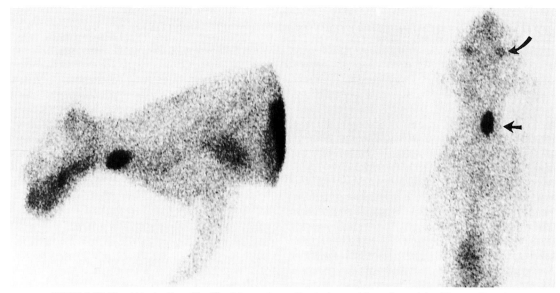

FIGURE 4-22 Thyroid technetium-99m (^{99mm}Tc) scan from a thyrotoxic cat with a unilateral thyroid tumor. Note the density of the thyroid *(straight arrow)* compared with that of the salivary glands *(curved arrow)*.

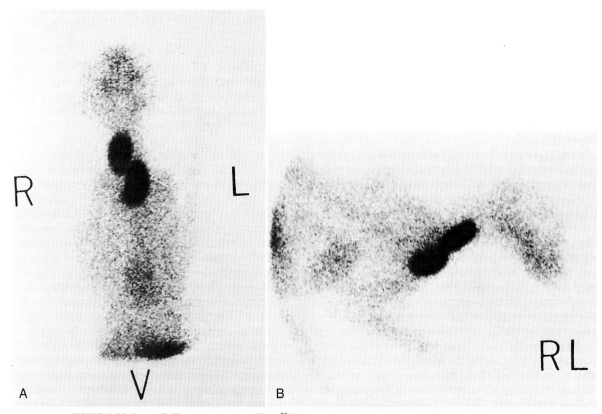

FIGURE 4-23 A and **B,** Thyroid technetium-99m (^{99m}Tc) scan from a thyrotoxic cat with bilaterally symmetric adenomatous hyperfunctional thyroids.

in the thorax. Although thyroid scintigraphy is an excellent diagnostic tool for locating ectopic or intra-thoracic thyroid tissue, it can be difficult to distinguish benign ectopic thyroid tissue from metastasis of thyroid carcinoma by scintigraphy (Figs. 4-26 to 4-29). There are no scintigraphic features that by themselves can distinguish benign from malignant disease (see discussion later), and in some cats with thyroid carcinoma, scintigraphic studies are identical to those of cats with benign disease.

Determine Presence of Functional Thyroid Carcinoma

The incidence of thyroid malignancy in hyperthyroid cats is believed to be approximately 3%, although it may be more common in hyperthyroid cats treated with medical therapy for long periods of time. Thyroid carcinoma should be suspected in hyperthyroid cats with large cervical masses, particularly when the masses are fixed or are attached to underlying or overlying tissues. Thyroid carcinoma should also be considered in cats with

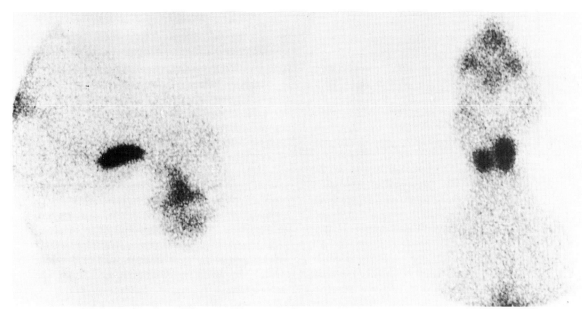

FIGURE 4-24 Thyroid technetium-99m (^{99m}Tc) scan from a thyrotoxic cat with bilaterally asymmetric adenomatous hyperfunctional thyroids. Note that on the lateral view one thyroid lobe overlies the other.

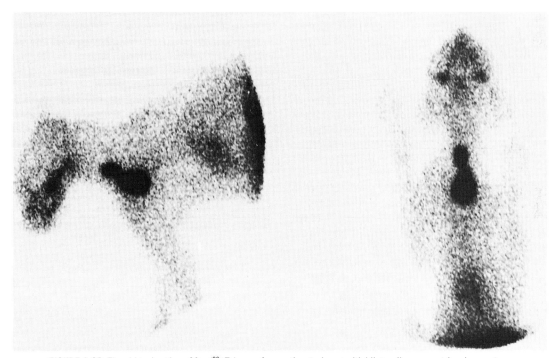

FIGURE 4-25 Thyroid technetium-99m (^{99m}Tc) scan from a thyrotoxic cat with bilaterally asymmetric adenomatous hyperfunctional thyroids. Note that this scan shows the larger thyroid below the smaller rather than the side-by-side location seen in Fig. 4-24.

ectopic tissue or a mediastinal mass on scintigraphy (see Figs. 4-27 to 4-29). Scintigraphic features such as distortion of the thyroid lobe, multiple foci of radionuclide uptake, heterogenous or irregular uptake with spiculated margins, extension caudally into the thoracic inlet, and the presence of linear multifocal patterns suggesting tumor extension along fascial planes, are considered suspicious for carcinoma, but definitive diagnosis requires histopathology (see Feline Thyroid Carcinoma). Some cats with thyroid carcinoma do not display these features, and some cats with benign thyroid disease have multifocal or irregular uptake of isotope (Harvey et al, 2009). Scintigraphy is also very helpful

to identify the presence of metastatic disease in cats with known thyroid carcinoma both before and after surgical resection.

Scintigraphy as a Diagnostic Aid in Cats with Nonthyroidal Illness

The thyroid scan may be used as a diagnostic test for cats with clinical signs of hyperthyroidism but normal or borderline serum total T_4 and fT_4 concentrations. Scintigraphy is particularly useful in suspected hyperthyroid cats with concurrent illness in which other tests do not perform well. The thyroid gland to salivary gland ratio in euthyroid cats should normally be 1:1 (see Fig. 4-21), but in hyperthyroid cats the ratio is higher (Broome et al, 2006). In this setting the thyroid scan has the potential for both diagnosing hyperthyroidism and locating the abnormal tissue.

Scintigraphy as an Aid to Planning Treatment

Scintigraphy can be useful in planning treatment, especially in cases in which thyroidectomy would be an option if the thyroid dysfunction was unilateral (see Treatment with Surgery). Some investigators have used scintigraphy to estimate thyroid mass volume and then utilized this information to determine the dose of radioactive iodine to be administered for treatment (Forrest et al, 1996). Unfortunately this approach has not proved to be reliable in predicting radioactive iodine uptake (RAIU) after treatment, because the biologic half-life of ^{131}I determined by tracer studies does not correlate well with the biologic half-life after administration of therapeutic doses of radioactive iodine. This is probably because of cellular necrosis and resultant changes in thyroid physiology after administration of large doses of [131]I.

Drugs That Cause Interference with Scintigraphy

Compounds that interfere with iodine uptake or thyroid hormone synthesis can influence the results of scintigraphy. Methimazole

has been documented to increase iodine trapping as measured by technetium and ^{123}I uptake in euthyroid cats (Nieckarz and Daniel, 2001). This effect was documented after 3 weeks of methimazole treatment, and iodine uptake was maximal 4 days after methimazole withdrawal. Uptake of radioisotope returned to baseline by 15 days after methimazole withdrawal. No effect of methimazole on pertechnetate uptake was documented in hyperthyroid cats after 30 days of methimazole treatment (Fischetti et al, 2005), presumably because TSH suppression was not relieved by methimazole treatment; in most of the cats, TSH concentration remained suppressed during methimazole treatment. Two cats with mild hyperthyroidism that had unilateral uptake before methimazole treatment developed bilateral uptake after methimazole treatment. For these reasons, when nuclear scintigraphy is used as a diagnostic tool to confirm hyperthyroidism, it is very important that methimazole treatment should be withdrawn at least 2 weeks prior to scintigraphy. Methimazole should also be discontinued prior to scintigraphy when it is used to identify the location of ectopic tissue, because it may cause errors in distinguishing unilateral from bilateral disease (Fischetti et al, 2005). Iodine and iodinated contrast agents (e.g., iohexol) may decrease uptake of radioiodine into the thyroid gland. Iohexol is often used to determine GFR in hyperthyroid cats prior to treatment with radioactive iodine. Studies suggest that treatment with iohexol within 24 hours of radioactive iodine administration decreases iodine uptake in the thyroid gland, although the effect was relatively small and the clinical outcome did not appear to be affected (Peremans et al, 2008). In a similar study, thyroid scintigraphy was performed in euthyroid cats before and after administration of iohexol (Lee et al, 2010). There was a significant decrease in technetium uptake on days 1, 3, and 14 after iohexol administration; however, uptake did not fall below the published reference ranges for euthyroid cats (Lee et al, 2010). Ideally concurrent administration of iohexol or other iodine containing compounds should be avoided prior to scintigraphy or treatment with [131]I. The protocol used

---

BOX 4-3   Indications for Thyroid Scintigraphy

1. Evaluation of the functional status of the thyroid glands
2. Determination of unilateral or bilateral thyroid lobe involvement
3. Detection and localization of ectopic thyroid tissue
4. Differentiation between benign and malignant thyroid diseases
5. Determination of the origin of a cervical mass
6. Detection of functional metastasis
7. Evaluation of the efficacy of therapy
8. Evaluation for residual tissue after thyroidectomy

From Daniel GB, Neelis DA: Thyroid scintigraphy in veterinary medicine, *Semin Nucl Med* 44(1):24-34, 2014.

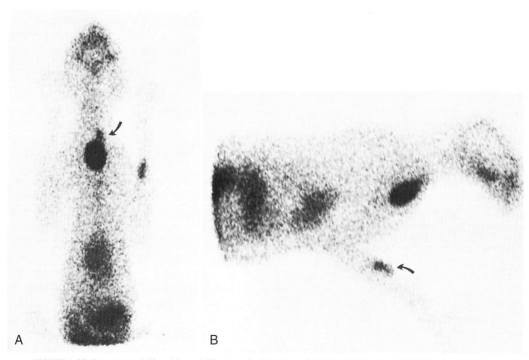

FIGURE 4-26 Dorsoventral **(A)** and lateral **(B)** views of a large intrathoracic anterior mediastinal thyroid mass with a small active gland just cranial to it (*arrow* in **A**). Also note that a small amount of pertechnetate leaked into the subcutaneous (SC) space during administration (*arrow* in **B**).

for sedation or anesthesia can also influence the results of scintigraphy, because drugs used commonly for sedation may increase or decrease salivation and thus influence the T:S ratio (Schaafsma et al, 2006). For example in a study of euthyroid cats, the T:S ratio for technetium was significantly higher at 40 minutes when ketamine-midazolam was used than when propofol or ketamine-midazolam-atropine protocols were used. Unfortunately this study did not include a control group without sedation. Although statistically significant changes were identified between the different sedation protocols, in most cats the T:S ratio was still within or close to the typical range of the normal T:S ratio of 0.8 to 1.2. It is recommended that a consistent protocol for sedation or

anesthesia is used when scintigraphy is performed and that each facility develop appropriate reference ranges for T:S ratios for the protocols used.

CERVICAL (THYROID) ULTRASONOGRAPHY/ COMPUTED TOMOGRAPHY

Although scintigraphy is the imaging procedure of choice for evaluation of the feline thyroid gland, cervical ultrasonography can also be used to evaluate feline thyroid glands and estimate thyroid gland volume. Cervical ultrasound usually requires no anesthesia or sedation, although more consistent positioning can be achieved

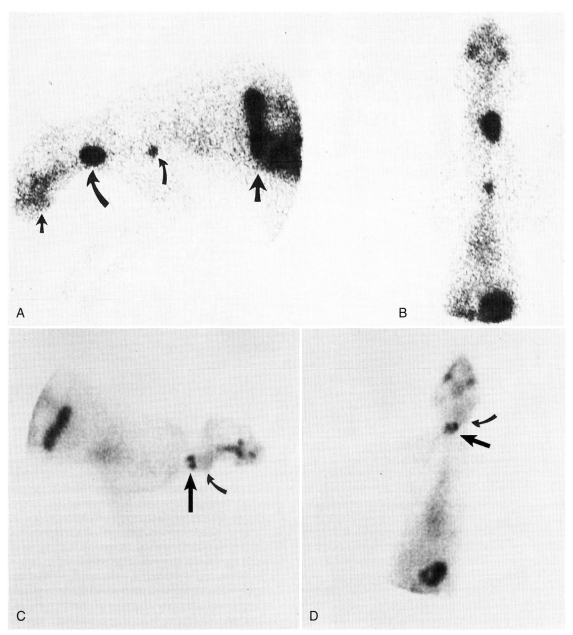

FIGURE 4-27 Lateral **(A)** and dorsoventral **(B)** views of a pertechnetate scan performed on a hyperthyroid cat. Note the large thyroid in the neck (*large curved arrow* on lateral view); the small, adenomatous thyroid tissue in the anterior mediastinum *(small curved arrow)*; the salivary glands and the saliva, which concentrates pertechnetate *(small straight arrow)*; and the gastric mucosa, which concentrates pertechnetate *(large straight arrow)*. In the lateral **(C)** and dorsoventral **(D)** views of the pertechnetate scans from another cat, note the large intracervical mass *(curved arrows)* that does not concentrate pertechnetate displacing the normal thyroid glands *(straight arrows)*. This mass was a salivary carcinoma, demonstrating that not all cervical masses are thyroid.

if cats are sedated for the procedure. As with any ultrasound evaluation, the value of cervical studies depends heavily on the skill of the operator.

In a study of six healthy cats and 14 cats with confirmed hyperthyroidism, a significant difference in the mean estimated thyroid volume of hyperthyroid cats compared with healthy cats was identified (Wisner et al, 1994). Although in most cases, there was good correlation between thyroid scintigraphy and ultrasound in regard to identifying unilateral versus bilateral thyroid dysfunction; thyroid lobes that could not be identified ultrasonographically were hyperfunctional on scintigraphy in two cats. Ultrasound cannot replace scintigraphy for locating ectopic or metastatic tissue, but it is considerably more available and less expensive.

Normal thyroid lobes are thin, fusiform-shaped structures that are moderately and uniformly echogenic (Fig. 4-30). The lobes are located adjacent and medial to the common carotid arteries and are surrounded by a thin, hyperechoic fascia. The cranial and caudal ends of each thyroid lobe usually taper within this sheath, which sometimes makes the exact margins difficult to discern. Linear measurements of each lobe are easiest to make in the long axis plane. Normal thyroid lobes are usually 15 to 25 mm long with calculated volumes of 40 to 140 mm^3 (Wisner et al, 1994; Table 4-12). Thyroid lobe parenchyma ranges from low to moderate echogenicity compared with surrounding tissue. Thyroid lobes from hyperthyroid cats are usually uniformly enlarged and are less echogenic than normal thyroid lobes. Some lobes have mildly or moderately lobulated outer margins and/or poor delineation from surrounding tissue. Although most abnormal glands are uniformly echogenic, a mottled echogenicity occasionally is seen. Cystic structures within the thyroid gland can be identified on ultrasound in a significant number of hyperthyroid cats. Cysts vary in shape and structure, some being unicameral and others containing one or several internal septae. It is not unusual for abnormal thyroid lobes to be "normal" in length but obviously rounder and thicker; this accounts for the abnormal volume, which usually ranges from 140 to 1000 mm^3 despite a length similar to that of the thyroid lobes of a healthy cat (see Fig. 4-30 and Table 4-12) (Wisner et al, 1994; Goldstein et al, 2001; Wells et al, 2001; Barberet et al, 2010).

Computed tomography (CT) has also been used to evaluate feline thyroid glands. Although the thyroid glands can be identified on CT and an estimate of thyroid lobe size obtained, CT is not able to reliably distinguish unilateral versus bilateral thyroid gland dysfunction and ectopic tissue cannot be identified (Lautenschlaeger et al, 2013).

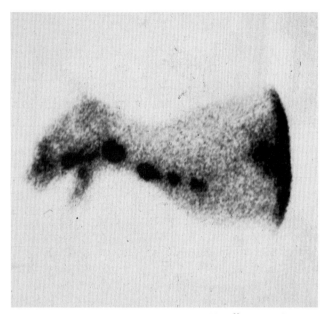

FIGURE 4-28 Lateral view of a thyroid technetium-99m (^{99m}Tc) scan from a thyrotoxic cat with multiple functioning hyperactive thyroid masses within the cervical region. This could be either ectopic adenomatous neoplasia or metastasis of thyroid carcinoma.

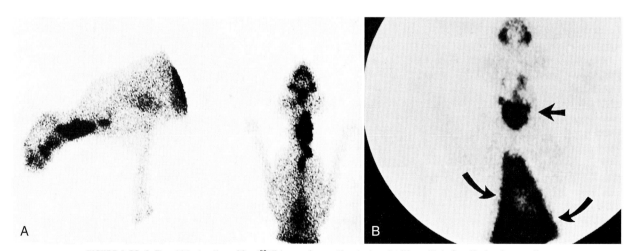

FIGURE 4-29 A, Thyroid technetium-99m (^{99m}Tc) scan from a thyrotoxic cat with multiple functioning hyperactive thyroid masses. This may be representative of a cat with a functioning thyroid carcinoma that has undergone massive local invasion throughout the neck and anterior mediastinum. This also could represent multiple adenomatous tissue—some of which is ectopic. **B,** Thyroid ^{99m}Tc scan from a thyrotoxic cat with multiple functioning thyroid masses. This cat had a thyroid carcinoma with massive local invasion throughout the neck *(straight arrow)* and diffuse functional carcinoma throughout the pulmonary parenchyma *(curved arrows).*

Nonfunctional Thyroid Nodules

In older cats, it is not uncommon to palpate an enlarged thyroid gland in an apparently healthy euthyroid cat. Possible differential diagnoses include early hyperthyroidism in which a goiter is present but the thyroid gland is not fully autonomous, thyroid cyst, thyroid cystadenoma, or nonfunctional thyroid adenoma or carcinoma (see Feline Thyroid Carcinoma). Nonfunctional thyroid carcinoma is very rare in the cat. If an obvious cervical nodule is palpated in a cat with a normal T_4 concentration, a fine needle aspirate should be considered to determine the tissue of origin. Unfortunately, thyroid cytology is not accurate for differentiation of benign from malignant thyroid disease.

 GENERAL CONCEPTS IN TREATMENT

Background

There are four methods of managing feline hyperthyroidism (Fig. 4-31). Each treatment modality has advantages and disadvantages (Table 4-13). Thyroid hormone synthesis can be inhibited by either anti-thyroid drugs or iodine restricted diets. Neither of these treatment methods results in permanent resolution of hyperthyroidism; however, medical therapy permits trial resolution of hyperthyroidism while the effect of reestablishing the euthyroid state on renal function is assessed. Definitive therapy includes either surgical thyroidectomy or administration of radioactive iodine.

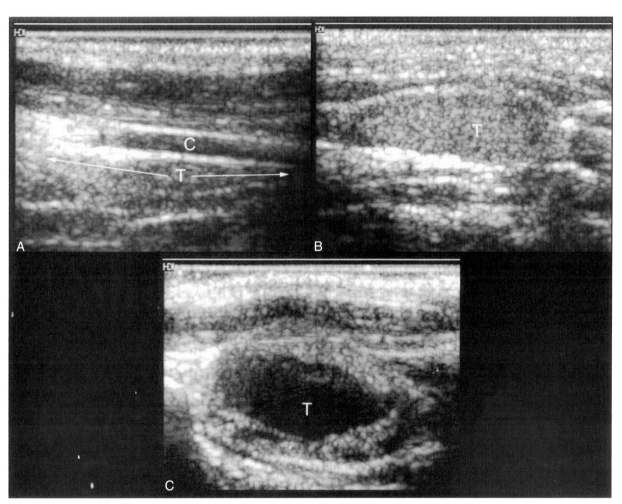

FIGURE 4-30 A, Cervical ultrasound of normal feline thyroid (*T,* thyroid; *C,* carotid artery). **B,** Abnormal enlarged thyroid in a cat with hyperthyroidism. **C,** Abnormal enlarged cystic thyroid in a cat with hyperthyroidism.

 TABLE 4-12 **LINEAR MEASUREMENTS (MM) AND VOLUMETRIC ESTIMATIONS (MM³) FOR LEFT AND RIGHT THYROID LOBES OF CONTROL AND HYPERTHYROID CATS**

	Left Lobe Mean ± Standard Deviation				Right Lobe Mean ± Standard Deviation			
	LENGTH	HEIGHT	WIDTH	VOLUME*	LENGTH	HEIGHT	WIDTH	VOLUME*
Control (n = 6)	20.5 ± 1.6	3.3 ± 0.8	2.5†	89 ± 23	20.3 ± 1.6	3.0 ± 0.6	2.5†	80 ± 19
Hyperthyroid (n = 14)	20.2 ± 3.6	5.5 ± 2.4	5.7 ± 2.1	382 ± 312	21.9 ± 4.4	8.1 ± 3.0	7.7 ± 2.4	782 ± 449

*Volume estimation calculated using the formula for a prolate ellipsoid, π/6 (length x height x width).
†Width measurements for normal thyroid lobes defaulted to 2.5 mm because they could not be seen ultrasonographically.

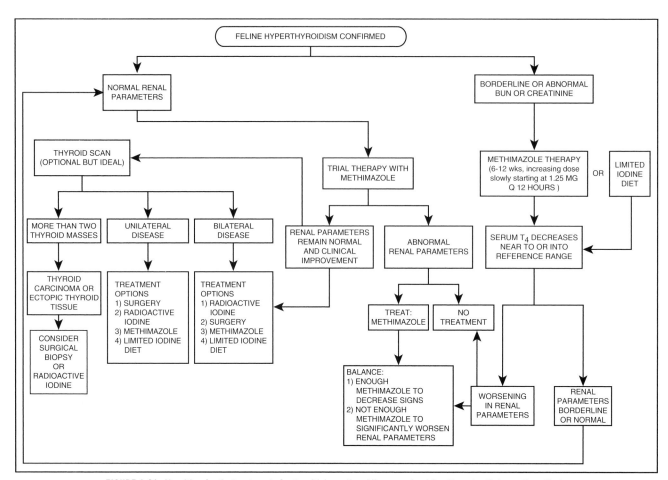

FIGURE 4-31 Algorithm for the treatment of cats with hyperthyroidism, emphasizing the potential negative effects of therapy on renal function.

The treatment chosen for an individual cat depends on various factors, including owner preference and financial constraints, the presence of nonthyroidal illness, the age of the cat, and availability of a skilled surgeon or a facility with nuclear medicine capability for administering radioactive iodine.

Treatment of Hyperthyroidism and Renal Function

Background

Clinical evaluation and management of geriatric cats with concurrent hyperthyroidism and CKD is challenging. The tendency of nonthyroidal illnesses such as CKD to lower serum T_4 concentrations may mask hyperthyroidism. On the other hand, hyperthyroidism can increase the GFR and thereby decrease the serum creatinine and BUN concentrations, masking underlying renal disease. The progressive weight loss and reduction in muscle mass associated with hyperthyroidism may further contribute to the reduction of serum creatinine concentrations, also obscuring evidence of concurrent renal disease. Finally if treatment of hyperthyroidism results in hypothyroidism, renal function may deteriorate further and exacerbate CKD. It has been estimated that as many as 40% of hyperthyroid cats have CKD. Whether CKD is more common in hyperthyroid cats than in the general geriatric cat population is unknown. Mechanisms by which hyperthyroidism could contribute to progression of renal disease in geriatric cats include induction of proteinuria, activation of the renin-angiotensin-aldosterone axis, hypertension and aberrations in calcium, and phosphate homeostasis.

Pathophysiology

Hyperthyroidism increases cardiac output and decreases peripheral vascular resistance, leading to increased renal plasma flow (RPF) and an increase in the GFR. Numerous studies have documented that GFR is increased in feline hyperthyroidism (Boag et al, 2007; Vandermeulen et al, 2008; van Hoek et al, 2008a; 2009a). In a study of 21 cats before and after treatment of hyperthyroidism using radioactive iodine, GFR was above the reference range for healthy cats in 80% of hyperthyroid cats (van Hoek et al, 2009a). In a study of geriatric cats followed until they became hyperthyroid, a decrease in creatinine was documented at the time of diagnosis of hyperthyroidism (Wakeling et al, 2011).

Worsening Renal Function after Resolution of Hyperthyroidism

Because restoration of euthyroidism normalizes the GFR, treatment of cats for hyperthyroidism usually results in an increase in serum creatinine, resulting in azotemia and overt renal failure in some cats (Graves et al, 1994; DiBartola et al, 1996; van Hoek et al, 2009a; Williams et al, 2010). Of 216 non-azotemic hyperthyroid cats, 41 (15%) developed azotemia within 240 days of diagnosis and treatment; the severity of azotemia and whether it was associated with clinical signs were not reported (Williams et al, 2010). As would be expected, a higher percentage of cats with well controlled hyperthyroidism became azotemic than cats that were poorly controlled (Williams et al, 2010). Pretreatment BUN and creatinine was positively correlated with development of azotemia, but posttreatment azotemia was not associated with decreased survival in this group of cats. The clinical effect of decreased GFR

TABLE 4-13	ADVANTAGES AND DISADVANTAGES OF DIFFERENT TREATMENTS FOR FELINE HYPERTHYROIDISM	
THERAPY	**ADVANTAGES**	**DISADVANTAGES**
Surgery	1. Usually corrects the thyrotoxicosis 2. Thyroids easily accessible 3. Relatively inexpensive 4. Sophisticated equipment not required 5. Definitive treatment 6. Rapid reduction in thyroid hormone concentrations	1. Risk of anesthesia in elderly and fragile cats 2. Anesthesia may decompensate other abnormal organ systems 3. Iatrogenic hypoparathyroidism 4. Iatrogenic hypothyroidism 5. Risk of surgical complications (recurrent laryngeal nerve damage) 6. Failure to remove all abnormal thyroid tissue 7. Effect on GFR irreversible

Oral anti-thyroid drugs	1. Usually corrects the thyrotoxicosis
	2. Inexpensive
	3. Small tablet size
	4. No anesthesia or surgery
	5. No expensive facilities
	6. No hospitalization required
	7. Effect on GFR reversible
		1. Side effects of the medication:
		  a. Anorexia
		  b. Vomiting
		  c. Depression/lethargy
		  d. Thrombocytopenia
		  e. Granulocytopenia
		  f. Hepatopathy
		2. Daily to twice daily medication required
		3. Iatrogenic hypothyroidism (reversible)
		4. Not definitive treatment
		5. Does not resolve underlying thyroid pathology

Radioactive iodine	1. Usually corrects the thyrotoxicosis 2. Only one treatment for most cats; no pills 3. No anesthesia or surgery 4. Rapid reduction in thyroid hormone concentrations 5. Definitive therapy	1. Need for sophisticated facilities 2. Radiation exposure to personnel and owners 3. Hospitalization after treatment to decrease risk of human exposure 4. Possibility of iatrogenic hypothyroidism 5. Re-treatment may be necessary in 2% to 5% 6. Irreversible
Nutritional management with iodine limited diets	1. Usually corrects the thyrotoxicosis 2. Inexpensive 3. No anesthesia or surgery required 4. No expensive facilities 5. No hospitalization required 6. Effect on GFR reversible	1. Cat can only eat one diet 2. Difficult to limit dietary intake in multi-cat households 3. Outdoor cats may have access to other dietary sources of iodine 4. Not palatable to all cats 5. Not definitive treatment 6. Does not resolve underlying thyroid pathology 7. Long-term consequences of limited iodine diet unknown

after treatment of hyperthyroidism is variable. Most cats have a modest increase in creatinine after treatment that may or may not be severe enough to result in azotemia. A smaller subset of cats has a clinically significant worsening of azotemia and developed overt signs of renal failure after treatment. Unfortunately there are no routine pretreatment clinical parameters that allow prediction of which cats will develop clinically significant failure. It has been stated that cats with a normal BUN and creatinine and a USG more than1.035 are unlikely to have clinically significant renal failure after treatment, but other studies and our clinical experience suggest that this is not always the case (Riensche et al, 2008). Cats that develop azotemia after treatment are likely to be older and have a higher total T_4, BUN, and creatinine; but measurement of GFR is believed to be a more sensitive predictor of renal failure after treatment (Adams et al, 1997; van Hoek et al, 2009a).

Predicting Emergence of Renal Failure by Determining the Glomerular Filtration Rate

Serum creatinine and BUN concentrations vary inversely with the GFR and are used as indirect measures of the GFR. However, these two commonly used parameters are relatively insensitive indicators of renal disease, because at least 75% of functional renal mass must be lost before changes are noted. Significant renal disease, therefore, can be present in the absence of serum biochemical abnormalities. In addition, BUN and serum creatinine are affected by factors other than functional renal mass and blood flow.

Methods to assess GFR include inulin or exogenous creatinine clearance, nuclear scintigraphy (using radiolabelled diethylenetriamine penta-acetic acid [DTPA] or ^{51}Cr- ethylenediaminetetraacetic acid [^{51}Cr-EDTA]), or measurement of plasma clearance of iohexol. Iohexol is an iodinated radiographic contrast agent, and the iohexol clearance test has been validated for determination of GFR in cats (van Hoek et al, 2008a). An IV catheter must be placed for administration of the iohexol. The research protocols that have been described require collection of blood samples at 0, 15, and 30 minutes and then at 1, 2, 3, 6, 8, and 10 hours after iohexol administration for measurement of either iodine or iohexol by high performance liquid chromatography (HPLC). An abbreviated protocol with collection of samples at 3, 4, and 5 hours after iohexol administration is recommended for clinical use, and the iohexol assay is commercially available (http://www.animalhealth.msu.edu). After assay of the iohexol concentration at these three time points, the diagnostic laboratory reports a calculated GFR.

In a study of 21 hyperthyroid cats in which GFR was measured before and 1, 4, 12, and 24 weeks after treatment of hyperthyroidism by radioactive iodine therapy, decreases in GFR occurred within 4 weeks of treatment and did not change thereafter. Maximum decrease in GFR could only be partially predicted by

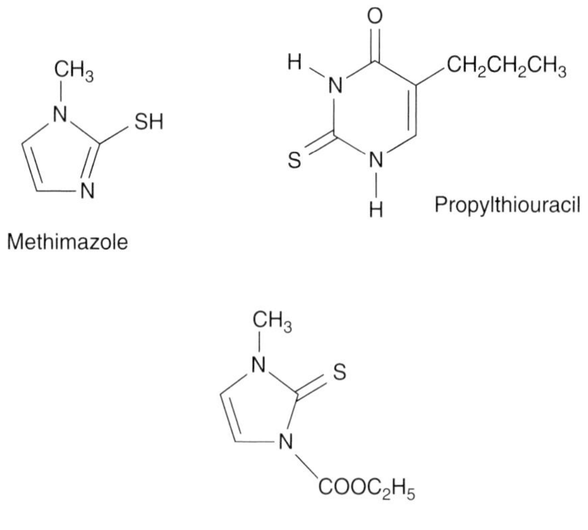

FIGURE 4-32 Chemical structures of the anti-thyroid drugs (thioureylenes), which inhibit thyroidal iodide organification.

a formula using the pretreatment GFR, serum total T_4, serum creatinine, BUN, and USG (van Hoek et al, 2009a). Although some studies have suggested that cats with a GFR more than 2.25 mL/kg/minute are unlikely to develop clinically significant renal failure after treatment of hyperthyroidism, other studies do not support this contention (Graves et al, 1994; Adams et al, 1997; Riensche et al, 2008).

Summary

There are no routine pretreatment parameters that reliably predict development of azotemia in cats after treatment of hyperthyroidism. Although measurement of pretreatment GFR is helpful, such studies do not consistently predict the development of renal failure after euthyroidism is restored. Therefore a methimazole trial with follow-up serum biochemical and urine analyses should be considered prior to definitive treatment of hyperthyroid cats with either thyroidectomy or radioactive iodine (Riensche et al, 2008). It is important to recognize that not all increases in serum creatinine concentration result in clinical signs of renal failure; mild increases in creatinine after treatment should be expected. Such changes do not preclude definitive treatment of hyperthyroidism. For cats that develop marked azotemia and overt clinical signs of renal failure after euthyroidism is established, medical therapy rather than definitive therapy is recommended long term, and the treatment should be tailored to balance the two disorders. Alternatively thyroid supplementation after definitive treatment of hyperthyroidism can be considered; however, most owners decline this option due to financial considerations.

TREATMENT WITH ANTI-THYROID DRUGS (THIOUREYLENES)

Mode of Action

The structures of the three available anti-thyroid drugs methimazole, carbimazole, and propylthiouracil (PTU) are shown in Fig. 4-32. After oral administration, carbimazole is rapidly converted to methimazole and has identical properties to methimazole. Ten milligrams of carbimazole is approximately equivalent to 6 milligrams methimazole. Methimazole and PTU are concentrated within the thyroid gland and inhibit the synthesis of thyroid hormones by inhibiting oxidation of iodide, organification of iodide, and coupling of iodothyronines to form T_4 and T_3 (Manna et al, 2013). Most studies suggest that the mode of action is via inhibition of thyroid peroxidase, although PTU also inhibits the type-I iodothyronine deiodinase (ID-I) thus impairing peripheral deiodination of T_4 to T_3 (Cooper, 2013). None of the anti-thyroid drugs affects the iodide pump, which concentrates iodide in the thyroid cells, or the secretion of thyroid hormone formed prior to treatment (Peterson and Becker, 1995). Although thioureylenes decrease thyroid hormone concentrations and thereby control the clinical signs of hyperthyroidism, they are not cytotoxic to the thyroid gland and do not resolve the underlying cause of hyperthyroidism.

When administered orally, anti-thyroid drugs are rapidly absorbed and have a volume of distribution close to that of total body water. Methimazole has a plasma half-life of 1.4 to 10 hours in cats; although because the drug is concentrated in the thyroid gland and the intrathyroidal turnover is low, the duration of the biologic effect exceeds the plasma half-life.

Propylthiouracil

Although PTU is effective in blocking the synthesis of thyroid hormones in cats and controlling hyperthyroidism, it has been reported to cause an unacceptable rate of mild to severe adverse effects. These include anorexia, vomiting, lethargy, immune-mediated hemolytic anemia, and thrombocytopenia (Peterson et al, 1984; Aucoin et al, 1985; 1988). Because of these side effects, PTU is not recommended for use in cats. It has been hypothesized that taurine deficiency, which impairs drug elimination, may have exacerbated the side effects of PTU when it was first used, but the drug is not currently recommended for use in cats.

Methimazole (Tapazole)

Indications

Methimazole has three indications in the treatment of hyperthyroidism. First, it can be used to normalize serum T_4 concentrations and allow assessment of the effect of resolution of hyperthyroidism on clinical signs, renal function, and other laboratory parameters prior to definitive treatment (see Fig. 4-31). Second, it can be used for short-term stabilization of hyperthyroidism in cats with severe clinical manifestations of hyperthyroidism prior to surgery or radioactive iodine treatment. Lastly, it can be used for long-term treatment of hyperthyroidism (Fig. 4-33 and Fig. 4-34).

Advantages

The advantages and disadvantages of oral methimazole therapy are shown in Table 4-13. Methimazole is relatively inexpensive and readily available, and it does not require sophisticated training, facilities, or prolonged hospitalization. The medication can be administered by owners, is relatively safe, and can be given to the oldest of hyperthyroid cats. Furthermore, the drug can also be administered topically (Hoffman et al, 2002; Sartor et al, 2004; Hill et al, 2011).

Methimazole reversibly inhibits thyroid hormone synthesis, and therefore there is no risk of permanent hypothyroidism. In general, the adverse effects are reversible after discontinuation. Methimazole is considered the anti-thyroid drug of choice in cats in the United States and is reported to be effective for control of hyperthyroidism in approximately 90% of hyperthyroid cats.

Oral Dosage Protocol. Methimazole is available as 2.5 mg and 5 mg sugar-coated tablets in a veterinary labelled product and in 5, 10, and 15 mg tablets in a human labelled product.

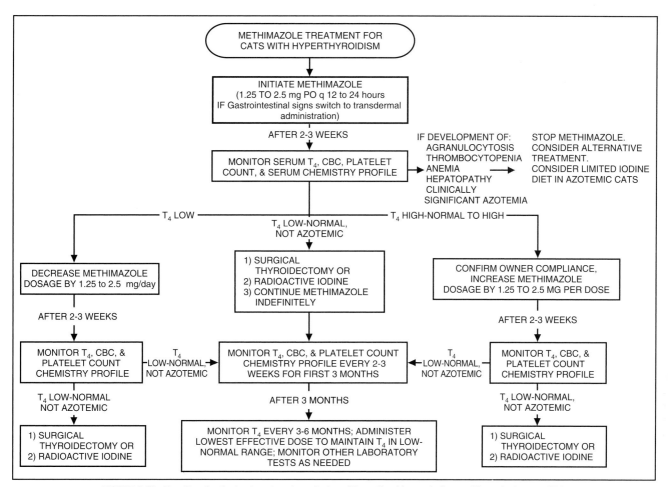

FIGURE 4-33 Algorithm for the treatment and monitoring of hyperthyroid cats during methimazole therapy. *CBC,* Complete blood count; T_4, thyroxine.

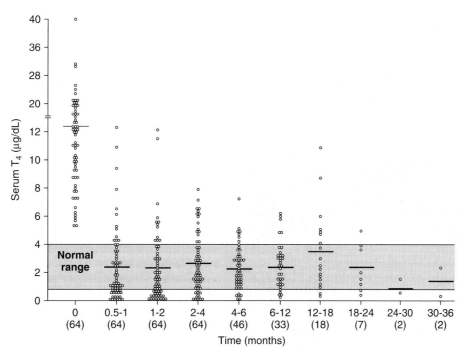

FIGURE 4-34 Serum thyroxine (T_4) concentrations in 64 cats with hyperthyroidism before and during long-term treatment with methimazole. The *horizontal lines* indicate mean values. The *numbers in parentheses* indicate the number of cats treated during each time period. (From Peterson ME, et al.: Methimazole treatment of 262 cats with hyperthyroidism, *J Vet Intern Med* 2[3]:150-157, 1988.)

The veterinary labelled sugar-coated tablets do not have the bitter taste of the uncoated human products, which reduces the risk of excessive salivation associated with methimazole administration in some cats. Whether oral methimazole can be absorbed through human skin has not been determined, but the sugar-coated tablets are less likely to result in systemic absorption.

The usual recommended starting dose for methimazole is 1.25 to 2.5 mg every 12 hours, with the more conservative dose recommended in very small and debilitated cats or those considered at high risk for adverse effects. The methimazole dose should be titrated every 2-3 weeks until the serum thyroid hormone concentration is within the lower half of the reference range (see Fig. 4-33). The total T_4 usually decreases within 1 week of treatment with oral methimazole, and the clinical signs improve within 2 to 3 weeks. Because the risk of adverse drug effects are highest during the initial 2 to 3 months of treatment, cats should be reassessed every 2-3 weeks with a history and physical examination, and blood should be obtained for a CBC, platelet count, serum biochemistry profile (BUN, creatinine, hepatic enzymes), and serum T_4 concentration in order to monitor for signs of toxicity and deterioration of renal function. Cats should be assessed in a similar way if they become clinically ill during treatment. Studies suggest that the length of time between drug administration and blood sample collection does not influence the serum thyroid hormone concentration during methimazole treatment; therefore a blood sample for therapeutic monitoring can be collected at any time of day (Rutland et al, 2009; Boretti et al, 2013a). If the serum T_4 concentration is within the lower half of the reference range, the dose should be maintained for an additional 2 to 6 weeks to allow determination of the need for any further dosage adjustments. If the serum T_4 concentration is below the reference range, the dose should be reduced. If the hyperthyroidism is not controlled, the dosage should continue to be increased every 2 weeks in increments of 2.5 mg a day until the measured total T_4 concentration is within the lower half of the reference range. If adverse effects are identified, methimazole should be discontinued. A decision can then be made to choose an alternative therapy, switch to transdermal methimazole, or reinitiate treatment using a lower dose of oral methimazole.

Most cats require 2.5 to 5 mg of methimazole every 12 hours to control hyperthyroidism, and total T_4 concentrations increase to pretreatment levels within 48 hours of discontinuing treatment (Peterson et al, 1988). Methimazole is more effective when administered twice a day than once a day at least for the first 4 weeks of treatment (Trepanier et al, 2003). Most cats require long-term twice daily treatment, but in some cats the frequency of dosing can be reduced to every 24 hours after a few weeks of treatment. The dose range of methimazole reported in the literature for long-term control of hyperthyroidism is 2.5 to 20 mg methimazole total mg dose per day. The most common reasons for treatment failure include problems with owner compliance and occurrence of adverse effects. Cats with very large goiters and those with thyroid carcinoma may be more resistant to treatment with methimazole.

Topical (Transdermal) Methimazole

Methimazole can also be administered to hyperthyroid cats as a topical gel. Methimazole is usually compounded in a pluronic lecithin organogel, which is a permeation enhancer that disrupts the stratum corneum and allows absorption into the systemic circulation (Sartor et al, 2004). Some methimazole may also be ingested by the oral route during grooming. Another novel lipophilic formulation has also been reported to result in effective absorption of methimazole (Hill et al, 2011). Methimazole for

transdermal application is usually dispensed in tuberculin syringes and can be formulated in a variety of concentrations (typically 2.5 or 5 mg/0.1 mL). The gel is applied to the non-haired pinna of the ear by the owners using a finger-cot. Dosing is alternated between ears and, if necessary, residual gel is removed from the ear prior to the next application using a cotton ball. In a study of 47 cats with newly diagnosed hyperthyroidism, randomized to receive either oral or transdermal methimazole, significantly more cats treated with oral methimazole were euthyroid than those treated with transdermal methimazole after 2 weeks of treatment, but by 4 weeks the difference was no longer significant. Nine of 11 cats treated with oral methimazole were euthyroid at 4 weeks, versus 14 of 21 cats receiving methimazole transdermally (Trepanier et al, 2003). Although the difference in efficacy at 4 weeks was not statistically significant, this may have been due to the smaller number of cats remaining in the study after 4 weeks. There is no difference in the incidence of hepatic, hematologic, or dermatologic side effects in cats treated with oral versus transdermal methimazole, but significantly fewer gastrointestinal side effects are observed with the transdermal form of treatment (Sartor et al, 2004). Some cats have mild inflammation and erythema of the pinnae where the drug is applied, and rarely these result in discontinuation of the drug. Other studies have confirmed that transdermal methimazole therapy can be very effective for long-term treatment of feline hyperthyroidism at doses ranging from 2.5 mg every 24 hours to 5 mg every 12 hours (Hill et al, 2011; Boretti et al, 2013a). In a long-term study of 60 cats treated with transdermal methimazole at doses ranging from 1 to 15 mg per day, clinical improvement was seen in all cats although higher doses were required after prolonged treatment, and several cats repeatedly had T_4 concentrations above or below the reference range during the study (Boretti et al, 2013b). Although most studies have evaluated transdermal methimazole administered every 12 hours, some cats are effectively managed with once daily administration (Fig. 4-35) (Boretti et al, 2013a).

The advantages of topical methimazole include the ease of administration and the decreased risk of gastrointestinal side effects. Disadvantages include the added expense, slightly slower onset of control of hyperthyroidism, and slightly lower efficacy. Care should be taken to ensure that children are not exposed to the methimazole gel. It is important to remember that there is little regulation of compounding pharmacies and care should be taken when choosing a pharmacy. Studies suggest that methimazole compounded in an organogel should be stored at room temperature and should be discarded after 60 days or earlier if there is visible separation of the components in the dosing syringe (Pignato et al, 2010).

Trial Methimazole Therapy to Assess Renal Function After Reestablishment of Euthyroid State

As discussed earlier, because it is not possible to accurately predict which cats will develop a clinically significant exacerbation of azotemia after therapy for hyperthyroidism, a clinical trial with methimazole is recommended in most cats prior to definitive treatment (see Figs. 4-31 and 4-33).

The recommended treatment protocol for a methimazole trial is to administer methimazole at an initial dose of 1.25 to 2.5 mg. A CBC, serum chemistry profile, and total T_4 is measured every 2 to 3 weeks, and the dose of methimazole adjusted until euthyroidism is achieved. If after 4 weeks of euthyroidism, the renal parameters are stable or only mildly increased, definitive treatment can be pursued. However, if the renal parameters worsen when the euthyroid state is reestablished, long-term treatment with a conservative

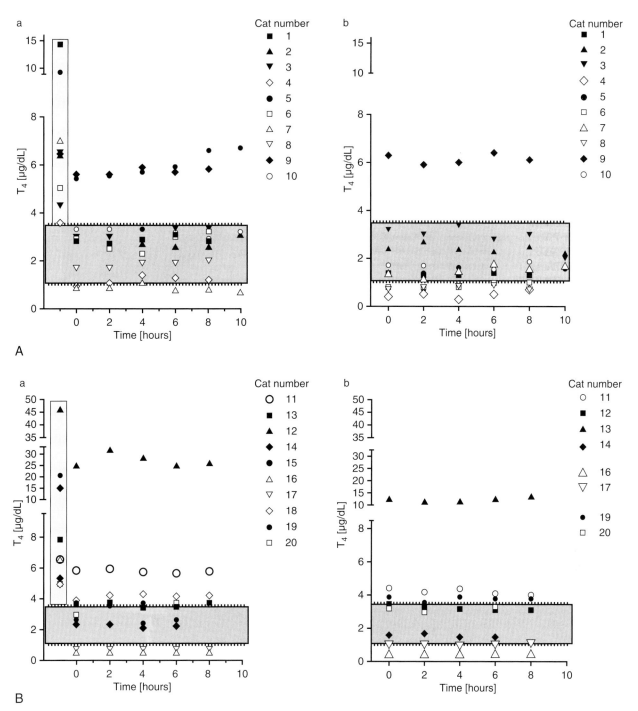

FIGURE 4-35 A, Change in serum T_4 concentrations during a 10-hour sampling period before and after twice daily transdermal methimazole application. Sustained T_4 suppression is evident during the whole observation period for most cats. *Dark gray shaded (horizontal area)* reference range T_4 concentrations, *light gray shaded (vertical area)* in **A:** T_4 concentrations before starting treatment. *a)* Week 1; *b)* Week 3. **B,** Change in serum T_4 concentrations during a 10-hour sampling period before and after once daily transdermal methimazole application. Sustained T_4 suppression is evident during the whole observation period for most cats. *Gray shaded (horizontal area)* reference range T_4 concentrations, *light-gray shaded (vertical area)* in **B:** T_4 concentrations before starting treatment. *a)* Week 1; *b)* Week 3. (From Boretti FS, et al.: Duration of T_4 suppression in hyperthyroid cats treated once and twice daily with transdermal methimazole, *J Vet Intern Med* 27[2]:377-381, 2013.)

TABLE 4-14   ADVERSE REACTIONS ASSOCIATED WITH DRUGS USED THERAPEUTICALLY IN FELINE HYPERTHYROIDISM

DRUG	REACTION	APPROXIMATE PERCENTAGE OF CATS AFFECTED	TIME AT OCCURRENCE	TREATMENT REQUIRED
Methimazole	Vomiting, anorexia, depression	15	< 4 weeks	Usually transient, decrease dose
	Eosinophilia, leukopenia, lymphocytosis	15	< 8 weeks	Usually transient
	Self-induced excoriations	2	< 4 weeks	Withdrawal and glucocorticoid therapy
	Agranulocytosis, thrombocytopenia	< 5	< 3 months	Withdrawal and symptomatic therapy
	Hepatopathy (anorexia,↑alanine aminotransferase, alkaline phosphatase)	< 2	< 2 months	Withdrawal and symptomatic therapy
	Positive antinuclear antibody	> 50	> 6 months	Decrease daily dosage
	Acquired myasthenia gravis	Rare	< 16 weeks	Withdrawal and appropriate treatment
Carbimazole	Vomiting, anorexia, depression	10	< 3 weeks	Usually transient, decrease dose
	Eosinophilia, leukopenia, lymphocytosis	5	< 2 weeks	Usually transient
	Self-induced excoriations	Rare	< 4 weeks	Withdrawal and glucocorticoid therapy
Stable iodine	Salivation and anorexia	Occasional	Immediate	Change formulation

dose of methimazole or alternatively nutritional management of hyperthyroidism should be considered. The goal is to minimize the clinical signs of hyperthyroidism as much as possible without causing escalation in renal failure.

Adverse Effects of Methimazole

Adverse effects of treatment with methimazole are common in cats (Table 4-14) and can occur whether methimazole is administered orally or transdermally.

Clinical Side Effects. Relatively mild clinical side effects from methimazole therapy are common, occurring in approximately 10% to 25% of cats (Peterson et al, 1988; Sartor et al, 2004). Most side effects are observed during the first 4 to 8 weeks of treatment; it is rare for a cat to develop methimazole-induced side effects after 2 to 3 months of treatment. The most common side effects include anorexia, vomiting, and lethargy (Peterson et al, 1988). These adverse reactions may be transient or may resolve after the dose is decreased. Gastrointestinal signs are managed by discontinuing the drug until all signs of toxicity have resolved for at least a week and then restarting the medication at a lower dose. The gastrointestinal side effects may result from direct gastric irritation, because they are much less common in cats treated with transdermal methimazole (Sartor et al, 2004).

Self-induced excoriation of the face and neck is an unusual reaction to methimazole seen in 2% to 3% of cats treated with methimazole. Like most of the drug's adverse effects, this problem usually occurs within the first 4 to 8 weeks of therapy. The characteristic scabbed lesions at the base of the pinna may improve after treatment with glucocorticoids, although drug discontinuation is usually necessary for complete resolution. Alternative treatment should be considered for these cats. Lymphadenopathy has also been reported in a cat treated with methimazole (Niessen et al, 2007), although other causes of lymphadenopathy were not completely ruled out.

Blood Dyscrasias. Mild hematologic changes caused by methimazole include eosinophilia, lymphocytosis, and mild leukopenia.

These changes are common in methimazole treated cats but do not usually require discontinuation of treatment. More severe hematologic reactions are much less common (3% to 9% cats) and include severe thrombocytopenia associated with bleeding (platelet count less than 75,000/µL), and neutropenia (less than 500/µL) associated with fever, anorexia, lethargy, and localized or systemic infections (Peterson et al, 1988). Any severe blood dyscrasia should prompt immediate cessation of treatment, and resolution usually occurs within 1 week. The mechanism for blood dyscrasias due to methimazole is unknown, but in humans these adverse effects are believed to be immune-mediated (Trepanier, 2006). Aplastic anemia was reported in a cat that had been treated with methimazole for 3 years, but the cat also had a mast cell tumor (Weiss 2006). In the largest case series of cats treated with methimazole, approximately 20% had had positive antinuclear antibody (ANA) test results, and 2% developed a positive direct Coombs test (Peterson et al, 1988). The risk of a positive antinuclear antibody (ANA) increased with duration of treatment and dose of methimazole. The importance of this finding is not known, because methimazole is not associated with development of lupus erythematosus or immune mediated hemolytic anima in cats.

Bleeding tendencies unassociated with thrombocytopenia have been rarely reported in methimazole treated cats, and in humans methimazole is reported to interfere with the vitamin K–dependent coagulation factors. In a study of 20 cats treated with methimazole, three cats had abnormal coagulation profiles characterized by prolongation of protein induced by vitamin K absence or antagonism (PIVKA) prior to treatment, and one cat developed prolongation of PIVKA bleeding time, unassociated with clinical signs of bleeding, 2 to 6 weeks after treatment (Randolph et al, 2000). No cats developed prolongation of prothrombin time (PT) or activated partial thromboplastin time (APTT). If a coagulopathy is suspected in a hyperthyroid cat treated with methimazole, testing of PIVKA may be more sensitive than the standard PT and APTT.

Hepatic toxicity occurs in a small number of cats treated with methimazole. The hepatopathy is characterized by systemic signs of illness (anorexia, vomiting, and lethargy), icterus, and marked increases in serum ALT and ALP activities. Days to weeks may be required for all clinical and biochemical abnormalities to resolve after discontinuation of the drug. Alternative therapies for hyperthyroidism should be considered for cats that develop these adverse reactions.

Myasthenia gravis has been reported to develop in hyperthyroid cats treated with methimazole (Shelton et al, 2000; Bell et al, 2012) and may be caused by the immunomodulatory effects of the drug. Methimazole has been associated with a number of different immune mediated diseases in humans, but the precise mechanism is unknown. Myasthenia gravis was reported to resolve in the two cats in which methimazole was withdrawn; interestingly one cat that was subsequently treated with carbimazole did not have recurrence of signs, but it was also treated with pyridostigmine (Bell et al, 2012). An adverse drug effect should be suspected in cats treated with methimazole that develop myasthenia gravis and potentially other immune mediated disorders.

Hypothyroidism. Although cats treated with methimazole rarely show clinical signs of hypothyroidism, overtreatment resulting in biochemical hypothyroidism is relatively common (Williams et al, 2010). Cats with iatrogenic hypothyroidism are at increased risk of azotemia and have a shorter survival time than euthyroid azotemic cats so it is important to avoid hypothyroidism by appropriate dose adjustment (Williams et al, 2010).

Methimazole administration should be discontinued and appropriate supportive care provided to any cat in which a clinically significant adverse effect of methimazole is suspected. Adverse reactions typically resolve within 7 days after discontinuation of the drug (Peterson et al, 1988). For severe or life-threatening adverse effects, alternative treatment should be considered rather than risking reexposure to the drug. It is unclear whether treatment with methimazole can interfere with response to treatment with ^{131}I; therefore it is recommended that treatment should be discontinued 1 to 2 weeks prior to treatment (see Treatment with Radioactive Iodine for more on this topic).

Carbimazole

Background

Carbimazole is a pro-drug of methimazole that is used in Europe and Australia for treatment of feline hyperthyroidism. Carbimazole is rapidly and almost completely converted to methimazole, either in the gastrointestinal tract or immediately after absorption, because drug concentrations of methimazole but not carbimazole are detected in the serum and thyroid gland after ingestion (Peterson et al, 1993). Carbimazole has a higher molecular weight than methimazole, so 5 mg of carbimazole is equivalent to 3 mg of methimazole. The starting dose for carbimazole is 5 mg every 8 to 12 hours. There is also a controlled release tablet formulation that can be administered once a day at a starting dose of 10 to 15 mg every 24 hours. In one study, the dose range required to achieve euthyroidism ranged from 10 mg every other day to 25 mg per day (Frénais et al, 2009). There have been no studies directly comparing the efficacy and adverse effects associated with carbimazole versus methimazole; however, anecdotally carbimazole is associated with a lower rate of adverse effects than methimazole, and severe blood dyscrasias have not yet been reported in association with carbimazole. The most common adverse effects associated with carbimazole administration are gastrointestinal signs (Bucknell, 2000). Other adverse effects that have been reported include excoriations of the head and neck, lymphadenopathy, pruritus, lymphocytosis, and leucopenia (Mooney et al, 1992). Despite the

suggestion that there are fewer side effects associated with carbimazole administration, carbimazole is rapidly converted to methimazole, so its use in cats that have adverse reactions to methimazole is probably unwise (Trepanier, 2007).

 ## TREATMENT WITH SURGERY

Although surgical thyroidectomy is an effective and usually permanent treatment for feline hyperthyroidism, over the last 20 years it has become less commonly performed because of the increasing availability of radioiodine treatment facilities, the potential for recurrence due to residual ectopic thyroid tissue, and the risk of adverse postoperative clinical consequences, such as hypoparathyroidism and hypothyroidism. These complications can occur because the functional status of the thyroid gland cannot be determined by visual inspection, and therefore it not always possible to determine at surgery whether one or both thyroid glands should be removed. Other less common complications of thyroidectomy include Horner's syndrome and damage to the laryngeal nerve. Despite these limitations, thyroidectomy is a very effective treatment for feline hyperthyroidism, and the concerns discussed earlier can be minimized by preoperative scintigraphy and good surgical technique. The advantages of thyroidectomy include a short hospital stay provided treatment for hypoparathyroidism is not required, and the opportunity to evaluate thyroid tissue by histopathology, which is important in cats with suspected thyroid carcinoma. In our opinion, scintigraphy should always be performed prior to surgical thyroidectomy to determine whether thyroid disease is unilateral or bilateral and to rule out the presence of ectopic thyroid tissue. Unfortunately many practitioners do not have ready access to scintigraphy, but understanding the benefit of this procedure and knowing when to refer for it is important. For cats that are determined to have unilateral thyroid disease, thyroidectomy is a simple and speedy surgical procedure that results in rapid resolution of hyperthyroidism. For cats with bilateral thyroid disease, thyroidectomy should be performed only if there are good reasons for avoiding radioactive iodine treatment. If bilateral thyroidectomy is chosen, owners need to be warned about the possibility of postoperative complications, such as hypoparathyroidism or hypothyroidism. In cats with ectopic tissue identified by scintigraphy, surgical treatment is not recommended because it is not always possible to readily identify the location of ectopic tissue at the time of surgery. Even if ectopic tissue is identified and removed surgically, recurrence is common (Naan et al, 2006). Thyroidectomy is most appropriate for cats that do not tolerate hospitalization and for owners who are concerned about use of radioactive iodine for treatment.

Presurgical Management

In an attempt to minimize perisurgical and postsurgical complications, hyperthyroid cats must be thoroughly evaluated for concurrent illness prior to surgery. Problems such as congestive heart failure, cardiac arrhythmias, hypertension, renal failure, and electrolyte abnormalities (e.g., hypokalemia) should be identified and treated prior to surgery (Naan et al, 2006). Depending on the severity of the thyrotoxicosis and the needs of the individual case, consideration should be given to controlling thyrotoxicosis with medical therapy prior to surgery, both to decrease risk of anesthetic complications and assess the effect of euthyroidism on renal function (see Treatment of Hyperthyroidism and Renal Function). The goal is to make the cat as stable as possible prior to surgery.

Treatment with beta blockers may be useful prior to surgery to control severe tachycardia and supraventricular tachyarrhthmias in cats that do not tolerate anti-thyroid drugs.

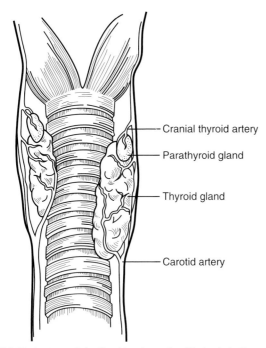

FIGURE 4-36 Anatomy of the thyroid and parathyroid glands in the cat. (From Panciera DL, Peterson ME, Birchard SJ: Diseases of the thyroid gland. In Birchard SJ, Sherding RG [eds]: *Saunders Manual of Small Animal Practice,* ed 3, St. Louis, 2006, Elsevier.)

Labels in figure:
- Cranial thyroid artery
- Parathyroid gland
- Thyroid gland
- Carotid artery

Anesthesia

The anesthetic protocol should be individualized based on the unique needs of each patient. Most cats undergoing anesthesia for thyroidectomy are fragile geriatric cats with concurrent medical problems. Particular attention should be paid to the renal and cardiovascular systems when planning anesthesia. Adequate fluid therapy is critical but overhydration must be avoided. Factors that should be taken into account include the body condition score, presence of concurrent illness, whether hyperthyroidism has been controlled with medical therapy prior to surgery, and how difficult the patient is to handle. The increased metabolic rate associated with hyperthyroidism increases the absorption, distribution, tissue uptake, and inactivation of anesthetic agents.

Premedication and Anesthesia Induction

Drugs that stimulate or potentiate adrenergic activity capable of inducing tachycardia and arrhythmias should be avoided. Anticholinergic agents (e.g., atropine) should also be avoided because they cause sinus tachycardia and enhance anesthetic-induced cardiac arrhythmias. The most common anesthetic protocol in our hospital is premedication with butorphanol (0.2 mg/kg) followed by induction with isoflurane in an anesthesia induction chamber. Induction with IV propofol (3 to 6 mg/kg to effect) with or without premedication is also an effective approach in cats in which an IV catheter can be placed prior to induction. Once anesthetized, the cat is intubated and inhalation anesthesia continued. In cats that are too fractious for placement of an IV catheter before induction, the catheter can be placed after use of an anesthesia induction chamber. It is important to minimize anesthesia/surgery time, and continuous monitoring of blood pressure, oxygen saturation, and the ECG is essential. Postoperative pain control should be routine. Buprenorphine (0.01 to 0.03 mg/kg every 6-8 hours IM IV or buccal) is a good choice for postoperative control of mild pain in cats.

Surgical Techniques

General Guidelines

Exploratory surgery of the ventrocervical region is relatively simple, quick, and inexpensive. The thyroid gland in the cat is divided into two lobes, which are usually located adjacent to the trachea and distal to the larynx, in close proximity to the carotid artery, jugular vein, and recurrent laryngeal nerve (Fig. 4-36). Normal thyroid lobes are pale tan, whereas a thyroid adenoma or adenomatous hyperplasia is typically brown to reddish brown. The area from above the normal location of the thyroids (hyoid region) down to the thoracic inlet should be examined with careful attention to hemostasis. After exposure and inspection of all visible thyroid tissue, the external parathyroid gland or glands should be identified (see Fig. 4-36). The external parathyroid glands are usually located in the loose fascia at the cranial pole of each lobe. The external parathyroids are much smaller than the thyroid lobes and can be distinguished from thyroid tissue by their lighter color and spherical shape (Birchard, 2006). The internal parathyroid glands are usually embedded in the thyroid lobe parenchyma and are variable in location.

Unilateral Versus Bilateral Involvement

Bilateral lobe involvement is present in more than 70% of hyperthyroid cats; however, in many cats, lobe enlargement is not symmetric. In unilateral cases, there is atrophy of the contralateral lobe, but the distinction between a small but hyperfunctional lobe and an atrophic lobe is not always obvious. For this reason, it is ideal to perform scintigraphy prior to surgery. If scintigraphy is not possible and a decision about whether to perform a unilateral or bilateral thyroidectomy has to be made at the time of surgery, the surgeon should determine whether the risk of persistence/recurrence of hyperthyroidism or the risk of hypoparathyroidism (and potentially hypothyroidism) are of the most concern. The decision depends upon the skill of the surgeon, the wishes of the owner, and whether or not the owners are able to administer oral medication for treatment of hypoparathyroidism and hypothyroidism.

Intracapsular Versus Extracapsular Thyroidectomy

Two surgical techniques have been described, and both have been successfully modified to enhance success rates for resolving hyperthyroidism and to preserve parathyroid tissue. The original intracapsular technique involved incision through the thyroid capsule and blunt dissection to separate and remove the thyroid lobe, leaving the capsule in situ. This technique did help preserve parathyroid tissue but was associated with recurrence due to regrowth of tissue adherent to the capsule (Swalec and Birchard, 1990). The original extracapsular technique involved removal of the intact thyroid lobe with its capsule, after ligation of the cranial thyroid artery, while attempting to preserve blood supply to the adjacent parathyroid gland. This technique reduced the recurrence rate but increased the risk of postsurgical hypoparathyroidism. Both these techniques have been modified (Fig. 4-37). The intracapsular modification involves removing most of the capsule after the thyroid tissue has been excised. The extracapsular modification involves use of bipolar electrocautery rather than ligatures, which minimizes blunt dissection around the parathyroid glands. The modified extracapsular technique is usually preferred, because it is quicker and is associated with less hemorrhage that could obscure the surgical field (Birchard, 2006; Welches et al, 1989).

Postsurgical Recurrence of Hyperthyroidism

Failure to remove all abnormal, adenomatous thyroid cells results in postsurgical recurrence of hyperthyroidism. In a study

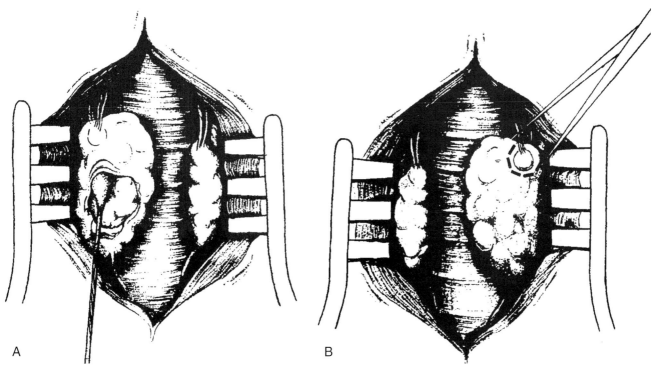

FIGURE 4-37 A, Intracapsular thyroidectomy. The thyroid capsule is incised and the thyroid lobe removed. (The modified technique involves excision of the capsule.) **B,** Extracapsular thyroidectomy. The thyroid lobe and capsule are removed, and the vascular supply to the external parathyroid glands is preserved. (The modified technique involves bipolar cautery rather than ligatures.) (From Mooney CT: Hyperthyroidism in cats, *Veterinary Practice* 22:103, 1990.)

of 101 cats undergoing thyroidectomy using a modified intracapsular technique, recurrence was reported in five cats (Naan et al, 2006). Three of these cats had had a previous thyroidectomy performed by the referring veterinarian, and four of the five cats had scintigraphic evidence of ectopic thyroid tissue that was removed at the time of surgery. Hyperthyroid cats with ectopic thyroid tissue had a significantly higher chance of recurrence even when the ectopic tissue was identified and removed at surgery. Recurrence of hyperthyroidism is uncommon in the absence of ectopic thyroid tissue (Swalec and Birchard, 1990; Naan et al, 2006).

Iatrogenic Hypoparathyroidism (Hypocalcemia)

One of the most serious complications associated with bilateral thyroidectomy is postsurgical hypocalcemia. Hypocalcemia has been reported in 6% to 82% of cats, depending on the surgical method (Birchard et al, 1984; Flanders et al, 1987; Welches et al, 1989; Naan et al, 2006). In most cats undergoing thyroidectomy, postoperative hypocalcemia is mild, transient, and attributed to local edema of the parathyroid gland and chronic depletion of bone calcium due to thyrotoxicosis. With successful surgery (even after unilateral tumor removal), the serum calcium concentration may decline below the reference range for several days as skeletal reserves are restored. This mild hypocalcemia (serum calcium concentration of 7.0 to 9.0 mg/dL) must be differentiated from the severe hypocalcemia associated with iatrogenic hypoparathyroidism. In a study of 86 cats undergoing bilateral thyroidectomy using the modified intracapsular technique, postoperative hypocalcemia required treatment in only five cats (Naan et al, 2006). Hypocalcemia in these five cats resolved after treatment with calcium and dihydrotachysterol within 3 to 6

days. The use of parathyroid transplantation in cats in which the parathyroid gland is accidentally removed or completely devascularized during surgery has been reported (Padgett et al, 1998). The parathyroid gland is cut into small 1 mm pieces and inserted into a pocket in the cervical musculature. This procedure may not prevent severe hypocalcemia from occurring in the first week after surgery but may prevent a long-term need for treatment of hypoparathyroidism.

Postsurgical Management

Management of Postoperative Hypocalcemia

The frequency of clinically significant hypocalcemia after bilateral thyroidectomy is variable and dependent upon the skills of the surgeon. If a bilateral thyroidectomy is performed, serum total or ionized calcium concentration should be assessed at least once daily for 4 to 7 days. As discussed earlier, it is common for mild and transient hypocalcaemia to develop after surgery. Clinically important hypocalcemia is usually associated with serum total calcium concentrations less than 7.0 mg/dL (ionized calcium less than 0.8 mmol/L). Cats should be carefully observed for clinical signs of hypocalcaemia (Box 4-4). Ideally, hypocalcemia should be documented by measurement of total or ionized calcium concentration before therapy is begun. If an acute crisis with clinical signs of tetany develops, a blood sample should be obtained for later evaluation and immediate treatment with IV calcium should be instituted. Management with oral vitamin D and calcium supplementation is initiated immediately after normalization of serum calcium by parenteral administration (see Chapter 16 for further discussion of management of hypocalcemia).

BOX 4-4   Signs Associated with Hypocalcemia in Cats

Anorexia
Restlessness
"Irritability"
Abnormal behavior
Muscle cramping or muscle pain
Muscle tremors, especially of face and ears
Tetany
Convulsions

Calcitriol (Rocaltrol; Roche, Nutley, NJ) is an analogue of activated vitamin D_3 (1,25 dihydroxycholecalciferol) and is the most effective vitamin D product for treatment of hypoparathyroidism. The advantages include quick onset of action, quick dissipation from the body if overdose occurs, and consistent effect. The recommended dose in cats is 0.02 to 0.03 µg/kg/day for 2 to 4 days; the dose is then tapered based on the serum calcium concentration. The maintenance dose is typically 0.005 to 0.015 µg/kg/day. Reformulation by a compounding pharmacy may be required for accurate dosing of calcitriol in cats.

Ergocalciferol (vitamin D_2) is a less expensive form of vitamin D that has to be converted to active vitamin D_3 and is not recommended for treatment of cats with postsurgical hypocalcemia. Ergocalciferol is available in a liquid solution suitable for administration to cats. Usually 10,000 IU given orally once daily increases serum calcium concentrations, but it can take from 5 to 21 days before an effect is seen. Because this vitamin preparation is fat soluble, tissue accumulation and subsequent hypercalcemia can occur. The ultimate dosage interval may be as infrequent as once every 7 to 14 days.

Dihydrotachysterol. Dihydrotachysterol is a synthetic analogue of vitamin D that has a more rapid onset of action than ergocalciferol and a shorter duration of activity; this reduces the risk of tissue accumulation and prolonged iatrogenic hypercalcemia. The starting dose is 0.03 mg/kg given orally once daily for 1 to 7 days until the serum calcium concentration increases into the reference range. The dose should then be decreased to 0.02 mg/kg and further dose adjustments made based on the serum calcium concentration. Unfortunately this product is currently not available commercially, although it can be obtained from some compounding pharmacies.

Calcium Supplementation. To control clinical signs of tetany, IV calcium gluconate should be administered slowly to effect (5 to 15 mg/kg), using ECG monitoring for detecting bradycardia or arrhythmias. Calcium gluconate mixed in an equal volume of saline can then be given subcutaneously two to four times a day, at a dose equal to that initially given intravenously, to control clinical signs of hypocalcemia. Calcium chloride should never be given subcutaneously, because it causes tissue irritation. Oral calcium supplementation can be accomplished with several over the counter calcium lactate or carbonate preparations. The dose is 0.5 to 1 g of calcium per cat/day.

Duration of Hypoparathyroidism. The persistence of hypoparathyroidism after thyroidectomy is variable and difficult to predict. Some cats may need medication for only a few days, whereas others require therapy for the rest of their lives. Recovery of parathyroid function may occur after days, weeks, or months of vitamin D and calcium supplementation. Whenever resolution of hypoparathyroidism is observed, it is assumed that reversible parathyroid damage occurred or that accessory parathyroid tissue has begun to compensate for glands damaged or removed at surgery. It is possible that accommodation of calcium-regulating mechanisms may occur despite absence of PTH (Flanders et al, 1991).

Replacement vitamin D therapy can suppress recovery of endogenous PTH secretion and cause hypercalcemia. After starting vitamin D therapy in any cat, the serum calcium concentration should be monitored prior to each planned dose reduction (every 2 weeks) and the dose gradually decreased if possible based on the results of these measurements. The tapering process can begin days to weeks after the start of vitamin D therapy and may take as long as 2 to 4 months. The goal is to maintain the serum calcium concentration within the low-normal range (8.5 to 9.5 mg/dL). In this range, clinical signs of hypocalcemia do not occur, but there is stimulation of growth and function of any atrophied parathyroid tissue. If accessory parathyroid tissue is present and functional, the medications may be completely discontinued within weeks to months of surgery. If hypocalcemia recurs, therapy with vitamin D and calcium must be reinstituted and is likely to be necessary lifelong.

Hypothyroidism

Subtotal Thyroidectomy. Cats that have undergone unilateral thyroidectomy may transiently develop low serum T_4 values. Thyroid hormone supplementation is not indicated in these cats. The remaining atrophied thyroid regains normal function within 1 to 3 months. Replacement thyroid medication only delays the growth and functional return of atrophied thyroid tissue.

Total Thyroidectomy. Plasma thyroid hormone concentrations decline, often to subnormal levels, within 24 to 72 hours of total thyroidectomy. However, not all cats become permanently hypothyroid, probably because of growth of accessory thyroid tissue in the neck or anterior mediastinum. Thyroid supplementation should only be initiated in the first few weeks after surgery if clinical signs of hypothyroidism (e.g., lethargy and obesity) are noted (see Chapter 3) or if there is a decline in renal function. Cats that are persistently hypothyroid 3 to 6 months after thyroidectomy should also be supplemented.

If thyroid replacement therapy is deemed necessary, L-T_4 at a dose of 0.05 mg to 0.1 mg once or twice a day is recommended. Not all cats will require thyroid supplementation long term, because some may recover endogenous thyroid function. Whether this represents the recovery of cellular function of cells left in situ or developing function in accessory tissue is not clear. Regardless, thyroid replacement therapy can suppress endogenous secretion of thyroid hormone; therefore the need for long-term treatment can only be determined after 8 to 12 weeks following discontinuation of thyroid replacement therapy.

Recurrence of Hyperthyroidism. Because of the potential for recurrence of hyperthyroidism, all cats treated surgically should have their serum thyroid hormone status monitored once or twice yearly (Welches et al, 1989; Swalec and Birchard, 1990). In cats with recurrence of hyperthyroidism, treatment with oral antithyroid medication or with radioactive iodine is recommended, because the incidence of surgical complications is considerably higher among cats undergoing a second surgery than among those undergoing their first surgery (Welches et al, 1989; Naan et al, 2006). Scintigraphy may be useful in these cats to document the location of functioning thyroid tissue and investigate for evidence of thyroid carcinoma.

Persistence of Hyperthyroidism. Rarely, clinical signs of hyperthyroidism persist despite unilateral or bilateral thyroidectomy.

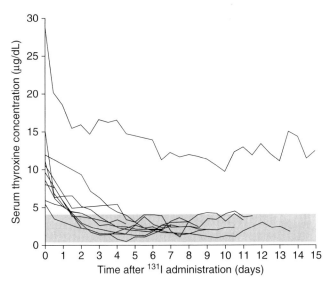

FIGURE 4-38 Serum thyroxine (T₄) concentrations in 10 hyperthyroid cats sampled every 12 hours following iodine-131 (¹³¹I) therapy. Note how quickly the T₄ concentrations decline. *Shaded region* represents the normal reference range. (From Meric S, et al.: Serum thyroxine concentrations after radioactive iodine therapy in cats with hyperthyroidism, *J Am Vet Med Assoc* 188[9]: 1038-1040, 1986.)

This is most common in cats undergoing thyroidectomy without prior scintigraphy and implies that not all abnormal thyroid tissue was removed surgically. Such ectopic tissue is most likely to be in the mediastinum, cranial to the heart. This complication can usually be avoided by preoperative thyroid scintigraphy.

Results of Surgery

In most veterinary hospitals, the results of surgery are excellent. Most treated cats respond well with resolution of the hyperthyroidism. Exceptions include cats with concurrent disease (e.g., renal failure), cats with unrecognized ectopic thyroid tissue, and cats that undergo unilateral thyroidectomy but that have adenomatous tissue in the contralateral gland. The major advantages of surgery are that the procedure can be performed by most practitioners; it is relatively inexpensive; it can result in a permanent cure; and morbidity and mortality can be minimized by appropriate presurgical and postsurgical management protocols.

TREATMENT WITH RADIOACTIVE IODINE

Thyroid cells concentrate radioactive iodine as they do stable iodine. Treatment with the radioisotope ¹³¹I is an effective and well-established treatment for hyperthyroidism in both cats and humans with a success rate of about 95% in both species. After IV or SC administration, radioactive iodine is transported into hyperplastic and neoplastic thyroid follicular cells and incorporated into thyroglobulin. The percentage uptake of iodide by the thyroid gland in hyperthyroid cats ranges from 10% to 60% (Broome et al, 1987; van Hoek et al, 2008b). The remainder of the administered iodine is excreted in the urine and feces. The isotope ¹³¹I emits both gamma rays and beta particles. It is the ionizing effects of the beta particles that are responsible for follicular cell death, manifested histopathologically as cell necrosis and inflammation. In humans, bizarre nuclear changes reminiscent of carcinoma are present cytologically after ¹³¹I treatment and may

persist for years. Care must thus be taken in interpreting thyroid cytology after radioiodine treatment.

Because beta particles travel only a short distance (1 to 2 mm) in tissue, surrounding tissues (e.g., the parathyroid glands) are spared the effects of ¹³¹I. In addition because atrophic thyroid tissue does not concentrate iodine, only functional thyroid tissue is affected by treatment. Thus, once hyperthyroidism is resolved and the normal feedback loops are reestablished, previously atrophic thyroid follicular cells return to function and long-term hypothyroidism is avoided.

Radioactive iodine therapy is now considered the treatment of choice for managing feline hyperthyroidism and is available in numerous locations throughout the United States and other countries. High dose treatment with ¹³¹I is also effective for treatment of cats with functional thyroid carcinoma (see Feline Thyroid Carcinoma).

Goal of Therapy

The goal of ¹³¹I therapy is to resolve hyperthyroidism and avoid hypothyroidism. In most cats, thyroid hormone concentrations normalize over a period of days to a few weeks (Meric et al, 1986; Peterson and Becker, 1995; Figs. 4-38 to 4-40). Various methods have been evaluated to determine a dose that results in a high success rate but does not induce hypothyroidism. Ideally the lowest effective dose should be used to minimize exposure to hospital personnel and family members.

Dose Determination

The radiation dose received by the thyroid gland is dependent on the dose administered, the thyroidal uptake of the isotope, and the duration of iodine retention by the thyroid gland. Three methods have been used to determine the appropriate dose of ¹³¹I for treatment of hyperthyroidism in cats. The dose can be determined by tracer studies, use of a scoring system, or a predetermined fixed dose can be administered. Interestingly all methods appear to result in the same clinical outcome in regard to both efficacy and rate of posttreatment hypothyroidism.

Iodine-131 Dose Determined by Tracer Studies

Prior to administration of therapeutic ¹³¹I, tracer studies can be performed to calculate RAIU and effective half-life of the radionuclide using a tracer dose of ¹³¹I (Broome, 1988b). The radiation dose is calculated based on the RAIU, tracer half-life, and estimated size of the thyroid gland based on technetium scans and digital palpation (Turrel et al, 1984; Meric et al, 1986; Theon et al, 1994). Using this approach, 94% of cats were euthyroid 1 year after treatment, and 84% were euthyroid 4 years after treatment, whereas 6% of cats became hypothyroid (Theon et al, 1994). Subsequent studies however have shown that the biologic half-life of ¹³¹I determined by tracer studies does not correlate well with the biologic half-life after administration of therapeutic doses of radioactive iodine, probably because of the changes in thyroid physiology after administration of large doses of ¹³¹I and resultant follicular cell necrosis.

Iodine-131 Dose Determined by Serum Thyroxine Concentration and Severity of Disease

This method of ¹³¹I dose determination uses a variety of scoring systems that use the severity of clinical signs, the subjective size of the abnormal thyroid(s), and the serum T₄ concentration

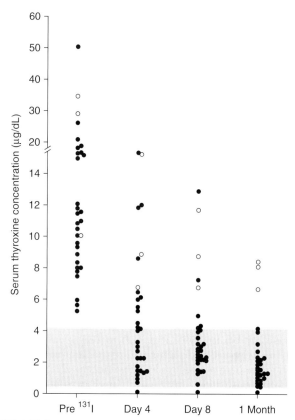

FIGURE 4-39 Serum thyroxine (T_4) concentrations in 31 hyperthyroid cats treated with iodine-131 (^{131}I). These cats were studied before therapy, 4 and 8 days after therapy, at the time of hospital discharge (variable), and 1 month after treatment. Note how quickly the T_4 concentrations decline. *Open circles* represent the three cats that remained hyperthyroid 1 month after treatment. *Shaded area* represents the normal reference range. (From Meric S, et al.: Serum thyroxine concentrations after radioactive iodine therapy in cats with hyperthyroidism, *J Am Vet Med Assoc* 188[9]:1038-1040, 1986.)

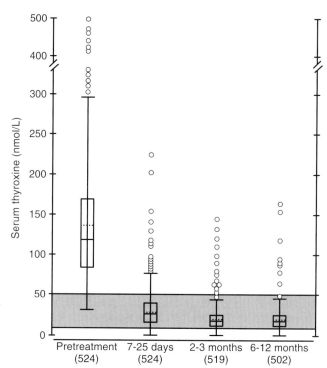

FIGURE 4-40 Box plots of serum thyroxine (T_4) concentrations in 524 cats before and at various times after administration of radioiodine for treatment of hyperthyroidism (see Fig. 4-10 for key). (From Peterson ME, Becker DV: Radioiodine treatment of 524 cats with hyperthyroidism, *J Am Vet Med Assoc* 207[11]:1422, 1995.)

	TABLE 4-15	**SCORING SYSTEM USED TO DETERMINE DOSE OF RADIOACTIVE IODINE IN CATS**

FACTOR	**CLASSIFICATION**	**SCORE**
Clinical Signs*	Mild	1
	Moderate	2
	Severe	3
Serum T_4 concentration	< 125 nmol/L (10 μg/dL)	1
	125-250 nmol/L (10-20 μg/dL)	2
	> 250 nmol/L (20 μg/dL)	3
Thyroid tumor size[†]	< 1.0 × 0.5 cm	1
	1.0 × 0.5 to 3.0 × 1.0 cm	2
	> 3.0 × 1.0 cm	3

From Peterson ME, Becker DV: Radioiodine treatment of 524 cats with hyperthyroidism, *J Am Vet Med Assoc* 207(11):1422-1428, 1995.
Cats with a total score of 3, 4, or 5 were treated with a low dose (2.0 to 3.4 mCi; 74 to 130 megabecquerels [MBq]), cats with a total score of 6 or 7 were treated with a moderate dose (3.5 to 4.4 mCi; 130 to 167 MBq), and cats with a total score of 8 or 9 were treated with a high dose (4.5 to 6.0 mCi; 167 to 222 MBq) of radioiodine.
*Severity of clinical signs determined on the basis of number and magnitude of clinical signs and the duration of illness.
†Thyroid tumor size estimated from digital palpation of the thyroid gland; if both thyroid lobes were enlarged, the sizes of both lobes were added together to determine the score.

to determine the dose administered (Jones et al, 1991; Mooney,1994; Peterson and Becker, 1995; Table 4-15). In the largest such study, a low (2.5 to 3.5 mCi), moderate (3.5 to 4.5 mCi), or high (4.5 to 6.5 mCi) dose of ^{131}I was administered to hyperthyroid cats (Peterson and Becker, 1995). The median dose administered was 3 mCi. The response to treatment was considered good in 94% of cats. Fewer than 2% of more than 500 cats remained hyperthyroid at 6 months and required a second dose of iodine (see Fig. 4-40). Only 2% developed signs and laboratory data consistent with a diagnosis of hypothyroidism. A similar number of cats (2%) had a relapse of hyperthyroidism within 1 to 6 years of treatment.

Administration of a Fixed Dose Iodine-131

Other investigators have evaluated the efficacy of administration if a fixed dose of ^{131}I for treatment of feline hyperthyroidism (Meric and Rubin, 1990; Chun, 2002; Forrest et al, 1996; Craig, 1993). The most commonly utilized dose reported was 4 mCi. Of 321 cats treated with 4 mCi, a good response to treatment was reported in 96% of cats and 7% were reported to become hypothyroid (Chun, 2002; Meric and Rubin, 1990; Craig, 1993).

There have been no studies that have directly compared these three methods of radioactive iodine dose estimation. All approaches have resulted in a high success rate and low incidence of hypothyroidism and therefore tracer studies are now rarely

performed. Whether dose estimation using a scoring system is superior to a fixed dose method requires further study. In theory, such an approach should decrease incidence of hypothyroidism, decrease hospitalization time, and decrease radiation exposure to personnel.

Treatment of Thyroid Carcinoma

Fewer than 2% to 3% of hyperthyroid cats are diagnosed with thyroid carcinoma. Findings that increase the likelihood of thyroid carcinoma include recurrence after surgery or low dose radioactive iodine treatment, a thyroid mass that is very large or irregular, "fixed" or attached to underlying tissues, or documentation of metastatic disease. On thyroid scintigraphy, some cats with thyroid carcinoma have scans indistinguishable from adenomatous hyperplasia or an adenoma, and some cats have large, irregular masses, more than two masses, or obvious distant metastases on scintigraphy. Confirmation of thyroid carcinoma requires histopathology; however, because some thyroid carcinomas are well differentiated, the diagnosis can be difficult to confirm unless there is evidence of metastasis or capsular or vascular invasion (Guptill et al, 1995). If thyroid carcinoma is confirmed, higher doses of radioactive iodine are required for effective treatment (10 to 30 mCi) (Turrel, 1988; Guptill et al, 1995; Hibbert, 2009). In our experience, the best outcomes are achieved with a combination of surgical debulking followed by administration of a high dose of radioactive iodine (Turrel et al, 1988; Guptill et al, 1995). Other investigators have relied on treatment with high dose radioactive iodine without prior debulking surgery with a good outcome reported in the majority of cases (Hibbert et al, 2009). The decision as to whether to perform debulking surgery depends on whether prior surgery has been performed, whether there is histopathologic confirmation of thyroid carcinoma, and the location of the neoplastic tissue. Risks of surgery include hypoparathyroidism, injury to structures (e.g., the recurrent laryngeal nerve), and the additional expense. Risks of treatment without surgery include the consequences of extensive tissue necrosis if there is a large volume of neoplastic tissue, especially if the thyroid tissue is intrathoracic, and the possibility of variable uptake of iodine by cells within the tumor such that not all neoplastic cells are destroyed. Ultimately the decision should be made on a case by case basis. Longer hospitalization can be anticipated if cats receive high doses of ^{131}I due to the additional time required for isotope excretion. Most cats treated with such high doses of radioactive iodine will become permanently hypothyroid.

Route of [131]-Iodine Administration

Although most early studies utilized the IV route of administration, ^{131}I can be safely administered subcutaneously, and studies have demonstrated that administration of radioactive iodine IV or SC is equally effective. Use of the SC route is safer for personnel and, subjectively, less stressful for the cat (Théon et al, 1994). Although commonly used in humans, oral ^{131}I is not recommended because of the increased risk of exposure to radiation by the personnel dosing the cats and the risk of vomiting after administration. Vomiting of the isotope not only results in inadequate dose administered but also could result in contamination of the nuclear medicine facility.

Prior Treatment with Methimazole

Methimazole inhibits synthesis of thyroid hormones but does not interfere with iodine trapping by follicular cells. In people, PTU lowers the efficacy of subsequent radioactive iodine treatment, and continuous treatment with methimazole during treatment decreases the final cure rate. Pretreatment with methimazole up to 7 days prior to radioactive iodine treatment does not influence either failure rate or rate of hypothyroidism (Andrade et al, 2001; Shi et al, 2009). The reasons for radioresistance due to treatment with anti-thyroid drugs are poorly understood. PTU may neutralize iodinated free radicals produced by radiation exposure. Both drugs may also decrease retention of radioactive iodine in the thyroid gland by inhibiting organification of iodine. Withdrawal of methimazole increases iodine uptake in the thyroid gland for up to 2 weeks. This could result in increased uptake of ^{131}I and mitigate the previous effects. Most clinical studies in cats have not demonstrated a difference in radioiodine efficacy in cats treated with methimazole prior to ^{131}I treatment (Peterson and Becker, 1995; Chun, 2002); however, most treatment centers still recommend that methimazole be withdrawn 1 to 2 weeks prior to treatment.

Prior Treatment with Limited Iodine Diets

Treatment with iodine-limited diets increases iodine uptake into the thyroid gland by 60% to 600% (Scott-Moncrieff, unpublished data). Theoretically this could increase thyroidal sensitivity to radioiodine treatment and increase the risk of hypothyroidism. Alternatively pretreatment with these diets could improve treatment response and, perhaps, reduce the dose of radioisotope required for a cure. This might reduce radiation exposure to the cat and personnel, and reduce cost. The increased iodine uptake returns to baseline by 2 weeks after withdrawal of the diet. Thus iodine limited diets should be discontinued 2 weeks prior to radioiodine treatment until further studies have evaluated this interaction.

Radiation Safety

In-Hospital

Radioactive iodine is a hazardous material with a long half-life (8 days). As such, ^{131}I-treated cats are a potential source of hazardous radiation to humans and to other animals due to gamma radiation released from ^{131}I trapped in the thyroid gland of the cat, as well as surface contamination of the cat's coat and paws by urine and feces containing radioactive iodine (so called "removable activity"; Chalmers, 2006). Any facility using radioactive iodine must adhere to national and state regulations regarding its use to minimize human exposure. Isolation of treated cats in an approved facility is required for a variable period that depends upon the dose administered and state regulations. Each animal is kept in an individual cage, and all urine and feces are disposed of as radioactive waste until the cat has a radioactivity level that is considered appropriate for release. Release criteria are based on measurement of gamma emissions measured with a survey meter either at the patient surface or at a specified distance from the neck (Chalmers, 2006). Surface emissions are correlated with urine concentrations of [131]I (Feeney, 2003). The principles of "as low as reasonably achievable" (ALARA) should be followed. Contact with hospital personnel should be limited to that required for adequate care of the cat. Attending personnel must wear protective clothing and gloves, be well trained in principles of radiation safety, and are required to carry regularly monitored dosimeters. The duration of hospitalization varies between facilities and ranges from 3 days to 3 weeks.

After Release from the Hospital

Owners should be given instructions on the proper care of their pet for the first few weeks after therapy (Fig. 4-41). Each cat should wear a collar with a "Caution Radioactive Material" label for 2 weeks and must be strictly confined to the home or kept on

RELEASE CRITERIA AND OWNER PRECAUTIONS
FOR ANIMALS TREATED WITH RADIOACTIVE IODINE-131

IN HOMES WITHOUT PREGNANT WOMEN AND WITHOUT CHILDREN UNDER 12 YEARS OF AGE

*The maximum exposure rate (dorsal to thyroid) at one foot from the pet shall not exceed **1 mR/hr.***

Animals released to their owners will contain a small amount of radioactivity and will continue to excrete low levels of radioactivity for a period. The amount of radiation exposure you may receive is well below levels that result in significant risk of harmful effects. The owners must sign a consent form to protect themselves and other members of the public. In this consent they will agree to the following:

Keep cats in their carriers for the drive home.

A.   Maintain a distance of six feet between you and your pet except for brief periods of necessary care.

B.   Children and pregnant or nursing women should have **NO** contact with the pet until the collar with radioactive label is removed.

C.   Minimize contact with the pet, including arrangement for a separate sleeping room away from people.

D.   The pet must wear a collar or tag with a "Caution Radioactive Material" label attached for 2 weeks.

Date for collar removal _____.

E.   Ensure that if the pet is a cat, it will remain indoors and use its litter box. The box should be lined with plastic. Change the litter frequently, disposing of it in the outside trash or by flushing it down the toilet.

F.   Care must be taken to wash hands after handling the animal, its food dishes, or litter pans.

G.   Ensure that your cat uses a litter box and line it with plastic.

H.   These restrictions will remain in force until the levels of activity decrease to insignificant levels.
      This time period will be 2 weeks.

Measured exposure		
(mR/hr at 1 foot):	Date:	Measured by:

As a condition for release of my pet following radioiodine therapy, I agree to the restrictions above:

I also understand the animal contains a small level of radioactivity and will excrete low-level radioactivity for a period of time. Minimizing contact with the pet, washing hands after contact, and arranging for the pet to sleep in another area will minimize my radiation exposure.

_____   _____
              Signed   Date

FIGURE 4-41 Example of a form used to inform cat owners about release criteria and owner precautions for animals treated with radioactive iodine.

a leash. Adults are recommended to stay 6 feet or farther away from the cat except for brief periods needed for necessary care, including arrangement for a separate sleeping area away from people. Children and pregnant women should have *no* contact with the cat until the collar has been removed. To further reduce any chance of unwanted exposure, it is recommended that owners line the litter pan with plastic. The used litter should be disposed of in the outside trash or by flushing flushable litter down the toilet. The hands should be washed thoroughly after handling of the cat, its food dishes, or the litter pan.

Rechecks and Hypothyroidism. Recheck evaluations are recommended 1, 3, 6, and 12 months following treatment for a complete history, physical examination (including weight and blood pressure measurement), serum biochemical profile, and measurement of serum T_4 concentrations. Most cats are euthyroid or have a serum T_4 concentration below the reference range at the time of hospital discharge. A small percentage of cats (15%) are still hyperthyroid at the time of discharge but become euthyroid within 6 months after treatment (Peterson and Becker, 1995). Some cats treated with radioactive iodine become transiently or permanently hypothyroid after radioactive iodine treatment. Persistent hypothyroidism after treatment is a risk factor for azotemia. Measurement of total T_4 together with TSH can help distinguish true hypothyroidism from NTIS (see Baseline Serum Thyrotropin Concentration). Cats that are still hypothyroid 6 months after treatment, those that develop clinical signs of hypothyroidism, and those that have progressive azotemia and a low serum T_4 concentration should be supplemented with L-T_4 at a dose of 0.05 to 0.1 mg of L-T_4 given orally once or twice daily. Cats that continue to have abnormally increased serum T_4 concentrations 6 months after radioiodine therapy may need to be retreated with ^{131}I. These cats are at higher risk of thyroid carcinoma, and this possibility should be investigated so that a higher dose of isotope can be administered if appropriate (see Feline Thyroid Carcinoma).

Prognosis for Resolution of Hyperthyroidism. More than 93% of cats treated with radioactive iodine become euthyroid after one treatment. Failure to respond to the first treatment is most common in cats that have large tumors, severe clinical signs, and very high serum T_4 concentrations (Peterson and Becker, 1995). Cats with thyroid carcinoma also fail to become euthyroid after low dose ^{131}I treatment. There are no reports of adverse effects on organs other than the thyroid glands after low dose ^{131}I therapy.

Need for Retreatment

Approximately 2% to 5% of ^{131}I-treated hyperthyroid cats require a second treatment (Peterson and Becker, 1995). Several factors, such as dose administered, thyroid gland size, thyroid gland pathology (adenoma, adenomatous hyperplasia, or carcinoma), and iodine excretion rate, may contribute to an incomplete response to an initial therapeutic dose of ^{131}I. Errors in radioisotope administration can also occur and explain a treatment failure. Prior to administration of a second treatment, the reason for failure should be evaluated. Although a second standard dose is effective in most cats, consideration should be given to obtaining an incisional or excisional thyroid biopsy in cats in which thyroid carcinoma is suspected. In cats with thyroid carcinoma, high dose radioactive iodine treatment may be necessary (see Feline Thyroid Carcinoma).

Recurrence

A small percentage of cats (less than 3%) develop recurrence of hyperthyroidism at a median time of 3 years (range 1 to 6 years) after treatment with radioactive iodine. No predictors of relapse have been identified. There was no difference between the T_4 concentration or the dose of radioactive iodine used between cats that did and did not relapse (Peterson and Becker, 1995). It is likely that relapse in these cats is due to development of new foci of autonomous tissue arising from new mutations.

NUTRITIONAL MANAGEMENT OF FELINE HYPERTHYROIDISM

In mammals, the only known function of iodine is incorporation into thyroid hormones; diets deficient in iodine cause

hypothyroidism and goiter. Published guidelines for iodine requirements for healthy cats have changed over the years, but current recommendations are that healthy cats should consume at least 0.46 mg/kg of dry food (Wedekind et al, 2010). There are no published guidelines for iodine requirements of hyperthyroid cats. Dietary iodine restriction to less than 0.3 mg/kg reduces the circulating thyroid hormone concentrations to the normal range in hyperthyroid cats (Melendez et al, 2011a; 2011b; Yu et al, 2011; van der Kooij et al, 2013), suggesting that dietary iodine restriction has potential as an alternative management strategy for feline hyperthyroidism.

Commercial cat foods are commonly supplemented with iodine using calcium iodate or potassium iodide. Studies suggest that there is huge variability in the concentration of iodine in commercial cat foods because of the variability of iodine content of individual ingredients. Ingredients that typically contain high concentrations of iodine include fish, shellfish, and fresh meats. The range of iodine content in commercial cat foods varies by a factor of 30, with the largest variation being found in canned cat food (Ranz et al, 2002; Mumma et al, 1986; Johnson et al, 1992; Edinboro et al, 2013).

Role of Dietary Iodine in the Pathogenesis of Disease

The variability in iodine content of commercial cat food and the similarities between feline hyperthyroidism and toxic nodular goiter in humans have prompted hypotheses, so far unsupported by research, that low iodine intake, high iodine intake, or wide variability in iodine content has contributed to the current increased prevalence of feline hyperthyroidism. Whether or not iodine content of the diet is important in the pathogenesis of feline hyperthyroidism, it is likely only one of many potential contributing factors. It is also clear that the final common pathway in the pathogenesis of feline hyperthyroidism is the presence of mutations in subsets of thyroid follicular cells that lead to autonomous thyroid hormone synthesis. Once thyroid follicular cells have become autonomous, the cellular changes are not reversible or likely to be influenced by dietary change. In other words, limiting the iodine content of the food can lead to normalization of thyroid hormone synthesis whether or not the iodine content of the diet is a factor in the underlying pathogenesis of feline hyperthyroidism.

Iodine-Limited Diets for Management of Feline Hyperthyroidism

In a series of studies involving 33 cats with naturally occurring hyperthyroidism, the effects of feeding diets containing from 0.15 mg/kg to 1.9 mg/kg dietary iodine concentration were investigated (Melendez et al, 2011a; 2011b; Yu et al, 2011). All cats studied were consuming commercial diets containing 1.9 mg/kg iodine at the time of diagnosis and were confirmed to be hyperthyroid by standard methods. The iodine content of the control and experimental diets was confirmed by epiboron neutron atomic activation—an extremely sensitive assay method. Four to 8 weeks after consumption of a diet containing 0.17 mg/kg or less of dietary iodine, all cats had a total T_4 within the reference range. Eight of nine cats consuming a diet of 0.28 mg/kg iodine were euthyroid within 3 to 12 weeks, whereas the proportion of cats becoming euthyroid was lower when consuming diets containing higher concentrations of iodine (0.39 mg/kg [7 of 9 cats] or 0.47 mg/kg [4 of 5 cats]). More extensive thyroid profiles were performed in 14 of the cats; fT_4, total T_3, free T_3, and TSH concentrations were within the laboratory reference range while consuming the iodine-restricted diet. There was no change in renal parameters after restoration of euthyroidism, which is surprising because decreased

CAT	PRE THYROXINE µG/DL (RR 2.5-4.6)	4-8 WEEK THYROXINE µG/DL (RR 2.5-4.6)	PRE CREATININE MG/DL	POST CREATININE MG/DL
1	13.3	2.8	1.2	1.4
2	6.4	1.7	1.0	0.7
3	12.4	6.5*	0.8	0.6
4	8.7	4.4	0.7	0.7
5	8.0	4.3	0.6	
6	8.9	3.4	0.6	0.4
7	13	2.6	0.8	0.7
8	8.7	2.8		
9	5.9	3.1	1.4	1.0
10	9.4	2.9		

TABLE 4-16   **RESPONSE TO TREATMENT WITH AN IODINE-LIMITED DIET IN 10 HYPERTHYROID CATS**

RR, Reference range.

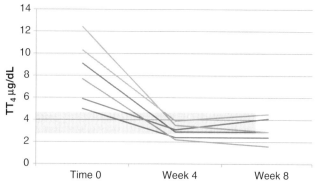

FIGURE 4-42 Change in total thyroxine (T$_4$) and free T$_4$ (fT$_4$) in six cats consuming an iodine-limited diet over an 8 week period (unpublished data).

GFR associated with reestablishment of euthyroidism results in azotemia in 15% to 49% of previously non-azotemic cats treated by other methods (Williams et al, 2010).

Clinical Experience

There is now a commercially available iodine-limited diet marketed for management of feline hyperthyroidism (Prescription Diet y/d). The diet is similar in formulation to Prescription g/d but has an iodine content of 0.2 mg/kg or less and is available as both canned and dry food. In a retrospective study of 49 client-owned hyperthyroid cats fed this diet exclusively, serum total T$_4$ became normal in 71% of cats between 21 and 60 days and 96% of cats between 61 and 180 days respectively. Cats with a higher starting total T$_4$ took longer to become euthyroid. The median heart rate, body weight, and serum creatinine did not change over the 6 months of the study (Scott-Moncrieff, unpublished data). The reasons for a lack of weight gain in these cats may reflect the influence of concurrent disease or subclinical hyperthyroidism in some cats.

Indications for Nutritional Management

Nutritional management is an alternate option for short-term management of hyperthyroidism or longer-term management of hyperthyroidism in cats that are not good candidates for definitive treatment of their hyperthyroidism. As with methimazole, limiting the intake of dietary iodine limits thyroidal synthesis of thyroid hormone, but the autonomous thyroid adenoma is still present. Therefore definitive treatment with ^{131}I or thyroidectomy should be recommended if possible; however, for cats that have concurrent nonthyroidal illness, for cats that have adverse effects of methimazole, for owners with financial constraints, or for owners who are unable to medicate their cats, nutritional management is a feasible alternative. Nutritional management is not a good option for cats that do not find the food to be palatable, for outdoor cats with access to other sources of dietary iodine, or for cats that need to be on a controlled diet to manage other concurrent illnesses, such as inflammatory bowel disease, allergic dermatitis, or heart disease. For cats in early renal failure, Prescription Diet y/d may be an acceptable diet because it is supplemented with omega-3 fatty acids and contains controlled amounts of phosphorus, sodium, and high-quality protein (36% dry matter basis). Cats with more severe renal failure may need to be fed a diet formulated for management of renal failure. Hyperthyroid cats in multicat households need to be fed individually, and access to food of other pets in the household must be prevented. Alternatively the iodine-limited diet can be fed to all cats in the household providing the euthyroid cats are supplemented daily with a food with higher iodine content.

Expected Outcome

More than 90 percent of hyperthyroid cats become euthyroid when fed a limited-iodine diet exclusively (Table 4-16; Fig. 4-42). The most common reason for failure to control the hyperthyroidism is access to iodine-containing food, such as treats, human food, or other pet foods. Even small amounts of other iodine-containing foods can result in an increase in the T$_4$ concentration. For this reason, cats being managed with an iodine-limited food need to be indoor cats, and the owner needs to feed the diet exclusively. For owners who consider it important to give their cats treats, one strategy is to feed the dry Prescription Diet y/d diet predominantly and give the canned Prescription Diet y/d as a treat. In cats that do not become euthyroid within 4 to 8 weeks of starting the limited-iodine diet, a detailed history should be investigated for evidence of other sources of iodine. Possible sources in addition to access to other pet foods include well water, medications or supplements, contaminated food bowls, and human food.

Long-Term Nutritional Management

Nutritional management of feline hyperthyroidism is an entirely new approach that does not have a parallel in people. In human medicine, low-iodine diets are only used for short periods of time prior to nuclear imaging to screen for metastasis in patients with thyroid carcinoma. For this reason the long-term consequences of dietary restriction of iodine are unknown. Iodine may have anti-oxidant and anti-inflammatory properties as well as playing a role in prevention of breast cancer and fibrocystic breast disease (Patrick, 2008). One concern is that cats managed long-term with iodine-limited diets might develop a clinically significant goiter due to continued follicular cell hyperplasia; additionally, management using an iodine-limited diet could increase the risk of transformation of adenomatous nodules into thyroid carcinoma. In a report of eight cats with thyroid carcinoma, two cases had both adenomatous changes and carcinoma cells contained within one gland, suggesting that the carcinoma could have arisen from a background of benign neoplasia (Hibbert et al, 2009). These potential risks are also of concern in cats treated chronically with methimazole. For these reasons, the thyroid gland should be palpated routinely in cats on a limited-iodine diet, and definitive therapy with radioactive iodine treatment should be recommended if clinically significant thyroid gland enlargement is identified.

Transitioning from Methimazole to a Limited-Iodine Diet

Iodine-limited diets should not be used concurrently with methimazole for management of feline hyperthyroidism because of the risk of severe hypothyroidism. Methimazole should be discontinued immediately prior to starting an iodine-limited diet. Transient hyperthyroidism may occur during the transition, but this is preferable to hypothyroidism because of the deleterious influence of hypothyroidism on the GFR.

Transitioning from a Limited-Iodine Diet to Other Treatments

If nutritional management fails to control hyperthyroidism despite investigation for other sources of iodine, another diet should be reinstituted and alternative treatment of the hyperthyroidism considered. A washout period is not necessary in cats started back on methimazole treatment, because thyroid hormone synthesis increases very rapidly once the limited iodine diet is discontinued. Little is known about the effect of a limited-iodine diet on response to radioactive iodine. In theory, increased iodine trapping by the thyroid gland due to the lack of iodine could make the normal atrophic thyroidal tissue more susceptible to the effects of radioactive iodine and increase the risk of hypothyroidism after ^{131}I treatment. Conversely consumption of a limited iodine diet could be used to decreased the required dose of ^{131}I needed to reestablish a euthyoid state. In eight hyperthyroid cats that were euthyroid after consumption of an iodine limited diet, radioisotope scans using ^{123}I revealed increased radio-isotope uptake of 60% to 600% (Scott-Moncrieff, unpublished data).

Recommended Monitoring

It is recommended that cats being managed with an iodine-limited diet be reevaluated by physical examination and measurement of a BUN, creatinine, USG, and total T_4 monthly until establishment of euthyroidism. As for methimazole treated cats the ideal range for the total T_4 is within the lower half of the reference range. Cats should then be monitored every 6 months if otherwise healthy; cats with concurrent illnesses may require more frequent monitoring.

FELINE THYROID CARCINOMA

Malignant thyroid neoplasia is diagnosed in approximately 1% to 3% of cats with hyperthyroidism (Peterson and Becker, 1995). Most malignant thyroid tumors in the cat are functional tumors with follicular carcinomas being most common. Nonsecretory thyroid tumors (tumors that do not produce excess concentrations of thyroid hormone but do concentrate iodine) and nonfunctional thyroid tumors (tumors that neither secret thyroid hormone nor concentrate iodine) have been described in cats but are rare (Turrel et al, 1988; Guptill et al, 1995).

Clinical Features

The signalment and clinical signs of cats with thyroid carcinoma are similar to those of cats with benign hyperthyroidism. Many cats have a history of prior thyroidectomy, and in addition to the typical clinical signs of hyperthyroidism, voice change has been reported. Palpable cervical mass masses are present in 71% of cases. In cats with thyroid carcinoma, thyroid gland palpation may be similar to that of a hyperthyroid cat with benign disease; however, in other cases, the masses associated with thyroid carcinoma are large and fixed rather than freely moveable and attached to underlying or overlying tissues.

Diagnosis

Common abnormalities on the minimum data base are similar to cats with benign thyroid disease with the exception of occasional hypercalcemia. Radiographic abnormalities may include cardiomegaly, evidence of congestive heart failure, mediastinal masses, and evidence of pulmonary metastasis. The majority of cats with thyroid carcinoma have increased basal serum T_4 concentrations. No differences have been identified in the range of serum T_4 concentrations in cats with benign and malignant thyroid tumors. A nonsecretory or nonfunctional tumor should be suspected if a thyroid tumor is identified but T_4 concentration is normal and there are no clinical signs of hyperthyroidism. Nuclear scintigraphy using sodium pertechnetate (technetium-99m [^{99m}Tc]) is valuable in the evaluation of cats with suspected malignant thyroid tumors. In cats with thyroid carcinoma, a ^{99m}Tc scan may demonstrate patchy or irregular uptake of isotope, extension of isotope uptake down the neck and into the mediastinum, and evidence of distant metastasis (see Fig. 4-29); however, in some cats with thyroid carcinoma scintigraphic findings may be similar to the scans of cats with thyroid adenomatous hyperplasia or adenoma. Conversely, scans that reveal uptake by multiple masses in the cervical region or masses extending into the cranial mediastinum in some cases may be benign ectopic tissue. Thus scintigraphy alone cannot definitively distinguish between adenomatous hyperplasia and thyroid carcinoma. Bronchogenic carcinoma may have scintigraphic findings that may be confused with those of thyroid tumors. Nonfunctional thyroid tumors may or may not take up ^{99m}Tc depending upon the degree of differentiation of the tumor.

Definitive diagnosis of thyroid carcinoma requires histopathologic examination of excised tissue. Because the majority of feline thyroid tumors are benign, thyroid carcinoma may not be suspected on the initial evaluation. Factors that should increase the index of suspicion for thyroid carcinoma include recurrence of hyperthyroidism after previous thyroidectomy(ies), failure to respond to low dose radioactive iodine treatment, presence of multiple palpable cervical nodules, and cervical nodules that are firmly attached to underlying or overlying structures. Large, palpable, thyroid masses that compress surrounding structures may be due either to thyroid carcinoma or benign thyroid cyst. Thyroid carcinoma should also be suspected if scintigraphy reveals multiple areas of radionuclide uptake and irregular or patchy isotope uptake.

Cytologic characteristics are usually unhelpful in differentiation of benign from malignant thyroid tumors, because pleomorphism, anaplasia, and increased mitotic rate are not consistent features. Features that distinguish malignant from benign tumors include local tissue invasion, regional lymph node involvement, and distant metastasis. Metastasis has been reported to occur in up to 71% of cats with thyroid carcinoma.

Treatment

Although cats with thyroid carcinoma may show clinical improvement when treated with anti-thyroid drugs, these drugs are not

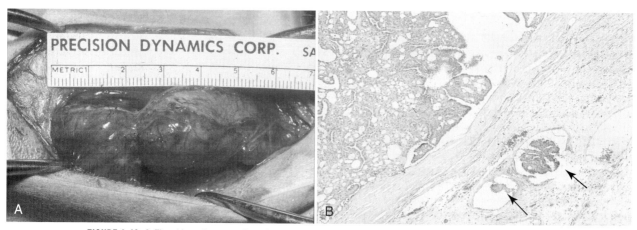

FIGURE 4-43 A, Thyroid carcinoma at time of cervical exploratory. Note the large size of the tumor and the irregular appearance. **B,** Photomicrograph of a thyroid follicular carcinoma in a different cat demonstrating extracapsular foci and possible lymphatic or blood vascular invasion *(arrows).*

recommended for several reasons. Anti-thyroid drugs may increase release of TSH from the anterior pituitary gland by decreasing secretion of T_4 and exacerbate tumor growth due to the tropic effects of TSH. Furthermore, anti-thyroid drugs are not cytotoxic and will neither slow progression of local tumor growth nor metastasis to distant organs. The only indication for using anti-thyroid drugs in the management of thyroid carcinoma is for the purpose of initial clinical stabilization prior to ^{131}I therapy or thyroidectomy. Beta blockers (e.g., propranolol or atenolol) are useful in hyperthyroid cats that require stabilization of cardiac disease prior to surgery or ^{131}I therapy.

Thyroidectomy is the initial treatment of choice in cats with suspected thyroid carcinoma, because the diagnosis must be confirmed by histopathology (Fig. 4-43) and because complete excision can be curative. Scintigraphy should always be performed prior to thyroidectomy. As much tumor as possible should be excised. Thyroid biopsy, followed by adjunctive therapy, may be more appropriate in cats with invasive or infiltrative masses. Preservation of the parathyroid glands is more difficult in cats with invasive thyroid carcinomas treated surgically, and postoperative monitoring of serum calcium concentrations is essential for cats undergoing bilateral thyroidectomy. A cat exhibiting signs of hypocalcemia after thyroidectomy (e.g., muscle tremors, tetany, or convulsions) should be treated with appropriate calcium and vitamin D supplementation (see Management of Postoperative Hypocalcemia for approach to treatment of hypocalcemia).

Even if all of the visible tumor is removed, many thyroid carcinomas will recur within weeks to months. Thus, in histopathologically confirmed thyroid carcinoma, thyroid scintigraphy should be repeated 4 to 8 weeks after thyroidectomy in order to evaluate the success of surgical removal. If tumor recurrence is confirmed, treatment with high dose ^{131}I is recommended. Following treatment with ^{131}I, reevaluation of serum T_4 concentrations and ^{99m}Tc scans should be performed every 3 to 6 months. If recurrence is not detected in these follow-up evaluations after 1 year, the period between evaluations can progressively be lengthened.

Treatment with ^{131}I is indicated in cats with non-resectable thyroid carcinoma and in cats with evidence of metastasis or recurrence after thyroidectomy, providing the neoplastic tissue concentrates iodine or technetium on scintigraphy. Higher doses of [131]I (10 to 30 mCi) are required to successfully treat cats with thyroid carcinoma than are required to treat cats with thyroid adenoma, because the thyroid tissue may concentrate iodine less

effectively and because there is often a larger mass of thyroid tissue present. A combination of surgical resection and postoperative treatment with high doses of ^{131}I is an effective approach to treatment. Surgical removal followed by administration of 30 mCi ^{131}I in seven cats with thyroid carcinoma resulted in survival times ranging from 10 to 41 months (Guptill et al, 1995), and none of the cats died due to thyroid carcinoma. Higher doses of ^{131}I necessitate a longer hospitalization time to allow the isotope time to decay to activity levels compatible with discharge to the home environment. The majority of cats treated with higher doses of ^{131}I become permanently hypothyroid and require supplementation with L-T_4. Treatment with 30 mCi ^{131}I as the sole mode of therapy has also been reported to result in a successful outcome in cats with feline thyroid carcinoma, although one of eight cats did not respond to treatment and one cat had recurrence 6 months after treatment (Hibbert et al, 2009). Adverse effects of high dose ^{131}I may include transient dysphagia and hypothyroidism. In one study, pancytopenia was identified 6 months after high dose ^{131}I treatment, but the relationship with the radioiodine treatment was unclear because the cat was also feline immunodeficiency virus (FIV) positive.

Thyroid Cysts

Thyroid cysts may occur associated with thyroid adenomatous hyperplasia, adenoma, or thyroid carcinomas. The cystic lesion may be palpated as a thin walled fluctuant mass that usually collapses and is non-palpable once the fluid has been removed (Fig. 4-44). The total T_4 concentration of the cystic fluid is typically high (Hofmeister et al, 2001). Diagnosis of thyroid cysts is best made by a combination of palpation and aspiration. Ultrasound examination can be helpful in evaluation of thyroid glands with cystic changes (Barberet, 2010). Treatment of large thyroid cysts is best accomplished by surgical resection of the cyst and associated thyroid tissue rather than radioactive iodine therapy.

MISCELLANEOUS THERAPIES

Percutaneous Ethanol and Heat Ablation Injection for Treatment of Feline Hyperthyroidism

Both ultrasound guided ethanol injection and percutaneous radio-frequency heat ablation have been evaluated for treatment of feline

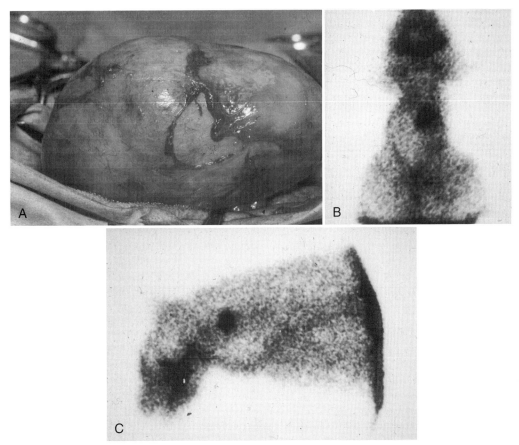

FIGURE 4-44 A, Photograph of a large thyroid cyst in a hyperthyroid cat during thyroidectomy and surgical resection of the thyroid cyst. **B** and **C,** Ventral and lateral thyroid technetium-99m (^{99m}Tc) scans from the same cat. Note that the cyst appears as a large "cold" area surrounded by a thin rim of tissue that takes up ^{99m}Tc. The majority of the thyroid gland is medial and dorsal to the cyst.

hyperthyroidism (Goldstein et al, 2001; Wells et al, 2001; Mallery et al, 2002). Problems with frequent recurrence and complications in cats with bilateral thyroid disease have limited the practicality of these approaches. For more information see Feldman and Nelson, *Canine and Feline Endocrinology and Reproduction,* ed 3.

Beta Blockers

Beta blockers may be useful to control tachycardia and other supraventricular tachyarrhythmias especially in cats that do not tolerate anti-thyroid drugs. Beta blockade results in slowing of the heart rate, lowers the end-diastolic pressure of the left ventricle, prolongs the ventricular filling time, decreases the oxygen demand of the myocardium, acts as an antiarrhythmic agent, and reduces outflow pressure gradients. Beta blockers may also reduce the systolic blood pressure and have been recommended for control of hypertension in hyperthyroidism; however, studies suggest that efficacy is limited in hyperthyroid cats with hypertension (Henik et al, 2008). More potent anti-hypertensive drugs (e.g., amlodipine) should be utilized in hyperthyroid cats with clinically significant hypertension.

Propranolol is a nonselective beta blocker that has the added advantage of also decreasing conversion of T_4 to T_3; however, propranolol can cause bronchospasm in cats with reactive airway disease because of blockade of beta$_2$ receptors in airway smooth muscle. Propranolol is rapidly absorbed from the gastrointestinal tract, and the plasma half-life is approximately 3 to 6 hours. The recommended dose of propranolol is 2.5 to 5 mg every 8 to 12 hours.

The dose should be started at the lower end of the range and then slowly increased until the goals of controlling tachycardia and arrhythmias are achieved. Propranolol is a potent myocardial depressant and should be used with extreme caution if heart failure is present. In a study of induced hyperthyroidism, the half-life of propranolol was not affected by hyperthyroidism (Jacobs et al, 1997). After oral administration, total body clearance was lower and the peak plasma propranolol concentration, fractional absorption, and area under the curve were higher in hyperthyroid cats compared with euthyroid cats. This indicated increased bioavailability in thyrotoxicosis, which was calculated to exceed 100% and suggested enterohepatic recycling of the drug. The findings of this study support starting at the lower end of the dose in hyperthyroid cats.

Atenolol is a selective beta$_1$ blocker with potential advantages over propranolol, including more selective β_1-adrenoreceptor blocking action and longer duration of action. Atenolol is rapidly absorbed from the gastrointestinal tract in cats and has a half-life of 3½ hours in cats. The duration of effect persists for at least 12 hours in healthy cats (Quiñones, 1996). Atenolol is used at a dosage of 6.25 to 12.5 mg per cat mg every 12 to 24 hours. The starting dose should be at the low end of the range, and the dose is then gradually increased depending upon the response.

Stable Iodine

Although the thyroid gland requires small amounts of iodide for hormone synthesis, large amounts given over a brief period

(1 to 2 weeks) may result in transient hypothyroidism in normal individuals due to the Wolff-Chaikoff effect. High doses of iodide inhibit organification of thyroid hormone, which results in reduced secretion. Iodide can be rapidly effective in ameliorating increased serum thyroid hormone concentrations associated with hyperthyroidism. Beneficial effects are seen in 7 to 14 days and include improvement in clinical signs, as well as reduction in the size and vascularity of the thyroid gland. Iodide has a role in the treatment of thyroid storm in humans. Unfortunately, it is rarely possible to achieve complete remission of hyperthyroidism or to maintain any degree of control for more than a few weeks with iodide, but it may be useful when used in conjunction with beta-blockers to control the disease preoperatively in cats that do not tolerate methimazole (Foster and Thoday, 1999). Potassium iodate (KI) at a dose of 21 to 42 mg every 8 hours was administered daily beginning 10 days prior to surgery in conjunction with propranolol. The KI was placed in a small gelatin capsule to avoid the aftertaste that may bother some cats. The most common side-effect of treatment with KI was gastrointestinal upset.

Iodinated Radiographic Contrast Agents

Oral cholecystographic agents (e.g., calcium ipodate and iopanoic acid) acutely inhibit peripheral conversion of T_4 to T_3 and may decrease T_4 synthesis. Blocking of the conversion of circulating thyroid hormone has been demonstrated in iatrogenic feline hyperthyroidism, and the drug appears to be well tolerated with few adverse side effects. In 12 cats with naturally occurring hyperthyroidism treated with calcium ipodate, eight exhibited a good response. The serum total T_3 concentrations decreased into the reference range within 2 weeks of the start of treatment and remained at those levels for a 14-week study period. In addition, improvement in clinical signs, body weight, heart rate, and blood pressure were documented. Four of the eight responders continued to do well for as long as 6 months, but two of them had relapses of hyperthyroidism by week 14. The serum total T_4 concentrations were not affected by treatment, and cats with severe disease were less likely to respond, even after the dose was doubled (Murray and Peterson, 1997). Unfortunately calcium ipodate is no longer commercially available. Iopanoic acid has been evaluated as an alternative agent and is also effective at decreasing T_3 concentration; however, in a study of 11 hyperthyroid cats, only five cats had partial and transient responses (Gallagher et al, 2011).

Treatment of Hypertension in Hyperthyroid Cats

As discussed earlier, the prevalence of hypertension in hyperthyroid cats is lower than previously believed, and only a small percentage of cats require specific treatment for hypertension. The criteria for initiating specific anti-hypertensive treatment include documentation of systolic blood pressure more than 160 mmHg on more than one occasion or evidence of end organ damage, such as retinal lesions due to hypertension. It is important that blood pressure is measured in as calm and non-stressful way as possible to minimize the white coat effect that hyperthyroid cats seem particularly susceptible to. In addition to specific management of the hypertension, underlying hyperthyroidism should be treated at the same time. Drugs that are used to control hypertension in hyperthyroid cats include beta-blockers (e.g., propranolol or atenolol), calcium

channel blockers (e.g., amlodipine), and angiotensin converting enzyme (ACE) inhibitors (e.g., benazepril and enalapril). As discussed earlier, beta blockers are effective at controlling tachycardia in hyperthyroid cats but are not as effective at controlling hypertension. In a study of 20 hyperthyroid cats with systolic blood pressure more than 160 mmHg treated with 1 to 2 mg/kg orally every 12 hours atenolol, the tachycardia was successfully controlled in most cats but systolic blood pressure only decreased below 160 mmHg in 30% of cats (Henik et al, 2008). Amlodipine (0.625 to 1.25 mg per cat every 24 hours) is a more effective antihypertensive drug in cats with hypertension and has the additional advantage of decreasing proteinuria in cats with CKD (Jepson et al, 2007). ACE inhibitors (e.g., benazepril) are less potent than amlodipine for control of feline hypertension but have both systemic and glomerular anti-hypertensive effects so are useful in cats with concurrent CKD. ACE inhibitors are typically used as a second drug in cats that do not have good control of systemic blood pressure with amlodipine alone (Stepien, 2011). As mentioned earlier, some cats with hyperthyroidism develop hypertension after control of the hyperthyroid state, so it is really important to continue to monitor blood pressure in all hyperthyroid cats after treatment.

Prognosis

A number of studies have evaluated the prognosis and predictors of survival for hyperthyroid cats treated with radioactive iodine. In a study of more than 200 cats, male cats were found to have a shorter life expectancy than females (Slater et al, 2001). Age at the time of treatment was also a prognostic factor, because older cats did not survive as long as younger cats. For example, 28% of 10-year-old male cats were alive 5 years after therapy and 4% of 16-year-old male cats were alive 5 years after treatment, whereas 42% of 10-year-old female cats were alive 5 years after treatment. The mean age of death was 15 years of age, with a range of 10 to 21 years. Clinical abnormalities documented just before death were renal disorders in 41% of cats and cancer in 16% of cats.

In a retrospective study of 300 hyperthyroid cats treated with methimazole, thyroidectomy, or radioactive iodine, median survival was 417 days; increasing age, presence of proteinuria, and hypertension were associated with decreased survival time (Williams et al, 2010). In another study, median survival time for feline hyperthyroidism after radioactive iodine was reported to be approximately 2 years (range 2 weeks to 7 years) (Peterson et al, 2001). In a retrospective study of 167 cats treated with methimazole and/or radioactive iodine, cats with pre-existing renal disease had significantly shorter survival times than cats without pre-existing renal disease (Milner et al, 2006; Fig. 4-45). When cats with pre-existing renal disease were excluded, cats treated with methimazole alone had a shorter median survival time (2 years) than cats treated with radioactive iodine alone or methimazole followed by radioactive iodine (4 years). The reasons for the difference in survival between the treatment groups may have been related to poorer control of the hyperthyroid state with long-term medical treatment as well as owner bias toward less aggressive management in methimazole treated cats. The prognosis for hyperthyroid cats managed by dietary iodine restriction is currently unknown, although some cats have reportedly been managed with this strategy for up to 6 years.

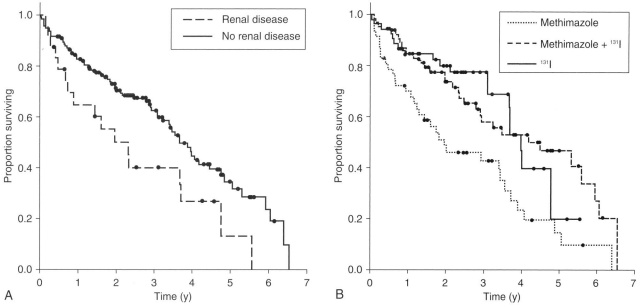

FIGURE 4-45 A, Kaplan-Meier curves of survival times for 167 hyperthyroid cats treated with methimazole, iodine-131 (^{131}I), or methimazole followed by ^{131}I, grouped according to whether they had evidence of renal disease prior to treatment. **B,** Kaplan-Meier curves of survival times for 167 hyperthyroid cats treated with methimazole, ^{131}I, or methimazole followed by ^{131}I, and grouped according to treatment. (**A,** From Milner RJ, et al.: Survival times for cats with hyperthyroidism treated with iodine 131, methimazole, or both: 167 cases [1996-2003], *J Am Vet Med Assoc* 228[4]:559-563, 2006. [Fig. 3; p. 562])

REFERENCES

Adams WH, et al.: Changes in renal function in cats following treatment of hyperthyroidism using ^{131}I, *Vet Radiol Ultrasound* 38:231, 1997.

Andrade VA, et al.: Methimazole pretreatment does not reduce the efficacy of radioiodine in patients with hyperthyroidism caused by Graves' disease, *J Clin Endocrinol Metab* 86:3488, 2001.

Archer FJ, Taylor SM: Alkaline phosphatase bone isoenzyme and osteocalcin in the serum of hyperthyroid cats, *Can Vet J* 37:735, 1996.

Aucoin DP, et al.: Propylthiouracil-induced immune-mediated disease in cats, *J Pharmacol Exp Ther* 234:13, 1985.

Aucoin DP, et al.: Dose dependent induction of anti-native DNA antibodies by propylthiouracil in cats, *J Arthr Rheum* 31:688, 1988.

Barber PJ, Elliott J: Study of calcium hemostasis in feline hyperthyroidism, *J Small Anim Pract* 37:575, 1996.

Barberet V, et al.: Pre- and posttreatment ultrasonography of the thyroid gland in hyperthyroid cats, *Vet Radiol Ultrasound* 51(3):324, 2010.

Beck KA, et al.: The normal feline thyroid: technetium pertechnetate imaging and determination of thyroid to salivary gland radioactivity ratios in 10 normal cats, *Vet Radiol* 26:35, 1985.

Beck-Peccoz P, et al.: Pituitary tumours: TSH-secreting adenomas, *Best Pract Res Clin Endocrinol Metab* 23(5):597, 2009.

Beleslin DB, et al.: Nature of salivation produced by thyrotropin-releasing hormone (TRH), *Brain Res Bull* 18:463, 1987a.

Beleslin DB, et al.: Studies of thyrotropin-releasing hormone (TRH)–induced defecation in cats, *Pharmacol Biochem Behav* 26:639, 1987b.

Belew AM, et al.: Evaluation of the white-coat effect in cats, *J Vet Intern Med* 13:134, 1999.

Bell ET, et al.: Immune-mediated myasthenia gravis in a methimazole-treated cat, *J Small Anim Pract* 53:661, 2012.

Berent AC, et al.: Liver function in cats with hyperthyroidism before and after ^{131}-I therapy, *J Vet Intern Med* 21:1217, 2007.

Biondi B, et al.: Subclinical hyperthyroidism: clinical features and treatment options, *Eur J Endocrinol* 152(1):1, 2005.

Birchard SJ: Thyroidectomy in the cat, *Clin Tech Small Anim Pract* 21(1):29, 2006.

Birchard SJ, et al.: Surgical treatment of feline hyperthyroidism: results of 85 cases, *J Am Anim Hosp Assoc* 20:705, 1984.

Boag AK, et al.: Changes in the glomerular filtration rate of 27 cats with hyperthyroidism after treatment with radioactive iodine, *Vet Rec* 161:711, 2007.

Boas M, et al.: Thyroid effects of endocrine disrupting chemicals, *Mol Cell Endocrinol* 355(2):240, 2012.

Bond BR, et al.: Echocardiographic findings in 103 cats with hyperthyroidism, *J Am Vet Med Assoc* 192:1546, 1988.

Boretti FS, et al.: Duration of T4 suppression in hyperthyroid cats treated once and twice daily with transdermal methimazole, *J Vet Intern Med* 27:377, 2013a.

Boretti FS, et al.: Transdermal application of methimazole in hyperthyroid cats: a long-term follow up study, *J Feline Med Surg* [Epub ahead of print], 2013b.

Branter E, et al.: Antioxidant status in hyperthyroid cats before and after radioiodine treatment, *J Vet Intern Med* 26:582, 2012.

Broome MR, et al.: Peripheral metabolism of thyroid hormones and iodide in healthy and hyperthyroid cats, *Am J Vet Res* 48:1286, 1987.

Broome MR, et al.: Serial determinations of thyroxine concentrations in hyperthyroid cats, *J Am Vet Med Assoc* 192:49, 1988a.

Broome MR, et al.: Predictive value of tracer studies for ^{131}I treatment in hyperthyroid cats, *Am J Vet Res* 49:193, 1988b.

Broome MR, et al.: Thyroid scintigraphy in hyperthyroidism, *Clin Tech Small Anim Pract* 21(1):10, 2006.

Broussard JD, et al.: Changes in clinical and laboratory findings in cats with hyperthyroidism from 1983 to 1993, *J Am Vet Med Assoc* 206:302, 1995.

Bucknell DG: Feline hyperthyroidism: spectrum of clinical presentations and response to carbimazole therapy, *Aust Vet J* 78:462, 2000.

Burch HB: Overview of the clinical manifestations of hyperthyroidism. In Braverman LE, Cooper DS, editors: *Werner and Ingbar's the thyroid: a fundamental and clinical text*, ed 10, Philadelphia, 2013, Lippincott Williams and Wilkins, p 434.

Chalmers HJ, et al.: Identifying removalbe radioactivity on the surface of cats during the first week after treatment with Iodine 131, *Vet Rad Ultrasound* 47:507, 2006.

Chiha M, et al.: Thyroid storm: an updated review, *J Intensive Care Med* [Epub ahead of print], 2013.

Christopher MM: Relation of endogenous Heinz bodies to disease and anemia in cats: 120 cases (1978-1987), *J Am Vet Med Assoc* 194:1089, 1989.

Chun R, et al.: Predictors of response to radioiodine therapy in hyperthyroid cats, *Vet Radiol Ultrasound* 43:587, 2002.

Combes A, et al.: Ultrasonographic measurements of adrenal glands in cats with hyperthyroidism, *Vet Radiol Ultrasound* 53(2):210, 2012.

Connolly DJ, et al.: Serum troponin I levels in hyperthyroid cats before and after treatment with radioactive iodine, *J Feline Med Surg* 7:289, 2005.

Cook AK, et al.: The prevalence of hypocobalaminemia in cats with spontaneous hyperthyroidism, *J Small Anim Pract* 52:101, 2011.

Cook SM, et al.: Radiographic and scintigraphic evidence of focal pulmonary neoplasia in three cats with hyperthyroidism: diagnostic and therapeutic considerations, *J Vet Intern Med* 7:303, 1993.

Cooper DS: Treatment of thyrotoxicosis. In Braverman LE, Cooper DS, editors: *Werner and Ingbar's the thyroid: a fundamental and clinical text*, ed 10, Philadelphia, 2013, Lippincott Williams and Wilkins, p 492.

Court MH, Freeman LM: Identification and concentration of soy isoflavones in commercial cat foods, *Am J Vet Res* 63:181, 2002.

Court MH, Greenblatt DJ: Molecular genetic basis for deficient acetaminophen glucuronidation by cats: UGT1A6 is a pseudogene, and evidence for reduced diversity of expressed hepatic UGT1A isoforms, *Pharmacogenetics* 10:355, 2000.

Craig A, et al.: A prospective study of 66 cases of feline hyperthyroidism treated with a fixed dose of intravenous ^{131}I, *Aust Vet Practit* 23:2, 1993.

Daniel GB, et al.: Quantitative thyroid scintigraphy as a predictor of serum thyroxine concentration in normal and hyperthyroid cats, *Vet Radiol Ultrasound* 43(4):374, 2002.

de Lange MS, et al.: High urinary corticoid/creatinine ratios in cats with hyperthyroidism, *J Vet Intern Med* 18(2):152, 2004.

De Wet CS, et al.: Prevalence of and risk factors for feline hyperthyroidism in Hong Kong, *J Feline Med Surg* 11(4):315, 2009.

DiBartola SP, et al.: Effects of treatment of hyperthyroidism on renal function in cats, *J Am Vet Med Assoc* 208:875, 1996.

Doerge DR, Sheehan DM: Goitrogenic and estrogenic activity of soy isoflavones, *Environ Health Perspect* 3:349, 2002.

Duyff RF, et al.: Neuromuscular findings in thyroid dysfunction: a prospective clinical and electrodiagnostic study, *J Neurol Neurosurg Psychiatry* 68:750, 2000.

Edinboro CH, et al.: Epidemiologic study of relationships between consumption of commercial canned food and risk of hyperthyroidism in cats, *J Am Vet Med Assoc* 224:879, 2004.

Edinboro CH, et al.: Feline hyperthyroidism: potential relationship with iodine supplement requirements of commercial cat foods, *J Feline Med Surg* 12:672, 2010.

Edinboro CH, et al.: Iodine concentration in commercial cat foods from three regions of the USA, 2008-2009, *J Feline Med Surg* 15:717, 2013.

Feeney DA, et al.: Relationship between orally administered dose, surface emission rate for gamma irradiation, and urine radioactivity in radioiodine treated hyperthyroid cats, *Am J Vet Res* 64:1242, 2003.

Feldman EC, Nelson RW: *Canine and feline endocrinology and reproduction*, ed 3, St Louis, 2004, Saunders/Elsevier.

Fischetti AJ, et al.: Effects of methimazole on thyroid gland uptake of ^{99m}TC-pertechnetate in 19 hyperthyroid cats, *Vet Radiol Ultrasound* 46:267, 2005.

Flanders JA, et al.: Feline thyroidectomy: a comparison of postoperative hypocalcemia associated with three different surgical techniques, *Vet Surg* 16:362, 1987.

Flanders JA, et al.: Functional analysis of ectopic parathyroid activity in cats, *Am J Vet Res* 52:1336, 1991.

Forrest LJ, et al.: Feline hyperthyroidism: efficacy of treatment using volumetric analysis for radioiodine dose calculation, *Vet Radiol Ultrasound* 37:141, 1996.

Foster DJ, Thoday KL: Use of propranolol and potassium iodate in the presurgical management of hyperthyroid cats, *J Small Anim Pract* 40:307, 1999.

Foster DJ, Thoday KL: Tissue sources of serum alkaline phosphatase in 34 hyperthyroid cats: a qualitative and quantitative study, *Res Vet Sci* 68:89, 2000.

Foster DJ, et al.: Selenium status of cats in four regions of the world and comparison with reported incidence of hyperthyroidism in cats in those regions, *Am J Vet Res* 62:934, 2001.

Fox PR, et al.: Electrocardiographic and radiographic changes in cats with hyperthyroidism: comparison of populations evaluated during 1992-1993 vs. 1979-1982, *J Am Anim Hosp Assoc* 35:27, 1999.

Frénais R, et al.: Clinical efficacy and safety of a once-daily formulation of carbimazole in cats with hyperthyroidism, *J Small Anim Pract* 50:510, 2009.

Gallagher AE, et al.: Efficacy of iopanic acid for treatment of spontaneous hyperthyroidism in cats, *J Feline Med Surg* 13:441, 2011.

Goldstein RE, et al.: Percutaneous ethanol injection for treatment of unilateral hyperplastic thyroid nodules in cats, *J Am Vet Med Assoc* 218:1298, 2001.

Gordon JM, et al.: Juvenile hyperthyroidism in a cat, *J Am Anim Hosp Assoc* 39:67, 2003.

Graves TK, et al.: Changes in renal function associated with treatment of hyperthyroidism in cats, *Am J Vet Res* 55:1745, 1994.

Guptill L, et al.: Response to high-dose radioactive iodine administration in cats with thyroid carcinoma that had previously undergone surgery, *J Am Vet Med Assoc* 207:1055, 1995.

Hammer KB, et al.: Altered expression of G proteins in thyroid gland adenomas obtained from hyperthyroid cats, *Am J Vet Res* 61:874, 2000.

Harvey AM, et al.: Scintigraphic findings in 120 hyperthyroid cats, *J Feline Med Surg* 11:96, 2009.

Hays MT, et al.: A multicompartmental model for iodide, thyroxine, and triiodothyronine metabolism in normal and spontaneously hyperthyroid cats, *Endocrinology* 122:2444, 1988.

Henik RA, et al.: Efficacy of atenolol as a single antihypertensive agent in hyperthyroid cats, *J Feline Med Surg* 10:577, 2008.

Hibbert A, et al.: Feline thyroid carcinoma: diagnosis and response to high-dose radioactive iodine treatment, *J Feline Med Surg* 11:116, 2009.

Hill KE, et al.: The efficacy and safety of a novel lipophilic formulation of methimazole for once daily transdermal treatment of cats with hyperthyroidism, *J Vet Intern Med* 25:1357, 2011.

Hoenig M, Ferguson DC: Impairment of glucose tolerance in hyperthyroid cats, *J Endocrinol* 121:249, 1989.

Hoffman SB, et al.: Bioavailability of transdermal methimazole in a pluronic lecithin organogel in healthy cats, *J Vet Pharmacol Ther* 25:189, 2002.

Hofmeister E, et al.: Functional cystic thyroid adenoma in a cat, *J Am Vet Med Assoc* 219:190, 2001.

Holtman JR Jr, et al.: Central respiratory stimulation produced by thyrotropin-releasing hormone in the cat, *Peptides* 7:207, 1986.

Holzworth J, et al.: Hyperthyroidism in the cat: ten cases, *J Am Vet Med Assoc* 46:345, 1980.

Ishii S, et al.: Triiodothyronine (T3) stimulates food intake via enhanced hypothalamic AMP-activated activity, *Regul Pept* 151:164, 2008.

Jacobs G, Panciera D: Cardiovascular complications of feline hyperthyroidism. In Kirk RW, Bonagura JD, editors: *Kirks' current veterinary therapy XI: small animal practice*, Philadelphia, 1992, WB Saunders, p 756.

Jacobs G, et al.: Congestive heart failure associated with hyperthyroidism in cats, *J Am Vet Med Assoc* 188:52, 1986.

Jacobs G, et al.: Pharmacokinetics of propranolol in healthy cats during euthyroid and hyperthyroid states, *Am J Vet Res* 58:398, 1997.

Jepson RE, et al.: Effect of control of systolic blood pressure on survival in cats with systemic hypertension, *J Vet Intern Med* 21:402, 2007.

Johnson LA, et al.: Iodine content of commercially-prepared cat foods, *NZ Vet J* 40:18, 1992.

Jones BR, Johnstone AC: Hyperthyroidism in an aged cat, *NZ Vet J* 29:70, 1981.

Jones BR, et al.: Radioiodine treatment of hyperthyroidism in cats, *NZ Vet J* 39:71, 1991.

Kang J-H, Kondo F: Determination of bisphenol A in canned pet foods, *Res Vet Sci* 73:177, 2002.

Kass PH, et al.: Evaluation of environmental, nutritional, and host factors in cats with hyperthyroidism, *J Vet Intern Med* 13:323, 1999.

Kobayashi DL, et al.: Hypertension in cats with chronic renal failure and hyperthyroidism, *J Vet Intern Med* 4:58, 1990.

Klein I, Ojamaa K: Thyroid hormone and the cardiovascular system, *N Engl J Med* 344:501, 2001.

Knowles S, et al.: Intraperitoneal ectopic thyroid carcinoma in a cat, *J Vet Diagn Invest* 22:1010, 2010.

Köhler B, et al.: Dietary hyperthyroidism in dogs, *J Small Anim Pract* 53:182, 2012.

Ladenson PW: Diagnosis of thyrotoxicosis. In Braverman LE, Cooper DS, editors: *Werner and Ingbar's the thyroid: a fundamental and clinical text*, ed 10, Philadelphia, 2013, Lippincott Williams and Wilkins, p 487.

Lapointe C, et al.: N-Acetyl-b-D-Glucosaminidase index as an early biomarker for chronic kidney disease in cats with hyperthyroidism, *J Vet Intern Med* 22:1103, 2008.

Laurberg P, et al.: High incidence of multinodular toxic goiter in the elderly population in a low iodine area vs. high incidence of Graves' disease in the young in a high iodine area: comparative surveys of thyrotoxicosis epidemiology in East-Jutland Denmark, and Iceland, *J Int Med* 229:415, 1991.

Lautenschlaeger IE, et al.: Comparison between computed tomography and ^{99m}Tc-pertechnetate scintigraphy characteristics of the thyroid gland in cats with hyperthyroidism, *Vet Radiol Ultrasound* 54:666, 2013.

Lee WR, et al.: The effects of iohexol administration on technetium thyroid scintigraphy in normal cats, *Vet Radiol Ultrasound* 51(2):182, 2010.

Liggert SB, et al.: Increased fat and skeletal muscle b-adrenergic receptors but unaltered metabolic and hemodynamic sensitivity to epinephrine in vivo in experimental human thyrotoxicosis, *J Clin Invest* 83:803, 1989.

Link KR, Rand JS: Changes in blood glucose concentration are associated with relatively rapid changes in circulating fructosamine concentrations in cats, *J Feline Med Surg* 10(6):583, 2008.

Liu S, et al.: Hypertrophic cardiomyopathy and hyperthyroidism in the cat, *J Am Vet Med Assoc* 185:52, 1984.

Lynn A, et al.: Caudal mediastinal thyroglossal cyst in a cat, *J Small Anim Pract* 50:147, 2009.

Mallery KF, et al.: Percutaneous ultrasound-guided radiofrequency heat ablation for treatment of hyperthyroidism in cats, *J Am Vet Med Assoc* 223:1602, 2003.

Manna D, et al.: Antithyroid drugs and their analogues: synthesis, structure, and mechanism of action, *Acc Chem Res* 46(11):2706, 2013.

Martin KM, et al.: Evaluation of dietary and environmental risk factors for hyperthyroidism in cats, *J Am Vet Med Assoc* 217:853, 2000.

Maxie MG: Neoplasms of the thyroid gland. In Maxie MG, editor: *Jubb, Kennedy, and Palmer's pathology of domestic animals*, ed 5, St Louis, 2007, Saunders/Elsevier, p 96.

Mayer-Roenne B, et al.: Urinary tract infections in cats with hyperthyroidism, diabetes mellitus, and chronic kidney disease, *J Feline Med Surg* 9:124, 2007.

McLoughlin MA, et al.: Influence of systemic nonthyroidal illness on serum concentrations of thyroxine in hyperthyroid cats, *J Am Anim Hosp Assoc* 29:227, 1993.

Melendez LD, et al.: Titration of dietary iodine for maintaining normal serum thyroxine concentrations in hyperthyroid cats (abstract), *J Vet Intern Med* 25:683, 2011a.

Melendez LM, et al.: Titration of dietary iodine for reducing serum thyroxine concentrations in newly diagnosed hyperthyroid cats (abstract), *J Vet Intern Med* 25:683, 2011b.

Mensching DA, et al.: The feline thyroid gland: a model for endocrine disruption by polybrominated dephenyl ethers (PBDEs)? *J Toxicol Environ Health A* 75(4):201, 2012.

Meric SM, Rubin SI: Serum thyroxine concentrations following fixed-dose radioactive iodine treatment in hyperthyroid cats: 62 cases (1986-1989), *J Am Vet Med Assoc* 197:621, 1990.

Meric SM, et al.: Serum thyroxine concentrations after radioactive iodine therapy in cats with hyperthyroidism, *J Am Vet Med Assoc* 188:1038, 1986.

Merryman JI, et al.: Overexpression of c-Ras in hyperplasia and adenomas of the feline thyroid gland: An immunohistochemical analysis of 34 cases, *Vet Pathol* 36(2):117, 1999.

Milner RJ, et al.: Survival times for cats with hyperthyroidism treated with iodine 131, methimazole, or both: 167 cases (1996-2003), *J Am Vet Med Assoc* 228:559, 2006.

Mooney CT: Radioactive iodine therapy for feline hyperthyroidism: effciacy and administration routes, *J Small Anim Pract* 35:289, 1994.

Mooney CT, et al.: Carbimazole therapy of feline hyperthyroidism, *J Small Anim Pract* 33:228, 1992.

Mooney CT, et al.: Effect of illness not associated with the thyroid gland on serum total and free thyroxine concentrations in cats, *J Am Vet Med Assoc* 208:2004, 1996a.

Mooney CT, et al.: Serum thyroxine and triiodothyronine responses of hyperthyroid cats to thyrotropin, *Am J Vet Res* 57:987, 1996b.

Mumma RO, et al.: Toxic and protective constituents in pet foods, *Am J Vet Res* 47:1633, 1986.

Murray LA, Peterson ME: Ipodate treatment of hyperthyroidism in cats, *J Am Vet Med Assoc* 211(1):63, 1997.

Naan EC, et al.: Results of thyroidectomy in 101 cats with hyperthyroidism, *Vet Surg* 35:287, 2006.

Nap AM, et al.: Quantitative aspects of thyroid scintigraphy with pertechnetate (^{99m}TcO$_4$) in cats, *J Vet Intern Med* 8:302, 1994.

Nelson LL, et al.: Pharyngeal pouch and cleft remnants in the dog and cat: a case series and review, *J Am Anim Hosp Assoc* 48:105, 2012.

Nemzek JA, et al.: Acute onset of hypokalemia and muscular weakness in four hyperthyroid cats, *J Am Vet Med Assoc* 205:65, 1994.

Nguyen LQ, et al.: Serum from cats with hyperthyroidism does not activate feline thyrotropin receptors, *Endocrinology* 143:395, 2002.

Nieckarz JA, Daniel GB: The effect of methimazole on thyroid uptake of pertechnetate and radioiodine in normal cats, *Vet Radiol Ultrasound* 42:448, 2001.

Niessen SJ, et al.: Generalized lymphadenomegaly associated with methimazole treatment in a hyperthyroid cat, *J Small Anim Pract* 48:165, 2007.

Norsworthy GD, et al.: Palpable thyroid and parathyroid nodules in asymptomatic cats, *J Feline Med Surg* 4:145, 2002.

Olczak J, et al.: Multivariate analysis of risk factors for feline hyperthyrodism in New Zealand, *NZ Vet J* 53:1, 2005.

Padgett SL, et al.: Efficacy of parathyroid gland autotransplantation in maintaining serum calcium concentrations after bilateral thyroparathyroidectomy in cats, *J Am Anim Hosp Assoc* 34:219, 1998.

Page RB, et al.: Accuracy of increased thyroid activity during pertechnetate scintigraphy by subcutaneous injection for diagnosing hyperthyroidism in cats, *Vet Radiol Ultrasound* 47(2):206, 2006.

Papasouliotis K, et al.: Decreased orocaecal transit time, as measured by the exhalation of hydrogen in hyperthyroid cats, *Res Vet Sci* 55:115, 1993.

Patrick L: Iodine: deficiency and therapeutic considerations, *Altern Med Rev* 13(2):116, 2008.

Pedersen IB, et al.: Large differences in incidences of overt hyper- and hypothyroidism associated with a small difference in iodine intake: a prospective comparative register-based population survey, *J Clin Endocrinol Metab* 87:4462, 2002.

Peremans K, et al.: Interference of iohexol with radioiodine thyroid uptake in the hyperthyroid cat, *J Feline Med Surg* 10:460, 2008.

Peter HJ, et al.: Autonomy of growth and of iodine metabolism in hyperthyroid feline goiters transplanted onto nude mice, *J Clin Invest* 80:491, 1987.

Peter HJ, et al.: Autonomous growth and function of cultured feline thyroid follicles from cats with spontaneous hyperthyroidism, *Thyroid* 1:331, 1991.

Peterson ME, Aucoin DP: Comparison of the disposition of carbimazole and methimazole in clinically normal cats, *Res Vet Sci* 54:351, 1993.

Peterson ME, Becker DV: Radioiodine treatment of 524 cats with hyperthyroidism, *J Am Vet Med Assoc* 207:1422, 1995.

Peterson ME, Gamble DA: Effect of nonthyroidal disease on serum thyroxine concentrations in cats: 494 cases (1988), *J Am Vet Med Assoc* 197:1203, 1990b.

Peterson ME, et al.: Spontaneous hyperthyroidism in the cat abstract, *Am Coll Vet Intern Med* 108, 1979.

Peterson ME: Hyperthyroidism in cats: what's causing this epidemic of thyroid disease and how can we prevent it? *J Feline Med Surg* 14:804, 2012.

Peterson ME, et al.: Feline hyperthyroidism: pretreatment clinical and laboratory evaluation of 131 cases, *J Am Vet Med Assoc* 103:103, 1983.

Peterson ME, et al.: Propylthiouracil-associated hemolytic anemia, thrombocytopenia, and antinuclear antibodies in cats with hyperthyroidism, *J Am Vet Med Assoc* 184:806, 1984.

Peterson ME, et al.: Serum thyroid hormone concentrations fluctuate in cats with hyperthyroidism, *J Vet Intern Med* 1:142, 1987.

Peterson ME, et al.: Methimazole treatment of 262 cats with hyperthyroidism, *J Vet Intern Med* 2:150, 1988.

Peterson ME, et al.: Triiodothyronine (T_3) suppression test: an aid in the diagnosis of mild hyperthyroidism in cats, *J Vet Intern Med* 4:233, 1990a.

Peterson ME, et al.: Use of the thyrotropin-releasing hormone (TRH) stimulation test to diagnose mild hyperthyroidism in cats, *J Vet Intern Med* 8:279, 1994.

Peterson ME, et al.: Measurement of serum concentrations of free thyroxine, total thyroxine, and total triiodothyronine in cats with hyperthyroidism and cats with nonthyroidal disease, *J Am Vet Med Assoc* 218:529, 2001.

Peterson ME, et al.: Accuracy of serum free thyroxine concentrations determined by a new veterinary chemiluminescent immunoassay in euthyroid and hyperthyroid cats [abstract]. Proceedings of the 21st ECVIM-CA Congress. Seville (Spain), September 8-10, 2011.

Pétervári E, et al.: Hyperphagia of hyperthyroidism: is neuropeptide Y involved? *Regul Pept* 131:103, 2005.

Phillips DE, et al.: Cystic parathyroid and parathyroid lesions in cats, *J Am Anim Hosp Assoc* 39:349, 2003.

Pignato A, et al.: Stability of methimazole in poloxamer lecithin organogel to determine beyond-use date, *Int J Pharm Compd* 14:522–525, 2010.

Quinones M, et al.: Pharmacokinetics of atenolol in clinically normal cats. *Am J Vet Res* 57:1050, 1996.

Ramspott S, et al.: Adrenal function in cats with hyperthyroidism, *J Feline Med Surg* 14:262, 2012.

Rand SJ, et al.: Acute stress hyperglycemia in cats is associated with struggling and increased concentrations of lactate and norepinephrine, *J Vet Intern Med* 16:123, 2002.

Randolph JF, et al.: Prothrombin, activated partial thromboplastin, and proteins induced by vitamin K absence or antagonists: clotting times in 20 hyperthyroid cats before and after methimazole treatment, *J Vet Intern Med* 14:56, 2000.

Ranz D, et al.: Estimation of iodine status in cats, *J Nutr* 132(Suppl 2):1751S, 2002.

Reed TP, et al.: Cystic ectopic lingual thyroid tissue in a male cat, *J Am Vet Med Assoc* 239:981, 2011.

Refsal KR, et al.: Use of the triiodothyronine suppression test for diagnosis of hyperthyroidism in ill cats that have a serum concentration of iodothyronines within normal range, *J Am Vet Med Assoc* 199:1594, 1991.

Reusch CE, Tomsa K: Serum fructosamine concentration in cats with overt hyperthyroidism, *J Am Vet Med Assoc* 215:1297, 1999.

Riensche MR, et al.: An investigation of predictors of renal insufficiency following treatment of hyperthyroidism in cats, *J Feline Med Surg* 10:160, 2008.

Roti E, Vagenakis G: Effect of excess iodide: clinical aspects. In Braverman LE, Cooper DS, editors: *Werner and Ingbar's the thyroid: a fundamental and clinical text*, ed 10, Philadelphia PA, 2013, Lippincott Williams and Wilkins, p 242.

Ruaux CG, et al.: Early biochemical and clinical responses to cobalamin supplementation in cats with signs of gastrointestinal disease and severe hypocobalaminemia, *J Vet Intern Med* 19:155, 2005.

Rutland BE, et al.: Optimal testing for thyroid hormone concentration after treatment with methimazole in healthy and hyperthyroid cats, *J Vet Intern Med* 23:1025, 2009.

Sabatino BR, et al.: Amino acid, iodine, selenium, and coat color status among hyperthyroid Siamese, and age-matched control cats, *J Vet Intern Med* 27(5):1049, 2013.

Sartor LL, et al.: Efficacy and safety of transdermal methimazole in the treatment of cats with hyperthyroidism, *J Vet Intern Med* 18:651, 2004.

Sassnau R: Epidemiological investigation on the prevalence of feline hyperthyroidism in an urban population in Germany, *Tierarztliche Praxis* 35:375, 2006.

Scarlett JM, et al.: Feline hyperthyroidism: a descriptive and case-control study, *Prev Vet Med* 6:295, 1988.

Schaafsma IA, et al.: Effect of four sedative and anesthetic protocols on quantitative thyroid scintigraphy in euthyroid cats, *Am J Vet Res* 67:1362, 2006.

Schlesinger DP, et al.: Use of breath hydrogen measurement to evaluate orocecal transit time in cats before and after treatment for hyperthyroidism, *Can Vet J* 57:89, 1993.

Scott-Moncrieff JC: Thyroid disorders in the geriatric veterinary patient, *Vet Clin Small Anim* 42:707, 2012.

Shelton GD, et al.: Risk factors for acquired myasthenia gravis on cats: 105 cases (1986-1998), *J Am Vet Med Assoc* 216:55, 2000.

Shi G-M, et al.: Influence of propylthiouracil and methimazole pre-treatment on the outcome of Iodine-131 therapy in hyperthyroid patients with Graves' disease, *J Int Med Res* 37(2):576, 2009.

Slater MR, et al.: Long-term health and predictors of survival for hyperthyroid cats treated with iodine-131, *J Vet Intern Med* 15:47, 2001.

Sparkes AK, et al.: Thyroid function in the cat: assessment by the TRH response test and the thyrotropin stimulation test, *J Small Anim Pract* 32:59, 1991.

Stegeman JR, et al.: Use of recombinant human thyroid-stimulating hormone for thyrotropin-stimulation testing of euthyroid cats, *Am J Vet Res* 64(2):149, 2003.

Stepien RL: Feline systemic hypertension: diagnosis and management, *J Feline Med Surg* 13:35, 2011.

Sullivan P, et al.: Altered platelet indices in dogs with hypothyroidism and cats with hyperthyroidism, *Am J Vet Res* 54:2004, 1993.

Swalec KM, Birchard SJ: Recurrence of hyperthyroidism after thyroidectomy in cats, *J Am Anim Hosp Assoc* 26:433, 1990.

Syme HM, Elliott J: The prevalence of hypertension in hyperthyroid cats at diagnosis and following treatment, *J Vet Intern Med* 17:754, 2003.

Syme HM: Cardiovascular and renal manifestations of hyperthyroidism, *Vet Clin North Am Small Anim Pract* 37(4):723, 2007.

Théon AP, et al.: A prospective randomized comparison of intravenous versus subcutaneous administration of radioiodine for treatment of feline hyperthyroidism: a study of 120 cats, *Am J Vet Res* 55:1734, 1994.

Thoday KL, Mooney CT: Historical, clinical and laboratory features of 126 hyperthyroid cats, *Vet Rec* 131:257, 1992.

Tolbert MK, Ward CR: Feline Thyroid storm. :Rapid recognition to improve patient survival, *Compend Contin Educ Vet*, Vol.32(12), p.E2-E2, 2010.

Tolbert K, et al.: Dermoid cysts presenting as enlarged thyroid glands in a cat, *J Feline Med Surg* 11:717, 2009.

Tomsa K, et al.: Thyrotropin-releasing hormone stimulation test to assess thyroid function in severely sick cats, *J Vet Intern Med* 15:89, 2001.

Trepanier LA: Medical management of hyperthyroidism, *Clin Tech Small Anim Pract* 21(1):22, 2006.

Trepanier LA: Pharmacologic management of feline hyperthyroidism, *Vet Clin North Am Small Anim Pract* 37(4):775, 2007.

Trepanier LA, et al.: Efficacy and safety of once versus twice daily administration of methimazole in cats with hyperthyroidism, *J Am Vet Med Assoc* 222:954, 2003.

Turrel JM, et al.: Radioactive iodine therapy in cats with hyperthyroidism, *J Am Vet Med Assoc* 184:554, 1984.

Turrel JM, et al.: Thyroid carcinoma causing hyperthyroidism in cats: 14 cases (1981-1986), *J Am Vet Med Assoc* 193:359, 1988.

van der Kooij M, et al.: Effects of an iodine-restricted food on client-owned cats with hyperthyroidism, *J Feline Med Surg* [Epub ahead of print], 2013.

Vandermeulen E, et al.: A single method for evaluating ^{51}chromium-ethylene diaminic tetraacetic acid clearance in normal and hyperthyroid cats, *J Vet Intern Med* 22:266, 2008.

van der Woerdt A, Peterson ME: Prevalence of ocular abnormalities in cats with hyperthyroidism, *J Vet Intern Med* 14(2):202, 2000.

van Hoek I, et al.: Plasma clearance of exogenous creatinine, exo-iohexol, and endo-iohexol in hyperthyroid cats before and after treatment with radioiodine, *J Vet Intern Med* 22:879, 2008a.

van Hoek I, et al.: Recombinant human thyrotropin administration enhances thyroid uptake of radioactive iodine in hyperthyroid cats, *J Vet Intern Med* 22:1340, 2008b.

van Hoek I, et al.: Short- and long-term follow-up of glomerular and tubular renal markers of kidney function in hyperthyroid cats after treatment with radioiodine, *Domest Anim Endocrinol* 36(1):45, 2009a.

van Hoek I, et al.: Retinol binding protein in serum and urine of hyperthyroid cats before and after treatment with radioiodine, *J Vet Intern Med* 23:1031, 2009b.

Wakeling J, et al.: Subclinical hyperthyroidism in cats: a spontaneous model of subclinical toxic nodular goiter in humans? *Thyroid* 17:12, 2007.

Wakeling J, et al.: Diagnosis of hyperthyroidism in cats with mild chronic kidney disease, *J Small Anim Pract* 49:287, 2008.

Wakeling J, et al.: Urinary iodide concentration in hyperthyroid cats, *Am J Vet Res* 70:741, 2009a.

Wakeling J, et al.: Risk factors for feline hyperthyroidism in the UK, *J Small Anim Pract* 50:406, 2009b.

Wakeling J, et al.: Evaluation of predictors for the diagnosis of hyperthyroidism in cats, *J Vet Intern Med* 25:1057, 2011.

Wang W, et al.: Polyuria of thyrotoxicosis: downregulation of aquaporin water channels and increased solute excretion, *Kidney Int* 72(9):1088, 2007.

Ward CR: Feline thyroid storm, *Vet Clin North Am Small Anim Pract* 37(4):745, 2007.

Ward CR, et al.: Thyrotropin-stimulated DNA synthesis and thyroglobulin expression in normal and hyperthyroid feline thyrocytes in monolayer culture, *Thyroid* 15:114, 2005a.

Ward CR, et al.: Expression of inhibitory G proteins in adenomatous thyroid glands obtained from hyperthyroid cats, *Am J Vet Res* 66:1478, 2005b.

Ward CR, et al.: Evaluation of activation of G proteins in response to thyroid stimulating hormone in thyroid gland cells from euthyroid and hyperthyroid cats, *Am J Vet Res* 71:643, 2010.

Watson SG, et al.: Somatic mutations of the thyroid-stimulating hormone receptor gene in feline hyperthyroidism: parallels with human hyperthyroidism, *J Endocrinol* 186(3):523, 2005.

Wedekind KJ, et al.: The feline iodine requirement is lower than the 2006 NRC recommended allowance, *J Anim Physiol Anim Nutr* 94(4):527, 2010.

Weichselbaum RC, et al.: Relationship between selected echocardiographic variables before and after radioiodine treatment in 91 hyperthyroid cats, *Vet Radiol Ultrasound* 46(6):506, 2005.

Weiss DJ: Aplastic anemia in cats-clinicopathologic features and associated disease conditions 1996-2004, *J Feline Med Surg* 8:203, 2006.

Welches CD, et al.: Occurrence of problems after three techniques of bilateral thyroidectomy in cats, *Vet Surg* 18:392, 1989.

Wells AL, et al.: Use of percutaneous ethanol injection for treatment of bilateral hyperplastic thyroid nodules in cats, *J Am Vet Med Assoc* 218:1293, 2001.

White HL, et al.: Effect of dietary soy on serum thyroid hormone concentrations in healthy adult cats, *Am J Vet Res* 65:586, 2004.

Williams GR: The skeletal system in thyrotoxicosis. In Braverman LE, Cooper DS, editors: *Werner and Ingbar's the thyroid: a fundamental and clinical text*, ed 10, Philadelphia, 2013, Lippincott Williams and Wilkins, p 468.

Williams TL, et al.: Association of iatrogenic hypothyroidism with azotemia and reduced survival time in cats treated for hyperthyroidism, *J Vet Intern Med* 24:1086, 2010a.

Williams TL, et al.: Survival and the development of azotemia after treatment of hyperthyroid cats, *J Vet Intern Med* 24:863, 2010b.

Williams TL, et al.: Calcium and phosphate homeostasis in hyperthyroid cats: associations with development of azotemia and survival time, *J Small Anim Pract* 53(10):561, 2012.

Williams TL, et al.: Investigation of the pathophysiological mechanism for altered calcium homeostasis in hyperthyroid cats, *J Small Anim Pract* 54:367, 2013.

Wisner ER, et al.: Ultrasonographic examination of the thyroid gland of hyperthyroid cats: comparison to ^{99m}Tc scintigraphy, *Vet Radiol Ultrasound* 35:53, 1994.

Wood ET, Kinlaw WB: Nondiabetic ketoacidosis caused by severe hyperthyroidism, *Thyroid* 14:628, 2004.

Yu S, et al.: A low selenium diet increases thyroxine and decreases 3,5,3′ triiodothyronine in the plasma of kittens, *J Anim Physiol and Anim Nutr* 86:36, 2002.

Yu S, et al.: Controlled level of dietary iodine normalizes serum total thyroxine concentrations in cats with naturally occurring hyperthyroidism, *J Vet Intern Med* 25:683, 2011.

CHAPTER 5

Canine Thyroid Tumors and Hyperthyroidism

J. Catharine Scott-Moncrieff

CHAPTER CONTENTS

Estimates for the prevalence of thyroid tumors in dogs range from 1% to 4% of all canine neoplasms (Brodey and Kelly, 1968; Birchard and Roesel, 1981; Harari et al, 1986). Although thyroid adenomas do occur in the dog, they are usually nonfunctional and too small to be palpable; they are therefore rarely identified clinically. Conversely thyroid carcinomas are usually large, nonfunctional, invasive, and malignant. For this reason approximately 90% of clinically detectable thyroid tumors in dogs are carcinomas. The thyroid gland is not normally palpable in dogs, and a palpable thyroid gland is therefore highly likely to be due to a malignant thyroid tumor.

TUMOR CLASSIFICATION

Although most thyroid tumors arise in the thyroid gland, tumors may also develop in vestigial thyroid tissue that may be present anywhere from the base of the tongue to the base of the heart (see Chapter 3; Capen, 2007). Benign thyroid tumors (adenomas) account for 30% to 50% of thyroid masses identified in studies published by veterinary pathologists (Brodey and Kelly, 1968; Leav et al, 1976). These benign tumors tend to be small, non-invasive, clinically silent, non-palpable tumors that involve one thyroid lobe and are incidental findings on necropsy. However, almost all clinically significant thyroid tumors in dogs are malignant and classified as carcinomas of varying types (Withrow and MacEwen, 2012). Malignant thyroid tumors in dogs are usually large fixed masses that are easily palpable. About two thirds of carcinomas are located in one lobe, whereas one third involve both lobes of the thyroid. Thyroid carcinomas are usually poorly encapsulated and commonly extend into or around the trachea, esophagus, and muscles of the neck. Thyroid tumors are usually highly vascular and may invade local blood vessels with resultant hemorrhage (Slensky et al, 2003).

THYROID ADENOMA/CARCINOMA

Most thyroid tumors are adenomas or carcinomas that arise from the epithelial cells that line the thyroid follicles. In dogs, most small solid thyroid adenomas are characterized by either small or large irregular follicles containing varying amounts of colloid (Leav et al, 1976). The cystic structures noted in some tumors are lined by dense fibrous capsules from which project fronds of uniform cells arranged in follicular and/or compact cellular patterns.

Thyroid follicular carcinomas are usually well differentiated and the distinction between benign and malignant is made based primarily on whether there is evidence of capsular or vascular invasion. Criteria such as cellular atypia and mitotic activity are not reliable markers of malignancy in thyroid tumors (Leav et al, 1976). Thyroid tumors of follicular cell origin may be further subclassified into follicular, compact (solid), papillary, compact-follicular, or undifferentiated (anaplastic) carcinomas depending on their pattern of growth (Box 5-1). In addition, veterinary oncologists use a clinical staging classification system initially developed by the World Health Organization Owen 1980 (Table 5-1). Most canine thyroid carcinomas contain both follicular and compact cellular patterns and are classified as compact follicular (mixed follicular-compact cellular) carcinomas. Slightly less common are pure follicular carcinomas. A smaller percentage of thyroid tumors are pure compact carcinomas. Undifferentiated (anaplastic) tumors are recognized in about 10% of dogs with thyroid tumors, whereas papillary carcinomas are rare (Leav et al, 1976). Although histologic subtype has prognostic significance in human thyroid tumors, it does not appear to influence outcome for well-differentiated tumors in dogs; however, high grade and anaplastic thyroid tumors do have a less favorable outcome.

In addition to tumors arising from follicular cells, medullary thyroid carcinomas may arise from the parafollicular C cells, which are

BOX 5-1 **Histologic Classification of Thyroid Tumors in Dogs**

Follicular adenoma
Compact follicular carcinoma
Follicular carcinoma
Compact (solid) carcinomas
Undifferentiated (anaplastic) carcinomas
Papillary carcinomas
Parafollicular (C-cell) carcinomas

TABLE 5-1 **CLINICAL STAGING OF CANINE THYROID TUMORS**

T: Primary Tumor

T0 No evidence of tumor

T1 Tumor < 2 cm maximum diameter: T1a, not fixed; T1b, fixed

T2 Tumor 2 to 5 cm maximum diameter: T2a, not fixed; T2b, fixed

T3 Tumor > 5 cm maximum diameter: T3a, not fixed; T3b, fixed

N: Regional Lymph Nodes*

N0 No evidence of RLN involvement†

N1 Ipsilateral RLN involved: N1a, not fixed; N1b, fixed

N2 Bilateral RLN involved: N2a, not fixed; N2b, fixed

M: Distant Metastasis

M0 No evidence of distant metastasis

M1 Distant metastasis detected

STAGE GROUPING	T	N	M
I	T1a, b	N0	M0
II	T0	N1	M0
	T1a, b	N1	M0
	T2a, b	N0 or N1a	M0
III	Any T3	Any N	M0
	Any T	Any N	M0
IV	Any T	Any N	M1

Modified from Owen LN, editor: *TNM classification of tumours in domestic animals*, Geneva, 1980, World Health Organization.
*The regional lymph nodes (RLNs) are the mandibular and the superficial cervical lymph nodes.
†Involvement implies histologic evidence of tumor invasion.

part of the amine precursor uptake decarboxylation (APUD) system and produce calcitonin (see Chapter 15). Although the tumors arise from different progenitor cells, the clinical presentation and treatment options for follicular and medullary carcinomas are similar.

 PATHOGENESIS OF THYROID TUMORS

As with most neoplastic conditions in dogs, the exact cause of thyroid tumors is not known. Studies in humans have suggested an association between thyroid neoplasia and (1) iodine deficiency or excess, (2) chronic excesses in thyroid-stimulating hormone (also known as thyrotropin; TSH) secretion, (3) ionizing radiation, and (4) gene abnormalities and oncogene expression. In dogs the only known risk factors for thyroid neoplasia are hypothyroidism due to thyroiditis (Benjamin et al, 1996) and ionizing radiation (Benjamin et al, 1997).

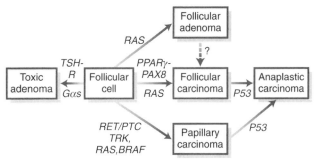

FIGURE 5-1 Genetic events in thyroid tumorigenesis. Activating point mutations of the RAS gene are found with a high frequency in follicular adenomas and carcinomas and are considered to be an early event in follicular tumorigenesis. The PPARγ-PAX8 rearrangement is found only in follicular tumors. Rearrangements of transmembrane receptors with tyrosine kinase activity (RET/PTC TRK genes) and activating point mutations of the BRAF gene are found only in papillary thyroid carcinomas (PTCs). Inactivating point mutations of the P53 gene are found only in poorly-differentiated and anaplastic thyroid carcinomas. Activation of the cyclic adenosine monophosphate pathway by point mutation of the thyrotropin receptor *(TSH-R)* or the alpha subunit of the G protein genes leads to the appearance of hyperfunctioning thyroid nodules. *Gαs*, Stimulatory guanyl nucleotide protein; *PPAR*, peroxisome proliferator-activated receptor. (Modified from Schlumberger M-J, et al.: Nontoxic diffuse and nodular goiter and thyroid neoplasia. In Melmed S, et al., editors: *Williams textbook of endocrinology*, ed 12, Philadelphia, 2011, Elsevier/Saunders, p. 452.)

Iodine Deficiency

Early epidemiologic studies suggested that thyroid cancer in humans was more frequent in iodine-deficient areas of the world. Although some of the evidence for an association between iodine intake and thyroid cancer is conflicting, the evidence for an association of iodine deficiency with an increased risk of follicular thyroid carcinoma (FTC) is quite strong (Schneider and Brenner, 2013). Studies in humans have demonstrated that when iodine supplementation is introduced into an iodine deficient area, the ratio of papillary to follicular carcinoma increases. These studies and others have suggested that iodine deficiency plays a role in the pathogenesis of follicular carcinoma, possibly due to prolonged TSH stimulation. Experimental data and clinical experience have neither confirmed nor denied the role of iodine in the pathogenesis of canine thyroid tumors.

Ionizing Radiation

The relationship between ionizing radiation and thyroid cancer is well established in humans. Radiation therapy of the cervical region and ingestion of radioactive iodine isotopes following nuclear accidents (e.g., at Chernobyl, Ukraine, in 1986) are associated with increased risk of thyroid neoplasia especially in children and adolescents. Thyroid neoplasia due to radiation exposure is usually well-differentiated thyroid papillary or papillary-follicular carcinomas (Schneider and Brenner, 2013). Ionizing radiation has also been demonstrated to be a cause of thyroid neoplasia in dogs (Benjamin et al, 1997).

Oncogenes

Genetic and epigenetic mutations have been shown to play a fundamental role in the pathogenesis of thyroid neoplasia in humans (Suarez et al, 2000; Schlumberger, 2011; Xing, 2013; Fig. 5-1). The progression of thyroid cancer occurs due to an accumulation of these mutations, which result in dysregulated activity of cellular signaling pathways that promotes the malignant transformation of normal tissue. Loss of radioiodine avidity of thyroid cancer promoted by the BRAF-V600E mutation is a cause of failure of radioiodine treatment in humans.

Studies investigating the molecular mechanisms of canine thyroid carcinoma are limited. In one study a p53 mutation was detected in one of 23 cases of thyroid carcinoma (Devilee et al, 1994). Trisomy 18 was the sole clonal cytogenetic abnormality found in a canine thyroid adenoma (Reimann et al, 1996). Aneuploidy is a common feature of canine thyroid carcinomas with hypoploidy being most common (Verschueren et al, 1991).

In a study of samples collected from 23 dogs with FTC, differential expression of 489 characterized transcripts were identified by microarray analysis between tissues from dogs with FTC and histologically normal thyroid tissue. Differentially expressed genes belonged to several gene categories including those regulating cell shape, cell adhesion, mitogen-activated protein (MAP) kinase activity, angiogenesis, and cell migration (Metivier et al, 2012). The expression of osteopontin was significantly increased in follicular carcinoma compared to normal thyroid tissue (Metivier et al, 2012). Osteopontin (secreted phosphoprotein I) is a promising marker for cancer detection and monitoring in humans and appears to also have potential in dogs.

Lymphocytic Thyroiditis/Hypothyroidism

Hypothyroidism due to lymphocytic thyroiditis was associated with the development of thyroid tumors in a colony of 276 Beagles that were allowed to live out their full life span without treatment of their thyroid disease. Lymphocytic thyroiditis was present in 26% of the beagles at the time of death and resulted in hypothyroidism in 16% of dogs in the colony. Hypothyroid dogs had an increased risk for thyroid follicular neoplasia, including follicular carcinoma. Fifty four percent of hypothyroid dogs had one or more thyroid neoplasms, whereas only 23% of euthyroid dogs had similar neoplasms (Benjamin et al, 1996). The authors hypothesized that chronic excess stimulation of residual follicular epithelium by TSH was responsible for the strong association between thyroiditis, hypothyroidism, and follicular neoplasia.

 BENIGN THYROID TUMORS

The majority of benign canine thyroid tumors (adenomas) are small, focal lesions that are not usually detected during life. When they are diagnosed, they are usually incidental findings identified by cervical ultrasonography. Much less commonly, a dog with a benign tumor may have a palpable mass or have clinical signs of hyperthyroidism (Leav et al, 1976; Lawrence et al, 1991). Canine thyroid adenomas are usually solitary masses and may be solid or cystic. Adenomas are typically round or ovoid and measure a few millimeters to several centimeters in diameter. They are usually cream to reddish brown in color and may compress adjacent normal thyroid tissue. Cystic adenomas can be turgid and filled with an amber or blood-tinged fluid (Leav et al, 1976).

 MALIGNANT THYROID TUMORS

Carcinomas of the canine thyroid are usually large solid masses that commonly invade into adjacent structures. Extension of malignant thyroid tumors into or around the esophagus, trachea, cervical musculature, nerves, and thyroidal vessels is fairly common. However, invasion into the lumen of structures, such as the esophagus or

ANATOMIC SITE	PERCENTAGE OF ANIMALS
Lung	77
Regional lymph node	51
Local incision†	49
Adrenal	14
Kidney	14
Heart muscle	9
Liver	6
Intestine	6
Skin	6
Brain	3
Spleen	3
Mesentery	3
Diaphragm	3

TABLE 5-2 FREQUENCY OF METASTATIC DISEASE IN DOGS WITH THYROID CARCINOMA*

From Leav I, et al.: Adenomas and carcinomas of the canine and feline thyroid, *Am J Pathol* 83:61, 1976.
*Data is based on 35 autopsied dogs with metastatic carcinoma of the thyroid.
†Includes invasion of thyroidal, jugular, and maxillary veins; esophagus; trachea; larynx; omohyoid muscle; and vertebra.

trachea, is unusual. Distant metastasis is common and is most frequent in the pulmonary parenchyma and the regional lymph nodes (retropharyngeal, mandibular, and superficial cervical). Lymphatic drainage of the thyroid gland is primarily in the cranial direction, so lymph node enlargement is most likely to be detected cranial and medial to the primary tumor. Occasionally, both ipsilateral and contralateral cervical lymph nodes may be involved. Other sites of metastasis include the jugular vein, liver, adrenal gland, kidneys, liver, heart base, spleen, bone and bone marrow, prostate, brain, skeleton, and spinal cord (Bentley et al, 1990; Harmelin et al, 1993; Theon et al, 2000; Tamura et al, 2007; Nadeau and Kitchell, 2011; Table 5-2). Approximately 30% to 40% of dogs with thyroid tumors have detectable distant metastases at time of diagnosis (Harari et al, 1986; Sullivan et al, 1987). Necropsy studies suggest that 60% to 80% of thyroid carcinomas had metastasized at the time of death (Leav et al, 1976). In one study, the risk of metastasis was correlated with the size of the tumor. In tumors with a volume of 20 cm³ or less, 14% of dogs had metastasis; whereas in tumors more than 100 cm³, 100% had metastasized (Leav et al, 1976; Table 5-3). The relation of size to metastasis likely reflects that larger or more aggressive tumors have escaped clinical detection longer, allowing for a greater probability of metastasis.

 CLINICAL APPROACH TO THYROID TUMORS

Signalment

Thyroid tumors in the dog typically develop in middle-aged and older individuals. The most common age range for dogs with thyroid tumors is 10 to 15 years (Wucherer et al, 2010). One study conducted within a small colony of Beagles demonstrated an age-specific incidence of thyroid tumors of 1.1% per year in dogs 8 to 12 years of age and 4.0 % per year in dogs 12 to 15 years of age (Haley et al, 1989).

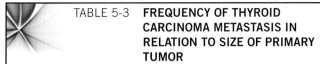

TABLE 5-3 FREQUENCY OF THYROID CARCINOMA METASTASIS IN RELATION TO SIZE OF PRIMARY TUMOR

TUMOR VOLUME (CU CM)	NUMBER OF ANIMALS AUTOPSIED*	PERCENT WITH METASTASIS
1-20	14	14
21-100	19	74
101-500	9	100
501-1000	4	100
1001-1500	3	100

From Leav I, et al.: Adenomas and carcinomas of the canine and feline thyroid, *Am J Pathol* 83:61, 1976.
*Measurements were not recorded in eight cases.

TABLE 5-4 OWNER-OBSERVED SIGNS IN 237 DOGS WITH THYROID TUMORS

SIGN	PERCENT OF DOGS
Visible mass in neck	78
Coughing	34
Rapid breathing (even at rest)	32
Dyspnea (difficulty breathing-distress)	28
Trouble swallowing (dysphagia)	23
Change in bark (dysphonia)	14
Weight loss	14
Listlessness/depression	13
No observed signs	12
Vomiting/regurgitation	11
Anorexia/decrease in appetite	11
Polydipsia/polyuria	10
Hyperactivity	9
Diarrhea	9
Increased appetite	3
Facial edema	2
Apparent cervical discomfort	2

There is no obvious gender predilection for thyroid neoplasia in the dog (Harari et al, 1986; Wucherer et al, 2010). By contrast, the incidence of human thyroid cancer is about four times greater in women than in men at most ages (Schneider and Brenner, 2013). Breeds thought to be at increased risk include Boxers, Beagles, Golden Retrievers, and Siberian Huskies (Leav et al, 1976; Harari et al, 1986; Verschueren et al, 1992; Wucherer et al, 2010).

Clinical Signs

Dogs with thyroid tumors that are not hyperthyroid are usually presented to veterinarians because of detection of a mid-cervical mass or because of clinical signs resulting from compression or invasion of surrounding tissues. The length of time between owner observation of the mass or clinical sign(s) and presentation for veterinary care is highly variable (days to years).

Because most benign thyroid tumors are clinically silent, it is very likely that a palpable thyroid mass is malignant, especially if it is not freely moveable. Most thyroid tumors are identified at or just below the level of the larynx, but larger tumors may extend closer to the thoracic inlet. Thyroid tumors are usually firm and non-painful and may be unilateral or bilateral. There is no predisposition for either the right or left thyroid lobes. In a study of 44 dogs with thyroid carcinoma, the lesion was unilateral in 64% of dogs and bilateral in 36% of dogs (Leav et al, 1976). In one study, bilateral tumors were much more likely to metastasize than unilateral tumors (Theon et al, 2000). It is usually not possible to determine whether bilateral tumors have arisen independently in each gland or whether metastasis from one lobe to the other has occurred. Other clinical signs of thyroid carcinoma include coughing, dyspnea or tachypnea, stridor or stertor, dysphagia, dysphonia, weight loss, listlessness/depression, vomiting, regurgitation, anorexia, facial edema, and apparent cervical pain or discomfort (Table 5-4). In one report, erosion of arterial blood vessels by a thyroid carcinoma resulted in acute severe hemorrhage into the tumor and rapid enlargement of the mass (Slensky et al, 2003). Dyspnea may be due to upper airway compression or pulmonary metastasis.

Additional clinical signs in dogs with functional thyroid tumors include signs of hyperthyroidism, such as weight loss, polydipsia, polyuria, polyphagia, vomiting, voluminous soft stools, increased activity or nervousness, weakness, poor hair coat, heat intolerance, panting, and shivering (Melián et al, 1996; Simpson and McCown, 2009). The clinical signs of hyperthyroidism may precede identification of a cervical mass and be the reason for initial patient evaluation.

Physical Examination

Most thyroid masses are firm, irregular in shape, and non-painful. Most thyroid tumors are located close to the typical location of the normal thyroid glands (at the level of or ventral to the larynx) and are not as ventral in location or as freely movable in the subcutaneous space as in cats (Fig. 5-2). Usually, the thyroid mass is non-moveable and obviously well embedded into surrounding tissue. It is usually not possible to palpate the interior or medial surface of the mass because of local invasion. An irregular shape is not always diagnostic of carcinoma, but an immovable mass usually implies local invasion and should raise a strong suspicion for malignancy. Submandibular lymph nodes may be enlarged as a result of tumor spread or lymphatic obstruction. Horner's syndrome may occur due to encroachment on the vagosympathetic trunk (Melián et al, 1996). Unfortunately palpation is not accurate for assessing extent of tumor invasion (Taeymans et al, 2013).

In addition to the presence of a palpable cervical mass, physical examination of dogs with functional thyroid tumors may reveal evidence of weight loss, muscle atrophy, or cachexia (Fig 5-3). Tachycardia with or without cardiac arrhythmias is common. Affected dogs may pant excessively and may be restless during the physical examination. Panting, respiratory distress, and swallowing difficulties may be the result of thyrotoxicosis or the tumor mass compressing the trachea and/or esophagus.

Minimum Data Base

The minimum data base is rarely helpful in diagnosis or management of dogs with thyroid tumors. Leukocytosis and a mild normocytic normochromic anemia are identified in some dogs. One report identified increased liver enzymes in 7 of 21 dogs, none of which were thyrotoxic (Harari et al, 1986). The cause of the enzyme increases was not determined. Hypercalcemia has also been identified in dogs with thyroid carcinoma and is attributed to a paraneoplastic condition (Lane and Wyatt, 2012). The urinalysis is usually unremarkable.

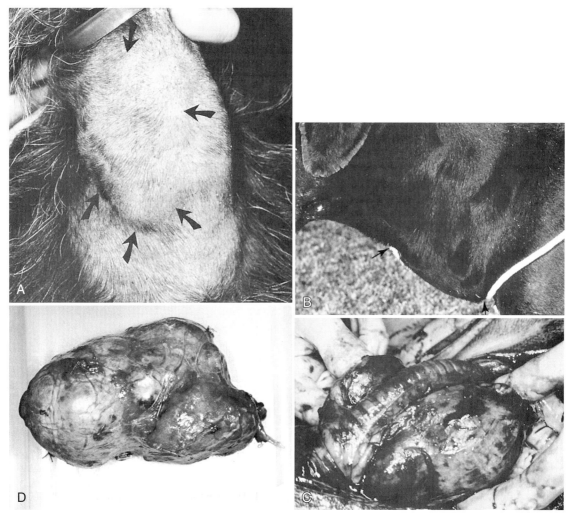

FIGURE 5-2 A, Photograph of the shaved ventral cervical area of a dog with a large, obvious goiter *(arrows).* **B,** Lateral view of the dog with a large thyroid tumor. The mass is delineated ventrally by the leash. **C,** Large thyroid tumor, at surgery, displacing the trachea. **D,** The thyroid tumor following excision. (**A,** Courtesy of Dr. Jane Turrel.)

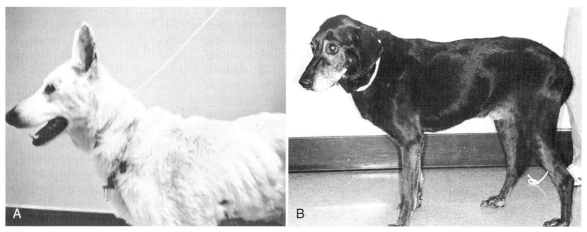

FIGURE 5-3 A, A cachectic 9-year-old German Shepherd dog with hyperthyroidism caused by a functioning thyroid carcinoma. **B,** A thin 12-year-old Labrador-mix with mild hyperthyroidism secondary to a functioning thyroid carcinoma.

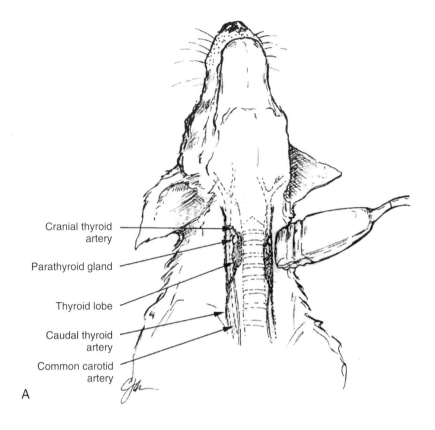

Cranial thyroid
artery

Parathyroid gland

Thyroid lobe

Caudal thyroid
artery

Common carotid
artery

A

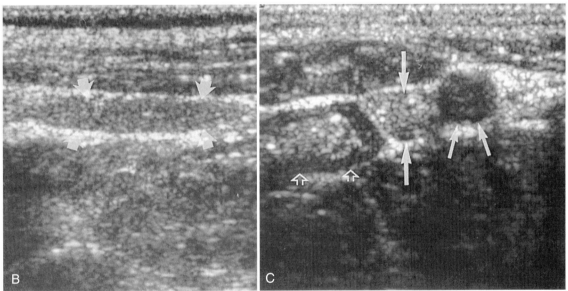

FIGURE 5-4 A, Ultrasound of the canine thyroid gland. For initial localization of the thyroid in long axis, the transducer is positioned on the jugular groove with the imaging plane directed midway between the frontal and parasagittal planes. The ipsilateral common carotid artery serves as an anatomic landmark. **B,** Ultrasound image of the normal canine thyroid gland (sagittal view). The normal canine thyroid lobe appears as a uniformly moderately echoic ellipsoid structure *(arrows)*. A thin hyperechoic fascial sheath surrounds and defines the thyroid lobe. **C,** Ultrasound image of the normal canine thyroid gland. In the short-axis view, the thyroid lobe *(large solid arrows)* appears as a roughly triangular structure adjacent and medial to the common carotid artery *(small solid arrows)*. The esophagus can be seen when imaging the left thyroid lobe and appears as an irregularly-shaped structure medial and dorsal to the thyroid lobe *(open arrows)*. (Modified from Wisner ER, Nyland TG: Ultrasonography of the thyroid and parathyroid glands, *Vet Clin N Amer Sm Anim Pract* 28:973, 1998. Used with permission.)

Radiography

Radiographs of the thorax should always be evaluated in a dog with a thyroid mass because of the high risk of pulmonary metastasis. In clinical studies, pulmonary metastasis is identified in 30% to 40% of dogs, which contrasts with histopathologic studies that report metastasis in up to 80% of dogs at time of death (Leav et al, 1976; Brodey and Kelly, 1968; Sullivan et al, 1987; Marks et al, 1994; Carver et al, 1995; Turrel et al, 2006). This discrepancy is likely due to the relative insensitivity of pulmonary radiographs for detection of pulmonary metastasis and due to progression of disease between diagnosis and time of death. Computed tomography (CT) is more sensitive for detection of pulmonary metastasis than is radiography (Armbrust et al, 2012) and should be done prior to treatment planning. Neoplastic transformation of ectopic thyroid tissue may result in identification of a cranial mediastinal mass on pulmonary radiographs (Liptak et al, 2008).

Radiography of the neck may identify a space-occupying mass caudal to the pharynx, which may contain areas of soft tissue mineralization (Taeymans et al, 2007). A mass in this location may cause an uneven or distorted laryngeal space and compress or displace the trachea ventrally. Esophageal displacement or focal dilatation may indicate esophageal invasion. Metastasis to the retropharyngeal lymph nodes may cause displacement of the pharynx, decreased size of the pharyngeal airspace, and loss of the fascial planes in the retropharyngeal area (Taeymans et al, 2007). Abdominal radiographs are usually normal, although dogs with hepatic metastasis may have an irregular hepatic silhouette.

Ultrasonography

Equipment and Positioning

Because the thyroid glands are very superficial structures, high frequency transducers of at least 10 MHz that result in high spatial resolution should be used to examine the thyroid glands (Taeymans et al, 2007). The ventral cervical area should be carefully clipped and the dog positioned as symmetrically as possible on a padded V-top table in dorsal recumbency. Dogs usually do not require sedation for cervical ultrasound; however, dogs that have cervical masses large enough to produce upper airway obstruction are at risk for developing severe dyspnea after being placed in dorsal recumbency. It may be safer to examine such dogs under general anesthesia with an endotracheal tube in place (Wisner and Nyland, 1998).

Normal Anatomy, Imaging Planes, and Indications

The thyroid lobes are normally located just caudal to the arch of the cricoid cartilage. Healthy medium-sized dogs have flattened lobes measuring approximately 6.0 cm × 1.5 × 0.5 cm (Fig. 5-4). The common carotid arteries are lateral and slightly superficial to the thyroid lobes, serving as an important internal landmark. Ultrasonography is a useful non-invasive and inexpensive screening tool for evaluation of cervical masses and is most useful for determining whether a mass is arising from the thyroid gland and if one or both the thyroid lobes are involved. The differential diagnosis of disorders resulting in a cervical mass is shown in Box 5-2.

When evaluating a dog with a neck mass of unknown etiology, the ultrasonographer should begin by attempting to identify both thyroid lobes. This usually allows quick identification of thyroid masses; however, large cervical masses can distort the normal anatomy and make identification of the origin of the mass more difficult. Lymph nodes and salivary masses are usually not difficult to distinguish from thyroid lobes based on location (usually cranial

and lateral to the thyroid lobes) and echogenicity. Salivary glands, for example, are typically uniformly hypoechoic with characteristic internal linear arborization that likely represents the salivary duct system (Wisner and Nyland, 1998).

Ultrasound Appearance of a Thyroid Carcinoma

Thyroid carcinomas are typically large nonhomogeneous masses that that may be poorly delineated (Fig. 5-5). The parenchyma may be complex, sometimes containing multiple cysts, or may have foci of mineralization. Thyroid carcinomas are highly vascular, and a large arterial vascular plexus is often distributed in and around these masses. The vascular plexus can be verified by pulsed or color-flow Doppler ultrasonographic evaluation. Some dogs develop arteriovenous malformations within the tumor; such abnormalities can also develop after surgery (Wisner et al, 1994; Wisner and Nyland, 1998). Invasion of surrounding structures (e.g., fascial sheaths, esophagus, and cervical vasculature) may also be detected by ultrasound. Although a tentative diagnosis of thyroid carcinoma can be made in most dogs based on localization to one or both thyroid lobes and qualitative ultrasonographic characteristics, the diagnosis must be confirmed by fine needle aspiration or biopsy. Because of the vascularity of thyroid tumors, needle aspiration or biopsy should be performed with ultrasound guidance to aid in avoiding larger blood vessels. Both aspiration and needle biopsy of a vascular tumor may only retrieve peripheral blood. Ultrasound may also be used to help stage a carcinoma, by documentation of tumor extent, invasiveness, and local metastasis; however, it is less accurate for tumor staging than are either CT or magnetic resonance imaging (MRI) (Taeymans et al, 2013).

Computed Tomography and Magnetic Resonance Imaging

Both CT and MRI have been used for preoperative diagnosis and staging of thyroid tumors. On CT, thyroid tumors have lower attenuation value than normal thyroid tissue. On MRI, thyroid carcinomas are hyperintense compared to surrounding musculature in both T1 and T2 imaging sequences (Taeymans et al, 2013). Characteristics that are important to evaluate by either modality are origin of the mass, mass size, tumor capsule disruption, local tissue invasion, lymphadenopathy, presence of metastatic disease, and parathyroid involvement in the tumor. Both CT and MRI are superior to ultrasound for establishing extent of invasion of thyroid tumors. CT is also useful for diagnosis and staging of thyroid tumors arising in ectopic locations (Rossi et al, 2013)

Scintigraphy

Thyroid gland scintigraphy in dogs is usually performed following intravenous (IV) administration of 2 to 4 mCi of technetium-99m pertechnetate ($^{99m}TcO_4$). Gamma camera imaging of the cervical

---

BOX 5-2	Differential Diagnosis for Cervical Masses in Dogs

Thyroid adenoma/carcinoma (see Box 5-1)
Secondary metastasis to thyroid gland
Carotid body tumor
Cellulitis/abscess/granuloma
Lymphadenopathy (submandibular, medial retropharyngeal, or cervical)
Salivary gland inflammation or neoplasia
Other neoplasia (e.g., rhabdomyosarcoma, leiomyosarcoma)

region and thorax is typically performed 20 to 60 minutes after isotope administration. The $^{99m}TcO_4$ is trapped by cells that concentrate iodine, including the thyroid gland, salivary glands, and gastric mucosa. Usually, static left lateral, right lateral, ventral, and dorsal images are acquired (Marks et al, 1994). The appearance of the normal canine thyroid glands is of paired spherical to ovoid lobes that have symmetrical isotope uptake (Fig. 5-6). The intensity

of isotope uptake in the thyroid gland is approximately equal to that of the parotid salivary tissue (thyroid-to-salivary ratio at 20 minutes 1.12:1 ± 0.13) (Daniel and Neelis, 2014). When a cervical mass arises from the thyroid gland, the scintigraphic appearance of the thyroid gland is abnormal (Fig. 5-7). If the mass arises from other tissues or ectopic thyroid tissue, the scintigraphic appearance of the thyroid glands should be normal, although concurrent

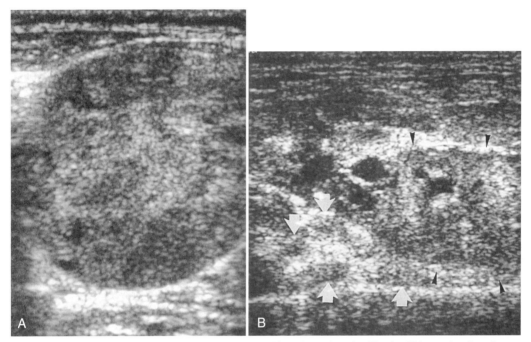

FIGURE 5-5 A, Cervical ultrasound of encapsulated thyroid carcinoma in a dog. The thyroid is grossly enlarged, and the thyroid parenchyma is heterogeneous, but the lesion appears to be well-marginated. **B,** Cervical ultrasound of poorly-marginated thyroid carcinoma in a dog. The thyroid is enlarged, and thyroid parenchyma is heterogeneous *(arrowheads)*. In addition, lesion margins are poorly defined and appear to extend into surrounding tissues *(arrows)*. (Modified from Wisner ER, Nyland TG: Ultrasonography of the thyroid and parathyroid glands, *Vet Clin N Amer Sm Anim Pract* 28:973, 1998. Used with permission.)

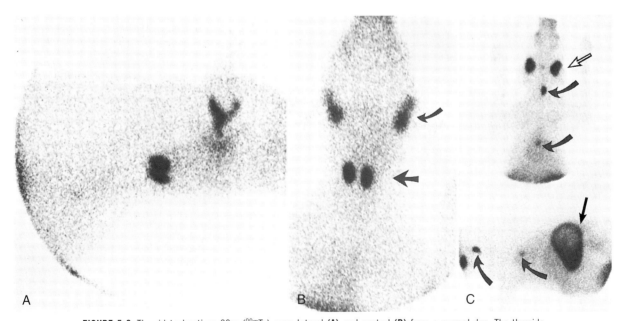

FIGURE 5-6 Thyroid technetium-99m (^{99m}Tc) scan lateral **(A)** and ventral **(B)** from a normal dog. The thyroids of a normal dog *(straight arrow)* are approximately the size of normal salivary glands *(curved arrow)*. **C,** Thyroid technetium-99m (^{99m}Tc) scan from a dog that had one thyroid lobe removed. One normal cervical thyroid and one ectopic anterior mediastinal thyroid *(curved arrows)* are identified. Salivary glands *(open arrow)* and stomach *(straight arrow)* are also visualized because these tissues concentrate pertechnetate.

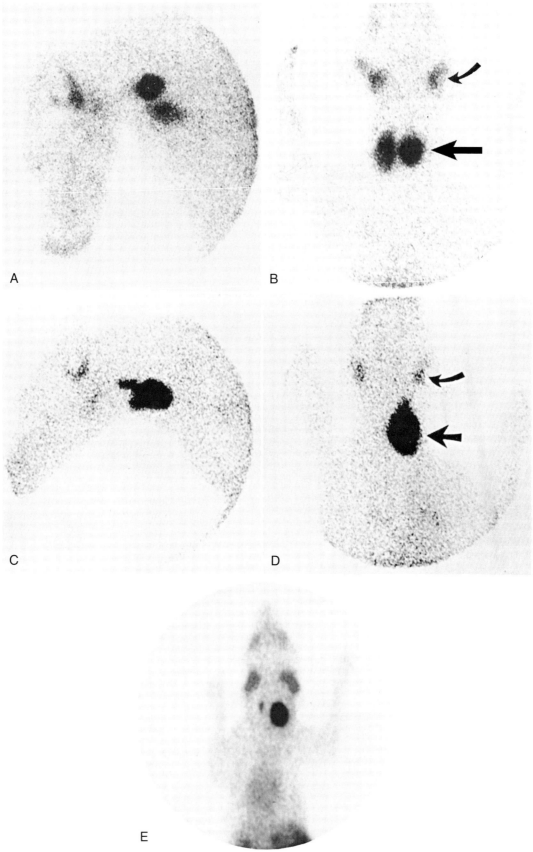

FIGURE 5-7 **A** to **D,** Thyroid technetium-99m (^{99m}Tc) scans from three dogs, each with thyroid tumors demonstrating well-circumscribed, homogeneous uptake. In the first two dogs (**B** and **D**) the thyroid tissue *(straight arrow)* and salivary tissue *(curved arrow)* are defined by uptake of the radioactive contrast. The first dog has bilateral thyroid follicular carcinomas, which were large (lateral **[A]** and dorsoventral **[B]** view) with partial ability to concentrate the radioactive material. The dog was euthyroid. Lateral **(C)** and dorsoventral **(D)** views of a pertechnetate thyroid scan from a dog with one large functioning thyroid follicular carcinoma *(straight arrow),* which concentrated the pertechnetate to a much greater degree than the salivary glands *(curved arrow).* This dog was hyperthyroid. **E,** Scan from a hypothyroid dog with a thyroid carcinoma.

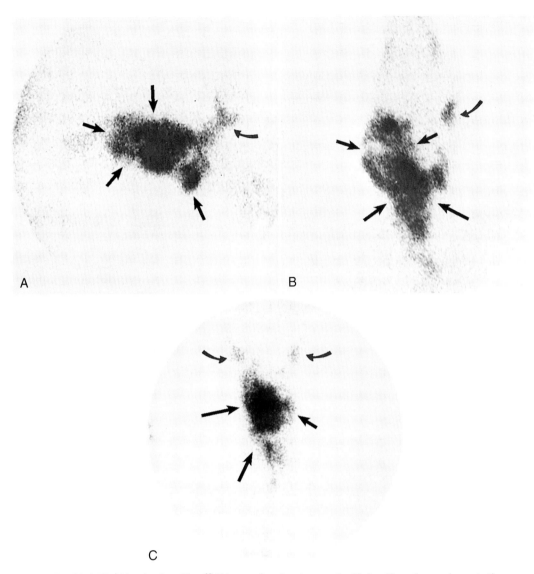

FIGURE 5-8 Thyroid technetium-99m (^{99m}Tc) scans from two dogs, each with thyroid carcinomas demonstrating poorly circumscribed, heterogeneous uptake in the cervical area (thyroid, *straight arrows;* salivary tissue, *curved arrows*). Lateral **(A)** and dorsoventral **(B)** views of a pertechnetate thyroid scan from a dog with typical local invasion of neoplastic cells throughout the cervical area. The dog was euthyroid despite the appearance of the thyroid on the scan. **C,** Thyroid technetium-99m (^{99m}Tc) scan (ventral view) from a dog with a thyroid tumor causing hyperthyroidism.

hypothyroidism can complicate interpretation of the scintigraphic image. The appearance of canine thyroid carcinoma on scintigraphy varies both in intensity and size. With a unilateral nonfunctional tumor, one thyroid lobe will appear abnormal and the other is usually normal in appearance. Some tumors have homogenous diffuse uptake of isotope, and some have diffuse but irregular uptake of isotope (see Fig. 5-7; Figs. 5-8, and 5-9). Poorly differentiated tumors have decreased uptake of isotope and are referred to as *cold nodules.* Some tumors have well-defined borders, whereas others have ill-defined or spiculated borders (see Fig. 5-8). Studies suggest that tumors with homogenous uptake and well-defined margins are more likely to be surgically resectable than those with heterogeneous uptake and poorly circumscribed margins (Marks et al, 1994). There is poor correlation between histologic type and scintigraphic pattern of thyroid tumors; however, tumors with homogenous diffuse uptake are more likely to be functional tumors that cause hyperthyroidism (Marks et al, 1994). Whether or not pulmonary metastasis is detected on scintigraphy depends upon whether

the metastatic cells retain the ability to trap iodine (see Fig. 5-9; Fig. 5-10). Even if the metastatic cells concentrate iodine, detection of metastasis may be less sensitive when the primary tumor is concentrating ("stealing") the majority of the radioactive isotope. In this situation, the metastatic lesion may only be visible after surgical resection of the primary tumor. Scintigraphy can also identify ectopic sites of thyroid tissue (neoplastic or normal) (see Fig. 5-6). Because of these variables, dogs with normal thoracic radiographs may have scintigraphic evidence of metastasis, whereas some dogs with pulmonary metastasis visible on radiography may not have scintigraphic evidence of metastasis (see Figs. 5-9 and 5-10).

Basal Serum Thyroxine Concentrations

The majority of dogs (55% to 60%) with thyroid tumors are euthyroid. Because most thyroid tumors are unilateral and more than 80% of both thyroid glands must be destroyed before clinical hypothyroidism results, hypothyroidism is rarely caused by thyroid

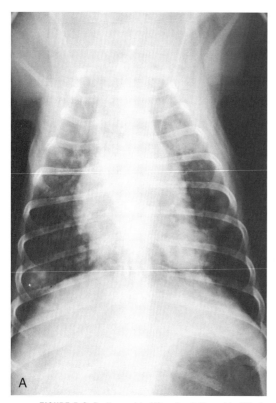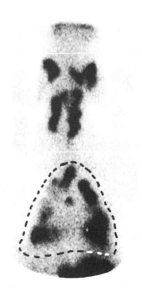

FIGURE 5-9 Radiographic (**A**) and scintigraphic (**B**) views of a dog with thyroid adenocarcinoma and pulmonary metastases. The location of the thorax is shown by dotted lines on the scintigraphic image.

tumors. In one study, 3 of 29 dogs with thyroid tumors were diagnosed as hypothyroid; however, interpretation of thyroid hormone concentrations in dogs with thyroid tumors is complicated by the effects of concurrent illness on serum thyroid hormone concentrations and because hypothyroidism may be a pre-existing condition (Benjamin et al, 1996). Hyperthyroidism has been reported in 10% to 20% of dogs with thyroid tumors (Verschueren et al, 1992; Marks et al, 1994; Rijnberk, 1996; Fig 5-11). Although functioning thyroid adenomas have been described, most tumors are malignant (Lawrence et al, 1991; Marks et al, 1994). A functional thyroid tumor is the only naturally occurring cause of hyperthyroidism in the dog other than consumption of diets containing thyroid tissue. Lymphocytic thyroiditis causing anti-triiodothyronine (T_3) and thyroxine (T_4) antibodies can result in the presence of spuriously increased thyroid hormone concentrations (see Chapter 3); but in dogs with thyroiditis, clinical signs of hyperthyroidism are absent and there is no palpable cervical mass.

Thyroid Biopsy

Thyroid tumors are highly vascular, and hemorrhage associated with any biopsy procedure is common. The hemorrhagic potential of these masses precludes routine large-bore needle biopsy procedures. Rather, we recommend fine-needle aspiration, using a 21- to 23-gauge needle ideally performed with ultrasound guidance. This technique is usually adequate for differentiating thyroid tumors from abscesses, cysts, salivary mucoceles, or lymph nodes. The number of neoplastic cells obtained by needle aspiration is variable, and the sample is almost always contaminated with blood. Because neoplastic follicular cells are fragile, many isolated nuclei may be seen, but intact cells found in clusters resemble glandular structures. A presumptive diagnosis of thyroid neoplasia

can often be made based on the presence of neuroendocrine cells in the sample, but definitive diagnosis requires histopathology. Samples for histopathology can be obtained by needle biopsy, incisional biopsy, or excisional biopsy. Large-bore needle biopsy is avoided when possible because of the risk of hemorrhage and the difficulty in obtaining a diagnostic biopsy sample. Incisional or excisional biopsy is preferred, and the choice is dependent upon the characteristics of the mass. If surgical excision is possible, then histopathology should be obtained at this time.

Differential Diagnosis

Common differential diagnoses for ventral cervical masses in dogs include thyroid adenoma or carcinoma, and submandibular, medial retropharyngeal, or cervical lymphadenomegaly. Lymphadenomegaly may result from tonsillar squamous cell carcinoma or spread from other tumors or non-tumor disorders that originate in the oral cavity or the neck such as cellulitis, abscess or granuloma or salivary gland tumor or inflammation (Wisner et al, 1994; see Box 5-2).

TREATMENT OF THYROID TUMORS

Treatment modalities used for treatment of thyroid tumors include surgical resection, radiation therapy, radioactive iodine treatment, and chemotherapy. In some cases, multiple treatment modalities are used together or sequentially. The choice of treatment depends upon a number of factors including size, vascularity, and mobility of the tumor, functional status of the tumor, severity of clinical signs particularly with regard to respiratory signs, presence or absence of metastatic disease, and financial constraints of the owner.

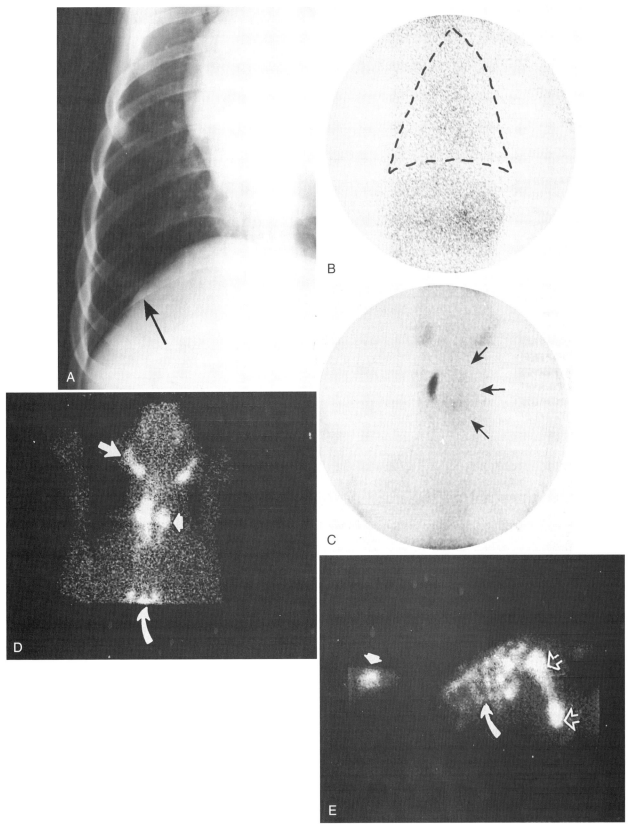

FIGURE 5-10 Radiographic **(A)** view of the thorax and scintiscan images of the thorax **(B)** and cervical region **(C)** in a dog with an undifferentiated thyroid carcinoma and pulmonary metastases. A metastatic nodule can be seen on the radiograph *(arrow)* but not on the thoracic scintiscan. The location of the thorax is shown by *dotted lines* on the scintigraphic image. The primary tumor had minimal pertechnetate uptake *(arrows)*. The dorsoventral area **(D)**, cervical area, and lateral thoracic area **(E)** on scintiscan of a hyperthyroid dog with a thyroid carcinoma and pulmonary metastases that concentrate pertechnetate. In this scan **(D** and **E)**, radioactive uptake is white. The salivary tissue *(straight arrow)*, stomach *(open arrowheads)*, cervical thyroid *(closed arrowheads)*, and pulmonary metastases *(curved arrows)* can be visualized.

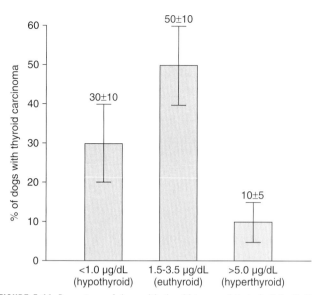

FIGURE 5-11 Percentage of dogs with thyroid tumors detected clinically that were hypothyroid, euthyroid, or hyperthyroid as determined from clinical signs and serum thyroxine (T_4) concentrations.

Surgical Resection

Surgical resection is most appropriate for the 25% to 50% of dogs with freely moveable non-invasive thyroid tumors (Carver et al, 1995; Klein et al, 1995). Mobility can be determined by deep palpation ideally under general anesthesia; however, ultrasound and ideally advanced imaging with CT or MR should be considered prior to surgery, because attachment to deep structures may be either under- or overestimated. Scintigraphy can also be useful to evaluate the suitability of a thyroid tumor for surgical resection. Surgical thyroidectomy is most appropriate for well-circumscribed tumors that have uniform uptake of pertechnetate (Fig. 5-12). Surgery is less likely to be a good choice in dogs with tumors that are poorly circumscribed or demonstrate patchy uptake of pertechnetate.

In one study of 82 dogs with thyroid carcinoma, 24% of dogs met the criteria of a freely moveable tumor with no evidence of metastasis. In this study, tumor resection resulted in long-term local control of the tumor with a median survival of more than 36 months and low incidence of metastasis (Klein et al, 1995). Metastasis was documented after surgery in only 2 of 20 dogs, suggesting that local tumor control had an impact on subsequent development of metastasis. Age, breed, and tumor histologic type were not associated with survival time (Klein et al, 1995). In a more recent study of 15 dogs with discrete mobile bilateral thyroid carcinomas that underwent thyroidectomy, median survival time was 38 months and de novo metastasis was not detected in any dog (Tuohy et al, 2012). In this study, tumor assessment of tumor mobility was based on documentation of mobility more than 1 cm in all planes by physical examination. Interestingly, in both of these studies, survival was not influenced by tumor histopathologic type, presence of bilateral thyroid gland involvement, tumor size, tumor volume, presence of gross tumor thrombi, histopathologic evidence of capsular or vascular invasion, preservation of parathyroid glands, or use of adjuvant chemotherapy. Indeed many dogs with evidence of gross tumor thrombi at surgery had long-term survival with no evidence of local tumor recurrence or metastasis, independent of whether adjuvant chemotherapy was administered. Based on these two studies, it appears that surgical resection alone may result in long-term survival for well-encapsulated mobile thyroid tumors in dogs without metastasis; the

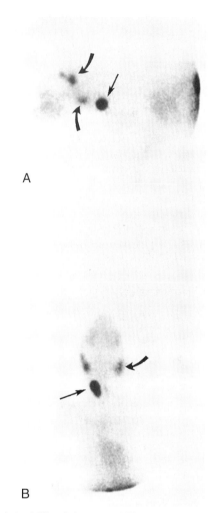

FIGURE 5-12 Lateral **(A)** and dorsoventral **(B)** scintiscans from a dog with hyperthyroidism secondary to a solitary functioning thyroid follicular adenoma. Note the parotid salivary glands *(curved arrows)* and the thyroid adenoma *(straight arrows)*. Surgical excision resulted in complete resolution of all clinical signs. Five-year follow-up was unremarkable.

merits of adjunctive therapy (even in dogs with evidence of capsular or vascular invasion or tumor thrombi) appear questionable in dogs with mobile tumors. Marginal resection at a plane adjacent to the tumor capsule does not appear to increase risk of recurrence and is associated with less postoperative complications than more aggressive approaches. Complications (e.g., hypocalcemia due to hypoparathyroidism and hypothyroidism) do occur but are easily treated and do not impact long-term survival. Approximately 50% of dogs require long-term calcitriol supplementation (Tuohy et al, 2012). If bilateral tumors are resected, iatrogenic hypoparathyroidism is likely and should be treated with calcitriol and calcium supplementation. In a study of 15 dogs undergoing bilateral thyroid tumor resection, 13 dogs required short-term calcitriol and calcium supplementation, 7 dogs required long-term calcitriol treatment, and 8 dogs required long-term thyroid hormone supplementation (Tuohy et al, 2012). Interestingly dogs treated for hypothyroidism had longer survival than those that were not supplemented. This could suggest that chronic stimulation by TSH led to more aggressive tumor growth (Tuohy et al, 2012). Other potential surgical complications associated with resection of thyroid tumors include laryngeal paralysis, hemorrhage, and need for short-term tracheostomy.

In dogs with invasive thyroid tumors, complete excision is usually not possible, and surgical thyroidectomy alone will not result in a cure. In these cases the pros and cons of surgical debulking should be carefully considered. In some dogs, careful tumor debulking may relieve clinical signs due to compression of the trachea and esophagus; however, further adjunctive therapy is required in such cases. Unless surgical debulking is required to relieve clinical signs due to cervical compression, consideration should be given to use of other non-surgical treatments (e.g., radiation therapy or chemotherapy) as the primary mode of treatment. If debulking surgery is attempted, heroic attempts to remove all malignant tissue are not recommended, because they result in a higher incidence of treatment related complications, such as hemorrhage, hypoparathyroidism, laryngeal paralysis, and the need for tracheostomy. Median survival times ranging from 8 to 20 months have been reported in studies that did not select for tumors that were freely mobile (Harari et al, 1986; Carver et al, 1995; Kent et al, 2002).

Postsurgical Monitoring

In dogs undergoing bilateral tumor removal, serum calcium concentrations should be measured at least once daily for 5 to 7 days after surgery. Although most dogs with iatrogenic hypoparathyroidism develop hypocalcemia within the first week following surgery, in some cases development of clinical hypocalcemia may be delayed by several weeks or precipitated by factors (e.g., chemotherapy) that decrease oral calcium intake (Tuohy et al, 2012). Vitamin D and calcium therapy should be instituted if clinical evidence of hypoparathyroidism (hypocalcemia) is present (see Chapter 16). Serum T_4 concentration should initially be assessed 4 weeks after surgery and, depending on clinical signs, replacement therapy implemented accordingly.

It is important that the excised tumor is examined histopathologically. If the tumor is a benign adenoma and the resection is complete, there is an excellent chance of a surgical cure and adjunctive treatment is unnecessary; however, follow up examinations should be scheduled 3, 6, and 12 months after surgery because of the possibility of missing a diagnosis of carcinoma. If the mass is malignant but excision is apparently complete with clean margins reported by the pathologist, close follow up including physical examination, thoracic radiographs, cervical and abdominal ultrasonography, and possibly scintigraphy should be performed every 3 months for the first year and every 6 months thereafter. If excision is not complete or there are tumor cells identified in the edges of the surgical field, adjunctive therapy with radiation or chemotherapy should be considered. Although it makes intuitive sense that radiation and chemotherapy are appropriate for treatment of dogs with histologic evidence of residual disease, the merits of such treatment for prolonging survival or quality of life have not yet been proven in dogs with thyroid carcinoma (Tuohy et al, 2012).

External Beam Radiation Therapy

Unfortunately there are limited prospective studies evaluating the efficacy of radiation therapy for treatment of thyroid tumors in dogs. In a study of 13 dogs with thyroid tumors treated with palliative external beam irradiation, the mean survival time was 96 weeks (range: 6 to 247 weeks; Brearley and Hayes, 1999). Another retrospective study of eight dogs with thyroid carcinoma treated with external beam irradiation resulted in a median survival time of more than 2 years (Pack et al, 2001). The largest study of thyroid tumors treated with curative intent external beam radiation therapy included 25 dogs with histologically confirmed thyroid carcinoma without metastasis (Theon

et al, 2000). The thyroid tumors in this study were categorized as compact-cellular (nine dogs), follicular (eight dogs), and follicular-compact-cellular (eight dogs) adenocarcinomas. The dogs ranged in age from 3 to 18 years (median, 10 years), and various breeds were represented. All had been referred for irradiation because the tumors were considered unresectable on the basis of clinical findings, such as palpation, ultrasonography, and radiography (11 dogs), or after unsuccessful attempts at resection (14 dogs). Of the 25 dogs, 6 had been diagnosed as hypothyroid, whereas the other 19 dogs were euthyroid. Imaging studies with sodium $^{99m}TcO_4$ were performed in 20 of the 25 dogs. Scintigraphy demonstrated that seven dogs had unilateral lobe involvement, eight had bilateral lobe involvement, and five had ventral midline masses with invasion of the laryngeal cartilages. A well-circumscribed area of homogeneous uptake was observed in seven dogs. Poorly-circumscribed areas of uptake were demonstrated in 13 dogs; 9 of these dogs had diffuse uptake throughout their masses, and 4 of them had mixed areas of no uptake together with some areas of uptake. Each dog in this study was treated with 48 Gy administered in 12 fractions on a 3-day-per-week schedule. The radiation treatment field included the primary thyroid tumor and the regional lymph nodes. Mean progression free survival time defined as time from completion of radiation therapy to local tumor recurrence or death from unrelated causes in the 25 dogs was 45 months. The progression free survival rate was 80% at 1 year and 72% at 3 years. Age, sex, tumor histologic type, tumor stage, gland involvement (right versus left), and pattern of $^{99m}TcO_4$ uptake were not associated with response to therapy. Interestingly the tumors were slow to regress, with time to maximum tumor size reduction ranging from 8 to 22 months. For this reason, radiation therapy is not a good choice when there is clinical evidence of cervical compression by the tumor. Patterns of failure were identified in 14 of the 25 dogs (11 did not have evidence of failure despite being followed for more than 4 years). In three dogs, local tumor progression was the first cause of failure. In four dogs with no clinical evidence of tumor progression, metastasis was the first cause of failure. Pulmonary metastases were detected in five dogs, one of which also had bone metastasis. In two dogs, metastases were found in abdominal viscera. Dogs with bilateral tumors had 16 times the risk for metastasis. Previous attempts at resection did not affect risk of metastasis (Theon et al, 2000). Adverse effects of radiation therapy develop during or after therapy and are usually reversible. Dry or moist desquamation of the skin, alopecia, and mucositis usually occur within the treatment field and are managed by supportive care and pain management. Hypothyroidism was reported in 2 of 19 hypothyroid dogs, 13 and 29 months after radiation, respectively, and 1 of these 2 dogs also developed hypoparathyroidism. This latent period for induction of hypothyroidism was longer than that previously reported for one dog that was treated with both radiation and surgery (Kramer et al, 1994). Whether there was an association between radiation therapy and development of hypothyroidism is unknown. In humans, subclinical hypothyroidism is a common complication following irradiation of the head and neck regions when the thyroid gland is in the radiation field (Nishiyama et al, 1996). The benefits of postoperative irradiation of the surgical field in dogs with incompletely resected tumors or when tumor cells are present in the surgical margins have not been conclusively demonstrated. Nevertheless, it is a good idea to consult with a radiation oncologist to obtain the latest data regarding treatment of malignant thyroid tumors.

Radioactive Iodine

Until recently, radioactive iodine treatment has been reserved for dogs with functional thyroid tumors. Recent studies however have reported good results after treatment of dogs with thyroid tumors that concentrated either $^{99m}TcO_4$ or radioactive iodine independent of the functional status of the tumor. In two retrospective studies that included a total of 82 dogs with thyroid carcinoma that were treated with either radioactive iodine alone or before or after incomplete thyroidectomy, median survival in dogs without documented metastasis ranged from 28 to 34 months (Worth et al, 2005; Turrel et al, 2006). Criteria for treatment with radioactive iodine included thyroid tumors that were surgically non-resectable or incompletely resected and documentation of $^{99m}TcO_4$ uptake by the tumor. In one study, iodine-deficient diets were fed for 3 weeks prior to radioactive iodine treatment for those dogs that were not functionally hyperthyroid in an attempt to increase iodine uptake by the tumor (Turrel et al, 2006). The dose of iodine-131 (^{131}I) was determined empirically and ranged from 11 to 191 mCi (4.2 mCi/kg). Factors taken into consideration when determining the treatment dose included body weight, technetium uptake, tumor size, and total T_4 concentration. The number of treatments administered ranged from one to three per dog. The only adverse effects documented were myelosuppression in three dogs in one study and hypothyroidism, which was documented and treated with T_4 supplementation in the majority of dogs in both studies. All of the dogs that developed myelosuppression were treated with doses of radioactive iodine above the median dose of 4 mCi/Kg, but other dogs treated with similar doses did not show myelosuppression. It is possible that transient myelosuppression unassociated with clinical consequences occurred in other dogs in these studies.

These studies together suggest that radioactive iodine has a place in treatment of thyroid carcinomas that are not amenable to complete surgical resection that concentrate iodine based on scintigraphy. Studies in humans suggest that assessment of tumor iodine trapping by either iodine-123 (^{123}I) or tracer ^{131}I may be superior to assessment based on uptake of $^{99m}TcO_4$, because iodine is not only trapped by follicular cells but also incorporated into thyroglobulin within follicular cells and thus is retained longer by the tumor. Although the superiority of radioactive iodine for detection of metastatic lesions was demonstrated in a dog with thyroid carcinoma, the higher cost of ^{123}I and the long-half-life of ^{131}I usually preclude their routine use for scintigraphy. In human studies, administration of recombinant human thyrotropin (rhTSH) prior to radioactive iodine treatment in patients with differentiated thyroid cancer enhances iodine uptake and decreases whole body radiation exposure. Preliminary studies of TSH administration in dogs with thyroid carcinoma showed no significant effect on iodine uptake (Campos et al, 2012). Whether this was due to the protocol used in the study (TSH dose, route of administration, timing of injection) or due to differences in concentration and affinity of TSH receptors in canine thyroid tumors is unknown. Advantages of radioactive iodine treatment include the low risk of adverse effects and the potential to effectively simultaneously treat both the primary tumor and metastatic lesions. The major disadvantage is the need for prolonged isolation after radioactive iodine treatment and the limited number of facilities that are licensed to administer the high doses required for treatment of canine tumors.

There are many unanswered questions that remain with regard to radioactive iodine treatment in dogs with malignant thyroid neoplasia. It is still unknown whether there is an advantage to surgical debulking or surgical resection either before or after radioactive iodine treatment. The ideal method for dose determination to maximize the therapeutic effect and minimize the risk of myelosuppression also still needs to be established.

In our clinical experience, the best outcome has been observed in dogs that have homogenous uptake of isotope on scintigraphy. This is likely because in dogs with heterogeneous isotope uptake, there are clones of cells with differing sensitivity to radioactive iodine. Careful case selection is recommended when considering radioactive iodine treatment so that the last few weeks of a patient's life are not spent in a radioactive iodine isolation facility.

Chemotherapy

A number of different chemotherapeutic agents have been used with varying degrees of success in dogs with thyroid carcinoma. Chemotherapeutic drugs are typically used in an adjunctive role for management of thyroid tumors. Chemotherapy is indicated when total surgical removal or destruction with external beam radiation is not successful, when distant metastatic lesions have been identified, or when local invasion or metastasis is suspected. Drugs that have been evaluated either alone or in combination for treatment of thyroid carcinoma include doxorubicin, cisplatin, carboplatin, mitoxantrone, toceranib phosphate, and chlorambucil.

The median survival time in 10 dogs with thyroid tumors treated with doxorubicin alone was 37 weeks (Jeglum and Whereat, 1983). In 13 dogs with thyroid carcinoma treated with cisplatin, one dog had complete remission, six dogs had partial remissions, and three dogs had stable disease; however, the median survival time was only 98 days (Fineman et al, 1998). In a retrospective study of dogs treated with either surgery alone or surgery in combination with chemotherapy using various combinations of carboplatin, cisplatin, gemcitabine, and doxorubicin, there was no difference in survival between the two groups, but the power to detect a difference was small (Nadeau and Kitchell, 2011). In a prospective trial evaluating metronomic chlorambucil chemotherapy in dogs with naturally occurring cancer, complete remission was documented in one dog with thyroid carcinoma and the duration of response was 114 weeks (Leach et al, 2011). The dosage of chlorambucil used in this study was 4 mg/m^2 daily. In a phase one study of the tyrosine kinase inhibitor toceranib phosphate, clinical benefit was reported in 12 of 15 dogs with thyroid carcinoma (four with partial remission; eight with stable disease; London et al, 2012). Most of the dogs in the study had been previously treated with a combination of surgery, other chemotherapeutic agents, and radiation therapy. A primary tumor was present in 13 dogs, and 10 dogs had metastatic disease. Dogs were treated with toceranib at a median dosage of 2.75 mg/kg every 2 to 3 days. The median duration of treatment for the 12 dogs that experienced a clinical benefit was 24½ weeks. Studies have demonstrated expression of potential targets for tyrosine kinase inhibitors, such as vascular endothelial growth factor receptor 2, platelet-derived growth factor receptors alpha and beta, and stem cell factor receptor in canine thyroid carcinoma (Urie et al, 2012). We urge consultation with a medical oncologist if chemotherapy is being considered.

TREATMENT OF HYPERTHYROIDISM

Approximately 10% to 20% of dogs with thyroid neoplasia are thyrotoxic based on measurement of serum T_4 concentration (Marks et al, 1994; Nadeau and Kitchell, 2011). Most dogs with thyrotoxicosis have clinical signs, such as weight loss, polyuria, polydipsia, and polyphagia, but some are asymptomatic (Marks et al, 1994; Kent et al, 2002; Worth et al, 2005; Tuohy et al, 2012). In most cases, the clinical signs are mild and resolve with surgical thyroidectomy. In dogs with functional thyroid carcinoma that is not amenable to surgical resection, therapeutic options are limited. Oral anti-thyroid drugs are not recommended as the primary mode of therapy, because they are not cytotoxic. However, we have used anti-thyroid drugs as palliative therapy to control clinical signs of hyperthyroidism in untreated dogs or those that had recurrence of hyperthyroidism after surgery or treatment with ^{131}I or chemotherapy. Our therapeutic approach is similar to that used in hyperthyroid cats—that is, 2.5 to 5 mg of methimazole twice daily with subsequent increases in the dosage as needed to control clinical signs and maintain serum T_4 concentrations between 1.0 and 3.0 g/dL. In rare cases, we have managed hyperthyroidism in dogs with thyroid neoplasia for prolonged periods of time with this approach. Because thyroid neoplasms may retain a stimulatory response to TSH, it is important to avoid hypothyroidism in dogs treated with methimazole.

PROGNOSIS IN CANINE THYROID NEOPLASIA

In dogs managed surgically, the degree of mobility of the tumor, histomorphologic criteria of malignancy (including the presence of capsular and vascular invasion, degree of cellular and nuclear polymorphism, and frequency of mitoses), and tumor stage are the only identified prognostic factors (Klein et al, 1995; Theon et al, 2000; Turrel et al, 2006; Tuohy et al, 2012). Histologic tumor classification, breed, gender, age, serum thyroid hormone concentrations, and serum thyroglobulin concentrations are not significant factors in determining prognosis. In one older study, bilateral tumors were much more likely to metastasize than unilateral tumors (Theon et al, 2000); however in a more recent study of 15 dogs with discrete mobile bilateral thyroid carcinomas that underwent thyroidectomy, median survival time was 38 months and de novo metastasis was not detected in any dog (Tuohy et al, 2012).

The influence of thyroid tumor size on prognosis is less clear. One study, Leav, et al. (1976), demonstrated that the likelihood of metastasis was related to tumor size and that smaller tumors carried a better prognosis. Other studies have not confirmed these findings however (Klein et al, 1995; Theon et al, 2000; Kent et al, 2002; Tuohy et al, 2012).

In general, the prognosis for dogs with malignant thyroid tumors is guarded to poor. Although long survival times have been reported for many dogs with mobile thyroid tumors following surgical resection, in most other cases the long-term prognosis is poor due to the invasiveness and high metastatic rate of most tumors. In humans, suppression of TSH by thyroid hormone supplementation is routinely recommended because differentiated thyroid tumors retain their response to TSH, and TSH is therefore a potential growth factor for thyroid neoplasia. This approach has not been routinely advocated in euthyroid dogs with thyroid neoplasia. Interestingly in one study of dogs with bilateral thyroid tumors, dogs that received thyroid supplementation after bilateral thyroidectomy had longer survival times (Tuohy et al, 2012). This approach requires further study in dogs.

REFERENCES

Armbrust LJ, et al.: Comparison of three-view thoracic radiography and computed tomography for detection of pulmonary nodules in dogs with neoplasia, *J Am Vet Med Assoc* 240:1088, 2012.

Benjamin SA, et al.: Associations between lymphocytic thyroiditis, hypothyroidism, and thyroid neoplasia in beagles, *Vet Pathol* 33:486, 1996.

Benjamin SA, et al.: Non-neoplastic and neoplastic thyroid disease in beagles irradiated during prenatal and postnatal development, *Radiat Res* 147:422, 1997.

Bentley JF, et al.: Metastatic thyroid solid-follicular carcinoma in the cervical portion of the spine of a dog, *J Am Vet Med Assoc* 197:1498, 1990.

Birchard SJ, Roesel OF: Neoplasia of the thyroid gland in the dog: a retrospective study of 16 cases, *J Am Anim Hosp Assoc* 17:369, 1981.

Brearley MJ, Hayes AM: Hypofractionated radiation therapy for invasive thyroid carcinoma in dogs: a retrospective analysis of survival, *J Am Anim Pract* 40:206, 1999.

Brodey RS, Kelly DF: Thyroid neoplasms in the dog: a clinicopathologic study of 57 cases, *Cancer* 22:406, 1968.

Campos M, et al.: Effect of recombinant human thyrotropin on the uptake of radioactive iodine (^{123}I) in dogs with thyroid tumors, *PLoS One* 7:e50344, 2012.

Capen CC: The endocrine glands. In Maxie MG, editor: *Jubb, Kennedy, and Palmer's pathology of domestic animals*, ed 5, St Louis, 2007, Saunders/Elsevier, p 379.

Carver JR, et al.: A comparison of medullary thyroid carcinoma and thyroid adenocarcinoma in dogs: a retrospective study of 38 cases, *Vet Surg* 24:315, 1995.

Daniel GB, Neelis DA: Thyroid scintigraphy in veterinary medicine, *Semin Nucl Med* 44:24, 2014.

Devilee P, et al.: The canine p53 gene is subject to somatic mutations in thyroid carcinoma, *Anticancer Res* 14:2039, 1994.

Fineman LS, et al.: Cisplatin chemotherapy for treatment of thyroid carcinoma in dogs: 13 cases, *J Am Vet Med Assoc* 34:109, 1998.

Haley PJ, et al.: Thyroid neoplasms in a colony of beagle dogs, *Vet Pathol* 26:438, 1989.

Harari J, et al.: Clinical and pathologic features of thyroid tumors in 26 dogs, *J Am Vet Med Assoc* 188:1160, 1986.

Harmelin A, et al.: Canine medullary thyroid carcinoma with unusual distant metastases, *J Vet Diagn Invest* 5:284, 1993.

Jeglum KA, Whereat A: Chemotherapy of canine thyroid carcinoma, *Compend Contin Educ Pract Vet* 5:96, 1983.

Kent MS, et al.: Computer assisted image analysis of neovascularization in thyroid neoplasms from dogs, *Am J Vet Res* 63:363, 2002.

Klein MK, et al.: Treatment of thyroid carcinoma in dogs by surgical resection alone: 20 cases (1981-1989), *J Am Vet Med Assoc* 206:1007, 1995.

Kramer RW, et al.: Hypothyroidism in a dog after surgery and radiation therapy for a functional thyroid adenocarcinoma, *Vet Radiol Ultrasound* 35:132, 1994.

Lane AE, Wyatt KM: Paraneoplastic hypercalcemia in a dog with thyroid carcinoma, *Can Vet J* 53:1101, 2012.

Lawrence D, et al.: Hyperthyroidism associated with a thyroid adenoma in a dog, *J Am Vet Med Assoc* 199:81, 1991.

Leach TN, et al.: Prospective trial of metronomic chlorambucil chemotherapy in dogs with naturally occurring cancer, *Vet Comp Oncol* 10:102, 2011.

Leav I, et al.: Adenomas and carcinomas of the canine and feline thyroid, *Am J Pathol* 83:61, 1976.

Liptak JM, et al.: Cranial mediastinal carcinomas in nine dogs, *Vet Comp Oncol* 6:19, 2008.

London C, et al.: Preliminary evidence for biologic activity of toceranib phosphate (Palladia) in solid tumors, *Vet Comp Oncol* 10:194, 2012.

Marks SL, et al.: ^{99m}Tc-pertechnetate imaging of thyroid tumors in dogs: 29 cases (1980-1992), *J Am Vet Med Assoc* 204:756, 1994.

Melián C, et al.: Horner's syndrome associated with a functional thyroid carcinoma in a dog, *J Small Anim Pract* 37:591, 1996.

Metivier KS, et al.: Gene expression profiling demonstrates differential expression of osteopontin in follicular thyroid carcinomas compared to normal thyroid tissue in dogs, *Vet Comp Oncol* 12:181, 2014.

Nadeau M-E, Kitchell BE: Evaluation of the use of chemotherapy and other prognostic variables for surgically excised canine thyroid carcinoma with and without metastasis, *Can Vet J* 52:994, 2011.

Nishiyama K, et al.: A prospective analysis of subacute thyroid dysfunction after neck irradiation, *Int J Radiat Oncol Biol Phys* 34:439, 1996.

Owen LN: Clinical stages (TNM) of canine tumours of the thyroid gland. In Owen LN, editor: *TNM classification of tumours in domestic animals*, Geneva, 1980, World Health Organization.

Pack LA, et al.: Definitive radiation therapy for infiltrative thyroid carcinoma in dogs, *Vet Radiol Ultrasound* 42:471, 2001.

Reimann N, et al.: Trisomy 18 in a canine thyroid adenoma, *Cancer Genet Cytogenet* 90:154, 1996.

Rijnberk A: Thyroids. In Rijnberk A, editor: *Clinical endocrinology of dogs and cats*, Dordrecht, The Netherlands, 1996, Kluwer Academic, p 35.

Rossi F, et al.: Computed tomographic features of basihyoid ectopic thyroid carcinoma in dogs, *Vet Radiol Ultrasound* 54:575, 2013.

Schlumberger MJ, et al.: Nontoxic diffuse and nodular goiter and thyroid neoplasia. In Melmed S, et al., editors: *Williams textbook of endocrinology*, ed 12, Philadelphia, 2011, Elsevier/Saunders.

Schneider AB, Brenner AV: Carcinomas of follicular epithelium: epidemiology and pathogenesis. In Braverman LE, Cooper DS, editors: *The thyroid: a fundamental and clinical text*, ed 10, Philadelphia, 2013, Saunders/Elsevier, p 665.

Simpson AC, McCown JL: Systemic hypertension in a dog with a functional thyroid gland adenocarcinoma, *J Am Vet Med Assoc* 235:1474, 2009.

Slensky KA, et al.: Acute severe hemorrhage secondary to arterial invasion in a dog with thyroid carcinoma, *J Am Vet Med Assoc* 223:649, 2003.

Suarez HG, et al.: Molecular basis of epithelial thyroid tumorigenesis, *C R Acad Sci III* 323:519, 2000.

Sullivan M, et al.: Thyroid tumours in the dog, *J Small Anim Pract* 28:505, 1987.

Taeymans O, et al.: Thyroid imaging in the dog: current status and future directions, *J Vet Intern Med* 21:673, 2007.

Taeymans O, et al.: Comparison between clinical, ultrasound, CT, MRI, and pathology findings in dogs presented for suspected thyroid carcinoma, *Vet Radiol Ultrasound* 54:61, 2013.

Tamura S, et al.: Multiple metastases of thyroid cancer in the cranium and pituitary gland in two dogs, *J Small Anim Pract* 48:237, 2007.

Theon AP, et al.: Prognostic factors and patterns of treatment failure in dogs with unresectable differentiated thyroid carcinomas treated with megavoltage irradiation, *J Am Vet Med Assoc* 216:1775, 2000.

Tuohy JL, et al.: Outcome following simultaneous bilateral thyroid lobectomy for treatment of thyroid gland carcinoma in dogs: 15 cases (1994-2010), *J Am Vet Med Assoc* 241:95, 2012.

Turrel JM, et al.: Sodium iodide I[131] treatment of dogs with non-resectable thyroid tumors: 39 cases (1990-2003), *J Am Vet Med Assoc* 229:542, 2006.

Urie BK, et al.: Evaluation of expression and function of vascular endothelial growth factor receptor 2, platelet derived growth factor receptors-alpha and -beta, KIT, and RET in canine apocrine gland anal sac adenocarcinoma and thyroid carcinoma, *BMC Vet Res* 8:67, 2012.

Verschueren CP, et al.: Flow-cytometric DNA ploidy analysis in primary and metastatic canine thyroid carcinoma, *Anticancer Res* 11:1755, 1991.

Verschueren CP, et al.: Thyrotropin receptors in normal and neoplastic (primary and metastatic) canine thyroid tissue, *J Endocrinol* 132:461, 1992.

Wisner ER, Nyland TG: Ultrasonography of the thyroid and parathyroid glands, *Vet Clin N Amer Sm Anim Pract* 28:973, 1998.

Wisner ER, et al.: Ultrasonographic evaluation of cervical masses in the dog and cat, *Vet Radiol Ultrasound* 35:310, 1994.

Withrow SJ, MacEwen EG: Tumors of the endocrine system. In Withrow SJ, et al., editors: *Withrow and MacEwen's small animal clinical oncology*, ed 5, St Louis, 2012, Saunders/Elsevier, p 423.

Worth AJ, et al.: Radioiodide (^{131}I) therapy for the treatment of canine thyroid carcinoma, *Aust Vet J* 83:208, 2005.

Wucherer KL, et al.: Thyroid cancer in dogs: an update based on 638 cases (1995-2005), *J Am Anim Hosp Assoc* 46:249, 2010.

Xing M: Molecular pathogenesis and mechanisms of thyroid cancer, *Nat Rev Cancer* 13:184, 2013.

CHAPTER 6

Canine Diabetes Mellitus

Richard W. Nelson

CHAPTER CONTENTS

The endocrine pancreas is composed of the islets of Langerhans, which are dispersed as "small islands" in a "sea" of exocrine-secreting acinar cells. Four distinct cell types have been identified within these islets on the basis of staining properties and morphology—alpha cells, which secrete glucagon; beta cells, which secrete insulin; delta cells, which secrete somatostatin; and pancreatic polypeptide (PP) cells, which secrete pancreatic polypeptide. Dysfunction involving any of these cell lines ultimately results

in either an excess or a deficiency of the respective hormone in the circulation. In the dog and cat, the most common disorder of the endocrine pancreas is diabetes mellitus, which results from an absolute or relative insulin deficiency due to deficient insulin secretion by the beta cells, often in conjunction with concurrent insulin resistance. The incidence of diabetes mellitus in dogs varies between countries. The largest study, to date, involved 180,000 insured dogs in Sweden and researchers estimated the cumulative proportion of dogs that would develop diabetes mellitus before 12 years of age at 1.2% (Fall et al, 2007). Davison, et al., (2005) reported from a UK insurance cohort a diabetes mellitus prevalence of 0.32%; Guptill, et al., (2003) reported a hospital prevalence of 0.64% in the United States; and Fracassi, et al., (2004) reported an Italian hospital prevalence of 1.33%.

CLASSIFICATION AND ETIOLOGY

Type 1 Diabetes Mellitus

The most common clinically recognized form of diabetes mellitus in the dog resembles type 1 diabetes mellitus in humans. In our hospital, virtually all dogs are insulin dependent at the time diabetes mellitus is diagnosed. Type 1 diabetes mellitus is characterized by permanent hypoinsulinemia, essentially no increase in endogenous serum insulin concentration following administration of an insulin secretagogue (e.g., glucose, glucagon), and an absolute necessity for exogenous insulin to maintain control of glycemia, avoid ketoacidosis, and survive. The etiology of type 1 diabetes has been poorly characterized in dogs but is undoubtedly multifactorial (Table 6-1). Genetic predispositions have been suggested by familial associations, pedigree analysis of Keeshonds, and genomic studies aimed at identification of susceptibility and protective major histocompatibility complex haplotypes in canine diabetes (Hess et al, 2000a; Guptill et al, 2003; Fracassi et al, 2004; Kennedy et al, 2006; Fall et al, 2007; Table 6-2). A number of genes linked with susceptibility to diabetes mellitus in humans are associated with an increased risk of diabetes mellitus in dogs (Catchpole et al, 2013). Diabetes mellitus in dogs has been associated with major histocompatibility complex class II genes, dog leucocyte antigen (DLA), with similar haplotypes and genotypes being identified in the most susceptible breeds. A region containing a variable number of tandem repeats and several polymorphisms have been identified in the canine insulin gene with some alleles associated with susceptibility or resistance to diabetes in a breed-specific manner (Catchpole et al, 2013).

Common histologic abnormalities in dogs include a reduction in the number and size of pancreatic islets, a decrease in the number of beta cells within islets, and beta cell vacuolation and degeneration. An extreme form of the disease may occur in juvenile dogs, represented by an absolute deficiency of beta cells and pancreatic islet hypoplasia or aplasia. Less severe changes of pancreatic islets and beta cells may predispose the adult dog to diabetes mellitus after it has been exposed to environmental factors, such as insulin-antagonistic diseases and drugs, obesity, and pancreatitis. Environmental factors may induce beta cell degeneration secondary to chronic insulin resistance or may cause release of beta cell proteins, which induce immune-mediated destruction of the islets (Nerup, 1994).

Studies suggest an immune-mediated component in the development of diabetes in some dogs. Immune-mediated insulitis has been described and antibodies directed against islet cells, insulin, proinsulin, intracellular glutamic acid decarboxylase 65 (GAD65), and insulinoma antigen 2 (IA-2) have been identified in diabetic dogs (Hoenig and Dawe, 1992; Alejandro et al, 1988; Davison et al, 2003a; 2008a; 2011; these are autoantibodies that are also identified in humans with type 1 diabetes. The presence of circulating autoantibodies against insulin, proinsulin, GAD65, and IA-2 usually precede the development of hyperglycemia or clinical signs in humans with type 1 diabetes. A similar sequence of events may also occur in dogs, although the onset of type 1 diabetes mellitus occurs in young humans versus older dogs. Canine

TABLE 6-1	**POTENTIAL FACTORS INVOLVED IN THE ETIOPATHOGENESIS OF DIABETES MELLITUS IN DOGS AND CATS**
DOG	**CAT**
Genetics	Islet amyloidosis
Immune-mediated insulitis	Obesity
Pancreatitis	Pancreatitis
Obesity	Concurrent hormonal disease
Concurrent hormonal disease	Hyperadrenocorticism
Hyperadrenocorticism	Acromegaly
Diestrus-induced excess of growth	Hyperthyroidism
hormone	Drugs
Hypothyroidism	Progestagens
Drugs	Glucocorticoids
Glucocorticoids	Infection
Progestagens	Concurrent illness
Infection	Renal insufficiency
Concurrent illness	Cardiac disease
Renal insufficiency	Hyperlipidemia (?)
Cardiac disease	Genetics (Burmese cat)
Hyperlipidemia	Immune-mediated insulitis (?)

diabetes more closely resembles latent autoimmune diabetes of adult humans (Andersen et al, 2010). Seemingly, autoimmune mechanisms in conjunction with genetic and environmental factors, insulin-antagonistic diseases and drugs, obesity, and pancreatitis all play a potential role in the initiation and progression of diabetes in dogs. The end result is a loss of beta-cell function, hypoinsulinemia, impaired transport of circulating glucose into most cells, and accelerated hepatic gluconeogenesis and glycogenolysis. The subsequent development of hyperglycemia and glycosuria causes polyuria, polydipsia, polyphagia, and weight loss. Ketoacidosis develops as the production of ketone bodies increases to compensate for the underutilization of blood glucose. Loss of beta-cell function is irreversible in dogs with type 1 diabetes, and lifelong insulin therapy is mandatory to maintain glycemic control of the diabetic state.

Clinically, pancreatitis is often seen in dogs with diabetes mellitus and has been suggested as a cause of diabetes after destruction of the islets (Watson et al, 2010; Bostrom et al, 2013). However, the incidence of histologically identifiable pancreatitis in diabetic dogs is only 30% to 40%. Although destruction of beta cells secondary to pancreatitis is an obvious explanation for the development of hypoinsulinemic diabetes mellitus, other perhaps more complex factors are involved in the development of diabetes mellitus in dogs without obvious exocrine pancreatic lesions.

Type 2 Diabetes Mellitus

In humans, type 2 diabetes mellitus is an obesity-associated disease characterized by insulin resistance, loss of beta cell function with or without loss of beta cell mass, impaired insulin secretion, and defects in insulin receptor function and insulin receptor-signal transduction (Porte, 1990; Haataja et al, 2008; Poitout and Robertson, 2008). Humans with type 2 diabetes are typically not dependent on insulin to control the disease. Control of the diabetic state is usually possible through diet, exercise, and oral hypoglycemic drugs—hence the term *non-insulin-dependent diabetes mellitus (NIDDM)*. However, insulin treatment may be necessary in some

TABLE 6-2	BREEDS WITH A SIGNIFICANTLY (*P* < 0.05) DECREASED OR INCREASED RISK OF DIABETES MELLITUS (VETERINARY MEDICAL DATA BASE, 1970-1999)		
BREED	**CASES**	**CONTROL**	**ODDS RATIO**
Australian Terrier	37	1	32.10
Standard Schnauzer	105	19	4.78
Samoyed	175	45	3.36
Miniature Schnauzer	624	172	3.13
Fox Terrier	91	26	3.02
Keeshond	57	20	2.45
Bichon Frise	50	18	2.40
Finnish Spitz	35	13	2.32
Cairn Terrier	67	28	2.07
Miniature Poodle	737	356	1.79
Siberian Husky	80	45	1.53
Toy Poodle	208	139	1.29
Mixed breed	**1860**	**1609**	**1.00 (Reference)**
Beagle	73	94	0.67
English Setter	30	42	0.61
Labrador Retriever	246	364	0.58
Basset Hound	33	50	0.57
Dalmatian	28	45	0.53
Doberman Pinscher	109	182	0.51
Irish Setter	68	121	0.48
Boston Terrier	31	68	0.39
Shih Tzu	31	69	0.38
Brittany	28	64	0.37
Old English Sheepdog	14	35	0.35
Norwegian Elkhound	10	26	0.33
Golden Retriever	108	294	0.31
English Pointer	11	36	0.26
Cocker Spaniel	90	307	0.25
Great Dane	15	54	0.24
Bulldog	7	26	0.23
Shetland Sheepdog	29	107	0.23
Collie	25	109	0.19
Pekingese	14	66	0.18
German Shepherd	70	365	0.16
Airedale Terrier	8	45	0.15
German Short-Hair Pointer	6	37	0.14
Boxer	7	82	0.07

The Veterinary Medical Data Base comprises medical records of 24 veterinary schools in the United States and Canada.
From Guptill L, et al.: Time trends and risk factors for diabetes mellitus in dogs: analysis of veterinary medical data base records (1970-1999), *Vet J* 165:240, 2003. Breeds were included in the analysis if there were at least 25 cases or 25 controls.

type 2 diabetics if insulin resistance, beta cell dysfunction, or both are severe. As such, humans with type 2 diabetes may be non-insulin dependent or insulin dependent depending on the severity of abnormalities affiliated with the disease. Obesity-associated diabetes also occurs in the cat and resembles type 2 diabetes mellitus in humans (Appleton et al, 2001; see Chapter 7).

Obesity-induced insulin resistance has been documented in dogs, but progression to type 2 diabetes does not occur (Verkest et al, 2012). Studies suggest that at least some of the etiopathogenic mechanisms responsible for development of obesity-associated type 2 diabetes in humans and cats do not occur in dogs. For example, beta-cell sensitivity to changes in glucose and the first-phase of the insulin secretory response by the beta cell are lost in humans and cats but not in dogs despite years of obesity-induced insulin resistance and compensatory hyperinsulinemia (Verkest et al, 2011a). In humans, loss of the first phase of insulin secretion is an important early marker of beta-cell failure (Gerich, 2002).

Islet amyloid polypeptide (amylin) forms toxic intracellular oligomers in beta cells in humans and cats but not in dogs, and amylin does not aggregate extracellularly as histologically visible amyloid in the pancreatic islets in dogs (Haataja et al, 2008; Scheuner and Kaufman, 2008). Circulating concentrations of the adipocyte-secreted hormone adiponectin are decreased in obese humans and low adiponectin concentrations predict progression to type 2 diabetes in humans (Li et al, 2009). In contrast, circulating adiponectin concentrations were not lower in chronically obese dogs compared with lean dogs, and adiponectin was not associated with insulin sensitivity in obese dogs (Verkest et al, 2011b). Although adiponectin does not appear to play a role in the development of canine obesity-associated insulin resistance, adiponectin receptors are present on pancreatic beta-cells, and adiponectin has been shown to protect beta-cells against fatty acid-induced apoptosis (Kharroubi et al, 2003; Rakatzi et al, 2004).

Other Specific Types and Diabetic Remission

The occurrence of diabetic remission after initiating insulin therapy is uncommon in the dog despite the presence of circulating C-peptide in a small percentage of dogs at the time diabetes is diagnosed (Montgomery et al, 1996; Fall et al, 2008a; German et al, 2009; Pöppl et al, 2013; Fig. 6-1). C-peptide is the connecting peptide found in the proinsulin molecule, is secreted into the circulation in equimolar concentrations as insulin, and is a marker for functional beta cells. The presence of circulating C-peptide suggests the presence of functional beta cells. Unfortunately, in our experience, these dogs have required insulin to control hyperglycemia, suggesting the increased C-peptide concentrations in these dogs is most likely due to residual beta-cell function in dogs with type 1 diabetes mellitus rather than a severe form of type 2 diabetes.

A transient increase in endogenous insulin secretion and reduced insulin dosage requirements may occur during the initial weeks to months after the diagnosis of type 1 diabetes mellitus in humans; this is called the *honeymoon period* (Rossetti et al, 1990). A syndrome similar to the honeymoon period occurs in some newly diagnosed diabetic dogs and is characterized by excellent glycemic control using dosages of insulin considerably less than what would be expected (i.e., less than 0.2 U/kg per injection; Fig. 6-2). Presumably, the existence of residual beta-cell function when diabetes is diagnosed (see Fig. 6-1) and possible correction of glucose toxicity (see Chapter 7) after initiating insulin therapy accounts for the initial ease of treating the diabetic state. Continuing progressive destruction of residual functioning beta cells results in worsening loss of endogenous insulin secretory capacity and a greater need for exogenous insulin to control the diabetes. As a result, glycemic control becomes more difficult to maintain, and insulin dosages increase to more commonly required amounts (0.5 to 1.0 U/kg per injection). This increase in insulin requirements usually occurs within the first 6 months of treatment.

When diabetic remission occurs, it is usually in older female dogs that are diagnosed with diabetes during diestrus or pregnancy when serum progesterone and growth hormone concentrations are increased (Fall et al, 2008b; 2010; Mared et al, 2012). Diabetic remission may also occur in spayed females with ovarian remnant syndrome and in diestrual bitches with concurrent pyometra (Pöppl et al, 2013). Documenting increased baseline serum insulin concentration supports the presence of functional beta cells and concurrent insulin resistance. Documenting an increase in serum progesterone concentration (2 ng/mL or higher) confirms the presence of functional corpora lutea and diestrus, regardless of the presence or absence of owner observed signs of a recent heat cycle. These dogs presumably have an adequate mass of functional beta cells to maintain carbohydrate tolerance when insulin resistance is not present (e.g., during anestrus), but they are unable to secrete an adequate amount of insulin to maintain euglycemia in the presence of insulin antagonism (Fall et al, 2008a). Early recognition and correction of the insulin resistance (e.g., following ovariohysterectomy) while some beta-cell function is still present may reestablish euglycemia without the long-term need for insulin therapy (Fig. 6-3). Failure to quickly correct insulin resistance often results in progressive loss of beta cells and a greater likelihood for permanent insulin dependency to control hyperglycemia

(Fall et al, 2010). Bitches that have undergone diabetic remission following diestrus have a high likelihood of developing permanent insulin dependent diabetes during the next estrus. For this reason, all female dogs that develop diabetes during diestrus should be spayed as soon as possible after diabetes is diagnosed.

A similar sequence of events may occur with the administration of insulin antagonistic drugs, most notably glucocorticoids and progestogens, and other insulin resistant disorders such as hyperadrenocorticism. Resolution of hyperglycemia is most likely to occur when the hyperglycemia is mild (less than 160 mg/dL; 9 mmol/L) and has not yet resulted in glycosuria. Dogs that become euglycemic after correction of insulin resistance presumably do not have a normal population of functional beta cells, should be considered subclinical diabetics, and may or may not progress to an insulin-requiring diabetic state in the future. Treatment with insulin antagonistic drugs should be avoided, and disorders causing insulin resistance should be treated quickly to prevent overt diabetes mellitus from developing.

PATHOPHYSIOLOGY

Diabetes mellitus results from a relative or absolute deficiency of insulin secretion by the beta cells. Insulin deficiency, in turn, causes decreased tissue utilization of glucose, amino acids, and fatty acids, accelerated hepatic glycogenolysis and gluconeogenesis, and accumulation of glucose in the circulation, causing hyperglycemia. As the blood glucose concentration increases, the ability of the renal tubular cells to resorb glucose from the glomerular ultrafiltrate

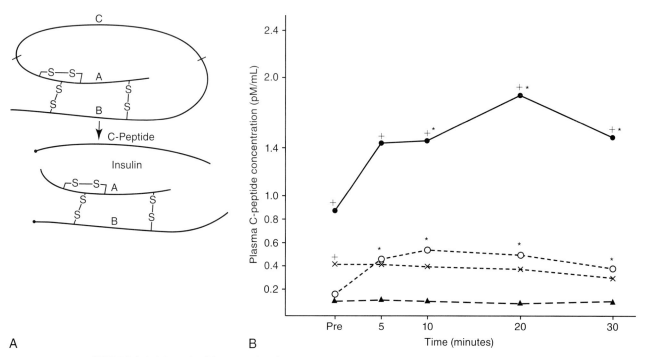

FIGURE 6-1 A, Schematic of the conversion of proinsulin *(top)* to insulin. Proteolytic cleavage of proinsulin forms equimolar concentrations of connecting peptide (C-peptide) and insulin, which are stored in secretory granules of beta cells. **B,** Mean plasma C-peptide concentration prior to and after intravenous (IV) administration of 1 mg glucagon in 24 healthy dogs *(broken line—open circles)*, 35 dogs with diabetes mellitus and low baseline C-peptide concentration *(broken line—triangles)*, 7 dogs with diabetes mellitus and increased baseline C-peptide concentration *(broken line—Xs)*, and 8 dogs with naturally acquired hyperadrenocorticism *(solid line—solid circles)*. **(B,** From Nelson RW: Diabetes mellitus. In Ettinger SJ, Feldman EC, editors: *Textbook of veterinary internal medicine,* ed 4, Philadelphia, 1995, WB Saunders Co, p. 1511.) * = significantly (*P* < 0.05) different from baseline value; + = significantly (*P* < 0.05) different from corresponding time in healthy dogs.

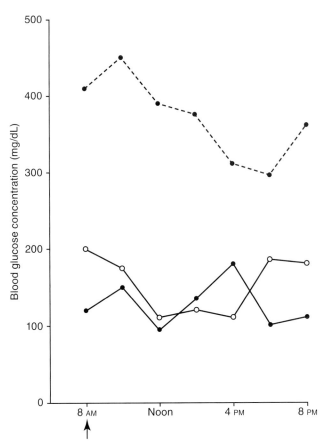

FIGURE 6-2 Blood glucose curve in a 32 kg male dog receiving 0.3 U/kg subcutaneously beef/pork source neutral protamine Hagedorn (NPH) insulin *(solid line—solid circles).* The blood glucose curve was obtained shortly after initiating insulin therapy. Five months later, glycemic control deteriorated and clinical signs recurred despite increasing the insulin dosage to 0.6 U/kg *(broken line—solid circles).* The dog was referred for possible insulin resistance. Insulin underdosage was pursued initially, and glycemic control was reestablished at an insulin dosage of 1.0 U/kg *(solid line—open circles).* ↑ = insulin injection and food.

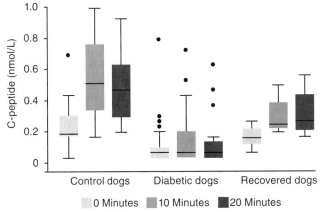

FIGURE 6-3 Box plots of the serum concentration of C-peptide before (0 minutes) and 10 and 20 minutes after the intravenous (IV) administration of a bolus dose of glucagon to 20 healthy dogs, 27 diabetic dogs, and 4 dogs that had recovered from diabetes. The *horizontal line* represents the median, the box represents the interquartile range (i.e., 25% to 75%), the *T-bars* represent the main body of data, and the *circles* represent outliers. (From Fall T, et al.: Glucagon stimulation test for estimating endogenous insulin secretion in dogs, *Vet Rec* 163:266, 2008.)

is exceeded, resulting in glycosuria. In dogs, this typically occurs whenever the blood glucose concentration exceeds 180 to 220 mg/dL (10 to 12 mmol/L). The threshold for glucose resorption appears more variable in cats, ranging from 200 to 280 mg/dL (11 to 16 mmol/L). Glycosuria creates an osmotic diuresis, causing polyuria. Compensatory polydipsia prevents dehydration. The diminished peripheral tissue utilization of ingested glucose results in weight loss as the body attempts to compensate for perceived "starvation."

The interaction of the "satiety center" in the ventromedial region of the hypothalamus with the "feeding center" in the lateral region of the hypothalamus is responsible for controlling the amount of food ingested (Barrett et al, 2012). The feeding center, responsible for evoking eating behavior, is chronically functioning but can be transiently inhibited by the satiety center after food ingestion. The amount of glucose entering the cells in the satiety center directly affects the feeling of hunger; the more glucose that enters these cells, the less the feeling of hunger and vice versa (Barrett et al, 2012). The ability of glucose to enter the cells in the satiety center is mediated by insulin. In diabetics with a relative or absolute lack of insulin, glucose does not enter satiety center cells, resulting in failure to inhibit the feeding center. Thus these individuals become polyphagic despite hyperglycemia.

The four classic signs of diabetes mellitus are polyuria, polydipsia, polyphagia, and weight loss. The severity of these signs is directly related to the severity of hyperglycemia. As these signs become obvious to the owner, the pet is brought to the veterinarian for care. Unfortunately, some dogs and cats are not identified by their owners as having signs of disease, and these untreated animals may ultimately develop diabetic ketoacidosis (DKA), systemic signs of illness, and potentially life-threatening derangements in fluid and acid/base balance. See Chapter 8 for a detailed discussion of the pathophysiology of DKA.

SIGNALMENT

Most dogs are 5 to 15 years old at the time diabetes mellitus is diagnosed (Table 6-3; Guptill et al, 2003). Juvenile-onset diabetes occurs in dogs younger than 1 year of age and is uncommon. One large epidemiologic study involving 6807 diabetic dogs and 6807 matched controls in the United States and Canada identified the following: female dogs were at increased risk for diabetes compared with male dogs, neutered male dogs were at increased risk compared with intact male dogs, mixed-breed dogs were at increased risk compared with pure breeds, and dogs weighing less than 22.7 kg were at increased risk compared with larger dogs (Guptill et al, 2003). A seasonal pattern in prevalence of diabetes was not identified. Breeds with a significantly increased or decreased risk for developing diabetes are listed in Table 6-2. Breed popularity and regions of the world may also impact breed predispositions. For example, breeds with the highest risk for diabetes in Italy include the Irish Setter, Poodle, Yorkshire Terrier, and English Setter (Fracassi et al, 2004). In Sweden, high risk breeds included Spitz type breeds (Samoyed, Swedish Elkhound, and Swedish Lapphund) and Scandinavian hound dogs (Finnish Hound, Hamilton Hound, and Drever) (Fall et al, 2007).

ANAMNESIS

The history in virtually all diabetic dogs includes the classic signs of polydipsia, polyuria, polyphagia, and weight loss. Owners will often bring their dog to the veterinarian because the dog can no longer make it through the night without having to be let outside to urinate or it begins urinating in the home. Occasionally an owner brings in a dog because of sudden blindness caused by cataract formation (Fig. 6-4). The classic signs of diabetes mellitus may have gone unnoticed or been considered irrelevant by the owner. If the clinical signs associated with uncomplicated diabetes are not observed by the owner and impaired vision caused by cataracts does not develop, a diabetic dog is at risk for the development of systemic signs of illness (i.e., lethargy, anorexia, vomiting, and weakness) as progressive ketonemia and metabolic acidosis develop. The time sequence from the onset of initial clinical signs to the development of DKA is unpredictable, ranging from days to weeks; an onset that is somewhat dependent on the type and severity of concurrent disease causing insulin resistance and accelerating the production of ketone bodies.

A complete history is extremely important even in the "obvious" diabetic dog to explore for concurrent disorders, which are almost always present at the time diabetes mellitus is diagnosed. The clinician should always ask, "Why has the dog developed clinical signs of diabetes now?" In many dogs the insulin antagonism caused by concurrent disorders (e.g., pancreatitis, bacterial infections, recent estrus, chronic kidney disease [CKD], or hyperadrenocorticism) is the final insult leading to overt diabetes. Identification and treatment of concurrent disorders plays an integral role in the successful management of the diabetic dog, and a thorough history is the first step toward identification of these disorders.

TABLE 6-3	**AGE AT TIME OF DIAGNOSIS OF DIABETES MELLITUS IN 6807 DOGS IDENTIFIED BETWEEN JANUARY 1, 1970, AND DECEMBER 31, 1999**

AGE (YEARS)	NUMBER OF DOGS	PERCENT OF DOGS
< 1	154	2.2%
1 to 2	46	0.7%
3 to 4	195	2.8%
5 to 7	1058	15.4%
8 to 10	2543	37.1%
11 to 15	2690	39.2%
> 15	121	1.8%

From Guptill L, et al.: Time trends and risk factors for diabetes mellitus in dogs: analysis of veterinary medical data base records (1970-1999), *Vet J* 165:240, 2003.

PHYSICAL EXAMINATION

Performance of a thorough physical examination is imperative in any dog suspected of having diabetes mellitus, in part, because of the high prevalence of concurrent disorders that can affect response to treatment. The physical examination findings in a dog with newly-diagnosed diabetes depend on whether DKA is present and its severity, on the duration of diabetes prior to its diagnosis, and on the nature of any other concurrent disorder. The nonketotic diabetic dog has no classic physical examination findings. Many diabetic dogs are obese but are otherwise in good physical condition. Dogs with prolonged untreated diabetes may have lost weight but are rarely emaciated unless concurrent disease (e.g., inflammatory bowel disease, pancreatic exocrine insufficiency) is present. Lethargy may be evident. The hair coat in newly-diagnosed or poorly-controlled diabetic dogs may be sparse; the hairs dry, brittle, and lusterless; and scales from hyperkeratosis may be present. Diabetes-induced hepatic lipidosis may cause hepatomegaly. Lenticular changes consistent with cataract formation are another common clinical finding in diabetic dogs. Anterior uveitis and keratoconjunctivitis sicca may also be present. In contrast to diabetic cats, clinical signs suggestive of diabetic neuropathy (e.g., rear limb weakness, ataxia) are uncommon in newly-diagnosed diabetic dogs. Additional abnormalities may be identified in the ketoacidotic diabetic.

ESTABLISHING THE DIAGNOSIS OF DIABETES MELLITUS

A diagnosis of diabetes mellitus requires the presence of appropriate clinical signs (i.e., polyuria, polydipsia, polyphagia, weight loss) and documentation of persistent fasting hyperglycemia and glycosuria. Measurement of the blood glucose concentration using a portable blood glucose monitoring (PBGM) device (see Serial Blood Glucose Curve) and testing for the presence of glycosuria using urine reagent test strips (e.g., KetoDiastix) allows the rapid confirmation of diabetes mellitus. The concurrent documentation of ketonuria establishes a diagnosis of diabetic ketosis or ketoacidosis.

It is important to document both persistent hyperglycemia and glycosuria to establish a diagnosis of diabetes mellitus. Hyperglycemia without glycosuria does not cause polyuria and polydipsia and may occur with causes of hyperglycemia that do not typically progress to a clinical diabetic state (Box 6-1). Glycosuria without

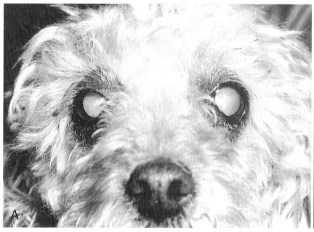
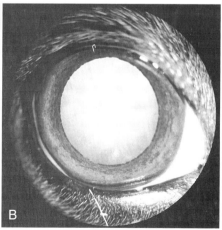

FIGURE 6-4 A, Bilateral cataracts causing blindness in a diabetic dog. **B,** Mature cataract with suture lines in a diabetic Collie.

hyperglycemia supports primary renal glycosuria or other renal tubular disorders, not diabetes mellitus.

Documenting an increase in the serum fructosamine concentration supports the presence of sustained hyperglycemia; however, a serum fructosamine concentration in the upper range of normal can occur in symptomatic diabetic dogs if the diabetes developed shortly before presentation of the dog to the veterinarian.

Mild hyperglycemia (i.e., 130 to 180 mg/dL; 7.3 to 10 mmol/L) is clinically silent and is usually an unexpected and unsuspected finding. If the dog with mild hyperglycemia is examined for polyuria and polydipsia, a disorder other than clinical diabetes mellitus should be sought. Mild hyperglycemia can occur shortly after consuming large quantities of easily digestible carbohydrates; in "stressed," hyperactive, aggressive, or extremely nervous dogs; in the early stages of development of diabetes mellitus (i.e., subclinical diabetes); and with disorders and drugs causing insulin resistance, most notably hyperadrenocorticism, glucocorticoids, and during diestrus in older intact female dogs. A diagnostic evaluation for disorders causing insulin resistance is indicated if mild hyperglycemia persists in the fasted, unstressed dog (see Concurrent Disorders Causing Insulin Resistance). Insulin therapy is usually not indicated in these animals, although some clinicians will initiate low-dose insulin therapy while searching for and treating the underlying cause of the insulin resistance in the hope that improving hyperglycemia will decrease the demand for insulin production and secretion by the beta cells and minimize further damage to the cells.

CLINICAL PATHOLOGIC ABNORMALITIES

Overview of Patient Evaluation

A thorough clinicopathologic evaluation is recommended once the diagnosis of diabetes mellitus has been established. The clinician must be aware of any disease that may be causing or contributing to the carbohydrate intolerance (e.g., hyperadrenocorticism), that may result from the carbohydrate intolerance (e.g., bacterial cystitis), or that may mandate a modification of therapy (e.g., pancreatitis) (Hess et al, 2000b; Peikes et al, 2001). The minimum laboratory evaluation in any newly-diagnosed diabetic dog should include a complete blood count (CBC), serum biochemical panel, and urinalysis with bacterial culture. Serum progesterone concentration should be determined if diabetes mellitus is diagnosed in an intact bitch, regardless of her cycling history. If available, abdominal ultrasound is indicated to assess for pancreatitis, adrenomegaly, pyometritis in an intact bitch, and abnormalities affecting the liver and urinary tract (e.g., changes consistent with pyelonephritis or cystitis). Because of the relatively high prevalence of pancreatitis in diabetic dogs, measurement of pancreatic lipase immunoreactivity (cPLI) should be considered, especially if abdominal ultrasound is not available. Additional tests may be warranted after obtaining the history, performing the physical examination, or identifying ketonuria. The laboratory evaluation of dogs with glycosuria and ketonuria is discussed in detail in Chapter 8. Potential clinical pathologic abnormalities are listed in Box 6-2.

BOX 6-1 Etiologic Classification of Diabetes Mellitus and Hyperglycemia

1. Type 1 diabetes mellitus
2. Type 2 diabetes mellitus
3. Other specific types
   A. Genetic defects
   B. Disease of the exocrine pancreas
      Pancreatitis
      Exocrine pancreatic neoplasia
   C. Endocrinopathies
      Hyperadrenocorticism
      Acromegaly (cat)
      Pheochromocytoma (dog)
      Hyperthyroidism (cat)
   D. Drug or chemical induced
      Glucocorticoids
      Progestagens
      Thyroid hormone
      Thiazide diuretics
      Beta adrenergic agonists
   E. Infections
      Pyometra
4. Gestational diabetes mellitus
   A. Diestrus (bitch)
   B. Ovarian remnant syndrome
5. Miscellaneous causes of hyperglycemia
   A. Head trauma
   B. Critical illness
   C. Stress, aggression, fright (cat)
   D. Dextrose-containing fluids
   E. Parenteral nutrition solutions
   F. Postprandial

Modified from the American Diabetes Association etiologic classification for humans.

BOX 6-2 Clinicopathologic Abnormalities Commonly Found in Dogs and Cats with Uncomplicated Diabetes Mellitus

Complete Blood Count
Typically normal
Neutrophilic leukocytosis, toxic neutrophils if pancreatitis or infection present

Biochemistry Panel
Hyperglycemia
Hypercholesterolemia
Hypertriglyceridemia (lipemia)
Increased alanine aminotransferase activity (typically < 500 U/L)
Increased alkaline phosphatase activity (typically < 500 U/L)

Urinalysis
Urine specific gravity (typically > 1.025)
Glycosuria
Variable ketonuria
Proteinuria
Bacteriuria

Ancillary Tests
Hyperlipasemia (canine pancreatic-specific lipase [cPL]) if pancreatitis present
Hyperamylasemia if pancreatitis present
Serum trypsin-like immunoreactivity (TLI) usually normal
   Low with pancreatic exocrine insufficiency
   High with acute pancreatitis
   Normal to high with chronic pancreatitis
Variable serum baseline insulin concentration
   Type 1 diabetes: Low, normal
   Type 2 diabetes: Low, normal, increased
   Insulin resistance induced: Low, normal, increased

Complete Blood Count

Results of a CBC are usually normal in the uncomplicated diabetic dog. A mild polycythemia may be present if the dog is dehydrated. An elevation of the white blood cell count may be caused by either an infectious or inflammatory disorder, such as pancreatitis. The presence of toxic or degenerative neutrophils or a significant shift toward immaturity of the cells supports the presence of an infectious process or severe necrotizing pancreatitis as the cause of the leukocytosis.

Serum Biochemical Panel

The prevalence and severity of abnormalities identified in the serum biochemistry panel are dependent on the duration of untreated diabetes and the presence of concurrent disease, most notably pancreatitis (Hess et al, 2000b). The serum biochemical panel is often unremarkable in "healthy" diabetic dogs without significant concurrent disease, aside from hyperglycemia and hypercholesterolemia. The most common abnormalities are an increase in serum alanine aminotransferase and alkaline phosphatase activities and hypercholesterolemia (see later). The increase in liver enzyme activities in "healthy" diabetic dogs is usually mild (less than 500 U/L) and presumed to be a result of hepatic lipidosis. Serum alkaline phosphatase activities in excess of 800 U/L should raise suspicion for concurrent hyperadrenocorticism, especially if other abnormalities consistent with hyperadrenocorticism are identified in the laboratory data (see Chapter 10). Serum alanine aminotransferase activities in excess of 600 U/L should raise suspicion for hepatopathy other than hepatic lipidosis, especially if additional abnormalities in endogenous liver function tests (e.g., low urea nitrogen, hypoalbuminemia, or increased serum bile acids) are identified. An increase in the serum total bilirubin concentration should raise suspicion for extrahepatic biliary obstruction caused by concurrent pancreatitis. When appropriate, abdominal ultrasound and histologic evaluation of a liver biopsy specimen may be indicated to establish concurrent liver disease.

The blood urea nitrogen (BUN) and serum creatinine concentrations are usually normal in the uncomplicated diabetic. An elevation in these parameters may be due to either primary renal failure or prerenal uremia secondary to dehydration. Primary renal failure as a result of glomerulosclerosis, which is damage specifically related to chronic hyperglycemia, is a well-recognized complication in humans but is uncommon in dogs (see Diabetic Nephropathy). Evaluation of urine specific gravity should help differentiate primary renal failure from prerenal uremia. Remember to consider the impact of glycosuria on results of urine specific gravity determined by refractometry (see later).

Alterations in serum electrolytes and acid-base parameters are common in dogs with DKA and are discussed in Chapter 8.

Urinalysis

Abnormalities identified in the urinalysis that are consistent with diabetes mellitus include glycosuria, ketonuria, proteinuria, and bacteriuria with or without associated pyuria and hematuria. The dog with uncomplicated diabetes usually has glycosuria without ketonuria. However, a relatively healthy diabetic may also have trace to small amounts of ketones in the urine. If large amounts of ketones are present in the urine—especially in an animal with systemic signs of illness (e.g., lethargy, vomiting, or dehydration), a diagnosis of DKA should be made and the animal treated appropriately.

The presence and severity of glycosuria should be considered when interpreting the urine specific gravity. Despite polyuria and polydipsia, urine specific gravities typically range from 1.025 to 1.035 in untreated diabetic dogs, in part, because of the large amount of glucose in the urine. In general, 2% or 4+ glycosuria as measured on urine reagent test strips will increase the urine specific gravity 0.008 to 0.010 when urine specific gravity is measured by refractometry. As such, identification of a urine specific gravity less than 1.020 in combination with 2% glycosuria suggests a concurrent polyuric/polydipsic disorder, most notably hyperadrenocorticism or CKD.

Proteinuria may be the result of urinary tract infection or glomerular damage secondary to disruption of the basement membrane (Struble et al, 1998). Identification of pyuria, hematuria, and bacteriuria suggests the presence of a urinary tract infection. However, failure to identify pyuria and hematuria does not rule out urinary tract infection (McGuire et al, 2002). Because of the relatively high prevalence of concurrent urinary tract infections in diabetic dogs, urine obtained by antepubic cystocentesis using aseptic technique should be submitted for bacterial culture and antibiotic sensitivity testing in all dogs with newly-diagnosed diabetes mellitus, regardless of the findings on urinalysis (Hess et al, 2000b).

Serum Cholesterol and Triglyceride Concentrations

Serum cholesterol and triglyceride concentrations are typically increased in newly-diagnosed diabetic dogs. Insulin is a powerful inhibitor of lipolysis and free fatty acid oxidation. During a state of insulin deficiency, lipoprotein lipase activity is reduced, hormone-sensitive lipase is activated, hepatic production of triglyceride-rich very–low-density lipoprotein (VLDL) particles is increased, and clearance of VLDL particles is decreased (Eckel, 1989; Massillon et al, 1997; Semenkovich et al, 2011). Activation of hormone-sensitive lipase results in the release of large quantities of free fatty acids from adipocytes into the blood. These free fatty acids are ultimately converted by the liver into triglycerides, packaged into VLDL particles, and secreted back into the circulation. Increased intrahepatic cholesterol concentration down-regulates the hepatocyte low-density lipoprotein (LDL) receptor, consequently reducing the clearance of circulating cholesterol-containing LDL and high-density lipoprotein (HDL) particles, which in turn causes hypercholesterolemia.

Chylomicrons and VLDLs are primarily involved in triglyceride metabolism, whereas HDLs and LDLs are primarily involved in cholesterol metabolism. In diabetic humans, circulating concentrations of LDLs and HDLs are increased and decreased, respectively. The combination of high LDL and low HDL cholesterol concentrations may play a role in the accelerated development of atherosclerotic vascular disease and coronary heart disease, which is the major long-term complication of diabetes in humans (Garg and Grundy, 1990). Similar vascular complications have been infrequently documented in diabetic dogs (Hess et al, 2002), presumably because HDLs predominate in dogs (as opposed to LDLs in humans), and dogs have a shorter life span that may limit development of atherosclerosis (Bauer, 2004). Fortunately, most lipid derangements in diabetic dogs can be improved with insulin and dietary therapy.

Pancreatic Enzymes

Blood tests to assess for the presence of pancreatitis should always be considered in the newly-diagnosed diabetic dog, especially if abdominal ultrasound is not available. Measurement of canine pancreatic-specific lipase (cPL) is currently the blood test of choice for identifying pancreatitis (Trivedi et al, 2011; McCord et al, 2012). Sensitivity and specificity of cPL varies between studies and is dependent on the severity of pancreatitis and the cutoff value (200 versus 400 µg/L) used to separate normal from pancreatitis (McCord et al, 2012; Bostrom et al, 2013). Serum cPL concentrations can be increased in dogs with a histologically confirmed normal pancreas and normal in dogs with histologically confirmed inflammation of the pancreas, especially when the inflammatory process is chronic and mild (Forman et al, 2004; Trivedi et al, 2011). Interpretation of serum cPL results should always be done in context with the history, physical examination findings, and additional findings on the laboratory tests. In our experience, abdominal ultrasound is the single best diagnostic test for identifying acute and chronic pancreatitis in the dog; however, results are equipment and operator dependent. Nevertheless, abdominal ultrasound should be considered if pancreatitis is suspected after evaluation of the history, physical examination, and laboratory test results. The concomitant presence of pancreatitis may necessitate the instigation of intensive fluid therapy and the initiation of diets aimed at treating pancreatitis rather than diabetes. Identification of chronic pancreatitis also has important prognostic implications regarding success of establishing and maintaining control of glycemia and long-term survival.

Measurement of serum trypsin-like immunoreactivity (TLI) is no longer recommended for identifying pancreatitis but is currently the blood test of choice to diagnose exocrine pancreatic insufficiency; an uncommon complication of diabetes mellitus that presumably develops as a sequela of chronic pancreatitis in most diabetic dogs (Wiberg et al, 1999; Wiberg and Westermarck, 2002). Exocrine pancreatic insufficiency should be suspected in diabetic dogs that are difficult to regulate with insulin, are thin or emaciated despite polyphagia, and defecate increased amounts of soft stools—not the voluminous, rancid stools considered classic for exocrine pancreatic insufficiency (EPI). Mild diffuse thickening of the small intestine may be evident during abdominal palpation. Serum TLI should be less than 2.5 µg/L in diabetic dogs with concurrent exocrine pancreatic insufficiency.

Serum Thyroxine Concentration

The veterinarian may periodically have to interpret a serum thyroxine (T_4) concentration in a diabetic dog, either because serum T_4 is a routine part of the serum biochemistry panel; because hypothyroidism is suspected after a review of the history, clinical signs, and physical examination findings; or because severe hyperlipidemia is identified or as part of the diagnostic evaluation for insulin resistance (Hofer-Inteeworn et al, 2012). Interpretation of serum T_4 results must be done cautiously, especially in a dog with newly-diagnosed diabetes mellitus and concurrent illness, such as pancreatitis or infection. "Healthy" diabetic dogs without concurrent illness usually have normal serum T_4 concentrations. However, the more poorly controlled the diabetic state and the more severe the concurrent illness, the more likely serum T_4 concentrations will be decreased into the hypothyroid range because of the suppressive effect of concurrent illness on the pituitary-thyroid axis rather than because of naturally-acquired hypothyroidism (see Chapter 3). As a general rule, in a newly-diagnosed diabetic dog with a concurrent low serum T_4 concentration, we treat the diabetes and reevaluate serum T_4 and thyroid-stimulating hormone (also known as thyrotropin; TSH) concentrations once control of glycemia has been established. If hypothyroidism is strongly

suspected at the time diabetes is diagnosed, we will evaluate serum free T_4 and TSH concentrations before initiating sodium levothyroxine treatment. See Chapter 3 for a more detailed discussion of the effects of concurrent lipemia, illness, and drug therapy on serum thyroid hormone concentrations and the tests used to diagnose hypothyroidism in dogs.

Serum Insulin Concentration

Measurement of serum insulin concentration (either baseline or after the administration of an insulin secretagogue) is not a routine part of our diagnostic evaluation of the newly-diagnosed diabetic dog. In theory, identifying increased endogenous serum insulin concentrations in a newly-diagnosed diabetic dog would suggest the presence of functioning beta cells and the presence of an underlying insulin antagonistic disorder. However, because the vast majority of dogs with newly-diagnosed diabetes have type 1 diabetes and serum insulin concentration is typically in the lower half of normal or undetectable, routine measurement of serum insulin concentration is not a cost-effective diagnostic procedure. The exceptions are older intact female dogs in diestrus and with newly-diagnosed diabetes mellitus (see Other Specific Types and Diabetic Remission). It is imperative that the insulin assay has been validated in dogs; that the reference interval has been determined using healthy, fasted dogs; and that the diabetic dog has not been recently treated with exogenous insulin. Most insulin assays will measure exogenously administered insulin, resulting in an increased serum insulin concentration and a misinterpretation of beta cell function in the diabetic dog. As a general rule, exogenous insulin should be withheld for at least 24 hours before blood is obtained for endogenous serum insulin measurement.

TREATMENT OF NONKETOTIC DIABETES MELLITUS

Goals of Therapy

There are two primary goals of therapy. The first goal is the elimination of the owner-observed signs occurring secondary to hyperglycemia and glycosuria. A persistence of clinical signs and the development of chronic complications (Table 6-4) are directly correlated with the severity and duration of hyperglycemia. Limiting blood glucose concentration fluctuations and maintaining near-normal glycemia will help minimize the severity of clinical signs and prevent the complications of poorly controlled diabetes. In the diabetic dog, this can be accomplished through proper insulin therapy, diet, exercise, and the prevention or control of concurrent inflammatory, infectious, neoplastic, and hormonal disorders.

Although it is worthwhile attempting to normalize the blood glucose concentration, the veterinarian must also guard against the animal developing of hypoglycemia, which is a serious and potentially fatal complication of therapy. Hypoglycemia is most apt to occur as the result of overzealous insulin therapy. The veterinarian must balance the benefits of tight glucose control obtainable with aggressive insulin therapy against the risk for hypoglycemia.

The second goal is to minimize the impact of therapy on the owner's lifestyle. A recent study evaluated the psychological and social impact of diabetes and its treatment on the quality of life of 101 owners of diabetic dogs living in the United Kingdom, United States, Canada, Australia, and Europe (Niessen et al, 2012). The top 10 negative impact items were associated mostly with the owner's quality of life rather than the pet's quality of

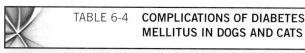

TABLE 6-4	**COMPLICATIONS OF DIABETES MELLITUS IN DOGS AND CATS**
COMMON	**UNCOMMON**
Iatrogenic hypoglycemia	Peripheral neuropathy (dog)
Persistent polyuria, polydipsia, weight loss	Glomerulonephropathy, glomerulosclerosis
Cataracts (dog)	Retinopathy
Bacterial infections, especially in the urinary tract	Exocrine pancreatic insufficiency
Pancreatitis	Gastric paresis
Ketoacidosis	Diabetic dermatopathy (dog) (i.e., superficial necrolytic dermatitis)
Hepatic lipidosis	
Peripheral neuropathy (cat)	

TABLE 6-5	**TOP TEN NEGATIVE PSYCHOLOGICAL AND SOCIAL IMPACTS OF DIABETES MELLITUS AND ITS TREATMENT ON THE QUALITY OF LIFE OF OWNERS OF A DIABETIC DOG**
ITEM	**MEAN ITEM WEIGHTED IMPACT SCORE**
Worry about pet's diabetes	-5.92
Interferes with visiting family and friends	-5.68
Worry about the dog developing cataracts	-5.58
Worry about boarding the dog	-5.18
Worry about dog developing hypoglycemia	-4.95
Having to fit the dog's needs into their social life	-4.82
Cost of treating the diabetes	-4.11
Worry about future ability to care for the dog	-4.07
Having to fit the dog's needs into their work schedule	-3.88
Restricting the owners' vacation and work activities	-3.88

Adapted from Niessen SJM, et al.: Evaluation of a quality-of-life tool for dogs with diabetes mellitus, *J Vet Intern Med* 26:953, 2012.
The quality of life survey was completed by 101 owners originating from the United Kingdom, United States, Canada, Australia, and Europe.

life (Table 6-5). The only positive items identified by the owners were related to more interactions and development of a special bond with their dog. Fortunately, 81% of diabetic dog owners rated their dog's quality of life as good despite 84% reporting a negative impact of diabetes on their dog's quality of life. Awareness of the impact of the treatment regimen, home monitoring, and frequency of evaluations by the veterinarian on the client and simplifying the overall management of the diabetic dog as much as possible without negatively impacting control of glycemia is important for the long-term success of treating diabetes.

Insulin Therapy

Overview of Insulin Preparations

Insulin preparations typically used for the home treatment of diabetes in dogs and cats include intermediate-acting insulin preparations (neutral protamine Hagedorn [NPH], Lente) and long-acting basal insulin preparations (protamine zinc insulin [PZI], insulin glargine, insulin detemir; Table 6-6). NPH (Humulin N, Novolin N) is a recombinant human insulin, Lente (Vetsulin, Caninsulin) is a purified pork-source insulin, PZI (Pro-Zinc) is a recombinant human insulin, and insulin glargine (Lantus) and insulin detemir (Levemir) are insulin analogues. NPH and PZI insulin preparations contain the fish protein protamine and zinc to delay insulin absorption and prolong the duration of insulin effect (Davidson et al, 1991). Lente insulin relies on alterations in zinc content and the size of zinc-insulin crystals to alter the rate of insulin absorption from the subcutaneous site of deposition. The larger the crystals are, the slower the rate of absorption and the longer the duration of effect. Lente insulin contains no foreign protein (i.e., protamine). Lente insulin is a mixture of three parts of short-acting, amorphous zinc insulin and seven parts of long-acting, crystalline zinc insulin. Lente insulin is considered an intermediate-acting insulin, although plasma insulin concentrations may remain increased for longer than 14 hours following subcutaneous administration in some dogs (Graham et al, 1997). The manufacturer of porcine Lente insulin now recommends vigorous shaking of the insulin vial until a homogeneous milky suspension is obtained prior to withdrawal of the insulin into the syringe.

NPH insulin, insulin glargine and insulin detemir are U100 insulin preparations (i.e., 100 units of insulin per mL of solution). Porcine-source Lente and protamine zinc insulin are approved by the Food and Drug Administration (FDA) for treatment of diabetes in dogs and cats, respectively and so are U40 insulin preparations (i.e., 40 units of insulin per mL of solution). The appropriate insulin syringe should be used for the insulin preparation being administered (i.e., U40 or U100 insulin syringe for a U40 or U100 insulin preparation). Insulin pens are also available for NPH insulin, porcine-source Lente insulin, insulin glargine, and insulin detemir.

Porcine-source Lente and recombinant human NPH insulin are effective for the treatment of diabetes in dogs (Lorenzen, 1992; Monroe et al, 2005). Problems with prolonged duration of insulin effect can occur with both insulin preparations but are not common (Hess and Ward, 2000; Fleeman et al, 2009a). Problems with short duration of insulin effect despite twice a day administration are more common than problems with prolonged duration of insulin effect, especially with NPH insulin (see Complications of Insulin Therapy; Palm et al, 2009). For this reason, porcine-source Lente insulin is considered the initial insulin of choice for the home treatment of diabetes in dogs. For a period of time, porcine-source Lente insulin was not available in the United States and veterinarians were forced to use alternative insulin preparations, most commonly NPH or insulin detemir. Fortunately porcine-source Lente insulin is once again available in the United States.

Recombinant human PZI insulin is commonly used for the treatment of diabetes in cats but published experiences with PZI in diabetic dogs is limited. In a recent study, PZI administered twice a day was effective in improving or maintaining control of glycemia in the majority of diabetic dogs enrolled in the study, and more than 80% of owners were satisfied with the results of treatment (Della-Maggiore et al, 2012). However, prolonged duration of PZI effect was a common problem that resulted in blood glucose nadirs often occurring at the beginning or end of the blood glucose cure, inconsistency in blood glucose results in

TABLE 6-6 COMMONLY-USED INSULIN PREPARATIONS FOR TREATING DIABETES IN DOGS AND CATS

			Administration		Typical Duration of Effect (hour)		
INSULIN	**ORIGIN**	**INDICATIONS**	**ROUTE**	**FREQUENCY**	**DOG**	**CAT**	**COMMON PROBLEMS**
Regular crystalline	Recombinant human	Treat DKA	IV	Continuous infusion	—	—	Rapid decrease in blood glucose concentration; may cause hypokalemia
			IM	Hourly initially	4-6	4-6	
			SC	Every 6 to 8 hours	6-8	6-8	
		Treat diabetes at home	SC	Every 8 hours	6-8	6-8	
Lispro	Recombinant human analog	Treat DKA	IV	Continuous infusion	—	—	Rapid decrease in blood glucose concentration; may cause hypokalemia
NPH	Recombinant human	Treat diabetes at home	SC	Every 12 hours	6-12	6-10	Short duration of effect in dogs and cats
Lente	100% pork	Treat diabetes at home; good initial insulin for dogs	SC	Every 12 hours	8-14	6-12	Short duration of effect in cats
PZI	Recombinant human	Treat diabetes at home; good initial insulin for cats	SC	Every 12 hours	10-16	10-14	Duration of effect too long for every-12-hour therapy in some dogs; unpredictable timing of glucose nadir in some dogs
Glargine	Recombinant human analog	Treat diabetes at home; good initial insulin for cats	SC	Every 12 to 24 hours	8-16	8-16	Duration of effect too long for every-12-hour therapy in some cats and dogs; weak glucose lowering effect and unpredictable timing of glucose nadir in some dogs
Detemir	Recombinant human analog	Treat diabetes at home	SC	Every 12 to 24 hours	8-16	8-16	Duration of effect too long for every-12-hour therapy in some cats and dogs; insulin dosage requirements considerably lower than with other insulin preparations

From Nelson RW, Couto CG: *Small animal internal medicine*, ed 5, St Louis, 2014, Mosby Elsevier, p. 784.

DKA, Diabetic ketoacidosis; *IM*, intramuscular; *IV*, intravenous; *NPH*, neutral protamine Hagedorn; *PZI*, protamine zinc insulin; *SC*, subcutaneous.

individual dogs, and difficulty in achieving ideal control of hyperglycemia within the time period of the study (60 days) in some dogs (Fig. 6-5). Problems with hypoglycemia and initiation of the Somogyi response may occur when an insulin preparation with a duration of effect longer than 12 hours is administered every 12 hours. Problems with prolonged duration of PZI effect precludes routine use of PZI in newly-diagnosed diabetic dogs but supports the potential use of PZI in diabetic dogs that are poorly controlled because of short duration of effect of NPH or Lente insulin.

Insulin Analogues. Recently, recombinant DNA technology has been applied for the production of insulin analogues that more closely duplicate the basal and meal-time components of endogenous insulin secretion. Rapid-acting insulin analogues include insulin lispro (Humalog), insulin aspart (Novolog) and insulin glulisine (Apidra). The relatively slow absorption of regular insulin is attributed to hexamer formation of insulin molecules that occurs when zinc is added to the solution that makes up regular insulin (Hirsch, 2005). The hexamers of insulin molecules slowly dissociate before absorption into the circulation occurs. By replacing certain amino acids in the insulin molecule, the tendency to self-associate can be reduced without affecting the insulin-receptor kinetics. Insulin lispro is produced by inverting the natural amino acid sequence of the B-chain at B28 (proline) and B29 (lysine), insulin aspart is produced by substituting aspartic acid for proline at position B28, and insulin glulisine is produced by substituting lysine for asparagine at position B3 and glutamic acid for lysine at position B29 (Lindholm et al, 2002; Home, 2012; Fig. 6-6). As a consequence of these alterations, insulin lispro, insulin aspart,

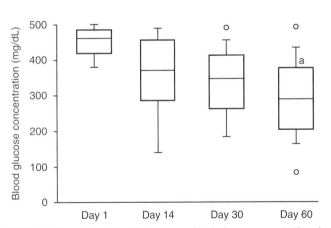

FIGURE 6-5 Box plots of the 10-hour mean blood glucose concentrations in 17 dogs with diabetes mellitus treated by the administration of various doses of recombinant human protamine zinc insulin (PZI) twice daily for 60 days. The 10-hour mean blood glucose concentration is the mean of the six blood glucose concentrations measured during a 10-hour period. The median time from insulin administration to the blood glucose nadir was 8 to 10 hours and occurred at the start or end of the 10-hour blood sampling interval in 54% of 68 blood glucose curves. The *horizontal line* represents the median, the *box* represents the interquartile range (i.e., 25% to 75%), the *T-bars* represent the main body of data, and the *circles* represent the outliers. (From Della-Maggiore A, et al.: Efficacy of protamine zinc recombinant human insulin for controlling hyperglycemia in dogs with diabetes mellitus, *J Vet Intern Med* 26:109, 2012.) *a,* P = 0.0003, compared with results on day 1.

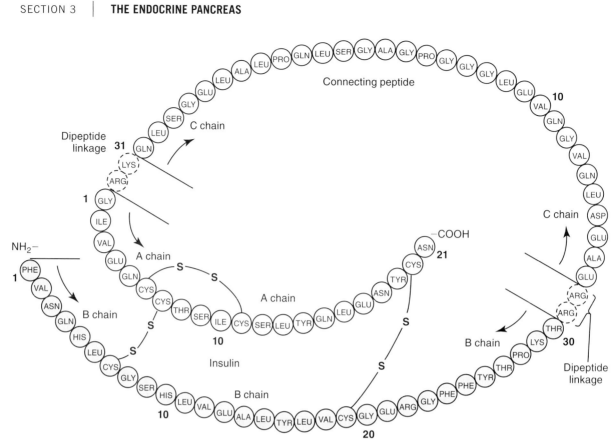

FIGURE 6-6 Amino acid structure of human proinsulin, connecting peptide (C-peptide) and insulin. The insulin molecule consists of an A and B chain connected by two disulfide bridges. (From Masharani U, Karam JH: Pancreatic hormones and diabetes mellitus. In Gardner DA, Shoback D, editors: *Greenspan's basic & clinical endocrinology*, ed 9, New York, 2011, McGraw-Hill, with permission.)

and insulin glulisine exhibit monomeric behavior in solution and display a rapid absorption, faster pharmacodynamic action, and shorter duration of effect than short-acting regular crystalline insulin (Howey et al, 1994; Home et al, 1999; Lindholm et al, 1999). Insulin lispro and insulin aspart are the current prandial insulins (i.e., insulin administered before each meal) commonly used for control of postprandial blood glucose concentrations in human diabetics and are typically administered three times a day before each of the three main meals (breakfast, lunch, and dinner). The role, if any, of these insulins for the home treatment of diabetic dogs remains to be determined. Because of their extremely short duration of effect, insulin lispro and insulin aspart would have to be used in conjunction with a longer-acting insulin preparation to maintain control of glycemia. A recent study documented similar effectiveness of insulin lispro and regular crystalline insulin for the treatment of DKA in dogs (Sears et al, 2012).

Insulin glargine (Lantus) and insulin detemir (Levemir) are long acting (basal) insulin analogues that have a slow, sustained absorption from the subcutaneous site of insulin deposition, are designed to inhibit hepatic glucose production, are typically administered once a day at bedtime, and are used in conjunction with rapid-acting (prandial) insulin analogues in diabetic humans. Insulin glargine has been modified by replacing the amino acid asparagine with glycine at position A21 of the A chain, and two arginines have been added to the C-terminus of the B chain of insulin; these modifications shift the isoelectric point from a pH of 5.4 toward a neutral pH (Pieber et al, 2000). This shift makes insulin glargine more soluble at a slightly acidic pH and less soluble at a physiological pH than native human insulin. The

solution in the bottle of glargine is acidic, which keeps glargine soluble and suspended in the solution (i.e., the solution is clear, and the bottle does not need to be shaken prior to drawing up the insulin into the syringe). Because of this dependency on pH, glargine should not be diluted or mixed with anything that may change the pH of the solution. Glargine forms microprecipitates in the subcutaneous tissue at the site of injection from which small amounts of insulin glargine are slowly released and absorbed into the circulation. In humans, the slow sustained release of insulin glargine from these microprecipitates results in a relatively constant concentration/time profile over a 24-hour period with no pronounced peak in serum insulin. The glucose-lowering effect of insulin glargine is similar to that of human insulin, the onset of action following subcutaneous administration is slower than NPH insulin, and the duration of effect is prolonged compared with NPH insulin (Owens et al, 2000). Insulin glargine is currently recommended as a basal insulin (i.e., sustained long-acting insulin used to inhibit hepatic glucose production) administered once a day at bedtime and used in conjunction with either rapid-acting insulin analogs or oral hypoglycemic drugs in human diabetics (Rosenstock et al, 2000; 2001).

Insulin glargine is commonly used for the treatment of diabetes in cats, but published experiences with insulin glargine in diabetic dogs are limited. Time-action profiles performed in three healthy dogs suggested the potential for prolonged duration of action of insulin glargine, a duration that could potentially cause problems if insulin glargine is administered twice a day (Mori et al, 2008; Fig. 6-7). In a recent study, insulin glargine administered twice a day was effective in improving or maintaining control of glycemia in

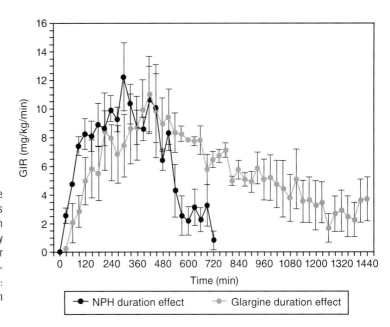

FIGURE 6-7 Time-action profile comparison between neutral protamine Hagedorn (NPH) insulin and insulin glargine for a 24-hour period. Results are presented as mean ± standard error of the mean glucose infusion rate (GIR) required to maintain euglycemia over time for three healthy non-diabetic dogs after subcutaneous (SC) administration of either 0.5 U/kg NPH insulin or 0.5 U/kg insulin glargine at time 0. Higher values of GIR indicate stronger insulin action. (Adapted from Mori A, et al.: Comparison of time-action profiles of insulin glargine and NPH insulin in normal and diabetic dogs, *Vet Res Commun* 32:563, 2008).

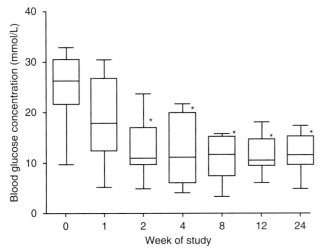

FIGURE 6-8 Box plots of 12-hour mean blood glucose concentrations in the blood glucose curves for 12 dogs with diabetes mellitus treated by various doses of insulin glargine administration twice daily for 24 weeks. Twelve-hour mean blood glucose concentration is the mean of the seven blood glucose concentrations measured during a 12-hour period. See Fig. 6-5 legend for interpretation of box plots. (From Fracassi F, et al.: Use of insulin glargine in dogs with diabetes mellitus, *Vet Rec* 170:52, 2012.) * = P < 0.05.

the majority of diabetic dogs enrolled in the study (Fracassi et al, 2012; Fig. 6-8). Fifty-eight (33%) of the dogs had attained good or moderate glycemic control by week 24 of the study. Insulin dosages required to attain glycemic control were similar to insulin dosages reported with NPH, Lente, and PZI insulin (Table 6-7). The timing of the glucose nadir was variable, suggesting that short and especially prolonged duration of action of insulin glargine occurs in diabetic dogs (Fig. 6-9). The authors speculated that the published success rate of other types of insulins (i.e., NPH and Lente) was somewhat better than insulin glargine. Our experiences with insulin glargine in dogs have been mixed and somewhat disappointing. We have been unable to attain good glycemic control in the majority of diabetic dogs treated with insulin glargine. We do not consider insulin glargine a first choice insulin for the treatment of

diabetes in dogs, but we do consider using insulin glargine in diabetic dogs with problems of short duration of effect of NPH and Lente insulin and problems with prolonged duration of effect of insulin detemir (see Complications of Insulin Therapy).

Insulin detemir is also a long-acting basal insulin analogue, in which the amino acid threonine has been removed at B30 and a 14 carbon fatty acid (myristic acid) has been bound to the lysine amino acid at position B29 of the B chain of the insulin molecule. Prolonged action results from strong self-association of the insulin molecules and binding of insulin detemir to albumin in the subcutaneous tissues and the systemic circulation through the fatty acid chain attached to lysine at B29. Binding to albumin resulted in reduced free insulin detemir concentrations in the circulation and slower distribution of insulin to peripheral target tissues (Hamilton-Wessler et al, 1999). Insulin detemir is a clear, colorless, aqueous neutral solution that does not need to be shaken prior to drawing up the insulin into the syringe. The manufacturer recommends that insulin detemir not be mixed or diluted with other insulin preparations. Insulin detemir can be diluted using the Insulin Diluting Medium for NovoRapid (insulin aspart) and Levemir (detemir) supplied by Novo Nordisk.

Published experiences with insulin detemir in diabetic dogs are limited. A recent study would suggest that insulin detemir is currently the longest acting insulin preparation for use in diabetic dogs. Time-action profiles performed in three healthy dogs identified a prolonged duration of action of insulin detemir with peak insulin action at 8 to 12 hours after the subcutaneous administration of insulin detemir and a duration of effect in excess of 16 hours (Sako et al, 2011; Fig. 6-10). In the same study, insulin detemir was more effective in attaining glycemic control in five diabetic dogs after 5 days of treatment than NPH or insulin glargine. Insulin dosages ranged from 0.41 to 0.63 U/kg, 0.34 to 0.54 U/kg, and 0.07 to 0.23 U/kg for NPH, insulin glargine, and insulin detemir, respectively. The lower dosage requirements for insulin detemir are presumably related to the prolonged duration of insulin action combined with twice a day administration. Sako, et al., (2011) speculated that insulin detemir carries a higher risk of inducing hypoglycemia as compared to either NPH insulin or insulin glargine. In an unpublished study, insulin detemir was effective in improving control of glycemia in thirteen diabetic

| | | **TABLE 6-7** | **COMPARISON OF INSULIN PREPARATION DOSAGES REQUIRED TO ATTAIN CONTROL OF GLYCEMIA IN DIABETIC DOGS** | |

| | | Insulin Dosage (U/kg/injection) | | |
INSULIN PREPARATION	NUMBER OF DOGS	MEDIAN	RANGE	STUDY
NPH	54	0.8* 0.4†	0.4-1.9 0.3-0.8	Lorenzen, 1992
Lente	35	0.8	0.3-1.4	Monroe et al, 2005
PZI	17	0.9	0.4-1.5	Della-Maggiore et al, 2012
Glargine	12	0.6	0.1-1.1	Fracassi et al, 2012
Detemir	13	0.2	NR	Ford, 2010
Detemir	15	0.3	0.1-0.6	UCD, 2013‡

NPH, Neutral protamine Hagedorn; *NR,* not reported; *PZI,* protamine zinc insulin.
*Dogs weighing < 15 kg
†Dogs weighing ≥ 15 kg
‡UCD, 2013: Insulin dosage required to attain glycemic control in 15 of 24 diabetic dogs treated with insulin detemir at UC Davis veterinary hospital; glycemic control could not be attained using detemir in 9 of the 24 dogs.

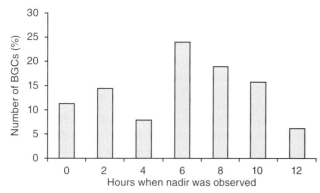

FIGURE 6-9 Histograms indicate the number of blood glucose curves (BGCs; %) from 12 dogs with diabetes mellitus treated by the administration of various doses of insulin glargine twice daily for 24 weeks where the glucose nadir was observed before (0) or 2, 4, 6, 8, 10, or 12 hours after insulin injection, respectively. (From Fracassi F, et al.: Use of insulin glargine in dogs with diabetes mellitus, *Vet Rec* 170:52, 2012.)

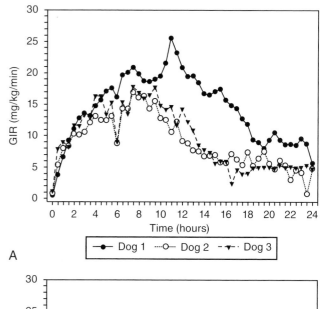

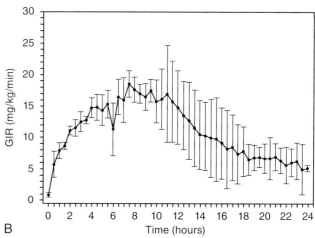

FIGURE 6-10 Time-action profile of insulin detemir over a 24-hour period in three individual healthy non-diabetic dogs **(A)** and mean ± standard deviation (SD) results in the three dogs **(B)**. Results are presented as glucose infusion rate *(GIR)* required to maintain euglycemia after the subcutaneous (SC) administration of 0.5 U/kg insulin detemir at time 0. Higher values of GIR indicate stronger insulin action. (From Sako T, et al.: Time-action profiles of insulin detemir in normal and diabetic dogs, *Res Vet Sci* 90:396, 2011.)

dogs managed with home blood glucose monitoring during a 4 to 24 month (median, 10 month) period (Ford et al, 2010). Ten of 13 dogs were previously treated with NPH or Lente insulin with poor results. The mean and median insulin dosage on the last week of evaluation was 0.45 and 0.22 U/kg/injection. Biochemical hypoglycemia (blood glucose less than 60 mg/dL; 3.4 mmol/L) was identified in approximately 2% of all blood glucose measurements and occurred on average 7.5 times per dog during the study. Our experiences with insulin detemir in dogs have been mixed but better than our experiences with insulin glargine. The absorption of insulin detemir from the subcutaneous site of injection is variable. In some diabetic dogs, the absorption is slow and sustained, resulting in relatively flat blood glucose curves (Fig. 6-11). In other dogs, the absorption is similar to that seen with intermediate-acting insulin preparations like Lente, resulting in U-shaped blood glucose curves (see Fig. 6-24). The most common problem with insulin detemir has been hypoglycemia and induction of glucose counterregulation (i.e., Somogyi response) when insulin detemir is given twice a day (see Insulin Overdosing and Glucose Counterregulation [Somogyi Response]). We do not consider insulin detemir a first choice insulin for the treatment of

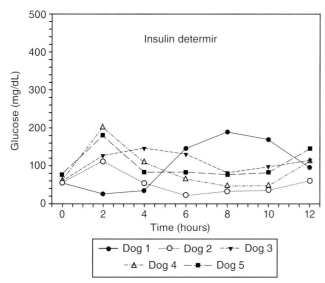

FIGURE 6-11 Results of 12-hour serum glucose curves after subcutaneous (SC) administration of various doses of insulin detemir twice a day for 5 days in five insulin-dependent diabetic dogs. Insulin detemir dosages administered at time 0 on day 5 were as follows: *Dog 1,* 0.23 U/kg; *Dog 2,* 0.19 U/kg; *Dog 3,* 0.09 U/kg; *Dog 4,* 0.18 U/kg; and *Dog 5,* 0.07 U/kg. (From Sako T, et al.: Time-action profiles of insulin detemir in normal and diabetic dogs, *Res Vet Sci* 90:396, 2011.)

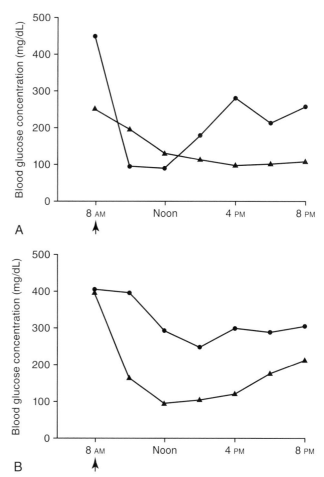

FIGURE 6-12 A, Blood glucose curve in a miniature poodle receiving recombinant human Lente insulin, 6 U/kg body weight *(solid line, triangles)* and recombinant human 70/30 neutral protamine Hagedorn (NPH)/regular insulin, 3 U/kg body weight *(solid line, circles)* subcutaneous (SC). **B,** Blood glucose curve in an 8 kg cat receiving 4 U recombinant human Ultralente insulin *(solid line, circles)* and 4 U of recombinant human 70/30 NPH/regular insulin *(broken line, triangles)* SC. (From Nelson RW: Diabetes mellitus. In Ettinger SJ, Feldman EC, editors: *Textbook of veterinary internal medicine,* ed 4, Philadelphia, 1995, Saunders, p. 1528.) ↑ = insulin injection and food.

diabetes in dogs but consider it the insulin of choice in diabetic dogs with problems of short duration of effect of NPH and Lente insulin. Our starting dosage for insulin detemir is 0.1 U/kg twice a day.

Insulin Mixtures. Mixtures of short- and long-acting insulin have been developed in an attempt to mimic the increase in portal insulin concentrations during and immediately following consumption of a meal, thereby minimizing postprandial hyperglycemia. NPH insulin can be mixed with regular crystalline insulin, and if injected immediately, the regular insulin remains rapid-acting. Stable premixed 75% NPH/25% regular, 70% NPH/30% regular, and 50% NPH/50% regular preparations are available (e.g., Humulin 70/30 and Mixtard 70/30). Similarly, mixtures of lispro and lispro protamine suspension (e.g., Humalog Mix 75/25 and Humalog Mix 50/50) and aspart and aspart protamine suspension (e.g., Novolog Mix 70/30) are available. In our experience, these premixed preparations are quite potent, causing a rapid decrease in blood glucose concentration within 60 to 90 minutes of subcutaneous administration (Fig. 6-12). In addition, the duration of effect has usually been short (less than 8 hours). We generally use these insulin mixtures only as a last resort when more conventional insulin preparations have been ineffective in establishing control of glycemia. Although regular insulin remains fast acting when added to NPH, when added to Lente insulin, regular insulin binds to excess zinc in the vial of Lente, blunting regular insulin's quick effect (Galloway, 1988).

Insulin Storage, Mixing, and Dilution

Freezing and heating the insulin bottle will inactivate insulin in the bottle. Historically, shaking the bottle of NPH, Lente, or PZI insulin was believed to inactivate the insulin, but recent studies performed by the pharmaceutical company have shown that shaking the bottle of Lente insulin does not impact insulin action, provides more uniform dispersal of insulin throughout the solution than rolling the bottle, and is currently recommended. Similar recommendations have not yet been reported for NPH and PZI

insulins. Although keeping the bottle of insulin at "room temperature" does not inactivate insulin, we routinely instruct clients to store the insulin bottle in the door of the refrigerator to maintain a consistent environment. Some veterinarians advocate replacing insulin with a new bottle every 1 to 2 months to prevent problems caused by loss of activity or sterility. This practice can create financial hardship for some clients and may not be necessary. The shelf life of a bottle of insulin that has been stored appropriately is longer than manufacturer recommendations. We have not appreciated a clinically significant loss of insulin action with time when insulin preparations, including glargine and detemir, are maintained in a constant environment (i.e., refrigerator) and handled appropriately. Routinely purchasing a new bottle of insulin every month may not be necessary, especially if the diabetic dog is doing well. However, development of cloudiness or discoloration suggest contamination, change in pH of the solution (glargine), and/or loss of insulin activity. The bottle of insulin should be discarded and replaced with a new bottle of insulin. Similarly, loss of insulin activity in the bottle should always be considered whenever clinical signs recur, regardless of the quantity of insulin remaining in the bottle.

Dilution of insulin is a common practice, especially in very small dogs and cats. Only diluting solutions provided by the respective company should be used. Although studies evaluating the shelf-life of diluted insulin have not been published, I recommend replacing diluted insulin preparations every 4 to 8 weeks. Even when these guidelines are observed, insufficient amounts of insulin are administered when diluted insulin is used in some dogs and cats, despite appropriate dilution and insulin administration techniques. These inadequacies are corrected when full-strength insulin is used. It is important to remember that insulin glargine is pH dependent and should not be diluted with solutions that may change the pH of the solution.

See Chapter 7 for additional information on insulin preparations, insulin handling, and owner instructions.

Initial Insulin Treatment Recommendations

Once the diagnosis of diabetes is established, dogs should be considered insulin dependent and treatment with insulin should be initiated. Porcine source Lente insulin (Vetsulin, Caninsulin) is the initial insulin of choice for treating newly-diagnosed diabetic dogs (see Table 6-6). Recombinant human NPH insulin is also effective but problems with short duration of effect are common with NPH insulin. Studies to date suggest that the median dosage of Lente and NPH insulin required to attain glucose control in most diabetic dogs is approximately 0.5 U/kg/injection, with a range of 0.2 to 1.0 U/kg (see Table 6-7). One important goal in the initial regulation of the diabetic dog is avoidance of symptomatic hypoglycemia, especially in the home environment. For this reason, the starting insulin dosage should be on the low end of the range (i.e., approximately 0.25 U/kg). Dietary therapy is initiated concurrently (see later). We routinely start with twice a day insulin administration because the overwhelming majority of diabetic dogs require Lente and NPH insulin twice a day (Hess and Ward, 2000; Monroe et al, 2005). Establishing control of glycemia is easier and problems with hypoglycemia and the Somogyi response (see Insulin Overdosing and Glucose Counterregulation [Somogyi Response]) are less likely when twice daily insulin therapy is initiated while the insulin dose is low (i.e., at the time insulin treatment is initiated).

Although recombinant human PZI, insulin glargine, and insulin detemir are effective in controlling glycemia in some diabetic dogs, problems with consistency of effect, variable and unpredictable timing of the glucose nadir, prolonged duration of effect, and suspected induction of the Somogyi response preclude recommending these insulin preparations in the newly-diagnosed diabetic dog. However, these insulin preparations should be considered when problems caused by short duration of insulin effect develop with Lente or NPH insulin (see Complications of Insulin Therapy).

Initial Adjustments in Insulin Therapy

Diabetic dogs require several days to equilibrate to changes in insulin dosage or preparation. Newly-diagnosed diabetic dogs are typically hospitalized for no more than 24 to 48 hours to finish the diagnostic evaluation and begin insulin therapy. During hospitalization, blood glucose concentrations are typically determined at the time insulin is administered and at 3, 6, and 9 hours later. The intent is to identify hypoglycemia (blood glucose less than 80 mg/dL; 4.5 mmol/L) in those dogs that are unusually sensitive to the actions of insulin. If hypoglycemia occurs, the insulin dosage is decreased prior to sending the dog home. A minor adjustment in the insulin dosage may be done in those dogs that remain hyperglycemic during these first few days of insulin therapy; however, the objective during this first visit is *not* to establish perfect

glycemic control before sending the dog home. Rather, the objective is to begin to reverse the metabolic derangements induced by the disease, allow the dog to equilibrate to the insulin and change in diet, teach the owner how to administer insulin, and give the owner a few days to become accustomed to treating the diabetic dog at home. Adjustments in insulin therapy are made on subsequent evaluations once the owner and pet have gotten used to the treatment regimen.

Diabetic dogs are typically evaluated once weekly until an effective insulin treatment protocol is identified. Glycemic control is attained when clinical signs of diabetes have resolved; the pet is healthy and interactive in the home; its body weight is stable (unless the dog is undergoing weight loss to correct obesity); the client is satisfied with the progress of therapy; and, if possible, the blood glucose concentrations range between 100 and 250 mg/dL (5.6 to 14 mmol/L) throughout the day. The client is informed at the time insulin therapy is initiated that it will take approximately 1 month to establish a satisfactory insulin treatment protocol, assuming unidentified insulin-antagonistic disease is not present. The goals of therapy are also explained to the client. During this month, changes in insulin dose and possibly insulin type are common and should be anticipated by the client. At each evaluation the client's subjective opinion of water intake, urine output, and overall health of the pet is discussed; a complete physical examination is performed; change in body weight noted; and serial blood glucose measurements obtained over a 10- to 12-hour period after insulin administration are assessed. Adjustments in insulin therapy are based on this information, the pet is sent home, and an appointment is scheduled for the next week to reevaluate the response to any change in therapy. If the dog remains poorly controlled, the dose of insulin is gradually increased by 1 to 5 U/injection (depending on the size of the dog) each week until control is attained. This gradual increase in dose helps prevent hypoglycemia and the Somogyi response. Control of glycemia can be established in most dogs using insulin doses in the range of 1.0 U of insulin/kg or less (median, 0.5 U/kg) administered twice each day. If the insulin dose exceeds 1.0 U/kg/injection without adequate glycemic control, then further investigations to determine the reason for treatment failure are indicated (see Complications of Insulin Therapy). If hypoglycemia is noted either clinically or biochemically at any time, the insulin dosage should be decreased and further adjustments in the insulin dose performed as needed to attain glycemic control.

Many factors affect the dog's glycemic control from day to day, including variations in insulin administration and absorption, dietary indiscretions and caloric intake, amount of exercise, and variables that affect insulin responsiveness (e.g., stress, concurrent inflammation, infection). As a consequence, the insulin dosage required to maintain glycemic control typically changes (increase or decrease) with time. Initially, a fixed dosage of insulin is administered at home during the first few months of therapy, and changes in insulin dosage are made only after the owner consults with the veterinarian. As the insulin dose range required to maintain glycemic control becomes apparent and as confidence is gained in the client's ability to recognize signs of hypoglycemia and hyperglycemia, the client is eventually allowed to make *slight* adjustments in the insulin dose at home on the basis of clinical observations of the pet's well-being. However, the client is instructed to stay within the agreed-upon insulin dose range. If the insulin dose is at the upper or lower end of the established range and the pet is still symptomatic, the client is instructed to call the veterinarian before making further adjustments in the insulin dose.

Dietary Therapy

Diet plays an important role in the management of the diabetic dog (Box 6-3). What diet is ultimately fed is dictated, in part, by the weight of the dog, concurrent disease, and owner and dog preferences. Correction of obesity is the most beneficial step that can be taken to improve control of glycemia. Obesity-induced insulin resistance has been documented in dogs and is an important factor accounting for variations in response to insulin therapy in diabetic dogs (Gayet et al, 2004; Yamka et al, 2006). Weight loss improves insulin resistance in obese diabetic dogs. Weight loss usually requires a combination of restricting caloric intake, feeding low calorie-dense diets, and increasing caloric expenditure through exercise. Diets specifically designed for weight loss should be considered for obese diabetic dogs to promote weight loss. Weight loss diets contain higher quantities of insoluble fiber than diabetic diets and lower fat content to decrease the caloric density of the food. High-fiber, low calorie-dense diets should not be fed to thin or emaciated diabetic dogs until control of glycemia is established and a normal body weight is attained using a higher-calorie-dense, lower-fiber diet designed for maintenance.

Most premium pet food companies offer diets designed for diabetic dogs (see Box 6-3). The composition of these diets varies but most contain fiber. Increasing the fiber content of the diet is beneficial for treating obesity and improving control of glycemia in diabetic dogs (Nelson et al, 1991; 1998; Graham et al, 1994; Fig. 6-13). The ability of the food fiber to form a viscous gel and thus impair convective transfer of glucose and water to the absorptive surface of the intestine appears to be of greatest importance in slowing intestinal glucose absorption. The more rapidly fermentable viscous soluble fibers (e.g., gums, citrus pectin) slow glucose diffusion to a greater degree than the slowly fermentable less viscous insoluble fibers (e.g., cellulose, hemicellulose) and, as such, are believed to be of greater benefit in improving control

of glycemia. Most diabetic diets contain a blend of soluble and insoluble fiber sources, including moderately fermentable fibers (e.g., rice bran, soy fiber, beet pulp) that have both soluble and insoluble fiber characteristics.

Complications of feeding diabetic diets containing high fiber content include excessive frequency of defecation, constipation, obstipation, soft stools, excessive flatulence, and refusal to eat the diet (Box 6-4). Most of these problems will resolve by changing the type or quantity of fiber consumed (i.e., a change in the diet). Problems with palatability are usually a result of too rapid of a switch from the dog's usual diet to the diabetic diet or a result of boredom after consuming the diabetic diet for months. If palatability is a problem initially, the dog can be gradually switched from its regular diet to a diabetic diet over a 2- to 4-week period. Periodic changes in the types of diabetic diets and mixtures of diabetic diets have been helpful in alleviating the problem of boredom with a diet. Palatability issues affiliated with feeding diets containing an increased amount of fiber should always be considered in the list of differential diagnoses for inappetence in a diabetic dog.

Type and quantity of carbohydrate in the diet may also affect post-prandial blood glucose concentrations. For example, sorghum and barley have a lower glycemic index (i.e., lower impact on postprandial blood glucose and insulin concentrations) than rice. Some diabetic diets for dogs use low glycemic index carbohydrates in an effort to minimize post-prandial hyperglycemia. Digestible carbohydrate content of the diet (i.e., percentage of metabolizable energy derived from carbohydrates) also affects post-prandial blood glucose concentrations (Nguyen et al, 1998). In a recent study, consumption of a lower carbohydrate-containing diet resulted in lower post-prandial blood glucose concentrations in healthy dogs, compared with a maintenance diet and a diabetic diet containing increased carbohydrate content (Elliott et al, 2012). Although diets with moderate versus high carbohydrate content may be preferred for diabetic dogs, a corresponding increase in the percent metabolizable energy derived from fat should be minimized to avoid an increase in blood lipid parameters, including cholesterol, triglycerides, free glycerol, and free fatty acids (Fleeman et al, 2009b). Derangements in fat metabolism are common in diabetic dogs and include increased serum concentrations of cholesterol, triglycerides, lipoproteins, chylomicrons, and free fatty acids, hepatic lipidosis, atherosclerosis, and a predisposition for development of pancreatitis (Hess et al, 2002). Dietary fat may also cause insulin resistance, promote hepatic glucose production, and in healthy dogs, suppress beta-cell function (Massillon et al, 1997; Kaiyala et al, 1999). Low fat highly digestible diets (e.g., Royal Canin Gastrointestinal Low Fat Diet) are an alternative to fiber-containing diabetic diets, especially if acute or chronic pancreatitis or persistent hyperlipidemia are concurrent problems or palatability is a problem with diabetic diets. A higher fat content may be needed for weight gain in thin or emaciated diabetic dogs. Feeding lower-fat diets may help minimize the risk of pancreatitis, control some aspects of hyperlipidemia, and reduce overall caloric intake to favor weight loss or maintenance (Remillard, 1999).

Feeding Schedule

The feeding schedule should be designed to enhance the actions of insulin and minimize postprandial hyperglycemia. The development of postprandial hyperglycemia depends, in part, on the amount of food consumed per meal, the rate at which glucose and other nutrients are absorbed from the intestine, and the effectiveness of exogenous insulin during the postprandial period. The daily caloric intake should be ingested when insulin is still present

---

BOX 6-3 Recommendations for Dietary Treatment of Diabetes Mellitus in Dogs

Correct obesity and maintain body weight in an acceptable range.
Control daily caloric intake.
Increase daily exercise.
Avoid excessive amounts of insulin.
Maintain consistency in the timing and caloric content of the meals.
Feed within the time frame of insulin action.
Feed one half the daily caloric intake at the time of each insulin injection with every 12-hour insulin therapy or at the time of the insulin injection and 6 to 10 hours later with every 24-hour insulin therapy.
Minimize the impact of food on postprandial blood glucose concentrations.
Avoid monosaccharides and disaccharides, propylene glycol, and corn syrup.
Let "nibbler" dogs nibble throughout the day and night; ensure that other pets do not have access to the food; provide one-half of total daily calories at time of each insulin injection.
Increase the fiber content of the diet.

Examples of Veterinary Diets Designed for Diabetic Dogs
Hill's Prescription Diet w/d
Hill's Prescription Diet r/d (obese diabetic dog)
Purina DCO
Purina OM (obese diabetic dog)
Royal Canin Diabetic

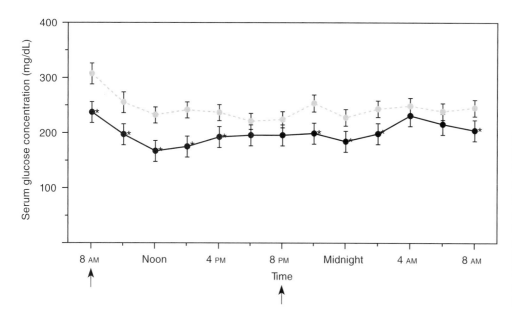

FIGURE 6-13 Mean (± standard error of the mean) serum concentrations of glucose in eleven dogs with naturally occurring diabetes mellitus fed high-insoluble fiber (i.e., cellulose; *solid line*) and low-fiber *(broken line)* diet. (From Nelson RW, et al.: Effect of dietary insoluble fiber on glycemic control in dogs with naturally-occurring diabetes mellitus, *J Am Vet Med Assoc* 212:380, 1998.) ↑ = Insulin administration and consumption of half of daily caloric intake; * = p < 0.05, compared with low fiber diet.

BOX 6-4	**Common Complications Associated with Feeding Diets Containing Increased Quantities of Fiber**

Inappetence caused by poor palatability or boredom with food
Increased frequency of defecation
Constipation and obstipation (insoluble fiber)
Soft stools and diarrhea (soluble fiber)
Increased flatulence (soluble fiber)
Weight loss
Hypoglycemia

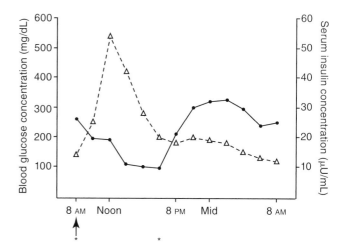

FIGURE 6-14 Mean blood glucose *(solid line)* and serum insulin *(broken line)* concentrations in eight dogs with diabetes mellitus treated with beef/pork source neutral protamine Hagedorn (NPH) insulin subcutaneously once daily. The duration of NPH effect is too short, resulting in prolonged periods of hyperglycemia beginning shortly after feeding the evening meal. (From Nelson RW: Diabetes mellitus. In Ettinger SJ, Feldman EC, editors: *Textbook of veterinary internal medicine*, ed 4, Philadelphia, 1995, Saunders, p. 1525.) ↑ = Insulin injection; * = equal-sized meals consumed.

in the circulation and is capable of disposing of glucose absorbed from the meal. If the meals are consumed while exogenous insulin is still metabolically active, the postprandial increase in blood glucose concentration is minimal or absent. In contrast, feeding the diabetic dog after insulin action has waned results in increasing blood glucose concentration beginning 1 to 2 hours postprandially (Fig. 6-14). If this occurs, either the type of insulin, frequency of insulin administration, or timing of the meals in relationship to the insulin injection should be adjusted.

Typically, dogs receiving exogenous insulin twice a day are fed equal-sized meals at the time of each insulin injection. If the dog is receiving exogenous insulin once a day, one half of the daily caloric intake is fed at the time of the insulin injection and the remaining half approximately 8 hours later. Unfortunately, the eating behavior of dogs varies considerably, from finicky eaters that nibble on food periodically throughout the day to gluttonous dogs that quickly consume everything placed in their food dish. Gluttonous dogs are fed as discussed earlier. Finicky dogs generally resist attempts by owners to convert them to a "gluttonous" type of eating behavior, which can be frustrating to the owner instructed to have their pet eat all of its food at the time of the insulin injection. However, if one adheres to the principle that feeding multiple small meals rather than one large meal within the time frame of insulin action helps minimize the hyperglycemic effect of each meal, then allowing a finicky eater to eat whenever it wants should help control fluctuations in blood glucose. For this reason, dogs that are finicky and nibble throughout the day should

be allowed to continue their pattern of eating. For these dogs, half of the total daily food intake should be available beginning at the time of each insulin injection and the dog allowed to choose when and how much to eat. The dog should have access to the food throughout the day and night, and other dogs in the household cannot have access to the food.

Modifications in Dietary Therapy

Concurrent disease in which diet is an important aspect of therapy also dictates the type of diet to be fed. For example, diabetic dogs with concurrent chronic pancreatitis or exocrine pancreatic insufficiency (pancreatic acinar atrophy) should be fed a low fat, low fiber, highly digestible diet. Diabetic dogs with CKD should be fed a lower protein diet designed for kidney failure. Diabetic dogs with concurrent inflammatory bowel disease may need a

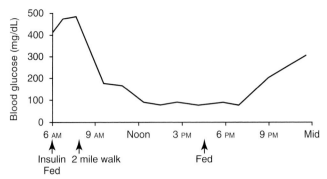

FIGURE 6-15 Serial blood glucose curve obtained by the owner at home after the administration of 1 U/kg porcine Lente insulin to a 35 kg male-castrate diabetic Labrador Retriever. The treatment regimen adopted by the owner included the administration of porcine Lente insulin once a day at 6 AM, equal-sized meals fed at 6 AM and 5 PM, and a 2-mile walk beginning at 9 AM. The owner was obtaining blood glucose curves almost every day and adjusting the insulin dose based on the results. The blood glucose concentration typically decreased 70 to 140 mg/dL after the walk as illustrated in this glucose curve, compared with days when the dog was not walked. The owner sought help because of persistence of polyuria and polydipsia, especially at night, despite increasing the insulin dose. Polyuria and polydipsia improved with initiation of twice a day administration of porcine Lente insulin and feeding the dog at the time of each insulin injection.

hypoallergenic diet to help control inflammation and clinical signs. Whenever possible, dietary therapy for all disorders should be "blended"; however, if this is not possible, dietary therapy for the most serious disorder should take priority. For example, dietary therapy for chronic renal failure, heart failure, or recurring pancreatitis is a higher priority than dietary therapy for diabetes mellitus. Dietary therapy for diabetes mellitus should be considered adjunctive; glycemic control can be maintained with insulin, regardless of the diet fed.

Exercise

Exercise plays an important role in maintaining glycemic control in the diabetic dog by helping promote weight loss and by eliminating the insulin resistance induced by obesity. Exercise also has a glucose-lowering effect by increasing the mobilization of insulin from its injection site, presumably resulting from increased blood and lymph flow, by increasing blood flow (and therefore insulin delivery) to exercising muscles, by stimulating translocation (i.e., upregulation) of glucose transporters (primarily GLUT-4) in muscle cells, and by increasing glucose effectiveness (i.e., ability of hyperglycemia to promote glucose disposal at basal insulin concentrations) (Fernqvist et al, 1986; Galante et al, 1995; Phillips et al, 1996; Nishida et al, 2001; Fig. 6-15). The daily routine for diabetic dogs should include exercise, preferably at the same time each day and not around the time of peak insulin effect. Strenuous and sporadic exercise can cause severe hypoglycemia and should be avoided. If unavoidable, the insulin dose should be decreased in dogs subjected to sporadic strenuous exercise on those days of anticipated increased exercise. The reduction in insulin dose required to prevent hypoglycemia is variable and determined by trial and error. Reducing the insulin dose by 50% initially is recommended, and further adjustments should be based on measurement of blood glucose concentration with a portable blood glucose monitor during exercise, the occurrence of symptomatic hypoglycemia, and the severity of polyuria and polydipsia that develops during the ensuing 24 to 48 hours. In addition, owners

must be aware of the signs of hypoglycemia and have a source of glucose (e.g., candy, food, sugar solution) readily available to give their dog should any of these signs develop.

Oral Hypoglycemic Drugs

Oral hypoglycemic drugs work by stimulating pancreatic insulin secretion (e.g., sulfonylureas, meglitinides, glucagon-like peptide-1 [GLP-1] receptor agonists, dipeptidyl peptidase-4 [DPP-4] inhibitors), inhibiting glucagon secretion (e.g., DPP-4 inhibitors or gliptins), enhancing tissue sensitivity to insulin (e.g., metformin, thiazolidinediones), or slowing postprandial intestinal glucose absorption (α-glucosidase inhibitors). Although controversial, chromium and vanadium are trace minerals that may also function as insulin sensitizers. Oral hypoglycemic drugs are primarily used for the treatment of type 2 diabetes; a form of diabetes that is not recognized in dogs. Oral sulfonylurea drugs (e.g., glipizide, glyburide) directly stimulate insulin secretion by beta cells and are the most commonly used oral hypoglycemic drugs for the treatment of diabetes mellitus in humans and cats but are ineffective in diabetic dogs, presumably because dogs have an inadequate mass of functional beta cells at the time diabetes is diagnosed.

Acarbose

Acarbose is a complex oligosaccharide of microbial origin that competitively inhibits pancreatic alpha-amylase and alpha-glucosidases (glucoamylase, sucrase, maltase, and isomaltase) in the brush border of the small intestinal mucosa, which delays digestion of complex carbohydrates, delays absorption of glucose from the intestinal tract, and decreases postprandial blood glucose concentrations. Placebo-controlled clinical studies completed in healthy and diabetic dogs documented a decrease in postprandial total glucose absorption and total insulin secretion when healthy dogs were treated with acarbose (compared with placebo) and a decrease in daily insulin dose, mean blood glucose concentration during an 8 hour blood sampling period, and blood glycated protein concentrations in diabetic dogs treated with acarbose (compared with placebo) (Robertson et al, 1999; Nelson et al, 2000; Fig. 6-16). Although acarbose may be beneficial in improving control of glycemia in some dogs with insulin-requiring diabetes, the high prevalence of adverse effects (diarrhea and weight loss) resulting from carbohydrate malassimilation and the expense of the drug limit its usefulness.

Chromium

Chromium is a ubiquitous trace element that exerts insulin-like effects in vitro. The exact mechanism of action is not known, but the overall effect of chromium is to increase insulin sensitivity, presumably through a post-receptor mechanism of action (Anderson, 1992; Striffler et al, 1995; Anderson et al, 1997). Chromium does not increase serum insulin concentrations. Chromium is an essential cofactor for insulin function, and chromium deficiency results in insulin resistance. In one study, dietary chromium picolinate supplementation improved results of an intravenous (IV) glucose tolerance test in healthy dogs, compared with healthy dogs not treated with chromium (Spears et al, 1998). Other studies failed to identify an effect of dietary chromium picolinate supplementation on glucose tolerance in obese dogs during weight reduction (Gross et al, 2000) nor did it improve control of glycemia in the diabetic dogs treated with 200 to 400 μg of chromium picolinate by mouth twice daily (Schachter et al, 2001; Fig. 6-17). Chromium picolinate is considered a nutraceutical in the United States and can be purchased in health food and drug stores. It is inexpensive, and there are no known toxic effects associated with its ingestion.

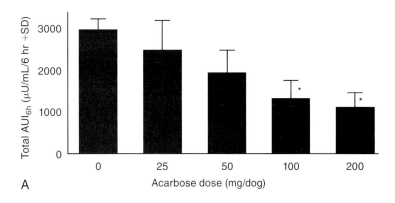

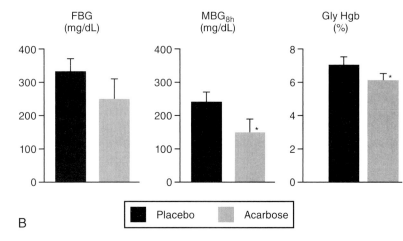

FIGURE 6-16 A, Mean total insulin secretion for five healthy dogs during the first 6 hours after consumption of a meal and a placebo or 25, 50, 100, or 200 mg of acarbose. *T-bars* represent standard error of the mean. **B,** Fasting blood glucose *(FBG),* mean blood glucose over an 8-hour time period *(MGB$_{8h}$),* and blood total glycosylated hemoglobin *(Gly Hgb)* in five dogs with insulin-dependent diabetes mellitus treated with insulin and placebo *(black bars)* and insulin and acarbose *(gray bars)* for 2 months each in a randomly assigned treatment sequence. *T-bars* represent standard deviation. (**A,** From Robertson J, et al.: Effects of the alpha-glucosidase inhibitor acarbose on postprandial serum glucose and insulin concentrations in healthy dogs, *Am J Vet Res* 60:541, 1999.) **A, B,** * = p < 0.05, compared with value obtained after treatment with placebo.

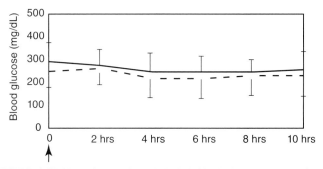

FIGURE 6-17 Mean (± standard deviation) blood glucose concentrations obtained from 13 dogs with insulin-dependent diabetes mellitus before insulin and feeding (8 AM = Time 0) and for 10 hours after insulin administration only *(broken line)* or after insulin and chromium tripicolinate administration *(solid line).* Dogs were treated for 3 months with insulin and then 3 months with insulin and chromium tripicolinate. Mean blood glucose concentrations are the mean of all corresponding blood glucose values obtained during the 10-hour blood sample collection period for each dog at 1, 2, and 3 months of each treatment period. (From Schachter S, et al.: Oral chromium picolinate and control of glycemia in insulin-treated diabetic dogs, *J Vet Intern Med* 15:379, 2001.) ↑ = time of insulin or insulin and chromium picolinate administration.

Herbs, Supplements, and Vitamins

Alternative therapies that include herbs, supplements, and vitamins in conjunction with or in lieu of the more conventional treatment options have been used by some individuals with type 2 diabetes. The goals for using herbs, supplements, and vitamins are primarily centered around decreasing blood glucose, triglyceride, and cholesterol concentrations; delaying the onset of long-term complications of diabetes (e.g., coronary artery disease, retinopathy); and improving the overall well-being of the patient (Roszler, 2001; Box 6-5). Proposed beneficial effects vary with the herb, supplement, or vitamin utilized and include delaying nutrient absorption from the gastrointestinal tract, stimulating insulin secretion, improving insulin sensitivity, altering lipid metabolism, improving circulation, and benefits attributed to antioxidant properties. Some herbs, supplements, and vitamins (e.g., ginseng, chromium, fish oils, and psyllium) have been critically evaluated for efficacy, whereas others are recommended based primarily on folklore and testimonials (Pastors et al, 1991; Striffler et al, 1995; Vuksan et al, 2001). Critical studies assessing the effects of herbs, supplements, and vitamins on diabetic control and complications are needed before these alternative therapies can be recommended in diabetic dogs. Intuitively, it seems doubtful that the herbs, supplements, and vitamins listed in Box 6-5 will have much of an impact in diabetic dogs—in part because these therapies are primarily used for treating type 2 diabetes, which is not recognized in diabetic dogs, and delaying chronic diabetic complications, which are uncommon in dogs.

Identification and Control of Concurrent Problems

Concurrent disease and administration of insulin-antagonistic drugs are commonly identified in the dog with newly-diagnosed diabetes mellitus (Hess et al, 2000b; Peikes et al, 2001). Concurrent disease and insulin-antagonistic drugs can interfere with tissue responsiveness to insulin, resulting in insulin resistance and poor control of the diabetes. Concurrent disease and insulin-antagonistic drugs typically cause insulin resistance by altering insulin metabolism (prereceptor problem), by decreasing the

---

BOX 6-5   Herbs, Supplements, and Vitamins that have been Used to Treat Diabetes Mellitus in Humans

Improve Hyperglycemia
Alpha-lipoic acid
Vitamin C
Vitamin E
Chromium
Vanadium
Fenugreek seeds
American and Asian ginseng
Gymnema sylvestre
Psyllium seeds
Cinnamon

Prevent Coronary Artery Disease
Vitamin C
Vitamin E
Quercetin

Improve Circulation
Gingko biloba
Pycnogenol

Prevent/Control Pain from Neuropathy
Alpha-lipoic acid
Vitamin B6

Capsaicin (cayenne pepper) (topical ointment)
Evening primrose oil

Improve Hyperlipidemia
Vitamin E
Evening primrose oil
Fish oils (e.g., omega-3 fatty acids)
Selenium

Prevent Cataracts
Alpha-lipoic acid
Vitamin C

Prevent Retinopathy
Vitamin E
Pycnogenol (pine bark extract)

Antioxidant
Alpha-lipoic acid
Vitamin A
Vitamin C
Vitamin E
Pycnogenol
Quercetin
Selenium

From Roszler J: Herbs, supplements and vitamins: what to try, what to buy, *Diabetes Interviews* August: 45, 2001.

---

concentration or binding affinity of insulin receptors on the cell membrane (receptor problem), by interfering with the insulin receptor signaling cascade (postreceptor problem), or by a combination of these. Depending on the etiology, insulin resistance may be mild and easily overcome by increasing the dose of insulin (e.g., obesity); may be severe, causing sustained and marked hyperglycemia regardless of the type and dose of insulin administered (e.g., hyperadrenocorticism); or may fluctuate in severity over time (e.g., chronic pancreatitis). Some causes of insulin resistance are readily apparent at the time diabetes is diagnosed, such as obesity and the administration of insulin-antagonistic drugs (e.g., glucocorticoids). Other causes of insulin resistance are not readily apparent and require an extensive diagnostic evaluation to be identified. In general, any concurrent inflammatory, infectious, hormonal, or neoplastic disorder can cause insulin resistance and interfere with the effectiveness of insulin therapy. Identification and treatment of concurrent disease plays an integral role in the successful management of the diabetic dog. A thorough history, physical examination, and complete diagnostic evaluation are imperative in the newly-diagnosed diabetic dog (see Clinical Pathologic Abnormalities).

TECHNIQUES FOR MONITORING DIABETIC CONTROL

The basic objective of insulin therapy is to eliminate the clinical signs of diabetes mellitus while avoiding or delaying the onset of common complications associated with the disease (Box 6-6). Blindness caused by cataract formation is inevitable for most diabetic dogs but can be delayed if good glycemic control can be established and wide fluctuations in the blood glucose concentration avoided (see Cataracts). Complications to avoid include poor hair coat and unthrifty appearance, weight loss, hypoglycemia,

---

BOX 6-6   Complications of Diabetes Mellitus

Common
Iatrogenic hypoglycemia
Persistent or recurring polyuria, polydipsia, weight loss
Cataracts
Lens-induced uveitis
Bacterial infections, especially involving the urinary tract
Chronic pancreatitis
Recurring ketosis, ketoacidosis
Hepatic lipidosis
Peripheral neuropathy
Systemic hypertension

Uncommon
Diabetic nephropathy
Significant proteinuria
Glomerulosclerosis
Retinopathy
Exocrine pancreatic insufficiency
Gastric paresis
Intestinal hypomotility and diarrhea
Diabetic dermatopathy (i.e., superficial necrolytic dermatitis)

---

recurring ketosis, and recurrence of polyuria and polydipsia. The devastating chronic complications of human diabetes (e.g., diabetic nephropathy, atherosclerosis) require years to develop and become clinically relevant, and are uncommon in diabetic dogs, in part, because diabetes is diagnosed in older dogs. As such, the need to establish nearly normal blood glucose concentrations is not necessary in diabetic dogs. Most clients are happy, and most dogs are healthy and relatively asymptomatic if most blood glucose concentrations are kept between 100 mg/dL and 250 mg/dL (5.6 to 14 mmol/L).

History and Physical Examination

The most important initial parameters for assessing control of glycemia are the owner's subjective opinion of severity of clinical signs and overall health of their pet, findings on physical examination, and stability of body weight. If the owner is happy with results of treatment, the physical examination is supportive of good glycemic control, and the body weight is stable, the diabetic dog is usually adequately controlled (Briggs et al, 2000). Measurement of serum fructosamine concentration can add further objective evidence for status of glycemic control (see Serum Fructosamine Concentration). Poor control of glycemia should be suspected and additional diagnostics (i.e., serial blood glucose curve, serum fructosamine concentration, tests for concurrent disorders) or a change in insulin therapy considered if the client reports clinical signs suggestive of hyperglycemia or hypoglycemia (i.e., polyuria, polydipsia, lethargy, weakness, ataxia), the physical examination identifies problems consistent with poor control of glycemia (e.g., thin appearance, poor hair coat), or the dog is losing weight.

Single Blood Glucose Determination

Measuring a single blood glucose concentration is helpful only if hypoglycemia is identified. Documenting hypoglycemia supports insulin overdosage and the need to decrease the insulin dose, especially if glycemic control is poor. In contrast, documenting an increased blood glucose concentration does not, *by itself,* confirm poor control of glycemia. Stress or excitement can cause marked hyperglycemia, which does not reflect the dog's responsiveness to insulin and can lead to the erroneous belief that the diabetic dog is poorly controlled. If a discrepancy exists between the history, physical examination findings, and blood glucose concentration or if the dog is fractious, aggressive, excited, or scared and the blood glucose concentration is known to be unreliable, measurement of serum fructosamine concentration should be done to further evaluate status of glycemic control. In addition, a single blood glucose concentration is not reliable for evaluating the effect of a given insulin type and dose in a poorly-controlled diabetic dog.

Serum Fructosamine Concentration

Serum fructosamines are glycated proteins found in blood that are used to monitor control of glycemia in diabetic dogs and cats (Reusch et al, 1993; Crenshaw et al, 1996; Elliott et al, 1999). Fructosamines result from an irreversible, non-enzymatic, insulin-independent binding of glucose to serum proteins. Serum fructosamine concentrations are a marker of the average blood glucose concentration during the circulating lifespan of the protein, which varies from 1 to 3 weeks depending on the protein (Kawamoto et al, 1992). The extent of glycosylation of serum proteins is directly related to the blood glucose concentration; the higher the average blood glucose concentration during the preceding 2 to 3 weeks, the higher the serum fructosamine concentration, and vice versa. Serum fructosamine concentrations increase when glycemic control of the diabetic dog worsens and decrease when glycemic control improves. Serum fructosamine concentration is not affected by acute increases in the blood

TABLE 6-8   SAMPLE HANDLING, METHODOLOGY, AND NORMAL VALUES FOR SERUM FRUCTOSAMINE CONCENTRATIONS MEASURED IN OUR LABORATORY IN DOGS

Blood sample	1 to 2 mL serum
Sample handling	Freeze until assayed
Methodology	Automated colorimetric assay using nitroblue tetrazolium chloride
Factors affecting results	Hypoalbuminemia (decrease), hypothyroidism (increase), hyperlipidemia (mild decrease), azotemia (mild decrease), prolonged storage at room temperature (decrease), hemolysis (decrease)
Normal range	225 to 365 µmol/L
Interpretation in diabetic dogs:	
Excellent control	350 to 400 µmol/L
Good control	400 to 450 µmol/L
Fair control	450 to 500 µmol/L
Poor control	> 500 µmol/L
Prolonged hypoglycemia	< 300 µmol/L
Diabetic remission	< 300 µmol/L

glucose concentration, as occurs with stress or excitement-induced hyperglycemia (Crenshaw et al, 1996). Serum fructosamine concentrations can be measured during the routine evaluation of the diabetic dog; to clarify the effect of stress or excitement on blood glucose concentrations; to clarify discrepancies between the history, physical examination findings, and serial blood glucose concentrations; and to assess the effectiveness of changes in insulin therapy.

Serum for fructosamine determination should be frozen and shipped on cold packs overnight to the laboratory. Although freezing does not cause a significant change in results, prolonged storage of serum at room temperature can decrease serum fructosamine results; storage of serum in the refrigerator can also decrease the serum fructosamine result (Jensen, 1992). An automated colorimetric assay using nitroblue tetrazolium chloride is used for measurement of fructosamine concentrations in serum. A linear relationship between serum total protein, albumin, and fructosamine concentration has been identified, and hypoproteinemia and hypoalbuminemia can decrease the serum fructosamine concentration below the reference range in healthy dogs and presumably diabetic dogs as well (Loste and Marca, 1999; Reusch and Haberer, 2001; Table 6-8). A decrease in serum fructosamine results has also been identified with hyperlipidemia, azotemia, hyperthyroidism (cats), and interfering substances such as hemolysis (Reusch and Haberer, 2001; Reusch and Tomsa, 1999). An increase in serum fructosamine concentration above the reference range has been identified in two dogs with hyperglobulinemia caused by multiple myeloma and in dogs with naturally-acquired hypothyroidism; an increase that decreased after initiation of sodium levothyroxine treatment (Zeugswetter et al, 2010; Reusch et al, 2002). A significant change in serum fructosamine results was not detected in healthy dogs with hyperproteinemia or hyperbilirubinemia or in healthy dogs treated with

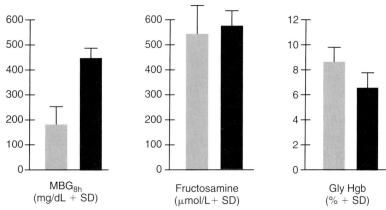

FIGURE 6-18 Mean blood glucose concentration determined over an 8-hour period *(MBG$_{8h}$)*, serum fructosamine concentration, and blood total glycosylated hemoglobin *(Gly Hgb)* in 10 diabetic dogs with poor control of glycemia caused by the Somogyi phenomenon *(gray bars)* and 12 diabetic dogs with poor control of glycemia caused by hyperadrenocorticism-induced insulin resistance *(black bars)*. Note the similar glycated protein results in both groups of dogs. Although the average blood glucose concentration is lower on the day hypoglycemia is identified in dogs with the Somogyi phenomenon, high blood glucose concentrations on subsequent days result in high glycated protein concentrations.

glucosamine-chondroitin sulfate (Lenox et al, 2010). Each laboratory should furnish its own reference range for serum fructosamine. In our laboratory, the normal reference range for serum fructosamine in dogs is 225 to 365 μmol/L, which is a range determined in healthy dogs with persistently normal blood glucose concentrations (Briggs et al, 2000). Serum fructosamine concentration in newly diagnosed diabetic dogs ranged from 320 to 850 μmol/L. The normal serum fructosamine concentration in a few diabetic dogs suggests hyperglycemia severe enough to cause clinical signs had only been present for a short time prior to diagnosis.

Interpretation of serum fructosamine in a diabetic dog must take into consideration the fact that hyperglycemia is common, even in well-controlled diabetic dogs (see Table 6-8). Most owners are happy with their pet's response to insulin treatment if serum fructosamine concentrations can be kept between 350 and 450 μmol/L. Values greater than 500 μmol/L suggest inadequate control of the diabetic state, and values greater than 600 μmol/L indicate serious lack of glycemic control. Serum fructosamine concentrations in the lower half of the reference range (i.e., < 300 μmol/L) or below the reference range should raise concern for significant periods of hypoglycemia in the diabetic dog or concurrent problems that decrease the serum fructosamine concentration (see Table 6-8). Increased serum fructosamine concentrations (i.e., > 500 μmol/L) suggest poor control of glycemia but do not identify the underlying problem (Fig. 6-18). Obtaining a serial blood glucose curve is usually the next diagnostic step to identify the problem (see Serial Blood Glucose Curve).

Serum fructosamine concentrations should not be used as the sole indicator of status of glycemic control but rather should be interpreted in conjunction with the history, findings on physical examination, and stability of body weight. A disconnect between interpretation of the serum fructosamine concentration and the clinical picture or, more commonly, results of blood glucose concentrations may occur in some diabetic dogs. When a low serum fructosamine concentration is identified in a dog with suspected poor control of the diabetic state, reasons for a low fructosamine test result (see Table 6-8) or an increase in serum glucose concentrations should be considered, and vice versa when a high serum fructosamine concentration is identified in a dog with suspected good control of the diabetic state. Whenever information used to assess glycemic control conflicts, reliance on the history, physical examination, and body weight is recommended when deciding if a change in insulin therapy is indicated.

Blood Glycated Hemoglobin Concentration

Glycated hemoglobin (Gly Hb) is a glycated protein that results from an irreversible, nonenzymatic, insulin-independent binding of glucose to hemoglobin in red blood cells. Blood Gly Hb is a marker of the average blood glucose concentration during the circulating lifespan of the red blood cell, which is approximately 110 days in the dog (Jain, 1993). The extent of glycosylation of hemoglobin is directly related to the blood glucose concentration; the higher the average blood glucose concentration during the preceding 3 to 4 months, the higher the blood Gly Hb, and vice versa. Gly Hb is used to monitor long-term effectiveness of treatment in human diabetics, in part, because diabetic humans self-monitor their blood glucose and adjust their insulin dose daily, and Gly Hb assesses a longer treatment interval than fructosamine (i.e., 3 to 4 months versus 2 to 3 weeks, respectively). In contrast, measurement of serum fructosamine is used to assess control of glycemia in diabetic dogs, in part, because the assay is readily available commercially and is better for assessing the impact of changes in insulin therapy on control of glycemia in fractious dogs because concentrations of fructosamine change more quickly than Gly Hb.

In dogs and cats, there are three fractions of Gly Hb—one major fraction (Gly HbA$_{1c}$) that binds glucose and two minor fractions (Gly HbA$_{1a}$ and Gly HbA$_{1b}$) that do not (Hasegawa et al, 1991; 1992). Measurement of Gly HbA$_{1c}$ is typically used to evaluate status of glycemic control in human diabetics, whereas studies in diabetic dogs have used assays that measure all three fractions—i.e., total Gly Hg (Elliott et al, 1997) or Gly HbA$_{1c}$ (Marca et al, 2000; Marca and Loste, 2001). Most techniques that measure total Gly Hg have been shown to be clinically valid for assessing degree of diabetic control (Elliott et al, 1997; Mahaffey and Cornelius, 1982).

Gly Hb is measured in whole blood collected in ethylenediaminetetraacetic acid (EDTA). Blood samples can be refrigerated up to a week without significant change in the Gly Hb concentration.

TABLE 6-9	SAMPLE HANDLING, METHODOLOGY, AND NORMAL VALUES FOR BLOOD TOTAL GLYCOSYLATED HEMOGLOBIN CONCENTRATIONS MEASURED IN OUR LABORATORY IN DOGS
Blood sample	1 to 2 mL whole blood in EDTA
Sample handling	Refrigerate until assayed
Methodology	Affinity chromatography and hemolysates derived from canine red blood cells
Factors affecting results	Storage at room temperature (decrease); storage at 4° C for longer than 7 days (decrease); anemia (Hct < 35%) (decrease)
Normal range	1.7% to 4.9%
Interpretation in diabetic dogs:	
Excellent control	4% to 5%
Good control	5% to 6%
Fair control	6% to 7%
Poor control	> 7%
Prolonged hypoglycemia	< 4%

EDTA, Ethylenediaminetetraacetic acid; *Hct,* hematocrit.

In dogs, blood Gly Hb has been measured by affinity chromatography (Wood and Smith, 1982; Elliott et al, 1997), colorimetric analysis (Mahaffey and Cornelius, 1981), ion-exchange high performance liquid chromatography (Hasegawa et al, 1991), and immunoturbidimetric assay (Marca and Loste, 2001). Assays for measuring Gly Hb are designed for use in humans. As such, it is important that the Gly Hb assay be validated for use in the dog and that a normal reference range is established for the dog. In our experience, several Gly Hb assays, especially in-house automated analyzers for rapid measurement of Gly HbA_{1c} in human diabetics, have not provided valid results in dogs or cats. Any condition that affects red cell life span may affect Gly Hb concentration. Anemia and polycythemia can falsely decrease and increase Gly Hb concentrations, respectively (Elliott et al, 1997). The hematocrit should be taken into consideration when interpreting Gly Hb concentrations.

In our laboratory, the normal reference range for total Gly Hb as measured by affinity chromatography in dogs was 1.7% to 4.9%, which is a range determined in healthy dogs with persistently normal blood glucose concentrations (Elliott et al, 1997). Blood total Gly Hb in newly diagnosed diabetic dogs ranged from 6.0% to 15.5%. Interpretation of blood Gly Hb in a diabetic dog must take into consideration the fact that hyperglycemia is common, even in well-controlled diabetic dogs (Table 6-9). Most owners were happy with their pet's response to insulin treatment if blood total Gly Hb was kept between 4% and 6%. Values greater than 7% suggest inadequate control of the diabetic state, and values greater than 8% indicate serious lack of glycemic control. Blood total Gly Hb less than 4% should raise concern for significant periods of hypoglycemia in the diabetic dog, assuming anemia is not present. Increased total Gly Hb (i.e., > 7%) suggests poor control of glycemia but does not identify the underlying problem (see Fig. 6-18). We no longer measure Gly Hg in diabetic dogs or

cats because, in our experience, blood Gly Hb did not have any diagnostic advantage over serum fructosamine determinations for assessing control of glycemia.

Urine Glucose Monitoring

Occasional monitoring of urine for glycosuria and ketonuria is helpful in diabetic dogs that have problems with recurring ketosis or hypoglycemia to identify ketonuria or persistent negative glycosuria, respectively. The client is instructed not to adjust daily insulin doses on the basis of morning urine glucose measurements, except to decrease the insulin dose in dogs with recurring hypoglycemia and persistent negative glycosuria. Many diabetic dogs develop complications because clients are misled by morning urine glucose concentrations and increase the insulin dose, which eventually results in the Somogyi response (see Insulin Overdosing and Glucose Counterregulation [Somogyi Response]). Persistent glycosuria throughout the day and night suggests inadequate control of the diabetic state and the need for a more complete evaluation of diabetic control using other techniques discussed in this section.

Serial Blood Glucose Curve

If an adjustment in insulin therapy is deemed necessary after reviewing the history, physical examination, changes in body weight, and serum fructosamine concentration, then a serial blood glucose curve should be generated to provide guidance in making the adjustment unless blood glucose measurements are unreliable because of stress, aggression, or excitement. The serial blood glucose curve provides guidelines for making rational adjustments in insulin therapy. Evaluation of a serial blood glucose curve is mandatory during the initial regulation of the diabetic dog and is necessary in the dog in which clinical manifestations of hyperglycemia or hypoglycemia have developed. Reliance on history, physical examination, body weight, and serum fructosamine concentration to determine when a serial blood glucose curve is needed help reduce the frequency of performing serial blood glucose curves, thereby minimizing the dog's aversion (and stress) to these evaluations and improving the chances of obtaining meaningful blood glucose results when a serial blood glucose curve is needed.

Protocol for Generating the Serial Blood Glucose Curve in the Hospital

When a blood glucose curve is being generated, the insulin and feeding schedule used by the client should be maintained and the dog dropped off at the hospital early in the morning. Owners of diabetic dogs who are finicky eaters should feed their pet at their home, not at the hospital. Inappetence can profoundly alter the results of a serial blood glucose curve (Fig. 6-19). The first blood sample for blood glucose measurement is obtained when the dog enters the hospital and subsequent blood samples are typically obtained every 2 hours throughout the day for glucose determination. Glucose measurements should be done more frequently than every 2 hours if the blood glucose is dropping quickly or hypoglycemia is identified. If there are concerns regarding the client's technique for administering insulin, the client can administer insulin (using his or her own insulin and syringe) in the hospital *after* the initial blood glucose is obtained or can demonstrate his or her technique using sterile saline after arriving to pick up the pet at the end of the day. The veterinarian or a veterinary technician should closely evaluate the entire insulin administration procedure. By measuring blood glucose concentration every 2 hours

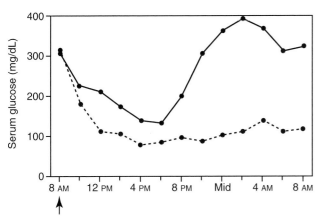

FIGURE 6-19 Mean blood glucose concentrations in eight diabetic dogs after administration of neutral protamine Hagedorn (NPH) insulin (↑) and feeding equal-sized meals at 8 AM and 6 PM *(solid line)* or feeding nothing *(broken line)* during the 24 hours of blood sampling. (From Nelson RW, Couto CG: *Essentials of small animal internal medicine,* St Louis, 1992, Mosby-Year Book, p. 572.)

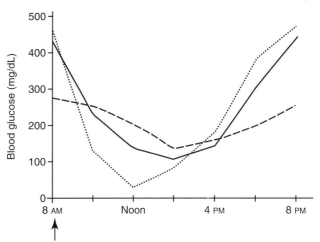

FIGURE 6-20 Blood glucose concentration curve in a Dachshund receiving 0.8 U of recombinant human Lente insulin per kilogram body weight twice a day *(solid line)*, a Miniature Poodle receiving 0.6 U of recombinant human Lente insulin per kilogram body weight twice a day *(broken line),* and a Terrier-mix receiving 1.1 U of recombinant human Lente insulin per kilogram body weight twice a day *(dotted line).* Insulin and food were given at 8 AM for each dog. Interpretation of the blood glucose curves suggest short duration of insulin effect in the Dachshund, insulin underdosage in the Miniature Poodle, and the Somogyi effect in the Terrier-mix. Notice that the blood glucose concentrations were similar in all dogs at 2 PM and 4 PM, and the glucose results at these times do not establish the diagnosis in any of the dogs. (From Nelson RW, Couto CG: *Small animal internal medicine,* ed 3, St Louis, 2003, Mosby, p. 741.)

throughout the day, the clinician will be able to determine if the insulin is effective and identify the glucose nadir, time of peak insulin effect, approximate duration of insulin effect, and range of blood glucose concentrations in that particular dog. Identifying the glucose nadir and the time of the glucose nadir in relation to the time of insulin administration is critical for assessing the duration of insulin effect. If the glucose nadir has not been identified by the time of the next insulin injection, the glucose curve should be continued, the scheduled insulin injection aborted, and the dog fed its evening meal (see Prolonged Duration of Insulin Effect). Obtaining only one or two blood glucose concentrations during the day has not been reliable for evaluating the effect of a given insulin dose (Fig. 6-20). Persistent poor control of the diabetic state often stems from misinterpretation of the effects of insulin that is based on assessment of only one or two blood glucose concentrations.

Changes in blood glucose concentrations are typically assumed to be comparable following the morning and evening administration of insulin, so most dogs receive the same dose of insulin morning and evening (Mori et al, 2013). This assumption is fine as long as the dog is doing well. However, different blood glucose results during the day versus the night should be suspected if polyuria and polydipsia persist despite blood glucose concentrations that are close to acceptable during the day, especially if polyuria and polydipsia are worse at night. For these cases, obtaining a 24-hour blood glucose curve or use of a continuous glucose monitoring (CGM) device should be considered.

Blood glucose concentrations are typically determined by either a point-of-care glucose analyzer or hand-held portable blood glucose meter (PBGM) device. The accuracy of commercially available PBGM devices designed for use in human diabetics varies considerably when used in diabetic dogs, compared with results using standard reference methods (i.e., glucose oxidase and hexokinase methods) (Cohn et al, 2000; Wess and Reusch, 2000a; Cohen et al, 2009; Table 6-10). Blood glucose values determined by most PBGM devices designed for use in human diabetics are typically lower than actual glucose values determined by reference methods, and the difference between the actual glucose value and value obtained from the PBGM increases as hyperglycemia worsens (Fig. 6-21). This bias may result in an incorrect diagnosis of hypoglycemia or the misperception that glycemic control is better than it actually is. Failure to consider this error could result in insulin underdosage and the potential for persistence of clinical

signs despite apparently acceptable blood glucose results. One exception is the AlphaTRAK by Abbott Laboratories, which is a PBGM device designed for use in diabetic dogs and cats. Accuracy of this PBGM device is very good, but glucose values may be higher or lower than glucose values measured by reference methodologies on the same blood sample, forcing the veterinarian to accept the blood glucose concentration at face value (Cohen et al, 2009). Hematocrit may also affect the results of PBGMs. In one study, results of the AlphaTRAK were less accurate compared with a laboratory reference method in blood samples with a lower hematocrit (< 30%) but not an increased hematocrit (> 50%), whereas results from a PBGM for use in humans was less accurate with increased hematocrit but not a decreased hematocrit (Paul et al, 2011).

Insulin therapy should be adjusted according to interpretation of a single serial blood glucose curve and the impact of the change initially assessed by client perceptions of clinical response and change in serum fructosamine concentration. If problems persist, the blood glucose curve can be repeated. If possible, performing blood glucose curves on multiple, consecutive days should be avoided, because it promotes stress-induced hyperglycemia and it takes time (several days) for derangements in hepatic glucose production and secretion to "reset." Information gained from a prior serial blood glucose curve should never be assumed to be reproducible on subsequent curves, especially if several weeks to months have passed or the dog has developed recurrence of clinical signs. The reproducibility of serial blood glucose curves varies from dog to dog. In some dogs, results of serial blood glucose curves may vary dramatically from day to day or month to month. Lack of consistency in the results of serial blood glucose curves is a source of frustration for many veterinarians. This lack of consistency is a direct reflection of all the variables that affect the blood glucose concentration in diabetics. Daily self-monitoring of blood glucose concentrations

TABLE 6-10 BIAS ASSOCIATED WITH BLOOD GLUCOSE CONCENTRATIONS OBTAINED WITH FIVE PORTABLE BLOOD GLUCOSE METERS DESIGNED FOR HUMAN DIABETICS AND ONE METER DESIGNED FOR DIABETIC DOGS VERSUS A REFERENCE ANALYZER

| | Glucose concentration obtained with the reference analyzer (mg/dL) | | | | |
METER	<100 N = 29	100-199 N = 31	200-299 N = 36	300-400 N = 36	> 400 N = 26
AlphaTRAK	8 (0-28)	12 (1-44)	18 (0-99)	32 (3-110)	58 (2-179)
PBGM 1	22 (2-37)	30 (6-53)	52 (4-112)	85 (24-152)	134 (48-234)
PBGM 2	20 (12-32)	34 (18-50)	46 (0-97)	64 (1-144)	82 (30-155)
PBGM 3	30 (22-52)	54 (38-76)	81 (7-141)	95 (5-182)	102 (5-197)
PBGM 4	21 (10-52)	34 (20-54)	47 (9-104)	72 (1-136)	121 (44-196)
PBGM 5	13 (2-29)	22 (4-43)	17 (0-80)	31 (1-113)	45 (2-118)

From Cohen TA, et al.: Evaluation of six portable blood glucose meters for measuring blood glucose concentration in dogs, *J Am Vet Med Assoc* 235:276, 2009.
N, Number of blood samples; *PBGM,* portable blood glucose meter.
Data are given as median bias (range) and represent results from 158 blood samples from 49 dogs. Bias was defined as the absolute value of the difference between blood glucose results obtained with the meter and the corresponding glucose value obtained with the reference analyzer (Roche/Hitachi 917 Chemistry Analyzer).

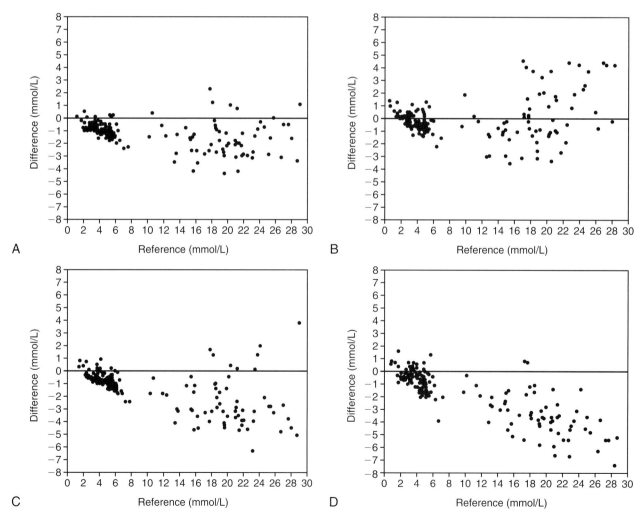

FIGURE 6-21 A to **D,** Scatterplots of the difference between blood glucose concentration obtained with four portable blood glucose meters and concentration obtained with a reference method versus concentration obtained with the reference method for blood samples from 170 dogs. (From Wess G, Reusch C: Evaluation of five portable blood glucose meters for use in dogs, *J Am Vet Med Assoc* 216:203, 2000.)

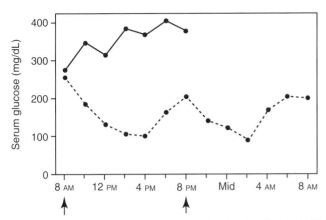

FIGURE 6-22 Blood glucose concentration curves in a fractious Terrier-mix. The same dose of neutral protamine Hagedorn (NPH) insulin was given for each curve. One glucose curve *(solid line)* was obtained with the dog in an agitated state requiring physical restraint each time a blood specimen was obtained; blood for the other glucose curve *(dotted line)* was obtained through a jugular catheter with minimal-to-no restraint and the dog in a quiet state. ↑ = Insulin administration and food.

and adjustments in insulin dose are used in human diabetics to minimize the effect of these variables on control of glycemia. A similar approach for diabetic dogs is becoming more common, as home blood glucose monitoring techniques are refined. For now, initial assessment of control of glycemia is primarily based on the client's perception of the diabetic pet's health combined with periodic examinations by the veterinarian. Serial blood glucose measurements are indicated if poor control of glycemia is suspected. The purpose of serial blood glucose measurements is to obtain a glimpse of the actions of insulin in that diabetic dog and identify a possible reason that the diabetic dog is poorly controlled.

Protocol for Generating the Serial Blood Glucose Curve at Home

Hyperglycemia induced by stress, aggression, or excitement is the single biggest problem affecting accuracy of the serial blood glucose curves (Fig. 6-22). The biggest factors causing stress-induced hyperglycemia are frequent hospitalizations and multiple venipunctures. An alternative to hospital-generated blood glucose curves is to have the client generate the blood glucose curve at home using the ear or metacarpal, metatarsal or foot pad prick technique and a PBGM device that allows the client to touch the drop of blood on the ear or foot pad with the end of the glucose test strip (Wess and Reusch, 2000b). There are several excellent websites on the Internet that demonstrate home blood glucose monitoring techniques for the owner of a diabetic dog, most notably the Abbott Laboratories website for the AlphaTRAK. This technique should be considered for diabetic dogs in which the reliability of blood glucose results generated in the veterinary hospital is questionable and is also becoming a routine monitoring technique used by clients. The biggest problem has been overzealous owners who monitor blood glucose concentrations too frequently and begin to interpret results and adjust the insulin dose without consulting their veterinarian, a practice that ultimately leads to insulin overdosage and the Somogyi response (see Fig. 6-27). See Chapter 7 for more information on home blood glucose monitoring.

Continuous Glucose Monitoring Systems

CGM systems are frequently used to monitor glucose concentrations in diabetic humans and are beginning to be used in diabetic dogs and cats (Wiedmeyer et al, 2008; Affenzeller et al, 2011).

CGM systems measure interstitial fluid glucose concentrations rather than blood glucose concentrations. The correlation between interstitial and blood glucose concentrations is good in diabetic dogs and cats (Davison et al, 2003b; Moretti et al, 2010). A commonly used CGM system (Guardian REAL-time) measures interstitial glucose with a small, flexible sensor inserted through the skin into the subcutaneous space and secured to the skin (Fig. 6-23). Interstitial glucose is detected via the glucose oxidase reaction, and detection occurs entirely at the electrode within the sensor component. Glucose results are transmitted by a wireless transmitter to a pager-sized monitor. The interstitial fluid glucose concentration is recorded and stored every 5 minutes, and the data can be downloaded to a computer for analysis (Fig. 6-24). Calibration of the CGM system is required at initiation of and periodically during glucose monitoring. The working glucose range for the CGM system is 40 to 400 mg/dL (2.2 to 22 mmol/L). Studies to date suggest that the primary advantage of continuous glucose monitoring is detection of hypoglycemic periods that are not detected with serial blood glucose curves and a PBGM device (Dietiker-Moretti et al, 2011). See Chapter 7 for more information on continuous glucose monitoring.

Interpreting the Serial Blood Glucose Curve

Results of the blood glucose curve allow the veterinarian to assess the effectiveness of the administered insulin to lower the blood glucose concentration and determine the glucose nadir and the approximate duration of insulin effect (Fig. 6-25). Ideally, all blood glucose concentrations should range between 100 and 250 mg/dL (5.6 to 14 mmol/L) during the time period between insulin injections, although many diabetic dogs do well despite blood glucose concentrations consistently in the high 100s to low 300s. The goal of insulin therapy is to have the highest blood glucose concentration less than 300 mg/dL (17 mmol/L), the glucose nadir between 80 and 130 mg/dL (4.5 and 7.3 mmol/L), and the mean of all the blood glucose values measured that day to be less than 250 mg/dL (14 mmol/L). Typically, the highest blood glucose concentrations occur at the time of each insulin injection, but this does not always occur. If the blood glucose nadir is greater than 130 mg/dL, the insulin dose may need to be increased, and if the nadir is less than 80 mg/dL, the insulin dose should be decreased.

Duration of insulin effect can be assessed if the glucose nadir is greater than 80 mg/dL (4.5 mmol/L) and there has not been a rapid decrease in the blood glucose concentration after insulin administration. Assessment of duration of insulin effect may not be valid when the blood glucose decreases to less than 80 mg/dL or decreases rapidly because of the potential induction of the Somogyi response, which can falsely decrease the apparent duration of insulin effect (see Insulin Overdosing and Glucose Counterregulation [Somogyi Response]). A rough approximation of the duration of effect of insulin can be gained by examining the time of the glucose nadir. For most well-controlled diabetic dogs, the initial blood glucose concentration near the time of insulin administration is less than 300 mg/dL (17 mmol/L) and the glucose nadir occurs approximately 8 hours after injection of insulin. An initial blood glucose concentration greater than 300 mg/dL (17 mmol/L), combined with a glucose nadir occurring 6 hours or less after insulin administration and subsequent blood glucose concentrations increasing to greater than 300 mg/dL is supportive of short duration of insulin effect. A glucose nadir occurring 12 hours or longer after insulin administration is supportive of prolonged duration of insulin effect. Dogs may develop hypoglycemia or the Somogyi response if the duration of insulin effect is 14 hours or longer and the insulin is being administered twice a day (Fig. 6-26).

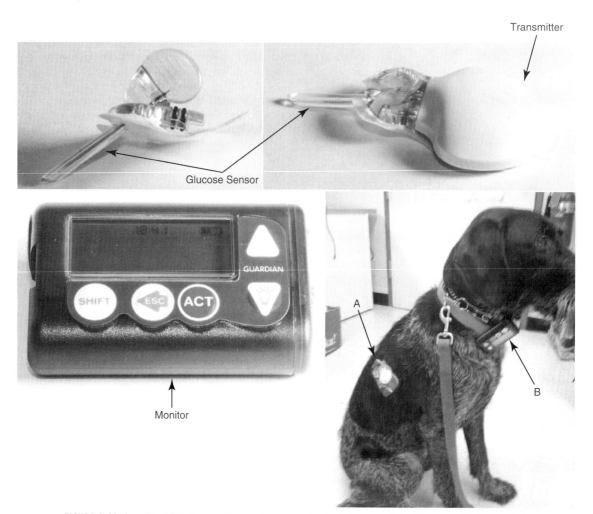

FIGURE 6-23 Guardian REAL-time continuous glucose monitor includes a small, flexible sensor that is inserted into the subcutaneous (SC) space, and interstitial glucose is measured by the glucose oxidase reaction within the sensor component. Glucose results are transmitted by a wireless transmitter to a pager-sized monitor. The interstitial fluid glucose concentration is recorded and stored every 5 minutes and the data can be downloaded to a computer for analysis. *A,* Glucose sensor and transmitter. *B,* Monitor attached to the dog's collar. The monitor can be kept in a basket next to the cage for cats.

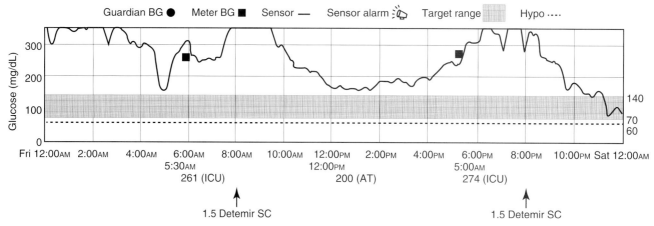

FIGURE 6-24 Example of results of continuous glucose monitoring using the Guardian REAL-time monitor in a 6 kg female-spayed diabetic Miniature Schnauzer with persistent polyuria, polydipsia, and weight loss despite various doses of insulin detemir twice daily. Hypoglycemia and possible glucose counterregulation was suspected, but blood glucose concentrations obtained by venipuncture were always increased. Stress-induced hyperglycemia was believed to be interfering with glucose results. Results of continuous glucose monitoring with minimal blood sampling documented efficacy of insulin detemir and the occurrence of hypoglycemia in the dog.

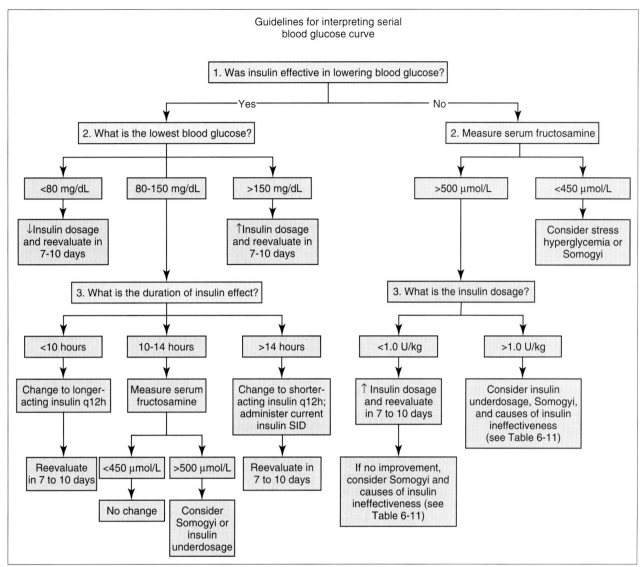

FIGURE 6-25 Algorithm for interpreting results of a serial blood glucose concentration curve. (From Nelson RW, Couto CG: *Small animal internal medicine,* ed 5, St Louis, 2014, Mosby, p. 792.)

Problems with loss of insulin activity in the bottle, insulin administration technique, insulin underdosage, and insulin resistance should be considered if the insulin is not effective in lowering the blood glucose concentration. In general, insulin underdosage should be considered if the insulin dosage is less than 1.0 U/kg per injection in the diabetic dog, and insulin resistance should be considered if the insulin dosage exceeds 1.0 U/kg per injection. The veterinarian should always be wary of the Somogyi response, especially in toy and miniature breeds, and the effect of stress on blood glucose results.

Stress Hyperglycemia

Transient hyperglycemia is a well-recognized problem in fractious, scared, or otherwise stressed cats and can also occur, albeit less frequently, in diabetic dogs. Hyperglycemia presumably develops as a result of increased catecholamine and glucocorticoid secretion and increased hepatic glucose production. Stress hyperglycemia can significantly increase blood glucose concentrations in diabetic dogs despite the administration of insulin—an effect that has serious consequences on the clinician's ability to accurately judge the effectiveness of the insulin injection. Failure to recognize the effect

of stress on blood glucose results may lead to the erroneous perception that the diabetic dog is poorly-controlled; insulin therapy is invariably adjusted, often by increasing the insulin dosage; and repetition of this cycle eventually culminates in induction of the Somogyi response, clinically-apparent hypoglycemia, or referral for evaluation of insulin resistance. Stress hyperglycemia should be suspected if the dog is visibly upset, excessively nervous or hyperactive, aggressive, or difficult to restrain during the venipuncture process. Stress hyperglycemia should also be suspected when there is disparity between assessment of glycemic control based on results of the history, physical examination and stability of body weight, and assessment of glycemic control based on results of blood glucose measurements.

Role of Serum Fructosamine in Aggressive, Excitable, or Stressed Dogs

Hyperglycemia induced by stress, aggression, or excitement is the single biggest problem affecting accuracy of the serial blood glucose curve. Stress can override the glucose-lowering effect of the insulin injection, causing high blood glucose concentrations

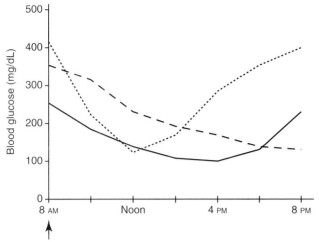

FIGURE 6-26 *Blood glucose concentration curves obtained from three diabetic dogs treated with recombinant human Lente insulin twice a day, illustrating a difference between dogs in the duration of insulin effect. The insulin is effective in lowering the blood glucose concentration in all dogs, and the blood glucose nadir is between 100 and 175 mg/dL for the dogs. However, the duration of insulin effect is approximately 12 hours (solid line) in one dog with good control of glycemia (ideal duration of effect), approximately 8 hours (dotted line) in one dog with persistently poor control of glycemia (short duration of effect), and greater than 12 hours (dashed line) in one dog with a history of good days and bad days of glycemic control (prolonged duration of effect)—a history suggestive of the Somogyi response (see Fig. 6-28). ↑ = Insulin injection and food.*

despite the presence of adequate amounts of insulin in the circulation and leading to a spiraling path of insulin overdosage, hypoglycemia, the Somogyi response, and poor control of glycemia. An alternative to hospital-generated blood glucose curves in dogs where the accuracy of blood glucose results is in question is to have the owner measure blood glucose concentrations at home as discussed previously. Alternatively, serum fructosamine concentrations can be used to assess control of glycemia and effectiveness of adjustments in insulin therapy. If a change in insulin therapy is deemed necessary, the clinician must make an educated guess as to where the problem lies (e.g., low insulin dose, short duration of insulin effect), make an adjustment in therapy, and rely on owner perception of response and the change in subsequent serum fructosamine concentration to assess the benefit of the change in treatment. Serum fructosamine concentrations should be measured prior to and 2 to 3 weeks after changing insulin therapy. If the change in insulin therapy improves control of glycemia, improvement in clinical signs and a decrease in serum fructosamine concentration of at least 50 μmol/L should occur. If the severity of clinical signs and the serum fructosamine concentration are the same or have worsened, the change was ineffective in improving glycemic control, another change in therapy should be done and the serum fructosamine measured again 2 to 3 weeks later.

 INSULIN THERAPY DURING SURGERY

Generally, elective surgery should be delayed in diabetic dogs until the animal's clinical condition is stable and the diabetic state is controlled with insulin. The exception is those situations in which surgery is required to eliminate insulin resistance (e.g., ovariohysterectomy in a diestrus bitch) or to save the dog's life. The surgery itself does not pose a greater risk in a stable diabetic dog than in a non-diabetic dog. The concern is the interplay between

insulin therapy and the lack of food intake during the perioperative period. The stress of anesthesia and surgery also cause the release of diabetogenic hormones, which in turn promotes ketogenesis. Insulin should be administered during the perioperative period to prevent severe hyperglycemia and minimize production of ketones. To compensate for the lack of food intake and to prevent hypoglycemia, the amount of insulin administered during the perioperative period is decreased and IV dextrose is administered, when needed. To correct marked hyperglycemia (i.e., blood glucose concentration greater than 300 mg/dL; 17 mmol/L), regular crystalline insulin is administered intramuscularly or by continuous IV infusion (see Chapter 8). Frequent blood glucose monitoring and appropriate adjustments in therapy are the key to avoiding hypoglycemia and severe hyperglycemia during the perioperative period.

We use the following protocol during the perioperative period in dogs undergoing surgery. The day before surgery, the dog is given its normal dose of insulin and fed as usual. Food is withheld after 10 PM. On the morning of the procedure, the blood glucose concentration is measured before the animal is given insulin. If the blood glucose concentration is less than 100 mg/dL (5.6 mmol/L), insulin is not given, and an IV infusion of 2.5% to 5% dextrose is initiated. If the blood glucose concentration is between 100 and 200 mg/dL (11 mmol/L), one-quarter of the animal's usual morning dose of insulin is given, and an IV infusion of dextrose is initiated. If the blood glucose concentration is more than 200 mg/dL, one-half of the usual morning dose of insulin is given, but the IV dextrose infusion is withheld until the blood glucose concentration is less than 150 mg/dL (8.4 mmol/L). In all three situations, the blood glucose concentration is measured every 30 to 60 minutes during the surgical procedure. The goal is to maintain the blood glucose concentration between 150 and 250 mg/dL (8.4 and 14 mmol/L) during the perioperative period. A 2.5% to 5% dextrose infusion is administered intravenously as needed to correct or prevent hypoglycemia. When the blood glucose concentration exceeds 300 mg/dL (17 mmol/L), the dextrose infusion should be discontinued and the blood glucose concentration evaluated 30 and 60 minutes later. If the blood glucose concentration remains greater than 300 mg/dL, regular crystalline insulin is administered intramuscularly at approximately 20% of the dose of the long-acting insulin being used at home. Subsequent doses of regular crystalline insulin should be given no more frequently than every 4 hours (6 hours if administered subcutaneously), and the dosage should be adjusted based on the effect of the first insulin injection on the blood glucose concentration.

On the day after surgery, the diabetic dog can usually be returned to the routine schedule of insulin administration and feeding. A dog that is not eating can be maintained with IV dextrose infusions and regular crystalline insulin injections given subcutaneously every 6 to 8 hours. Once the animal is eating regularly, it can be returned to its normal insulin and feeding schedule.

 COMPLICATIONS OF INSULIN THERAPY

Hypoglycemia

Hypoglycemia is a common complication of insulin therapy. Signs of hypoglycemia are most apt to occur after sudden large increases in the insulin dose, with excessive overlap of insulin action in dogs receiving insulin twice a day, after prolonged inappetence, during unusually strenuous exercise, and following sudden improvement in concurrent insulin resistance. In these situations severe hypoglycemia may occur before glucose counterregulation (i.e., secretion of glucagon, epinephrine, cortisol, and growth hormone) is able to compensate for and reverse hypoglycemia. Signs of hypoglycemia include lethargy, weakness, head tilting, ataxia, seizures, and coma. The occurrence and severity of clinical signs is dependent on the rate of blood glucose decline and the severity of hypoglycemia. Symptomatic hypoglycemia is treated with glucose administered as food, sugar water, or dextrose IV (see Chapter 9). Whenever signs of hypoglycemia occur, the owner should be instructed to stop insulin therapy until hyperglycemia and glycosuria recur. Urine glucose testing by the owner with the dog in its home environment is useful for identifying when glycosuria recurs. The adjustment in the subsequent insulin dosage is somewhat arbitrary; as a general rule of thumb, the insulin dosage initially should be decreased 25% to 50%, and subsequent adjustments in the dosage should be based on clinical response and results of blood glucose measurements. Failure of glycosuria to recur following a hypoglycemic episode is very uncommon in diabetic dogs and suggests diabetic remission (see Other Specific Types and Diabetic Remission) or impaired glucose counterregulation (see later).

In many diabetic dogs, signs of hypoglycemia are not apparent to clients, and hypoglycemia is identified during evaluation of a serial blood glucose curve or suspected when a low serum fructosamine concentration is identified. Failure to identify hypoglycemia during a blood glucose curve or low-normal serum fructosamine concentration does not rule out asymptomatic hypoglycemia, in part, because of hypoglycemia-induced glucose counterregulation (Somogyi response). Clinical signs of hyperglycemia, transient asymptomatic hypoglycemia, and high serum fructosamine concentrations dominate the clinical picture in diabetic dogs with the Somogyi response.

Treatment of asymptomatic hypoglycemia involves decreasing the dose of insulin (typically 10% to 20%) and assessing the clinical response, change in serum fructosamine concentration, and blood glucose concentrations. If hypoglycemia remains a reoccurring problem despite reductions in the insulin dose, problems with prolonged duration of insulin effect should be considered.

Impaired Glucose Counterregulation

Secretion of the diabetogenic hormones, most notably epinephrine and glucagon, stimulates hepatic glucose secretion and helps counter severe hypoglycemia. A deficient counterregulatory response to hypoglycemia has been identified as early as 1 year after diagnosis of type 1 diabetes in humans (White et al, 1983). As a consequence, when the blood glucose concentration approaches 60 mg/dL (3.4 mmol/L), there is no compensatory response by the body to increase the blood sugar, and prolonged hypoglycemia ensues. An impaired counterregulatory response to hypoglycemia has also been documented in diabetic dogs (Duesberg et al, 1995). Dogs with impaired counterregulation had more problems with hypoglycemia than diabetic dogs without impaired counterregulation. Impaired counterregulation should be considered in a diabetic dog exquisitely sensitive to small doses of insulin or with problems of prolonged hypoglycemia after administration of an acceptable dose of insulin.

Inappetence

A healthy, well-regulated diabetic dog should maintain an excellent appetite. Occasional inappetence at mealtime is not, by itself, an indication to stop insulin therapy. Most diabetic dogs eat within a couple of hours of the insulin injection, as the blood glucose begins to decline. If the inappetence persists or if other signs of gastrointestinal dysfunction develop (e.g., vomiting), insulin therapy should be modified or discontinued until the veterinarian has examined the dog. Common causes of inappetence in diabetic dogs include pancreatitis, ketoacidosis, hepatopathy, inflammatory bowel disease, bacterial infection, finicky eaters, and boredom with high fiber diets. Appropriate diagnostic and therapeutic steps should be initiated, depending on results of the physical examination.

Recurrence or Persistence of Clinical Signs

Recurrence or persistence of clinical signs (i.e., polyuria, polydipsia, polyphagia, weight loss) is perhaps the most common complication of insulin therapy in diabetic dogs. Recurrence or persistence of clinical signs is usually caused by problems with biologic activity of the insulin or with owner technique in administering insulin; problems with the insulin treatment regimen; or problems with responsiveness to insulin caused by concurrent inflammatory, infectious, neoplastic, or hormonal disorders (i.e., insulin resistance). The most common problems with the insulin treatment regimen in the dog include insulin underdosage, induction of the Somogyi response, short duration of effect of Lente or NPH insulin, and once a day insulin administration. Discrepancies in the parameters used to assess glycemic control, resulting in an erroneous belief that the diabetic dog is poorly controlled, should also be considered. This is usually caused by erroneously high blood glucose concentrations induced by stress that suggest insulin ineffectiveness or presence of a concurrent unrecognized disorder that also causes polyuria and polydipsia, such as early renal insufficiency. When evaluating a diabetic dog for suspected insulin ineffectiveness, it is important that all parameters used to assess glycemic control be critically analyzed, most notably the owners' perceptions of how their dog is doing in the home environment, findings on physical examination, and changes in body weight. If the history, physical examination, change in body weight, and serum fructosamine concentration suggest poor control of the diabetic state, a diagnostic evaluation to identify the cause is warranted, beginning with evaluation of the owner's insulin administration technique and the biologic activity of the insulin preparation.

Problems with Owner Administration and Activity of the Insulin Preparation

Failure to administer an appropriate dose of biologically active insulin results in recurrence or persistence of clinical signs. Common reasons include administration of biologically inactive insulin (e.g., outdated, previously heated or frozen; see Insulin Storage, Mixing, and Dilution), administration of diluted insulin, use of inappropriate insulin syringes for the concentration of insulin (e.g., U100 syringe with U40 insulin), or problems with insulin administration technique (e.g., failure to correctly read the insulin syringe, inappropriate injection technique). These problems are identified by evaluating the client's insulin administration technique and by administering new, undiluted insulin and measuring several blood glucose concentrations throughout the day. In addition, the skin and subcutaneous tissues should be assessed in the area where insulin injections are given. Some diabetic dogs develop low-grade inflammation, edema, and thickening of the dermis and subcutaneous tissues in areas of chronic insulin administration and these changes can interfere with insulin absorption following subcutaneous administration (see Allergic Reactions to Insulin).

Problems with the Insulin Treatment Regimen

The most common problems causing poor control of glycemia in this category include insulin underdosage, the Somogyi phenomenon, short duration of effect of Lente and NPH insulin, and once a day insulin administration. The insulin treatment regimen should be critically evaluated for possible problems in these areas, and appropriate changes should be made to try to improve insulin effectiveness, especially if the history and physical examination do not suggest a concurrent disorder causing insulin resistance.

Insulin Underdosage

Control of glycemia can be established in most dogs using 1.0 U or less of insulin/kg of body weight administered twice each day (see Table 6-7). An inadequate dose of insulin in conjunction with once a day insulin therapy is a common cause for persistence of clinical signs. In general, insulin underdosing should be considered if the insulin dosage is less than 1.0 U/kg and the dog is receiving insulin twice a day. If insulin underdosing is suspected, the dose of insulin should be gradually increased by 1 to 5 U/injection (depending on the size of the dog) per week. The effectiveness of the change in therapy should be evaluated by client perception of clinical response and measurement of serum fructosamine or serial blood glucose concentrations. Although some dogs require insulin dosages as high as 1.5 U/kg to attain control of glycemia, other causes for insulin ineffectiveness, most notably the Somogyi response and concurrent insulin resistance, should be considered once the insulin dose exceeds 1.0 U/kg/injection, the insulin is being administered every 12 hours, and control of glycemia remains poor.

Insulin Overdosing and Glucose Counterregulation (Somogyi Response)

The Somogyi response results from a normal physiologic response to impending hypoglycemia induced by excessive insulin. When the blood glucose concentration declines to less than 65 mg/dL (3.6 mmol/L) or when the blood glucose concentration decreases rapidly regardless of the glucose nadir, direct hypoglycemia-induced stimulation of hepatic glycogenolysis and secretion of diabetogenic hormones (most notably epinephrine and glucagon) increase the blood glucose concentration, minimize signs of hypoglycemia, and cause marked hyperglycemia within 12 hours of glucose counterregulation. The marked hyperglycemia that occurs after hypoglycemia is due, in part, to an inability of the diabetic dog to secrete sufficient endogenous insulin to dampen the rising blood glucose concentration in conjunction with insufficient concentrations of circulating insulin derived from the injected insulin (Fig. 6-27; see Hypoglycemia and the Counterregulatory Response in Chapter 9; Cryer and Polonsky, 1998; Karam, 2001). By the next morning, the blood glucose concentration can be extremely elevated (greater than 400 mg/dL; 22 mmol/L), and the morning urine glucose concentration is consistently 1 to 2 gm/dL as measured with urine glucose test strips.

Unrecognized short duration of insulin effect combined with insulin dose adjustments based on morning urine glucose concentrations is historically the most common cause for the Somogyi response in dogs. Currently, the most common cause for the Somogyi response are clients who monitor their pet's blood glucose concentration at home and adjust the insulin dose (i.e., increase the dose) without consulting their veterinarian. The increasing use of longer-acting insulin preparations (i.e., insulin glargine, insulin detemir) that have the potential to last longer than 12 hours may

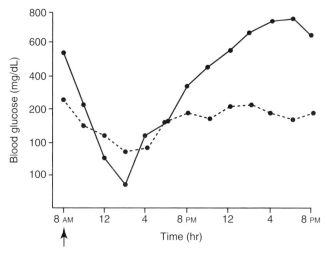

FIGURE 6-27 Blood glucose concentrations in a 6.1 kg Cairn terrier after receiving beef/pork source neutral protamine Hagedorn (NPH) insulin at 8 AM. The dog was fed at 8 AM and 6 PM. *Solid line,* 20 units; *broken line,* 4 units; (From Feldman EC, Nelson RW: Insulin-induced hyperglycemia in diabetic dogs, *J Am Vet Med Assoc* 180:1432, 1982.) ↑ = insulin injection.

dampen the severity of the post-hypoglycemic hyperglycemia historically affiliated with the Somogyi response, presumably because insulin derived from the injected insulin is still present in the circulation. The diabetogenic hormonal response to hypoglycemia is still intact, and persistently increased concentrations of these hormones will still negatively impact control of glycemia, especially if hypoglycemia and the diabetogenic hormonal response reoccur frequently.

Clinical signs of hypoglycemia are typically mild or not recognized by the client; clinical signs caused by hyperglycemia tend to dominate the clinical picture. The insulin dose that induces the Somogyi response is variable and unpredictable. The Somogyi response should be suspected in poorly-controlled diabetic dogs in which insulin dosage exceeds 1.0 U/kg body weight/injection but can also occur at insulin dosages less than 0.5 U/kg/injection (see Table 6-7). Toy and miniature breeds of dogs are especially susceptible to development of the Somogyi response with lower-than-expected doses of insulin. The Somogyi response should always be suspected in any poorly-controlled diabetic dog, regardless of the amount of insulin being administered. Induction of the Somogyi response typically leads to high insulin doses as the veterinarian reacts to the persistence of clinical signs, absence of clinical hypoglycemia, and high blood glucose and serum fructosamine concentrations by increasing the insulin dose and perpetuating the problem.

The diagnosis of the Somogyi response requires demonstration of hypoglycemia (less than 65 mg/dL; 3.6 mmol/L) followed by hyperglycemia (greater than 300 mg/dL; 17 mmol/L) after insulin administration (Feldman and Nelson, 1982; Fig. 6-28). The Somogyi response should also be suspected when the blood glucose concentration decreases rapidly regardless of the glucose nadir (e.g., a drop from 400 to 100 mg/dL [22 to 5.6 mmol/L] in 2 to 3 hours). If the duration of insulin effect is greater than 12 hours, hypoglycemia often occurs at night after the evening dose of insulin, and the serum glucose concentration is typically greater than 300 mg/dL the next morning. Unfortunately, the diagnosis of the Somogyi response can be elusive, in part because of the effects of the diabetogenic hormones on blood glucose concentrations after an episode of glucose counterregulation.

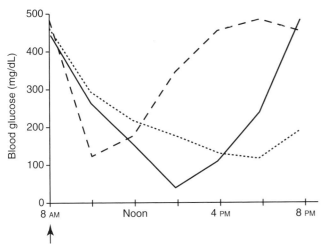

FIGURE 6-28 Blood glucose concentration curves obtained from three poorly-controlled diabetic dogs treated with recombinant human Lente insulin twice a day, illustrating the typical blood glucose curves suggestive of the Somogyi response. In one dog *(solid line)* the glucose nadir is less than 80 mg/dL and is followed by a rapid increase in the blood glucose concentration. In one dog *(dashed line)* a rapid decrease in the blood glucose concentration occurs within 2 hours of insulin administration and is followed by a rapid increase in the blood glucose concentration; the rapid decrease in blood glucose stimulates glucose counterregulation, despite maintaining the blood glucose nadir above 80 mg/dL. In one dog *(dotted line)* the blood glucose curve is not suggestive of the Somogyi response, per se. However, the insulin injection causes the blood glucose to decrease by approximately 300 mg/dL during the day, and the blood glucose concentration at the time of the evening insulin injection is considerably lower than the 8 am blood glucose concentration. If a similar decrease in the blood glucose occurs with the evening insulin injection, hypoglycemia and the Somogyi response would occur at night and would explain the high blood glucose concentration in the morning and the poor control of the diabetic state. (From Nelson RW, Couto CG: *Small animal internal medicine,* ed 5, St Louis, 2014, Mosby, p. 794.) ↑ = Insulin injection and food.

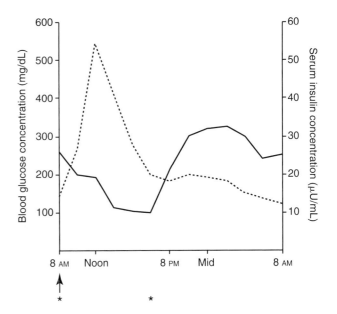

FIGURE 6-29 Mean blood glucose *(solid line)* and serum insulin *(dotted line)* concentrations in eight dogs with diabetes mellitus treated with a beef/pork source neutral protamine Hagedorn (NPH) insulin subcutaneously once daily. The duration of NPH effect is too short, resulting in prolonged periods of hyperglycemia beginning shortly after the evening meal. (From Nelson RW, Couto CG: *Small animal internal medicine,* ed 5. St Louis, 2014, Mosby, p. 795.) ↑ = Insulin injection; * = equal-sized meals consumed.

However, if the client reports no change or improvement in polyuria and polydipsia, continued gradual reduction of the insulin dose should be pursued until polyuria and polydipsia worsen again, which identifies an inadequate dose of insulin for the dog. Alternatively, glycemic regulation of the diabetic dog could be started over using an insulin dose of 0.25 U/kg given twice daily.

Short Duration of Insulin Effect

For most dogs, the duration of effect of recombinant human Lente and NPH insulin is 10 to 14 hours, and twice a day insulin administration is effective in controlling blood glucose concentrations. However, in some diabetic dogs, the duration of effect of Lente and NPH insulin is less than 10 hours; a duration that is too short to prevent periods of hyperglycemia and persistence of clinical signs (Fig. 6-29; see Fig. 6-14). Diabetic dogs with the problem of short duration of insulin effect have persistent morning glycosuria (> 1 g/dL on urine glucose test strips) regardless of the insulin dose being administered. Owners of these pets usually mention continuing problems with evening polyuria and polydipsia, or weight loss. If owners are adjusting the daily insulin dosage based on the morning urine glucose concentration, they usually induce the Somogyi response as the insulin dosage is gradually increased in response to persistent morning glycosuria. Serum fructosamine concentrations are variable but typically greater than 500 µmol/L. A diagnosis of short duration of insulin effect is made by demonstrating an initial blood glucose concentration greater than 300 mg/dL combined with a glucose nadir above 80 mg/dL (4.5 mmol/L) that occurs less than 8 hours after insulin administration and recurrence of hyperglycemia (greater than 300 mg/dL; 17 mmol/L) within 12 hours of the insulin injection (see Fig. 6-26). Diabetic dogs that have a short duration of insulin effect can be diagnosed only by determining serial blood glucose

Secretion of diabetogenic hormones during the Somogyi response may induce insulin resistance, which can last 24 to 72 hours after the hypoglycemic episode. If a serial blood glucose curve is obtained on the day glucose counterregulation occurs, hypoglycemia will be identified and the diagnosis established. However, if the serial blood glucose curve is obtained on a day when insulin resistance predominates, hypoglycemia will not be identified and the insulin dose may be incorrectly increased in response to the high blood glucose values. A cyclic history of 1 or 2 days of good glycemic control followed by several days of poor control should raise suspicion for insulin resistance caused by glucose counterregulation. Serum fructosamine concentrations are unpredictable but are usually increased >500 µmol/L, results that confirm poor glycemic control but do not identify the underlying cause (see Fig. 6-18).

Establishing the diagnosis may require several days of hospitalization and serial blood glucose curves, an approach that eventually leads to problems with stress-induced hyperglycemia. An alternative, preferable approach is to arbitrarily gradually reduce the insulin dose 1 to 5 units (depending on the size of the dog and dose of insulin) and have the client evaluate the dog's clinical response over the ensuing 2 to 5 days, specifically as it relates to changes in polyuria and polydipsia. If the severity of polyuria and polydipsia worsens after an initial reduction in the insulin dose, another cause for the insulin ineffectiveness should be pursued.

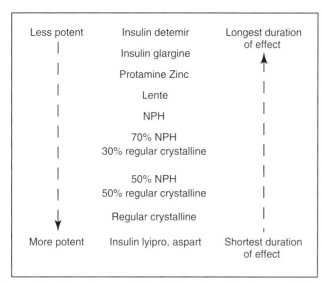

FIGURE 6-30 Types of commercial insulin based on their potency and duration of effect. An inverse relationship exists between the potency and duration of effect. (From Nelson RW, Couto CG: *Small animal internal medicine,* ed 5, St Louis, 2014, Mosby, p. 793.)

concentrations. One or two afternoon blood glucose determinations consistently fail to identify the problem. They may identify normal glucose concentrations or mild hyperglycemia, findings that are not consistent with the worries of the owner and do not identify the underlying problem. Alternatively, one or two afternoon blood glucose determinations may reveal severe hyperglycemia, findings that do not differentiate short duration of insulin effect from the Somogyi response or insulin resistance. Treatment involves changing to a longer-acting insulin (Fig. 6-30). Although PZI, insulin glargine, and insulin detemir all have the potential to be effective in diabetic dogs, my preference is to switch to insulin detemir when Lente and NPH are ineffective because of short duration of insulin effect. Insulin detemir is a potent insulin with the potential for prolonged duration of effect (greater than 14 hours), which can create issues with hypoglycemia and the Somogyi response when insulin detemir is given twice a day. Regardless, most diabetic dogs require insulin detemir twice a day to attain diabetic control, recognizing that the insulin dosage can be quite small to compensate for the potency and prolonged duration of effect of the insulin. The recommended starting dosage for insulin detemir is 0.1 U/kg administered every 12 hours.

Prolonged Duration of Insulin Effect

In some diabetic dogs, the duration of effect of Lente and NPH insulin is greater than 12 hours, and twice a day insulin administration creates problems with hypoglycemia and the Somogyi response. In these dogs, the glucose nadir following the morning administration of insulin typically occurs near or after the time of the evening insulin administration, and the morning blood glucose concentration is usually greater than 300 mg/dL (17 mmol/L) (see Fig. 6-26). Gradually decreasing blood glucose concentrations measured at the time of sequential insulin injections is another indication of prolonged duration of insulin effect. The effectiveness of insulin in lowering the blood glucose concentration is variable from day to day, presumably because of varying concentrations of diabetogenic hormones whose secretion was induced by prior hypoglycemia. Serum fructosamine concentrations are variable but typically greater than 500 μmol/L. An

effective treatment depends, in part, on the duration of effect of the insulin. An extended blood glucose curve should be generated after administration of insulin once in the morning and feeding the dog at the normal times of the day. This allows the clinician to evaluate the effect of the evening meal on postprandial blood glucose concentrations and estimate whether insulin from the morning injection is still present in the blood and capable of preventing a postprandial increase in the blood glucose. If the postprandial blood glucose increases (typically 75 mg/dL [4.2 mmol/L] or more) within 2 hours of feeding, the duration of effect is close to 12 hours and manipulation of the insulin dose, the timing of the meals in relation to the timing of the insulin injections, or both, should be tried before switching to a longer acting insulin. Failure of the blood glucose to increase 2 hours or longer after eating the evening meal suggests a prolonged duration of effect (i.e., longer than 14 hours). Switching to a longer acting insulin (e.g., insulin detemir) administered once a day can be tried initially (see Fig. 6-30).

Inadequate Insulin Absorption

Slow or inadequate absorption of insulin from the subcutaneous site is uncommon in diabetic dogs treated with NPH or Lente insulin. Impaired absorption of insulin may occur as a result of thickening of the skin and inflammation of the subcutaneous tissues caused by chronic injection of insulin in the same area of the body (see Allergic Reactions to Insulin). Rotation of the injection site helps prevent this problem, and avoidance of regions that have become thickened should improve insulin absorption.

Circulating Insulin-Binding Antibodies

Insulin antibodies result from repeated injections of a foreign protein (i.e., insulin). The structure and amino acid sequence of the injected insulin relative to the native endogenous insulin influence the development of insulin antibodies. The presence of substances in the insulin preparation designed to prolong insulin effect (e.g., protamine) may also play a role in inducing antibody formation (Kurtz et al, 1983). Conformational insulin epitopes are believed to be more important in the development of insulin antibodies than differences in the linear subunits of the insulin molecule, per se (Thomas et al, 1985; 1988; Nell and Thomas, 1989; Davison et al, 2008b). The more divergent the insulin molecule being administered from the species being treated is, the greater the likelihood that significant amounts of insulin antibodies will be formed. Canine, porcine, and recombinant human insulin are similar, and development of a clinically relevant amount of insulin antibodies is uncommon in dogs treated with porcine or recombinant human insulin. In contrast, canine and beef insulin differ and serum insulin antibodies have been identified in 40% to 65% of dogs treated with beef/pork or beef insulin (Haines, 1986; Davison et al, 2008b).

Insulin-binding antibodies can enhance and prolong the pharmacodynamic action of insulin by serving as a carrier, or they can reduce insulin action by excessive binding and reduction of circulating unbound "free" insulin (Bolli et al, 1984; Marshall et al, 1988; Lahtela et al, 1997). Antibodies may also have no apparent clinical effect on insulin dosage or status of glycemic control (Lindholm et al, 2002). In our experience, the presence of significant amounts of insulin-binding antibodies is associated with erratic and often poor control of glycemia, an inability to maintain control of glycemia for extended periods of time, frequent adjustments in insulin dose, and occasional development of severe insulin resistance (Fig. 6-31). Insulin-binding antibodies can also

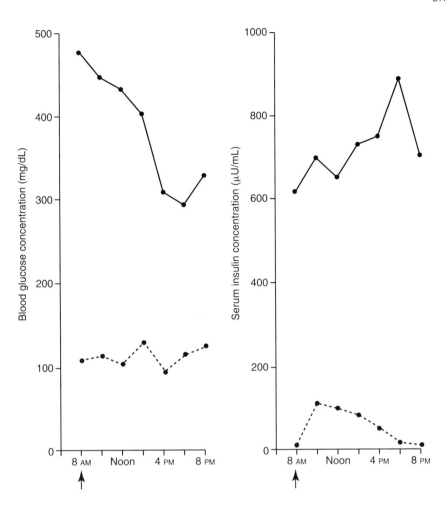

FIGURE 6-31 Blood glucose and serum insulin concentrations in a 7.6 kg, spayed dog receiving 1.1 U/kg beef/pork source Lente insulin (solid line) subcutaneously. The dog had severe polyuria, polydipsia, and weight loss. A baseline serum insulin concentration was greater than 1000 μU/mL 48 hours after discontinuing insulin therapy. Interference from anti-insulin antibodies was suspected, and the source of insulin was changed to recombinant human insulin. Clinical signs improved within 2 weeks, and a blood glucose curve was obtained 4 weeks later with the dog receiving 0.9 U/kg recombinant human Lente insulin (broken line), showed excellent glycemic control. Presumably, loss of anti-insulin antibody interference with the insulin radioimmunoassay (RIA) allowed a more accurate assessment of changes in the serum insulin concentration after recombinant human insulin administration. (From Nelson RW, Couto CG: *Small animal internal medicine*, ed 5. St Louis, 2014, Mosby, p. 795.) ↑ = Insulin injection and food.

cause erratic fluctuations in the blood glucose concentration with no correlation between the timing of insulin administration and changes in blood glucose concentration (Fig. 6-32). Presumably, fluctuations in blood glucose concentration result from erratic and unpredictable changes in the circulating free (i.e., non–antibody-bound) insulin concentration (Bolli et al, 1984). This phenomenon causes inappropriate and potentially life-threatening hypoglycemia at unexpected times in human diabetics. We have observed a similar syndrome in diabetic dogs treated with beef/pork insulin preparations. Problems with glycemic control typically improve or resolve with the initiation of porcine-source or recombinant human insulin preparations. Although uncommon, insulin antibodies can develop in dogs treated with recombinant human insulin and should be suspected as the cause of poor glycemic control when another cause cannot be identified.

Documentation of serum insulin-binding antibodies should make use of assays that have been validated in diabetic dogs. A radioimmunoassay (RIA) for identifying insulin antibodies in dogs is currently available at the Diagnostic Center for Population and Animal Health, Michigan State University, East Lansing, Mich. Although the finite range of possible results with this assay is 0% to 100%, normal results are typically 15% or less and significant positive results are greater than 40% to 50%.

Circulating insulin-binding antibodies may interfere with some RIA techniques used to measure serum insulin concentration in a manner similar to the effects of thyroid hormone antibodies on RIA techniques for serum triiodothyronine (T_3) and T_4 concentrations (see Chapter 3). The presence of insulin-binding antibodies in the serum sample causes spuriously high insulin values when a single-phase separation system utilizing antibody-coated tubes is used to measure serum insulin concentration. This interference can be used to raise the clinician's index of suspicion for insulin-binding antibodies as a cause for insulin resistance. The serum insulin concentration is typically less than 50 μU/mL (360 pmol/L) 24 hours after insulin administration in diabetic dogs without antibodies causing interference with the RIA. In contrast, serum insulin concentrations are typically greater than 400 μU/mL (2800 pmol/L) 24 hours after insulin administration when insulin-binding antibodies interfere with the RIA results—an interaction that causes spurious results (see Fig. 6-31).

A switch to porcine-source or recombinant human insulin preparation, a switch to an insulin preparation that does not contain protamine, or both should be considered if insulin-binding antibodies are identified in a poorly-controlled diabetic dog. Studies evaluating the antigenicity of insulin analogues (i.e., glargine, detemir) in diabetic dogs have not been reported. In our experience, insulin antibody results greater than 15% using the Michigan State University insulin antibody assay are uncommon in diabetic dogs treated with insulin analogues.

Allergic Reactions to Insulin

Significant reactions to insulin occur in as many as 5% of human diabetics treated with insulin and include erythema, pruritus, induration, and lipoatrophy at the injection site. Allergic reactions to insulin have been poorly documented in diabetic dogs. Pain on injection of insulin is usually caused by inappropriate injection

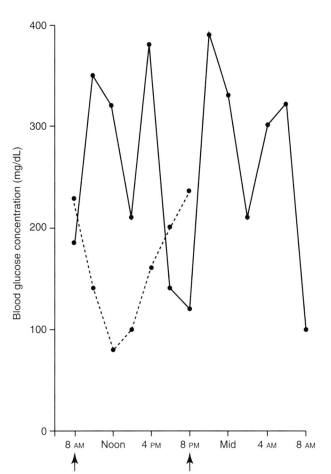

FIGURE 6-32 Blood glucose curve in a 50 kg male dog receiving 0.7 U/kg beef/pork source Lente insulin *(solid line)* subcutaneously. Note the erratic fluctuations in the blood glucose concentration. The dog had polyuria, polydipsia, and weight loss and was blind from cataract formation. A baseline serum insulin concentration was 825 μU/mL 24 hours after discontinuing insulin therapy. Interference from anti-insulin antibodies was suspected, and the source of insulin was changed to recombinant human insulin. Clinical signs improved within 1 month, and a blood glucose curve was obtained 8 weeks later with the dog receiving 0.5 U/kg recombinant human Lente insulin *(broken line),* showing excellent glycemic control and loss of erratic fluctuations in the blood glucose concentration.

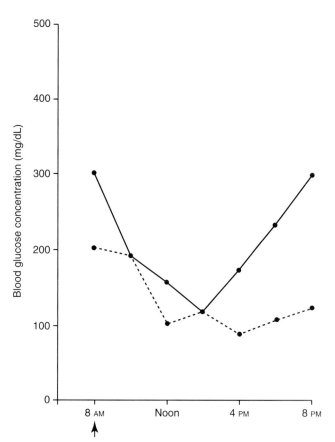

FIGURE 6-33 Blood glucose curve in a 12 kg male diabetic dog with untreated hypothyroidism receiving 2.2 U/kg recombinant human Lente insulin *(solid line).* The large amount of insulin required to lower the blood glucose concentration suggests insulin resistance. Glycemic control was improved, and the insulin dosage was decreased to 0.9 U/kg after sodium levothyroxine therapy was initiated *(broken line).* ↑ = Subcutaneous (SC) insulin injection and food.

technique, inappropriate site of injection, a reaction to the cold temperature of insulin stored in the refrigerator, the acidic pH of insulin glargine, or issues with behavior and not an adverse reaction to insulin, per se. Chronic injection of insulin in the same area of the body may cause inflammation and thickening of the skin and subcutaneous tissues and may be caused by an immune reaction to insulin or some other protein (e.g., protamine) in the insulin bottle. Inflammation and thickening of the skin and subcutaneous tissues may impair insulin absorption, resulting in recurrence of clinical signs of diabetes. Rarely, diabetic dogs develop acute focal subcutaneous edema and swelling at the site of an insulin injection. Insulin allergy is suspected in these animals. Treatment includes switching to a less antigenic insulin and to a more purified insulin preparation. Systemic allergic reactions to insulin in dogs have yet to be identified.

Concurrent Disorders Causing Insulin Resistance

Insulin resistance is a condition in which a normal amount of insulin produces a subnormal biologic response. Insulin resistance may

result from problems occurring prior to the interaction of insulin with its receptor (e.g., circulating insulin-binding antibodies), at the receptor (e.g., altered insulin receptor binding affinity or concentration), or at steps distal to the interaction of insulin and its receptor (e.g., block in insulin signal transduction). Prereceptor problems reduce free metabolically active insulin concentration and include increased insulin degradation and insulin-binding antibodies. Receptor problems include alterations in insulin-receptor binding affinity and concentration and insulin-receptor antibodies. Postreceptor problems are difficult to differentiate clinically from receptor problems, and both often coexist. In dogs, receptor and postreceptor abnormalities are usually attributable to obesity, circulating acute phase proteins, and inflammatory cytokines (e.g., tumor necrosis factor alpha [TNFα], interleukin-1, interleukin-6) that interfere with insulin signal transduction or a disorder causing excessive or deficient secretion of an insulin-antagonistic hormone, such as cortisol, growth hormone, progesterone, or thyroid hormone (Tilg and Moschen, 2006; Vick et al, 2008).

No insulin dose clearly defines insulin resistance. For most diabetic dogs, control of glycemia can usually be attained using 1.0 U or less of Lente or NPH insulin per kilogram of body weight given twice daily (see Table 6-7). Insulin resistance should be suspected if control of glycemia is poor despite an insulin dosage in excess of 1.5 U/kg, when excessive amounts of insulin (i.e., insulin dosage >1.5 U/kg) are necessary to maintain the blood glucose concentration below 300 mg/dL (Fig. 6-33), and when control of glycemia

| | TABLE 6-11 | **RECOGNIZED CAUSES OF INSULIN INEFFECTIVENESS OR INSULIN RESISTANCE IN DIABETIC DOGS** |

CAUSED BY INSULIN THERAPY	DISORDERS TYPICALLY CAUSING SEVERE INSULIN RESISTANCE	DISORDERS TYPICALLY CAUSING MILD OR FLUCTUATING INSULIN RESISTANCE
Inactive insulin	Hyperadrenocorticism	Obesity
Diluted insulin	Diestrus in intact female	Infection
Improper administration technique	Progesterone secreting adrenocortical tumor	Chronic inflammation
Inadequate dose	Diabetogenic drugs	Chronic pancreatitis
Somogyi response	Glucocorticoids	Chronic inflammatory bowel disease
Inadequate frequency of insulin administration	Progestagens	Disease of the oral cavity
Impaired insulin absorption		Chronic kidney disease (CKD)
Insulin-binding antibodies		Hepatobiliary disease
		Cardiac disease
		Hypothyroidism
		Hyperthyroidism
		Pancreatic exocrine Insufficiency
		Hyperlipidemia
		Neoplasia
		Glucagonoma
		Pheochromocytoma

is erratic and insulin requirements are constantly changing in an attempt to maintain control of glycemia. Failure of the blood glucose concentration to decrease below 300 mg/dL (17 mmol/L) during a serial blood glucose curve is suggestive of, but not definitive for, the presence of insulin resistance. An insulin resistance–type blood glucose curve can also result from stress-induced hyperglycemia, the Somogyi response, and other problems with insulin therapy (Table 6-11), and a decrease in the blood glucose concentration below 300 mg/dL can occur with disorders causing relatively mild insulin resistance (e.g., obesity, inflammation). Serum fructosamine concentrations are typically greater than 500 μmol/L in dogs with insulin resistance and can exceed 700 μmol/L if resistance is severe. Unfortunately, an increased serum fructosamine concentration is merely indicative of poor glycemic control not insulin resistance, per se.

The severity of insulin resistance is dependent, in part, on the underlying etiology. Insulin resistance may be mild and easily overcome by increasing the dosage of insulin or may be severe, causing marked hyperglycemia regardless of the type and dosage of insulin administered. Some causes of insulin resistance are readily apparent at the time diabetes is diagnosed, such as obesity and the administration of insulin-antagonistic drugs (e.g., glucocorticoids, progestogens). Other causes of insulin resistance are not readily apparent and require an extensive diagnostic evaluation to be identified. In general, any concurrent inflammatory, infectious, hormonal, neoplastic, or organ system disorder can cause insulin resistance and interfere with the effectiveness of insulin therapy (see Table 6-11). In our experience, the most common concurrent disorders interfering with insulin effectiveness in diabetic dogs include diabetogenic drugs (glucocorticoids), severe obesity, hyperadrenocorticism, diestrus, chronic pancreatitis, CKD, inflammatory bowel disease, oral cavity disease, infections of the urinary tract, hyperlipidemia, and insulin-binding antibodies in dogs receiving beef insulin. Obtaining a complete history and performing a thorough physical

examination is the most important initial step in identifying these concurrent disorders. If the history and physical examination are unremarkable, a CBC, serum biochemical analysis, serum cPL, serum progesterone concentration (intact female dog), abdominal ultrasound, and urinalysis with bacterial culture should be obtained to further screen for concurrent illness. Additional tests will be dependent on results of the initial screening tests (Box 6-7).

Treatment and reversibility of insulin resistance is dependent on the etiology. Insulin resistance is reversible with treatable disorders—for example, sodium levothyroxine treatment in a diabetic dog with concurrent hypothyroidism (Ford et al, 1993) or ovariohysterectomy in an intact female diabetic dog in diestrus (see Other Specific Types and Diabetic Remission; Fall et al, 2008b). In contrast, insulin resistance often persists with disorders that are difficult to treat, such as chronic recurring pancreatitis. In some situations, measures can be taken to prevent insulin resistance, such as avoidance of glucocorticoids in diabetic dogs and an ovariohysterectomy at the time diabetes mellitus is diagnosed in an intact female dog.

Insulin Dosage Adjustments

Adjustments in the insulin dosage should always be considered at the time treatment of the insulin-resistant disorder is initiated. How much to decrease the insulin dosage is variable and dependent, in part, on the severity of insulin resistance, the amount of insulin being administered, and the expected rapidity of improvement in insulin resistance after treatment of the disorder. For example, poorly-controlled diabetic dogs with newly diagnosed hypothyroidism will have a rapid improvement in insulin resistance after initiating thyroid hormone treatment (see Fig. 6-33; Ford et al, 1993). Failure to decrease the insulin dosage may result in symptomatic hypoglycemia within days of starting thyroid hormone treatment. In contrast, correction of obesity and subsequent improvement in insulin resistance is a relatively slow

---

BOX 6-7　Diagnostic Tests to Consider for the Evaluation of Insulin Resistance in Diabetic Dogs

CBC, serum biochemistry panel, urinalysis
Bacterial culture of the urine
Serum cPL (pancreatitis)
Serum TLI (exocrine pancreatic insufficiency)
Adrenocortical function tests
　Urine cortisol-to-creatinine ratio (spontaneous hyperadrenocorticism)
　Low-dose dexamethasone suppression test (spontaneous hyperadrenocorticism)
　ACTH stimulation test (iatrogenic hyperadrenocorticism)
Thyroid function tests
Baseline serum total and free T_4 (hypothyroidism or hyperthyroidism)
Endogenous serum TSH (hypothyroidism)
TSH stimulation test (hypothyroidism)
Serum progesterone concentration (diestrus in intact female dog)
Plasma growth hormone or serum IGF-1 concentration (acromegaly)
Serum insulin antibody test (see Circulating Insulin-Binding Antibodies)
Fasting serum triglyceride concentration (hyperlipidemia)
Abdominal ultrasonography (adrenomegaly, adrenal mass, pancreatitis, pancreatic mass)
Thoracic radiography (cardiomegaly, neoplasia)
CT or MRI (pituitary mass)

ACTH, Adrenocorticotropic hormone; *CBC,* complete blood count; *cPL,* canine pancreatic-specific lipase; *CT,* computed tomography; *IGF-1,* insulin-like growth factor-1; *MRI,* magnetic resonance imaging; *T₄,* thyroxine; *TLI,* trypsin-like immunoreactivity; *TSH,* thyroid-stimulating hormone (also known as thyrotropin).

process affiliated with a gradual reduction in the insulin dosage over a period of time as obesity improves. Avoiding hypoglycemia is the primary goal when adjusting the insulin dosage. Always err on the side of decreasing the insulin dose too much rather than too little, recognizing that hyperglycemia is not life-threatening but severe hypoglycemia can be. Monitoring urine for ketonuria identifies those dogs in which the reduction in insulin combined with insulin resistance resulted in ketone formation and the need for more insulin (see Chapter 8). When in doubt, I decrease the insulin dose to approximately 0.5 U/kg per injection for diabetic dogs and rely on owner observations regarding the overall health of their pet and the presence of clinical signs suggestive of hypoglycemia. Home blood glucose monitoring and monitoring random urine samples for negative glycosuria may also be considered.

Glucocorticoids and Hyperadrenocorticism

Diabetic dogs are often treated with glucocorticoids for treatment of concurrent disease (e.g., allergic skin disease). Glucocorticoids have the potential to cause severe insulin resistance, creating a tendency for large amounts of insulin to be administered in an attempt to control hyperglycemia (Tiley et al, 2008). If glucocorticoids are required for treatment of a concurrent disease, the glucocorticoid dose should be kept as low as possible and administered as infrequently as possible to minimize the severity of insulin resistance. Insulin dosage requirements will be higher in the presence of insulin resistance to maintain some semblance of glycemic control. It is important to remember the interplay between dosage adjustments of glucocorticoids and the impact of the adjustment on severity of insulin resistance and insulin dosage requirements. Appropriate adjustments in the insulin dose should be done whenever the glucocorticoid dose is increased or decreased to minimize hyper- and hypoglycemia, respectively.

Naturally occurring hyperadrenocorticism and diabetes mellitus are common concurrent diseases in dogs. For most dogs, glycemic control remains poor despite insulin therapy and good glycemic control is generally not possible until the hyperadrenocorticism is controlled. The initial focus should be on treating the hyperadrenal state in a poorly-controlled diabetic dog diagnosed with hyperadrenocorticism. Insulin treatment is indicated; however, aggressive efforts to control hyperglycemia should not be attempted. Rather, a conservative dose (approximately 0.5 U/kg) of intermediate-acting insulin (i.e., Lente or NPH) should be administered twice a day to prevent ketoacidosis and severe hyperglycemia. Monitoring water consumption and frequency of urination is not reliable because both diseases cause polyuria and polydipsia; polyuria and polydipsia may persist if poor control of hyperglycemia persists despite attaining control of hyperadrenocorticism. As control of hyperadrenocorticism is achieved, insulin resistance resolves and tissue sensitivity to insulin improves. Home blood glucose monitoring and testing urine for the presence of glucose can be done by the owner to help prevent hypoglycemia and identify when insulin resistance is resolving. Any blood glucose concentration less than 150 mg/dL (8.4 mmol/L) or urine sample found to be negative for glucose should be followed by a 20% to 25% reduction in the insulin dose and evaluation of control of the hyperadrenocorticism. Critical assessment of glycemic control and adjustments in insulin therapy should be initiated once hyperadrenocorticism is controlled. The ability to establish consistent glycemic control seems more problematic for dogs treated with trilostane versus mitotane (lysodren), presumably because of differences in their mechanism of action and ability to maintain decreased cortisol concentrations (see Chapter 10).

Chronic Pancreatitis

Chronic pancreatitis is the most significant concurrent inflammatory disorder in diabetic dogs. Chronic pancreatitis is identified at necropsy in approximately 35% of diabetic dogs (Alejandro et al, 1988). Most of these animals have a similar history, characterized by poorly controlled diabetes, fluctuating insulin requirements, blood glucose concentrations often greater than 300 mg/dL (17 mmol/L), intermittent lethargy and inappetence, and owner concerns that their pet is "just not doing well." An inability to correct these problems ultimately leads to euthanasia for many dogs. Establishing a diagnosis relies on a combination of clinical signs, physical examination findings, serum cPL, ultrasound evaluation of the pancreas, and clinical suspicion for the disorder (see Pancreatic Enzymes). Feeding a low-fat highly digestible diet is the cornerstone of treatment.

Chronic Kidney Disease

CKD and diabetes mellitus are common geriatric diseases and often occur concurrently. Abnormal kidney function may result from the deleterious effects of the diabetic state (i.e., diabetic nephropathy) or may be an independent problem that has developed in conjunction with diabetes in the geriatric dog. As kidney function declines, human diabetics with concurrent nephropathy are at increased risk for severe hypoglycemia as a result of decreased renal clearance of insulin and decreased renal glucose production by gluconeogenesis (Stumvoll et al, 1997; Rave et al, 2001). Tissue responsiveness to insulin (i.e., insulin sensitivity) is also attenuated, resulting in poorer metabolic control of the diabetic state (Eidemak et al, 1995). Prolonged duration of insulin effect, insulin resistance, and less commonly hypoglycemia are recognized problems in diabetic dogs with concurrent CKD. The interplay between progression and severity of CKD, severity of insulin resistance, and impairment of insulin clearance creates unpredictable fluctuations in control of glycemia and insulin requirements and frustration for the owner and veterinarian. In addition, reliance on an important indicator of diabetic control (i.e., severity of polyuria and polydipsia) is no longer reliable because of the concurrent CKD. Indicators for possible mild (i.e., non-azotemic) concurrent CKD include persistent polyuria and polydipsia despite good glycemic control of the diabetic state and urine specific gravities less than 1.020 despite 1% to 2% glycosuria. In most cases, treatment for CKD and failure takes priority and insulin therapy is modified, as needed, to attain the best possible control of the diabetic state while trying to avoid hypoglycemia, recognizing that attainment of good control may be difficult and polyuria and polydipsia will persist regardless of the status of glycemic control.

Hypertriglyceridemia

Increased serum concentrations of cholesterol and triglycerides are common in newly diagnosed diabetic dogs and usually resolve after initiation of insulin treatment (see Serum Cholesterol and Triglyceride Concentrations). Persistent hypertriglyceridemia may impair insulin receptor-binding affinity, promote downregulation of insulin receptors, and cause a postreceptor defect in insulin action (Berlinger et al, 1984; Bieger et al, 1984) Hypertriglyceridemia may be secondary to other disorders or may be a primary hyperlipidemic disorder (Box 6-8). The insulin resistance caused by hypertriglyceridemia is most commonly appreciated in diabetic dogs that develop hypothyroidism and in diabetic Miniature Schnauzers with idiopathic hyperlipidemia but should be considered in any poorly-controlled diabetic dog with persistent lipemia (Xenoulis et al, 2011). Unfortunately, hypertriglyceridemia is common in poorly-regulated diabetic dogs, and the differentiation between hypertriglyceridemia caused by poorly controlled diabetes versus hypertriglyceridemia that has developed independent of the diabetic state can be difficult. As a general rule, serum triglyceride concentrations in poorly-controlled diabetics are usually less than 500 mg/dL. Serum triglyceride concentrations in excess of 500 mg/dL, especially 800 mg/dL, should raise suspicion for a concurrent disorder causing the hypertriglyceridemia, most notably pancreatitis, hypothyroidism, and primary hyperlipidemic disorders. Restriction of dietary fat is the cornerstone of therapy for hypertriglyceridemia.

CHRONIC COMPLICATIONS OF DIABETES MELLITUS

Complications resulting from diabetes, its treatment, or affiliated disorders are common in diabetic dogs and include blindness and anterior uveitis resulting from cataract formation, diabetic retinopathy (retinal hemorrhage, microaneurysms), hypoglycemia, chronic pancreatitis, recurring infections, poor glycemic control, and ketoacidosis (see Table 6-4). Many owners are hesitant to treat their newly diagnosed diabetic dog because of knowledge regarding chronic complications experienced in human diabetics and concern that a similar fate awaits their pet. However, clients should be assured that the devastating chronic complications of human diabetes (e.g., nephropathy, neuropathy, vasculopathy) require years to develop and become clinical and therefore are uncommon in diabetic dogs. Diabetes mellitus is a disease of older dogs and most do not live beyond 5 years from the time of diagnosis (Fall et al, 2007). In our experience, owners are usually willing to "tackle" the care of their diabetic dog once the fears related to chronic complications seen in human diabetics are alleviated and assurances are made that administering insulin is easy and dogs are very tolerant of insulin injections.

BOX 6-8   Causes of Hyperlipidemia in Dogs and Cats

Postprandial hyperlipidemia
Primary hyperlipidemia
   Idiopathic hyperlipoproteinemia (Miniature Schnauzers)
   Idiopathic hyperchylomicronemia (cats)
   Lipoprotein lipase deficiency (cats)
   Idiopathic hypercholesterolemia
Secondary hyperlipidemia
   Hypothyroidism
   Diabetes mellitus
   Hyperadrenocorticism
   Pancreatitis
   Cholestasis
   Hepatic insufficiency
   Nephrotic syndrome
   Drug-induced hyperlipidemia
     Glucocorticoids
     Progestagens (cats)

Chronic hyperglycemia is the central initiating factor for all types of microvascular complications in diabetic humans. The duration and severity of hyperglycemia is strongly correlated with the extent and progression of diabetic microvascular disease. Although all cells are exposed to hyperglycemia, hyperglycemic damage is limited to those cell types (e.g., endothelial cells in the retina, glomerulus, and nerve vasa nervosum) that develop intracellular hyperglycemia (Brownlee et al, 2011). The common pathophysiologic feature of diabetic microvascular disease is progressive narrowing and eventual occlusion of vascular lumina, which results in inadequate perfusion and function of affected tissues and microvascular cell loss.

Four major hypotheses for how hyperglycemia causes diabetic complications have been extensively studied and are listed here: (1) increased polyol pathway flux involving aldose reductase and sorbitol, (2) increased intracellular formation of advanced glycation end products, (3) activation of protein kinase C, and (4) increased hexosamine pathway flux with increased shunting of glucose into the hexosamine pathway (Brownlee et al, 2011). All four of these different pathogenic mechanisms reflect a single hyperglycemia-induced process: overproduction of superoxide by the mitochondrial electron transport chain. Hyperglycemia increases the production of reactive oxygen species, which inhibits the activity of a key glycolytic enzyme (glyceraldehyde-3-phosphate dehydrogenase). Inhibition of this enzyme results in the upstream accumulation of glycolytic intermediates which, in turn, activate each of the four proposed mechanisms. The pathophysiologic mechanisms for chronic complications in diabetic dogs have been poorly characterized but are assumed to be comparable to those in diabetic humans.

Cataracts

Cataract formation is the most common long-term complication of diabetes mellitus in the dog (see Fig. 6-4). A retrospective-cohort study on the development of cataracts in 132 diabetic dogs referred to a university referral hospital found cataract formation in 14% of dogs at the time diabetes was diagnosed and a time interval for 25%, 50%, 75%, and 80% of the study population to develop cataracts at 60, 170, 370, and 470 days, respectively (Beam et al, 1999). The pathogenesis of diabetic cataract formation is thought to be related to altered osmotic relationships in the lens induced by the accumulation of sorbitol and galactitol, which are sugar alcohols that are produced following reduction of glucose and galactose by the enzyme aldose reductase in the lens. Sorbitol and galactitol are potent hydrophilic agents and cause an influx of water into the lens, leading to swelling and rupture of the lens fibers and the development of cataracts (Richter et al, 2002). Cataract formation is an irreversible process once it begins, and it can occur quite rapidly. Diabetic dogs that are poorly controlled and have problems with wide fluctuations in the blood glucose concentration seem especially at risk for rapid development of cataracts. Good glycemic control and minimal fluctuation in the blood glucose concentration prolongs the onset of cataract formation. Once blindness occurs as a result of cataract formation, the need for stringent blood glucose control is reduced.

Blindness may be eliminated by removing the abnormal lens. Vision is restored in approximately 80% of diabetic dogs that undergo cataract removal (Appel et al, 2006; Sigle and Nasisse, 2006). Factors that affect the success of surgery include the degree of glycemic control preceding surgery, presence of retinal disease, and presence of lens-induced uveitis. Acquired retinal degeneration affecting vision is more of a concern in older diabetic dogs than is diabetic retinopathy. Fortunately, acquired retinal degeneration is unlikely in an older diabetic dog with vision immediately before cataract formation. If available, electroretinography should be performed before surgery to evaluate retinal function.

In a study by Kador, et al., (2010), the topical administration of the aldose reductase inhibitor Kinostat significantly delayed the onset and/or progression of cataracts in dogs with diabetes mellitus during a 12-month period. If Kinostat becomes available commercially, it may offer a medical option for preventing or slowing the formation of cataracts in diabetic dogs.

Lens-Induced Uveitis

During embryogenesis, the lens is formed within its own capsule and its structural proteins are not exposed to the immune system. Therefore, immune tolerance to the crystalline proteins does not develop (van der Woerdt et al, 1992). During cataract formation and reabsorption, lens proteins are exposed to local ocular immune system, resulting in inflammation and uveitis. Uveitis that occurs in association with a reabsorbing, hypermature cataract may decrease the success of cataract surgery and must be controlled before surgery (Bagley and Lavach, 1994). The treatment of lens-induced uveitis focuses on decreasing the inflammation and preventing further intraocular damage. Topical ophthalmic glucocorticoids (e.g., prednisone acetate) are the most commonly used drugs for the control of ocular inflammation. However, systemic absorption of topically applied glucocorticoids may cause insulin resistance and interfere with glycemic control of the diabetic state, especially in toy and miniature breeds. An alternative is the topical administration of nonsteroidal anti-inflammatory agents, such as diclofenac (Voltaren) or flurbiprofen ophthalmic (Ocufen). Although not as potent an anti-inflammatory agent as glucocorticoids, nonsteroidal anti-inflammatory drugs should not interfere with glycemic control.

Corneal Ulceration

Diabetes mellitus has been associated with pathologic changes in the corneas of dogs, which are directly related to the degree of diabetic control (Yee et al, 1985), and a significant reduction in corneal sensitivity in all regions of the cornea has been documented in diabetic dogs, compared with non-diabetic normoglycemic dogs (Good et al, 2003). Corneal nerves are critical for eliciting and regulating corneal protection via their role in the mediation of tear production and eyelid closure and regulation of corneal collagen expression and epithelial cell function and integrity (Baker et al, 1993; Marfurt, 2000). Corneal sensory deficits are thought to be a component of the diffuse neuropathy affecting the peripheral sensorimotor nervous system of diabetic humans and animals and may have important implications regarding corneal healing and the development of recurrent or nonhealing corneal ulcers in diabetic dogs.

Diabetic Retinopathy

Diabetic retinopathy in the dog is characterized histologically by damage to the retinal vasculature and retinal neurons, specifically degeneration of retinal ganglion cells (Howell et al, 2013). Ophthalmoscopically identifiable retinal hemorrhages and microaneurysms are considered the maker for diabetic retinopathy in dogs. Additional ophthalmoscopic findings include dilatation and tortuosity of retinal venules, hyper-reflectivity of the tapetal portion of the retina, and chorioretinal exudates. In one study, 11 of 52 (21%) diabetic dogs developed ophthalmoscopic signs of retinal hemorrhages or microaneurysms, compared with 1 of 17 (0.6%) non-diabetic dogs (Landry et al, 2004). Median time from diagnosis of diabetes to diagnosis of retinopathy was 1.4 years (range, 0.5 to 3.2 years). Histologic changes include an increased thickness of the capillary basement membrane, loss of pericytes, capillary shunts, and microaneurysms. The cause of diabetic retinopathy is probably multifactorial and may involve biochemical changes secondary to hyperglycemia and increased aldose reductase activity, advanced glycation end products, hemodynamic alterations, and vascular endothelial and pericyte loss (Merimee, 1990; Stitt, 2003). Risk factors for development of diabetic retinopathy have been poorly characterized in diabetic dogs, although status of glycemic control may be associated with progression of diabetic retinopathy (Engerman and Kern, 1987). Retinal ganglion cell degeneration is significantly inhibited by good to moderate glycemic control in diabetic dogs (Howell et al, 2013). Loss of vision is uncommon in dogs with diabetic retinopathy.

Unfortunately, the rapid development of cataracts often inhibits the ability to evaluate the retina in the dog with diabetes mellitus. Because of the high incidence of cataract formation, the retinas should always be evaluated in the newly-diagnosed diabetic pet to ensure normal function and lack of grossly visible disease should cataract formation and subsequent lens removal become necessary in the future. Lens removal would be unwarranted in a diabetic dog with retinal changes sufficiently severe to result in blindness itself. An electroretinogram can also be used to evaluate the function of the retina prior to cataract surgery.

Diabetic Neuropathy

Although a common complication in diabetic cats, diabetic neuropathy is infrequently recognized in the diabetic dog (Braund and Steiss, 1982; Johnson et al, 1983; Katherman and Braund, 1983; Morgan et al, 2008). Diabetic neuropathy in the dog is primarily a distal polyneuropathy, characterized by segmental demyelination and remyelination and axonal degeneration. Subclinical neuropathy is more common than severe neuropathy resulting in clinical signs. Clinical signs consistent with diabetic neuropathy are most commonly recognized in dogs that have been diabetic for a long period of time (i.e., 5 years or longer), although dogs have been diagnosed with diabetic neuropathy shortly after the diagnosis of diabetes is established (Morgan et al, 2008). Clinical signs and physical examination findings suggestive of diabetic neuropathy include pelvic limb paresis, abnormal gait, decreased muscle tone, muscle atrophy, depressed limb reflexes, and deficits in postural reaction testing. Electrodiagnostic abnormalities include spontaneous sharp waves and fibrillation potentials and decreased M-wave amplitude on electromyogram, suggestive of axonal disease, and decreased motor and sensory nerve conduction velocities, suggestive of demyelinating disease (Steiss et al, 1981; Boulton et al, 2005; Morgan et al, 2008). There is no specific treatment for diabetic neuropathy besides meticulous metabolic control of the diabetic state. See Chapter 7 for more information on diabetic neuropathy.

Diabetic Nephropathy

Diabetic nephropathy has occasionally been reported in the dog. Diabetic nephropathy is a microvascular disease involving the capillary and precapillary arterioles and is manifested mainly by thickening of the capillary basement membrane. Histopathologic findings include membranous glomerulonephropathy, glomerular and tubular basement membrane thickening, an increase in the mesangial matrix material, the presence of subendothelial deposits, glomerular fibrosis, and glomerulosclerosis (Steffes et al, 1982; Jeraj et al, 1984). Glucose plays a central role in the development of microvascular damage. Clinical signs depend on the severity of glomerulosclerosis and the functional ability of the kidney to excrete metabolic wastes. Initially, diabetic nephropathy is manifested as proteinuria, primarily albuminuria. As glomerular changes progress, glomerular filtration becomes progressively impaired, resulting in the development of azotemia and eventually uremia. With severe fibrosis of the glomeruli, oliguric and anuric kidney failure develop.

Monitoring urine for the presence of microalbuminuria is used as an early marker for development of diabetic nephropathy in diabetic humans. Microalbuminuria occurs in diabetic dogs and increased urine albumin-to-creatine ratios precede increased urine protein-to-creatinine ratios. In one study, 11 (55%) of 20 diabetic dogs had an increase in the urine albumin-to-creatinine ratio and only 6 of these 11 dogs also had an increase in urine protein-to-creatinine ratio, suggesting that monitoring urine albumin-to-creatinine ratio may be of value as an early marker for kidney disease in diabetic dogs (Mazzi et al, 2008). However, the predictive value of microalbuminuria for diabetic nephropathy and the clinical relevance of microalbuminuria in diabetic dogs remains to be clarified. Diabetic nephropathy is a significant chronic complication in diabetic humans that takes years to progress to chronic end-stage kidney disease; a time line that may explain why clinically relevant diabetic nephropathy is uncommon in diabetic dogs. Presumably in most dogs, diabetes mellitus and CKD develop as independent events in aged dogs.

Regardless, proteinuria, kidney function, and systemic blood pressure should be monitored in diabetic dogs that have developed microalbuminuria. There is no specific treatment for diabetic nephropathy apart from meticulous metabolic control of the diabetic state, conservative medical management of the kidney disease, administration of angiotensin converting enzyme (ACE) inhibitors to minimize proteinuria, and control of systemic hypertension.

Systemic Hypertension

Diabetes mellitus and hypertension commonly coexist in dogs. Struble et al. (1998) found the prevalence of hypertension to be 46% in 50 insulin-treated diabetic dogs, in which hypertension was defined as systolic, diastolic, or mean blood pressure greater than 160, 100, and 120 mm Hg, respectively. Median (range) systolic, diastolic, and mean blood pressure in the hypertensive diabetic dogs were 175 (160 to 205) mmHg, 112 (101 to 150) mmHg, and 132 (120 to 186) mmHg, respectively. The development of hypertension was associated with the duration of diabetes and an increased albumin-to-creatinine ratio in the urine. Diastolic and mean blood pressure were higher in dogs with longer duration of disease. A correlation between control of glycemia and blood pressure was not identified. Systemic hypertension may result from existing subclinical kidney disease or develop secondary to the effects of diabetes on vascular compliance, glomerular function, or some other mechanism (Dukes, 1992). Treatment for hypertension should be initiated if the systolic blood pressure is consistently greater than 160 mm Hg.

 PROGNOSIS

The prognosis for dogs diagnosed with diabetes mellitus depends, in part, on owner commitment to treating the disorder, ease of glycemic regulation, presence and reversibility of concurrent disorders, avoidance of chronic complications associated with the diabetic state, and minimization of the impact of treatment on the quality of life of the owner (see Table 6-5). In a large study involving insured dogs in Sweden, the median survival time after the first diabetes mellitus claim (686 dogs) was 57 days and for dogs surviving at least 1 day (463 dogs) was 2.0 years (Fall et al, 2007). For dogs surviving at least 30 days after the first diabetes mellitus claim (347 dogs), the proportion of dogs surviving 1, 2, and 3 years was 40%, 36%, and 33%, respectively. However, survival times vary between countries and between socioeconomic regions within a country, and survival time is somewhat skewed because dogs are often 8 to 12 years old at the time of diagnosis; a relatively high mortality rate exists during the first 6 months because of concurrent life-threatening or uncontrollable disease (e.g., ketoacidosis, acute pancreatitis, kidney failure). In our experience, diabetic dogs that survive the first 6 months can easily maintain a good quality of life for longer than 5 years with proper care by the owners, timely evaluations by the veterinarian, and good client-veterinarian communication.

REFERENCES

Affenzeller N, et al.: Home-based subcutaneous continuous glucose monitoring in 10 diabetic dogs, *Vet Rec* 169:206, 2011.

Alejandro R, et al.: Advances in canine diabetes mellitus research: etiopathology and results of islet transplantation, *J Am Vet Med Assoc* 193:1050, 1988.

Andersen MK, et al.: Latent autoimmune diabetes in adults differs genetically from classical type 1 diabetes diagnosed after the age of 35 years, *Diabetes Care* 33:3062, 2010.

Anderson RA: Chromium, glucose tolerance, and diabetes, *Biol Trace Element Res* 32:19, 1992.

Anderson RA, et al.: Elevated intakes of supplemental chromium improve glucose and insulin variables in individuals with type 2 diabetes, *Diabetes* 46:1786, 1997.

Appel SL, et al.: Evaluation of client perceptions concerning outcome of cataract surgery in dogs, *J Am Vet Med Assoc* 228:870, 2006.

Appleton DJ, et al.: Insulin sensitivity decreases with obesity, and lean cats with low insulin sensitivity are at greatest risk of glucose intolerance with weight gain, *J Feline Med Surg* 3:211, 2001.

Bagley LH, Lavach JD: Comparison of postoperative phacoemulsification results in dogs with and without diabetes mellitus: 153 cases (1991-1992), *J Am Vet Med Assoc* 205:1165, 1994.

Baker KS, et al.: Trigeminal ganglion neurons affect corneal epithelial phenotype: influence of type VII collagen expression in vitro, *Invest Ophthalmol Vis Sci* 34:137, 1993.

Barrett KE, et al.: *Ganong's review of medical physiology*, ed 24, New York, 2012, McGraw-Hill Lange.

Bauer JE: Lipoprotein-mediated transport of dietary and synthesized lipids and lipid abnormalities of dogs and cats, *J Am Vet Med Assoc* 224:668, 2004.

Beam S, et al.: A retrospective-cohort study on the development of cataracts in dogs with diabetes mellitus: 200 cases, *Vet Ophthalmology* 2:169, 1999.

Berlinger JA, et al.: Lipoprotein-induced insulin resistance in aortic endothelium, *Diabetes* 33:1039, 1984.

Bieger WP, et al.: Diminished insulin receptors on monocytes and erythrocytes in hypertriglyceridemia, *Metabolism* 33:982, 1984.

Bolli GB, et al.: Abnormal glucose counterregulation after subcutaneous insulin in insulin-dependent diabetes mellitus, *N Engl J Med* 310:1706, 1984.

Bostrom BM, et al.: Chronic pancreatitis in dogs: a retrospective study of clinical, clinicopathological, and histopathological findings in 61 cases, *Vet J* 195:73, 2013.

Boulton AJM, et al.: Diabetic neuropathies: a statement by the American Diabetes Association, *Diabetes Care* 28:956, 2005.

Braund KG, Steiss JE: Distal neuropathy in spontaneous diabetes mellitus in the dog, *Acta Neuropathol (Berl)* 57:263, 1982.

Briggs C, et al.: Reliability of history and physical examination findings for assessing control of glycemia in dogs with diabetes mellitus: 53 cases (1995-1998), *J Am Vet Med Assoc* 217:48, 2000.

Brownlee M, et al.: Complications of diabetes mellitus. In Melmed S, Polonsky KS, Larsen PR, Kronenberg HM, editors: *Williams textbook of endocrinology*, ed 12, St Louis, 2011, Elsevier Saunders, p 1462.

Catchpole B, et al.: Genetics of canine diabetes mellitus: are the diabetes susceptibility genes identified in humans involved in breed susceptibility to diabetes mellitus in dogs? *Vet J* 195:129, 2013.

Cohen TA, et al.: Evaluation of six portable blood glucose meters for measuring blood glucose concentrations in dogs, *J Am Vet Med Assoc* 235:276, 2009.

Cohn LA, et al.: Assessment of five portable blood glucose meters, a point-of-care analyzer, and color test strips for measuring blood glucose concentration in dogs, *J Am Vet Med Assoc* 216:198, 2000.

Crenshaw KL, et al.: Serum fructosamine concentration as an index of glycemia in cats with diabetes mellitus and stress hyperglycemia, *J Vet Intern Med* 10:360, 1996.

Cryer PE, Polonsky KS: Glucose homeostasis and hypoglycemia. In Wilson JD, Foster DW, Kronenberg HM, Larsen PR, editors: *Williams textbook of endocrinology*, ed 9, Philadelphia, 1998, WB Saunders, p 939.

Davidson JK, et al.: Insulin therapy. In Davidson JK, editor: *Clinical diabetes mellitus: a problem oriented approach*, New York, 1991, Thieme Medical Publishers, p 266.

Davison LJ, et al.: Anti-insulin antibodies in dogs with naturally occurring diabetes mellitus, *Vet Immunol Immunopath* 91:53, 2003a.

Davison LJ, et al.: Evaluation of a continuous glucose monitoring system in diabetic dogs, *J Small Anim Pract* 44:435, 2003b.

Davison LJ, et al.: Study of 253 dogs in the United Kingdom with diabetes mellitus, *Vet Rec* 156:467, 2005.

Davison LJ, et al.: autoantibodies to GAD65 and IA-2 in canine diabetes mellitus, *Vet Immunol Immunopath* 126:83, 2008a.

Davison LJ, et al.: Anti-insulin antibodies in diabetic dogs before and after treatment with different insulin preparations, *J Vet Intern Med* 22:1317, 2008b.

Davison LJ, et al.: Autoantibodies to recombinant canine proinsulin in canine diabetic patients, *Res Vet Sci* 91:58, 2011.

Della-Maggiore A, et al.: Efficacy of protamine zinc recombinant human insulin for controlling hyperglycemia in dogs with diabetes mellitus, *J Vet Intern Med* 26:109, 2012.

Dietiker-Moretti S, et al.: Comparison of a continuous glucose monitoring system with a portable blood glucose meter to determine insulin dose in cats with diabetes mellitus, *J Vet Intern Med* 25:1084, 2011.

Duesberg C, et al.: Impaired counterregulatory response to insulin-induced hypoglycemia in diabetic dogs (abstract), *J Vet Intern Med* 9:181, 1995.

Dukes J: Hypertension: a review of the mechanisms, manifestations and management, *J Small Anim Pract* 33:119, 1992.

Eckel RH: Lipoprotein lipase: a multifunctional enzyme relevant to common metabolic diseases, *N Engl J Med* 320:1060, 1989.

Eidemak I, et al.: Insulin resistance and hyperinsulinaemia in mild to moderate progressive chronic renal failure and its association with aerobic work capacity, *Diabetologia* 38:565, 1995.

Elliott DA, et al.: Glycosylated hemoglobin concentrations in the blood of healthy dogs and dogs with naturally developing diabetes mellitus, pancreatic beta-cell neoplasia hyperadrenocorticism, and anemia, *J Am Vet Med Assoc* 211:723, 1997.

Elliott DA, et al.: Comparison of serum fructosamine and blood glycosylated hemoglobin concentrations for assessment of glycemic control in cats with diabetes mellitus, *J Am Vet Med Assoc* 214:1794, 1999.

Elliott KF, et al.: A diet lower in digestible carbohydrate results in lower postprandial glucose concentrations compared with a traditional canine diabetes diet and an adult maintenance diet in healthy dogs, *Res Vet Sci* 93:288, 2012.

Engerman RL, Kern TS: Progression of incipient diabetic retinopathy during good glycemic control, *Diabetes* 36:808, 1987.

Fall T, et al.: Diabetes mellitus in a population of 180,000 insured dogs: incidence, survival, and breed distribution, *J Vet Intern Med* 21:1209, 2007.

Fall T, et al.: Glucagon stimulation test for estimating endogenous insulin secretion in dogs, *Vet Rec* 163:266, 2008a.

Fall T, et al.: Gestational diabetes mellitus in 13 dogs, *J Vet Intern Med* 22:1296, 2008b.

Fall T, et al.: Diabetes mellitus in Elkhounds is associated with diestrus and pregnancy, *J Vet Intern Med* 24:1322, 2010.

Feldman EC, Nelson RW: Insulin-induced hyperglycemia in diabetic dogs, *J Am Vet Med Assoc* 180:1432, 1982.

Fernqvist E, et al.: Effects of physical exercise on insulin absorption in insulin-dependent diabetics: a comparison between human and porcine insulin, *Clin Physiol* 6:489, 1986.

Fleeman LM, et al.: Pharmacokinetics and pharmacodynamics of porcine insulin zinc suspension in eight diabetic dogs, *Vet Rec* 164:232, 2009a.

Fleeman LM, et al.: Lack of advantage of high-fibre, moderate-carbohydrate diets in dogs with stabilised diabetes, *J Small Anim Pract* 50:604, 2009b.

Ford SL, et al.: Insulin resistance in three dogs with hypothyroidism and diabetes mellitus, *J Am Vet Med Assoc* 202:1478, 1993.

Ford SL, et al.: *Evaluation of detemir insulin in diabetic dogs managed with home blood glucose monitoring, Proceedings*, ACVIM Forum, Anaheim, CA, 2010, p 442.

Forman MA, et al.: Evaluation of serum pancreatic lipase immunoreactivity and helical computed tomography versus conventional testing for the diagnosis of feline pancreatitis, *J Vet Intern Med* 18:807, 2004.

Fracassi F, et al.: Breed distribution of canine diabetes mellitus in Italy, *Vet Res Commun* 28:339, 2004.

Fracassi F, et al.: Use of insulin glargine in dogs with diabetes mellitus, *Vet Rec* 170:52, 2012.

Galante P, et al.: Acute hyperglycemia provides an insulin-independent inducer for GLUT4 translocation in C_2C_{12} myotubes and rat skeletal muscle, *Diabetes* 44:646, 1995.

Galloway JA: Chemistry and clinical use of insulin. In Galloway JA, et al., editors: *Diabetes mellitus*, Indianapolis, 1988, Eli Lilly, p 105.

Garg A, Grundy SM: Management of dyslipidemia in NIDDM, *Diabetes Care* 13:153, 1990.

Gayet C, et al.: Insulin resistance and changes in plasma concentration of TNF, IGF-1, and NEFA in dogs during weight gain and obesity, *J Anim Physiolo Anim Nutr* 88:157, 2004.

Gerich JE: Is reduced first-phase insulin release the earliest detectable abnormality in individuals destined to develop type 2 diabetes? *Diabetes* 51(suppl):S117, 2002.

German AJ, et al.: Improvement in insulin resistance and reduction in plasma inflammatory adipokines after weight loss in obese dogs, *Domest Anim Endocrinol* 37:214, 2009.

Good KL, et al.: Corneal sensitivity in dogs with diabetes mellitus, *Am J Vet Res* 64:7, 2003.

Graham PA, et al.: Canned high fiber diet and postprandial glycemia in dogs with naturally occurring diabetes mellitus, *J Nutri* 124:2712S, 1994.

Graham PA, et al.: Pharmacokinetics of a porcine insulin zinc suspension in diabetic dogs, *J Small Anim Pract* 38:434, 1997.

Gross KL, et al.: Dietary chromium and carnitine supplementation does not affect glucose tolerance in obese dogs (abstr), *J Vet Intern Med* 14:345, 2000.

Guptill L, et al: Time trends and risk factors for diabetes mellitus in dogs: analysis of veterinary medical data base records (1970-1999), *Vet J* 165:240, 2003.

Haataja L, et al.: Islet amyloid in type 2 diabetes, and the toxic oligomer hypothesis, *Endocr Rev* 29:303, 2008.

Haines DM: A re-examination of islet cell cytoplasmic antibodies in diabetic dogs, *Vet Immunol Immunopathol* 11:225, 1986.

Hamilton-Wessler M, et al.: Mechanism of protracted metabolic effects of fatty acid acylated insulin, NN304, in dogs: retention of NN304 by albumin, *Diabetologia* 42:1254, 1999.

Hasegawa S, et al.: Glycated hemoglobin fractions in normal and diabetic dogs measured by high performance liquid chromatography, *J Vet Med Sci* 53:65, 1991.

Hasegawa S, et al.: Glycated hemoglobin fractions in normal and diabetic cats measured by high performance liquid chromatography, *J Vet Med Sci* 54:789, 1992.

Hess RS, Ward CR: Effect of insulin dosage on glycemic response in dogs with diabetes mellitus: 221 cases (1993-1998), *J Am Vet Med Assoc* 216:217, 2000.

Hess RS, et al.: Breed distribution of dogs with diabetes mellitus admitted to a tertiary care facility, *J Am Vet Med Assoc* 216:1414, 2000a.

Hess RS, et al.: Concurrent disorders in dogs with diabetes mellitus: 221 cases (1993-1998), *J Am Vet Med Assoc* 217:1166, 2000b.

Hess RS, et al.: Association between hypothyroidism, diabetes mellitus, and hyperadrenocorticism and development of atherosclerosis in dogs (abstract), *J Vet Intern Med* 16:360, 2002.

Hirsch IB: Insulin analogues, *N Engl J Med* 352:174, 2005.

Hoenig M, Dawe DL: A qualitative assay for beta cell antibodies: preliminary results in dogs with diabetes mellitus, *Vet Immunol Immunopathol* 32:195, 1992.

Hofer-Inteeworn N, et al.: Effect of hypothyroidism on insulin sensitivity and glucose tolerance in dogs, *Am J Vet Res* 73:529, 2012.

Home PD: The pharmacokinetics and pharmacodynamics of rapid-acting insulin analogues and their clinical consequences, *Diabetes Obes Metab* 14:780, 2012.

Howell SJ, et al.: Degeneration of retinal ganglion cells in diabetic dogs and mice: relationship to glycemic control and retinal capillary degeneration, *Mol Vision* 19:1413, 2013.

Howey DC, et al.: [Lys(B28), Pro(B29)]-human insulin: a rapidly absorbed analog of human insulin, *Diabetes* 43:396, 1994.

Jain NC: Erythrocyte physiology and changes in disease. In Jain NC, editor: *Essentials of veterinary hematology*, Philadelphia, 1993, Saunders.

Jensen AL: Serum fructosamine in canine diabetes mellitus: an initial study, *Vet Res Commun* 16:1, 1992.

Jeraj K, et al.: Immunofluorescence studies of renal basement membranes in dogs with spontaneous diabetes, *Am J Vet Res* 45:1162, 1984.

Johnson CA, et al.: Peripheral neuropathy and hypotension in a diabetic dog, *J Am Vet Med Assoc* 183:1007, 1983.

Kador PF, et al.: Topical KINOSTAT™ ameliorates the clinical development and progression of cataracts in dogs with diabetes mellitus, *Vet Ophthalmol* 13:363, 2010.

Kaiyala KJ, et al.: Reduced beta-cell function contributes to impaired glucose tolerance in dogs made obese by high-fat feeding, *Am J Physiol* 277:E659–E667, 1999.

Karam JH: Hypoglycemic disorders. In Greenspan FS, Gardner DG, editors: *Basic and clinical endocrinology*, ed 6, New York, 2001, Lange Medical Books/McGraw-Hill, p 699.

Katherman AE, Braund KG: Polyneuropathy associated with diabetes mellitus in a dog, *J Am Vet Med Assoc* 182:522, 1983.

Kawamoto M, et al.: Relation of fructosamine to serum protein, albumin, and glucose concentrations in healthy and diabetic dogs, *Am J Vet Res* 53:851, 1992.

Kennedy LJ, et al.: Identification of susceptibility and protective major histocompatibility complex haplotypes in canine diabetes mellitus, *Tissue Antigens* 68:467, 2006.

Kharroubi I, et al.: Expression of adiponectin receptors in pancreatic beta cells, *Biochem Biophys Res Commun* 312:1118, 2003.

Kurtz AB, et al.: Circulating IgG antibody to protamine in patients treated with protamine insulins, *Diabetologia* 25:322, 1983.

Lahtela JT, et al.: Severe antibody-mediated human insulin resistance: successful treatment with the insulin analog lispro, *Diabetes Care* 20:71, 1997.

Landry MP, et al.: Funduscopic findings following cataract extraction by means of phacoemulsification in diabetic dogs: 52 cases (1993-2003), *J Am Vet Med Assoc* 225:709, 2004.

Lenox CE, et al.: Effects of glucosamine-chondroitin sulfate supplementation on serum fructosamine concentration in healthy dogs, *J Am Vet Med Assoc* 236:183, 2010.

Li S, et al.: Adiponectin levels and risk of type 2 diabetes: a systematic review and meta-analysis, *J Am Vet Med Assoc* 302:179, 2009.

Lindholm A, et al.: Improved postprandial glycemic control with insulin aspart: a randomized double-blind cross-over trial in type 1 diabetes, *Diabetes Care* 22:801, 1999.

Lindholm A, et al.: Immune responses to insulin aspart and biphasic insulin aspart in people with type 1 and type 2 diabetes, *Diabetes Care* 25:876, 2002.

Lorenzen FH: The use of isophane insulin for the control of diabetes mellitus in dogs, *Acta Vet Scand* 33:219, 1992.

Loste A, Marca MC: Study of the effect of total serum protein and albumin concentrations on canine fructosamine concentration, *Can J Vet Res* 63:138, 1999.

Mahaffey EA, Cornelius LM: Evaluation of a commercial kit for measurement of glycosylated hemoglobin in canine blood, *Vet Clin Path* 10:21, 1981.

Mahaffey EA, Cornelius LM: Glycosylated hemoglobin in diabetic and nondiabetic dogs, *J Am Vet Med Assoc* 180:635, 1982.

Marca MC, Loste A: Glycosylated haemoglobin in dogs: study of critical difference value, *Res Vet Sci* 71:115, 2001.

Marca MC, et al.: Blood glycated hemoglobin evaluation in sick dogs, *Can J Vet Res* 64:141, 2000.

Mared M, et al.: Evaluation of circulating concentrations of glucose homeostasis biomarkers, progesterone, and growth hormone in healthy Elkhounds during anestrus and diestrus, *Am J Vet Res* 73:242, 2012.

Marfurt C: Nervous control of the cornea. In Burnstock G, Sillito AM, editors: *Nervous control of the eye*, Amsterdam, 2000, Harwood Academic Publishers, p 41.

Marshall MO, et al.: Development of insulin antibodies, metabolic control and B-cell function in newly diagnosed insulin dependent diabetic children treated with monocomponent human insulin or monocomponent porcine insulin, *Diabetes Res* 9:169, 1988.

Massillon D, et al.: Induction of hepatic glucose-6-phosphatase gene expression by lipid infusion, *Diabetes* 46:153, 1997.

Mazzi A, et al.: Ratio of urinary protein to creatinine and albumin to creatinine in dogs with diabetes mellitus and hyperadrenocorticism, *Vet Res Commun* 32:S299, 2008.

McCord K, et al.: A multi-institutional study evaluating the diagnostic utility of the spec cPL™ and SNAP® cPL™ in clinical acute pancreatitis in 84 dogs, *J Vet Intern Med* 26:888, 2012.

McGuire NC, et al.: Detection of occult urinary tract infections in dogs with diabetes mellitus, *J Am Anim Hosp Assoc* 38:541, 2002.

Merimee TJ: Diabetic retinopathy: a synthesis of perspectives, *N Engl J Med* 322:978, 1990.

Monroe WE, et al.: Efficacy and safety of a purified porcine insulin zinc suspension for managing diabetes mellitus in dogs, *J Vet Intern Med* 19:675, 2005.

Montgomery TM, et al.: Basal and glucagon-stimulated plasma C-peptide concentrations in healthy dogs, dogs with diabetes mellitus, and dogs with hyperadrenocorticism, *J Vet Intern Med* 10:116, 1996.

Moretti S, et al.: Evaluation of a novel real-time continuous glucose-monitoring system for use in cats, *J Vet Intern Med* 24:120, 2010.

Morgan MJ, et al.: Clinical peripheral neuropathy associated with diabetes mellitus in 3 dogs, *Can Vet J* 49:583, 2008.

Mori A, et al.: Comparison of time-action profiles of insulin glargine and NPH insulin in normal and diabetic dogs, *Vet Res Commun* 32:563, 2008.

Mori A, et al.: Comparison of glucose fluctuations between day- and night-time measured using a continuous glucose monitoring system in diabetic dogs, *J Vet Med Sci* 75:113, 2013.

Nell LJ, Thomas JW: Human insulin autoantibody fine specificity and H and L chain use, *J Immunol* 142:3063, 1989.

Nelson RW, et al.: Effects of dietary fiber supplementation on glycemic control in dogs with alloxan-induced diabetes mellitus, *Am J Vet Res* 52:2060, 1991.

Nelson RW, et al.: Effect of dietary insoluble fiber on control of glycemia in dogs with naturally acquired diabetes mellitus, *J Am Vet Med Assoc* 212:380, 1998.

Nelson RW, et al.: Effect of the alpha-glucosidase inhibitor acarbose on control of glycemia in dogs with naturally acquired diabetes mellitus, *J Am Vet Med Assoc* 216:1265, 2000.

Nerup J: On the pathogenesis of IDDM, *Diabetologia* 37(suppl 2):S82, 1994.

Nguyen P, et al.: Glycemic and insulinemic responses after ingestion of commercial foods in healthy dogs: influence of food composition, *J Nutr* 128:2654S, 1998.

Niessen SJM, et al.: Evaluation of a quality-of-life tool for dogs with diabetes mellitus, *J Vet Intern Med* 26:953, 2012.

Nishida Y, et al.: Effect of mild exercise training on glucose effectiveness in healthy men, *Diabetes Care* 24:1008, 2001.

Owens DR, et al.: Pharmacokinetics of ^{125}I-labeled insulin glargine (HOE901) in healthy men-comparison with NPH insulin and the influence of different subcutaneous injection sites, *Diabetes Care* 23:813, 2000.

Palm CA, et al.: An investigation of the action of neutral protamine Hagedorn human analogue insulin in dogs with naturally occurring diabetes mellitus, *J Vet Intern Med* 23:50, 2009.

Pastors JG, et al.: Psyllium fiber reduces rise in postprandial glucose and insulin concentrations in patients with non-insulin-dependent diabetes, *Am J Clin Nutr* 53:1431, 1991.

Paul AEH, et al.: Effect of hematocrit on accuracy of two point-of-care glucometers for use in dogs, *Am J Vet Res* 72:1204, 2011.

Peikes H, et al.: Dermatologic disorders in dogs with diabetes mellitus: 45 cases (1986-2000), *J Am Vet Med Assoc* 219:203, 2001.

Phillips SM, et al.: GLUT-1 and GLUT-4 after endurance training in humans, *Am J Physiol* 270:E456, 1996.

Pieber TR, et al.: Efficacy and safety of HOE 901 versus NPH insulin in patients with type 1 diabetes, *Diabetes Care* 23:157, 2000.

Poitout V, Robertson RP: Glucolipotoxicity: fuel excess and β-cell dysfunction, *Endocr Rev* 29:351, 2008.

Pöppl AG, et al.: Diabetes mellitus remission after resolution of inflammatory and progesterone-related conditions in bitches, *Res Vet Sci* 94:471, 2013.

Porte D: Beta-cells in type II diabetes mellitus, *Diabetes* 40:166, 1991.

Rakatzi I, et al.: Adiponectin counteracts cytokine- and fatty acid-induced apoptosis in the pancreatic beta-cell line INS-1, *Diabetologia* 47:249, 2004.

Rave K, et al.: Impact of diabetic nephropathy on pharmacodynamic and pharmacokinetic properties of insulin in type 1 diabetic patients, *Diabetes Care* 24:886, 2001.

Remillard RL: Nutritional management of diabetic dogs, *Compend Contin Educ Pract Vet* 21:699, 1999.

Reusch CE, Haberer B: Evaluation of fructosamine in dogs and cats with hypo- or hyperproteinaemia, azotaemia, hyperlipidaemia and hyperbilirubinaemia, *Vet Rec* 148:370, 2001.

Reusch CE, Tomsa K: Serum fructosamine concentration in cats with overt hyperthyroidism, *J Am Vet Med Assoc* 215:1297, 1999.

Reusch CE, et al.: Fructosamine: a new parameter for diagnosis and metabolic control in diabetic dogs and cats, *J Vet Int Med* 7:177, 1993.

Reusch CE, et al.: Serum fructosamine concentrations in dogs with hypothyroidism, *Vet Res Comm* 26:531, 2002.

Richter M, et al.: Aldose reductase activity and glucose-related opacities in incubated lenses from dogs and cats, *Am J Vet Res* 63:1591, 2002.

Robertson J, et al.: Effects of the alpha-glucosidase inhibitor acarbose on postprandial serum glucose and insulin concentrations in healthy dogs, *Am J Vet Res* 60:541, 1999.

Rosenstock J, et al.: Basal insulin glargine (HOE901) versus NPH insulin in patients with type 1 diabetes on multiple daily insulin regimens, *Diabetes Care* 23:1137, 2000.

Rosenstock J, et al.: Basal insulin therapy in type 2 diabetes: 28-week comparison of insulin glargine (HOE901) and NPH insulin, *Diabetes Care* 24:631, 2001.

Rossetti L, et al.: Glucose toxicity, *Diabetes Care* 13:610, 1990.

Roszler J: Herbs, supplements and vitamins: what to try, what to buy, *Diabetes views*, August:45, 2001.

Sako T, et al.: Time-action profiles of insulin detemir in normal and diabetic dogs, *Res Vet Sci* 90:396, 2011.

Schachter S, et al.: Oral chromium picolinate and control of glycemia in insulin-treated diabetic dogs, *J Vet Intern Med* 15:379, 2001.

Scheuner D, Kaufman RJ: The unfolded protein response: a pathway that links insulin demand with β-cell failure and diabetes, *Endocr Rev* 29:317, 2008.

Sears KW, et al.: Use of lispro insulin for treatment of diabetic ketoacidosis, *J Vet Emerg Critic Care* 22:211, 2012.

Semenkovich CF, et al.: Disorders of lipid metabolism. In Melmed S, Polonsky KS, Larsen PR, Kronenberg HM, editors: *Williams textbook of endocrinology*, ed 12, St Louis, 2011, Elsevier Saunders, p 1633.

Sigle SJ, Nasisse MP: Long-term complications after phacoemulsification for cataract removal in dogs: 172 cases (1995-2002), *J Am Vet Med Assoc* 228:74, 2006.

Spears JW, et al.: Influence of chromium on glucose metabolism and insulin sensitivity. In Reinhart GA, Carey DP, editors: *Recent advances in canine and feline nutrition*, Vol II. Wilmington, Ohio, 1998, Orange Frazer Press, p 97.

Steffes MW, et al.: Diabetic nephropathy in the uninephrectomized dog: microscopic lesions after one year, *Kidney Int* 21:721, 1982.

Steiss JE, et al.: Electrodiagnostic analysis of peripheral neuropathy in dogs with diabetes mellitus, *Am J Vet Res* 42:2061, 1981.

Stitt AW: The role of advanced glycation in the pathogenesis of diabetic retinopathy, *Exp Mol Pathol* 75:95, 2003.

Striffler JS, et al.: Chromium improves insulin response to glucose in rats, *Metabolism* 44:1314, 1995.

Struble AL, et al.: Systemic hypertension and proteinuria in dogs with naturally occurring diabetes mellitus, *J Am Vet Med Assoc* 213:822, 1998.

Stumvoll M, et al.: Renal glucose production and utilization: new aspects in humans, *Diabetologia* 40:749, 1997.

Thomas JW, et al.: Heterogeneity and specificity of human anti-insulin antibodies determined by isoelectric focusing, *J Immunol* 134:1048, 1985.

Thomas JW, et al.: Spectrotypic analysis of antibodies to insulin A and B chains, *Mol Immunol* 25:173, 1988.

Tiley HA, et al.: Effects of dexamethasone administration on insulin resistance and components of insulin signaling and glucose metabolism in equine skeletal muscle, *Am J Vet Res* 69:51, 2008.

Tilg H, Moschen AR: Adipocytokines: mediators linking adipose tissue, inflammation and immunity, *Nat Rev Immunol* 6:772, 2006.

Trivedi S, et al.: Sensitivity and specificity of canine pancreas-specific lipase (cPL) and other markers for pancreatitis in 70 dogs with and without histopathologic evidence of pancreatitis, *J Vet Intern Med* 25:1241, 2011.

van der Woerdt A, et al.: Lens-induced uveitis in dogs: 151 cases (1985-1990), *J Am Vet Med Assoc* 201:921, 1992.

Verkest KR, et al.: Evaluation of beta-cell sensitivity to glucose and first-phase insulin secretion in obese dogs, *Am J Vet Med* 72:357, 2011a.

Verkest KR, et al.: Distinct adiponectin profiles might contribute to differences in susceptibility to type 2 diabetes in dogs and humans, *Domest Anim Endocrinol* 41:67, 2011b.

Verkest KR, et al.: Spontaneously obese dogs exhibit greater postprandial glucose, triglyceride, and insulin concentrations than lean dogs, *Domest Anim Endocrinol* 42:103, 2012.

Vick MM, et al.: Effects of systemic inflammation on insulin sensitivity in horses and inflammatory cytokine expression in adipose tissue, *Am J Vet Res* 69:130, 2008.

Vuksan V, et al.: American ginseng (Panax quinquefolius L.) attenuates postprandial glycemia in a time-dependent but not dose-dependent manner in healthy individuals, *Am J Clin Nutr* 73:753, 2001.

Watson PJ, et al.: Observational study of 14 cases of chronic pancreatitis in dogs, *Vet Rec* 167:968, 2010.

Wess G, Reusch C: Evaluation of five portable blood glucose meters for use in dogs, *J Am Vet Med Assoc* 216:203, 2000a.

Wess G, Reusch C: Capillary blood sampling from the ear of dogs and cats and use of portable meters to measure glucose concentration, *J Small Anim Pract* 41:60, 2000b.

White NH, et al.: Identification of type I diabetic patients at increased risk for hypoglycemia during intensive therapy, *N Engl J Med* 308:485, 1983.

Wiberg ME, Westermarck E: Subclinical exocrine pancreatic insufficiency in dogs, *J Am Vet Med Assoc* 220:1183, 2002.

Wiberg ME, et al.: Serum trypsinlike immunoreactivity measurement for the diagnosis of subclinical exocrine pancreatic insufficiency, *J Vet Intern Med* 13:426, 1999.

Wiedmeyer CE, et al.: Continuous glucose monitoring in dogs and cats, *J Vet Intern Med* 22:2, 2008.

Wood AW, Smith JE: Elevation rate of glycosylated hemoglobins in dogs after induction of experimental diabetes mellitus, *Metab* 31:906, 1982.

Yamka RM, et al.: Identification of canine markers related to obesity and the effects of weight loss on the markers of interest, *Int J Apl Res Vet Med* 4:282, 2006.

Xenoulis PG, et al: Association of hypertriglyceridemia with insulin resistance in healthy Miniature Schnauzers, *J Am Vet Med Assoc* 238:1011, 2011.

Yee RW, et al.: Corneal endothelial changes in diabetic dogs, *Curr Eye Res* 4:759, 1985.

Zeugswetter F, et al.: Elevated fructosamine concentrations caused by IgA paraproteinemia in two dogs, *J Vet Sci* 11:359, 2010.

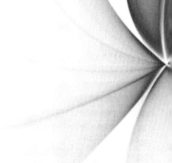

| # Feline Diabetes Mellitus

Claudia E. Reusch

CHAPTER CONTENTS

Diabetes mellitus in dogs and cats differs in a number of ways, which are important to consider for work-up and therapy. The majority of cats suffer a type of diabetes similar to type 2 in humans; in dogs, this type is extremely rare or may not exist at all. Unlike dogs, obesity is an important risk factor for the development of diabetes in cats; the difference is most likely associated with the different types of diabetes in the two species, because obesity and type 2 diabetes are closely related. A substantial percentage of cats with type 2 diabetes experience diabetic remission, and achievement of remission is nowadays one of the major treatment goals in diabetic cats. In dogs, however, remission is a very rare event, it usually only occurs after castration of a bitch with diestrus-associated diabetes. In cats, other endocrine disorders (e.g., hypersomatotropism and hyperadrenocorticism) are associated with the development of diabetes in most cases, whereas concurrent diabetes is relatively rare in dogs with

hyperadrenocorticism and variable in the case of hypersomatotropism. Cats are prone to stress hyperglycemia, which may cause difficulties in diagnosis and monitoring of the disease, whereas in dogs, stress associated increase in blood glucose is of minor importance. The so-called renal threshold for glucose absorption is higher in cats than in dogs, rendering measurement of urine glucose for monitoring purposes in diabetic cats even more problematic than in the dog. Diabetes-associated complications differ between the two species: diabetic cataract is rare in cats and common in dogs, whereas gait abnormalities due to diabetic neuropathy are common in cats and rare in dogs. Of note, both cataract and diabetic neuropathy also exist in the respective counterpart, however, usually at a subclinical level. Cats, but not dogs are obligate carnivores and therefore, dietary management is different. Last but not least, duration of effect of exogenous insulin in cats is often shorter than in dogs.

PREVALENCE AND RISK FACTORS IN HUMANS AND CATS

In humans, diabetes mellitus is one of the most common chronic diseases in nearly all countries (Whiting et al, 2011). Type 2 diabetes is the predominant form, which accounts for approximately 90% of cases worldwide. Type 2 has long been the disease of elderly people; however, this has changed substantially and nowadays more and more children and young adults are affected. Due to the dramatic increases in prevalence during the last few decades, diabetes has also been called a "new epidemic" (Kaufman, 2002). The International Diabetes Federation routinely publishes estimates of diabetes prevalence every 3 years starting in the year 2000. In 2011, there were 366 million people with diabetes, and the number is expected to rise to 552 million by 2030. Although the number differs between countries, every region of the world will have an increase well in excess of adult population growth (Whiting et al, 2011). Excessive caloric intake leading to obesity and sedentary lifestyle are known to be the major risk factors in humans; an increase in the incidence of obesity has always been paralleled by an increase in diabetes incidence. Aging, female sex, and belonging to certain racial and ethnic groups are additional critical factors. There is no doubt that diabetes has become one of the most important global health problems (Kaufman, 2002; Buse et al, 2011; Whiting et al, 2011).

As in humans, diabetes is a common disorder in cats. Different from human medicine, however, there are only limited data on the prevalence of the disease. Some recent publications provide a general overview of the current situation, although the methods of data collection differ. Most numbers reflect the proportion of diabetic cats in a particular practice or a hospital ("hospital prevalence") and not the situation in the field. A study from the United States reported an increase in hospital prevalence over 30 years from 0.08% in 1970 to 1.2% in 1999. At the same time, case fatality at the first visit decreased from 40% to 10% suggesting either improvement in treatment regimens or an increased willingness of owners to undertake long-term management (Prahl et al, 2007). Studies from Australia showed overall hospital prevalence (i.e., all cat breeds) of 0.55% and 0.74%; prevalence in the Burmese cats was much higher with 1.8% and 2.2%, respectively (Baral et al, 2003; Lederer et al, 2009). Recently, a non-hospital prevalence was evaluated in a large population of insured cats in the United Kingdom and was found to be 0.43%. Prevalence of diabetes in the Burmese cats was again higher with 1.8%, which compared well with the studies from Australia (McCann et al, 2007). As in humans, obesity is a major risk factor for diabetes in cats, and overweight cats are several times more likely to develop diabetes than optimal weight cats (Scarlet and Donoghue, 1998). Physical inactivity and indoor confinement, which is most likely associated with obesity ("sedentary lifestyle") as well as advancing age, have also been identified as important risk factors in cats. The overrepresentation of male cats within the feline diabetic population has been known for a long time and has been confirmed by various studies (Panciera et al, 1990; Crenshaw and Peterson, 1996; McCann et al, 2007; Prahl et al, 2007; Slingerland et al, 2009). The exception is the Burmese cat, for which a gender predisposition is less clear. A study performed in the United Kingdom did not identify male gender as a risk factor in the Burmese breed, whereas in the study from Australia, male Burmese cats were twice as likely to develop diabetes as were female Burmese cats (McCann et al, 2007; Lederer et al, 2009). The reason for the male predominance in most breeds has not yet been clarified. What is known is that insulin sensitivity is generally lower in normal male than in normal female cats and that cats with reduced insulin sensitivity have a higher risk of becoming glucose intolerant after weight gain. Male cats tend to gain more weight when fed ad libitum than female cats (Appleton et al, 2001). It is not clear if neutering is an independent risk factor, as one study found neutering (in both sexes) to be associated with an increased risk of diabetes, whereas another study did not find this association (McCann et al, 2007; Prahl et al, 2007). Neutered cats are at greater risk of gaining weight, and it is probably the increased risk of obesity that contributes to the development of diabetes (McCann et al, 2007). In the United States, no particular breed of cats appears to be associated with an increased risk for diabetes; in Australia, New Zealand, and the United Kingdom, however, the Burmese breed is known to be at increased risk (Panciera et al, 1990; Crenshaw and Peterson, 1996; Rand et al, 1997; Wade et al, 1999; McCann et al, 2007; Lederer et al, 2009). In a study using a large insured cat population in the United Kingdom, Burmese cats were approximately four times more likely to develop diabetes than non-pedigree cats. Data from New Zealand point to a genetic predisposition; the differences between the countries are most likely the result of different breeding programs and different lines within the Burmese breed (Wade et al, 1999; McCann, et al, 2007). Treatment with glucocorticoids or progestagens also increases the likelihood of the development of diabetes (Slingerland et al, 2009). In summary, many of the risk factors for development of diabetes are similar in humans and cats, including obesity, physical inactivity, and increasing age. Interestingly, however, the predominance in the male gender is unique to the cat. Although data are scarce, it is the impression of most endocrinologists that the incidence of diabetes in cats is increasing, which is most likely associated with the increased incidence of obesity, physical inactivity, and longevity.

CLASSIFICATION OF DIABETES MELLITUS

Traditionally, the classification of diabetes mellitus in cats has more or less followed the scheme used in human medicine. Although the etiopathogenic mechanisms may not be completely identical, the "human model" provides a guide for identification and differentiation of the various forms of the disease.

The first real attempt to classify human diabetes in a uniform way was done in 1965 by the World Health Organization (WHO) Expert Committee, recognizing that without a clear classification, it is difficult to take a systematic epidemiological approach to clinical research and develop evidence-based guidelines for therapy and prevention (George et al, 2011). At that time, little was known about the etiology of diabetes and the classification scheme contained somewhat confusing categories. The second report of the WHO Expert Committee in 1980 offered a classification that was widely accepted. Two main classes were introduced: insulin-dependent diabetes mellitus (IDDM) and non-insulin-dependent diabetes mellitus (NIDDM). Additional classes were other types and gestational diabetes mellitus. During the following years, understanding of the complex facets of the diabetic disease improved, leading to a new classification scheme that included both etiology and clinical stages. The categories were named type 1, type 2, other specific types, and gestational diabetes. It was suggested that the terms *insulin-dependent* and *non-insulin-dependent diabetes mellitus (IDDM, NIDDM)* should be abandoned, because they were considered confusing and frequently resulted in patients being classified on the basis of treatment rather than on etiopathogenesis (World Health Organization, 1999). Up until now, a few updates were made; however, there are no fundamental changes compared with the report in 1999 (George et al, 2011; American

Diabetes Association, 2013). Although the scheme is helpful, it is recognized that assigning a type of diabetes to an individual often depends on the circumstances present at the time of diagnosis, and individuals may not easily fit into one class. For instance, a person who becomes diabetic after receiving exogenous steroids may regain normoglycemia after the discontinuation of the drug, but may again develop diabetes after episodes of pancreatitis.

Similarly, a woman with gestational diabetes may continue to be diabetic after delivery and may in fact suffer from type 2 diabetes (American Diabetes Association, 2013). Box 7-1 lists the classification scheme according to etiology currently used in human medicine. Fig. 7-1 displays the clinical stages and their dynamics within the four types of diabetes.

Types of Diabetes in Humans

The discussion of the various types of diabetes is done separately for humans and cats; this will enable a better overview over the current state of knowledge in the two species. Many of the findings in humans may also be of importance for feline diabetes, and it is recommended to read the sections on humans prior to reading the feline sections.

Type 1 Diabetes Mellitus

Type 1 diabetes mellitus accounts for 5% to 10% of human cases and was previously known as IDDM or juvenile-onset diabetes. Although it is commonly seen in childhood and adolescence, it can occur at any age, even in the 8th or 9th decade of life. It most commonly (> 90%) results from cellular-mediated autoimmune destruction of the β-cells leading to failure of insulin synthesis (American Diabetes Association, 2013). The characteristic pathological lesion in the pancreas is the presence of mononuclear immune cells around and within the islets. This infiltration, also called *insulitis,* is dominated by T lymphocytes, in particular "cytotoxic" (cluster of differentiation 8 [CD8]) T lymphocytes; others are "helper" (cluster of differentiation 4 [CD4]) T lymphocytes and macrophages. The destructive process is limited to the β-cells, all other endocrine cells of the islets are spared (Peakman, 2011). The rate of β-cell destruction is variable; rapid destruction is often seen in children, whereas the destructive process often is prolonged in adults (American Diabetes Association, 2013). Interestingly, the pattern of β-cell destruction is markedly heterogenous, and an intact pancreatic islet can be located next to an

---

BOX 7-1   Etiological Classification of Diabetes Mellitus in Humans

I. Type 1 diabetes
 (β-cell destruction, usually leading to absolute insulin deficiency)
 a. Immune-mediated
 b. Idiopathic
II. Type 2 diabetes
 (ranging from predominantly insulin resistance with relative insulin deficiency to predominantly an insulin secretory defect with insulin resistance)
III. Other specific types of diabetes
 a. Genetic defects of β-cell function
 b. Genetic defects in insulin action
 c. Diseases of the exocrine pancreas
  (e.g., pancreatitis, neoplasia, trauma, pancreatectomy)
 d. Endocrinopathies
  (e.g., hypersomatotropism, hyperadrenocorticism, pheochromocytoma, hyperthyroidism, hyperaldosteronism)
 e. Drug- or chemical-induced
 f. Infection
 g. Uncommon forms of immune-mediated diabetes
 h. Other genetic syndromes sometimes associated with diabetes
IV. Gestational diabetes mellitus

Modified from American Diabetes Association: Diagnosis and classification of diabetes mellitus, *Diabetes Care* 36 (suppl 1):67, 2013.

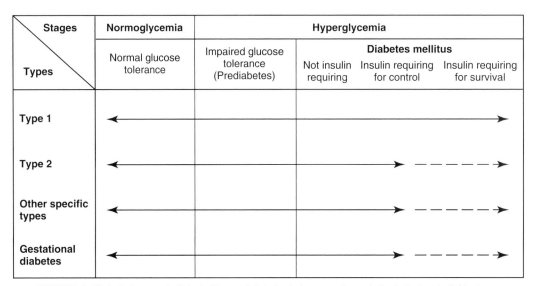

Stages / Types	Normoglycemia	Hyperglycemia		
	Normal glucose tolerance	Impaired glucose tolerance (Prediabetes)	Diabetes mellitus		
			Not insulin requiring	Insulin requiring for control	Insulin requiring for survival
Type 1	←——————————————————————————————→				
Type 2	←————————————————————————————→ – – – – →				
Other specific types	←————————————————————————————→ – – – – →				
Gestational diabetes	←————————————————————————————→ – – – – →				

FIGURE 7-1 Clinical stages and etiological types of diabetes in humans. *Arrows* indicate that an individual may move between the clinical stages; *broken arrows* illustrate that individuals in one category who would by definition not require insulin for survival may develop the need for insulin under certain circumstances (e.g., disease progression, development of diabetic ketoacidosis [DKA]). (Modified from George K, et al.: Classification and diagnosis of diabetes mellitus. In Wass JAH, Stewart PM, Amiel SA, Davies MC, editors: *Oxford textbook of endocrinology and diabetes,* ed 2, Oxford, 2011, Oxford University Press; and American Diabetes Association: Diagnosis and classification of diabetes mellitus, *Diabetes Care* 36[suppl 1]:67, 2013.)

islet with completely destroyed β-cells (Klinke, 2008). Recently, the widely-held belief that the disease only becomes clinically apparent when 80% to 90% of the individual's β-cells are destroyed has been challenged. It was suggested, that the extent of β-cell destruction at which hyperglycemia develops is age-dependent. In younger humans (at age 20) a reduction of 40% of β-cell mass was sufficient to precipitate clinical signs (Klinke, 2008). A major marker of autoimmune type 1 diabetes is the presence of circulating autoantibodies against glutamic acid decarboxylase 65 (GAD65), islet antigen-2 (IA-2), insulin, and zinc transporter 8 (ZnT8). One or more of these islet-related autoantibodies can be detected months to years before the clinical onset of the disease in most human patients. Their measurement is useful to differentiate type 1 diabetes from other types in newly diagnosed individuals and to follow individuals at risk to predict the development of the disease. Although their predictive value is very high, not all subjects with autoantibodies will develop diabetes, most likely because of protective genes. With time, autoantibodies tend to decline (Delli et al, 2010; Masharani and German, 2011). What exactly triggers the autoimmune process has not yet been unraveled. It has been known for quite some time that genetic factors increase the predisposition for the disease and that genetic susceptibility is most closely associated with allelic variants within the human leukocyte antigen (HLA) region that lie on the short arm of chromosome 6. High and lower risk haplotypes as well as protective haplotypes have been identified. Genes outside of the HLA region also contribute to the risk of type 1 diabetes, however, to a much smaller extent (Erlich et al, 2008; Concannon et al, 2009). Although genetics play an important role, studies in monozygotic twins revealed that the concordance rate is only approximately 50%, indicating that other causes are at least as important. Environmental factors, assumed to be associated with increased risk of type 1 diabetes, are virus infections (e.g., mumps virus, rubella virus, and the Cocksackie B virus), dietary factors (short breast-feeding/bovine milk), and toxic substances. The incidence of type 1 diabetes increases steadily, in particular in Western societies. It has been suggested that the sharp rise is due to a change in environmental factors operating early in life. According to the "hygiene hypothesis," the lack of exposure to common pathogens (in particular parasites) in a clean, more sterile environment may result in an exaggerated immune response (Bilous and Donelly, 2010; Masharani and German, 2011).

Type 2 Diabetes Mellitus

Type 2 diabetes mellitus was previously referred to as NIDDM or adult-onset diabetes and accounts for up to 90% of human cases (American Diabetes Association, 2013). Type 2 diabetes is a complex and heterogeneous disease resulting from a large number of genetic and environmental insults. The genetic association is stronger than for type 1 diabetes, and the concordance rate in monozygotic twins is much higher. Depending on the population studied, the latter may be as high as 90%; however, it has been assumed that part of the high rate may also be due to similar environmental factors (Bilous and Donnelly, 2010; Masharani and German, 2011).

Type 2 diabetes is characterized by two defects, namely insulin resistance and relative insulin deficiency due to β-cell dysfunction (as opposed to absolute deficiency in type 1 diabetes) (American Diabetes Association, 2013) (Fig. 7-2). It has long been assumed that insulin resistance was the primary and most important defect. However, most humans with insulin resistance do not develop diabetes, because their β-cells are able to compensate by augmenting insulin production and secretion. It is now generally agreed

that individuals cannot develop type 2 diabetes without having dysfunctional β-cells. Therefore, at the time of diagnosis, both insulin resistance and β-cells abnormalities are present (Robertson, 2009; Masharani and German, 2011). The term *insulin resistance* describes the inability of insulin to exert its normal biological effects at concentrations that are effective in normal individuals. The main sites of insulin resistance are liver, muscle, and adipose tissue. The defects seem to involve the insulin receptor binding only to a minor extent; most abnormalities are at post-receptor levels in the insulin-signaling cascade. Insulin resistance leads to impaired suppression of hepatic gluconeogenesis (under basal conditions as well as after meals) and impaired glucose uptake of peripheral tissues (Yki-Järvinen, 2010). A large number of genes associated with the disease have been identified, the majority of which are associated with reduction in β-cell function; only a few are related to insulin sensitivity (De Silva and Frayling, 2010; Schäfer et al, 2011; Kahn et al, 2012). Besides genetics, insulin sensitivity is negatively influenced by various factors, including obesity, physical inactivity, some drugs, and high glucose levels. Obesity is recognized as the major critical factor worldwide. With an increase in obesity, there has been a parallel global increase in the incidence of type 2 diabetes mellitus. Approximately 80% of humans with type 2 diabetes are obese, and the risk of diabetes increases with body fat mass. The pattern of obesity is important, as central (intra-abdominal) fat carries a much higher risk than fat deposition at other sites. Individuals with type 2 diabetes with a body mass index not meeting the definition for obesity may still have an excessive

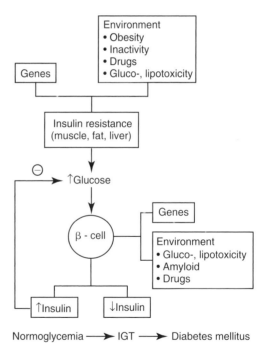

FIGURE 7-2 Simplified model of etiopathogenesis of type 2 diabetes mellitus. Although this graph is taken from human medicine, it is currently assumed that the principal factors are similar in cats. At the time of diagnosis of type 2 diabetes the two defects, insulin resistance and β-cell dysfunction, are present. Initially, β-cells are able to compensate for insulin resistance by increasing insulin synthesis and normoglycemia is maintained. With time, however, dysfunctional β-cells are not able to meet the increased demand, leading to impaired glucose tolerance and thereafter, to overt diabetes. In individuals without β-cell defect, diabetes mellitus will not develop because β-cells are able to compensate. (Modified from Bilous R, Donnelly R: *Handbook of diabetes,* ed 4, 2010, Wiley-Blackwell.) *IGT,* Impaired glucose tolerance.

intra-abdominal fat accumulation (Bilous and Donnelly, 2010). The discovery that adipose tissue (in particular the central visceral stores) is an active endocrine organ, and part of the innate immune system has sparked intense research on obesity. Factors secreted by adipose tissue play a major role in the regulation of metabolism. These factors include non-esterified fatty acids (NEFAs) and proteins, called *adipocytokines,* which act in an autocrine, paracrine, or endocrine fashion. Adipose tissue in lean subjects secretes relatively high levels of the adipocytokine adiponectin, which has anti-inflammatory actions and is associated with an increase in insulin sensitivity and therefore with a favorable metabolic status. With obesity, adiponectin secretion decreases considerably and instead, large amounts of NEFA, leptin, and pro-inflammatory cytokines, such as tumor necrosis factor alpha (TNFα), interleukin-6 (IL-6), monocyte chemotactic protein-1 (MCP-1) and others, are secreted by adipocytes and/or activated macrophages within the adipose tissue. These factors impair insulin signaling and therefore induce or worsen insulin resistance. Additionally, inflammatory factors are released into the systemic circulation and may promote inflammation in other tissues, including the islets (Rasouli and Kern, 2008; Donath and Shoelson, 2011).

Dysfunction of β-cells is crucial in the development of type 2 diabetes mellitus. Initially, the β-cells are able to increase insulin synthesis and release to meet the increased demand caused by the insulin resistance. With time, however, β-cells start to fail, first leading to glucose intolerance, which is usually followed by overt diabetes mellitus. It is currently assumed that the primary defect is a genetic predisposition and that additional acquired or environmental factors amplify the genetic damage, ultimately worsening the hyperglycemia (Robertson, 2009). By the time of diagnosis, β-cell function is reduced by approximately 50% and continues to decline. Beta-cell mass will also decrease during type 2 diabetes, however, not to an extent that would fully explain the extent of dysfunction. Therefore, besides morphological defects (reduction in number of β-cells), important functional defects contribute to the disease. The latter may be, at least in part, reversible and are therefore an interesting topic for new drug therapies (Robertson, 2009). Characteristic reflections of β-cell defects include disruption of the normal basal oscillatory pattern of insulin release, reduced or absent first phase insulin secretion in response to intravenous (IV) glucose (and with time reduced second phase release), reduced insulin response to a mixed-meal, and insufficient conversion of proinsulin to insulin. The other cells of the islets remain intact (Alsahli and Gerich, 2010). Type 2 is a polygenic disease, and many genetic variants contribute to the susceptibility of the disease. As already mentioned, most of the risk genes affect β-cell function, in particular glucose-stimulated insulin secretion, incretin-stimulated insulin secretion, and proinsulin-to-insulin conversion. So far, the most important type 2 risk gene is the gene encoding transcription factor 7-like 2 (TCF7L2); mutations are mainly associated with an impairment of the incretin effect (Schäfer et al, 2011) (incretins are discussed in Oral Hypoglycemic Agents and Non-Insulin Injectables). Acquired or environmental factors that worsen the damage of the β-cells in genetically predisposed individuals include glucotoxicity, lipotoxicity, oxidative stress, pro-inflammatory cytokines derived from adipose tissues, and increased deposition of amyloid. They may induce an inflammatory reaction within the islets, as suggested by the presence of infiltrating macrophages and increased IL-1 β (Donath and Shoelson, 2011). Gluco- and lipotoxicity are covered in the Remission of Diabetes in Cats section, and amyloid deposition is covered in the Types of Diabetes in Cats section. In brief, glucotoxicity describes the phenomenon that hyperglycemia per se impairs insulin secretion and possibly leads to β-cell death; similarly free fatty acids increase during the course of diabetes and in turn may cause β-cell damage. Amyloid derives from islet amyloid polypeptide (IAPP), which is co-secreted from the β-cell with insulin. Either the mature insoluble amyloid fibrils lying outside the β-cell or, more likely, small oligomers within the cell may contribute to the progressive β-cell damage (Alsahli and Gerich, 2010).

Other Specific Types of Diabetes and Gestational Diabetes

The category "other specific types" refers to diabetes that develops in association with diseases or factors other than those described under type 1 or type 2 diabetes mellitus. A large number of genetic syndromes, which have not been described in animals, are listed in this category. One example is the maturity-onset of diabetes of the young (MODY), which is inherited in an autosomal dominant pattern. Diabetes may occur secondary to disorders of the exocrine pancreas, and any process that diffusely injures the pancreas can cause diabetes (e.g., pancreatitis, trauma, infection, or pancreatic carcinoma). Several endocrinopathies (e.g., hypersomatotropism, hyperadrenocorticism, hyperthyroidism, pheochromocytoma, hyperaldosteronism, and glucagonoma) are associated with excessive secretion of hormones that antagonize the insulin effect. Similarly, the administration of diabetogenic drugs may result in glucose intolerance or overt disease. Diabetes mellitus usually only occurs in humans with pre-existing β-cell defect. A fourth category in the human model is *gestational diabetes*, which is defined as carbohydrate intolerance with onset or first recognition during pregnancy (American Diabetes Association, 2013).

Types of Diabetes in Cats

Type 1 Diabetes Mellitus

Type 1-like diabetes is generally considered to be rare in cats. Lymphocytic infiltration into the islets (insulitis) as a marker of immune-mediated disease has only been described in a few cases (Minkus et al, 1991; Hall et al, 1997). In a recent study, when examining islet lesions in a larger group of diabetic cats against a control population (matched in age, sex, and body weight), a tendency of lymphocytes to be more frequent in diabetic cats was found (in 20% of diabetic cats and in 5% of control cats). The infiltration was usually mild and may reflect an inflammatory situation also known to be present in type 2 diabetes. Only one of the 27 diabetic cats had severe lymphocytic infiltration, which was similar in severity to those described in the two studies mentioned earlier (Zini et al, 2012; Fig. 7-3, *A*). Beta cell and insulin antibodies have so far not been demonstrated in newly diagnosed diabetic cats (Hoenig et al, 2000a).

Type 2 Diabetes Mellitus

It is currently assumed that approximately 80% of diabetic cats suffer from a type 2-like diabetes mellitus, although there are no thorough studies to support this assumption. Nevertheless, most endocrinologists would agree that type 2-like diabetes is the most frequent form in cats. Similar to human type 2 diabetes mellitus, feline type 2 diabetes is a heterogeneous disease attributable to a combination of impaired insulin action in liver, muscle, and adipose tissue (insulin resistance), and β-cell failure. Environmental as well as genetic factors are thought to play a role in the development of both defects (see Fig. 7-2).

Genetic Factors. Genetic factors have just started to be investigated (Forcada et al, 2010). However, most likely similar to humans, diabetes in the cat is a polygenic disease, and many genes will be associated with an increased risk for the disease. The most convincing evidence of a genetic basis comes from studies

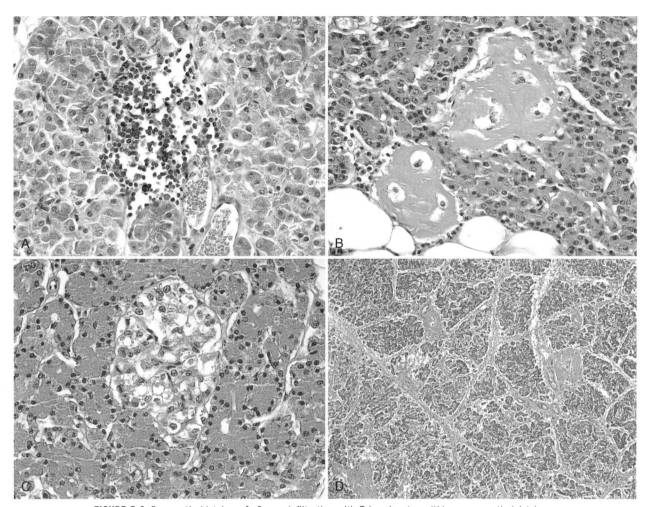

FIGURE 7-3 Pancreatic histology. **A,** Severe infiltration with T lymphocytes within a pancreatic islet in an 18-year-old Domestic Short-Hair (DSH) cat with diabetes mellitus. This is a rare finding, because usually only few or no lymphocytes are found in islets of diabetic cats. Immunohistochemistry for cluster of differentiation 3 (CD3), hematoxylin and eosin (H&E) counterstain (× 40). **B,** Islet amyloidosis in a 16-year-old, spayed female, DSH cat with diabetes mellitus (H&E, × 40). **C,** Vacuolar degeneration of an islet in a 9-year-old, castrated male, DSH with diabetes (H&E, × 40). **D,** Fibrosis in exocrine pancreas in an 8-year-old Siamese cat with diabetes mellitus (H&E, × 40). (From Zini E, et al.: Histological investigation of endocrine and exocrine pancreas in cats with diabetes mellitus, *J Vet Intern Med* 26 (abstract):1519, 2012.)

in the Burmese cat. In breeding lines from Australia, New Zealand, and the United Kingdom, the frequency of diabetes mellitus was shown to be about four times higher in Burmese cats than in domestic cats. In some families of Burmese cats, more than 10% of the offspring were affected by diabetes (Rand et al, 1997; Wade et al, 1999; McCann et al, 2007; Lederer et al, 2009).

Obesity, Gender, and Other Risk Factors. One of the major risk factors for the development of diabetes in cats is obesity. Others are male gender, physical inactivity and indoor confinement, increasing age, and the administration of glucocorticoids and progestagens (Panciera et al, 1990; Crenshaw and Peterson, 1996; Scarlet and Donoghue, 1998; McCann et al, 2007; Prahl et al, 2007; Slingerland et al, 2009). It has been shown that obese cats are 3.9 times more likely to develop diabetes mellitus than were cats with an optimal weight (Scarlett and Donoghue, 1998). Experimental studies in healthy cats showed that an average weight gain of 1.9 kg during a feeding trial was associated with a decrease in insulin sensitivity of more than 50% (Appleton et al, 2001). Similar results were reported in another trial in which each kilogram increase in weight led to approximately

30% loss in insulin sensitivity (Hoenig et al, 2007). Insulin sensitivity differs considerably between individuals, and it was suggested that cats with intrinsically low insulin sensitivity are at increased risk of developing glucose intolerance with weight gain. Male cats tended to have lower insulin sensitivity prior to the feeding trial and gained more weight than female cats, which might explain in part why male cats are at increased risk of developing diabetes mellitus (Appleton et al, 2001). The mechanisms of insulin resistance on a cellular level and the interrelations of the different findings are not yet understood in cats. Most of the research to date has focused on glucose transporters (GLUTs), insulin signaling genes in insulin-sensitive tissues, and secretion of adipocytokines from adipose tissue. In cats that became obese, the expression of the insulin-sensitive GLUT-4 in muscle and fat was significantly lower than in lean cats, whereas the expression of GLUT-1, which is not insulin-sensitive, remained unchanged (Brennan et al, 2004). Expression of several insulin signaling genes in liver and skeletal muscles were significantly lower in obese cats than in lean cats, which is similar in humans with insulin resistance (Mori et al, 2009a).

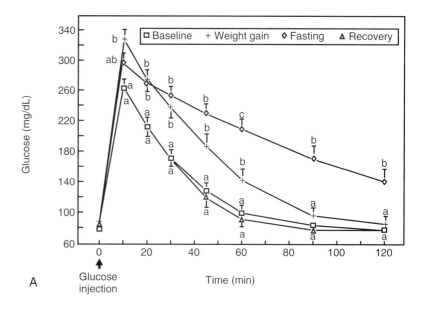

A

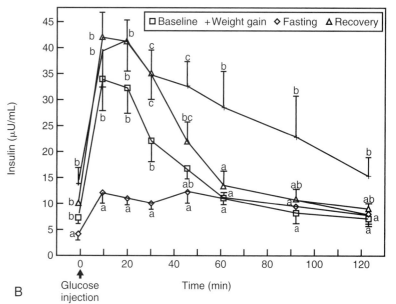

B

FIGURE 7-4 Mean glucose **(A)** and insulin **(B)** concentrations (± standard error of the mean [SEM]) in 12 cats after intravenous (IV) administration of 0.5 g of glucose per kilogram of body weight at entry into the study (baseline), after 9 ± 2 months of weight gain, after a voluntary fast of 5 to 6 weeks (weight loss), and 5 weeks after the end of fasting (recovery). *a* to *c*, Points with a different letter are significantly different ($p < 0.05$) among periods. Note the development of impaired glucose tolerance despite increased insulin secretion with weight gain and improvement in glucose tolerance and the exaggerated insulin secretory response with weight loss. (From Biourge V, et al.: Effect of weight gain and subsequent weight loss on glucose tolerance and insulin response in healthy cats, *J Vet Intern Med* 11:86, 1997).

Adipokines and Proinflammatory Cytokines. Also similar to humans, it is now recognized in cats that adipose tissue is an active and complex endocrine organ. It was shown that adiponectin, which is almost exclusively produced in adipose tissue, decreases with obesity and diabetes mellitus in cats (Brömel et al, 2004; Hoenig et al, 2007). Adiponectin belongs to the large group of molecules synthesized in adipose tissue and collectively termed *adipokines*. Adiponectin enhances insulin sensitivity and has anti-inflammatory properties; a decrease, therefore, contributes to insulin resistance and inflammation. Leptin, the "prototypic" adipokine, is involved in appetite suppression and energy expenditure and plays a role in modulation of insulin sensitivity (Radin et al, 2009). Obese cats have been found to be leptin-resistant (i.e., they have much higher leptin levels than lean cats without causing an appropriate physiological response) (Hoenig, 2012). As described earlier, it is known in humans that adipose tissue secretes a number of proinflammatory cytokines, and obesity is now considered a state of low-grade chronic inflammation. TNFα was the first adipose-derived factor suggested to represent a link between obesity and the insulin resistance seen in human type 2 diabetes; this cytokine exerts a strong negative influence on insulin signaling. Today, various additional cytokines and chemokines (e.g., IL-6, MCP-1) are known also to be involved in the inflammatory process in humans (Kanaya and Vaisse, 2011). Adipose tissue in cats may behave in a similar manner, because the level of TNFα (in fat) was significantly higher in obese than in lean cats (Hoenig et al, 2006). Further studies, in particular in naturally acquired diabetes, are needed to substantiate those findings. The interested reader is referred to the reviews of Radin, et al., (2009) and German, et al., (2010) for more details on obesity, adipokines, and inflammation. For everyday practice, it is important to know that insulin resistance evolving during weight gain is reversible after weight loss. When healthy cats were fed ad libitum, weight gain was associated with a significant increase in glucose, and insulin concentrations during an intravenous glucose tolerance test (IVGTT) compared to baseline and the total amount of insulin secretion was significantly higher. Several weeks after weight loss was achieved by low caloric intake, the results of the IVGTT were similar to those at baseline (Biourge et al, 1997; Fig. 7-4). The study underscores the importance of weight management throughout life and in particular in cats with diabetes.

Beta-Cell Dysfunction, Amyloid, and Glucotoxicity. It is important to note that although obesity induces insulin resistance, not all obese cats develop diabetes mellitus. Healthy β-cells adapt to obesity and insulin resistance by increasing insulin secretion to maintain normal glucose tolerance (see also Fig. 7-2). Additionally, cats also seem to be able to lower their glucose output from the liver in case of peripheral insulin resistance (Hoenig, 2012). For diabetes to develop, there must be β-cell dysfunction leading to impaired glucose tolerance and eventually type 2 diabetes. Unfortunately, there are nearly no data on β-cell function and insulin secretion in cats during the natural development of diabetes. Most studies were done in healthy cats in which obesity was induced within a short period of time by ad libitum feeding. In one study, cats were made diabetic by pancreatectomy and administration of insulin antagonistic drugs (Hoenig et al, 2000b). From this study one can conclude that in the early stage of diabetes the first phase of insulin release becomes delayed and smaller, whereas insulin secretion during the second phase is more pronounced; during this stage, baseline glucose is still normal. With time, the first phase of insulin secretion disappears almost completely, insulin secretion becomes erratic, and the total amount of insulin during the 2-hour IVGGT decreases substantially. At this time, baseline glucose concentration is increased (i.e., overt diabetes is present). As a reminder: Healthy lean cats have a biphasic insulin secretion pattern when stimulated with glucose during an IVGGT (Hoenig et al, 2000b; Hoenig, 2012).

The big question, "What exactly leads to β-cell failure under natural conditions?" is unanswered until today. One long-known hypothesis concerns β-cell destruction by amyloid deposition. Islet amyloid derives from a hormone named IAPP also known as *amylin*. IAPP is a normal product of the β-cells, which is stored together with insulin in secretory vesicles and is co-secreted with insulin into the circulation. IAPP levels are elevated in conditions associated with insulin resistance (e.g., in cats with obesity) (Henson et al, 2011). Only cats, humans, and nonhuman primates have an amyloidogenic amino acid structure of IAPP with the potential to form amyloid depositions within the islets of the pancreas (O'Brien, 2002; Hull et al, 2004). Amyloid depositions have been found in many cats with diabetes; it is, however, also a frequent finding in non-diabetic cats. In a recent study, 56% of diabetic cats and 42% of control cats matched for age, sex, and body weight had amyloid depositions, the amount of which was also comparable (Zini et al, 2012; see Fig. 7-3, *B*). The situation is similar in humans, because many of the type 2 diabetics, but also a substantial percentage of non-diabetics, have amyloid depositions in the pancreatic islets (Alshali and Gerich, 2010).

The open questions are: "Why aren't all individuals with an amyloidogenic structure of amylin forming amyloid depositions?" and "Is amyloid a cause or consequence of the disease?" It has been shown that disturbed protein folding and/or trafficking of amylin within the β-cells lead to the formation of so-called toxic oligomers. These intracellular molecules induce cytotoxicity and may lead to a decline in β-cell function and to β-cell apoptosis. The extracellular amyloid deposits seem to be less toxic and represent the end point of misfolding (Costes et al, 2013). Loss of β-cell function may therefore be present before amyloid depositions are visible. Opinions on the importance of IAPP/amyloid in the pathogenesis of β-cell failure differ between research groups (in particular in human medicine). It is likely that the misfolding is a reflection of another defect within the β-cells and not the primary cause of β-cell dysfunction. When present, however, these abnormalities may accelerate further damage. An additional factor, which has a negative impact on β-cell function and survival, is high blood glucose concentrations—a phenomenon known as *glucotoxicity*. There

is little doubt that glucotoxicity is a secondary event, because hyperglycemia becomes apparent only after β-cells start to fail. However, improving glycemic control by insulin therapy will reverse some of the negative effects, and reversal of glucotoxicity is an important mechanism to explain diabetic remission. *Lipotoxicity* is the term used for the damaging effect of high levels of free fatty acids; in cats, however, lipotoxicity may not be as important as glucotoxicity (Zini et al, 2009a). Details are discussed in the section on remission of diabetes. In humans with type 2 diabetes, inflammatory changes within the islets have been reported, potentially contributing to β-cell apoptosis (Robertson, 2009; Donath and Shoelson, 2011). As mentioned in the beginning of this section, more lymphocytes were found in the islets of diabetic cats than in a matched control population. It was speculated that they may have contributed to the loss of β-cells (Zini et al, 2012). Clearly, more studies are needed to define the role of islet inflammation.

Other Specific Types of Diabetes (Secondary Diabetes Mellitus)

Diabetes in cats may develop as a consequence of another disease or the administration of diabetogenic drugs, such as glucocorticoids and progestins. In humans, this category encompasses various disorders (in particular genetic disorders), which are so far unknown in cats. Some of the subcategories, such as diabetes associated with pancreatic diseases or other endocrinopathies, are known to occur also in cats. These diseases may account for approximately up to 20% of diabetic cases in cats. Diabetes induced by glucocorticoids or progestins is relatively common (see also Concurrent Disorders Causing Insulin Resistance and Drug-Induced Diabetes). The interrelationships of the endocrine and exocrine parts of the pancreas are complex. For instance, acinar tissue is in close contact with the islets without surrounding capsule or basement membrane, and an islet-acinar portal system communicates between both parts (Chen et al, 2011). It is, therefore, easy to understand that a disease in one part will also affect the other one. Pancreatitis has gained a lot of attention during the past years, and it is now known that it is a relatively common disease in cats. The cause and effect of pancreatitis and diabetes in cats, however, is difficult to define and is largely unknown. In previous studies, histological abnormalities consistent with pancreatitis were found in 22% and 51% of diabetic cats. Findings included neutrophilic infiltration and necrosis considered consistent with acute pancreatitis and diffuse lymphocytic and lymphoplasmacytic infiltration considered consistent with chronic pancreatitis (Kraus et al, 1997; Goossens et al, 1998). However, recent histological studies also revealed a high prevalence of pancreatitis in cats without diabetes. De Cock, et al., (2007) performed histological examinations of the pancreas of 115 cats that had been euthanized for various reasons; 41 of them had been clinically healthy. The overall prevalence of pancreatitis was 67%, evidence for chronic pancreatitis was found in 50.4%, for acute pancreatitis in 6.1% of cases, and approximately 10% of cases had both acute and chronic pancreatitis. We recently studied pancreatic tissue of 37 diabetic cats in comparison to tissue from 20 matched control cats using the same histological criteria as De Cock, et al. The findings in control cats were similar to their study, and interestingly, the prevalence of pancreatic lesions in diabetic cats was as high as in the non-diabetic control cats. The overall prevalence of pancreatitis in diabetic cats was 57% and in control cats 60%. Diabetic cats had a trend for more severe lesions and higher prevalence of acute pancreatitis; however, the difference was not significant (Zini et al, 2012). As suggested by De Cock, et al., (2007), the pancreas generally seems to be very sensitive to drugs, stress, metabolic derangements, or ischemia associated with a wide variety of diseases. According to the currently available data and the impression of the author, pancreatitis is not a frequent cause of diabetes mellitus. Although in principle, severe pancreatitis with extensive tissue destruction may result in damage of the pancreatic islets and β-cell loss, but this seems to be a rare event. Pancreatitis, however, seems to be a frequent comorbidity, and it is very likely that pancreatitis emerges during the course of the diabetic disease. In a substantial percentage of cats, it seems to be a clinical insignificant bystander; in others, it causes clinical signs and may render diabetic regulation at times very difficult. Pancreatitis may also play a role in the development of diabetic ketoacidosis (DKA) (Goossens et al, 1998; Armstrong and Williams, 2012). Diabetes mellitus may also be seen with pancreatic adenocarcinoma; in humans, there is debate as to which diabetes is due to direct effects of the tumor or induced by diabetogenic substances produced by the cancer cells (Chen et al, 2011). Among the endocrinopathies listed under "Other specific types of diabetes" in Box 7-1, hypersomatotropism (acromegaly) and hyperadrenocorticism are the most relevant in cats. Nearly all cats with hypersomatotropism and approximately 80% of cats with hyperadrenocorticism will develop diabetes, which oftentimes is difficult to regulate due to severe insulin resistance. Whereas hyperadrenocorticism is a rare disorder, hypersomatotropism may be present in 10% to 15% of diabetic cats. See Chapters 2 and 11 for more details. In cats, hyperthyroidism and hyperaldosteronism are rarely associated with overt diabetes and pheochromocytoma is extremely uncommon.

In summary, diabetes mellitus in cats is a heterogeneous disease caused by a large number of different factors; the exact etiopathogenic mechanisms are unknown at the moment. The main histological findings within the islets are reduced numbers of β-cells, whereas the other endocrine cells are unaffected; amyloid deposition and vacuolar degeneration, in some of the cats lymphocytic infiltration may be found (see Fig. 7-3, *A* to *D*). Necrosis and fibrosis as well as neutrophilic or lymphocytic infiltration may be present in the exocrine pancreas reflecting acute or chronic pancreatitis.

 ## REMISSION OF DIABETES IN CATS

Remission of diabetes is defined as a situation in which clinical signs disappear, blood glucose concentration normalizes, and insulin treatment (or other antidiabetic drugs) can be discontinued. In human medicine, the duration of normoglycemia has to be at least 1 year to be labelled remission, and prolonged remission is a period of normoglycemia of at least 5 years (Buse et al, 2009). In cats, a cut-off of 4 weeks of normoglycemia has been used (i.e., the disease-free interval should last for at least 4 weeks before the diabetes is considered to be in remission; Sieber-Ruckstuhl et al, 2008; Zini et al, 2010; Tschuor et al, 2011). Prolonged remission may be in duration of at least 1 year. The first publication on 10 cats that had experienced diabetic remission appeared about 15 years ago; at that time the phenomenon was termed *transient diabetes* (Nelson et al, 1999). Interestingly, at the time of diagnosis of the diabetes, baseline insulin concentrations were undetectably low or within the reference range and did not increase after IV glucagon administration, mimicking type 1 diabetes. The cats were treated with insulin or glipizide for 4 to 16 weeks, after which treatment could be discontinued. A second glucagon test, performed after remission had occurred, showed an immediate and significant increase in insulin concentration, insulin peak response, and total insulin secretion compared with initial values; the results of the glucagon test after remission were

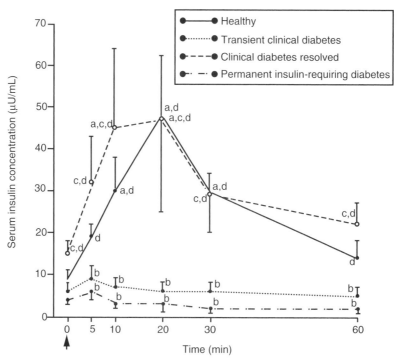

FIGURE 7-5 Mean (± standard deviation [SD]) serum insulin concentrations before and after intravenous (IV) administration of 0.5 mg of glucagon per cat in ten healthy cats—10 cats with transient clinical diabetes at the time clinical diabetes was diagnosed and after clinical diabetes resolved, and six cats with permanent insulin-requiring diabetes at the time diabetes was diagnosed. *a,* Significantly (p < 0.05) different compared with baseline value. *b,* Significantly (p < 0.05) different compared with corresponding time in healthy cats. *c,* Significantly (p < 0.05) different compared with corresponding time when clinical diabetes was diagnosed. *d,* Significantly (p < 0.05) different compared with corresponding time in cats with permanent insulin-requiring diabetes. *Arrow* indicates glucagon administration. (From Nelson RW, et al.: Transient clinical diabetes mellitus in cats: 10 cases (1989–1991), *J Vet Intern Med* 13:28, 1999).

similar to test results in healthy cats (Fig. 7-5). Histological evaluation of the pancreas was possible in some of the cats and revealed decreased numbers of islets, islet amyloidosis, and vacuolar degeneration of islet cells. This study demonstrates that initial insulin secretion is severely impaired even in cats with the potential of remission and that the glucagon test performed at the time of diagnosis does not allow differentiation between cats with reversible and cats with irreversible β-cell function. Treatment can lead to improvement of β-cell function, most likely due to abolishment of the damaging effects of high blood glucose on β-cell function (glucotoxicity). The study also showed that cats experiencing diabetic remission are not "cured," because they have islet cell pathology, potentially predisposing them to a relapse of clinical diabetes (Nelson et al, 1999). Since this first report, remission is increasingly recognized, and it is now well accepted that good glycemic control improves β-cell function and that diabetic remission can be achieved in a substantial percentage of cats. Those cats most likely have a type 2-like diabetes resulting from insulin resistance and β-cell dysfunction and some degree of β-cell loss. Their remaining β-cells, however, have the capacity to recover, at least in part, during treatment. Cats that do not experience diabetic remission may be in a more advanced stage of their disease with more pronounced β-cell loss and/or a more pronounced functional defect. Diabetic remission most often occurs during the first 3 to 4 months of therapy; however, remission 1 year and longer after start of therapy may occasionally be seen. The currently available studies, which have included information on remission, are difficult to compare, because they differ with regard to definition of remission, inclusion criteria of cats, blood glucose targets, and monitoring protocols, as well as type of insulin and type of diet. Published remission rates vary between 13% and 100% (Nelson et al, 1999; Bennett et al, 2006; Martin and Rand, 2007; Boari et al, 2008; Michiels et al, 2008; Marshall et al, 2009; Roomp and Rand, 2009; 2012; Hall et al, 2009; Zini et al, 2010; Hafner et al, 2011; Tschuor et al, 2011). It has been suggested that remission rates are higher in cats when treated with newer types of insulin (e.g., insulin analogues such as glargine or detemir) than with other/older types of insulin (e.g., Lente type) (Marshall et al, 2009; Roomp and Rand, 2009; 2012). Although type of insulin and improved time-action profiles of newer insulins may have an important effect on glycemic control and remission rates, other factors such as glucose targets and intensity of monitoring certainly contribute to the high remission rates in some of the studies. For instance, in two recent studies using insulin glargine and detemir respectively, overall remission rates of 64% and 67% were achieved (Roomp and Rand, 2009; 2012). Those studies, however, used an extremely intensive treatment and monitoring protocol: Glucose targets were set very low (50 to 200 mg/dL and 50 to 100 mg/dL respectively; 2.8 to 11.1 mmol/L, 2.8 to 5.5. mmol/L); the owners had to measure blood glucose at home at least three times daily and adapt the insulin dosage accordingly. Those treatment protocols can only be used under very close supervision, because there is an increasing risk of hypoglycemia the lower the glucose targets are set. Low-carbohydrate diets may also contribute to good glycemic control and possible diabetic remission, although data are slim. One study found that remission rate was higher in cats fed a low-carbohydrate diet compared to a moderate carbohydrate diet, whereas in another study, remission rates were similar (Bennet et al, 2006; Hall et al, 2009). However, as mentioned earlier, the studies are difficult to compare because diet composition, type of insulin, and treatment protocols differed. In our own institution, remission rate has varied between 40% and 50% over the years under the following conditions:

- Cats are newly diagnosed with diabetes and have no severe concurrent diseases.
- They are treated according to a standardized treatment protocol, which includes administration of insulin glargine b.i.d. and feeding a low-carbohydrate–high-protein diet.
- Frequent reevaluations are done during the first 4 months of therapy.

Home monitoring of blood glucose has been shown to be advantageous because it allows close supervision and more frequent dose amendments. Remission rates are influenced substantially by which cats are evaluated. In cats with severe concurrent disease or in cats with long duration of diabetes, remission rate will be lower. In cats with previous steroid treatment, remission rates will usually be relatively high. A recent survey among primary practitioners in the United States revealed an approximate remission rate of 26% (Smith et al, 2012). This seems to be a realistic number under an "everyday" condition, in which cats are not preselected and treatment as well as monitoring is more difficult to standardize than in an university environment.

Recently, the question if the capacity of β-cells can be assessed by the time of diagnosis was investigated with the rationale if remission of diabetes can be predicted before initiating therapy. As shown some time ago by Nelson, et al., (1999), no difference in insulin response during glucagon test was seen in cats with and without remission. Studies in humans have demonstrated that the first defect in the early phase of diabetes is a loss response to IV glucose, followed by a loss of response to IV glucagon, whereas response to arginine persists the longest. It was therefore hypothesized that cats that experience remission at some time after starting treatment have less severe β-cell defects than cats with permanent disease and would therefore show normal or at least some degree of insulin response after IV arginine. However, the expectations were not met. In both groups of cats (remission and no remission) insulin concentrations increased mildly after IV arginine, but there was no significant difference between the two groups, similar to what has been shown with the glucagon test (Tschuor et al, 2011; Fig. 7-6). Therefore, none of the tests used so far allows discrimination between cats with and without the chance of remission. A few other studies have evaluated clinical parameters that may be associated with the likelihood of diabetic remission. Interestingly, in a study including 90 cats with newly-diagnosed diabetes, remission rate was shown to increase with increasing age at diagnosis (Fig. 7-7). This finding was unexpected, because it is known that generally β-cell mass decreases with age in healthy individuals. It is possible that in case of diabetes, β-cell destruction is slower in elderly cats, which is similar to what is known from human diabetics (Zini et al, 2010). Other factors shown to be associated with higher likelihood of remission are early treatment of diabetes and prior steroid therapy (Roomp and Rand, 2009). Some factors such as presence of peripheral neuropathy and increased cholesterol have been identified to be associated with reduced likelihood of remission (Roomp and Rand, 2009; Zini et al, 2010). Both may reflect a more advanced state of the disease with more pronounced β-cell loss; hypercholesterolemia may also be a contributing factor to β-cell dysfunction (lipotoxicity). Of note, DKA has not been identified as a negative predictive factor and remission may also occur in cats presented with DKA (Sieber-Ruckstuhl et al, 2008). In many cats, remission lasts for months to years and may even be life-long. Roughly 30% of cats with remission will have a relapse with recurrence of clinical signs and hyperglycemia and will again

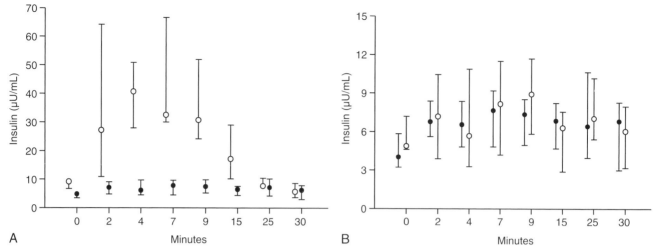

FIGURE 7-6 A, Insulin concentration after intravenous (IV) arginine administration in 7 healthy cats *(open circles)* and 17 cats with newly-diagnosed diabetes *(closed circles).* Insulin concentrations in healthy cats were significantly higher 2, 4, 7, 9, and 15 minutes after arginine administrations, where no difference was found between the groups at baseline and after 25 and 30 minutes. **B,** The insulin concentrations of the 17 newly-diagnosed cats shown in **A** were divided into two groups. *Open circles,* 7 cats that experienced diabetic remission during subsequent therapy; *closed circles,* 10 cats with permanent diabetes. The insulin concentrations did not differ at any time point. (Data from Tschuor F, et al.: Remission of diabetes mellitus cannot be predicted by the arginine stimulation test, *Am J Vet Res* 25:83, 2011).

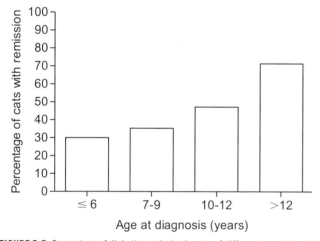

FIGURE 7-7 Percentage of diabetic remission in cats of different ages. It is obvious that remission rates increases with age at the time of diagnosis. Remission rate was approximately 30% when the cats were ≤ 6 years at the time of diabetes diagnosis and remission rate was approximately 70% in cats that were 12 years and older. (Data from Zini E, et al.: Predictors of clinical remission in cats with diabetes mellitus, *J Vet Int Med* 24:1314, 2010).

require insulin therapy. In some of them, a second remission is possible. More often, however, permanent insulin therapy is required. The latter situation most likely reflects deterioration of β-cell function and reduction of β-cell mass.

The damaging effects of chronic hyperglycemia have been known for a long time; nowadays those effects are usually summarized under the umbrella term of *glucotoxicity.* In 1948, Dohan and Lukens administered large doses of glucose to normal cats and induced permanent hyperglycemia, hydropic degeneration of the islets of Langerhans, and ketonuria. It took nearly 50 years for those findings to be recognized in veterinary medicine

when Link and Rand (1996) performed a similar experiment. They showed that insulin levels in healthy cats decreased within days when high blood glucose levels were maintained by glucose infusion. Several cats even became ketonuric and required 1 to 2 weeks of insulin therapy after cessation of the glucose infusion (Link and Rand, 1996; Link et al, 2013). The cellular mechanisms by which chronic hyperglycemia affects insulin secretion and insulin sensitivity are poorly understood. In humans, it has been proposed that oxidative stress and inflammatory cytokines play an important role (Robertson, 2009; Donath and Shoelson, 2011).

In a recent study, glucose-induced lesions in β-cells were investigated in cats. After 10 days of IV glucose infusion, healthy cats had 50% fewer β-cells per islet area than control cats. Islet cells showed apoptotic features and were caspase-3 (a marker for apoptosis) positive (Fig. 7-8). Interestingly, hyperglycemia induced a systemic inflammatory response, characterized by an increased plasma concentration of α1-acid glycoprotein. Systemic inflammation has also been described in human type 2 diabetes. Another potential acquired cause of beta-cell dysfunction is lipotoxicity (i.e., the deleterious effects of fatty acids on β-cells). However, in contrast to the 10-day glucose infusion, lipid infusion over the same time period did not affect plasma insulin or glucose levels or result in β-cell apoptosis. In human medicine, it has been proposed that glucotoxicity occurs independently of lipotoxicity, whereas lipotoxicity requires increased blood glucose levels to fully manifest. This may also apply to cats (Zini et al, 2009a).

The concept of glucotoxicity (and possibly lipotoxicity) is very important to understand because immediate treatment of diabetes may reverse the negative effects of glucose on β-cells and increase the chance of remission. Of note, islet cell pathology is present in cats in diabetic remission and remission should not be confused with cure of the disease. Recurrence of clinical overt diabetes is always possible and may be triggered by stressors (increase in body weight, concurrent disease, diabetogenic drugs) or without any obvious event.

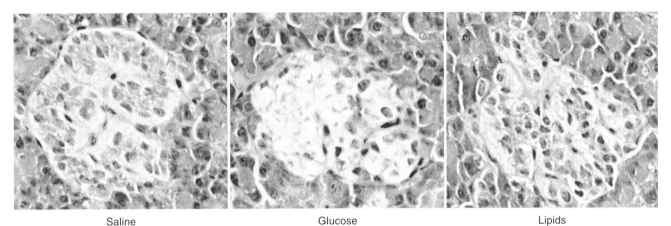

Saline   Glucose   Lipids

FIGURE 7-8 Pancreatic islets of healthy cats after receiving 0.9% NaCl, intravenous (IV) glucose infusion and IV lipids for 10 days. No lesions were seen in the control cat and in the cat that received lipids. In the glucose-infused cat, a large area of the islet appeared devoid of nuclei and included several vacuoles, which is suggestive of hydropic degeneration. Hydropic degeneration of islet cells indicates accumulation of glycogen. The remaining islet nuclei appear larger than in the control cat. (H&E, × 40) (From Zini E, et al.: Hyperglycemia but not hyperlipidemia causes beta-cell dysfunction and loss in the domestic cat, *Diabetologia* 52:336, 2009a [with permission].)

INSULIN, METABOLIC EFFECTS, AND PATHOPHYSIOLOGY*

Insulin Synthesis, Structure, and Regulation

Glucose homeostasis is maintained by a complex system of regulating and modulating hormones and factors, the most important of which is insulin. Insulin is the only hormone capable of decreasing blood glucose levels.

Insulin synthesis begins in the rough endoplasmic reticulum with the formation of preproinsulin, which is then converted to proinsulin by removal of a small peptide fragment. Proinsulin is further processed to insulin in the Golgi apparatus by removing another peptide, called *connecting peptide (C-peptide)*. Insulin and C-peptide are packed and stored in secretory granules and released in equimolar amounts by the process of exocytosis. Within the granules, insulin co-precipitates with zinc ions to form hexamers and microcrystals, whereas in the circulation, insulin exists as monomer.

Normally, proinsulin conversion is largely completed before secretion and is therefore not encountered in the circulation in appreciable quantities. In human diabetics, increased proinsulin concentrations may be found in plasma, which is considered to be an indicator of β-cell dysfunction (Breuer et al, 2010; Wang and Osei, 2011). Knowledge in cats is limited to obese individuals, which revealed abnormal proinsulin to insulin ratios during IVGTTs (Kley et al, 2008).

Insulin consists of two polypeptide chains: an A chain with 21 amino acids and a B chain with 30, which are connected by two disulfide bridges. The insulin molecule has been highly conserved during evolution, and the differences between species are small. Feline insulin is most similar to bovine insulin, differing by only

*The section on insulin, metabolic effects and pathophysiology has been published in a similar form in two other book chapters: Reusch CE, et al.: Endocrine pancreas. In Rijnberk A, Kooistra HG, editors: *Clinical endocrinology of dogs and cats,* ed 2, Hannover, Germany, 2010, Schluetersche, pp. 155-185; Reusch CE: Feline diabetes mellitus. In Ettinger SJ, Feldman EC, editors: *Textbook of veterinary internal medicine,* ed 7, St Louis, 2010, Saunders/Elsevier, pp. 1796-1816.

TABLE 7-1	DIFFERENCES IN AMINO ACID SEQUENCE OF THE INSULIN MOLECULE BETWEEN SPECIES		
	A8	**A10**	**A18**	**B30**
Human	Thr	Ile	Asn	Thr
Pig/dog	Thr	Ile	Asn	Ala
Cattle	Ala	Val	Asn	Ala
Cat	Ala	Val	His	Ala

one amino acid; it differs from canine and human insulin at three and four positions, respectively (Table 7-1).

Insulin circulates almost entirely unbound in the blood, has a half-life of about 5 to 8 minutes, and is mainly metabolized by the liver and the kidneys (Sjaastad et al, 2010). Continuous availability of insulin and moment-to-moment adjustments are crucial for normal carbohydrate, protein, and lipid metabolism. The body exhibits complex mechanisms to ensure adequate basal insulin secretion between meals as well as increased insulin secretion after a meal. The most important regulator is the glucose concentration in the blood, and there is a positive feedback mechanism between blood glucose concentration and insulin secretion rate.

Glucose is transported into β-cells via the glucose transporter protein GLUT-2, which allows rapid equilibration of extra- and intracellular glucose concentrations. Glucose is metabolized (phosphorylation by glucokinase and production of pyruvate) within the β-cells to produce adenosine triphosphate (ATP). The increase in the ATP/adenosine diphosphate (ADP) ratio is followed by the closure of ATP-sensitive potassium channels in the β-cell membrane, preventing potassium ions from leaving the β-cell. This in turn causes membrane depolarization and opening of voltage-dependent calcium channels in the membrane. The increase in cytosolic calcium then triggers insulin release.

Oral glucose induces a more pronounced insulin secretion than glucose given intravenously. This phenomenon is due to the actions of so-called incretin hormones—the most important being glucagon-like peptide-1 (GLP-1) and glucose-dependent insulinotropic polypeptide, previously called *gastric inhibitory polypeptide (GIP)*. Incretins are secreted by endocrine cells in the gastrointestinal tract in response to nutrients. They are then carried in the bloodstream to the pancreatic islets where they interact with specific β-cell receptors to amplify insulin secretion. GLP-1 has additional effects, which include reduction of glucagon secretion, stimulation of beta-cell differentiation and proliferation, delayed gastric emptying, and induction of satiety (Reusch and Padrutt, 2013).

In addition to glucose and other sugars, amino acids and fatty acids are also stimulators of insulin secretion; stimulation may be direct or potentiated by incretins. The autonomous nervous system modulates islet hormone release; secretion of insulin is stimulated by vagal nerve fibers and inhibited by sympathetic nerve fibers. Several other pancreatic and extra-pancreatic hormones, such as IAPP, glucagon, somatostatin, cortisol, and growth hormone (GH), affect insulin secretion directly or indirectly (Flatt, 2003; Persaud and Howell, 2003; Utzschneider et al, 2004).

Metabolic Effects of Insulin

Insulin regulates numerous metabolic processes through binding to high-affinity cell surface receptors. Like the receptors for other protein hormones, the receptor for insulin is embedded in the plasma membrane. It is a tetrameric protein, composed of two α- and two β-subunits linked by disulfide bonds. The α-subunits are extracellular and house insulin binding domains, whereas the β-subunits penetrate through the cell membrane (Fig. 7-9). The insulin receptor belongs to the large group of tyrosine kinase receptors.

Binding of insulin to the α-subunits triggers the tyrosine kinase activity of the β-subunits leading to autophosphorylation, thus activating the catalytic activity of the receptor. The "substrate" proteins, which are phosphorylated by the insulin receptor, are called *insulin-receptor substrate (IRS) molecules.* They are key mediators in the insulin signaling pathway and act as docking proteins between the insulin receptor and a complex network of intracellular molecules. Dysregulation within the signaling cascade may lead to insulin resistance, and in this context, IRS molecules seem to play a major role.

Within seconds after insulin binds to its receptor, the so-called rapid insulin actions lead to the uptake of glucose, amino acids, potassium, and phosphate into cells. After a few minutes, intermediate actions occur, mainly effecting protein and glucose metabolism, followed several hours later by delayed actions, which mainly include effects on lipid metabolism.

Glucose is a polar molecule and cannot diffuse across cell membranes. Transport of glucose is facilitated by a family of GLUT proteins or by active transport with sodium in the intestine and kidney. Currently, 14 different GLUTs are known for humans, which are named in order of discovery—GLUT 1 to 14. GLUT-4 is the major insulin-responsive transporter and is found almost exclusively in muscle and adipose tissue. Insulin stimulates glucose transport in those two tissues by causing the translocation of GLUT-4 from the cytosol to the cell membrane with which they fuse. There, they function as pores enabling glucose entry. When insulin levels decrease, GLUT-4 is removed from the cell membrane (see Fig. 7-9). In various other tissues (e.g., brain, liver, kidney, and intestinal tract), glucose uptake is insulin-independent and occurs by other GLUT proteins (Garvey, 2004; Thorens and Mueckler, 2010; Barrett et al, 2012).

Insulin is the most important anabolic hormone in the body and prevents catabolism of nutrient stores. Its main function is to ensure storage of glucose as glycogen, amino acids as protein and fatty acids as fat. The primary target tissues for insulin are liver, muscle, and fat. Insulin facilitates the oxidation of glucose to pyruvate and lactate through the induction of enzymes, such as glucokinase, some hexokinases, phosphofructokinase, and pyruvate kinase. Insulin promotes glycogen synthesis in liver, adipose tissue, and muscle by increasing glycogen synthase activity. Gluconeogenesis is decreased by insulin because of the promotion of protein synthesis in peripheral tissues, thus decreasing the amount of amino acids available for gluconeogenesis. Additionally, insulin decreases the activity of hepatic enzymes that are involved in the conversion of amino acids to glucose.

In adipose tissue, insulin promotes the synthesis of lipids and inhibits their degradation. Insulin activates the enzymes pyruvate dehydrogenase and acetyl coenzyme A (acetyl-CoA) carboxylase, which promote the synthesis of fatty acids from acetyl-CoA. Insulin also increases the activity of lipoprotein lipase, an enzyme that is located in the endothelium of capillaries of extrahepatic tissues and promotes the entry of fatty acids into adipose tissue. Inhibition of lipolysis is mediated through the inhibition of the enzyme hormone-sensitive lipase.

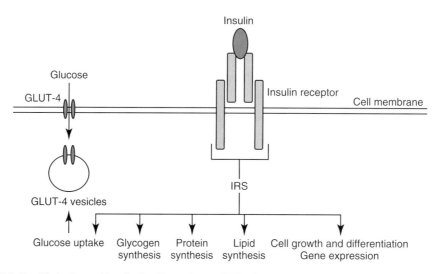

FIGURE 7-9 Simplified scheme of insulin signaling pathways. *GLUT-4,* Glucose transporter 4; *IRS,* insulin receptor substrate.

Insulin stimulates protein synthesis and inhibits protein degradation, therefore promoting a positive nitrogen balance. Glucagon is the main antagonist of insulin. It acts predominantly on the liver where it increases gluconeogenesis and glycogenolysis and decreases glycogen synthesis. It is also a ketogenic hormone, because of its ability to enhance lipolysis. Insulin and glucagon act in concert after ingestion of protein. Both hormones are released when the concentration of amino acids increases in the plasma. Insulin leads to a decrease in blood glucose concentration in concert with a decrease in amino acid levels. Glucagon counterbalances the decrease in glucose concentration by stimulation of hepatic gluconeogenesis. This interaction allows growth and survival with diets containing almost exclusively protein and fat.

Pathophysiology

Hyperglycemia develops when insulin secretion is absent or inadequate for the degree of insulin resistance. Absolute or relative lack of insulin has profound effects on carbohydrate, fat, and protein metabolism. Hyperglycemia results in part from reduced glucose entry into muscle, adipose tissue, and liver. Intestinal absorption of glucose and glucose entry into brain, kidney, and erythrocytes are not affected. The second and perhaps most important cause of hyperglycemia is unopposed glucose production in the liver (by gluconeogenesis and glycogenolysis). Glucagon contributes to increased production of glucose, as do other (stress) hormones. When the renal capacity for glucose reabsorption is exceeded, glucose is lost in the urine. The resulting osmotic diuresis is compensated by increased water intake, which may lead to severe polydipsia. Diabetic polyphagia is regulated by central mechanisms, in which ghrelin-signaling and other pathways are important. Derangement of lipid metabolism plays a major role in the development of diabetes mellitus and its complications. Intracellular deficits of glucose and lack of insulin lead to acceleration of lipid catabolism. Increased levels of NEFA are transported to the liver, where they undergo β-oxidation to produce acetyl-CoA, the amount of which may exceed the capacity for further oxidation. This results in a shift to ketone body production and may lead to the development of ketoacidosis. An increased hepatic concentration of fatty acids also results in enhanced hepatic synthesis of triglycerides and very–low-density lipoproteins (VLDLs). The consequences are hepatic steatosis and hyperlipidemia.

Protein metabolism shifts towards decreased protein synthesis and increased proteolysis. The increased availability of amino acids further accelerates hepatic gluconeogenesis. Consequences are negative nitrogen balance, loss of muscle mass, and possibly cachexia (Fig. 7-10).

 SIGNALMENT

Most cats with diabetes mellitus are older than 4 years of age at the time of diagnosis, although the disease may occur at any age. Juvenile onset of diabetes (i.e., diabetes during the first year of age) is a rare event. In a recent study involving 2576 cats with diabetes mellitus in the United States, only 1.3% of cats were 1 year old or younger, another 1.3% were between 1 and 2 years old, whereas nearly 50% of the cats were between 10 and 15 years old (Prahl et al, 2007; Table 7-2). There is a male predominance; in two large studies from the United States and the United Kingdom, 63% and 65% of diabetic cats were male. It is not yet clear if neutering (in both sexes) is associated with an increased risk of diabetes; in the study performed in the United Kingdom, neutered cats were more likely to be diabetic than intact ones, whereas this was not the case in the study performed in the United States (McCann et al, 2007; Prahl et al, 2007). The vast majority of diabetic cats are mixed-breed cats (i.e., Domestic Short-Hair and Domestic Long-Hair). In some countries (e.g., Australia, New Zealand, and the United Kingdom), the Burmese breed has been shown to be at increased risk (Wade et al, 1999; McCann et al, 2007; Lederer et al, 2009), whereas this risk seems not to be present in breeding lines of other countries. In our own population of diabetic cats, approximately 50% to 60% are overweight, 30% to 40% are normal weight, and 5% to 10% are underweight (Reusch, 2010). For more details on prevalence and risk factors, see Prevalence and Risk Factors in Humans and Cats at the beginning of the chapter.

TABLE 7-2	AGE OF 2576 CATS WITH DIABETES MELLITUS FROM THE VETERINARY MEDICAL DATA BASE JANUARY 1, 1970, THROUGH DECEMBER 31, 1999

AGE (YEARS)	NUMBER OF CATS	PERCENT
≤ 1	32	1.3
1 to 2	34	1.3
2 to 4	83	3.3
4 to 7	288	11.3
7 to 10	570	22.5
10 to 15	1220	48.1
> 15	311	12.2

From Prahl A, et al.: Time trends and risk factors for diabetes mellitus in cats presented to veterinary teaching hospitals, *J Feline Med Surg* 9:351, 2007.

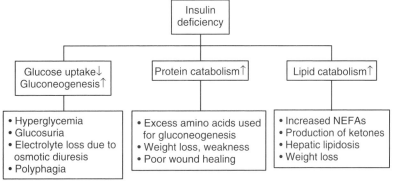

FIGURE 7-10 Effects of insulin deficiency (simplified overview). *NEFAs,* Non-esterified fatty acids.

ANAMNESIS

The typical history includes the classic signs of polydipsia, polyuria, polyphagia, and weight loss. A common complaint of cat owners is the need to frequently change the litter and an increase in the size of the litter clumps, indicating polyuria. Oftentimes, additional clinical signs are present, such as lethargy, decreased interaction with family members, lack of regular grooming, and the development of a dry, lusterless, and unkempt hair coat. Generally, severity of clinical signs ranges between mild/moderate to severe depending on the duration and extent of the diabetic disease. Approximately 10% of diabetic cats have overt signs of diabetic neuropathy, which include hind limb weakness, decreased ability to jump, and a plantigrade posture while standing or walking. Usually, those signs are restricted to the hind limbs; on rare occasion, additional weakness and plantigrade stance may be seen in the front legs. Some owners may overlook the more typical signs of diabetes and the cat is presented because of "lameness" or difficulty to walk and jump. Different to dogs, cats with diabetes are almost never presented because of sudden blindness caused by diabetic cataract. Interestingly, however, the vast majority of diabetic cats reveal some degree of cataract when a specific ophthalmic examination is performed (for details see Chronic Complications of Diabetes Mellitus; Williams and Heath, 2006). In diabetic cats with concurrent disease, additional or other than the classical signs may be reported by the owner. For instance, cats with concurrent pancreatitis may show reduced appetite or complete lack of food intake, some show vomiting, whereas diarrhea is rare. If the clinical signs of uncomplicated diabetes go unnoticed by the owner, a diabetic cat may be at risk to develop DKA. In such a case, the classical clinical signs of diabetes usually are no longer present at the time of presentation. Cats with DKA have similar signs as cats with pancreatitis (both problems often occur in concert), such as lethargy, anorexia, and vomiting; water intake may also be reduced. The time sequence from the onset of diabetes to the development of DKA is unpredictable, ranging from weeks to months and depends in part on the type and severity of any concurrent disease. A complete history is of utmost importance, and the clinician should always consider the possibility of concurrent disorders. Any disorder may reduce insulin sensitivity and may potentially lead to overt diabetes in predisposed animals. Similarly, a detailed medical history should be taken as glucocorticoids (systemic and topical) and progestagens have diabetogenic effects (see Fig. 7-2). Identification and treatment of concurrent disorders and cessation of diabetogenic drugs play major roles in the successful management of the diabetic cats. Dietary history and feeding management (meal or continuous feeding) should also be taken.

 PHYSICAL EXAMINATION

The findings during the physical examination depend on the duration and severity of the diabetic disease as well as the presence or absence of DKA and the nature of any concurrent diseases. Cats with recent onset of diabetes or in which severity of diabetes is mild may appear clinically normal and physical examination may be more or less unremarkable. In contrast, cats with long-duration of untreated diabetes may appear seriously ill, in particular if DKA is present. Many newly diagnosed diabetic cats are overweight, although they usually have lost weight. They are rarely emaciated unless a serious concurrent disease (e.g., exocrine pancreatic insufficiency, pancreatic neoplasia,

inflammatory bowel disease, or hyperthyroidism) is present. It is helpful to characterize the cats according to one of the currently available body scoring systems (e.g., a 5- or 9-point scale) at initial evaluation and during all rechecks (Fig. 7-11). The same system should be consistently used by all doctors and staff of the hospital. It should be noted that the commonly-used body condition scoring (BCS) focuses mainly on the determination of body fat through evaluation of body silhouette and palpation of adipose tissue (Laflamme, 1997; Michel et al, 2011). Loss of muscle mass may be missed or underestimated or only detected in seriously underweight cats. Assessing muscle condition, however, is important, because loss of muscle adversely affects strength and immune function and has been shown to be independently associated with mortality in humans (Baldwin et al, 2010). Evaluation of muscle mass should be done additionally to the determination of the BCS. It includes visual inspection and palpation over the temporal bones, scapulae, lumbar vertebrae, and pelvic bones. Currently, a 4-point scale is used to assess muscle mass, ranging from normal muscle mass, to mild, moderate, and marked muscles wasting (Baldwin et al, 2010; Michel et al, 2011). See the "AAHA Nutritional Assessment Guidelines for Dogs and Cats" for further details (Baldwin et al, 2010). Diabetic cats may be lethargic, although this may not be obvious immediately if the cat is severely stressed in the examination room. Cats with newly diagnosed or poorly controlled diabetes often stop grooming and develop a dry, lusterless, and unkempt hair coat. The vast majority of diabetic cats show nerve lesions similar to those seen in humans with diabetic neuropathy when histological examinations of peripheral nerves are performed. Obvious clinical signs, however, are present only in approximately 10% of cases. Abnormalities include weakness in the hind limbs, inability to jump, ataxia, muscle atrophy, and a plantigrade posture when standing and walking (Fig. 7-12). A palmigrade posture may also be seen in rare cases. Cats may be object to touching and palpation limbs or feet, presumably because of pain associated with the neuropathy. Findings during neurological examination include postural reaction deficits and decreased tendon reflexes of different severity. Subtle neurological changes may go unnoticed if the cat's gait is not evaluated carefully and no thorough neurological examination is performed. See Box 7-2 and Chronic Complications of Diabetes Mellitus for further details.

Abdominal palpation may reveal hepatomegaly due to diabetes-induced hepatic lipidosis. In cats with concurrent pancreatitis, a mass in the cranial abdomen, consisting of pancreas and inflamed peripancreatic fat, can sometimes be palpated. This mass can easily be misdiagnosed as another intraabdominal structure (e.g., neoplasia within the intestinal tract, enlarged mesenteric lymph node). Palpation may or may not elicit a response of pain. Severe acute or acute on chronic pancreatitis may be associated with dehydration, tachycardia, tachypnea, and icterus; cats may be hypothermic; fever is also possible but less common (Armstrong and Williams, 2012; Caney, 2013). For more details on pancreatitis, see Types of Diabetes in Cats and the discussion on pancreatic enzymes in Clinical Pathology. Similarly, in cats with DKA, severe lethargy, dehydration, abdominal pain, and icterus may be present. Pancreatitis and DKA oftentimes occur in concert.

Lens opacities associated with diabetic cataract are usually mild and only visible by ophthalmoscopy in most cases. More severe cataracts may be present in diabetic kittens compared with adult cats with diabetes (Thoresen et al, 2002; Williams and Heath, 2006).

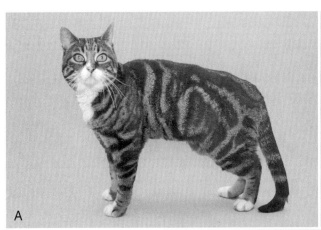
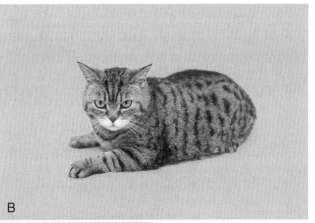
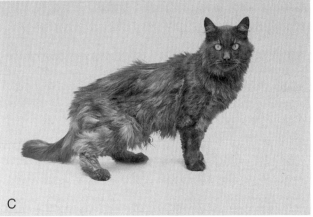

FIGURE 7-11 Three cats with newly-diagnosed diabetes mellitus and different body condition scores using a 9-point scale. **A,** An example of a relatively normal looking diabetic cat. **B,** A severely overweight cat. **C,** An underweight cat. **A,** Domestic Short-Hair (DSH), spayed female, 13 years old with a body weight of 4.2 kg and a body condition score (BCS) of 5/9. The cat suffered from polyuria/polydipsia, polyphagia, and some weight loss for approximately 4 weeks before presentation. The cat was clinically well, initial blood glucose concentration was 468 mg/dL (26 mmol/L), and fructosamine concentration was 636 µmol/L. **B,** British Shorthair cat, castrated male, 12 years old with a body weight of 8 kg and a BCS of 9/9. The presenting complaint was polydipsia. The cat was slightly lethargic, initial blood glucose was 223 mg/dL (12.4 mmol/L), and fructosamine was 615 µmol/L. **C,** Norwegian Forest cat, castrated male, 14 years old with a body weight of 4.8 kg and a BCS of 3/9. The cat had lost 2 kg of body weight during the previous 2 months, and more recently, the owner had noticed polyuria and polydipsia and reduced appetite. He was dehydrated and had a poor hair coat, initial blood glucose concentration was 509 mg/dL (28.3 mmol/L), and fructosamine concentration was 706 µmol/L. Lipase activity and feline pancreas-specific lipase (Spec fPL) were slightly increased, and ultrasonographic findings were consistent with chronic pancreatitis of moderate severity. After initiating insulin therapy the clinical condition improved and body weight increased.

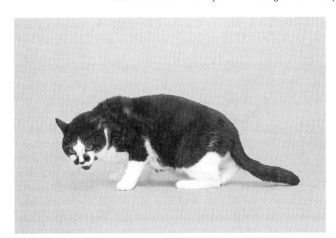

FIGURE 7-12 Plantigrade stance due to diabetic neuropathy in a 15-year-old, castrated male, Domestic Short-Hair (DSH) with diabetes mellitus. The gait improved slightly during insulin therapy.

 ESTABLISHING A DIAGNOSIS OF DIABETES MELLITUS

A diagnosis of diabetes mellitus is based on the presence of appropriate clinical signs (i.e., polyuria, polydipsia, polyphagia, weight loss) and documentation of persistent fasting hyperglycemia and glycosuria. In contrast to human medicine, no precise diagnostic criteria for feline diabetes have so far been established. Therefore, the cut-off value for blood glucose concentration, above which the animal is considered diabetic, is somewhat vague. The vast majority of cats are not presented until blood glucose concentrations exceed the renal capacity for glucose reabsorption (approximately 270 mg/dL, 15 mmol/L). It is usually only at this stage of the disease that clinical signs become apparent. Glycosuria alone is insufficient to diagnose diabetes, because it may also occur with primary renal defects and some of the commercially available urine reagent test strips and tablets may show false positive results associated with

BOX 7-2	Criteria for Neurological Assessment of Severity of Signs and Determination of Severity Rank of Nondiabetic and Diabetic Cats

Severity of Neurological Signs	Criteria
Very mild	• Walks with base-narrow gait • Difficulty in jumping • No evidence of plantigrade stance • Normal postural reactions and reflexes
Mild	• Irritable when touching and manipulating feet • Partially plantigrade, partially crouched limb position • Mild postural reaction deficits • Normal tendon reflexes
Mild/moderate	• Irritable when touching and manipulating feet • Base-narrow gait • Partially plantigrade when walking and standing • Moderately decreased postural reactions and reflexes • Normal tendon reflexes
Moderate	• Irritable when touching and manipulating feet • Plantigrade when walking and standing • Mild generalized muscle atrophy • Decreased postural reactions • Mildly to moderately decreased tendon reflexes
Moderate/severe	• Irritable when touching and manipulating feet • Obvious ataxia and paresis, especially in pelvic limbs • Palmigrade and plantigrade when standing • Plantigrade when walking • Generalized muscle atrophy • Severe postural reaction deficits • Hyporeflexia to areflexia
Severe	• Irritable when touching and manipulating feet • Obvious generalized ataxia and paresis • Palmigrade and plantigrade when standing • Fully palmigrade and plantigrade when walking • Generalized muscle atrophy • Severe postural reaction deficits • Hyporeflexia to areflexia

Modified from Mizisin AP, et al.: Neurological complications associated with spontaneously occurring feline diabetes mellitus, *J Neuropathol Exp Neurol* 61:872, 2002.

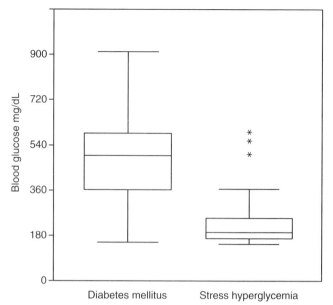

FIGURE 7-13 Blood glucose concentrations in cats with diabetes mellitus and in cats with stress hyperglycemia. Diabetic cats had significantly higher glucose concentrations; however, substantial overlap was seen, and in 20% of the cats with stress hyperglycemia, blood glucose concentrations were increased above the renal threshold. To convert mg/dL to mmol/L multiply by 0.056. (Data from Laluha P, et al.: Stress hyperglycemia in sick cats: a retrospective study over 4 years, *Schweiz Arch Tierheilkd* 146:375, 2004.)

Fig. 7-13). In cats with mild to moderate stress hyperglycemia, glycosuria usually does not occur. However, if stress induces an increase of blood glucose above the renal threshold for some time (hours), glycosuria may be present as in cats with diabetes. Stress hyperglycemia may be diagnosed by repeated blood glucose measurements and the demonstration of normalized glucose levels. Some cats, however, are stressed throughout the period of hospitalization, and glucose levels remain high. In those cases, the measurement of serum fructosamine may be helpful (see Serum Fructosamine Concentration).

Recently, the term *prediabetes* has started to be used in veterinary medicine. In humans, the term describes individuals whose glucose levels do not meet the criteria for diabetes, yet they are higher than those considered normal (American Diabetes Association, 2013; Table 7-3). So far, there is no officially recognized definition in dogs and cats and the term is somewhat arbitrarily used for any degree of mild hyperglycemia. Cats that have blood glucose concentrations below the renal threshold usually do not have clinical signs of diabetes, and therefore, glucose concentrations between approximately 120 and 270 mg/dL (6.7 to 15 mmol/L) may be considered to represent mild hyperglycemia. Differential diagnosis includes blood glucose increase after a carbohydrate-rich meal, stress hyperglycemia, and mild/beginning diabetes mellitus. Postprandial hyperglycemia may be ruled out by repeating the measurement in a fasted state. Stress hyperglycemia and mild/beginning diabetes mellitus, however, are difficult to differentiate, because fructosamine may be normal in both instances. Normalization of blood glucose concentrations over time is indicative for stress hyperglycemia. Mild/beginning diabetes may have various causes; one of them is the previous or current administration of glucocorticoids or progestagens. In principle, any disease may lead to some degree of insulin resistance and some cats may not be able to compensate by increasing their insulin production (see Fig. 7-2). Cats with mild hyperglycemia should undergo a thorough evaluation and repetitive blood glucose measurements in a fasted state.

the administration of drugs (e.g., some antimicrobials) (Rees and Boothe, 2004). Cats are prone to stress-induced hyperglycemia, which may be difficult to differentiate from hyperglycemia due to diabetes. Increases in blood glucose caused by stress are often only mild to moderate. However, in some cats, blood glucose may increase to levels higher than 270 mg/dL (15 mmol/L) (Rand et al, 2002; Laluha et al, 2004). In a recent study, blood glucose levels in 106 cats with stress hyperglycemia ranged from 146 to 592 mg/dL with a median of 192 (8.1 to 32.9 mmol/L, median 10.7), 21 of the 106 cats (20%) had glucose levels higher than 270 mg/dL (15 mmol/L). Although blood glucose concentrations in cats with stress hyperglycemia were significantly lower than in cats with diabetes, substantial overlap was seen (Laluha et al, 2004;

	CRITERIA FOR DIAGNOSIS OF PREDIABETES IN HUMANS	CRITERIA FOR DIAGNOSIS OF DIABETES IN HUMANS
TABLE 7-3 CRITERIA FOR THE DIAGNOSIS OF PREDIABETES AND DIABETES IN HUMANS		
Fasting blood glucose	100 to 125 mg/dL (5.6 to 6.9 mmol/L)	≥ 126 mg/dL (7.0 mmol/L)
2-hour glucose in the 75-g oral glucose tolerance test	140 to 199 mg/dL (7.8 to 11.0 mmol/L)	≥ 200 mg/dL (11.1 mmol/L)

From American Diabetes Association: Diagnosis and classification of diabetes mellitus, *Diabetes Care* 36 (suppl 1):67, 2013.

If no treatable cause is identified, regular reevaluations should be performed to determine if overt diabetes develops. In the stage of "prediabetes," weight reduction and feeding a low-carbohydrate–high-protein diet should be recommended, and insulin treatment should be initiated if blood glucose concentrations begin to rise.

In cats with DKA or severe concurrent disease (e.g., acute pancreatitis), the typical clinical signs of diabetes may not be present at the time of diagnosis, and instead signs of systemic illness will dominate the clinical picture. In those cases, confirmation of diabetes relies on the documentation of hyperglycemia, glycosuria, and increased fructosamine concentration. Immediate further work-up is required, because the animal may be in a life-threatening condition. The finding of ketone bodies in urine by use of urine test strips or increased β-hydroxybutyrate concentration in blood by a handheld meter (Precision Xtra or Precision Xceed, Abbott) is indicative for DKA. Please see Chapter 8 for further details. Diagnosis of pancreatitis is discussed later in this chapter.

CLINICAL PATHOLOGY

After establishing the diagnosis of diabetes, it is important to evaluate the cat for the presence of concurrent diseases. Any disease can worsen insulin resistance and has the potential to render insulin therapy difficult. In some cases, it is only because a concurrent problem occurred that the diabetic disease progressed from a subclinical to a clinically overt state. Reducing insulin resistance by treating the concurrent problem(s) is an important part of diabetic management. The minimum laboratory evaluation in a newly diagnosed diabetic cat should include a complete blood count (CBC), a serum biochemical panel, and an urinalysis with bacterial culture. If available, abdominal ultrasonography should also be performed as part of the routine work-up (see later).

Complete Blood Count, Serum Biochemical Panel, Urinalysis, and Urine Culture

Cats and dogs with diabetes mellitus have similar clinical pathological abnormalities. See Chapter 6 for more details.

In cats with uncomplicated diabetes, a CBC usually does not reveal major abnormalities. Mild normochromic, normocytic anemia (packed cell volume [PCV] 25% to 30%) is a relatively frequent finding, most likely reflecting chronic disease. In dehydrated cats, mild polycythemia may be present, which is frequently associated with an increase in total protein concentrations. Cats with uncomplicated diabetes oftentimes have a normal white blood cell count or a so-called stress leukogram (mature neutrophilia, lymphopenia, eosinopenia). Pronounced neutrophilia, in particular when associated with an increase in immature neutrophils as well as the finding of toxic neutrophils (with or without neutrophilia), points to an inflammatory or infectious process. In the latter situation, the clinician should consider acute pancreatitis as one of the major differential diagnosis. The most common biochemical abnormalities include hyperglycemia, hypercholesterolemia, and increased liver enzyme activities. The vast majority of newly diagnosed diabetic cats have blood glucose concentrations above 300 mg/dL (17 mmol/L); on rare occasions, blood glucose may be as high as 900 mg/dL (50 mmol/L) or even higher. Extremely elevated blood glucose concentrations in diabetic cats are often associated with concurrent chronic renal failure. Between 40% and 50% of diabetic cats have increased serum alanine aminotransferase (ALT) and/or alkaline phosphatase (ALP) activities, which is presumably due to diabetes-associated hepatic lipidosis. The increases are typically up to five times the upper limit of normal in cases of ALT and up to three times the upper limit of normal in cases of ALP. More pronounced increases should raise suspicion for hepatic lipidosis being more severe than what is consistent with uncomplicated diabetes, other liver diseases, or pancreatitis. Increased cholesterol and triglyceride concentrations are present in roughly one-third of diabetic cats, which is usually up to three times the upper limit of normal.

A mild increase in total bilirubin concentration (up to two times the upper limit of normal) is quite common and most likely caused by the typical diabetes-associated hepatic lipidosis. If moderate to severe hyperbilirubinemia is present, severe hepatic lipidosis, other liver diseases, or extrahepatic biliary obstruction by pancreatitis should be considered as the most likely causes. Some diabetic cats reveal hypocalcemia, potentially associated with the presence of pancreatitis. Blood urea nitrogen (BUN) and serum creatinine are usually normal in cats with uncomplicated diabetes. An elevation in these parameters may either be due to a prerenal cause (most likely dehydration) or renal disease. In humans, nephropathy is a common complication of diabetes mellitus, whereas in cats, diabetes-associated kidney lesions seem to be rare (see Chronic Complications of Diabetes Mellitus). Chronic renal failure in diabetic cats should therefore be considered a coincidence, because both diseases are relatively frequent in the elderly cat population.

The most typical finding in the urinalysis is moderate to marked glycosuria. Cats with uncomplicated diabetes usually do not have ketonuria; however, trace to small amounts of ketone bodies may occasionally be found. Moderate to large amounts of ketones are indicative of DKA, in particular in cats with signs of systemic illness. In the majority of cats, urine specific gravity is more than 1.020; approximately 50% to 70% of cases have proteinuria, which is usually mild to moderate with a urine protein-to-creatinine ratio less than 2.0. Hematuria, pyuria, and bacteriuria in the urine sediment have been shown to correlate strongly with a positive urine culture. However, in some cats with bacterial urinary tract infection, the urine sediment is unremarkable. Therefore, urine culture should be performed in all cats with diabetes, irrespective of urine specific gravity, presence or absence of proteinuria, and abnormal sediment findings. In two recent studies, urinary tract infection was identified in 12% and 13.2% of diabetic cats, with *Escherichia coli* being the most common isolate (Bailiff et al, 2006; Mayer-Roenne et al, 2007). Urinary tract infections with *Candida spp.* have been reported sporadically in diabetic cats (Pressler et al, 2003; Jin and Lin, 2005).

Pancreatic Enzymes

Pancreatitis has been recognized as a common concurrent disease in cats with diabetes mellitus. Feline pancreatitis is classified into acute and chronic forms, the latter being more common. Some cats suffer from both acute and chronic pancreatitis, and recurrent bouts of acute phases may occur. The cause and effect relationship between pancreatitis and diabetes is largely unknown and very difficult to explore due to the lack of longitudinal studies, which would include histopathology of the pancreas. Severe pancreatitis may result in damage not only of the exocrine but also of the endocrine part of the pancreas, which then would lead to diabetes. Most likely, however, this is a relatively rare event. In the opinion of the author, it is more common for pancreatitis to develop during the course of the diabetic disease. The clinical presentation of pancreatitis varies widely. In some cats, pancreatitis is clinically insignificant with no obvious clinical signs. Other cats suffer from recurrent bouts of pancreatitis ranging from mild lethargy and reduced appetite of a few days' duration to severe illness with complete lack of food intake, vomiting, and dehydration and again others may be constantly unwell. Another subset of diabetic cats suffers from a single episode of severe pancreatitis, which may be severe and life-threatening. Pancreatitis (and/or DKA) should be considered in any diabetic cat presented with lethargy, reduced appetite or anorexia, vomiting, and dehydration. Pancreatitis is also an important differential diagnosis in a difficult to regulate diabetic cat, in particular if the course of the disease is waxing and waning (i.e., times of good glycemic control or hypoglycemia alter with times of poor control). Diagnosis of pancreatitis, however, is challenging, because all available tests have major limitations. Serum amylase activity is often low or normal in cats with pancreatitis and therefore considered to be of no diagnostic value (Kitchell et al, 1986; Parent et al, 1995; Zoran, 2006). Similarly, traditional assays of lipase activity are widely described to be unreliable due to poor sensitivity and specificity. During the recent years, assays that specifically measure the pancreatic lipase activity (known as *fPLI* or *Spec fPL*) became available and are currently considered to be the most accurate blood tests for diagnosing pancreatitis in cats (Steiner et al, 2004; Forman et al, 2009; Armstrong and Williams, 2012). One study reported an overall sensitivity of fPLI for pancreatitis of 67% (100% for moderate to severe pancreatitis and 54% for mild pancreatitis). Overall specificity was 91% (100% in healthy cats and 67% in symptomatic cats with normal pancreatic histology) (Forman et al, 2004). Another study evaluated the Spec fPL and also found 100% sensitivity for severe chronic pancreatitis; specificity, however, was only 54% (Oppliger et al, 2013a). These numbers nicely demonstrate the problems associated with the measurement of the fPLI/Spec fPL test: In cats with severe pancreatitis, the test will usually be positive, whereas it may be negative in mild disease. A positive test result, however, does not mean that the cat has pancreatitis, as specificity is low (67% and 54%). A few studies evaluated fPLI/Spec fPL in cats with diabetes mellitus so far. Prevalence of increased fPLI or Spec fPL was 30%, 43%, and 83% (Forcada et al, 2008; Zini et al, 2011; Schäfer et al, 2013). Interestingly, none of the more than 200 cats showed any clinical signs suggestive of pancreatitis. It is possible that those cats had pancreatic lesions that were not severe enough to cause clinical signs; histopathology, however, was not performed. We do not recommend measuring Spec fPL in cats with uncomplicated diabetes, because any increased value will be difficult to interpret. In diabetic cats with clinical signs suggestive of pancreatitis, diagnosis should be based on the careful assessment of history, physical examination, Spec fPL (or DGGR lipase, see later), additional laboratory findings, and abdominal ultrasonography. In some cats, however, pancreatitis remains a diagnosis by exclusion.

Very recently, the belief that the "normal" serum lipase activity is of no diagnostic utility has been challenged. It was shown in a large number of cats that a particular lipase assay (DGGR assay) agrees substantially with the Spec fPL. The DGGR assay can be performed by routine autoanalysis and therefore be incorporated into a serum biochemical panel rendering lipase measurement more readily available and less expensive (Oppliger et al, 2013b).

Increase in serum fTLI is only very short lived in cats after the onset of pancreatitis and its sensitivity is therefore low. Its measurement is mainly recommended for the diagnosis of exocrine pancreatic insufficiency in the cat, which may develop as a sequela of chronic pancreatitis. Exocrine pancreatic insufficiency should be considered as differential diagnosis in cats with weight loss, polyphagia, and loose stools; a low fPLI would support the diagnosis (Steiner, 2012).

Serum Thyroxine Concentration

Hyperthyroidism is a common endocrine disorder and its prevalence has increased continuously over the last decades. A recent study performed in more than 200 diabetic cats treated with insulin for at least 1 month revealed that 4.5% of them had increased serum thyroxine (T_4) concentrations. This number was considered to approximate the prevalence of hyperthyroidism in the general elderly cat population (Schaefer et al, 2013). Natural occurring and experimentally induced hyperthyroidism has been shown to cause insulin resistance. (Hoenig and Ferguson, 1989; Hoenig et al, 1992). Insulin resistance and possibly impaired insulin secretion is also a well-known phenomenon in humans with hyperthyroidism (Hanley, 2010). The presence of concurrent hyperthyroidism is therefore important to recognize, and the thyroid status should be evaluated in every diabetic cat. When interpreting the laboratory results, the veterinarian should remember that poor glycemic control and any other concurrent diseases may lower the T_4 concentration ("euthyroid sick syndrome") and the diagnosis may be missed. Similarly, in newly diagnosed diabetic cats, T_4 concentrations often are quite low and increase during insulin therapy. This is true for diabetic cats with and without concurrent hyperthyroidism. The latter may therefore be overlooked if T_4 measurements are not repeated after insulin therapy has been performed for some weeks (Fig. 7-14).

In our hospital, we routinely measure T_4 concentrations in newly-diagnosed diabetic cats. Increased T_4 levels support hyperthyroidism and appropriate therapy is initiated additionally to the treatment of diabetes. If the T_4 concentration is normal or low, initial measures are restricted to diabetic management. T_4 measurements are repeated after a few weeks, in particular in cats in which we do not successfully regulate the diabetic disease. We have seen quite a number of diabetic cats in which T_4 measurement had to be repeated several times before hyperthyroidism could be demonstrated. T_4 is also routinely evaluated in all diabetic cats with poor glycemic control, including cats in which glycemic control suddenly deteriorates during therapy. As mentioned earlier, hyperthyroidism lowers serum fructosamine concentrations due to accelerated protein metabolism. Therefore, a low or normal fructosamine concentration or a sudden decrease in fructosamine concentration in a cat with poor glycemic control should alert the veterinarian to the possibility of concurrent hyperthyroidism. Chapter 4 presents a detailed discussion on diagnosis of hyperthyroidism. It also includes information on diagnostic tests that may

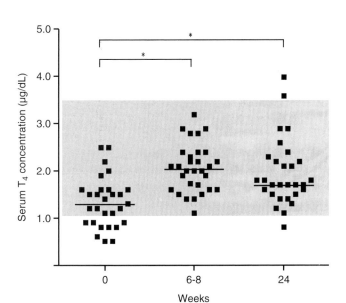

FIGURE 7-14 Serum thyroxine (T_4) concentrations in 30 cats with newly-diagnosed uncomplicated diabetes mellitus. At the time of diagnosis of diabetes, nine of the cats (30%) had T_4 concentrations below the reference range, which normalized after 6 to 8 weeks of insulin therapy. After 24 weeks of insulin therapy, two cats revealed increased T_4 concentrations; those cats were considered hyperthyroid and medical treatment was started. Their initial T_4 concentrations were 2.2 and 2.5 µg/dL, respectively. Reference range: 1.0 to 3.5 µg/dL. To convert µg/dL to nmol/L multiply by 12.87. (Unpublished data from Hafner M, University of Zurich, Switzerland.) * = Significant difference.

be performed in questionable cases (i.e., cats suspected of hyperthyroidism but have normal T_4 concentrations).

Serum Insulin Concentration

Measurement of the serum insulin concentration is not part of the routine work-up in our hospital. In newly-diagnosed diabetic cats, baseline insulin and insulin concentrations after the administration of a secretagogue (e.g., glucagon, arginine) are usually low or low-normal and do not differ between cats in which diabetic remission occurs during subsequent therapy and cats with permanent diabetes (Nelson et al, 1999; Tschuor et al, 2011). Insulin measurements therefore are not helpful to differentiate between an irreversible β-failure and β-cells that have the potential to recover after the negative effects of high blood glucose concentrations (glucotoxicity) have been reversed by insulin treatment. In theory, a high insulin concentration in a newly diagnosed diabetic cat suggests the presence of functioning β-cells and the presence of an insulin-antagonistic disorder. However, as insulin concentrations are low or low-normal in the vast majority of cats at the time of diagnosis, this is not a cost-effective diagnostic procedure. In cases in which insulin measurements are performed, it is of utmost importance that the insulin assay is validated for the cat and that species-specific reference ranges are available. Most commercially available assays are designed to measure human insulin and do not work in the cat due to amino acid differences between human and feline insulin. Recently, an enzyme-linked immunosorbent assay (ELISA) designed to measure feline insulin was validated (Strage et al, 2012). Most assays will cross-react with exogenously administered insulin; therefore, treatment should be withheld for at least 24 hours in cats already undergoing insulin therapy. Insulin withdrawal may, however, put the cat at risk for DKA, in particular in a stressful environment (i.e., in the hospital). The risk should be

weighed carefully against any potential benefit. See Remission of Diabetes in Cats earlier and Figs. 7-5 and 7-6 for more details.

DIAGNOSTIC IMAGING

Thoracic and abdominal radiographs play a limited role in the work-up of cats with newly diagnosed diabetes. In uncomplicated cases, hepatomegaly usually is the only relevant finding. Loss of detail or a mass-like effect would raise suspicion for pancreatitis or pancreatic neoplasia. We perform survey radiographs cats in which we suspect the presence of concurrent disease (e.g., cardiorespiratory, skeletal, urolithiasis); this includes cats that are difficult to regulate and cats presented with DKA. In contrast, abdominal ultrasonography is part of our routine work-up in any cat presented with diabetes. Ultrasonography is helpful to investigate size and parenchyma of abdominal organs and abdominal lymph nodes, the bile duct for obstruction, the renal pelvis for dilatation (e.g., in case of pyelonephritis), and the wall thickness and layering of the intestinal tract. In diabetic cats, the pancreas is of particular interest, and ultrasonography is one of the major tools to diagnose pancreatitis. However, visualization of the pancreas is quite difficult and therefore dependent on the experience of the operator and the ultrasonographic equipment. The normal sonographic appearance of the pancreas in cats is isoechoic to slightly hyperechoic to the adjacent liver and nearly isoechoic to the surrounding mesenteric fat. Pancreatitis has various ultrasonographic appearances, depending on the severity, duration of the disease, and extent of pancreatic and peripancreatic inflammation (Penninck, 2008; Fig. 7-15).

Findings associated with acute pancreatitis include enlargement of the pancreas, irregular pancreatic margins, hypoechoic irregular parenchyma, pancreas surrounded by hyperechoic mesentery and/or hyperechoic fat as a result of fat saponification, dilation of the biliary duct, peripancreatic fluid accumulation, and thickening of gastric and duodenal wall, and altered wall layering. Some cats show signs of pain associated with the pressure of the ultrasound probe. Hyperechoic or mixed echogenicity, nodular echotexture, and acoustic shadowing due to mineralization and scarring may be found in cases with chronic pancreatitis. Pancreatic pseudocysts and abscesses may be seen as a sequela to pancreatitis, appearing as round to irregularly marginated fluid-filled mass lesions (Hecht and Henry, 2007). Findings of acute and chronic pancreatitis may overlap, because cats may have acute or chronic disease. The most useful criteria appear to be thickening of the pancreas, severely irregular pancreatic margins, and hyperechoic peripancreatic fat (Williams et al, 2013). It is important to note, however, that the pancreas may also look unremarkable in cats with pancreatitis and that ultrasonographic findings may not correlate with clinical disease. Additionally, the appearance of different pancreatic diseases overlap (e.g., a mass may represent an inflammatory lesion, nodular hyperplasia, or neoplasia). Therefore, ultrasonographic findings need to be interpreted in the light of the clinical situation and laboratory abnormalities.

Reported sensitivity of ultrasonography differs widely between studies; in part this is certainly due to differences in technical equipment and study design. In a study with histological confirmation of pancreatitis, overall sensitivity of abdominal ultrasound was 67% (80% for moderate to severe pancreatitis, 62% for mild pancreatitis) and overall specificity was 73% (88% in healthy cats and 33% in symptomatic cats without pancreatic histology) (Forman et al, 2004). Ultrasonography is also used to guide fine-needle aspiration (FNA), particularly in cats with pancreatic masses. FNA cytology awaits studies to investigate its diagnostic accuracy for

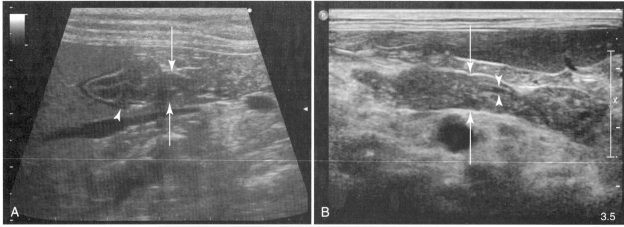

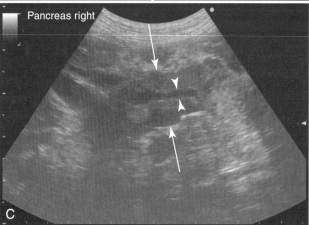

FIGURE 7-15 Ultrasonographic images of the pancreas in three cats with diabetes mellitus at initial presentation. **A,** Siamese cat, castrated male, 7 years old. The pancreas was of normal size, echogenicity was homogenous with smooth margins, and the pancreatic duct was of homogenous width. The pancreas was considered unremarkable. *White arrows* indicate the right branch of the pancreas; *white arrow heads* indicates the papilla duodeni. **B,** Norwegian Forest cat, castrated male, 14 years old (same cat as in Fig. 7-11, *C*). The pancreas was slightly enlarged, echogenicity was heterogenous and slightly hypoechoic, and the pancreatic duct was of homogenous width. Organ margins were slightly irregular. The findings were considered consistent with chronic pancreatitis of moderate intensity. *White arrows* indicate the pancreas; *white arrow heads* indicates the pancreatic duct. **C,** Domestic Short-Hair (DSH), castrated male, 16 years old. Severe diffuse enlargement of the pancreas with mixed echogenicity and irregular margins surrounded by hyperechoic fat was present. The diameter of the pancreatic duct was variable and appeared mildly dilated. The findings were consistent with pancreatitis, which was most likely an overlap between acute and chronic disease. *White arrows* indicate pancreas; *white arrow heads* indicates pancreatic duct. (Courtesy of Dr. Matthias Dennler and Prof. Patrick Kircher, Division of Diagnostic Imaging, Vetsuisse Faculty Zurich, Switzerland.)

the diagnosis of pancreatitis. Knowledge on the value of computed tomography (CT) in the diagnosis of pancreatitis is still scarce. According to currently available studies, its sensitivity seems to be very low (Gerhardt et al, 2001; Forman et al, 2004). We routinely evaluate the adrenal glands in diabetic cats during abdominal ultrasound. Symmetrical enlargement may suggest acromegaly or pituitary-dependent hyperadrenocorticism. An unilateral nodule or a mass may have various causes (see Table 13-5).

TREATMENT OF NONKETOTIC DIABETES MELLITUS

Goals of Therapy

The primary goal in treating nonketotic diabetes mellitus is to eliminate the clinical signs of diabetes, such as polyuria, polydipsia, polyphagia, and weight loss by good glycemic control, to prevent complications (e.g., hypoglycemia, DKA) and thereby enable a good quality of life. Early treatment and good glycemic control is important to increase the chance of diabetic remission. However, this issue requires special attention and one should remember that aggressive insulin therapy and aiming for normal or near normal blood glucose concentrations increases the risk of hypoglycemia. We routinely discuss the possibility of diabetic remission with owners of newly diagnosed diabetic cats. However, we do not stress remission as the major treatment goal for two reasons: to avoid treatment that is too aggressive (i.e., autonomous increase of insulin dose by the owner) and to avoid frustration of the owner if remission does not occur.

Successful treatment requires that the owner is highly motivated, able, and willing to adapt his or her daily routine to the cat's treatment plan and to work in close collaboration with the veterinarian. It may be difficult for some of the owners to understand the nature of the diabetic disease and the various treatment and monitoring options. Therefore, treatment should follow a precise and comprehensive protocol, and the owner should receive written information on all relevant aspects of the disease and the insulin injection. Short videos demonstrating handling and injection of insulin are also helpful (provided on websites of insulin manufacturers or diabetes forums). Another goal is to minimize the potential negative impact of the cat's disease on the owner and thereby avoid cessation of therapy or euthanasia. Recently, a study evaluated the psychological and social impact of diabetes and its daily treatment regimen on quality of life of both owner and diabetic cat. 221 cat owners from the United States, Canada, Australia, and various countries in Europe completed the survey. The factors with the most negative impact on quality of life were boarding difficulties, owners wanting more control on diabetes, difficulties leaving cat with friends or family, general worry about the cats' diabetes, worried about hypoglycemia, adapting social life, diabetes-related costs, and adapting work life (Niessen et al, 2010). The results of this study may help the veterinarian to address those issues and to make amendments to the treatment and monitoring protocol according to the needs of the individual owner (e.g., simplification of treatment if social life, work life, or costs are the major problems, access to home monitoring of blood glucose if owner wants more control, and avoidance of tight glucose regulation if owner is worried about hypoglycemia).

Treatment of a diabetic cat consists of medical therapy (usually insulin therapy), dietary management (including weight reduction if the cat is overweight), cessation of diabetogenic drugs, and prevention or control of any concurrent disease.

Initial Insulin Therapy

The administration of insulin is the most important part of the treatment regimen in diabetic cats and should be initiated as soon as possible after the diagnosis is established. In humans with type 2 diabetes, initial treatment usually consists of lifestyle modification and oral hypoglycemic drugs. Because many of the cat owners are either diabetic themselves or have diabetic relatives or friends, they tend to ask for those treatment modalities. We then explain our reason for using insulin as first line choice, which is mainly that insulin therapy is superior to the currently available oral hypoglycemic drugs to reverse the negative effects of glucose toxicity and to increase the chance of diabetic remission. In overt diabetes mellitus, dietary management alone is insufficient and may lead to deterioration of the disease and potentially to DKA. Diet, however, is an important part of the treatment.

In the last two decades, the manufacture and development of insulin for human use has undergone revolutionary changes, which have had important implications in veterinary medicine. First, insulins derived from animal sources are being more and more replaced by recombinant human preparations and will eventually disappear from the market. Although there are differences in the amino acid sequences (see Table 7-1) human insulins (and their analogues) are fortunately biologically active in cats. Second, insulin preparations for human use containing 40-IU/mL have largely been replaced by 100-IU/mL insulins. It is important that owners understand the difference, because two insulin preparations for veterinary use (Vetsulin/Caninsulin and ProZinc) are supplied as 40-IU/mL, and using the wrong syringe size would lead to substantial dosing errors. Third, new classes of insulins called *insulin analogues* have been developed. They were designed to improve the pharmacodynamic properties of insulin and render insulin absorption or insulin delivery to tissues more predictable. The currently available insulin analogues are certainly just the start of a whole new area of insulin preparations. The market for

insulin can be confusing because insulin availability (particularly if animal-derived) differs between countries as do the names for the same kind of insulin (e.g., Vetsulin is called Caninsulin outside of the United States). Insulin preparations available today may be withdrawn from the market tomorrow. The Internet is helpful to determine the status of a particular insulin (e.g., announcement of withdrawal of Vetsulin starting in 2009 and announcement of its re-approval in April 2013 in the United States).

Insulin preparations are classified as short-acting, intermediate-acting, long-acting, and so-called premixed or biphasic insulins. In principle, more potent insulin preparations have a shorter duration of action than less potent ones (see Fig. 6-30). Short-acting insulin (regular insulin, short-acting analogues such as aspartate, lispro, glulisine) is typically used in cats with DKA, hyperglycemic hyperosmolar state, or with extremely unstable glycemic control. Intermediate and long-acting preparations are used for long-term control of cats with uncomplicated diabetes. The longer duration of action is achieved by slowing the rate of absorption from the subcutaneous tissue. Delayed absorption is due either to the addition of substances that are virtually inert and do not have therapeutic properties themselves (e.g., protamine and zinc) or to a modification of the insulin molecule (as in insulin glargine and insulin detemir). Insulin detemir has some additional protracting effect because it binds to albumin not only in the subcutaneous and extracellular compartment but also in the systemic circulation (Havelund et al, 2004; Owens, 2011). A number of premixed or biphasic insulin formulations are available to facilitate treatment regimens in humans. They are designed to provide a more convenient approach to cover both basal and prandial insulin requirements and consist of a mixture of a short-acting and an intermediate/long-acting component. Ratios of the two components vary (e.g., 75:25, 70:30, and 50:50 intermediate-/long-acting-to-short-acting), premixed preparations are available as insulin analogues or as mixtures of conventional insulin preparations (Bilous and Donnelly, 2010). The use of premixed insulins has so far not been studied in cats. It is likely, however, that they will not be beneficial because cats do not have the same type of postprandial hyperglycemia as humans. See the section on insulin therapy in Chapter 6 for more details on insulin preparations.

Neutral Protamine Hagedorn Insulin

Neutral protamine Hagedorn (NPH) insulin preparations are potent insulins with a marked peak. Unfortunately, duration of action is considerably less than 12 hours in most cats, often resulting in hyperglycemia for several hours during the day. Additionally, the strong peak action increases the risk of hypoglycemia a few hours after administration. The use of NPH insulin is therefore not recommended.

Lente Insulin

A porcine-derived Lente-type insulin (Vetsulin/Caninsulin, Merck/MSD Animal Health) is licensed for use in cats in many countries. It is identical to canine insulin and differs from feline insulin by three amino acids (see Table 7-1). Vetsulin/Caninsulin is available at a concentration of 40 IU/mL, and should be administered twice a day (b.i.d.). Recently, a pen specifically designed to be used with this insulin has been marketed under the name of Vet-Pen. The pen comes in two sizes (0.5 to 8 IU and 1 to 16 IU); the smaller of the two allows insulin dosing in steps of 0.5 units. The pen is used with cartridges containing 2.7 mL (= 108 units) of insulin. Several studies have shown that Vetsulin/Caninsulin is effective and safe for the treatment of diabetes in cats. They are, however, difficult to compare due to the different study designs. As a rough summary, one may state that approximately 70% to 80% of cats were adequately controlled or diabetic remission was achieved and remission rates varied between 15% and 43%. Clinical hypoglycemia was seen in up to 25% of cats, and biochemical hypoglycemia was seen in more than 40% of cats. The time until the glucose nadir was reached varied substantially and ranged between 2 and 12 hours, and mean/median nadir was reached between 4 and 6 hours (Martin and Rand, 2001; 2007; Weaver et al, 2006; Michiels et al, 2008; Marshall et al, 2009). Vetsulin/Caninsulin is a mixture of 30% to 35% short-acting amorphous and 65% to 70% long-acting crystalline insulin; in theory, this combination should result in a relatively fast onset of action and duration of action of approximately 12 hours. However, in a substantial percentage of cats, the duration of action is considerably shorter, and adequate control cannot be achieved. The recently published American Animal Hospital Association (AAHA) guidelines therefore do not recommend Vetsulin/Caninsulin as the initial insulin option for diabetic cats (Rucinsky et al, 2010). Of note, the manufacturer has recently changed the label and now recommends vigorous shaking the vial prior to first use until a homogenous, uniformly milky suspension is obtained. This should ensure adequate homogenization of the two parts of the insulin, which obviously was a problem with the former recommendation of gently rolling the vial.

Protamine Zinc Insulin

Protamine zinc insulin (PZI) is insulin combined with protamine and zinc. It contains more protamine than NPH and therefore has a longer duration of action. Duration of action is also longer than in Lente insulin (Marshall et al, 2008a). The previous PZI product often used for diabetic cats, which was made from bovine and porcine insulin (PZI-Vet, IDEXX Laboratories), was discontinued some years ago. PZI-Vet was considered a good treatment option; a study reported that 90% of cats had good glycemic control after 45 days of therapy based on owner assessment (Nelson et al, 2001). The gap was filled by the release of ProZinc (Boehringer Ingelheim), which is a recombinant human insulin, formulated as protamine zinc insulin. The level of glycemic control was shown to be similar between the animal-derived and the recombinant product. Good glycemic control was achieved in 85% of cases by the end of the study (day 45). The final median insulin dose was 0.59 IU/kg b.i.d. (range 0.1 to 1.4). The glucose nadir occurred between 1 and 9 hours (mean 4.6); of note in 24% of cats, the lowest blood glucose concentration was at the last blood sampling, and the nadir presumably was later than 9 hours after the insulin administration. A long duration of effect may result in a substantial overlap and potentially hypoglycemia. Clinical hypoglycemia was rare and seen in only 1.5% of cases; biochemical hypoglycemia, however, was a frequent event and seen in 64% of cats at some time during the study period (Nelson et al, 2009). So far, knowledge on remission rates with PZI is scarce. One study reported a remission rate of 38% (Marshall et al, 2009). The AAHA Diabetes Management Guidelines lists ProZinc and Lantus (Insulin glargine, Sanofi) as the two insulin preparations of choice to initiate insulin therapy in cats (Rucinsky et al, 2010). ProZinc contains 40 IU insulin/mL. Contrary to the recommendation for Vetsulin/Caninsulin, the manufacturer of ProZinc recommends mixing by gently rolling the vial. It should be used b.i.d.; in some cats with very long duration of effect, once a day (s.i.d.) administration may be also be effective.

Long-Acting Insulin Analogues

Lantus (insulin glargine, Sanofi) has been the focus of attention in veterinary medicine for several years because of its theoretical benefits, namely a more constant rate of absorption and longer duration

of effect compared with several other insulin preparations. Initial studies confirmed that its duration of action is clearly longer than that of Lente insulin and comparable to PZI (Marshall et al, 2008a; 2008b). Recently, the pharmacodynamics of insulin glargine was compared to insulin detemir (Levemir, Novo Nordisk), which is another long-acting insulin analogue. The study was performed using an isoglycemic clamp method, which is considered to be the gold standard method in humans. Performance of the two insulin analogues was similar, the only significant difference was a faster onset of action of insulin glargine (mean of 1.3 hours versus mean of 1.8 hours). Mean time to peak action was 5.3 hours in glargine and 6.9 hours in detemir, and end of action was reached after a mean of 11.3 hours in glargine and 13.5 hours in detemir (Table 7-4). Interestingly, there were considerable variations in the shape of glucose curves; some cats had a flat curve whereas others revealed a pronounced peak (Gilor et al, 2010a). The results from this study compare quite well with our clinical experience made over the past years. Although duration of insulin glargine is quite long, b.i.d. administration is usually required to achieve adequate control or diabetic remission; shape of the glucose curves differ considerably between cats and also within the same cat. So far, insulin glargine has not been evaluated systematically in large clinical trials. A few pilot studies showed that it is safe and effective in diabetic cats and adequate glycemic control can be achieved in many cases. Insulin glargine used over a 4-month period resulted in diabetic remission in 8 of 8 cats (100%), whereas only 3 of 8 cats (38%) treated with PZI and 2 of 8 cats (25%) treated with Lente insulin achieved remission (Marshall et al, 2009). Other studies using insulin glargine were not able to repeat the high treatment success: remission rates ranged between 17% and 47% (Boari et al, 2008; Hall et al, 2009; Hafner et al, 2011). In an Internet-based study using 55 diabetic cats from a German diabetes forum, a remission rate of 64% was achieved (Roomp and Rand, 2009). However, owners were required to measure blood glucose at least three times per day, and insulin dosage was constantly adjusted, which is a regimen suitable for only a selected group of owners. The occurrence of hypoglycemia in glargine treated cats has also not yet been evaluated systematically. In the study by Roomp and Rand (2009), clinical hypoglycemia was reported in only 1 of 55 cats (1.8%), whereas 93% of cats revealed biochemical hypoglycemia at various levels of severity. The latter is certainly mostly associated with the intensive treatment protocol used in the particular study and not with the type of insulin.

There is so far little experience with insulin detemir in diabetic cats. Roomp and Rand (2012) performed a similar study with insulin glargine, again using the intensive treatment protocol and an online German diabetes forum for owners of diabetic cats. The results were similar, remission rate was 67% with insulin detemir;

TABLE 7-4	PHARMACODYNAMIC PARAMETERS OF INSULIN GLARGINE AND INSULIN DETEMIR		
	INSULIN GLARGINE (Lantus) n = 10	**INSULIN DETEMIR** (Levemir) n = 10	p-value
Onset of action (h)	1.3 (0.9 to 1.6)	1.8 (1.1 to 2.3)	0.03
Time to peak action (h)	2.5 to 8.0 (5.3)	4.7 to 9.2 (6.9)	0.31
End of action (h)	8.0 to 14.5 (11.3)	11.0 to 16.0 (13.5)	0.18

Modified from Gilor C, et al.: Pharmacodynamics of insulin detemir and insulin glargine assessed by an isoglycemic clamp method in healthy cats, *J Vet Intern Med* 24:870, 2010a.

clinical hypoglycemia was seen in 1 of the 18 cats (6%), whereas biochemical hypoglycemia was common. The starting dose of insulin detemir was similar to the starting dose of insulin glargine in the two studies (0.25 IU/kg of ideal body weight); however, maximal dose of detemir was lower than the maximal dose of insulin glargine (0.5 to 4.0 IU, median 1.75 versus 1.0 to 9.0 IU, median 2.5). Another difference was the relatively frequent development of chronic renal failure in cats treated with insulin detemir. It is unknown so far if this is related to the insulin itself or to the fact that the cats in the detemir study were slightly older than the cats in the glargine study.

Insulin Choice and Initial Dose

The initial insulin of choice depends on personal preference and availability. Cats are unpredictable in their response to insulin and none of the insulin preparations described above are routinely effective to control the disease. We nowadays start treatment in diabetic cats with insulin glargine (Lantus). PZI (ProZinc) would also be a good first choice. Both, insulin glargine and PZI are recommended by the AAHA Diabetes Management Guidelines (Rucinsky et al, 2010). In previous years, we achieved good glycemic control in many diabetic cats using Lente insulin (Vetsulin/Caninsulin), and therefore it may in principle also be used. As mentioned earlier, however, duration of action is often shorter than 12 hours (i.e., shorter than the duration of action of insulin glargine and PZI). If a diabetic cat is well regulated with Vetsulin/Caninsulin, there is no reason to switch it to one of the other insulins preparations. Nearly all cats require insulin twice daily, therefore we always start with b.i.d. administration. The initial dose in cats weighing ≤ 4 kg is 1 IU/cat b.i.d., and in cats weighing > 4 kg it is usually 1.5 IU/cat (–2.0 IU/cat) b.i.d. In cats with a blood glucose concentration < 350 mg/dL (20 mmol/L) at the time of diagnosis, no more than 1 IU/cat b.i.d. is given, independent of the body weight. The starting dose should not exceed 2.0 IU/cat b.i.d., even in a very large cat. It is better to start conservatively (e.g., maximum dose of 1.5 IU/cat b.i.d.), than to risk hypoglycemia during the first few days, which may lead to owner frustration and potentially cessation of therapy. Very small cats (≤ 2 kg) are started on no more than 0.5 IU/cat b.i.d. (Box 7-3).

BOX 7-3 Protocol for the Management of Non-Ketotic Diabetic Cats

Initial Presentation

- Diagnosis of diabetes mellitus (clinical signs, hyperglycemia, glucosuria, increased fructosamine)
- Routine laboratory evaluation (CBC, serum biochemistry panel* urine analysis, urine culture)
- Abdominal ultrasonography
- Cessation of diabetogenic drugs (glucocorticoids, progestagens)
- Start with intermediate-/long-acting insulin
  - First-line: Lantus, ProZinc; second-line: Vetsulin/Caninsulin
  - Initial dose
    - Depends on severity of clinical signs and degree of hyperglycemia; initial dose should not exceed 1.5 to 2.0 IU/cat b.i.d., even in very large cats
    - 0.5 IU/cat b.i.d. if body weight is ≤ 2 kg
    - 1.0 IU/cat b.i.d. if body weight is 2.5 to 4 kg
    - 1.5 IU/cat (– 2.0 IU/cat) b.i.d. if body weight is > 4 kg
- Treatment of concurrent problems (e.g., urinary tract infection, stomatitis/gingivitis)
- Dietary management
  - High protein, low carbohydrate diet; provided that no other disease has priority
  - 45 to 60 kcal/kg/day
  - If overweight, aim for 1% weight loss per week
- Owner instruction (requires at least 1 hour)
- Written instructions for owners

Reevaluation 1 Week after Diagnosis

- Administration of insulin and food at home, and then bring cat to hospital as soon as possible
- History, physical examination, and body weight
- Generation of a BGC (glucose measurement every 2 hours for the remainder of the day, preferentially until next insulin injection, or even thereafter if nadir is not reached)
- Fructosamine measurement
- Adjustment of insulin dosage if required: 0.5 IU/injection. In case of Somogyi effect or overt hypoglycemia, dose reduction of 25% to 50%, depending on the insulin dosage used

Reevaluation 2 to 3 Weeks after Diagnosis

- Repeat all procedures as during first reevaluation
- Introduction to home monitoring, and instruction on all relevant technical aspects (requires at least ½ hour)
- Frequency of home monitoring
  - During initial phases of therapy approximately one BGC per week
  - After stabilization (i.e., when adequate glycemic control is achieved), approximately one BGC every 3 to 4 weeks
  - BGC results should be sent to hospital and dose changes discussed with the veterinarian

Reevaluation 6 to 8 Weeks after Diagnosis

- All procedures as during first reevaluation; BGC may not be required if pet appears clinically well, blood glucose measured close to the time of insulin administration is 10 to 15 mmol/L (180 to 270 mg/dL) and fructosamine is 350 to 450 µmol/L
- Home monitoring results should be assessed and owner technique evaluated
- If glycemic control is inadequate and insulin dose is close to 1 IU/kg b.i.d. or above, further work-up should be pursued

Reevaluation 10 to 12 Weeks and 14 to 16 Weeks after Diagnosis, Then Every 4 Months

- Repeat all procedures done 6 to 8 weeks after diagnosis (except further work-up if not needed)

Goals of Therapy

- Good glycemic control
  - Clinical signs: Resolution of pu/pd, polyphagia, normal body weight
  - Blood glucose: Highest concentration between 180 to 270 mg/dL (10 to 15 mmol/L) and nadir between 80 to 140 mg/dL (4.5 to 7.8 mmol/L)
  - Fructosamine: Ideally between 350 and 450 µmol/L
- Diabetic remission
  - May be achieved in 25% to 50% of newly-diagnosed diabetic cats

---

*1,2-0-dilauryl-rac-glycero-glutaric acid-ester (DGGR) lipase (part of routine biochemistry panel in some laboratories) or Spec fPL should be measured if clinically indicated.
b.i.d., Bis in die (twice a day); *BGC,* blood glucose curve; *CBC,* complete blood count; *pu/pd,* polyuria/polydipsia.

After diagnosing diabetes mellitus, the cat may be kept in the hospital for 1 to 2 days to complete the work-up. During this time, blood glucose concentration should be measured three to four times throughout the day and the insulin dosage reduced if a low glucose concentration (< 90 mg/dL, 5 mmol/L) is detected. If the blood glucose concentration decreases only slightly, we do not increase the insulin dose because it takes a few days for full insulin action to develop (so-called equilibration). Adjustments in insulin dosage are made on subsequent evaluations. The initial work-up and start of treatment may also be done on an outpatient basis.

The approach is similar in cats that already receive insulin therapy but in which the disease is not adequately controlled. If we consider the type of insulin to be the problem, we switch to a different type, using the same dosing schedule as for the newly-diagnosed diabetic cats. The exception are cats that were shown to be prone to hypoglycemia with the previous insulin, those would not receive more than 0.5 U/cat b.i.d. of the new insulin as a starting dose.

Insulin Handling and Owner Instruction

One of the most important periods in the owner's care of a diabetic pet is the time during which the veterinarian or the technician teaches the technical aspects of the treatment and explains the monitoring protocol. The owner should be instructed to mix the insulin correctly: the manufacturer of ProZinc recommends gently rolling of the vial, whereas Vetsulin/Caninsulin should be vigorously shaken. Lantus (and Levemir) are clear solutions and need no mixing. It should be demonstrated how to load a syringe without air bubbles, and the veterinarian may also refer the owner to one of the many administration videos available through the Internet. We recommend injecting the insulin over the lateral chest wall because perfusion is better there than in the neck area, which increases absorption of insulin. The spot should rotate each time. The owner must understand the differences between U-40 and U-100/mL insulins: ProZinc and Vetsulin/Caninsulin are U 40/mL, whereas Lantus and Levemir are U-100/mL preparations. The use of the correct size of syringe is imperative. The use of non-matching syringes based on conversion tables or the owner's own calculations is discouraged, because the risk of confusion is high. The administration of small doses of insulin is difficult and requires particular attention. For the administration of Lantus (and Levemir) we routinely use 0.3 mL syringes, designed for the application of U-100 insulin preparations in 0.5 IU increments (BD Micro-Fine+Demi U 100 syringes, 0.3 mL, Becton Dickenson); however, for some people a pen designed to deliver 0.5 IU increments may be an alternative. Lantus must not be diluted because dilution changes the time/action profile; Levemir may be diluted with Insulin Diluting Medium for NovoRapid and Levemir supplied by Novo Nordisk (unfortunately it is not available in all countries). Dilution of other insulin preparations has been common practice; however, there are no studies on potential changes of pharmacokinetics and stability. We avoid dilution whenever possible and never dilute Lantus.

Unopened vials should generally be stored in the refrigerator, distant from the freezer compartment. Freezing and heating inactivates the insulin; similarly direct exposure to sun light must be avoided. We also recommend storage of in-use vials in the refrigerator to ensure a consistent environment. However, insulin is also stable at room temperature (as long as it is < 86° F, < 30° C, and light-protected) for approximately 4 weeks, which may be important for travelling. Insulin stored in the refrigerator should be allowed to warm up a bit before injection. Manufacturers declare that opened (in use) vials have to be replaced after

28 (Lantus), 42 (Vetsulin/Caninsulin, Levemir) or 60 days (ProZinc); however, true shelf-life is certainly longer and often owners use the insulin for longer times. We routinely inform owners about the potential risk of contamination and loss of activity and that cloudy or discolored vials should be discarded. Similarly the vial should be replaced if glycemic controls inexplicably deteriorate.

Reevaluations and Adjustment of Insulin Dose

After the initial work-up, the cat is discharged with insulin, syringes, diet, and, if needed, treatment for any concurrent disease. We inform the owner about the fact that during the next 3 months, frequent reevaluations and close monitoring are needed. Reevaluations are scheduled as a minimum after weeks 1, 2 to 3, 6 to 8, 10 to 12, 14 to 16, and then approximately every 4 months (see Box 7-3). Additional appointments may be necessary in some cats. It usually takes between 1 and 3 months until adequate glycemic control is achieved, and it is also during the first 3 months that the likelihood of diabetic remission is greatest. The latter should not be overlooked, because serious hypoglycemia may occur. We also introduce the general concept of home monitoring after initial work-up, and our written instructions contain some more information and pictures about the technical aspects. However, we usually wait for 2 to 3 weeks until teaching the technique. We first want to ensure that the owner is able to handle the other parts of the disease (regular insulin injections, change in diet, weight management) until moving on to the next step. The exceptions are highly motivated owners or diabetic owners being familiar with capillary glucose measurements. Ideally, insulin injections should be given every 12 hours; however, this may not be possible for all owners. Therefore, we "allow" shifts of 1 to 2 hours. We always start with the same insulin dose in the morning and in the evening. In some cats, "different" doses may be required during long term management (e.g., a lower dose in the evening if recurrent episodes of hypoglycemia occur at night).

Clinical signs of diabetes usually resolve when blood glucose concentrations can be kept below the renal threshold, ideally the lowest glucose concentration (glucose nadir) should be between 80 and 140 mg/dL (4.5 to 7.8 mmol/L), the highest glucose concentration between 180 and 270 mg/dL (10 to 15 mmol/L). At each reevaluation, the owner is questioned about his/her opinion on the cat's overall health, water intake, urine output, a thorough physical examination is performed, body weight is recorded, and a serial blood glucose curve (BGC) is generated. Fructosamine measurement may also be informative. If glycemic control is considered unsatisfactory, the insulin dose is increased in steps of 0.5 IU/cat per injection. It is possible that the insulin dose has to be increased several times until a reaction (clinically and with regard to blood glucose concentration) is seen. We usually make dose changes no more often than every 5 to 7 days. It is also possible that the type of insulin has to be changed. If duration of action is too short, a longer acting insulin should be used and vice versa. As mentioned earlier, Vetsulin/Caninsulin usually has a shorter duration of action than ProZinc and Lantus; in some cats, ProZinc may have a longer duration of action than Lantus, although there is variability between cats. Levemir seems to have a slightly longer duration of action than Lantus. However, there are substantial differences between diabetic cats, and the insulin dose has to be adapted according to the need of the individual cat. If hypoglycemia is noted at any time, the insulin dose should be reduced and another reevaluation scheduled soon thereafter. Most diabetic cats can be adequately controlled with insulin doses between 0.5 and 3 IU/cat b.i.d. (i.e., usually with less than 1.0 IU/kg b.i.d.). If the insulin requirement increases to 1 IU/kg b.i.d. or more without achieving adequate control, further work-up for any disease causing insulin resistance is indicated.

Diabetic remission may occur in approximately 25% to 50% of cases, usually during the first 3 months of therapy. Therefore, an "extended" treatment goal is to increase the chance of diabetic remission. We do not use a specific remission protocol (meaning to aim for lower glucose targets), because more aggressive insulin treatment is associated with a greater risk of hypoglycemia. However, we always start insulin therapy immediately after diagnosis and aim for good glycemic control. All of our owners are aware of the blood glucose targets mentioned earlier. If those targets are reached and the owner is willing to perform home monitoring of blood glucose, we consider "to push" treatment a bit further to see if diabetic remission is possible (see details in the sections Home-Monitoring of Blood Glucose, Frequency of Monitoring, and Interpretation of Blood Glucose Curves and Adjustment of Insulin Doses). The target for the glucose nadir, however, is not altered (i.e., blood glucose concentration should not decrease to less than 80 to 120 mg/dL [4.5 to 6.7 mmol/L]). If remission occurs unnoticed and the administration of insulin is not discontinued, serious hypoglycemia may result.

Oral Hypoglycemic Agents and Non-Insulin Injectables

In humans with newly-diagnosed type 2 diabetes, initial therapeutic measures consist of lifestyle interventions and prescription of an oral hypoglycemic agent. According to the latest position statement of the American Diabetes Association and the European Association for the Study of Diabetes, metformin is the initial drug of choice. If the glycemic target is not reached after approximately 3 months of metformin therapy, another antidiabetic drug should be added. This may be a sulfonylurea, thiazolidinedione, dipeptidyl peptidase-4 (DPP-4) inhibitor, GLP-1 receptor agonist, or insulin. In newly-diagnosed human patients with severe diabetic symptoms and severe hyperglycemia (blood glucose > 300 to 350 mg/dL, 16.7 to 19.4 mmol/L), insulin therapy should be started immediately (Inzucchi et al, 2012). In short, this means that if β-cell function has deteriorated beyond the capacity of oral agents to provide adequate glycemic control, the introduction of insulin should not be delayed (Bailey and Krentz, 2010). It is currently assumed that the majority of diabetic cats suffer a type 2-like

diabetes, and therefore, oral hypoglycemic drugs and non-insulin injectables may theoretically be of use. However, those classes have not gained wide popularity, certainly due to two main reasons. First, it may be as difficult (or even more difficult) for a cat owner to give life-long oral medication as to inject insulin. Secondly, for those drugs investigated in the cat, efficacy has been poor or moderate at best. Diabetic cats usually have symptoms of severe hyperglycemia and insulin secretion is low. As in humans with severe disease, oral drugs and non-insulin injectables are usually unable to combat the profound metabolic derangements. Immediate and effective treatment should be initiated with the aim of preserving the remaining β-cell mass and reversing the effects of glucotoxicity on β-cell function. We consider insulin treatment superior to any other currently available antidiabetic drug to increase the chance of diabetic remission. Insulin therapy is therefore highly recommended to owners of cats with newly diagnosed diabetes. Oral drugs and non-insulin injectables (e.g., the GLP-1 agonists) may play a role in cats with mild forms of diabetes or as add-on treatment. The latter are also used when the owner absolutely refuses to inject insulin or is unable to do so.

The currently available oral agents and non-insulin injectables can be divided by their mechanism of action into several groups: insulin secretagogues (sulfonylureas, glinides), insulin sensitizers with predominant action on the liver (metformin), insulin sensitizers with predominant action in peripheral insulin-sensitive tissues (glitazones), carbohydrate absorption inhibitors (α-glucosidase inhibitors), incretin-related therapies (DPP-4 inhibitors, GLP-1 agonists), and others/novel agents with less clear mechanisms (Buse et al, 2011; Table 7-5). Not all agents are available in all countries, and the same drug may be named differently in different countries.

Sulfonylureas

Sulfonylureas were introduced into human medicine in the 1950s and are the oldest oral hypoglycemic agents. Early sulfonylureas are referred to as "first generation" and include tolbutamide, carbutamide, acetohexamide, tolazamide, and chlorpropamide. They have largely been replaced by the more potent "second generation" sulfonylureas, such as glipizide, glyburide (glibenclamide), gliclazide, and glimepiride. They act directly on the β-cell to induce insulin secretion; they do so by binding to the cytosolic surface of the sulfonylurea receptor, which causes closure of ATP-sensitive potassium channels, followed by depolarization of the plasma membrane, opening of calcium channels, and exocytosis of insulin

TABLE 7-5	CLASSES OF ORAL HYPOGLYCEMIC AGENTS AND NON-INSULIN INJECTABLES AND THEIR MAIN MODES OF ACTION	
CLASS OF ANTIDIABETIC DRUG WITH EXAMPLES	**MAIN MODE OF ACTION**	**PREDOMINANT SITE OF ACTION**
Sulfonylureas (glipizide, glyburide/glibenclamide, gliclazide, glimepiride)	Stimulate insulin secretion	β-cells
Glinides/meglitinides (repaglinide, nateglinide)	Stimulate insulin secretion (faster onset and shorter duration of action than sulfonylureas)	β-cells
Biguanide (metformin)	Decrease of hepatic gluconeogenesis and glycogenolysis, increase of glucose-uptake	Liver (muscle)
Glitazones/thiazolidinediones (pioglitazone, rosiglitazone)	Increase insulin sensitivity	Adipose tissue, muscle, (liver)
α-glucosidase inhibitors (acarbose, miglitol, voglibose)	Slow digestion of carbohydrate	Small intestine
GLP-1 receptor agonists (exenatide, liraglutide, albiglutide) DPP-4 inhibitors/gliptins (sitagliptin, saxagliptin, vildagliptin, linagliptin, alogliptin)	Enhance glucose-dependent insulin secretion (see also Table 7-10)	β-cells

DPP-4, Dipeptidyl peptidase-4; *GLP-1,* glucagon-like peptide-1.

(Bailey and Krentz, 2010). Sulfonylureas can only exert their effect if there is a sufficient reserve of β-cells function left, and they usually become ineffective as β-cell function declines during the progression of the diabetic disease. They are contraindicated in individuals with an absolute insulin deficiency. Sulfonylureas can stimulate insulin release even if blood glucose concentrations are low (< 90 mg/dL, 5 mmol/L), rendering hypoglycemia the most serious adverse effect. Another negative effect of sulfonylurea therapy is weight gain.

Glipizide is the drug in this class most often used in cats and which has been studied best (Nelson et al, 1993; Feldman et al, 1997). There are no parameters to help the clinician identify cats that will respond to glipizide therapy, and selection of patients therefore relies on assessing the severity of disease. Glipizide should only be used in diabetic cats that are in good physical condition, non-ketotic, have only mild to moderate signs of diabetes, and can be monitored closely. The starting dose of glipizide is 2.5 mg/cat b.i.d. in conjunction with a meal. The dose is increased to 5 mg/cat b.i.d. after 2 weeks provided that no adverse effects have occurred and hyperglycemia is still present. The cat should be reevaluated after another 1 to 2 weeks and at regular intervals thereafter. Therapy is continued as long as the drug provides good glycemic control, i.e., resolution of clinical signs, stable body weight, blood glucose concentrations between 180 to 270 mg/dL (10-15 mmol/L) and 80 to 140 mg/dL (4.5-7.8 mmol/L). The dose should be reduced or discontinued if normoglycemia or hypoglycemia occurs, and the cat should be reevaluated after a few days. If hyperglycemia is again present, glipizide at a lower dose should be reintroduced. Glipizide should be discontinued and insulin therapy started when clinical signs and hyperglycemia are not under control or worsen after a few weeks of treatment or ketoacidosis develops. The dose of glipizide should not be increased above 5 mg/cat b.i.d. Adverse effects (besides hypoglycemia) occur in approximately 15% of cats and include anorexia, vomiting, increased liver enzymes, and increased bilirubin with icterus. Please see Box 7-4

for recommendations in case those adverse effects occur. One should be aware that glipizide is only effective in approximately 30% of cases. In some of them, glipizide becomes ineffective after a few weeks to months; in others, good glycemic control can be maintained for a long period (years). Glipizide may have negative effects on islets and may accelerate β-cell loss. Under experimental conditions, increased amyloid deposition has been found in islets of cats treated with glipizide compared to cats treated with insulin; this is most likely due to the stimulatory effect of glipizide on both insulin and amylin secretion (Hoenig et al, 2000b). This finding is comparable to studies using human cell cultures, in which sulfonylureas lead to increased β-cell apoptosis (Maedler et al, 2005). One study investigated the efficacy of transdermal glipizide; unfortunately absorption was low and inconsistent (Bennet et al, 2005).

There is very little to no experience with other sulfonylureas in diabetic cats. Glyburide (glibenclamide) has a longer duration of action than glipizide and may be suitable for once daily use in some cats. Initial dose is 0.625 mg/cat b.i.d., which may be increased to 1.25 mg/cat b.i.d., if no effect is seen. Guidelines and adverse effects are similar to those described for glipizide. Glimepiride is the most recently developed sulfonylurea for once daily use in humans. So far, it has been investigated only in healthy cats, in which a significant glucose lowering effect was demonstrated (Mori et al, 2009b).

Because sulfonylureas (e.g., glipizide) do not offer any medical advantage over insulin, we only use them if owners are unable or unwilling to inject insulin. During the following weeks, confidence and willingness of owners often increase and a transition to insulin will eventually be possible.

Glinides/Meglinides

Glinides/meglinides are insulin secretagogues, which also bind to the sulfonylurea receptors, but on a different site from sulfonylureas. They induce a prompt, albeit short-lived insulin secretion and are specifically designed to counteract postprandial hyperglycemia. As such, they are also termed *short-acting prandial insulin releasers*. Adverse effects include hypoglycemia and weight gain; severity of both, however, is less than with sulfonylureas (Bailey and Krentz, 2010). Recently, nateglinide (one of the two members of this class) was evaluated in healthy cats. It induced a more rapid and more pronounced increase in insulin secretion than the sulfonylurea glimepiride, resulting in an earlier decrease in blood glucose concentrations (Mori et al, 2009b). There are no reports on their use in diabetic cats, and because cats have unique nutritional characteristics (see Dietary Management), they may not be helpful for glycemic control.

Biguanides

Metformin is the only drug of the biguanide class in most countries. According to the guidelines for the treatment of humans with type 2 diabetes, metformin should be considered as first line medical therapy, provided that there are no contraindications (Inzucchi et al, 2012). Its mechanisms of action are complex and not fully understood. Some of the actions are achieved through enhanced insulin sensitivity, whereas others are independent of insulin, including activation of adenosine monophosphate-activated protein kinase (AMPK) (Bailey and Davies, 2011). The primary site of action is the liver, where it reduces gluconeogenesis and glycogenolysis. Metformin also enhances glucose uptake and glycogenesis in skeletal muscle and promotes glycogen synthesis. The glucose-lowering effect requires the presence of at least some circulating insulin, and therefore metformin is ineffective in patients with complete lack of insulin. Metformin does not stimulate insulin

BOX 7-4	**Adverse Reactions to Glipizide Treatment in Diabetic Cats**
Adverse Reaction	**Recommendation**
Vomiting within 1 hour of administration	Vomiting usually subsides after 2 to 5 days of glipizide therapy; decrease dose or frequency of administration if vomiting is severe; discontinue if vomiting persists longer than 1 week.
Increased serum hepatic enzyme activities	Continue treatment and monitor enzymes every 1 to 2 weeks initially; discontinue glipizide if cat becomes ill (lethargy, inappetence, vomiting) or the alanine aminotransferase activity exceeds 500 IU/L.
Icterus	Discontinue glipizide treatment; reinstitute glipizide therapy at lower dose and frequency of administration once icterus has resolved (usually within 2 weeks); discontinue treatment permanently if icterus recurs.
Hypoglycemia	Discontinue glipizide treatment; recheck blood glucose concentration in 1 week; reinstitute glipizide therapy at lower dose or frequency of administration if hyperglycemia recurs.

release, and although it reduces hepatic glucose production, the risk of hypoglycemia is minimal. Weight gain is also not a relevant adverse effect. The main adverse effects in humans are gastrointestinal symptoms (anorexia, nausea, vomiting, abdominal discomfort, diarrhea), and they are usually dose-related and may be reduced in most patients by dose-titration or switching to a slow-release formula. There are various contraindications, such as impaired renal function, cardiac or respiratory insufficiency, liver disease, and others. Metformin may also reduce vitamin B_{12} absorption (Bailey and Krentz, 2010; Bailey and Davies, 2011). The most frightening and serious potential adverse effect is lactic acidosis. An increase in blood lactate concentration is a consequence of the effect of metformin to inhibit hepatic gluconeogenesis, for which lactate is an important substrate. Lactic acidosis, however, is a rare event and mostly associated with the use of metformin in patients with comorbidities and risk factors (e.g., renal insufficiency) (Krentz and Nattrass, 2003; Renda et al, 2013). So far only very few studies have been performed in cats. Doses suggested to be necessary to reach plasma concentrations known to be effective in human diabetics varied between 2 mg/kg b.i.d. and 50 mg/cat b.i.d. (Michels et al, 1999; Nelson et al, 2004). Unfortunately, results achieved in a small number of diabetic cats are not encouraging, because only one of five cats with diabetes responded to treatment. Clinical signs improved 3 weeks after the metformin dose had been increased to 50 mg/cat b.i.d. (from 10 mg/cat s.i.d., 10 mg/cat b.i.d., 25 mg/cat b.i.d.). Three diabetic cats failed to respond and one diabetic cat died unexpectedly some days after initiating therapy. The responder was the only diabetic cat that had detectable insulin concentrations prior to treatment, supporting the concept that some circulating insulin has to be present for metformin to be effective (Nelson et al, 2004).

Glitazones

Glitazones are also known as *thiazolidinediones (TZDs)*. Most of their antidiabetic effect is achieved through stimulation of a nuclear receptor, the peroxisome proliferator-activated receptor-γ (PPAR-γ). PPAR-γ is highly expressed in adipose tissue and to a lesser extent in muscle and liver. Stimulation results in differentiation of preadipocytes into small, insulin-sensitive adipocytes that take up fatty acids and reduce their availability for gluconeogenesis. TZDs also increase insulin-mediated glucose uptake ("insulin sensitizer") into skeletal muscle and adipose tissue, reduce the production of several proinflammatory cytokines (e.g., TNFα) and increase the production of adiponectin in adipose tissue. They may also be of benefit in early stages of the disease and may slow the progression of β-cell destruction. TZDs, like metformin, require the presence of some circulating insulin to be effective; it may take 2 to 4 months until the full effect is seen. They do not stimulate insulin secretion and do not cause hypoglycemia. They are often taken in combination with other antidiabetic drugs (e.g., metformin) to achieve an additive effect, but they may also be used as monotherapy. Adverse effects include weight gain due to fluid retention and accumulation of subcutaneous fat; they may be associated with an increased risk of heart failure and bone fractures (Bailey and Krentz, 2010; Bailey and Davies, 2011; Buse et al, 2011). So far, no studies describe the use of TZDs in cats with diabetes. The potential for this drug for the treatment of diabetic cats is currently unknown. Healthy cats had significantly lower cholesterol, triglyceride, and leptin concentrations after 6 weeks of darglitazone treatment (2 mg/kg s.i.d., orally) compared with control cats. A significant decrease in the area under the curve for NEFAs, glucose, and insulin during an IVGTT was demonstrated; the latter suggested an increase in insulin sensitivity induced by the drug

(Hoenig and Ferguson, 2003). Recently, the pharmacokinetics of pioglitazone, another member of the TZD class, was evaluated in healthy cats. It was suggested that 1 to 3 mg/kg of pioglitazone would be an appropriate oral dose for further studies on its efficacy (Clark et al, 2011).

Alpha-Glucosidase Inhibitors

Drugs of this class are competitive inhibitors of α-glucosidase enzymes in the brush border of enterocytes, lining the intestinal villi. Thereby, they prevent the final step of carbohydrate digestion (i.e., cleavage of disaccharides and oligosaccharides into monosaccharides). As a result, glucose absorption is delayed. It is not inhibited per se but moved distally in the gastrointestinal tract. These drugs can only be effective in the presence of a substantial amount of complex carbohydrate and when given with a meal. The main adverse effects are gastrointestinal signs (e.g., abdominal discomfort, flatulence, and diarrhea), which often limit their use in humans. In humans, they may be used as monotherapy in patients with postprandial hyperglycemia but only slightly increased fasting hyperglycemia. More often, however, they are considered as additive therapy with other antidiabetic drugs (Bailey and Krentz, 2010; Bailey and Davies, 2011). In cats, α-glucosidase inhibitors may be useful in cases in which a high-carbohydrate diet is fed. In diabetic cats, the α-glucosidase inhibitor acarbose (12.5 mg/cat b.i.d. with a meal) had no apparent positive effect when given with a low-carbohydrate diet (Mazzaferro et al, 2003). This observation is consistent with the results of a study comparing the effects of acarbose in healthy cats fed low- and high-carbohydrate diets. Cats on a high-carbohydrate diet had significantly lower blood glucose concentrations when acarbose was added, although the same glucose-lowering effect was seen with the low-carbohydrate diet. The acarbose dose was 25 mg/cat s.i.d. for cats fed once daily, and 25 mg/cat b.i.d. if fed several meals (Singh et al, 2006; Rand, 2012; Palm and Feldman, 2013). As in humans, gastrointestinal side effects may occur, the severity of which may be reduced by slow dose titration. In diabetic cats fed low-carbohydrate diets, acarbose is of no or negligible use. Acarbose has been suggested for diabetic cats in which a low-carbohydrate–high-protein diet may not be appropriate (e.g., in cats with concurrent renal failure). It should be noted, however, that acarbose is considered contraindicated in humans with impaired renal function (Yale, 2005; Tschöpe et al, 2013); the issue has not yet been investigated in cats.

Incretin-Related Therapeutics

Incretins are hormones that are released from the gastrointestinal tract during food intake and that potentiate insulin secretion from the β-cells. GIP and GLP-1 are the two currently known incretin hormones. GIP is ineffective in diabetic individuals, whereas GLP-1 retains its stimulatory effect provided that there is still an adequate mass of β-cells present. It also has beneficial effects on glucagon, gastric emptying, and satiety. GLP-1 is mainly produced in the L-cells in the intestinal tract. In the cat, the highest density of L-cells was recently shown to be in the ileum (Gilor et al, 2013). Native GLP-1 is quickly degraded by the enzyme DPP-4, which has led to the development of GLP-1 agonists with resistance to degradation and to inhibitors of DPP-4 activity (Mudaliar and Henry, 2012). Although both classes improve glycemic control, various differences exist between them. From a practical standpoint, a major difference is the route of application: GLP-1 agonists have to be injected subcutaneously, whereas DPP-4 inhibitors are oral agents. For both GLP-1 agonists and DPP-4 inhibitors, the risk of hypoglycemia

TABLE 7-6	COMPARISON OF GLP-1 RECEPTOR AGONISTS AND DPP-4 INHIBITORS	
	GLUCAGON-LIKE PEPTIDE-1 RECEPTOR AGONISTS	**DIPEPTIDYL PEPTIDASE-4 INHIBITORS**
Administration	Subcutaneous injection	Orally
Glucose-dependent insulin secretion	Enhanced	Enhanced
Glucose-dependent glucagon secretion	Reduced	Reduced
Postprandial hyperglycemia	Reduced	Reduced
Risk of hypoglycemia	Low	Low
Gastric emptying	Decelerated	No effect
Appetite	Suppressed	No effect
Satiety	Induced	No effect
Body weight	Reduced	Neutral
Main adverse effects	Nausea, vomiting	Headache, nasopharyngitis, urinary tract infection

From Reusch CE, Padrutt I: New incretin hormonal therapies in humans relevant to diabetic cats, *Vet Clin North Am Small Anim Pract* 43:417, 2013 (with permission).

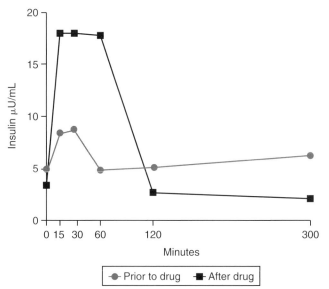

FIGURE 7-16 Insulin secretion before and 5 weeks after once weekly subcutaneous injection of exenatide long-acting (Bydureon). Samples for insulin measurement were taken before and 15, 30, 60, 120, and 300 minutes after feeding a test meal. Results are mean values of three healthy cats. *Prior to drug,* Insulin secretion before the start of the study. *After drug,* Insulin secretion after weekly administration of 200 μg/kg exenatide long-acting for 5 weeks. (From Padrutt I, et al.: Comparison of the GLP-1 analogues exenatide short-acting, exenatide long-acting and the DPP-4 inhibitor sitagliptin to increase insulin secretion in healthy cats, *J Vet Int Med* 26:1520, abstract, 2012.)

is low (Reusch and Padrutt, 2013; Table 7-6). In humans with type 2 diabetes, incretin based therapy is currently used as monotherapy, as well as in combination with other antidiabetic drugs. In the rat and mouse, it has been shown that GLP-1 analogues preserve β-cell mass by inducing β-cell proliferation. There is hope that the same may be true for humans, because this would then be of great benefit to slow progression of the diabetic disease (Rutti et al, 2012). The same would be of course true for the cat.

GLP-1 agonists and DPP-4 inhibitors have thus far been investigated only in healthy cats. The GLP-1 agonist exenatide was shown to potentiate insulin secretion in association with a glucose load, similar to its effect in other species (Gilor et al, 2011). In a dose escalation study, the application of 0.2, 0.5, 1.0, and 2.0 μg/kg exenatide b.i.d. for 5 days resulted in pronounced insulin increase (area under the curve after a meal-response test) of 320%, 364%, 547%, and 198%. Exenatide is also available as long-acting or extended-release preparation, which allows less frequent application (once per week instead of twice daily). Once weekly injection of exenatide long-acting (200 μg/kg) for 5 weeks, resulted in a very efficient increase of meal-induced insulin secretion (Fig. 7-16). The application of the DPP-4 inhibitor sitagliptin in a dose-escalation manner (1, 3, 5, and 10 mg/kg s.i.d. for 5 days) resulted in a less pronounced increase of insulin (43%, 101%, 70%, and 56%). Transient gastrointestinal side effects were seen with all three drugs; however, well-being and appetite were unaffected (Padrutt et al, 2012; Reusch and Padrutt, 2013). Clinical studies in diabetic cats are under way, although the currently high costs of the drugs may be prohibitive for the routine use in practice.

Other Therapies

Chromium is an essential trace element, required for normal glucose metabolism. It is assumed that it may modulate insulin signaling; its precise mode of action, however, is unclear. Trivalent (3+) chromium is found in a wide range of foods and is available as an inexpensive nutritional supplement. Chromium chloride, chromium nicotinate, and chromium picolinate are formulations of trivalent chromium; the absorption of the latter seems to be the most consistent. There is controversy as to whether chromium supplementation should be routinely recommended in diabetic humans without documented deficiency. Some studies have found evidence in favor, others against a beneficial effect (Wang and Cefalu, 2010). In cats, the effect of chromium was so far investigated only in healthy animals and results also differ. In one study, using 100 μg chromium picolinate for 6 weeks, no effect on glucose tolerance was found (Cohn et al, 1999); in another study, a small, but significant improvement in glucose tolerance was seen after chromium picolinate was supplemented for 6 weeks at mean concentrations of 22.9 μg and 44.9 μg (Appleton et al, 2002). Adverse effects were not identified in any of the studies. It is not known if diabetic cats with adequate dietary intake would benefit from additional chromium supplementation.

Vanadium is another trace element, which does have insulin-mimetic properties in liver, skeletal muscle, and adipose tissue; most likely it plays an activating role in the insulin signaling cascade. The effects are similar, regardless of the type of vanadium salts used. Several clinical trials in human diabetics have documented improvement in glycemic control; there is, however, a high incidence of gastrointestinal adverse effects (Smith et al, 2008; Clark et al, 2014). There is very little experience with vanadium supplementation in diabetic cats. Cats treated with insulin (PZI) and oral vanadium dipicolinate (45 mg orally, s.i.d.) had a slightly better glycemic control than cats treated with insulin alone. Adverse effects included anorexia and vomiting (Fondacaro et al, 1999). Further studies are needed to define the role of chromium and vanadium supplementation in diabetic cats. So far, no dose recommendation can be made due to the lack of dose finding studies. See Herbs, Supplements, and Vitamins in Chapter 6 for a discussion on further "alternative" therapies.

Oral hypoglycemic agents and non-insulin injectables are an area of intensive research in human medicine, and many new drugs have recently been developed. Amongst them are amylin analogues (pramlintide), dopamine agonists (bromocriptine), and sodium-glucose-transporter-2 inhibitors. None of them have been studied in cats so far. Many more will come, and the big challenge will be to critically evaluate them in a sufficient number of diabetic cats.

Dietary Management

Diet is an important component of the treatment plan. The goal of dietary therapy is to provide a nutritionally complete and palatable food that is readily consumed. Regular eating is of particular importance in the diabetic cat, because lack of food intake may lead to hypoglycemia. In addition, the diet should provide day-to-day consistency with regard to composition, ingredients, and calories so that an optimal body condition can be achieved and maintained. The diet should also reduce postprandial hyperglycemia and minimized fluctuations in blood glucose. Choosing an appropriate diet will also increase the chance of diabetic remission.

Obesity

Obesity is an important risk factor for the development of diabetes and the prevalence of both obesity and diabetes is increasing. Obesity is the result of excessive caloric intake, decreased energy expenditure, or both. Neutering and physical inactivity (indoor confinement) lead to a reduction in energy expenditure. Unfortunately, those events are often combined with feeding highly palatable, energy-dense diets in high amounts. Other factors, such as genetic background, epigenetic modulation of gene expression, and the nature of the environment may also contribute (Zoran and Buffington, 2011).

There is some debate on which macronutrients (fat or carbohydrates) play the most important role in the development of obesity. Recent studies showed that diets high in fat result in weight gain and increase in body fat when fed ad libitum (Nguyen 2004; Backus et al, 2007). Body fat increased with increasing dietary fat and an obesity-promoting effect was seen when dietary fat exceeded 25% of metabolizable energy (ME). Because dietary fat was exchanged for carbohydrates, those diets low in fat were high in carbohydrates (and vice versa), providing evidence that diets high in fat pose a greater risk for obesity than diets high in carbohydrates (Backus et al, 2007; Laflamme, 2010). However, consumption of carbohydrates in excess of energy needs will also contribute to obesity, meaning that any excess of calories poses a risk for obesity (Laflamme, 2010). Cats are strict carnivores and need larger amounts of dietary protein than dogs and humans. Although it is the restriction of calories that ultimately leads to weight loss, it is important to minimize loss of lean body mass. Therefore, a weight-loss diet should be calorie-restricted but provide an adequate amount of protein. The minimum daily protein requirement for an adult cat was recently reported to be at least 5.2 g/kg body weight per day. Dietary fiber is a helpful component of weight loss diets. It provides little dietary energy and thereby reduces the caloric density of the diet, and it also has a satiety effect (Laflamme, 2012; Laflamme and Hannah, 2013).

Dietary Carbohydrate and Protein

Several of the commonly manufactured cat foods (in particular dry foods) contain high amounts of carbohydrates (up to 50% of ME). It has been debated whether long-term feeding of those diets contributes to the development of diabetes in cats. The reason behind those debates is the fact that the natural diet of cats in the wild includes mice and birds and is low in carbohydrates and that the feline carbohydrate metabolism has some specifics. For instance, cats have low amylase activity in saliva and the small intestinal tract, and their liver lacks glucokinase, which is an enzyme responsible for phosphorylation of glucose for subsequent oxidation or storage. Glucokinase operates when the liver receives large amounts of glucose from the portal vein. Other glycolytic enzymes, such as hexokinase (a constitutive enzyme), however, were found to be present in even higher concentrations than in the liver of dogs (Washizu et al, 1999; Tanaka et al, 2005). Cats have a rather limited capacity to metabolize simple sugars, and experimental diets containing up to 40% of glucose and sucrose resulted in hyperglycemia and glucosuria (Kienzle, 1994). After eating a glucose enriched meal, healthy cats reveal significant higher blood glucose concentrations than dogs with a later glucose peak and a later return to baseline. More "physiological" dietary studies used different levels of starch instead of adding simple sugars. Using a high-starch diet (43% ME), blood glucose was significantly higher compared to baseline after 11 hours and remained significantly elevated until the end of the trial (19 hours after the meal) in cats; in dogs, blood glucose increased only minimally. After feeding a low or moderate starch diet (12% and 30% ME), glucose concentrations did not increase in both species (Hewson-Hughes et al, 2011a; 2011b). Another study confirmed the finding that cats may have a long postprandial increase in blood glucose concentration. Hyperglycemia, albeit mild, was already seen after feeding a diet with moderate carbohydrate content (25% of ME). Mean baseline glucose concentration was 90 mg/dL (5 mmol/L) and increased to a mean of 130 mg/dL (7.2 mmol/L) after feeding. The median time until blood glucose reached its peak was 6 hours after feeding, and the median time until glucose returned to baseline was 12.2 hours. Insulin concentrations returned to baseline after a median of 12.3 hours (Farrow et al, 2012). Interestingly, the use of a moderate starch diet lead to a postprandial glucose increase in one of the studies, whereas no increase was seen in the other study (Hewson-Hughes et al, 2011b; Farrow et al, 2012). It is possible that the differences are due to the use of different carbohydrate sources in the diets.

De-Oliveira, et al., (2008) fed diets containing 35% of starch from six different carbohydrate sources. Digestibility of the various carbohydrates varied slightly, but was generally very high. The time until the peak blood glucose was reached was quite different between the diets and ranged between 2.5 and 7.2 hours. Interestingly, the overall maximum blood glucose concentration was only 93.3 mg/dL (5.2 mmol/L) (i.e., none of the cats had blood glucose concentrations above the normal range). The highest blood glucose was seen when corn was used as carbohydrate source, followed by brewers rice, and the lowest was with lentil and cassava flour. From the studies mentioned, one may conclude the following: healthy cats seem to be able to digest carbohydrate if properly processed; blood glucose and insulin concentrations increase after dietary carbohydrate intake, the extent of which probably correlates with the carbohydrate concentration and carbohydrate source; the increase of blood glucose, if present, is usually mild, and it is unclear if this slight increase has any negative impact. Currently, there are no studies showing that consumption of high dietary carbohydrates causes diabetes mellitus in cats. It is more likely that excess intake of those diets leads to obesity, which in turn is a risk factor. Other factors associated with the change in the lifestyle of cats also play a role. Slingerland, et al., (2009) showed that indoor confinement and physical inactivity was significantly correlated with the development of diabetes, whereas the percentage of dry food (high in carbohydrates) was not.

The topic of diet is less controversial in cats with overt diabetes and there is current agreement that a high-protein–low-carbohydrate diet should be fed (Laflamme, 2010; Rucinsky et al, 2010; Zoran and Rand, 2013). High-fiber diets are no longer recommended as diets of first choice in diabetic cats, because they usually do not have a low carbohydrate content. They may, however, be used if cats do not tolerate high-protein–low-carbohydrate diets or if weight loss is insufficient. It should be noted that the current dietary recommendation is based on a relatively small number of clinical studies (Frank et al, 2001; Mazzaferro et al, 2003; Bennett et al, 2006). The most comprehensive study compared a moderate carbohydrate/high-fiber diet (26% carbohydrate [CHO] ME) and a low carbohydrate/low fiber diet (12% CHO ME) randomly assigned to cats with diabetes. After 4 months, significantly more cats fed the low carbohydrate diet were in diabetic remission compared with cats fed the moderate carbohydrate diet (68% versus 41%); of the cats still requiring insulin, more cats on the low carbohydrate diet were well regulated (40% versus 26%) (Bennett et al, 2006). The positive effect on glycemic control occurs before there is apparent loss of body weight. The exact mechanisms involved remain to be investigated (e.g., if low carbohydrate or high protein is the key factor and what roles the different sources of proteins and carbohydrates play).

Current recommendations state that the protein content in a diet for diabetic cats should be more than 40% to 45% ME and the carbohydrate content should be less than 12% to 15% ME, or as low as the cat will eat (Rucinsky et al, 2010; Zoran and Rand, 2013). No clear statements are made with regard to fat content.

It has been shown that healthy cats may tolerate high amounts of fat (up to 66% ME) well without negative impact on plasma lipid concentrations (Butterwick et al, 2012). In diabetic cats, however, it seems reasonable to avoid high fat diets (e.g., growth diets), because they may be associated with further weight gain and possibly with increased risk of pancreatitis. Canned food has some advantages over dry food, such as a lower calorie density (the cat can eat more for the same caloric intake), and usually a lower carbohydrate content and provision of additional water, which increases hydration as well as satiety (Rucinsky et al, 2010; Zoran and Rand, 2013). Many diets (in particular canned diets) fulfill the aforementioned criteria. Most premium pet food companies offer diets specifically designed for diabetic cats (Table 7-7). We routinely prescribe canned food with high protein and very low carbohydrate content to the owners of diabetic cats. If palatability is a problem with our first choice diet, we switch to another diet with comparable characteristics. In cats in which diabetic remission is achieved after some time and insulin therapy is discontinued, we recommend that the high-protein–low-carbohydrate diet is fed life-long. Similarly, in cats with prediabetes, weight reduction and feeding a high-protein–low-carbohydrate diet is recommended.

Calculation of Energy Requirement and Feeding Schedule

Energy requirement differs between individuals, and therefore, guidelines should only be used as a rough estimate. The maintenance energy requirement of typical sized (4 to 5 kg), neutered indoor cats is 45 to 55 kcal/kg body weight per day. For neutered male cats, the lower number should be used (Zoran and Buffington, 2011). In obese cats, the calculation of energy requirement should be based on ideal body weight. It is, however, possible that this amount is still too high and energy intake must be reduced much further. A reduction of calories in steps of 10% to 15% every few weeks may be necessary. To avoid loss of lean

		PROTEIN (% ME)	FAT (% ME)	CH (% ME)	FIBER (g/100 kcal ME)	PROTEIN (g/100 kcal ME)
TABLE 7-7	**APPROXIMATE NUTRIENT CONTENT OF SOME COMMERCIALLY-AVAILABLE DIETS USED FOR DIETARY MANAGEMENT OF DIABETES AND/OR WEIGHT LOSS IN CATS***					
Purina DM (canned)		46.0	47.3	7.7	0.9	13.1
Purina DM (dry)		46.2	38.1	17.9	0.4	13.2
Hill's Prescription Diet m/d (canned)		45.7	40.7	15.6	1.5	13.1
Hill's Prescription Diet m/d (dry)		42.5	40.9	19.0	0.9	12.1
Royal Canin Diabetic DS (wet)		47.2	38.2	16.8	2.2	13.5
Royal Canin Diabetic DS 46 (dry)		45.2	28.6	30.0	1.0	12.9
Hill's Prescription Diet w/d (canned)		39.2	37.9	26.1	2.9	11.2
Hill's Prescription Diet w/d (dry)		39.2	37.9	26.1	2.3	11.2
Hill's Prescription Diet r/d (canned)		41.0	24.3	39.6	4.8	11.7
Hill's Prescription Diet r/d (dry)		40.7	27.9	35.9	4.1	11.6
Purina OM (canned)		51.1	36.8	13.9	1.9	14.6
Purina OM (dry)		53.7	21.7	28.1	2.4	15.3
Royal Canin Obesity Management (wet)		48.5	31.4	22.9	2.8	13.9
Royal Canin Obesity Management (dry)		45.4	26.2	32.5	2.1	13.0

Courtesy of Prof. Annette Liesegang, Institute of Animal Nutrition, Vetsuisse Faculty, Zurich, Switzerland.
*Metabolizable energy (ME) content was determined using the modified Atwater factors on the basis of data provided by the pet food companies. Results are calculated estimates and the total energy in percent may therefore slightly deviate from 100%.

muscle mass, the diet has to meet the minimum daily protein requirement. It is important to set realistic goals and avoid frustration of the owner. Weight should decrease slowly; a loss of 1% per week is considered optimal. Severely overweight cats may never reach optimal body weight; however, a moderate weight loss may improve glycemic control. A small percentage of diabetic cats are underweight. If insulin therapy does not lead to the desired weight gain, calories should be increased in steps of 10% to 15%. Diabetic cats should be weighted once per week, providing that their owners have a precise scale. At each veterinary visit, the notes of the owners should be reviewed, body weight as well as body and muscle scoring should be evaluated, and amounts of calories should be amended if needed. It should be remembered that cats with untreated diabetes lose weight, which is stopped with adequate insulin therapy. Many cats gain some weight with the start of insulin therapy (when calories are not restricted) as the body aims for its original weight. Persistent weight gain, however, should alert the clinician to consider high caloric intake, insulin overdose, or acromegaly as possible causes. Persistent weight loss may be caused by low caloric intake, inadequate insulin therapy, or any concurrent disease (e.g., pancreatitis, pancreatic insufficiency, hyperthyroidism, inflammatory bowel disease, or lymphoma). The best feeding pattern for diabetic cats is unknown at the moment. We currently recommend to offer half of the cat's daily calorie intake at the time of each insulin injection; any leftovers should remain available to the cat until the next meal (Box 7-5).

Modifications in Dietary Therapy

In cats with concurrent disease (e.g., pancreatitis, food allergy, or chronic renal failure) diets designed for diabetes management may not be appropriate. Dietary therapy for the most serious disease should take priority. Please see Modifications in Dietary Therapy in Chapter 6.

BOX 7-5 Recommendations for Dietary Treatment of Cats with Diabetes Mellitus

Dietary Composition
- First choice: High-protein and low-carbohydrate diet (protein > 40 to 45 ME, carbohydrate < 12% to 15% ME)
- Second choice: High-fiber and moderate carbohydrate diet

Type of Food
- First choice: Canned food
- Second choice: Mixture of canned and dry food

Calculation of Quantity
- Energy requirement for an average sized indoor neutered cat is 45 to 55 kcal/kg body weight per day (use lower number for neutered male cats)
- If cat is overweight, aim for loss of 1% of body weight per week
- Adjust daily caloric intake on individual basis
  - Reduce in steps of 10% to 15% if cat is overweight and no weight loss is achieved
  - Increase in steps of 10% to 15% if cat is underweight and no weight gain is achieved during insulin therapy
- Avoid loss of lean body mass by providing adequate amount of protein (5.2 g/kg body weight per day)

Feeding Schedule
- Half of daily caloric intake at time of each insulin injection; any leftover should remain available for the rest of the day or the night

ME, Metabolizable energy.

Exercise

In humans, the positive effect of physical activity on glycemic control is well known. Exercise is associated with improved insulin sensitivity through various mechanisms (e.g., increased postreceptor insulin-signaling, increased GLUT protein, increased delivery of glucose to muscle, and decrease in body fat; Yardley et al, 2010). According to the current recommendations of the American Diabetes Association, adult humans should perform at least 150 min/week of moderate intensity aerobic physical activity with no more than 2 consecutive days without exercise (American Diabetes Association, 2013). In dogs, comparable physical activity can be achieved by daily walks of similar intensity; this kind of therapeutic intervention is limited in the cat. However, so-called environmental enrichment may increase the level of activity and may also have positive psychological effects on the diabetic cat. Enrichment strategies include structured play, use of toys (e.g., wire toys mimicking air-borne prey), food balls, cat trees, play tunnels, and others (Ellis, 2009; Hoyumpa Vogt et al, 2010).

Concurrent Problems

Any concurrent disease (inflammatory, infectious, metabolic, or neoplastic) can cause insulin resistance and can have a negative impact on the management of diabetes. Insulin resistance may range from mild to severe or may fluctuate over time. A thorough evaluation of newly-diagnosed diabetic cats is of great importance, and any concurrent problem should be addressed appropriately. Similarly, glucocorticoids and progestagens have a negative influence on insulin sensitivity, and their administration should be stopped immediately. If a concurrent disease requires immunomodulatory medication, alternative drugs should be used if possible (e.g., Ciclosporin). If glucocorticoids are absolutely required, the dose should be kept as low as possible and administration as infrequent as possible. Insulin dose will be higher in those cases and need to be adjusted whenever the glucocorticoid dose is changed. Successful treatment of concurrent problems (e.g., oral care, eradication of urinary tract infection) and/or cessation of diabetogenic drugs oftentimes result in improved glycemic control and improve the chance of diabetic remission. Some diseases, such as chronic renal failure and chronic pancreatitis, cannot be cured and require long-term management. Treatment of diabetes in those situations is often very difficult because there may be substantial fluctuations in insulin sensitivity. Owners should be made aware that treatment may be very challenging and more frequent monitoring and dose amendments than in the usual diabetic cat may be required. The presence of hyperadrenocorticism and acromegaly is oftentimes not suspected until large doses of insulin are required (see Concurrent Disorders Causing Insulin Resistance and Drug-Induced Diabetes in this chapter and Concurrent Disorders Causing Insulin Resistance in Chapter 6.

 TECHNIQUES FOR MONITORING DIABETIC CONTROL

The primary goals of therapy are to eliminate the clinical signs of diabetes while preventing short-term complications (hypoglycemia, DKA). Concurrent problems also need to be controlled, because they may render glycemic control difficult. See Reevaluation and Adjustment of Insulin Dose and Box 7-3 for further details on treatment goals, blood glucose targets, and times of reevaluations. The monitoring techniques are similar for dogs and cats. Different from dogs, however, cats may develop stress hyperglycemia when brought to an unfamiliar environment and/or manipulated by a veterinarian. Stress hyperglycemia may render the interpretation of blood glucose concentrations and BGCs generated in the hospital difficult. Measurement of blood glucose at home is less stressful or even stress-free when done by experienced owners, and results of home monitoring are usually more reliable than results generated in the hospital.

History and Physical Examination

The most important parameters to assess glycemic control are the clinical signs observed by the owner: the stability of the body weight and the findings during physical examination. Cats, in which the initial clinical signs (e.g., polyuria, polydipsia, polyphagia, lethargy, and/or poor hair coat) have resolved, the body weight stays within the desired range, and physical examination reveals a good clinical condition are usually well controlled. In those cases, measurement of serum fructosamine concentration and generation of BGCs will help to confirm the status of good glycemic control and are useful for the "fine-tuning" of insulin therapy. The measurements also help to determine if diabetic remission has occurred. Persistence or reoccurrence of clinical signs and unwanted weight loss is suggestive of inadequate glycemic control or the presence of another disease. Serum fructosamine and in particular generation of BGCs help to characterize the exact problem and to guide the amendment of therapy. Additional tests may be needed in cases in which history or physical examination suggests the presence of a concurrent disease.

Serum Fructosamine Concentration

Fructosamine is the product of an irreversible reaction between glucose and the amino groups of plasma proteins. Its concentration mainly depends on the blood glucose concentration (e.g., extent and duration of hyperglycemia) and the lifespan of plasma proteins; it is generally assumed that fructosamine reflects the mean blood glucose concentration of the preceding 1 to 2 weeks. The reference ranges differ slightly between laboratories but are usually between approximately 200 and 360 μmol/L. To enable comparison between consecutive measurements, serum samples should always be sent to the same laboratory. Fructosamine is measured in serum using commercially-available test kits adapted to autoanalysis. Shipping should be on cold packs if samples will be in transit for more than 24 hours. Lean cats have lower fructosamine concentrations than normal weight or obese cats, whereas age has no influence. In two older studies, fructosamine did not differ between male and female cats, whereas in the most recent study, fructosamine was higher in male cats (Thoresen and Bredal, 1995; Reusch and Haberer, 2001; Gilor et al, 2010b). In the vast majority of newly diagnosed diabetic cats, fructosamine levels are more than 400 μmol/L and may be as high as 1500 μmol/L. Fructosamine is not affected by short-term increases in blood glucose concentration and thus is usually normal in cats with stress hyperglycemia (Reusch et al, 1993; Lutz et al, 1995; Crenshaw et al, 1996).

However, fructosamine is not a foolproof parameter, and certain aspects need to be considered. In cats with a very recent onset of diabetes or with mild diabetes, serum fructosamine may be in the normal range, rendering the differentiation between stress and diabetic hyperglycemia impossible. In a recent study, two groups of healthy cats were infused with glucose to maintain either a marked or a moderate hyperglycemia (540 mg/dL, 30 mmol/L; or 300 mg/dL, 17 mmol/L) for 42 days. In the group with marked hyperglycemia, it took 3 to 5 days until fructosamine exceeded the upper limit of the reference range; in the group with moderate hyperglycemia, fructosamine concentrations mostly fluctuated just below the upper limit of the reference range (Link and Rand, 2008).

Fructosamine is also influenced by plasma protein concentration and by protein turnover. It has been shown that cats suffering from hypoproteinemia or hyperthyroidism have significantly lower levels of fructosamine than healthy cats (Reusch and Tomsa, 1999; Graham et al, 1999; Reusch and Haberer 2001). It is possible that diabetic cats with concurrent hypoproteinemia or uncontrolled hyperthyroidism may have normal (or even low) fructosamine levels, which would then be misinterpreted as indicative for stress hyperglycemia. In those situations (e.g., cats with concurrent hyperthyroidism or hypoproteinemia), fructosamine should be interpreted only if it is increased, which then indicates diabetes mellitus. There are arguments for and against correction of fructosamine for the serum protein level. Correction, however, may lead to falsely high concentrations and is not recommended. In the majority of situations, fructosamine is a helpful parameter to differentiate between stress- and diabetes-related hyperglycemia.

After initiating insulin therapy, blood glucose concentrations usually start to decrease, which is followed by a decrease in fructosamine after a few days. We consider 50 μmol/L to be the so-called critical difference (i.e., the difference between two consecutive fructosamine measurements has to exceed 50 μmol/L to reflect a change in glycemic control; Reusch, 2013). Another study found a lower critical difference of 33 μmol/L (Link and Rand, 2008). Generally, fructosamine concentrations increase when glycemic control worsens and decrease when glycemic control improves. As mentioned earlier, serum fructosamine concentration is not affected by a short term increase in blood glucose concentration, which may be seen in cats in the hospital. It is also not affected by lack of food intake, which is common in hospitalized cats and often leads to much lower blood glucose concentrations than what is seen with food intake. Routine measurement of fructosamine is therefore helpful to clarify the effects of stress or lack of food intake (e.g., to clarify discrepancies between history and physical examination and blood glucose measurements). Most well-controlled diabetic cats are slightly hyperglycemic for some time during a 24-hour period, and consequently, fructosamine concentrations will not become completely normal during therapy. In cats that achieve diabetic remission, however, fructosamine concentrations decrease into the normal range (Fig. 7-17).

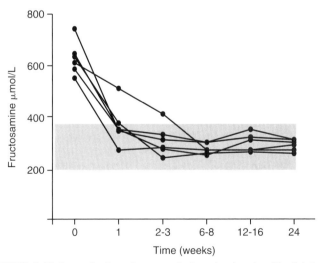

FIGURE 7-17 Serum fructosamine concentrations in six cats with diabetes mellitus experiencing diabetic remission. Remission occurred during the first 12 weeks of therapy, and diabetes of all cats was still in remission after 24 weeks. *0,* Initial presentation; *gray area,* reference range (200 to 340 μmol/L).

As long as fructosamine is elevated (even if only slightly), we do not consider cats to be in diabetic remission. In those cases, insulin therapy is continued under close supervision. Fructosamine concentrations between approximately 350 and 450 µmol/L reflect good glycemic control, concentrations between 450 and 550 µmol/L suggest moderate, and concentrations above 550 to 600 µmol/L suggest poor glycemic control. In the latter situation, fructosamine is not helpful to identify the underlying problem because the various possible reasons for poor regulation (e.g., application error, insulin underdose, too short duration of insulin effect, diseases causing insulin resistance, or Somogyi phenomenon) are associated with high blood glucose concentrations and therefore have the same impact. Generation of one or several BGCs and revision of the owner's injection technique are usually the next steps in those cases. Fructosamine concentrations less than 350 µmol/L suggest diabetic remission, hypoglycemia or concurrent hypoproteinemia, or hyperthyroidism (Reusch, 2010). It is important to note that there are substantial differences in glycation between individuals. In healthy cats in which blood glucose was maintained at 540 mg/dL (30 mmol/L), fructosamine concentrations ranged between 400 and 633 µmol/L when the plateau was reached (Link and Rand, 2008). The study underscores that diabetic cats with similar quality of glycemic regulation may have quite different fructosamine concentrations. The ranges of interpretation listed earlier therefore should only be used as rough guidelines. Fructosamine is useful if followed in individual cats over time; however, it should never be used as the sole indicator of the quality of metabolic control. The parameter is less important than the evaluation of clinical signs and body weight and generation of BGCs.

DKA, dehydration, acidosis, and other unidentified factors may influence fructosamine concentrations. If a diabetic cat is hospitalized for any reason, fructosamine levels measured at the time of admission may be considerably different from concentrations measured a few days later. It is therefore reasonable to repeat the measurement at the time of discharge and to use this concentration as a reference point. See Serum Fructosamine Concentration in Chapter 6 for additional information.

Glycated Hemoglobin Concentration

Glycated hemoglobin is formed by non-enzymatic, irreversible binding of glucose to amino groups of the globin part of the hemoglobin molecule. Its concentration reflects the average blood concentration over the lifespan of the erythrocytes, which is approximately 70 days in the cat. In human diabetics, glycated hemoglobin is one of the cornerstones of glycemic control, and its measurement in regular intervals is strongly recommended (American Diabetes Association, 2013). The matter is somewhat confusing because many different measuring methods are available that measure different species of the molecule. Currently, considerable effort is made in human medicine for an international standardization of glycated hemoglobin measurement (John, 2012). In humans, HBA_{1c} is the component present in largest amounts and results from binding of glucose to the N-terminal amino acid valine of the β-chain of hemoglobin. HBA_1 is a series of glycated variants resulting from the binding of different carbohydrates to valine and includes HBA_{1a} and HBA_{1b}, as well as HBA_{1c}. Total glycated hemoglobin denotes the binding of all carbohydrates at any site of the hemoglobin molecule. High-performance liquid chromatography (HPLC) mainly measures HBA_{1c} as do the newer immunoassays, whereas affinity chromatography methods measure total glycated hemoglobin (Pickup, 2003).

Feline hemoglobin differs considerably from human and canine hemoglobin, which limits the use of some of the human assays. Successful measurement of glycated hemoglobin has been achieved by HPLC and affinity chromatography (Hasegawa et al, 1992; Hoyer-Ott et al, 1995; Elliott et al, 1997; 1999; Haberer and Reusch, 1998; Hoenig and Ferguson, 1999). Glycated hemoglobin was shown to be significantly higher in diabetic cats compared to healthy cats and to cats with stress hyperglycemia. It was also higher in poorly-controlled than in well-controlled diabetic cats. Its concentration decreased significantly after initiating insulin therapy or after improvement of glycemic control respectively. Glycated hemoglobin is measured in ethylenediaminetetraacetic acid (EDTA) whole blood; the molecule is stable at 4° C for at least 1 week. As stability at room temperature differs between assays, the instructions of the laboratory should be followed for shipping. We no longer use glycated hemoglobin mainly because of the limited availability of assays validated for the cat and the lack of advantage over fructosamine, which is very easy to measure. Additionally, glycated hemoglobin in cats is substantially lower than in dogs and humans, and the increase in case of diabetes is less pronounced. Consequently, the difference between well-, moderately-, and poorly-controlled cats is quite small, and the interpretation of results therefore is more difficult.

Urine Glucose Monitoring

Glucose is freely filtered by the glomerulus and reabsorbed in the proximal tubules by the sodium-glucose cotransporter 2 (SGLT2). The reabsorption capacity is limited, and when the blood glucose concentration exceeds the so-called renal threshold (approximately 17 mmol/L, 300 mg/dL in cats), glucose is excreted in the urine. The higher the blood glucose concentration is, the more glucose is found in the urine, which would render the urine test a valuable monitoring tool in theory. However, measurement of urine glucose may be misleading for several reasons: (1) the result does not reflect the actual blood glucose concentration, but is an average over the time of urine accumulation in the bladder; (2) a negative urine test does not differentiate between hypoglycemia, normoglycemia, or mild hyperglycemia; and (3) hydration status and urine concentration may affect the result. It should also be noted that the renal threshold mentioned earlier is only an approximate number. It is known from humans that there are substantial differences between individuals and the threshold may also change within the same individual. Therefore, marked hyperglycemia may exist without glycosuria, or glycosuria may occur with a normal blood glucose concentration (Pickup, 2003; Rave, 2006). Very few studies have investigated the analytical aspects of urine glucose testing in cats. Recently, a commonly used test strip (Bayer Multistix) was compared with a litter additive designed for monitor urine glucose at home (Purina Glucotest). The Multistix inaccurately classified the degree of glycosuria in 24.2 of samples (19% overestimation, 5.2% underestimation). The Glucotest was read immediately after exposure to urine and at different time points thereafter over the course of 8 hours. At the initial reading, the test was inaccurate in 22 % of samples (21% overestimation, 1% underestimation); the inaccuracy decreased to 10% and 3% when the test was read at 30 minutes and 8 hours, respectively (Fletcher et al, 2011).

In summary, numerous biological and analytical factors render urine glucose testing unreliable. In our hospital, we do not adjust insulin dosages based on urine glucose measurements, and we strongly discourage owners from doing so. Owners who are unable to measure blood glucose but still want to do some type of monitoring may be advised to use urine glucose measurements in all urine

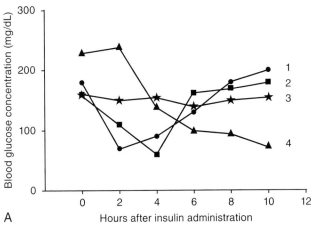

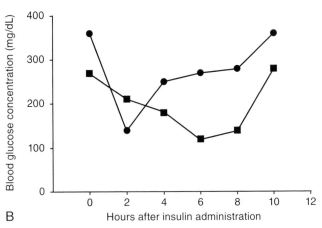

FIGURE 7-18 A, Variable glucose nadirs during blood glucose curves (BGCs) in four diabetic cats treated with insulin glargine (Lantus) between 1 to 2.5 U/cat b.i.d. In cat 1 and 2, the nadirs are 2 and 4 hours, respectively, after insulin administration. Cat 3 does not display an obvious nadir, and in cat 4, the nadir has not been reached during the time of blood glucose measurements (e.g., the nadir is ≥ 10 hours after insulin administration). Insulin glargine has been designed as a peakless insulin for humans. However, in a substantial percentage of cats, a clear peak of action (associated with a clear nadir) is seen during BGCs. Some cats, in particular well-regulated cats, do not show a nadir, and the BGC resembles a flat line as in cat 3. **B,** Two BGCs generated 4 weeks apart from each other in the same cat at home showing different times of glucose nadirs (after 2 and 6 hours respectively). The cat was treated with 1.5 U/cat insulin glargine (Lantus) at both points in time. *0,* Time of insulin administration. To convert mg/dL into mmol/L, multiply blood glucose concentration by 0.056.

samples voided throughout 1 day per week. Replacement of litter by nonabsorbable material (e.g., aquarium gravel) facilitates urine collection. Persistent glycosuria would suggest inadequate glycemic control and the need for thorough evaluation in the hospital. If no glucose is detected in any of the samples, the cat is either very well controlled, is in diabetic remission, or is overdosed with insulin and should be evaluated by a veterinarian. In cats prone to develop DKA, we recommend that the owners check the urine for ketone bodies on a regular basis (e.g., once to twice per week).

Single Blood Glucose Determination

Measurement of a single blood glucose concentration is usually insufficient to assess glycemic control. The exception may be cats with long-standing diabetes in which clinical signs of diabetes mellitus have disappeared, physical examination is unremarkable, and serum fructosamine concentration ranges between 350 and 450 μmol/L. In these cases, the finding of a blood glucose concentration between 180 and 270 mg/dL (10 to 15 mmol/L) around the time of insulin injection is usually consistent with good glycemic control and may render further glucose measurements unnecessary. In cats with more recent onset of diabetes, achievement of diabetic remission is potentially possible and generation of a BGC should be pursued. It is the glucose nadir measured during a BGC that mainly determines if there is room for further (slight) increase in insulin dose. Of note, the time of the glucose nadir varies between cats and also within the same cat (Fig. 7-18). Therefore, determination of a single glucose concentration at the time of the assumed nadir may be misleading.

A single low blood glucose concentration most often is due to insulin overdose, but may also be seen if there is lack of food intake.

Blood Glucose Curve

In addition to evaluation of clinical signs, serial measurement of blood glucose throughout the day (known as *blood glucose curve,*

BGC) is the most important monitoring tool for diabetic cats. BGCs are particular important during the initial phases of therapy. During the first weeks to months, insulin doses usually need to be adjusted several times; it is also most often during the first 3 months of therapy that diabetic remission occurs. During long-term management regular, albeit less frequent generation of BGCs is helpful to ensure that the animal is still well-regulated. If clinical signs of diabetes reappear at any time during long-term management, generation of BGCs helps to identify the underlying problem and allows informed dose amendments.

Generation of Blood Glucose Curves in the Hospital

We prefer that owners give insulin and food at home, and then bring the cat to the hospital as soon as possible (within 2 hours) for a BGC. This approach eliminates the effect of lack of food intake on blood glucose levels—at least in those cats that are fed only at the time of insulin administration. When technical difficulties are suspected, owners are asked to bring the cat to the hospital before insulin application and to carry out the entire administration procedure under supervision of a veterinarian or a technician. We generate BGCs by measuring the glucose concentration on average every 2 hours throughout the day until the next insulin administration is due. Shorter intervals (i.e., 1 hour) are chosen in cats with suspected hypoglycemia, and longer intervals (i.e., 3 hours) are sufficient in patients with stable disease. If the glucose nadir is not reached during this time, insulin administration should be delayed and glucose measurements continued. The cat should be handled as carefully as possible and any unnecessary manipulation should be avoided to reduce stress. Blood samples are not obtained by venipuncture but by collecting capillary blood from the ear or the footpad using the same PBGM meter as the owner at home. Usually, the cat can stay in the cage, and when performed by an experienced technician, the procedure is usually well tolerated. With these precautions, we often achieve meaningful measurements (i.e., blood glucose concentrations that match

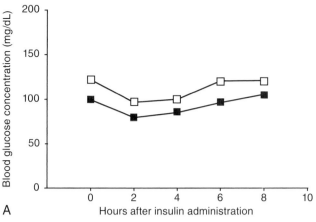
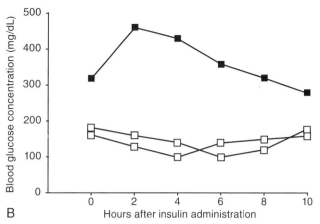

FIGURE 7-19 A, Example of a good correlation between blood glucose curves (BGCs) generated in the hospital and at home by the owner. The two curves were generated 3 days apart from each other. The cat (Domestic Short-Hair [DSH], castrated male, 7 kg, 15 years old) received 1 U/cat insulin glargine (Lantus) b.i.d. at both points in time. Clinical signs were well controlled and serum fructosamine concentration was 346 μmol (reference range 200 to 340 μmol/L). *Open squares,* BGC generated at home; *closed squares,* BGC generated in the hospital. **B,** Example of a poor correlation between BGCs generated in the hospital and at home by the owner. The owner generated BGCs at home for 2 consecutive days; another BGC was generated in the hospital 1 week thereafter. The cat (DSH, castrated male, 4.4 kg, 11 years old) received 0.5 U/cat Lente-type insulin (Vetsulin/Caninsulin) b.i.d. at all three points in time. Clinical signs of diabetes were well controlled, and serum fructosamine concentration was 358 μmol/L (reference range 200 to 340 μmol/L). The two home-BGCs show good agreement with each other and support the clinical assessment of good glycemic control. The blood glucose concentrations in the hospital are substantially higher and were attributed to stress. Insulin dose was not changed and the cat continued to do well. *Open squares,* BGCs generated at home; *closed squares,* BGC generated in the hospital. *0,* Time of insulin administration. To convert mg/dL into mmol/L, multiply blood glucose concentration by 0.056.

very well with our clinical impression and the serum fructosamine concentration; Fig. 7-19).

Generally, however, BGCs generated in the hospital are prone to be affected by stress, abnormal housing conditions (small cage compared to free-roaming in the house), and decreased food intake. Cats are particularly sensitive to stress caused by an unfamiliar environment and manipulation by the veterinarian or technician. Consequently, blood glucose concentrations may rise during the BGC and never decrease again while the cat is in the hospital, or glucose levels may be high from the beginning. Blood glucose concentrations in stressed cats in excess of 300 mg/dL (17 mmol/L) are common and may even be higher than 400 mg/dL (22 mmol/L). Stress hyperglycemia should be suspected if the cat is obviously upset or aggressive, although it may also occur in cats appearing calm. The most reliable indicator of stress hyperglycemia is a discrepancy between the clinical impression, body weight, and fructosamine concentration on the one hand and results of the BGC on the other. Lack of food intake has the opposite effect because it may result in low blood glucose concentrations, a situation which is difficult to differentiate from insulin overdose. In addition, BGCs are time-consuming and expensive, and therefore they are often not performed as often as required. It is easy to overlook diabetic remission if blood glucose concentrations are not measured frequently. The veterinarian may also be more reluctant to increase the insulin dose in cats in which BGCs are performed only sporadically, which may hamper achievement of good glycemic control or diabetic remission. Close monitoring of blood glucose is also indicated in diabetic patients with concurrent diseases, which may require frequent adjustments of the insulin dose. See the sections Home Monitoring of Blood Glucose, Frequency of Monitoring, and Interpretation of Blood Glucose Curves and Adjustment of Insulin Doses for more details.

Home Monitoring of Blood Glucose

Treatment success depends largely on the active participation of the owner and on how well he or she is trained for this task by the veterinarian or the technician. The owner should assess the cat for clinical signs of diabetes on a daily basis, and body weight should be measured at least once per week. Home monitoring of blood glucose by the owner was developed approximately 15 years ago and since then has been a routine part of our diabetic treatment and monitoring protocol (Wess and Reusch, 2000). Home monitoring enables frequent blood glucose measurements, and consequently the insulin dose can be amended more often and more precisely. The technique is of particular value in cats because stress hyperglycemia and the potential of diabetic remission renders diabetic monitoring even more challenging than in dogs.

All of our cat owners are introduced to the option of home monitoring of blood glucose, and many of them are willing and able to generate BGCs on a long-term basis (e.g., for several years). Once owners are familiar with the technique, they highly appreciate having more control over the disease. Major points mentioned by owners were that they could monitor blood glucose frequently and were able to assess if changes in the cats well-being are associated with hypo- or hyperglycemia. Owners also appreciate that home BGCs are less stressful for the cat than in-hospital BGCs (Kley et al, 2004).

Introduction of Technique to Cat Owners

Owners are often worried when they learn that their cat is diabetic. At first they need to gain confidence that they will be able to manage the disease, get some basic understanding about diabetes, and learn how to inject insulin and they need to adapt their own lifestyle to the new needs of their cat. The immediate introduction to home monitoring may overburden many owners and should therefore be delayed until the owner feels confident. We usually introduce the general concept of home monitoring by the time of discharge from the hospital after the diagnosis of diabetes has been made. Our written instructions on the various aspects of therapy also contain pictures on how capillary blood glucose can be taken. During the first reevaluation (approximately 1 week later), the importance of BGCs in the control of the disease is emphasized, and the owner is informed that the procedure of home monitoring can be started after the next reevaluation (2 to 3 weeks after diagnosis). Owners who are very keen to perform home monitoring and those who are familiar with capillary blood sampling (e.g., have another diabetic pet or are diabetics themselves) may start home monitoring earlier.

Teaching capillary blood sampling and the use of the PBGM device takes at least 30 minutes and should be performed by an experienced veterinarian or technician who has performed the procedure many times. The owner is taught how to use the lancing device and all relevant technical aspects of the PBGM device. Some PBGM devices come with very detailed information and an instructional DVD (e.g., the AlphaTRAK); the veterinarian can also refer the owner to one of the many websites demonstrating the technique. The owner should not leave the hospital before being able to generate a blood drop and to work the PBGM device correctly. Along with the PBGM device and test strips, we provide forms for recording the blood glucose values and show how the glucose concentration should be plotted. It is important that owners performing home monitoring have ready access to veterinary support if required.

Sampling Site, Lancing Device, and Portable Blood Glucose Monitoring Device

Capillary blood can be obtained from various sites. Initial studies showed that blood glucose concentrations obtained from the ear correlated very well with those from venous blood (Wess and Reusch, 2000). Recent comparison of blood glucose concentrations between different sampling sites (ear, metacarpal, and metatarsal pads) revealed only minor, insignificant differences (Zeugswetter et al, 2010). Sampling sites may therefore be rotated (i.e., if no blood can be obtained at one site, another one can be used). Our preferred site of sampling is the inner aspect of the pinna. The tip of the ear is held between thumb and index finger, and the entire surface of the outer pinna is held flat using the remaining fingers of the same hand. One may also place a cotton ball on the outside of the pinna. With the other hand, the lancing device is placed on a non-haired area of the pinna and triggered. We aim for capillary, not for venous blood, and therefore avoid lancing a vein. No bleeding is expected after capillary sampling, and therefore no pressure is needed after the puncturing procedure. Shaving, warming, or any other preparation is hardly ever needed (Wess and Reusch, 2000; Casella et al, 2002; Reusch, 2013). If the cat dislikes being touched at the ears, we use the metacarpal, metatarsal, or digital pads (Fig. 7-20). Others prefer to sample from the lateral ear margin on the outside of the pinna or use non–weight-bearing pads (wrist pads) instead of weight-bearing pads to avoid discomfort when walking or risk of infection with use of a litter box (Ford and Lynch, 2013). Several starter kits not only provide the PBGM device with test strips but also a lancing device with a certain number of lancets. Pharmacies offer devices of different gauge sizes and various depth settings. Which lancing device is used is a question of personal preference. The most important point is that the veterinarian or technician is familiar with the device and is able to convincingly demonstrate

its use. Unfortunately, the lancing device Microlet Vaculance (Bayer Diagnostics) designed for use on alternative sites (i.e., not the fingertip) in humans is no longer available. The Microlet Vaculance developed a vacuum after lancing, which helped to suck out blood.

The first PBGM device was the Ames Reflectance Meter, patented in 1971 by the Ames company. It was almost 20 cm long and required a very large drop of blood. Since then, numerous models have been developed that are smaller, lighter, faster, and easier to handle. Modern PBGM devices have a memory capacity for the test results, and some allow data to be transferred to a personal computer. Various models require coding or calibration, which is the process of matching the PBGM device with the test strips. Usually, this is done by inserting a code strip or a code number into the meter each time a new batch of test strips is used. If done incorrectly, the readings may be inaccurate. Some models use a "no coding technology," meaning that the device is automatically calibrated and coded whenever a test strip is inserted. In human medicine, the quality control of PBGM devices is of continuous concern because the success of diabetes management depends largely on the reliability of the blood glucose measurements. The analytical quality of measurements can be compromised by operator and other procedural errors (e.g., dirty meters), hematocrit, altitude, humidity, ambient temperature, and lot-to-lot variability of test strips (Farmer, 2010; Nerhus et al, 2011; Baumstark et al, 2012). A number of accuracy standards have been proposed over the past decades. The most recent International Organization for Standardization (ISO) accuracy standards for PBGM devices used in humans (known as ISO 15197 criteria) state that 95% of the PBGM device measurements should fall within ± 15 mg/dL (0.84 mmol/L) of the reference method at blood glucose concentrations < 100 mg/dL (5.6 mmol/L) and within ± 15% of the reference method at blood glucose concentrations ≥ 100 mg/dL (Garg et al, 2013; International Organization for Standardization, 2013). However, those requirements are often not met. A recent study in humans showed that only 18 of 34 PBGM devices (52.9%) fulfilled those ISO standards (Freckmann et al, 2012).

A huge number of different PBGM devices are currently available, and most of them are made for use in humans. Unilke earlier times, most human PBGM devices are nowadays plasma-calibrated (i.e., they read the blood glucose concentrations from capillary [whole] blood as if they were plasma glucose concentrations). The reason behind this calibration is to enable better comparison between laboratory and PBGM device measurements. As the amount of glucose within erythrocytes in cats (and dogs) is lower than in humans, those PBGM devices may underestimate the "true" blood glucose concentration.

Several companies are now marketing devices for veterinary use, claiming that they give more accurate results in dogs and cats. We are currently using the PBGM meter, AlphaTRAK 2 (Abbott Animal Health), in the hospital and recommend its use to owners. This PBGM meter is also plasma-calibrated, taking into account the difference of glucose distribution in whole blood in dogs and cats (see www.alphatrakmeter.com for more information). So far, a small number of studies have compared the performance of the AlphaTRAK meter with those of several human PBGM devices and demonstrated that quality parameters were better for the AlphaTRAK (Cohen et al, 2009; Zini et al, 2009b). However, glucose readings from the AlphaTRAK may still differ considerably from the reference method, and differences increase as blood glucose concentrations increase. In contrast to many human PBGM devices, which usually give readings in dogs and cats that are lower than the reference method, the AlphaTRAK

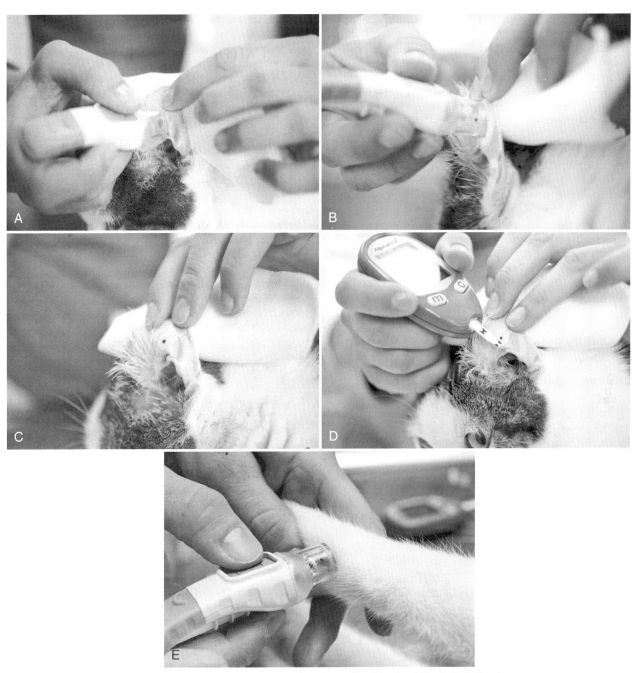

FIGURE 7-20 Capillary blood sampling from the ear (**A** to **D**) and pad (**E**) of a diabetic cat.

may either under- or overestimate the "true" glucose concentrations. Therefore, unlike earlier times when the veterinarian could assume the "true" glucose level to be a bit higher than what is measured with the PBGM device, we now have to accept the concentration at face value. In most cases, the differences are small; in rare instances, however, hypoglycemia may be overlooked. In our most recent evaluation, using 78 feline samples, no difference between the AlphaTRAK reading and the reference method was found in 7 samples (9%). In 40 samples (51%), the Alpha-TRAK overestimated the glucose concentration; the differences to the reference method ranged between 1.8 to 72 mg/dL, median 4.4 mg/dL (0.1 to 4.0 mmol/L, median 0.8 mmol/L). In 31 samples (40%), the AlphaTRAK underestimated the glucose concentration by (–1.8) to (–122) mg/dL, median (–12.6) mg/dL ([–0.1] to [–6.8] mmol/L, median [–0.7]). Table 7-8 shows the differences

in the glucose categories < 100 mg/dL (5.6 mmol/L) and ≥ 100 mg/dL. Fortunately, precision of the AlphaTRAK is better at blood glucose concentrations < 100 mg/dL (5.6 mmol/L), where exact measurements are most important, and approximately 90% of values fall within ± 15 mg/dL (0.85 mmol/L) of the reference method. At blood glucose above 100 mg/dL (5.5 mmol/L) imprecision is higher but is less serious. It is usually of lesser importance to distinguish a blood glucose concentration of 200 mg/dL from 250 mg/dL (11 and 14 mmol/L) because treatment decision does not change or is minor.

The bottom line is that according to currently available data, the AlphaTRAK performs reasonably well in cats and dogs. Additional advantages are the very small sample volume (0.3 µL) and the wide measurement range of 20 to 750 mg/dL (1.1 to 42 mmol/L). The influence of factors (e.g., hematocrit, ambient temperature, and others) known to have an impact on the precision of human PBGM devices have not yet been investigated for the AlphaTRAK with feline blood. Other "veterinary" PBGM devices are on the market, and many more will certainly come. It is very important that the veterinarian ensures that independent quality control studies have been performed before using them. A certain degree of deviation from the reference method, however, has to be accepted.

Problems and Long-Term Compliance

Many of our clients call for advice one or more times after the start of home monitoring. Some have specific questions regarding the procedure, and others just need reassurance that they are performing the procedure correctly. If support via telephone is insufficient, additionally, demonstration of the techniques should be provided. By watching an owner perform the procedure, the veterinarian or technician can identify and correct errors immediately. The most frequently encountered problem is failure to generate an adequate amount of blood. If repeated demonstration is unsuccessful, an alternative sampling site (e.g., switching form pinna to footpad) may be helpful. Handling the PBGM device is usually not a problem for owners, and most report that their cat tolerates the procedure quite well. As little restraint as possible should be used to avoid the cat becoming stressed. Usually, cats become accustomed to the procedure with time and increasing experience of the owner. Many owners try different strategies for easier restraint and report that their cats tolerate blood collection better when placed in a favorite spot, such as bed, window sill, and/or a confined area such as a sink.

Most owners are able to measure blood glucose without help, but a second person may be required initially. The skin puncture

does not seem to be painful, and the puncture sites are barely visible, even after numerous blood collections. The exceptions are cats with very thin ears in which we have seen aural hematomas. In those cats, blood samples should be collected from the footpads. Long-term compliance with home monitoring is usually good, and many owners measure blood glucose on a regular basis for many years. The vast majority of owners highly appreciate their active participation in the management of the disease. Periodic reassessment of the entire procedure (capillary blood sampling, use of the PBGM device, and correct reading and interpretation of the measurements) in the hospital is highly recommended (Casella et al, 2002; 2005; Kley et al, 2004; Reusch et al, 2006a). However, home monitoring is an additional burden to owners that should not be underestimated. The veterinarian must carefully determine whether an owner is able (psychologically and time-wise) to cope with home monitoring and should keep in mind that owners may opt for euthanasia if they feel stressed. Owners should understand that home monitoring is an additional tool in the management of diabetes, which provides valuable information. It is not an absolute requirement. On the other hand, there are also "overmotivated" owners who absolutely want to have a perfectly regulated cat. Those owners tend to contact the hospital whenever a blood glucose value is outside the target range, even if the deviation is only slight. They need to understand that the blood glucose concentration in a diabetic individual is influenced by numerous factors and can vary from day to day. It is important that those owners learn to look at the general picture (well-being, stability of body weight, and most but not all glucose measurement within the target range) than on single glucose values. The exception is the finding of a very low glucose concentration, which requires an immediate reduction of the insulin dose. It has been assumed that cat owners who perform home monitoring would visit the hospital less frequently. However, our experience over the past 15 years does not support this assumption. Frequency of veterinary visits does not differ to a relevant degree among cats with and without home monitoring.

Frequency of Monitoring

Our protocol for generation of a BGC at home is to have the owner measure the glucose concentration before the morning insulin injection and every 2 hours thereafter until the evening insulin injection is due. One of the several advantages of home monitoring is the fact that the veterinarian can ask for further blood glucose measurements in cats in which the glucose nadir is not reached during this time (e.g., generation of a 14- or 16-hour BGC) without interfering with working hours of the practice. More frequent measurement (hourly) may be suggested in cases with suspected hypoglycemia so that the lowest glucose concentration is not missed. In cats in which the diabetes is well controlled, the intervals may be prolonged to approximately every 3 hours—in particular during long-term management. Opinions on the question, "How often owners should check their cat's blood glucose?" differ. Some investigators have suggested that owners should perform measurements several times per day and adjust the insulin dose accordingly following a very tight dosing algorithm. Those algorithms are sometimes called *remission protocols,* and it has been claimed that following those protocols lead to higher remission rates (Roomp and Rand, 2009; 2012). There is little doubt that early and adequate treatment results in better diabetic control, fewer complications, and potentially to a higher remission rate compared with situations in which treatment is delayed and poorly done. However, those intensive protocols require owners who have the time to measure several times per day, and they bear a high risk of hypoglycemia,

TABLE 7-8	COMPARISON OF GLUCOSE CONCENTRATIONS MEASURED BY THE PORTABLE BLOOD GLUCOSE MONITORING DEVICE, ALPHATRAK, AND THE REFERENCE ANALYZER*

	Glucose Concentration Obtained with Reference Analyzer	
	< 100 mg/dL (5.6 mmol/L)	≥ 100 mg/dL (5.6 mmol/L)
AlphaTRAK		
Number of samples with no difference	4 (11%)	3 (7%)
Overestimation		
Number of samples	17 (49%)	23 (53%)
Range (median)	1.8 to 27 mg/dL (7.2) 0.1 to 1.5 mmol/L (0.4)	1.8 to 72 mg/dL (36) 0.1 to 4.0 mmol/L (2.0)
Underestimation		
Number of samples	14 (40%)	17 (40%)
Range (median)	(−1.8) to (−18) mg/dL (−5.4 mg/dL) (−0.1) to (−1.0) mmol/L (−0.3)	(−3.6) to (−122) mg/dL (−22 mg/dL) (−0.2) to (−6.8) mmol/L (−1.2 mmol/L)

*Data are given for glucose concentrations < 100 mg/dL (5.6 mmol/L) and ≥ 100 mg/dL. A total of 78 feline samples were analyzed; in 35 samples, blood glucose measured with the reference analyzer was < 100 mg/dL, and in 43 samples, blood glucose was ≥ 100 mg/dL.

even when performed under close supervision. The remission rate in our hospital using the protocol described here ranges between 40% to 50% over the years; this is only slightly lower than the rate of 51%, which was achieved with a "remission protocol" (Roomp and Rand, 2009), provided that cats with prior steroid treatment were excluded from the analysis. In cats that develop diabetes during steroid treatment, remission is often easily achieved after cessation of the drug and initiating insulin therapy, and remission rates may therefore appear to be high if many of those cats are included in a study. Our protocol foresees that owners generate a BGC once a week during the first months of therapy. After stabilization (and if no remission is achieved), the time intervals are prolonged to approximately every 3 to 4 weeks. We also ask owners to measure the fasting blood glucose (pre-insulin glucose) twice weekly and to perform a spot glucose check whenever they feel uncertain about the well-being of the cat. Although many of our owners work full-time, this protocol is feasible for most of them, because they generate the BGC during the weekend. There are cases in which we ask for additional BGCs (e.g., in an extremely unstable diabetic), but those are rare exceptions.

Interpretation of Blood Glucose Curves and Adjustment of Insulin Doses

Owners can certainly be taught how to interpret BGCs and to make adjustments in insulin dose. However, we prefer that decisions are made by the veterinarian and BGCs be sent to the hospital, especially during the first 3 months of therapy. This initial treatment period needs particular attention, because most cats require several dose adjustments. It is also during this time that either diabetic remission occurs or the presence of insulin resistance becomes apparent, requiring further work-up. During long-term management, owners may take more responsibility and make (slight) dose adjustments on their own.

BGCs are extremely helpful for the titration of the insulin dose, either upward or downward. Interpretation of BGCs generated at home follows the same rules as BGCs generated in the hospital. Our goal is to achieve blood glucose concentrations that are below the renal threshold by avoiding hypoglycemia. The highest glucose concentration, which is usually (but not always) the fasting/pre-insulin concentration, should not exceed 180 to 270 mg/dL (10 to 15 mmol/L); the lowest glucose concentration (glucose nadir) should ideally be between 80 and 140 mg/dL (4.5 to 7.8 mmol/L). Lower nadirs may be due to insulin overdose (including sudden improvement of insulin-resistant states), excessive overlap of insulin actions, or lack of food intake. They may also be found in cats in which diabetes is ready to go into remission or is already in remission. Finding a nadir below 70 mg/dL (3.9 mmol/L) should always lead to a reduction of the insulin dose. We tolerate the occasional occurrence of a nadir between 70 and 80 mg/dL (3.9 to 4.5 mmol/L) if the cat is doing well and is monitored closely. In general and in the long-run, however, nadirs should not be lower than 80 mg/dL (4.5 mmol/L). The dose reduction should be 0.5 to 1.0 U/cat b.i.d. if the cat is on a low to moderate dose of insulin (0.5 to 3/cat b.i.d.) or 25% to 50% if the cat is on a higher dose.

BGCs allow assessment of the insulin efficacy, the glucose nadir, and duration of the insulin effect. *Insulin efficacy* means the effectiveness of insulin to lower the blood glucose concentration, and it may be evaluated by determining the difference between the highest and lowest glucose concentration of a BGC. A small difference is acceptable when all blood glucose concentrations are well within the target range; however, it is not acceptable if this is not the case. Of note, the shape of BGCs differs considerably

between cats and also within the same cat. Additionally, the type of insulin influences the shape of a BGC. With Lente-type insulins (Vetsulin/Caninsulin) and PZI oftentimes more or less bell-shaped BGCs with a pronounced peak are seen (i.e., the fasting glucose concentrations are substantially higher than the glucose nadirs). Long-acting insulin analogues (insulin glargine/Lantus, insulin detemir/Levemir) are so-called peakless insulins, which in theory should keep the blood glucose concentration at a fairly constant level. In fact, in some cats treated with insulin glargine, the BGC is flat. In others, however, a clear peak is seen. The shape of the BGC may change with time in the same cat. Initially, when glycemic control is still poor, blood glucose concentrations may just fluctuate in the high glycemic range; with improved glycemic control, a "true" curve is often seen, which again changes into a more or less flat line when good glycemic control or diabetic remission is achieved (Fig. 7-21).

The glucose nadir is an important parameter because it is the major determinant of dose adjustment. We titrate the insulin dose in steps of 0.5 U/cat b.i.d. until the glucose nadir is between 80 to 140 mg/dL (4.5 to 7.8 mmol/L). Dose requirements differ substantially between cats. Some are adequately controlled with an insulin dose as low as 0.5 U/cat b.i.d., and others need up to 1 U/kg b.i.d. or more. The majority of diabetic cats need between 0.5 and 3.0/cat b.i.d. Insulin requirements > 1.0 U/kg should raise suspicion for the presence of concurrent disease, and further work-up should be considered. However, some diabetic cats without concurrent disease may need quite high insulin doses (1.0 to 1.5 U/kg b.i.d.) during the initial phases of treatment, and oftentimes the dose can be cut back after some time. The reason is unclear; it is possible that those cats suffer from more serious glucose toxicity and/or insulin resistance, which may be

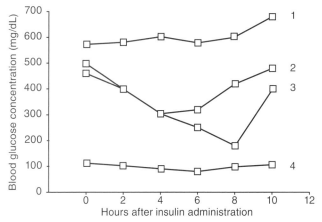

FIGURE 7-21 Change of blood glucose curve (BGC) shape in a diabetic cat (Devon Rex, castrated male, 9 years old, 4.5 kg) during treatment with insulin glargine (Lantus). *BGC 1:* 1 week after initiating treatment, insulin dose was 2.0 U/cat b.i.d.; *BGC 2:* 6 weeks after start of therapy, insulin dose was 4.5 U/cat b.i.d.; *BGC 3:* 10 weeks after start of therapy, insulin dose was 6.0 U/cat b.i.d.; *BGC 4:* 20 weeks after start of therapy, insulin dose was 0.5 U/cat s.i.d. Insulin administration was stopped at that time; diabetes is still in remission (2 years after cessation of insulin administration). The increase and decrease in insulin dose was done in steps of 0.5 U/cat b.i.d., and before each step, a BGC curve was generated. Here, only four BGCs are shown to demonstrate that the shape of the BGC may change during treatment. All BGCs were generated by the owner at home. Generally, although insulin glargine is considered a peakless insulin, some cats display a clear glucose nadir, whereas in others, the BGC resembles more a flat line. *0*, Time of insulin administration. To convert mg/dL into mmol/L, multiply blood glucose concentration by 0.056.

overcome with treatment. The duration of effect is defined as the time from the insulin injection through the glucose nadir until the blood glucose concentration exceeds 180 to 270 mg/dL (10 to 15 mmol/L), and it should be evaluated when the glucose nadir is within the target range and be ideally approximately 12 hours. If the duration is less than 8 to 10 hours, the cat usually reveals signs of diabetes; and if the duration is longer than 14 hours, the risk of hypoglycemia or the occurrence of the Somogyi effect increases (see Complications of Insulin Therapy).

Dose adjustments are generally done once a week after receiving the weekly BGC from the owner. The numbers of dose adjustments differ widely between diabetic cats. In some, one or two adjustments are sufficient to achieve the target glucose range, and in others, it takes several weeks. It is not uncommon that the need to increase the dose alternates with the need of dose reduction. In cats that continue to be severely hyperglycemic after the first 2 to 3 weeks, the process of dose increase is hastened slightly, and the intervals are shortened to approximately every 5 days. We do not change the dose more often than every 5 to 7 days (except in the case of hypoglycemia) because the insulin needs some time to equilibrate. Insulin glargine, which is currently our preferred insulin, is designed as intermediate/long-acting insulin. In humans, it is very often used in a treatment regimen, called *basal-bolus* or *multiple daily injection regimen*. Therewith, it is attempted to mimic the normal physiological secretion of insulin as close as possible by providing background basal insulin coverage (with insulin glargine) along with a bolus injection of short-acting insulin at each mealtime. In humans, it is recommended not to make changes more frequently than every 3 days, particularly for the basal insulin (Gough and Narendran, 2010). This means that intermediate/long-acting insulins are not designed for daily dose changes.

Basal-bolus regimens are usually not suitable for cats, and treatment is limited to the use of the basal insulin preparation. Due to the small size of our feline patients, the percentage of dose adjustment (even when done in small steps such as 0.5 U) is much bigger than what is done in humans. We therefore include a safety margin to avoid hypoglycemia by using a somewhat longer equilibration phase. When the blood glucose targets are reached in a particular cat, the question arises whether remission of the disease can be achieved or not. One may decide to leave the situation as it is and "wait and see." We sometimes consider to "push" it a bit further, and we discuss the pros and cons (chance of remission versus risk of hypoglycemia) with the owner. The decision mainly depends on the glucose nadir. If the nadir is in the lower range of what we regard ideal (e.g., 80 to 90 mg/dL, 4.5 to 5.0 mmol/L), we do not increase the dose. However, if the nadir is 95 to 140 mg/dL (5.3 to 7.8 mmol/L), we suggest increasing the dose by 0.5 U/cat b.i.d. The cat should be supervised closely during the following days, fasting blood glucose concentrations should be measured, and a BGC should be generated within a few days. If hypoglycemia occurs (blood glucose < 70 mg/dL, 3.9 mmol/L), the insulin dose is cut back again to the previous one.

The next challenge is to decide if remission has occurred. *Remission* is defined as the situation in which the clinical signs of diabetes have resolved, serum fructosamine and blood glucose concentration are in the normal range, and insulin therapy can be ceased. In cats in which all blood glucose measurements of a BGC range between 80 and 120 mg/dL (4.5 to 6.7 mmol/L) and serum fructosamine concentration is < 350 µmol/L, we start to reduce the insulin dose in steps of 0.5 U/cat b.i.d. every 5 to 7 days. The owner is advised to monitor the cat closely with regard to reappearance of clinical signs, and a BGC is performed prior to each reduction step. The insulin is reduced until a dose of

0.5 U/cat s.i.d. is reached; if the blood glucose is still normal, insulin administration is terminated.

Close clinical monitoring and regular glucose measurement (e.g., fasting blood glucose twice per week) is recommended to ensure that there is no relapse of the disease. Reduction is done in larger steps than 0.5 U/cat if hypoglycemia is seen. Besides the nadir, the fasting/pre-insulin blood glucose concentration is an important variable. Fasting blood glucose below the target range may be due to insulin overdose, improvement of an insulin-resistant state, overlap of insulin actions, or in case of diabetic remission. In those situations, we use the following as a rough guideline. If the fasting blood glucose is between 140 and 180 mg/dL (7.8 to 10 mmol/L), the cat should be fed, and in case the cat can be monitored throughout the day, the normal insulin dose should be administered; otherwise, the dose should be reduced by 0.5 U/cat. If the fasting blood glucose is between 80 and 140 mg/dL (4.5 to 7.8 mmol/L), the cat should be fed and the insulin dose reduced by 0.5 U/cat. If the fasting blood glucose is < 80 mg/dL (4.5 mmol/L), the cat should be fed and no insulin be given. Another glucose measurement should be performed after 1 to 2 hours. If the blood glucose is still < 80 mg/dL (4.5 mmol/L), no insulin should be given; if the blood glucose is > 80 mg/dL, a small dose ($\frac{1}{3}$ of the normal dose) should be administered. It should be understood that those cats need to be evaluated with regard to the cause of the low fasting blood glucose and to decide on the further insulin dose. It also needs to be understood that the protocol is a guideline and all decisions have to be made on an individual basis. Insulin sensitivity varies between cats and therefore some cats may require a more pronounced dose reduction. Reduction may also be more pronounced in cats receiving high doses of insulin.

Variability of Blood Glucose Curves

In humans, it is well known that blood glucose concentrations can vary markedly from day to day. These variations are associated with different levels of activity, emotional stress, and differences in meal size and composition. However, even when these factors are held constant, day-to-day variability may persist. Causes include variable rate of insulin absorption, variation in length of insulin activity, variation in insulin sensitivity, and remaining β-cell function. There is also substantial variability among BGCs of diabetic cats. When BGCs generated at home were compared with those generated in the hospital within the same week under the same conditions (i.e., same insulin dose and diet, same blood sampling conditions), treatment decisions would have been identical regardless of the BGC used in approximately 60% of cases, whereas in approximately 40% of cases, the decisions would have been different (Casella et al, 2005).

In a follow-up study, BGCs generated on 2 consecutive days at home and on 1 day in the hospital within the same week were compared. In some cats differences between the consecutive home BGCs were also relatively high and often not smaller than between home and clinic BGC. In cats with good glycemic control, variability between BGCs was less than in cats with moderate or poor glycemic control (Alt et al, 2007; see Fig. 7-19, *B*; Fig. 7-22). The bottom line is that single BGCs may not be totally reliable for treatment decisions, even when they are generated at home. However, one of the major advantages of home monitoring is that the veterinarian can ask the owner for more than one BGC before a treatment decision is made. This is of particular importance in cats that are difficult to regulate. Treatment decisions should never be made on the basis of glucose measurements alone, but they should always include the interpretation of the clinical situation.

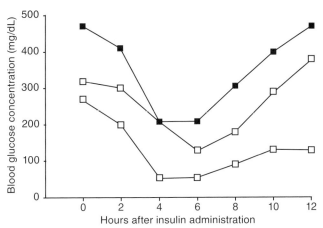

FIGURE 7-22 Variability of blood glucose curves (BGCs) generated at home and in the hospital in a cat (Siamese, castrated male, 14 years old, 6.1 kg) receiving 3.0 U Lente-type insulin (Vetsulin/Caninsulin) b.i.d. The two home-BGCs were generated on 2 consecutive days; the clinic-BGC was generated within the same week. The nadir in one of the home-BGCs was 54 mg/dL, which is too low. The nadir of the other home-BGC was 130 mg/dL, which is acceptable; however, several of the glucose concentrations measured throughout the day were too high. The nadir of the clinic-BGC was too high (210 mg/dL), as were all the other glucose concentrations. The cat was suffering from chronic pancreatitis, which may have been the cause of the variability. At the time the BGCs were generated, the cat had polyuria and polydipsia and reduced appetite, and serum fructosamine concentration was 560 μmol/L. The dose was not changed at this point in time, but had to be amended thereafter a few times (dose increase and decrease). With time, the clinical situation stabilized, blood glucose concentrations became more consistent, and serum fructosamine decreased to 427 μmol/L. In this case, a change to an insulin with a different activity profile (e.g. insulin glargine /Lantus) may have been a good alternative. These BGCs demonstrate that blood glucose concentrations should always be interpreted in conjunction with clinical signs. The advantage of home monitoring is that one or more additional BGCs can be generated before a treatment decision is made. *0,* Time of insulin administration. To convert mg/dL into mmol/L, multiply blood glucose concentration by 0.056.

Continuous Glucose Monitoring

Continuous glucose monitoring (CGM) systems were developed approximately two decades ago, and they have been introduced more recently into veterinary medicine (Davison et al, 2003; Wiedmeyer et al, 2003; Ristic, 2005). Those systems measure glucose concentrations in the subcutaneous interstitial fluid by using transcutaneous sensors. Interstitial fluid is easily accessible with transcutaneous sensors and has rapid equilibration with the blood, resulting in a good correlation of interstitial and blood glucose concentrations. Various different CGM systems are currently available, and as with the PBGM devices, many more are expected to become available in the future. The first systems (and some of the systems used until today) offered only retrospective analysis of the glucose concentrations after disconnecting the sensor and uploading the data, whereas newer generations measure and display the data immediately—real-time continuous glucose monitoring (RT-CGM). Immediate availability of results is a major advantage because it allows direct intervention. We evaluated various aspects of one of those real-time systems (Guardian REAL-Time system) and consider it to be a highly valuable additional monitoring tool. The system uses a small electrode, which is inserted in the subcutaneous tissue by means of a 22 G needle and fixed with tape after clipping and disinfecting a small area of skin.

Thereafter, the sensor is connected to a transmitter that is also fixed to the patient with tape, and that sends data in a wireless fashion to a pager-sized monitor. Data are collected every 10 seconds, and a mean glucose value in the sensor is computed every 5 minutes and seen on the monitor (Figs. 7-23 and 7-24). Wireless transmission of data is only possible if the monitor is within 2 to 3 meters of the patient (e.g., is fixed to the cage). This is the major limiting factor of the device, because it limits the use for home monitoring. Theoretically, one could affix the monitor to the patient; however, the well-being of the cat would most likely be compromised. There are a few other limitations of the system. It requires a 2-hour period for initialization, and no data are provided during this time. The system then has to be calibrated; however, only glucose concentrations between 40 and 400 mg/dL (2.2 to 22.4 mmol/L) can be used for calibration. If the glucose is higher or lower, calibration has to be postponed until the blood glucose concentration is within the working range. Changes of blood glucose are followed by changes in interstitial blood glucose with a delay of approximately 11 minutes in cats (Moretti et al, 2010). Therefore, calibration should not be performed during times when blood glucose changes rapidly. Further calibration is needed 6 hours after initial calibration and then every 12 hours thereafter, which requires capillary or venous blood sampling. The sensor, which is quite expensive, has a limited sensor life; however, a complete restart of the system after the official lifespan of 72 hours allows another 72 hours of monitoring. Recently, a new sensor generation was marketed (Enlite Sensor, used with a different transmitter), which has a lifespan of 144 hours. The monitor displays glucose concentrations between 40 and 400 mg/dL (2.2. to 22.4 mmol/L); concentrations outside this range are correctly recorded but have to be downloaded to be seen.

Cats usually tolerate sensor placement and the bandage well, and usually no adverse skin reactions occur. Accuracy of measurements is an important issue, and none of the systems provides 100% accuracy. With the Guardian REAL-Time system, underestimation of blood glucose is more frequent than overestimation. Fig. 7-25 shows scatterplots of the differences between measurements with the CGM system and the PBGM device, AlphaTRAK, derived from 448 samples from diabetic (n = 39) and healthy cats (n = 5). Almost all measurements in the normo- and hyperglycemic range are clinically accurate (i.e., CGM system readings do not lead to a treatment error). In the hypoglycemic range, CGM system measurements deviate to a slightly larger extent from the reference measurement (Moretti et al, 2010). When simultaneous BGCs were generated with the Guardian REAL-Time system and the AlphaTRAK and analyzed in a blinded fashion by three internal medicine specialists, treatment decisions did not differ, supporting adequate accuracy for clinical use (Dietiker-Moretti et al, 2011). Readings differ depending on the site of the sensor placement. In cats, readings from the neck area have been shown to be more accurate than those from the lateral chest area or the knee fold. Additionally, initial calibration is more often successful when the neck is used. Technical problems include failure to successfully calibrate after the initialization period, discontinuation of recordings at some time during the long-term measurement (usually due to calibration errors) and loss of proper placement of the sensor underneath the skin (Hafner et al, 2013).

Currently, our main indication for the use of CGM system is blood glucose monitoring in diabetic cats that are hospitalized for several days (e.g., in case of DKA). The costs of the sensor and the 2-hour initialization period are major limitations for generation of BGCs on a routine basis. The great potential of those systems, however, is the possibility to continuously record blood glucose at home and thereby giving valuable information on the glycemic

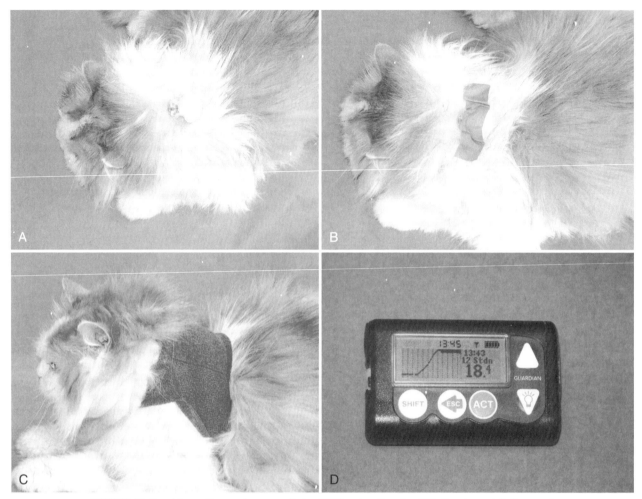

FIGURE 7-23 Use of the continuous glucose monitoring (CGM) system Guardian REAL-Time in a cat. **A,** Placement of the sensor in the subcutaneous neck area; the sensor is connected to the transmitter *(white)*. **B** and **C,** Attachment with tape and bandage. **D,** Glucose concentrations are transmitted wirelessly to the monitor and displayed in real time. Here, the glucose given is 18.4 mmol/L (331 mg/dL).

situation during the night. With the current Guardian REAL-Time device, home monitoring is difficult, because the monitor has to be within 2 to 3 meters away from the patient. Various other wireless CGM systems also have a limited transmission range. The iPro system uses the same electrochemical sensor; however, the wireless transmitter used with the Guardian REAL-Time system is replaced by a recording device for data storage. Data are not recorded real-time but have to be downloaded. The device might be suitable for home monitoring, but it has not yet been evaluated in cats or dogs (Surman and Fleeman, 2013).

Insulin Therapy During Surgery

The approach to managing diabetic dogs and cats is similar and is discussed in Chapter 6 (see Insulin Therapy During Surgery).

 COMPLICATIONS OF INSULIN THERAPY

Although the majority of diabetic cats can be adequately stabilized during the first 3 months of therapy, problems may occur any time during management. They usually fall within one of the following categories: stress hyperglycemia, hypoglycemia, technical errors, insulin underdose, insulin overdose with glucose counterregulation (Somogyi effect), short duration of insulin effect, prolonged

duration of insulin effect, inadequate absorption of insulin, circulating insulin antibodies, fluctuating insulin requirements, and concurrent diseases causing insulin resistance.

Recurrence or persistence of clinical signs is a common problem requiring a logical and stepwise approach. The first step is to confirm that the cat indeed is poorly regulated (i.e., has clinical signs of diabetes such as polyuria, polydipsia, polyphagia, progressive weight loss, lethargy and decreased interaction with family members, lack of grooming behavior, and poor hair coat). High blood glucose levels may have been incorrectly interpreted to be the result of poor glycemic control when, in fact, they were stress induced. Fructosamine concentration is also not always a reliable parameter and is sometimes moderately or even markedly increased, although the cat is clinically well. Box 7-6 gives a stepwise approach to the work-up. Complications of insulin therapy are similar for diabetic dogs and cats; see Chapter 6 for a more comprehensive discussion.

Stress Hyperglycemia

Cats are prone to stress hyperglycemia, which develops as a result of an increase in catecholamines or may be due to increased gluconeogenesis stimulated by lactate release in struggling cats (Rand et al, 2002). Stress-induced hyperglycemia not only renders

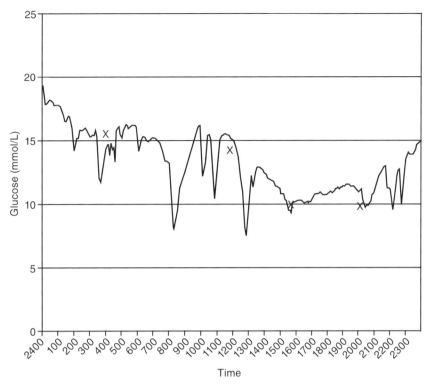

FIGURE 7-24 Blood glucose curve (BGC) over 24 hours generated by the continuous monitoring system Guardian REAL-time in a newly diagnosed diabetic cat after the start of insulin therapy. The curve is generated by the continuous glucose monitoring (CGM) system; X marks the glucose concentrations measured by the AlphaTRAK. To convert mmol/L to mg/dL, multiply by 18.

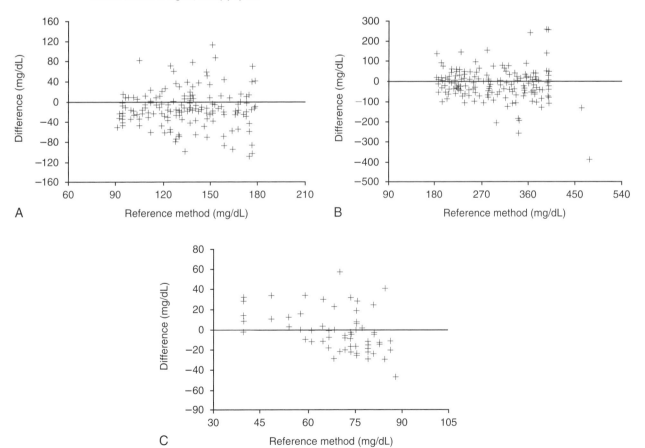

FIGURE 7-25 Scatterplots of the differences between blood glucose concentrations obtained by the use of the Guardian REAL-Time continuous glucose monitoring (CGM) system versus concentration obtained with the reference portable blood glucose monitoring (PBGM) meter AlphaTRAK at **(A)** normal, **(B)** high, and **(C)** low glucose concentrations in cats. To convert from mg/dL to mmol/L, multiply by 0.056. (From Moretti S, et al.: Evaluation of a novel real-time continuous glucose-monitoring system for use in cats, *J Vet Intern Med* 24:120, 2010 [with permission].)

BOX 7-6   Stepwise Work-Up in Diabetic Cats with Persistence or Recurrence of Clinical Signs

Step 1
- Confirm that the cat has clinical signs of diabetes.
- Determine whether work-up and previous treatment has been done according to the protocol (see Box 7-3).

Step 2
- Determine whether insulin used by owner is outdated, has been diluted, frozen, or heated.
- Determine whether appropriate syringes are being used (U 40/mL vs. U 100/mL).
- Assess owner's method of mixing, drawing up the correct dose, and injecting insulin.
- Review diet regimen.
  These points in problem-solving are often overlooked. However, technical errors are a frequent cause of difficulty in regulating a diabetic pet.

Step 3
- Increase insulin dose every 5 to 7 days until the cat receives a dose of approximately 1.0 U/kg twice daily (intermediate/long-acting insulin).

Step 4
- Generate blood glucose curves (BGCs) to determine whether there is the Somogyi effect or short duration of insulin effect. Blood glucose should be measured at home every 1 to 2 hours for at least 12 hours.

Step 5
- If no problem has been identified thus far, carry-out work-up for diseases causing insulin resistance. In principle, any other concurrent disease (e.g., inflammatory, infectious, or neoplastic) may cause insulin resistance. The most relevant problems are pancreatitis, pancreatic neoplasia, hyperadrenocorticism, hypersomatotropism (acromegaly), infections (e.g., of oral cavity or urinary tract), chronic renal failure, and obesity.
- As a last resort, poor absorption of insulin and circulating insulin antibodies should be considered. The relevance of the latter is controversial. Although insulin antibodies are produced (in particular when insulin of a different species is used), it is not yet clear to what extent they interfere with the action of the injected insulin. At this stage of the work-up, however, a switch to insulin of a different species is indicated.

---

diagnosis of diabetes difficult but also complicates the accurate evaluation of blood glucose concentrations measured during long-term management. Increases in blood glucose can range from mild to severe. Blood glucose levels may remain extremely elevated throughout the day despite insulin therapy or may start in an acceptable range and then steadily increase. Blood sampling can be extremely stressful for cats and is, therefore, a common cause of stress hyperglycemia. Failure to recognize the effect of stress on the blood glucose concentrations may lead to the erroneous assumption that the diabetic cat is poorly controlled. If insulin therapy is adjusted by increasing the dose, hypoglycemia or the Somogyi effect may result.

Stress hyperglycemia should be suspected, if there is a disparity between the assessment of glycemic control based on the owner's observations, body weight, results of physical examination, and the results of BGCs. Evaluation of serum fructosamine can provide additional valuable information, because the parameter is not influenced by a short-term increase of blood glucose. A fructosamine concentration within an acceptable range in a cat with no or little clinical signs is consistent with adequate glycemic control. If such a cat has highly elevated blood glucose concentrations, they are most likely stress-induced. In those cats, treatment decisions cannot be based on blood glucose levels. In our hospital, blood glucose is usually obtained from the pinna (as described earlier for home monitoring) by an experienced technician. The technique is usually well tolerated, and it is our impression that stress hyperglycemia is less of a problem with this technique. Stress hyperglycemia may also occur in the home environment if the owner has difficulty performing the procedure. However, in most cases, home monitoring is a good alternative to generation of BGCs in the hospital. See Establishing a Diagnosis of Diabetes Mellitus for more details on stress hyperglycemia.

Hypoglycemia

Hypoglycemia is the most serious complication of insulin therapy. It is the major factor that prevents achievement of near normoglycemia in diabetic patients with more tight glycemic control (i.e., increase of insulin dose), the risk of hypoglycemia increases. In humans, it is well established that the risk of hypoglycemia increases in proportion to the reduction of glycated hemoglobin. The positive effect of tight glycemic control is counterbalanced by fear and anxiety of hypoglycemia, reduction in quality-of-life, reduced productivity, and increased healthcare costs (Bilous and Donnelly, 2010; Fidler et al, 2011). Similarly, cat owners worry about hypoglycemia, and a survey identified fear of hypoglycemia as one of the main factors having a negative impact on the quality of the owner's life (Niessen et al, 2010). In a physiological state, hypoglycemia is prevented by inhibition of insulin secretion from the β-cells that occurs when the blood glucose declines in the postabsorptive phase. If the glucose level falls just below the normal range, secretion of counterregulatory hormones (in particular glucagon and epinephrine) is triggered. In humans, the threshold for the latter is a blood glucose concentration between 65 to 70 mg/dL (3.6 to 3.9 mmol/L). If these defenses fail to abort an episode of developing hypoglycemia, lower blood glucose levels lead to a more intense sympatho-adrenal response that causes neurogenic symptoms. Those symptoms cause awareness of hypoglycemia that prompts the behavioral defense mechanism of carbohydrate ingestion. In humans with diabetes, all of those defense mechanisms are typically compromised, a phenomenon known as *hypoglycemia unawareness* or *hypoglycemia-associated autonomic failure* (Cryer, 2010; 2013). An impaired counterregulatory response has also been documented in diabetic dogs (see Insulin Overdosing and Glucose Counterregulation [Somogyi Response]). If this phenomenon exists in diabetic cats, it has not yet been investigated. However, quite a substantial percentage of diabetic cats do not seem to sense hunger even if the blood glucose concentration decreases to quite low levels (e.g., < 50 mg/dL, 2.8 mmol/L); therefore, one should bear the possibility of failing defense mechanisms in mind. Hypoglycemia in diabetic cats is caused by an absolute or relative insulin excess. It results from insulin overdose, sudden increase in insulin sensitivity due to cure or improvement of concurrent disorders, diabetic remission that goes unnoticed, long duration of insulin action resulting in excessive overlap (mainly with PZI or insulin glargine, insulin detemir), or lack of food intake. Hypoglycemia may be a recurrent problem, most often seen in cats with concurrent disease in which phases of insulin sensitivity and insulin resistance alternate. Diabetic cats with chronic renal failure are notoriously difficult to regulate because insulin resistance due to uremic toxins coexists with reduced insulin clearance by the kidneys.

Hypoglycemia may be asymptomatic (biochemical) or symptomatic (clinical). There is no well-defined cutoff of blood glucose below which hypoglycemia will become symptomatic. The lower the blood glucose and the more rapid the glucose level drops, the more likely clinical signs will be apparent. In cats, clinical hypoglycemia is more difficult to identify than in dogs. Hypoglycemic cats oftentimes just become quiet, withdraw from family life, and hide away. More obvious signs include restlessness, aggression, hunger, lethargy, weakness, salivation, muscle twitching, ataxia, seizures, and coma. Severe hypoglycemia may be fatal. Owners should be advised to treat symptomatic hypoglycemia depending on its severity either by offering food or administration of any of the various oral glucose gels (over-the-counter medication) or sugar water. Our owners do not inject glucagon in case of suspected hypoglycemia, although this option may be worth exploring (Niessen, 2012). If signs do not resolve immediately, the cat should be brought to the hospital and treatment performed as described in Chapter 9. Owners should also be advised to measure the blood glucose concentration in any of those situations. Documentation by the owner that hypoglycemia was present is very helpful for the veterinarian, because it may have resolved when the cat arrives in the hospital.

We consider blood glucose concentrations < 70 mg/dL (3.9 mmol/L) as too low, although clinical signs usually only occur when glucose levels are lower than 50 to 60 mg/dL (2.8 to 3.4 mmol/L). In cats showing symptomatic hypoglycemia, insulin administration should be discontinued until the blood glucose levels are > 180 mg/dL (10 mmol/L). Thereafter, insulin should be restarted with a dose reduced by approximately 50% per injection. In the case of asymptomatic hypoglycemia (e.g., hypoglycemia found by chance), the calculation of the dose reduction depends on the previous dose. If the cat was on a low to moderate insulin dose (0.5 to 3.0 U/cat b.i.d.), the dose should be reduced by 0.5 to 1.0 U/cat b.i.d.; if the cat was on a higher dose, reduction should be somewhat arbitrarily between 25% to 50%. Further monitoring and glucose measurements are mandatory to ensure that there are no further episodes of hypoglycemia and for the fine-tuning of the insulin dose. Some cats only need an insulin dose as low as 0.5 U/cat s.i.d.

Insulin Overdose and Glucose Counterregulation (Somogyi Effect)

The Somogyi effect is defined as rebound hyperglycemia due to hypersecretion of counter-regulatory hormones (mainly epinephrine, glucagon) during hypoglycemia, induced by a (slight) overdose of insulin. The phenomenon received its name after Michael Somogyi, a Hungarian biochemist. He postulated in 1959 that nocturnal hypoglycemia provokes rebound hyperglycemia and fasting hyperglycemia on the following morning in diabetic humans (Somogyi, 1959). In cats, the first description of the phenomenon was published in 1986 (McMillan and Feldman, 1986). Thereafter not much work on the Somogyi effect has been done, although it is frequently mentioned as an important cause of poor glycemic control. For the effect to occur, blood glucose levels must decrease to less than 65 mg/dL (3.6 mmol/L); however, it may also occur when the blood glucose concentration decreases rapidly regardless of the nadir (Fig. 7-26). Clinical signs of hyperglycemia are obvious, whereas signs of hypoglycemia often go unnoticed. Owners may report that days of good glycemic control are followed by several days of poor control, which should raise the suspicion of the Somogyi effect. Diagnosis requires the documentation of hypoglycemia or a very rapid drop in blood glucose concentration followed by hyperglycemia (blood glucose > 300 mg/dL, 17 mmol/L) within a 12-hour period.

The hyperglycemic period can last 24 to 72 hours; the diagnosis may therefore be missed with a single BGC and accordingly, the incorrect assumption is made that the insulin dose is too low. Rebound hyperglycemia and the Somogyi effect should always be considered as a differential diagnosis when BGCs show persistently elevated blood glucose levels. To identify the problem, a series of BGCs is often needed, which may be best performed by home monitoring. If the Somogyi effect is documented or is assumed to be present, the insulin dose should be reduced—the degree of which is somewhat arbitrarily (0.5 to 1.0 U/cat b.i.d. in cats on a low to moderate dose, approximately 25% in cats on a higher dose of insulin). If no change is seen, a further slight dose reduction may be pursued. If clinical signs worsen, the approach was incorrect. Of note, classic glucose changes affiliated with this problem are not as apparent today as they were two to three decades ago, and this may reflect the changes in type of insulin used. We have seen a substantial number of cats in which the Somogyi effect was assumed to be the cause of the problem, but the cats were in fact suffering from a short duration of insulin effect. Lente-type insulins in particular may exert a pronounced peak with a quite fast decline in blood glucose concentration, but the effect is short lasting. In the latter situation, the shape of the BGC resembles a BGC showing the Somogyi effect. Close monitoring and generation of BGCs after the change of the insulin dose is therefore important. See the discussion on the Somogyi effect in Chapter 6 and the discussion on counterregulation in response to hypoglycemia in Chapter 9.

Technical Problems

Errors in injecting and handling insulin are frequent causes of poor glycemic control and include failure to mix the insulin correctly (if it is a suspension such as Vetsulin/Caninsulin or ProZinc), diluting, freezing or heating, use of outdated insulin, drawing up air instead of insulin, inappropriate insulin dose and timing, poor injection technique, and use of the wrong syringe size (U-40 mL vs. U-100/mL—a frequent error). Careful history taking, asking the owners to bring their own insulin and syringes, and watching the owner during the procedure will usually unravel the problem.

Insulin Underdose

Most cats are well regulated with insulin doses between 0.5 and 3.0 U b.i.d. (usually with ≤ 1 U/kg b.i.d.). Some diabetic cats may need insulin doses > 1.0 U/kg b.i.d.; however, this is oftentimes only temporarily during the initial phases of therapy and requirement decreases thereafter, which is most likely due to improvement of glucose toxicity. In general, insulin underdose should be considered if the insulin dose is considerably less than 1.0 U/kg b.i.d., and the dose should be increased. As mentioned earlier, we increase the insulin dose in steps of 0.5 U/cat b.i.d. every 5 to 7 days, and a BGC is generated before each step. The higher the insulin requirement, the more likely a concurrent disease is present, which causes insulin resistance. Further work-up should be pursued when the dose requirement is > 1.0 U/kg b.i.d.

Insulin underdose should always be considered if the cat receives the insulin only once daily. Duration of effect is usually never as long as 24 hours, independent of the type of insulin used, leaving the hepatic glucose production unopposed for a long time. In those cats, administration should be changed from s.i.d. to b.i.d., starting with a dose as recommended for the initial treatment (see Box 7-3).

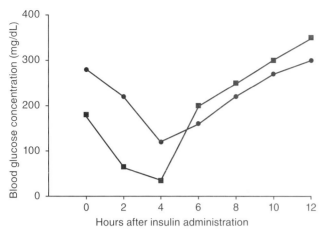

FIGURE 7-26 Blood glucose curve (BGC) 1 *(squares):* Suspected Somogyi effect in a diabetic cat (Domestic Short-Hair [DSH], spayed female, 12 years old, 5.9 kg) receiving 4.5 U/cat insulin glargine (Lantus) b.i.d. The blood glucose dropped to a nadir of 46 mg/dL within 4 hours of insulin administration, followed by an increase to 350 mg/dL within 8 hours. The effect did not reappear after reduction of the insulin dose to 3.5 U/cat b.i.d. BGC 2 *(dots):* Short duration of insulin effect in a diabetic cat (DSH, castrated male, 12 years old, 4.3 kg) receiving 1 U/cat Lente-type insulin (Vetsulin/Caninsulin) b.i.d. Short duration of effect is quite common in cats using this type of insulin. The change to another type of insulin with longer duration of action (e.g., insulin glargine) should be considered. Please note that BGCs displaying short duration of effect or the Somogyi effect may look quite similar. It is important to reevaluate the patient soon after amendment of treatment (e.g., dose reduction, change to another type of insulin) to make sure that the decision was correct. *0,* Time of insulin administration. To convert mg/dL into mmol/L, multiply blood glucose concentration by 0.056.

Short Duration of Insulin Effect

A short duration of insulin effect is a common cause of difficult to regulate diabetes in cats. It is almost always seen if the insulin is given once daily; however, it is also frequently encountered when given twice daily. NPH insulin preparations are notorious for their short duration of effect, and their use in cats is not recommended. However, short duration is also quite common in cats treated with Lente-type insulin (Vetsulin/Caninsulin). PZI insulin (ProZinc) and the long-acting insulin analogues (insulin glargine/Lantus, insulin detemir/Levemir) have longer duration of action, although twice daily administration is needed in the vast majority of cases (see also Long-Acting Insulin Analogues and Table 7-4). If duration of action is less than 8 to 10 hours, the cat usually has signs of diabetes. Diagnosis of duration of action requires generation of one or several BGCs, which is best done by home monitoring. Stress and reduced food intake in the hospital have a major impact on glucose values, rendering determination of duration of action nearly impossible. Duration of action should be assessed only if the blood glucose nadir is within the target range (80 to 140 mg/dL, 4.5 to 7.8 mmol/L), and should ideally be 10 to 12 hours. Diagnosis of short duration of action is confirmed by demonstrating blood glucose concentrations more than 180 to 270 mg/dL (10 to 15 mmol/L) within less than 10 hours of the insulin injection (see Fig. 7-26). Single glucose measurements (e.g., in the morning) are unsuitable and may lead to the erroneous assumption of insulin underdose. Fructosamine levels are usually moderately to severely increased. Treatment consists of changing to an insulin preparation with a longer duration of effect. For instance, if the cat is treated with Lente-type insulin (Vetsulin/Caninsulin), switching to PZI (ProZinc) or insulin glargine (Lantus) may solve

the problem; if the cat is on insulin glargine and duration is too short, a change to PZI (ProZinc) or insulin detemir (Levemir) should be considered. Lente-type insulin is more potent than PZI and the long-acting insulin analogues, and therefore the change should be accompanied by a slight dose reduction (0.5 to 1.0 U/cat b.i.d.).

Prolonged Duration of Insulin Effect

Prolonged duration of insulin effect is a rather uncommon problem in diabetic cats. It is usually not seen with NPH or Lente-type insulin (Vetsulin/Caninsulin). It may, however, occur occasionally in cats treated with twice daily application of PZI, insulin glargine, or detemir. If duration of effect is longer than 12 hours, an overlap in insulin action results, which eventually leads to the Somogyi effect or to overt hypoglycemia. Indications for a prolonged duration of effect are a glucose nadir occurring 10 or more hours after insulin administration and constantly decreasing glucose concentrations beyond the time of the next insulin administration. An extended BGC (glucose measurements every 2 hours for 14 to 18 hours) will usually unravel the problem. In some cats, a slight dose reduction can counterbalance the prolonged effect. If this is unsuccessful or results in worsening of glycemic control, one should switch to an insulin preparation with shorter duration of effect. In exceptional cases, switching from twice daily to once daily administration is possible; however, duration of effect should be at least 20 hours.

Impaired Absorption of Insulin

Slow absorption was a frequent problem with Ultralente insulin, which is no longer available. The problem is not considered to be important with the insulin preparations used today.

However, insulin absorption is influenced by various factors, including hydration status, local blood flow in the area where the insulin is injected, obesity, size of the insulin dose, exercise, and environmental temperature. The unpredictability of insulin absorption was the stimulus for development of the new generation of insulins, the insulin analogues. Insulin analogues were designed for humans mainly to provide more consistent absorption kinetics. The currently available insulin analogues are still not perfect, and new analogues are under development. Repeated injection of insulin at the same location are known to result in local hypertrophy of adipose tissue in humans (called *lipohypertrophy*) (Gough and Narendran, 2010). The same may be true for cats and therefore, the injection sites should be rotated. However, as blood flow differs, we advise that the body region should be held constant (e.g., lateral thoracic wall).

Binding of Insulin by Insulin Antibodies

Because the amino acid sequence of feline insulin differs to a varying extent from human, porcine, and bovine insulin (see Table 7-1), it is logical to assume that treatment will result in the production of anti-insulin antibodies. In principle, those antibodies are capable of binding circulating insulin and reducing its free concentration. If the antibody-insulin complex is subsequently removed by the reticuloendothelial system, the requirement for exogenous insulin may be extremely high. Alternatively, insulin may dissociate from the complex in an unpredictable manner, resulting in erratic concentrations of free insulin. Humans with diabetes produce anti-insulin antibodies even if they are treated with human insulin. According to a comprehensive review, there is little proof that the development of insulin antibodies in humans affects glycemic control, insulin dose requirement, or the incidence of hypoglycemia, although the matter is somewhat controversial (Fineberg et al, 2007).

The relevance of anti-insulin antibodies in the management of diabetic cats has not been extensively investigated. Two studies identified antibodies in 14% and 37% of cats treated with recombinant human, beef, and beef/pork insulins. There was no correlation between glycemic control and the presence or absence of antibodies (Harb-Hauser et al, 1998; Hoenig et al, 2000a). Studies evaluating potential antibody production during therapy with the long-acting insulin analogues have not yet been performed in cats. The currently available data allow the assumption that problems in regulating diabetic cats are only rarely (if at all) due to anti-insulin antibodies. We consider the possibility that anti-insulin antibodies are the reason for the difficulty to regulate diabetes only as a last resort (i.e., we switch to an insulin preparation of a different species only after excluding the other causes of poor control).

Allergic Reaction to Insulin

Allergic reactions to insulin have not been documented in the cat. See Allergic Reaction to Insulin in Chapter 6.

Concurrent Disorders Causing Insulin Resistance and Drug-Induced Diabetes

Most diabetic cats can be regulated with insulin doses (intermediate-/long-acting insulin) between 0.5 and 3.0 U b.i.d. (usually with doses ≤ 1.0 U/kg b.i.d.). In cats with insulin requirements above this "threshold," concurrent disorders should be suspected provided that the problems discussed earlier (i.e., technical problems, short duration of effect) have been excluded. No insulin dose clearly defines insulin resistance. Insulin resistance should be suspected when glycemic control is poor despite insulin doses of more than 1.0 U/kg b.i.d., high doses (> 1.5 U/kg) are required to maintain blood glucose less than 270 mg/dL (15 mmol/L), and when glycemic control is erratic and insulin requirements constantly change. It is important to note that severity of insulin resistance can vary widely. Resistance can be mild and easily counterbalanced by some increase in insulin dose; however, it can also be severe requiring very high insulin doses or can fluctuate with time. See Concurrent Disorders Causing Insulin Resistance in Chapter 6 for more details on mechanism of insulin resistance and on insulin dose adjustment. Any inflammatory, infectious, neoplastic, and endocrine disorder can cause insulin resistance, as well as obesity and administration of insulin-antagonistic drugs. In cats, insulin resistance is most commonly caused by severe obesity, chronic renal failure, chronic pancreatitis, stomatitis/oral infections, hyperadrenocorticism, and hypersomatotropism (acromegaly). The latter two diseases are the ones with the potential of the most severe insulin resistance. Some of the causes will be obvious after obtaining a detailed history (e.g., administration of progestagens or glucocorticoids) and performing a thorough physical examination (obesity, stomatitis/oral infection). If history and physical examination are fruitless, CBC, serum biochemical panel, lipase/fPLI serum T_4 concentration, measurement of insulin-like growth factor-1 (IGF-1), urinalysis and urine culture, and abdominal ultrasonography should be the next steps. Additional tests (e.g., biopsy of a mass or organ abnormality, low-dose dexamethasone test) may be required. Insulin resistance may, at least in

part, be reversible. Therefore, the administration of progestagens or glucocorticoids should be ceased. In case of obesity, a weight-reduction program should be instituted, and all treatable diseases should be managed as well as possible. Close monitoring is mandatory, because the insulin requirement may decrease substantially. With some disorders, such as chronic renal failure and chronic pancreatitis, insulin resistance persists or continues to fluctuate, and glycemic control usually remains challenging. In those cases, teaching the owner about the latter will help to avoid frustration. The glucose targets should be set less tight, and the insulin dose chosen with the aim of avoiding hypoglycemia, very severe hyperglycemia, and DKA. Home monitoring of blood glucose is helpful to amend the insulin dose during acute flares or worsening of the disease.

Obesity

See Obesity under Dietary Management, and also see Obesity, Gender, and Other Risk Factors.

Chronic Pancreatitis

Acute flares of chronic pancreatitis may need in-hospital treatment including IV fluid therapy (with potassium supplementation), plasma transfusions, pain management, nutritional support (tube feeding), antiemetic, and antibiotic therapy. Long-term treatment of chronic pancreatitis is difficult, and a complete cure is often not possible. Suggested measures include the use of appetite stimulators (mirtazapine, cyproheptadine), cobalamin supplementation (if deficient), and supplementation with antioxidants (S-adenosyl-methionine [SAMe], vitamin C, vitamin E, and/or selenium). In humans with acute pancreatitis, the use of glucocorticoids is currently under investigation. There are anecdotal reports on clinical improvement when used in cats with chronic or chronic relapsing pancreatitis (Armstrong and Williams, 2012). However, there are currently no criteria that would help the clinician to decide which cat would potentially benefit from a short-term steroid administration and in which cases it would cause harm.

Chronic Kidney Disease

See Concurrent Disorders Causing Insulin Resistance in Chapter 6.

Hyperthyroidism

See Serum Thyroxine Concentration.

Exogenous Glucocorticoids and Progestins

Glucocorticoids were named for their hyperglycemic effects, and they have the potential to exert strong diabetogenic properties. They may induce hyperglycemia in previously normoglycemic patients as well as worsen glycemic control in patients already known to have diabetes mellitus. Glucocorticoids induce or worsen diabetes mellitus by increasing insulin resistance in peripheral tissues (muscle, fat) and by increasing hepatic glucose production. Additionally, they may inhibit insulin release from the β-cells (Delaunay et al, 1997; Gittoes et al, 2010; Lowe et al, 2009). In humans, overt diabetes or impaired glucose tolerance is seen in 14% to 28% of individuals receiving long-term glucocorticoids. Humans who are not able to increase their insulin secretion to counterbalance the effects of the glucocorticoid (i.e., have an intrinsically low insulin secretion capacity) are particularly susceptible (Wajngot et al, 1992; Gittoes et al, 2010). In cats, the prevalence of overt diabetes during glucocorticoid therapy has not yet been systematically evaluated. Steroid diabetes can occur after oral or parenteral as well as after topical administration of any of the currently available glucocorticoids. Glucocorticoid sensitivity varies between individual cats and therefore dose, duration, and frequency of application that will ultimately lead to hyperglycemia, cannot be predicted. Experimental studies have shown that abnormalities may already become apparent after short-term therapy. Administration of 2 mg/kg prednisolone s.i.d. for 8 days resulted in reduced glucose tolerance after an IV glucose load in all six cats, and three of the six developed hyperglycemia (Middleton and Watson, 1985). It has been suggested that dexamethasone has greater diabetogenic effects than equipotent doses of prednisolone (Lowe et al, 2008; 2009). Steroid diabetes often goes into remission, provided that the glucocorticoid application is ceased immediately and insulin treatment is initiated. Careful monitoring of blood glucose levels is important. After the effect of the glucocorticoid on insulin sensitivity wears off, the insulin requirement decreases, resulting in the need to also decrease the insulin dose. Remission may fail to appear if treatment is inadequate or if the cat has substantial islet pathology. If glucocorticoid therapy cannot be terminated and no alternative drug can be used, the insulin dose has to be adjusted on the severity of the insulin resistance. In those cases, glycemic control oftentimes remains difficult.

Progestins are known to exert glucocorticoid activity, and they have similar effects to glucocorticoids on insulin sensitivity. Treatment with progestins (e.g., megestrol acetate) may therefore also result in glucose intolerance or overt diabetes (Peterson, 1987; Middleton and Watson, 1985; Middeleton et al, 1987). Other glucocorticoid-like side effects including skin atrophy, alopecia, and skin lacerations may be seen as well. Similar to glucocorticoids, it is not possible to predict which cat will develop diabetes, and therefore, regular reevaluations are mandatory. Remission of diabetes may occur after discontinuation of progestin administration and the initiation of insulin therapy.

Hypersomatotropism (Acromegaly)

Hypersomatotropism is a disease that is almost always associated with diabetes mellitus. It has the potential to cause very severe insulin resistance and requirements of insulin doses more than 2 U/kg b.i.d. are no exception. Insulin resistance, however, can also be quite mild, in particular in the initial phases of the disease. Hypersomatotropism in cats is caused by a GH-producing tumor (usually an adenoma) in the pars distalis of the pituitary gland. GH has catabolic and anabolic effects; the latter are in part mediated by IGF-1. The catabolic effects are mainly due to insulin antagonism and are the reason for the diabetes mellitus. The anabolic effects include proliferation of bone, cartilage, soft tissue, and organs resulting in a large body size, broad head and large paws, weight gain, prognathia inferior, respiratory difficulties because of thickening of pharyngeal tissues, degenerative arthropathy, and organomegaly with potential organ dysfunction. Growth of the tumor may lead to signs of a central nervous system (CNS) disease. Of note, clinical signs may also be very subtle or even absent, and the disease may therefore be overlooked. Acromegaly has long been considered a rare disorder. However, it was recently suggested that acromegaly occurs more frequently than previously thought and is most likely underdiagnosed (Niessen et al, 2007). Because the availability of a validated GH assay for cats is a problem, diagnosis is usually based on the finding of a high IGF-1 concentration. A few important points should be kept in mind. First, circulating IGF-1 is bound to proteins, which must be removed before measurement. Not all methods are equally effective, and intra-assay inference of binding proteins may lead to falsely high IGF-1 levels (Tschuor et al, 2012). Therefore, only assays validated for the cat should be used. Second, IGF-1 concentrations are often low in newly diagnosed diabetic cats and increase markedly after initiating insulin therapy. Low IGF-1 levels have also been seen initially in untreated diabetic cats with acromegaly (Reusch et al, 2006b). In our hospital, IGF-1 is measured 6 to 8 weeks after initiating insulin therapy. Because IGF-1 measurements are not 100% reliable, the final diagnosis requires documentation of a pituitary mass by CT or magnetic resonance imaging (MRI) scan. See Chapter 2 for more details.

Hyperadrenocorticism

Hyperadrenocorticism is considered to be a rare disease and is associated with diabetes mellitus in approximately 80% of cats. Pituitary-dependent disease is present in 75% to 80%, and 20% to 25% suffer from a cortisol-secreting adrenocortical tumor. In rare circumstances, adrenocortical tumors secrete steroid hormones other than cortisol. Progesterone-producing tumors result in clinical signs that are identical to those caused by hypercortisolism, and they may also be associated with diabetes mellitus (Boord and Griffin, 1999; Rossmeisl et al, 2000; Quante et al, 2009). In addition to polyuria/polydipsia (pu/pd) and weight loss, which are usually due to concurrent diabetes mellitus, typical clinical signs are abdominal enlargement, an unkempt seborrheic hair coat, thinning of the hair coat, failure of hair to regrow or alopecia, and muscle weakness. Severe cases may have thin fragile skin that tears easily. Cats with large pituitary masses may have CNS disturbances. However, clinical signs may also be mild, and hyperadrenocorticism is often not suspected until it becomes evident that the diabetes is difficult to regulate. The dexamethasone suppression test is the preferred screening test. Whether poorly-regulated diabetics have hyperactivity of the hypothalamus-pituitary-adrenal gland axis that leads to false positive test results is controversial. We recently investigated the dexamethasone test in a group of diabetic cats 6 weeks after initiating insulin therapy. In 20 of 22 cats, the cortisol concentration was completely suppressed at 4 and 8 hours after the application of 0.1 mg/kg dexamethasone IV. The results did not differ between cats with good glycemic control and those with moderate to poor control. In two cats, the test was abnormal and hyperadrenocorticism was confirmed by histopathology (Kley et al, 2007). Based on our results, the dexamethasone test appears to be a suitable part of the diagnostic work-up in diabetic cats suspected of having hyperadrenocorticism. In our hospital, we perform testing for hyperadrenocorticism in cats in which glycemic control remains difficult after several weeks of therapy and other problems have been excluded. Usually, the test is carried out 6 to 8 weeks after initiating insulin therapy. Further details on feline hyperadrenocorticism can be found in Chapter 11.

Fluctuating Insulin Requirements (Glycemic Instability)

One of the most frustrating problems encountered with insulin therapy is the inability to maintain glycemic control. For instance, previously well-regulated cats on a stable dose of insulin suddenly develop clinical signs of diabetes and severe hyperglycemia; an increase in insulin dose may solve the problem for a short time, after which further dose amendments (either increase or decrease) are required. Other cats suffer from recurrent flares of DKA, despite being closely monitored, and have to be brought to the hospital as an emergency frequently. Another subset of diabetic cats suffers from frequent episodes of hypoglycemia that alternate with phases of adequate control or hyperglycemia. In humans, the same problems occur and the term *brittle diabetes* is used for individuals with glycemic instability sufficient to disrupt the patient's lifestyle. Causes of "brittleness" are numerous and include failure to follow treatment regimen correctly, inappropriate lifestyle and dietary management, recurrent infections, gastrointestinal diseases, chronic pancreatitis, concurrent endocrinopathies or administration of diabetogenic drugs, impaired counterregulatory hormone secretion, delayed gastric emptying due to autonomic neuropathy, genetic defects in or beyond the insulin receptor, and psychiatric and psychological problems. In some patients, no obvious cause is found, which is then called *idiopathic brittle diabetes* (Voulgari et al, 2012). Most of those causes are also known to cause difficulties regulating diabetes in cats and have already been discussed. Most commonly, glycemic instability in cats is due to acute flares of chronic pancreatitis or the development of another concurrent disease (infections, neoplasia, chronic renal disease), severity of which can range from mild (and may be overlooked) to severe. Any disease may increase insulin resistance, and if insulin dose is not adequately increased, signs of diabetes reoccur and DKA may develop. After improvement or resolution of the concurrent disease, insulin resistance decreases, which may result in hypoglycemia if the insulin dose is not amended. Cats with glycemic instability need a thorough work-up as discussed earlier (see also Box 7-6). If a cause cannot be identified, close monitoring is mandatory, and regular home monitoring of blood glucose is of great help to decide on insulin dose amendments.

CHRONIC COMPLICATIONS OF DIABETES MELLITUS

Systemic Hypertension

There is currently no convincing evidence that diabetes in cats is associated with clinically relevant hypertension. Of eight cats with recently-diagnosed diabetes, two had increased systolic blood pressure of 170 and 180 mm Hg. However, values of 170 and 180 mm Hg were also found in two of 20 healthy control cats (Sander et al, 1998). Similar findings were described in 14 cats with a median diabetes duration of 18 months. None of the cats had systolic blood pressures more than 180 mm Hg, and blood pressures of healthy controls and diabetic cats did not differ. None of the cats had proteinuria or retinopathy (Senello et al, 2003). These findings are in agreement with two other studies, in which the duration of diabetes was not specified; however, none of the 13 cats examined had hypertension (Bodey and Sansom, 1998; Norris et al, 1999). In a more recent study, the prevalence of hypertension was not different in diabetic cats compared to control cats (Al-Ghazlat et al, 2011). Nevertheless, there may be exceptional cases. In one study, two diabetic cats with hypertensive retinopathy were described; one had evidence of renal dysfunction, which may have been the cause of hypertension, but the other cat had no other concurrent disease (Maggio et al, 2000). Further studies using larger cohorts of diabetic cats are needed to evaluate questions, such as the definitive prevalence of hypertension and the risk of kidney-damage when blood pressure is in the upper end of normal (Reusch et al, 2010).

Diabetic Cataracts

For a long time it was believed, that diabetic cataract does not develop in cats. A recent study demonstrated, however, that cataract formation is in fact a frequent event in feline diabetics. Forty-eight of 50 cats (96%) with diabetes had some degree of lens opacification. In 22 of them (46%), the findings were limited to linear posterior cortical opacification, which is similar to what is seen in normal, elderly cats. Twenty-six cats (54%), however, had more pronounced cortical cataracts or posterior subcapsular plaques. Severity of diabetic cataracts differs substantially between dogs and cats, as none of the cats was blind (Williams and Heath, 2006). Therefore, different from diabetic dogs, cataract formation in diabetic cats is usually of limited clinical relevance. More severe cataract with potential blindness may develop in diabetic kittens (Thoresen et al, 2002). The enzyme aldose reductase and the sorbitol pathway seem to play an important role in formation of diabetic cataract. (See Chronic Complications of Diabetes Mellitus in Chapter 6.) It has been shown that aldose reductase activity is significantly lower in lenses of older cats than in younger cats and dogs, which may prevent serious cataract formation (Richter et al, 2002).

Diabetic Nephropathy

In humans, diabetic nephropathy is a well-known and extremely serious complication of diabetes. It is a chronic disease developing over many years and is characterized by gradually increasing urine protein excretion and blood pressure, which is later followed by a decline in glomerular filtration rate and azotemia. Urine protein excretion itself gradually increases from microalbuminuria to overt proteinuria, and the development of overt nephropathy takes many years (Marshall and Flyvberg, 2010). Histopathological lesions affect predominantly the glomeruli, but there may also be severe interstitial and vascular involvement. Findings include thickening of the glomerular basement membrane, mesangial expansion, nodular sclerosis (Kimmelstiel-Wilson lesions), tubular basement membrane thickening, mononuclear cell infiltrates in the interstitium, interstitial fibrosis and atrophy, and arteriolar hyalinosis (Tervaert et al, 2010). Chronic renal disease is common in the elderly, non-diabetic cat population, and its cause is usually unknown. Diabetes is also relatively common in elderly cats. So far, it is unclear if diabetes in cats leads to kidney damage and chronic renal failure or if the coexistence of the two diseases is just coincidence. In recent studies, the prevalence of chronic renal disease in diabetic cats ranged between 17% and 63% (Roomp and Rand, 2009; 2012; Callegari et al, 2013). In a group of newly diagnosed diabetic cats, 13.3% developed chronic renal failure during a 6-month follow-up study (Hafner et al, 2013).

Proteinuria is assumed to be a marker for progression of chronic renal disease and high urine protein-to-creatinine (UPC) ratios have been shown to predict the development of azotemia in non-diabetic cats (Jepson et al, 2009; Chakrabarti et al, 2012). In diabetic cats, the prevalence of proteinuria was recently shown to be significantly higher than in healthy and sick, non-diabetic controls (75%, 18%, 34%). None of the cats were azotemic by the time of urinalysis, and no follow-up information with regard to potential progression to chronic renal failure was given (Al-Ghazlat et al, 2011). One small study reported histopathological findings in six diabetic cats, which consisted of mesangial proliferation in two cats, and glomerular sclerosis and interstitial inflammation in one cat each (Nakayama et al, 1990). We recently compared histopathological findings in 32 diabetic cats to those of 20 matched control cats. Glomerular lesions were observed in 17 (53%) of diabetic cats and 12 (60%) of the controls and consisted mainly of increased mesangial matrix, glomerular basement membrane thickening, and thickening of the Bowman capsule. Tubulointerstitial lesions were demonstrated in 26 (81%) of the diabetic and 16 (80%) of the controls and included interstitial fibrosis, inflammation, atrophy, and necrosis; vascular abnormalities were found in 3 (9.4%) of the diabetic and 2 (10%) of the controls. Statistical analysis revealed no difference between the groups. Of note, tubule-interstitial necrosis tended to be more frequent in diabetic cats than in controls (50% and 25%); however, the difference did not reach significance. Based on those results, it is very likely that cats do not develop diabetes-induced nephropathy. The short life expectancy of diabetic cats and the low prevalence of hypertension may be main reasons for the difference from human diabetics (Zini et al, 2014). If proteinuria is found in a diabetic cat, the next step is to exclude urinary tract infection and hypertension as possible causes. Thereafter, one should aim for good glycemic control and perform regular reevaluations. If severity of proteinuria increases, treatment with angiotensin converting enzyme (ACE) inhibitors may be considered, although data on their benefit in cats are scarce. Treatment of chronic renal failure in diabetic cats should follow the same guidelines as in non-diabetic cats.

Diabetic Neuropathy

Diabetic neuropathy is one of the most common chronic complications of diabetes in cats. The vast majority (90%) of diabetic cats reveal nerve abnormalities if peripheral nerves are examined by electron microscopy (Dahme et al, 1989). Overt neurological signs, however, are seen in only approximately 10% of cats. Clinical signs range from very mild to severe and include hind limb weakness, difficulty or inability to jump, a base-narrow gait, ataxia, muscle atrophy most noticeable in the distal pelvic limbs, and a plantigrade posture when standing and walking, postural reaction deficits and decreased tendon reflexes, and irritability when the feet are touched or manipulated. Clinical signs may progress to include the front legs with a palmigrade stance and gait (Mizisin et al, 2002; see Box 7-2). By means of electrophysiological testing, decreased motor and sensory nerve conduction velocities can be demonstrated with more severe decrease in diabetic cats with severe clinical neuropathy. Thoracic limbs tend to be less severely affected than the pelvic limbs, and sensory nerve conduction is less severely affected than motor nerve conduction. Electromyographic abnormalities are usually absent or if identified, are consistent with denervation (Mizisin et al, 2002; 2007).

Histological evaluations of nerve biopsies display concurrent injury to both Schwann cells and axons of myelinated fibers, which is remarkably similar to lesions in human diabetic neuropathy. Schwann cell injury is mainly characterized by splitting and ballooning of the myelin sheath and subsequent demyelination. Additionally, disproportionally thin myelin sheath can be found, being indicative of episodes of remyelination following demyelination and suggests ongoing metabolic dysfunction. Axonal injury consists of axoplasmic dystrophic accumulation of membranous debris and glycogen as well as degenerative fibre loss. Similar axonal injuries can be found in unmyelinated fibers (Dahme et al, 1989; Mizisin et al, 1998; 2002; 2007). Recently, it was shown that nerve fibre injury in diabetic cats is also associated with endoneurial microvascular abnormalities, some of which parallel those in human diabetic neuropathy (Estrella et al, 2008).

The pathogenesis of diabetic neuropathy is only incompletely understood and most likely multifactorial. Most data are derived from studies with diabetic rodent models. Potential mechanisms include increased flux through the polyol pathway, accumulation of advanced glycation end products on nerve and/or vessel proteins, disturbances in n-6 essential fatty acids and prostaglandin metabolism resulting in abnormal nerve membranes and microvasculature, depletion of nerve growth factors, and inflammatory as well as immunological processes (Ziegler, 2010). Data in cats are scarce. One study demonstrated an increase in nerve glucose and nerve fructose suggesting increased polyol pathway activity (Mizisin et al, 2002). The first step in the polyol-pathway is the reduction of glucose to sorbitol by the enzyme aldose reductase; thereafter, the enzyme sorbitol dehydrogenase oxidizes sorbitol to fructose. It is currently assumed, that those enzymatic steps consume NADPH, which is an important cofactor to regenerate reduced glutathione. The latter in turn is an important scavenger of reactive oxygen species (ROS); thus reduction in NADPH could induce or worsen oxidative stress (Giacco and Brownlee, 2010). Interestingly, in humans with type 1 diabetes, intensive treatment and enhanced glycemic control significantly reduces the risk for developing diabetic neuropathy, whereas in type 2 diabetics, glucose control has only small effects on the prevention of neuropathy (Callaghan et al, 2012). These data suggest that other factors (e.g., obesity, hyperlipidemia, and hypertension) are important contributors to the risk of diabetic neuropathy. Once diabetic neuropathy is established, intensive treatment and even diabetic remission does not result in significant improvement in humans. Various drugs have been studied (including aldose reductase inhibitors), but no major breakthrough has been achieved. Treatment is therefore mainly limited to pain relief; reduction in neuropathic pain has been seen with the use of antioxidants, such as alpha lipoic acid, acetyl-L carnitine, and benfotiamine (Smith and Singleton, 2012; Singleton and Smith, 2012). There is currently no recommended treatment for neuropathy in diabetic cats. In some cats, good glycemic control results in improvement of neurological signs, in others, however, no effect is seen. Complete reversal of diabetic neuropathy is a rare event. Lipoic acid may also show some effects in diabetic cats, however, it is associated with an increased risk of hepatotoxicity and should not be used until further studies on dosing regimens are available (Hill et al, 2004).

PROGNOSIS

The prognosis depends in part on owner commitment to treat the diabetes, presence of concurrent diseases (e.g., pancreatitis, chronic renal disease, and acromegaly), and the ease of glycemic control including the avoidance of complications such as DKA. In a recent study, survival time and prognostic factors were evaluated in 114 cats with newly diagnosed diabetes (Callegari et al, 2013). Mortality rate during the first 10 days was 16.7%, and the main causes of death were severe concurrent diseases. The rate compares quite well with mortality rates of 11% seen during the first weeks in previous studies (Kraus et al, 1997; Goossens et al, 1998). Median survival time was 516 days (range 1 to 3468 days), 70%, 64%, and 46% lived longer than 3, 6, and 24 months, respectively. Survival time was shorter for cats with concurrent diseases; increased serum creatinine concentrations at diagnosis was significantly associated with a poor outcome. Cats that achieved diabetic remission had longer survival times than cats that were persistently diabetic (Callegari et al, 2013). From those data, one may conclude that prognosis of diabetes in cats is moderate at best. However, two points have to be considered. First, cats are usually already quite old when diabetes is diagnosed, and second, the studies mentioned earlier were performed in referral centers, and data therefore are most likely associated with a negative selection bias. In cats without severe concurrent diseases, good quality of life can often be achieved for several years.

REFERENCES

Al-Ghazlat SA, et al.: The prevalence of micro-albuminuria and proteinuria in cats with diabetes mellitus, *Top Companion Anim Med* 26:154, 2011.

Alsahli M, Gerich JE: Abnormalities of insulin secretion and β-cell defects in type 2 diabetes. In Holt RIG, Cockran CS, Flyvbjerg A, Goldstein B, editors: *Textbook of diabetes*, ed 4, Chichester, 2010, Wiley-Blackwell.

Alt N, et al.: Day-to-day variability of blood glucose concentration curves generated at home in cats with diabetes mellitus, *J Am Vet Med Assoc* 230:1011, 2007.

American Diabetes Association: Standards of medical care in diabetes—2013, *Diabetes Care* 36(Suppl. 1):11, 2013.

Appleteon DJ, et al.: Insulin sensitivity decreases with obesity, and lean cats with low insulin sensitivity are at greatest risk of glucose intolerance with weight gain, *J Feline Med Surg* 3:211, 2001.

Appleton DJ, et al.: Dietary chromium tripicolinate supplementation reduces glucose concentrations and improves glucose tolerance in normal-weight cats, *J Feline Med Surg* 4:13, 2002.

Armstrong PJ, Williams DA: Pancreatitis in cats, *Topics in Compan An Med* 27:140, 2012.

Backus RC, et al.: Gonadectomy and high dietary fat but not high dietary carbohydrate induce gains in body weight and fat of domestic cats, *Br J Nutr* 98:641, 2007.

Bailey CJ, Krentz AJ: Oral antidiabetic agents. In Holt RIG, Cockran CS, Flyvbjerg A, Goldstein B, editors: *Textbook of diabetes*, ed 4, Chichester, 2010, Wiley-Blackwell.

Bailey CJ, Davies MJ: Pharmacological therapy of hyperglycemia in type 2 diabetes mellitus. In Wass JAH, Stewart PM, Amiel SA, Davies MJ, editors: *Oxford textbook of endocrinology and diabetes*, ed 2, Oxford, 2011, Oxford University Press.

Bailiff NL, et al.: Frequency and risk factors for urinary tract infection in cats with diabetes mellitus, *J Vet Intern Med* 20:850, 2006.

Baldwin K, et al.: AAHA nutritional assessment guidelines for dogs and cats, *J Am Anim Hosp Assoc* 46:285, 2010.

Baral RM, et al.: Prevalence of feline diabetes mellitus in a feline private practice (abstract), *J Vet Intern Med* 17:433, 2003.

Barrett KE, et al.: Endocrine functions of the pancreas & regulation of carbohydrate metabolism. In Ganong WF, editor: *Review of medical physiology*, ed 24, McGraw Hill Lange, 2012.

Baumstark A, et al.: Lot-to-lot variability of test strips and accuracy assessment of systems for self-monitoring of blood glucose according to ISO 15197, *J Diabetes Sci Technol* 6:1076, 2012.

Bennett N, et al.: Evaluation of transdermal application of glipizide in a pluronic lecithin gel to healthy cats, *Am J Vet Res* 66:581, 2005.

Bennett N, et al.: Comparison of a low carbohydrate-low fiber diet and a moderate carbohydrate-high fiber diet in the management of feline diabetes mellitus, *J Feline Med Surg* 8:73, 2006.

Bilous R, Donnelly R, editors: *Handbook of diabetes*, ed 4, Wiley-Blackwell, 2010.

Biourge V, et al.: Effect of weight gain and subsequent weight loss on glucose tolerance and insulin response in healthy cats, *J Vet Intern Med* 11:86, 1997.

Boari A, et al.: Glargine insulin and high-protein-low-carbohydrate diet in cats with diabetes mellitus, *Vet Res Commun* 32(Suppl. 1):243, 2008.

Bodey AR, Sansom J: Epidemiological study of blood pressure in domestic cats, *J Small Anim Pract* 39:567, 1998.

Boord M, Griffin C: Progesterone secreting adrenal mass in a cat with clinical signs of hyperadrenocorticism, *J Am Vet Med Assoc* 214:666, 1999.

Brennan CL, et al.: GLUT4 but not GLUT1 expression decreases early in the development of feline obesity, *Domest Anim Endocrinol* 26:291, 2004.

Breuer TG, et al.: Proinsulin levels in patients with pancreatic diabetes are associated with functional changes in insulin secretion rather than pancreatic beta-cell area, *Eur J Endocrinol* 163:551, 2010.

Brömel, et al.: Determination of adiponectin, a novel adipocytes hormone, in healthy and diabetic normal weight and obese cats (abstract), *J Vet Intern Med* 18:403, 2004.

Buse JB, et al.: How do we define cure of diabetes? *Diabetes Care* 32:2133, 2009.

Buse JB, et al.: Type 2 diabetes mellitus. In Melmed S, Polonsky KS, Larsen P, Kronenberg HM, editors: *Williams textbook of endocrinology*, ed 12, Philadelphia, 2011, Saunders Elsevier.

Butterwick RF, et al.: Effects of increases in dietary fat intake on plasma lipid and lipoprotein cholesterol concentrations and associated enzyme activities in cats, *Am J Vet Res* 73:62, 2012.

Callaghan BC, et al.: Diabetic neuropathy: one disease or two? *Curr Opin Neurol* 25:536, 2012.

Callegari C, et al.: Survival time and prognostic factors in cats with newly diagnosed diabetes mellitus: 114 cases (2000-2009), *J Am Vet Med Assoc* 243:91, 2013.

Caney SM: Pancreatitis and diabetes in cats, *Vet Clin North Am Small Anim Pract* 43:303, 2013.

Casella M, et al.: Measurement of capillary blood glucose concentrations by pet owners: a new tool in the management of diabetes mellitus, *J Am Anim Hosp Assoc* 38:329, 2002.

Casella M, et al.: Home-monitoring of blood glucose in cats with diabetes mellitus: evaluation over a 4-month period, *J Feline Med Surg* 7:163, 2005.

Chakrabarti S, et al.: Clinicopathological variables predicting progression of azotemia in cats with chronic kidney disease, *J Vet Intern Med* 26:275, 2012.

Chen N, et al.: The complex exocrine-endocrine relationship and secondary diabetes in exocrine pancreatic disorders, *J Clin Gastroenterol* 45:850, 2011.

Clark MH, et al.: Pharmacokinetics of pioglitazone in lean and obese cats, *J Vet Pharmacol Therap* 35:428, 2011.

Clark TA, et al.: Alternative therapies for diabetes and its cardiac complications: role of vanadium, *Heart Fail Rev*, 2014.

Cohen TA, et al.: Evaluation of six portable blood glucose meters for measuring blood glucose concentration in dogs, *J Am Vet Med Assoc* 235:276, 2009.

Cohn LA, et al.: Effects of chromium supplementation on glucose tolerance in obese and nonobese cats, *Am J Vet Res* 60:1360, 1999.

Concannon P, et al.: Genetics of type 1A diabetes, *N Engl J Med* 360:16, 2009.

Costes S, et al.: β-cell failure in type 2 diabetes: a case of asking too much of too few? *Diabetes* 62:327, 2013.

Crenshaw KL, Peterson ME: Pretreatment clinical and laboratory evaluation of cats with diabetes mellitus: 104 cases (1992-1994), *J Am Vet Med Assoc* 209:943, 1996.

Crenshaw KL, et al.: Serum fructosamine concentration as an index of glycemia in cats with diabetes mellitus and stress hyperglycemia, *J Vet Intern Med* 10:360, 1996.

Cryer PE: Hypoglycemia in diabetes. In Holt RIG, Cockran CS, Flyvbjerg A, Goldstein B, editors: *Textbook of diabetes*, ed 4, Chichester, 2010, Wiley-Blackwell.

Cryer PE: Mechanisms of hypoglycemia-associated autonomic failure in diabetes, *N Engl J Med* 369:362, 2013.

Dahme E, et al.: Diabetic neuropathy in dogs and cats—a bioptic electron microscopic study, *Tierarztl Prax* 17:177, 1989.

Davison LJ, et al.: Evaluation of a continuous glucose monitoring system in diabetic dogs, *J Small Anim Pract* 44:435, 2003.

De Cock HE, et al.: Prevalence and histopathologic characteristics of pancreatitis in cats, *Vet Pathol* 44:39, 2007.

Delaunay F, et al.: Pancreatic beta cells are important targets for the diabetogenic effects of glucocorticoids, *J Clin Invest* 100:2094, 1997.

Delli AJ, et al.: autoimmune type 1 diabetes. In Holt RIG, Cockran CS, Flyvbjerg A, Goldstein B, editors: *Textbook of diabetes*, ed 4, Chichester, 2010, Wiley-Blackwell.

De-Oliveira LD, et al.: Effects of six carbohydrate sources on diet digestibility and postprandial glucose and insulin responses in cats, *J Anim Sci* 86:2237, 2008.

De Silva NM, Frayling TM: Novel biological insights emerging from genetic studies of type 2 diabetes and related metabolic traits, *Curr Opin Lipidol* 21:44, 2010.

Dietiker-Moretti S, et al.: Comparison of a continuous glucose monitoring system with a portable blood glucose meter to determine insulin dose in cats with diabetes mellitus, *J Vet Intern Med* 25:1084, 2011.

Dohan FC, Lukens FD: Experimental diabetes produced by the administration of glucose, *Endocrinol* 42:244, 1948.

Donath MY, Shoelson SE: Type 2 diabetes as an inflammatory disease, *Nat Rev Immunol* 11:98, 2011.

Elliott DA, et al.: Glycosylated hemoglobin concentration for assessment of glycemic control in diabetic cats, *J Vet Intern Med* 11:161, 1997.

Elliott DA, et al.: Comparison of serum fructosamine and blood glycosylated hemoglobin concentrations for assessment of glycemic control in cats with diabetes mellitus, *J Am Vet Med Assoc* 214:1794, 1999.

Ellis S: Environmental enrichment. Practical strategies for improving feline welfare, *J Feline Med Surg* 11:901, 2009.

Erlich H, et al.: HLA DR-DQ haplotypes and genotypes and type 1 diabetes risk, *Diabetes* 57:1084, 2008.

Estrella JS, et al.: Endoneurial microvascular pathology in feline diabetic neuropathy, *Microvasc Res* 75:403, 2008.

Farmer AJ: Monitoring diabetes. In Holt RIG, Cockran CS, Flyvbjerg A, Goldstein B, editors: *Textbook of diabetes*, ed 4, Chichester, 2010, Wiley-Blackwell.

Farrow H, et al.: Postprandial glycaemia in cats fed a moderate carbohydrate meal persists for a median of 12-hours—female cats have higher peak glucose concentrations, *J Feline Med Surg* 14:706, 2012.

Feldman EC, et al.: Intensive 50-week evaluation of glipizide administration in 50 cats with previously untreated diabetes mellitus, *J Am Vet Med Assoc* 210:772, 1997.

Fidler C, et al.: Hypoglycemia: an overview of fear of hypoglycemia, quality-of-life, and impact on costs, *J Med Econ* 14:646, 2011.

Fineberg SE, et al.: Immunological responses to exogenous insulin, *Endocrine Reviews* 28:625, 2007.

Flatt PR: The hormonal and neural control of endocrine pancreatic function. In Pickup JC, Williams G, editors: *Textbook of diabetes*, ed 3, Blackwell Publishing, 2003.

Fletcher JM, et al.: Glucose detection and concentration estimation in feline urine samples with the Bayer Multistix and Purina Glucotest, *J Feline Med Surg* 13:705, 2011.

Fondacaro JV, et al.: Treatment of feline diabetes mellitus with protamine zinc analine insulin (PZI) alone compared with PZI and oral vanadium dipicolinate, *J Vet Intern Med* 13:244, 1999. abstract.

Forcada Y, et al.: Determination of serum fPLI concentrations in cats with diabetes mellitus, *J Feline Med Surg* 10:480, 2008.

Forcada Y, et al.: A missense mutation in the coding sequence of MC4R (MC4R:c.92 C > T) is associated with diabetes mellitus in DSH cats, *J Vet Intern Med* 24:1567, 2010. abstract.

Ford SL, Lynch H: Practical use of home blood glucose monitoring in feline diabetics, *Vet Clin North Am Small Anim Pract* 43:283, 2013.

Forman MA, et al.: Evaluation of serum feline pancreatic lipase immunoreactivity and helical computed tomography versus conventional testing for the diagnosis of feline pancreatitis, *J Vet Intern Med* 18:807, 2004.

Forman MA, et al.: Evaluation of feline pancreas-specific lipase (SPEC fPL™) for the diagnosis of feline pancreatitis (abstract), *J Vet Intern Med* 23:733, 2009.

Frank G, et al.: Use of a high-protein diet in the management of feline diabetes mellitus, *Vet Ther* 2:238, 2001.

Freckmann G, et al.: System accuracy evaluation of 43 blood glucose monitoring systems for self-monitoring of blood glucose according to DIN EN ISO 15197, *J Diabetes Sci Technol* 6:1060, 2012.

Garg SK, et al.: Possible impacts of new accuracy standards of self-monitoring of blood glucose, *US Endocrinology* 9:16, 2013.

Garvey WT: Mechanisms of insulin signal transduction. In DeFronzo RA, Ferrannini E, Kne H, Zimmet P, editors: *International textbook of diabetes mellitus*, ed 3, Wiley, 2004.

George K, et al.: Classification and diagnosis of diabetes mellitus. In Wass JAH, Stewart PM, Amiel SA, Davies MJ, editors: *Oxford textbook of endocrinology and diabetes*, ed 2, Oxford, 2011, Oxford University Press.

Gerhardt A, et al.: Comparison of the sensitivity of different diagnostic tests of pancreatitis in cats, *J Vet Intern Med* 15:329, 2001.

German AJ, et al.: Obesity, its associated disorders and the role of inflammatory adipokines in companion animals, *Vet J* 185:4, 2010.

Giacco F, Brownlee M: Pathogenesis of microvascular complications. In Holt RIG, Cockran CS, Flyvbjerg A, Goldstein B, editors: *Textbook of diabetes*, ed 4, Chichester, 2010, Wiley-Blackwell.

Gilor C, et al.: Pharmacodynamics of insulin detemir and insulin glargine assessed by an isoglycemic clamp method in healthy cats, *J Vet Intern Med* 24:870, 2010a.

Gilor C, et al.: The effects of body weight, body condition score, sex, and age on serum fructosamine concentrations in clinically healthy cats, *Vet Clin Pathol* 39:322, 2010b.

Gilor C, et al.: The GLP-1 mimetic exenatide potentiates insulin secretion in healthy cats, *Domest Anim Endocrinol* 41:42, 2011.

Gilor C, et al.: Distribution of K and L cells in the feline intestinal tract, *Domest Anim Endocrinol* 45:49, 2013.

Gittoes NJL, et al.: Drug-induced diabetes. In Holt RIG, Cockran CS, Flyvbjerg A, Goldstein B, editors: *Textbook of diabetes*, ed 4, Chichester, 2010, Wiley-Blackwell.

Goossens MM, et al.: Response to insulin treatment and survival in 104 cats with diabetes mellitus (1985-1995), *J Vet Intern Med* 12:1, 1998.

Gough S, Narendran P: Insulin and insulin treatment. In Holt RIG, Cockran CS, Flyvbjerg A, Goldstein B, editors: *Textbook of diabetes*, ed 4, Chichester, 2010, Wiley-Blackwell.

Graham PA, et al.: Serum fructosamine concentrations in hyperthyroid cats, *Res Vet Sci* 67:171, 1999.

Haberer B, Reusch CE: Glycated haemoglobin in various pathological conditions: investigations based on a new, fully automated method, *J Small Anim Pract* 39:510, 1998.

Hafner M, et al.: Intensive intravenous insulin therapy in diabetic cats, *J Vet Intern Med* 25:1493, 2011. abstract.

Hafner M, et al.: Evaluation of sensor sites for continuous glucose monitoring in cats with diabetes mellitus, *J Feline Med Surg* 15:117, 2013.

Hall DG, et al.: Lymphocytic inflammation of pancreatic islets in a diabetic cats, *J Vet Diagn Invest* 9:98, 1997.

Hall TD, et al.: Effects of diet on glucose control in cats with diabetes mellitus treated with twice daily insulin glargine, *J Feline Med Surg* 11:125, 2009.

Hanley NA: Endocrine disorders that cause diabetes mellitus. In Holt RIG, Cockran CS, Flyvbjerg A, Goldstein B, editors: *Textbook of diabetes*, ed 4, Chichester, 2010, Wiley-Blackwell.

Harb-Hauser M, et al.: Prevalence of insulin antibodies in diabetic cats, *J Vet Intern Med* 12:245, 1998. abstract.

Hasegawa S, et al.: Glycated hemoglobin fractions in normal and diabetic cats measured by high performance liquid chromatography, *J Vet Med Sci* 54:789, 1992.

Havelund S, et al.: The mechanism of protraction of insulin detemir, a long-acting, acylated analog of human insulin, *Pharm Res* 21:1498, 2004.

Hecht S, Henry G: Sonographic evaluation of the normal and abnormal pancreas, *Clin Tech Small Anim Pract* 22:115, 2007.

Henson MS, et al.: Evaluation of plasma islet amyloid polypeptide and serum glucose and insulin concentrations in nondiabetic cats classified by body condition score and in cats with naturally occurring diabetes mellitus, *Am J Vet Res* 72:1052, 2011.

Hewson-Hughes A, et al.: Postprandial glucose and insulin profiles following a glucose-loaded meal in cats and dogs, *Br J Nutr* 106:101, 2011a.

Hewson-Hughes AK, et al.: The effect of dietary starch level on postprandial glucose and insulin concentrations in cats and dogs, *Br J Nutr* 106(Suppl. 1):105, 2011b.

Hill AS, et al.: Lipoic acid is 10 times more toxic in cats than reported in humans, dogs or rats, *J Anim Physiol Anim Nutr (Berl)* 88:150, 2004.

Hoenig M: The cat as a model for human obesity and diabetes, *J Diabetes Sci Technol* 6:525, 2012.

Hoenig M, Ferguson DC: Impairment of glucose tolerance in hyperthyroid cats, *J Endocrinol* 121:249, 1989.

Hoenig M, Ferguson DC: Diagnostic utility of glycosylated hemoglobin concentrations in the cat, *Domest Anim Endocrinol* 16:11, 1999.

Hoenig M, Ferguson DC: Effect of darglitazone on glucose clearance and lipid metabolism in obese cats, *Am J Vet Res* 64:1409, 2003.

Hoenig M, et al.: Glucose tolerance and insulin secretion in spontaneously hyperthyroid cats, *Res Vet Sci* 53:338, 1992.

Hoenig M, et al.: Beta cell and insulin antibodies in treated and untreated diabetic cats, *Vet Immunol Immunopathol* 77:93, 2000a.

Hoenig M, et al.: A feline model of experimentally induced islet amyloidosis, *Am J Pathol* 157:2143, 2000b.

Hoenig M, et al.: Activity and tissue-specific expression of lipases and tumor-necrosis factor α in lean and obese cats, *Domest Anim Endocrinol* 30:333, 2006.

Hoenig M, et al.: Insulin sensitivity, fat distribution, and adipocytokine response to different diets in lean and obese cats before and after weight loss, *Am J Physiol Regul Integr Comp Physiol* 292:227, 2007.

Hoyer-Ott MA, et al.: Glycosylated hemoglobin in the cat: affinity chromatography determination in healthy, permanent diabetes mellitus and transient hyperglycemic cats, *Tierartzl Prax* 23:155, 1995.

Hoyumpa Vogt A, et al.: AAFP-AAHA: feline life stage guidelines, *J Feline Med Surg* 12:43, 2010.

Hull RL, et al.: Islet amyloid: a critical entity in the pathogenesis of type 2 diabetes, *J Clin Endocrinol Metab* 89:3629, 2004.

International Organization for Standardization: In vitro diagnostic test systems—requirements for blood-glucose monitoring systems for self-testing in managing diabetes mellitus, *ISO* 15197, 2013 (E).

Inzucchi SE, et al.: Management of hyperglycaemia in type 2 diabetes: a patient-centered approach. Position statement of the American Diabetes Association (ADA) and the European Association for the Study of Diabetes (EASD), *Diabetologia* 55:1577, 2012.

Jepson RE, et al.: Evaluation of predictors of the development of azotemia in cats, *J Vet Intern Med* 23:806, 2009.

Jin Y, Lin D: Fungal urinary tract infections in the dog and cat: a retrospective study (2001-2004), *J Am Anim Hosp Assoc* 41:373, 2005.

John WG: Global standardisation of haemoglobin A(1c) using metrological principles, *Clin Biochem* 45:1048, 2012.

Kahn SE, et al.: Interactions between genetic background, insulin resistance and β-cell function, *Diabetes Obes Metab* 14(Suppl. 3):46, 2012.

Kanaya AM, Vaisse C: Obesity. In Gardner DG, Shoback D, editors: *Greenspan's basic & clinical endocrinology*, ed 9, San Francisco, 2011, McGraw Hill.

Kaufman FR: Type 2 diabetes in children and young adults: a "new epidemic," *Clinical Diabetes* 20:217, 2002.

Kienzle E: Blood sugar levels and renal sugar excretion after the intake of high carbohydrate diets in cats, *J Nutr* 124:2563, 1994.

Kitchell BE, et al.: Clinical and pathologic changes in experimentally induced acute pancreatitis in cats, *Am J Vet Res* 27:1170, 1986.

Kley S, et al.: Evaluation of long-term home monitoring of blood glucose concentrations in cats with diabetes mellitus: 26 cases (1999-2002), *J Am Vet Med Assoc* 225:261, 2004.

Kley S, et al.: Evaluation of the low-dose dexamethasone suppression test and ultrasonographic measurements of the adrenal glands in cats with diabetes mellitus, *Schweiz Arch Tierheilkd* 149:493, 2007.

Kley S, et al.: Development of a feline proinsulin immunoradiometric assay and a feline proinsulin enzyme-linked immunosorbent assay (ELISA): a novel application to examine beta cell function in cats, *Domest Anim Endocrinol* 34:311, 2008.

Klinke DJ 2nd: Extent of beta cell destruction is important but insufficient to predict the onset of type 1 diabetes mellitus, *PLoS ONE* 3:e1374, 2008.

Kraus MS, et al.: Feline diabetes mellitus: a retrospective mortality study of 55 cats (1982-1994), *J Am Anim Hosp Assoc* 33:107, 1997.

Krentz AJ, Nattrass M: Acute metabolic complications of diabetes: diabetic ketoacidosis, hyperosmolar non-ketotic hyperglycemia and lactic acidosis. In Pickup JC, Williams G, editors: *Textbook of diabetes*, ed 3, Blackwell Publishing, 2003.

Laflamme DP: Development and validation of a body condition score system for cats: a clinical tool, *Feline Pract* 25:13, 1997.

Laflamme DP: Focus on nutrition: cats and carbohydrates: implications for health and disease, *Compend Contin Educ Vet* 32:E1, 2010.

Laflamme DP: Nutritional care for aging cats and dogs, *Vet Clin Small Anim* 42:769, 2012.

Laflamme DP, Hannah SS: Discrepancy between use of lean body mass or nitrogen balance to determine protein requirements for adult cats, *J Feline Med Surg* 15:691, 2013.

Laluha P, et al.: Stress hyperglycemia in sick cats: a retrospective study over 4 years, *Schweiz Arch Tierheilkd* 146:375, 2004.

Lederer R, et al.: Frequency of feline diabetes mellitus and breed predisposition in domestic cats in Australia, *Vet J* 179:254, 2009.

Link KR, Rand JS: Glucose toxicity in cats (abstract), *J Vet Intern Med* 10:185, 1996.

Link KR, Rand JS: Changes in blood glucose concentration are associated with relatively rapid changes in circulating fructosamine concentrations in cats, *J Feline Med Surg* 10:583, 2008.

Link KR, et al.: The effect of experimentally induced chronic hyperglycaemia on serum and pancreatic insulin, pancreatic islet IGF-1 and plasma and urinary ketones in domestic cat (Felis felis), *Gen Comp Endocrinol* 188:269, 2013.

Lowe AD, et al.: Clinical, clinicopathological and histological changes observed in 14 cats treated with glucocorticoids, *Vet Rec* 162:777, 2008.

Lowe AD, et al.: A pilot study comparing the diabetogenic effects of dexamethasone and prednisolone in cats, *J Am Anim Hosp Assoc* 45:215, 2009.

Lutz TA, et al.: Fructosamine concentrations in hyperglycemic cats, *Can Vet J* 36:155, 1995.

Maedler K, et al.: Sulfonylurea induced β-cell apoptosis in cultured human islets, *J Clin Endocrinol Metab* 90:501, 2005.

Maggio F, et al.: Ocular lesions associated with systemic hypertension in cats: 69 cases (1985-1998), *J Am Vet Med Assoc* 217:695, 2000.

Marshall RD, et al.: Glargine and protamine zinc insulin have a longer duration of action and result in lower mean daily glucose concentrations than lente insulin in healthy cats, *J Vet Pharmacol Ther* 31:205, 2008a.

Marshall RD, et al.: Insulin glargine has a long duration of effect following administration either once daily or twice daily in divided doses in healthy cats, *J Feline Med Surg* 10:488, 2008b.

Marshall RD, et al.: Treatment of newly diagnosed diabetic cats with glargine insulin improves glycaemic control and results in higher probability of remission than protamine zinc and lente insulins, *J Feline Med Surg* 11:683, 2009.

Marshall SM, Flyvbjerg A: Diabetic nephropathy. In Holt RIG, Cockran CS, Flyvbjerg A, Goldstein B, editors: *Textbook of diabetes*, ed 4, Chichester, 2010, Wiley-Blackwell.

Martin GJ, Rand JS: Pharmacology of a 40 IU/ml porcine lente insulin preparation in diabetic cats: findings during the first week and after 5 or 9 weeks of therapy, *J Feline Med Surg* 3:23, 2001.

Martin GJ, Rand JS: Control of diabetes mellitus in cats with porcine insulin zinc suspension, *Vet Rec* 161:88, 2007.

Masharani U, German MS: Pancreatic hormones and diabetes mellitus. In Gardner DG, Shoback D, editors: *Greenspan's basic & clinical endocrinology*, ed 9, San Francisco, 2011, McGraw Hill.

Mayer-Roenne B, et al.: Urinary tract infections in cats with hyperthyroidism, diabetes mellitus and chronic kidney disease, *J Feline Med Surg* 9:124, 2007.

Mazzaferro EM, et al.: Treatment of feline diabetes mellitus using an alpha-glucosidase inhibitor and a low-carbohydrate diet, *J Feline Med Surg* 5:183, 2003.

McCann TM, et al.: Feline diabetes mellitus in the UK: the prevalence within an insured cat population and a questionnaire-based putative risk factor analysis, *J Feline Med Surg* 9:289, 2007.

McMillan FD, Feldman EC: Rebound hyperglycemia following overdosing of insulin in cats with diabetes mellitus, *J Am Vet Med Assoc* 12:1426, 1986.

Michel KE, et al.: Correlation of a feline muscle mass score with body composition determined by dual-energy X-ray absorptiometry, *Br J Nutr* 106:57, 2011.

Michels GM, et al.: Pharmacokinetics of the antihyperglycemic agent metformin in cats, *Am J Vet Res* 60:738, 1999.

Michiels L, et al.: Treatment of 46 cats with porcine lente insulin—a prospective, multicentre study, *J Feline Med Surg* 10:439, 2008.

Middleton DJ, Watson AD: Glucose intolerance in cats given short-term therapies of prednisolone and megestrol acetate, *Am J Vet Res* 46:2623, 1985.

Middleton DJ, et al.: Suppression of cortisol responses to exogenous adrenocorticotrophic hormone, and the occurrence of side effects attributable to glucocorticoid excess, in cats during therapy with megestrol acetate and prednisolone, *Can J Vet Res* 51:60, 1987.

Minkus G, et al.: Pathological changes of the endocrine pancreas in dogs and cats in comparison with clinical data, *Tierartzl Prax* 19:282, 1991.

Mizisin AP, et al.: Myelin splitting, Schwann cell injury and demyelination in feline diabetic neuropathy, *Acta Neuropathol* 95:171, 1998.

Mizisin AP, et al.: Neurological complications associated with spontaneously occurring feline diabetes mellitus, *J Neuropathol Exp Nerol* 61:872, 2002.

Mizisin AP, et al.: Comparable myelinated nerve pathology in feline and human diabetes mellitus, *Acta Neuropathol* 113:431, 2007.

Moretti S, et al.: Evaluation of a novel real-time continuous glucose-monitoring system for use in cats, *J Vet Intern Med* 24:120, 2010.

Mori A, et al.: Decreased gene expression of insulin signaling genes in insulin sensitive tissues of obese cats, *Vet Res Comm* 33:315, 2009a.

Mori A, et al.: Effect of glimepiride and nateglinide on serum insulin and glucose concentration in healthy cats, *Vet Res Commun* 33:957, 2009b.

Mudaliar S, Henry RR: The incretin hormones: from scientific discovery to practical therapeutics, *Diabetologia* 55:1865, 2012.

Nakayama H, et al.: Pathological observation of six cases of feline diabetes mellitus, *Nihon Juigaku Zasshi* 52:819, 1990.

Nelson RW, et al.: Effect of an orally administered sulfonylurea, glipizide, for treatment of diabetes mellitus in cats, *J Am Vet Med Assoc* 203:821, 1993.

Nelson RW, et al.: Transient clinical diabetes mellitus in cats: 10 cases (1989-1991), *J Vet Intern Med* 13:28, 1999.

Nelson RW, et al.: Efficacy of protamine zinc insulin for treatment of diabetes mellitus in cats, *J Am Vet Med Assoc* 218:38, 2001.

Nelson R, et al.: Evaluation of the oral antihyperglycemic drug metformin in normal and diabetic cats, *J Vet Intern Med* 18:18, 2004.

Nelson RW, et al.: Field safety and efficacy of protamine zinc recombinant human insulin for treatment of diabetes mellitus in cats, *J Vet Intern Med* 23:787, 2009.

Nerhus K, et al.: Effect of ambient temperature on analytical performance of self-monitoring blood glucose systems, *Diabetes Technol Ther* 13:883, 2011.

Nguyen PG: Effect of dietary fat and energy on body weight and composition after gonadectomy in cats, *Am J Vet Res* 65:1708, 2004.

Niessen SJ, et al.: Feline acromegaly: an underdiagnosed endocrinopathy? *J Vet Intern Med* 21:899, 2007.

Niessen SJ, et al.: Evaluation of a quality-of-life tool for cats with diabetes mellitus, *J Vet Intern Med* 24:1098, 2010.

Niessen SJM: Glucagon: Are we missing a (life-saving) trick? *J Vet Emerg Crit Care* 22:523, 2012.

Norris CR, et al.: Serum total and ionized magnesium concentrations and urinary fractional excretion of magnesium in cats with diabetes mellitus and diabetic ketoacidosis, *J Am Vet Med Assoc* 215:1455, 1999.

O'Brien TD: Pathogenesis of feline diabetes mellitus, *Mol Cell Endocrinol* 197:213, 2002.

Oppliger S, et al.: Evaluation of serum spec FPL™ and 1,2-o-dilauryl-rac-glycero-3-glutaric acid-(6'-methylresorufin) ester (DGGR) lipase in 40 cats with standardized pancreatic histopathological assessment (abstract), *J Vet Intern Med* 27:696, 2013a.

Oppliger, et al.: Agreement of the serum Spec fPL™ and 1,2-o-dilauryl-rac-glycero-3-glutaric acid-(6'-methylresorufin) ester lipase assay for the determination of serum lipase in cats with suspicion of pancreatitis, *J Vet Intern Med* 27:1077, 2013b.

Owens DR: Insulin preparations with prolonged effect, *Diabetes Technol Ther* 13(Suppl.1):5, 2011.

Padrutt I, et al.: Comparison of the GLP-1 analogues exenatide (short-acting), exenatide (long-acting) and the DPP-4 inhibitor sitagliptin to increase insulin secretion in healthy cats (abstract), *J Vet Intern Med* 26:1520, 2012.

Palm CA, Feldman EC: Oral hypoglycemics in cats with diabetes mellitus, *Vet Clin North Am Small Anim Pract* 43:407, 2013.

Panciera DL, et al.: Epizootiologic patterns of diabetes mellitus in cats: 333 cases (1980-1986), *J Am Vet Med Assoc* 197:1504, 1990.

Parent C, et al.: Serum trypsin-like immunoreactivity, amylase and lipase in the diagnosis of feline acute pancreatitis (abstract), *J Vet Intern Med* 9:194, 1995.

Peakman M: Immunology of type 1 diabetes. In Wass JAH, Stewart PM, Amiel SA, Davies MJ, editors: *Oxford textbook of endocrinology and diabetes*, ed 2, Oxford, 2011, Oxford University Press.

Penninck D: Pancreas. In Penninck D, d'Anjou M-A, editors: *Atlas of small animal ultrasonography*, Blackwell Publishing, 2008.

Persaud SJ, Howell SL: The biosynthesis and secretion of insulin. In Pickup JC, Williams G, editors: *Textbook of diabetes*, ed 3, Blackwell Publishing, 2003.

Peterson ME: Effects of megestrol acetate on glucose tolerance and growth hormone secretion in the cat, *Res Vet Sci* 42:354, 1987.

Pickup JC: Diabetic control and its measurement. In Pickup JC, Williams G, editors: *Textbook of diabetes*, ed 3, Blackwell Publishing, 2003.

Prahl A, et al.: Time trends and risk factors for diabetes mellitus in cats presented to veterinary teaching hospitals, *J Feline Med Surg* 9:351, 2007.

Pressler, et al.: Candida spp. urinary tract infections in 13 dogs and seven cats: predisposing factors, treatment, and outcome, *J Am Anim Hosp Assoc* 39:263, 2003.

Quante S, et al.: Hyperprogesteronism due to bilateral adrenal carcinomas in a cat with diabetes mellitus, *Schweiz Arch Tierheilkd* 151:437, 2009.

Radin MJ, et al.: Adipokines: a review of biological and analytical principles and an update in dogs, cats, and horses, *Vet Clin Pathol* 38:136, 2009.

Rand J: Feline diabetes mellitus. In Mooney CT, Peterson ME, editors: *BSAVA Manual of canine and feline endocrinology*, ed 4, British Small Animal Veterinary Association, 2012.

Rand JS, et al.: Over representation of Burmese cats with diabetes mellitus, *Aust Vet J* 75:402, 1997.

Rand JS, et al.: Acute stress hyperglycemia in cats is associated with struggling and increased concentrations of lactate and norepinephrine, *J Vet Intern Med* 16:123, 2002.

Rasouli N, Kern PA: Adipocytokines and the metabolic complications of obesity, *J Clin Endocrinol Metab* 93:64, 2008.

Rave K: Renal glucose excretion as a function of blood glucose concentration in subjects with type 2 diabetes—results of a hyperglycaemic glucose clamp study, *Nephrol Dial Transplant* 21:2166, 2006.

Rees CA, Boothe DM: Evaluation of the effect of cephalexin and enrofloxacin on clinical laboratory measurements of urine glucose in dogs, *J Am Vet Med Assoc* 224:1455, 2004.

Renda F, et al.: Metformin-associated lactic acidosis requiring hospitalization. A national 10 year survey and a systemic literature in review, *Eur Rev Med Pharmacol Sci* 17(Suppl. 1):45, 2013.

Reusch CE: Feline diabetes mellitus. In Ettinger SJ, Feldman EC, editors: *Textbook of veterinary internal medicine*, ed 7, St Louis, 2010, Saunders/Elsevier.

Reusch CE: Diabetic monitoring. In Bonagura JD, Twedt DC, editors: *Kirk's current veterinary therapy XV*, ed 1, St Louis, 2013, Saunders/Elsevier.

Reusch CE, Haberer B: Evaluation of fructosamine in dogs and cats with hypo- or hyperproteinaemia, azotaemia, hyperlipidaemia and hyperbilirubinaemia, *Vet Rec* 148:370, 2001.

Reusch CE, Padrutt I: New incretin hormonal therapies in humans relevant to diabetic cats, *Vet Clin North Am Small Anim Pract* 43:417, 2013.

Reusch CE, Tomsa K: Serum fructosamine concentration in cats with overt hyperthyroidism, *J Am Vet Med Assoc* 215:1297, 1999.

Reusch CE, et al.: Fructosamine. A new parameter for diagnosis and metabolic control in diabetic dogs and cats, *J Vet Intern Med* 7:177, 1993.

Reusch CE, et al.: Home monitoring of the diabetic cat, *J Feline Med Surg* 8:119, 2006a.

Reusch CE, et al.: Measurements of growth hormone and insulin-like growth factor 1 in cats with diabetes mellitus, *Vet Rec* 158:195, 2006b.

Reusch CE, et al.: Endocrine hypertension in small animals, *Vet Clin North Am Small Anim Pract* 40:335, 2010.

Richter M, et al.: Aldose reductase activity and glucose-related opacities in incubated lenses from dogs and cats, *Am J Vet Res* 63:1591, 2002.

Ristic JM: Evaluation of a continuous glucose monitoring system in cats with diabetes mellitus, *J Feline Med Surg* 7:153, 2005.

Robertson RP: β-cell deterioration during diabetes: what's in the gun? *Trends in Endocrinol Metabol* 20:388, 2009.

Roomp K, Rand J: Intensive blood glucose control is safe and effective in diabetic cats using home monitoring and treatment with glargine, *J Feline Med Surg* 11:668, 2009.

Roomp K, Rand J: Evaluation of detemir in diabetic cats managed with a protocol for intensive blood glucose control, *J Feline Med Surg* 14:566, 2012.

Rossmeisl JH, et al.: Hyperadrenocorticism and hyperprogesteronemia in a cat with an adrenocortical adenocarcinoma, *J Am Anim Hosp Assoc* 36:512, 2000.

Rucinsky R, et al.: AAHA diabetes management guidelines, *J Am Anim Hosp Assoc* 46:215, 2010.

Rutti S, et al.: In vitro proliferation of adult human beta-cells, *PLoS ONE* 7:1, 2012.

Sander C, et al.: Indirect blood pressure measurement in cats with diabetes mellitus, chronic nephropathy and hypertrophic cardiomyopathy, *Tierarztl Prax Ausg K Kleintiere Heimtiere* 26:110, 1998.

Scarlett JM, Donoghue S: Associations between body condition and disease in cats, *J Am Vet Med Assoc* 212:1725, 1998.

Schäfer SA, et al.: New type 2 diabetes risk genes provide new insights in insulin secretion mechanisms, *Diabetes Res Clin Pract* 93:9, 2011.

Schäfer S, et al.: Evaluation of insulin-like growth factor 1 (IGF-1), thyroxine (T4), feline pancreatic lipase immunoreactivity (FPLI) and urinary corticoid creatinine ratio (UCCR) in cats with diabetes mellitus in Switzerland and the Netherlands, *ECVIM-CA congress Liverpool*, 2013.

Senello KA, et al.: Systolic blood pressure in cats with diabetes mellitus, *J Am Vet Med Assoc* 223:198, 2003.

Sieber-Ruckstuhl NS, et al.: Remission of diabetes mellitus in cats with diabetic ketoacidosis, *J Vet Intern Med* 22:1326, 2008.

Singh R, et al.: Switching to an ultra-low carbohydrate diet has a similar effect on postprandial blood glucose concentrations to administering acarbose to healthy cats fed a high carbohydrate diet, *J Vet Intern Med* 20:726, 2006. abstract.

Singleton JR, Smith AG: The diabetic neuropathies: practical and rational therapy, *Semin Neurol* 32:196, 2012.

Sjaastad OV: The endocrine system. In Sjaastad OV, Sand O, Hove K, editors: *Physiology of domestic animals*, Oslo, 2010, Scandinavian Veterinary Press.

Slingerland LI, et al.: Indoor confinement and physical inactivity rather than the proportion of dry food are risk factors in the development of feline type 2 diabetes mellitus, *Vet J* 179:247, 2009.

Smith AG, Singleton JR: Diabetic neuropathy, *Continuum Lifelong Learning Neurol* 18:60, 2012.

Smith DM, et al.: A systematic review of vanadium oral supplements for glycaemic control in type 2 diabetes mellitus, *Q J Med* 101:351, 2008.

Smith JR, et al.: A survey of southeastern United States veterinarians' preferences for managing cats with diabetes mellitus, *J Feline Med Surg* 14:716, 2012.

Somogyi M: Exacerbation of diabetes by excess insulin action, *Am J Med* 26:169, 1959.

Steiner JM: Exocrine pancreatic insufficiency in the cat, *Top Companion Anim Med* 27:113, 2012.

Steiner JM, et al.: Development and analytical validation of a radioimmunoassay for the measurement of feline pancreatic lipase immunoreactivity in serum, *Can J Vet Res* 23:476, 2004.

Strage EM, et al.: Validation of an enzyme-linked immunosorbent assay for measurement of feline serum insulin, *Vet Clin Pathol* 41:518, 2012.

Surman S, Fleeman L: Continuous glucose monitoring in small animals, *Vet Clin North Am Small Anim Pract* 43:381, 2013.

Tanaka A, et al.: Comparison and expression of glucokinase gene and activities of enzymes related to glucose metabolism in livers between dog and cat, *Vet Res Commun* 29:477, 2005.

Tervaert TW, et al.: Pathologic classification of diabetic nephropathy, *J Am Soc Nephrol* 21:556, 2010.

Thorens B, Mueckler M: Glucose transporters in the 21st century, *Am J Physiol Endocrinol Metab* 298:141, 2010.

Thoresen SI, Bredal WP: Determination of a reference range for fructosamine in feline serum samples, *Vet Res Commun* 19:353, 1995.

Thoresen SI, et al.: Diabetes mellitus and bilateral cataracts in a kitten, *J Feline Med Surg* 4:115, 2002.

Tschöpe D, et al.: The role of co-morbidity in the selection of antidiabetic pharmacotherapy in type-2 diabetes, *Cardiovascular Diabetology* 12:62, 2013.

Tschuor F, et al.: Remission of diabetes mellitus in cats cannot be predicted by the arginine stimulation test, *J Vet Intern Med* 25:83, 2011.

Tschuor F, et al.: Evaluation of four methods used to measure plasma insulin-like growth factor 1 concentrations in healthy cats and cats with diabetes mellitus or other diseases, *Am J Vet Res* 73:1925, 2012.

Utzschneider KM, et al.: Normal insulin secretion in humans. In DeFronzo RA, Ferrannini E, Kne H, Zimmet P, editors: *International textbook of diabetes mellitus*, ed 3, Chichester, West Sussex, 2004, John Wiley & Sons Ltd.

Voulgari C, et al.: "Brittleness" in diabetes: easier spoken than broken, *Diabetes Technol Ther* 14:835, 2012.

Wade C, et al.: Evidence of a genetic basis for diabetes mellitus in Burmese cats (abstract), *J Vet Intern Med* 13:269, 1999.

Wajngot A, et al.: The diabetogenic effects of glucocorticoids are more pronounced in low- than in high-insulin responders, *Proc Natl Acad Sci USA* 89:6035, 1992.

Wang J, Osei K: Proinsulin maturation disorder is a contributor to the defect of subsequent conversion to insulin in β-cells, *Biochem Biophys Res Commun* 411:150, 2011.

Wang ZQ, Cefalu WT: Current concepts about chromium supplementation in type 2 diabetes and insulin resistance, *Curr Diab Rep* 10:145, 2010.

Washizu T, et al.: Comparison of the activities of enzymes related to glycolysis and gluconeogenesis in the liver of dogs and cats, *Res Vet Sci* 67:203, 1999.

Weaver KE, et al.: Use of glargine and lente insulins in cats with diabetes mellitus, *J Vet Intern Med* 20:234, 2006.

Wess G, Reusch C: Capillary blood sampling from the ear of dogs and cats and use of portable meters to measure glucose concentration, *J Small Anim Pract* 41:60, 2000.

Whiting DR, et al.: IDF diabetes atlas: global estimates of the prevalence of diabetes for 2011 and 2030, *Diabetes Res Clin Pract* 94:311, 2011.

Wiedmeyer CE, et al.: Evaluation of a continuous glucose monitoring system for use in dogs, cats, and horses, *J Am Vet Med Assoc* 223:987, 2003.

Williams DL, Heath MF: Prevalence of feline cataract: results of a cross-sectional study of 2000 normal animals, 50 cats with diabetes and one hundred cats following dehydrational crises, *Vet Ophthalmol* 9:341, 2006.

Williams JM, et al.: Ultrasonographic findings of the pancreas in cats with elevated serum pancreatic lipase immunoreactivity, *J Vet Intern Med* 27:913, 2013.

World Health Organization: *Diabetes mellitus report of a WHO expert committee* (Tech. Rep. Ser., no 310), (PDF online): Geneva, 1965, World Health Org. http://whqlibdoc .who.int/trs/WHO_TRS_310.pdf. Accessed May 22, 2014.

World Health Organization: *WHO expert committee on diabetes mellitus: second report* (Tech. Rep. Ser., no 646), (PDF online): Geneva, 1980, World Health Org. http://w hqlibdoc.who.int/trs/WHO_TRS_646.pdf. Accessed May 22, 2014.

World Health Organization: *Definition, diagnosis, and classification of diabetes mellitus and its complications: report of a WHO consultation. Part 1: diagnosis and classification of diabetes mellitus* (WHO/NCD/ NCS/99.2), (PDF online): Geneva, 1999, World Health Org. http://whqlibdoc.who.int /hq/1999/who_ncd_ncs_99.2.pdf. Accessed May 22, 2014.

Yale JF: Oral antihyperglycemic agents and renal disease: new agents, new concepts, *J Am Soc Nephrol* 16:S7, 2005.

Yardley JE, et al.: Lifestyle issues: exercise. In Holt RIG, Cockran CS, Flyvbjerg A, Goldstein B, editors: *Textbook of diabetes*, ed 4, Chichester, Wiley-Blackwell, 2010.

Yki-Järvinen HE: Insulin resistance in type 2 diabetes. In Holt RIG, Cockran CS, Flyvbjerg A, Goldstein B, editors: *Textbook of diabetes*, ed 4, Chichester, 2010. Wiley-Blackwell.

Zeugswetter FK, et al.: Alternative sampling site for blood glucose testing in cats: giving the ears a rest, *J Feline Med Surg* 12:710, 2010.

Ziegler D: Diabetic peripheral neuropathy. In Holt RIG, Cockran CS, Flyvbjerg A, Goldstein B, editors: *Textbook of diabetes*, ed 4, Chichester, 2010, Wiley-Blackwell.

Zini E, et al.: Hyperglycaemia but not hyperlipidaemia causes beta cell dysfunction and beta cell loss in the domestic cat, *Diabetologia* 52:336, 2009a.

Zini E, et al.: Evaluation of a new portable glucose meter designed for the use in cats, *Schweiz Arch Tierheilkd* 151:448, 2009b.

Zini, et al.: Predictors of clinical remission in cats with diabetes mellitus, *J Vet Intern Med* 24:1314, 2010.

Zini E, et al.: Pancreatic enzymes activity and ultrasonographic findings in diabetic cats at diagnosis and during follow-up (abstract), *J Vet Intern Med* 25:1491, 2011.

Zini, et al.: Histological investigation of endocrine and exocrine pancreas in cats with diabetes mellitus (abstract), *J Vet Intern Med* 26:1519, 2012.

Zini E, et al.: Renal morphology in cats with diabetes mellitus, *Vet Pathol* Feb 24, 2014 (Epub ahead of print).

Zoran DL: Pancreatitis in cats: diagnosis and management of a challenging disease, *J Am Anim Hosp Assoc* 42:1, 2006.

Zoran DL, Buffington CAT: Effects of nutrition choices and lifestyle changes on the well-being of cats, a carnivore that has moved indoors, *J Am Vet Med Assoc* 239:596, 2011.

Zoran DL, Rand JS: The role of diet in the prevention and management of feline diabetes, *Vet Clin North Am Small Anim Pract* 43:233, 2013.

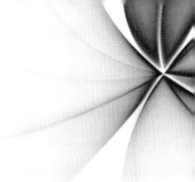

CHAPTER 8 | Diabetic Ketoacidosis

Richard W. Nelson

CHAPTER CONTENTS

Diabetic ketoacidosis (DKA) is a serious complication of diabetes mellitus. Before the availability of insulin in the 1920s, DKA was a uniformly fatal disorder. Even after the discovery of insulin, DKA continued to carry a grave prognosis with a reported mortality rate in humans ranging from 10% to 30%. However, with the expanding knowledge regarding the pathophysiology of DKA and the application of new treatment techniques for the complications of DKA, the mortality rate for this disorder has decreased to less than 5% in experienced human medical centers (Kitabchi et al, 2008). We have experienced a similar decrease in the mortality rate for DKA in our hospital over the past two decades. DKA remains a challenging disorder to treat, in part because of the deleterious impact of DKA on multiple organ systems and the frequent occurrence of concurrent often serious disorders that are responsible for the high mortality rate of DKA. In humans, the incidence of DKA has not decreased, appropriate therapy remains controversial, and patients continue to succumb to this complication of diabetes mellitus. This chapter summarizes current concepts regarding the pathophysiology and management of DKA in dogs and cats.

PATHOGENESIS AND PATHOPHYSIOLOGY

Generation of Ketone Bodies

Ketone bodies are derived from oxidation of nonesterified or free fatty acids (FFAs) by the liver and are used as an energy source by many tissues during periods of glucose deficiency. FFAs released from adipose tissue are assimilated by the liver at a rate dependent on their plasma concentration. Within the liver, FFAs can be incorporated into triglycerides, can be metabolized via the tricarboxylic acid (TCA) cycle to CO_2 and water, or can be converted to ketone bodies (Hood and Tannen, 1994; Kitabchi et al, 2001; Fig. 8-1). Oxidation of FFAs leads to the production of acetoacetate. In the presence of NADH, acetoacetate is reduced to β-hydroxybutyrate. Acetone is formed by spontaneous decarboxylation of acetoacetate (see Fig. 8-1). These ketone bodies—acetoacetate, β-hydroxybutyrate, and acetone—are substrates for energy metabolism by most tissues. The metabolism of ketone bodies is integrated with that of other substrates of energy metabolism, both in peripheral tissues and in the liver. However, excessive production of ketone bodies, as occurs in uncontrolled diabetes, results in their accumulation in the circulation and development of the ketosis and acidosis of ketoacidosis.

Role of Insulin Deficiency

The most important regulators of ketone body production are FFA availability and the ketogenic capacity of the liver (McGarry et al, 1989; Zammit, 1994). For the synthesis of ketone bodies to be enhanced, there must be two major alterations in intermediary metabolism: (1) increased mobilization of FFAs from triglycerides stored in adipose tissue and (2) a shift in hepatic metabolism from fat synthesis to fat oxidation and ketogenesis (Hood and Tannen, 1994; Kitabchi et al, 2001). Insulin is a powerful inhibitor of lipolysis and FFA oxidation (Groop et al, 1989). A relative or absolute deficiency of insulin results in increased activity of hormone sensitive lipase in adipocytes, which increases FFA release from adipocytes—thus increasing the availability of FFAs to the liver and in turn promoting ketogenesis. Insulin deficiency also reduces peripheral utilization of glucose and ketones. The combination of increased production and decreased utilization leads to an accumulation of glucose and ketones in blood. Virtually all dogs and cats with DKA have a relative or absolute deficiency of insulin (Fig. 8-2). In established diabetic animals after insulin is discontinued and in newly-diagnosed diabetic animals that are diagnosed with ketoacidosis on initial examination, circulating insulin levels are low or undetectable. Some dogs and cats have serum insulin concentrations similar to those observed in healthy, fasted dogs and cats (i.e., within the reference range; Durocher et al, 2008). However, such insulin concentrations are inappropriately low ("relative" insulin deficiency) for the severity of hyperglycemia encountered.

Some diabetic dogs and cats develop ketoacidosis despite receiving daily injections of insulin, and circulating insulin concentrations may even be increased. Insulin deficiency per se cannot be the sole physiologic cause for the development of DKA. In this group, a "relative" insulin deficiency is present. Presumably these dogs and cats have insulin resistance potentially resulting from an increase in circulating glucose counterregulatory hormones (i.e., glucagon, epinephrine, cortisol, growth hormone), an increase in proinflammatory cytokines (e.g., tumor necrosis factor alpha [TNFα] and interleukin-6 [IL-6]), an increase in plasma FFAs and amino acids, and development of metabolic acidosis (Tilg and

Moschen, 2006; Vick et al, 2008). The ability to maintain normal glucose homeostasis represents a balance between the body's sensitivity to insulin and the amount of insulin secreted by the beta-cell or injected exogenously. With the development of insulin resistance, the need for insulin may exceed the daily injected insulin dose, and this leads to a predisposition for the development of DKA (Fig. 8-3).

Role of Glucose Counterregulatory Hormones

Circulating levels of glucagon, epinephrine, cortisol, and growth hormone are typically markedly increased in humans with DKA, as are plasma FFA and amino acid concentrations (Luzi et al,

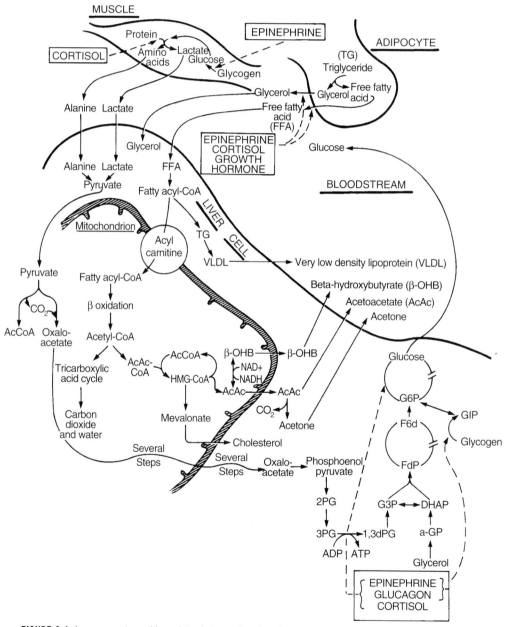

FIGURE 8-1 In response to a wide variety of stress situations (e.g., sepsis, heart failure, and pancreatitis), the body increases its production of the glucoregulatory hormones—insulin, glucagon, epinephrine, cortisol, and growth hormone. In diabetes, the lack of insulin allows the glucogenic effects of the stress hormones to be unopposed in liver, muscle, and adipose tissue. This results in excess ketone formation, fat and muscle breakdown, and a classic catabolic state. *ADP,* Adenosine diphosphate; *ATP,* adenosine triphosphate; *DHAP,* dihydroxyacetone phosphate; *GIP,* gastric inhibitory polypeptide; *HMG,* hydroxymethylglutaryl; *NAD+,* nicotinamide adenine dinucleotide; *NADH,* nicotinamide adenine dinucleotide (reduced form).

1988; Fig. 8-4). Increased circulating concentrations of these counterregulatory hormones cause insulin resistance, stimulate lipolysis and the generation of FFAs in the circulation, and shift hepatic metabolism of FFAs from fat synthesis to fat oxidation and ketogenesis (McGarry et al, 1989; Zammit, 1994). Glucagon is considered the most influential ketogenic hormone. Increased concentrations accompany ketotic states, and low concentrations blunt ketogenesis in ketogenic conditions (Hood and Tannen, 1994). Glucagon can directly influence hepatic ketogenesis. A low insulin-glucagon ratio has a direct effect on the liver that promotes increased production of ketones (Durocher et al, 2008). However, glucagon's effects still depend on substrate availability, and ketogenesis can occur in the absence of glucagon. Catecholamines are

also important modulators of ketogenesis, primarily through stimulation of lipolysis. Both epinephrine and glucagon contribute to insulin resistance by inhibiting insulin-mediated glucose uptake in muscle and by stimulating hepatic glucose production through an augmentation of both glycogenolysis and gluconeogenesis (Cherrington et al, 1987; Cryer, 1993). Cortisol and growth hormone enhance lipolysis in the presence of a relative or absolute deficiency of insulin (see Fig. 8-1), block insulin action in peripheral tissues (Bratusch-Marrain, et al, 1982; Boyle, 1993), and potentiate the stimulating effect of epinephrine and glucagon on hepatic glucose output (Sherwin et al, 1980). An elevation in plasma FFA concentration and FFA oxidation inhibits insulin-mediated glucose uptake in muscle and stimulates hepatic gluconeogenesis (Thiebaud et al, 1982; Ferrannini et al, 1983). The combination of insulin deficiency and excesses in counterregulatory hormones also stimulates protein catabolism. Increased plasma amino acid concentrations impair insulin action in muscle and provide substrate to drive gluconeogenesis (Tessari et al, 1985). The net effect of these hormonal disturbances is accentuation of insulin deficiency through the development of insulin resistance, stimulation of lipolysis leading to ketogenesis, and stimulation of gluconeogenesis, which worsens hyperglycemia. All of these factors lead to the eventual onset of clinical manifestations associated with DKA.

The body increases its production of the glucose counterregulatory hormones in response to a wide variety of diseases and stress situations. Although this response is usually beneficial, in DKA the activity of these hormones as insulin antagonists usually worsens hyperglycemia and ketonemia, provoking acidosis, fluid depletion, and hypotension. This condition progresses in a self-perpetuating spiral of metabolic decompensation (Fig. 8-5). It is rare for the dog or cat with DKA not to have some coexisting disorder, such as pancreatitis, infection, chronic kidney disease, or concurrent hormonal disorder. These disorders have the potential for increasing glucose counterregulatory hormone secretion. For example, infection causes a marked increase in the secretion of cortisol and glucagon, heart failure and trauma result in increased circulating levels of glucagon and catecholamines, and fever induces secretion of glucagon, growth hormone, catecholamines, and cortisol (Kandel and Aberman, 1983; Feldman and Nelson, 1987). The recognition and treatment of disorders that coexist with DKA are critically important for successful management of DKA (see Fig. 8-3).

Physiologic Consequences of Enhanced Ketone Body Production

The physiologic derangements that accompany DKA are a direct result of relative or absolute insulin deficiency, hyperketonemia, and hyperglycemia (Box 8-1). In a short-term situation,

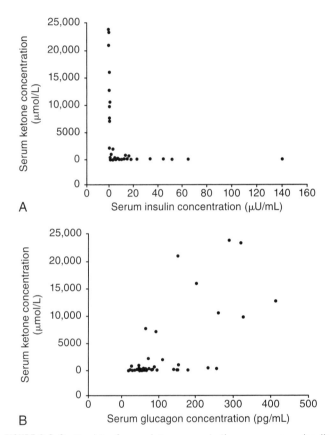

FIGURE 8-2 Scatterplots of serum ketone concentrations versus serum insulin concentration **(A)** and serum glucagon concentration **(B)** in 48 dogs with diabetes mellitus. There was a significant (P < 0.001) linear relationship between serum ketone concentration and serum glucagon concentration. (From Durocher LL, et al.: Acid-base and hormonal abnormalities in dogs with naturally occurring diabetes mellitus, *J Am Vet Med Assoc* 232:1310, 2008.)

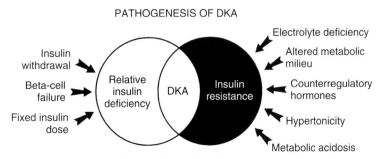

PATHOGENESIS OF DKA

FIGURE 8-3 The pathogenesis of diabetic ketoacidosis *(DKA),* illustrating the interaction of insulin deficiency and insulin resistance necessary in the development of the ketoacidotic state.

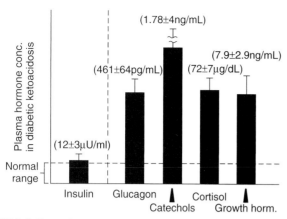

FIGURE 8-4 Plasma insulin and counterregulatory hormone concentrations in diabetic ketoacidosis (DKA) (mean ± standard error of the mean [SEM]). DKA is characterized by relative insulin deficiency and stress hormone excess. Plasma cortisol concentration is characteristically elevated in all humans admitted to the hospital in severe DKA. Although the mean growth hormone concentration also tends to be elevated in ketoacidosis, in many humans this hormone does not become elevated until therapy is begun with insulin and fluids. (Reprinted from Schade DS, et al.: Diabetic ketoacidosis: pathogenesis, prevention, and therapy. In Schade DS, et al, editors: *Diabetic coma,* Albuquerque, 1981, University of New Mexico Press, p. 84.)

the conversion of FFAs to ketone bodies is actually a positive metabolic development. Diabetes mellitus is interpreted physiologically as a state of starvation. With glucose deficiency, ketone bodies can be used as an energy source by many tissues. However, increasing plasma glucose and ketone concentrations eventually surpass the renal tubular threshold for complete reabsorption and spill into the urine, inducing an osmotic diuresis. Each gram of glucose excreted via the kidneys adds a solute load of approximately 6 mOsm. The lower molecular weight of ketones accounts for a greater osmotic load per gram, and excretion of ketones is responsible for one-third to one-half of the osmotic diuresis in humans with DKA (DeFronzo et al, 1994; Kitabchi et al, 2001). The anionic charge on the ketones, even at a maximally acid urine pH, obligates the excretion of positively charged ions (e.g., sodium, potassium, calcium, and magnesium) to maintain electrical neutrality. This increased solute excretion impairs the reabsorption of water throughout the proximal tubule and loop of Henle, lowering the concentration of sodium and chloride in the tubular lumen, creating an increased concentration gradient for their reabsorption, and thereby inhibiting their transport from lumen to blood. The result is an excessive loss of electrolytes and water with depletion of water roughly twice that of solutes, leading to volume contraction, underperfusion of tissues, and hypertonicity of the extracellular fluid (ECF) compartment. Insulin deficiency per se also contributes to the excessive renal losses of water and electrolytes. Physiologic increases in plasma insulin concentration augment salt and water reabsorption in both the proximal and distal portions of the nephron and enhance proximal tubular phosphate reabsorption (DeFronzo et al, 1994). Conversely, insulin deficiency leads to enhanced water and electrolyte excretion.

The formation of ketones by the liver is associated with the production of an equivalent number of hydrogen ions, which titrate the plasma bicarbonate concentration. As ketones continue to accumulate in the blood, the body's buffering system becomes overwhelmed, causing an increase in arterial hydrogen ion concentration, a decrease in serum bicarbonate, and development of metabolic acidosis. Further loss of water and electrolytes occurs

as a result of repeated bouts of vomiting, diarrhea, or both combined with a lack of fluid intake; problems that often develop as the metabolic acidosis worsens (see Fig. 8-5). The excessive loss of electrolytes and water leads to further volume contraction, underperfusion of tissues, decline in the glomerular filtration rate (GFR), and worsening prerenal azotemia and dehydration. Hyperglycemic dogs and cats with reduced GFR lose the ability to excrete glucose and, to a lesser degree, hydrogen ions. Glucose and ketones then accumulate in the vascular space at a more rapid rate. The result is increasing hyperglycemia and ketonemia and worsening metabolic acidosis (see Fig. 8-5). The increase in blood glucose concentration increases plasma osmolality, and the resulting osmotic diuresis further aggravates the increase in plasma osmolality by causing water losses in excess of salt loss. The increase in plasma osmolality causes water to shift out of cells, leading to cellular dehydration and the eventual development of obtundation and coma. The severe metabolic consequences of DKA, which include severe acidosis, obligatory osmotic diuresis, hyperosmolality, dehydration, and electrolyte derangements, ultimately become life-threatening.

SIGNALMENT

DKA is a serious complication of diabetes mellitus that occurs most commonly in dogs and cats with previously undiagnosed diabetes. Less commonly, DKA develops in an insulin-treated diabetic dog or cat that is receiving an inadequate dosage of insulin, which is often in conjunction with a concurrent infectious, inflammatory, or insulin-resistant hormonal disorder. Because of the close association between DKA and newly-diagnosed diabetes mellitus, the signalment for DKA in dogs and cats is similar to that for non-ketotic diabetics (see Chapters 6 and 7). For the most part, DKA appears to be a disease of middle-aged and older dogs and cats, although DKA can be diagnosed at any age. In dogs, DKA is diagnosed more commonly in females, whereas in cats it is more common in males. Any breed of dog or cat can develop DKA.

HISTORY AND PHYSICAL EXAMINATION

The history and findings on physical examination are variable, in part because of the progressive nature of the disorder and the variable time between the onset of DKA and owner recognition of a problem. The spectrum ranges from ketonuric dogs and cats that are otherwise healthy, eating, and have not yet developed metabolic acidosis (i.e., diabetic ketosis [DK]) to ketonuric dogs and cats that have developed severe metabolic acidosis (i.e., DKA), have severe signs of illness, and are moribund.

Polyuria, polydipsia, polyphagia, and weight loss develop initially but are either unnoticed or considered insignificant by the owner. Systemic signs of illness (i.e., lethargy, anorexia, vomiting) ensue as progressive ketonemia and metabolic acidosis develop, the severity of systemic signs being directly related to the severity of metabolic acidosis, hyperosmolality, and dehydration and the nature of concurrent disorders (e.g., pancreatitis, infection) that are often present. The time interval from the onset of initial clinical signs of diabetes to development of systemic signs of illness caused by DKA is unpredictable and ranges from a few days to several months. Once ketoacidosis begins to develop, however, severe illness typically becomes evident within a week.

When a severely ill dog or cat is brought to a veterinarian, the owner may not mention signs that were present prior to those most

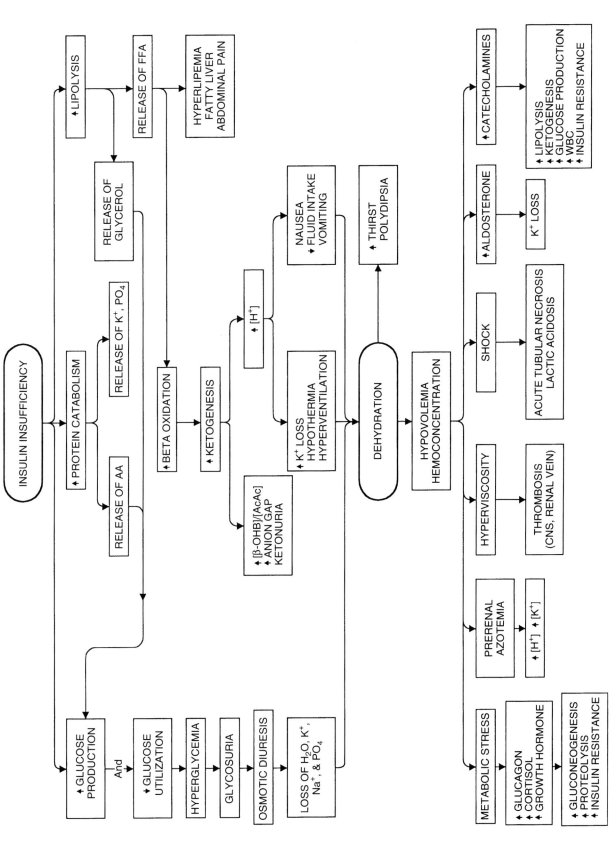

FIGURE 8-5 The interrelationship of the pathophysiologic mechanisms that result in diabetic ketoacidosis (DKA). *AA*, Amino acids; *AcAc*, acetoacetate; *β-OHB*, beta-hydroxybutyrate; *CNS*, central nervous system; *FFAs*, free fatty acids; *K*, potassium; *WBC*, white blood cells.

BOX 8-1   **Pathophysiologic Derangements in Diabetic Ketoacidosis**

Hyperglycemia	Hyperketonemia	Insulin Deficiency
Osmotic diuresis	Osmotic diuresis	Electrolyte and fluid losses
Sodium	Sodium	
Potassium	Potassium	Sodium
Water	Water	Water
Calcium	Calcium	Phosphate
Phosphate	Phosphate	Negative nitrogen balance
Intracellular dehydration	Metabolic acidosis	

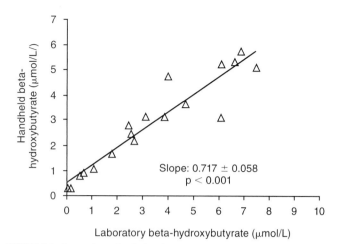

FIGURE 8-6 Comparison of β-hydroxybutyrate measurements using a laboratory-based enzymatic assay and a handheld ketone meter in 16 dogs and 3 cats. (From Hoenig M, et al.: Use of a hand-held meter for the measurement of blood beta-hydroxybutyrate in dogs and cats, *J Vet Emerg Crit Care* 18:86, 2008.)

obvious and worrisome at the moment. If the owner is questioned closely with regard to the past history, the changes noted before severe illness include the classic history for diabetes mellitus (i.e., polyuria, polydipsia, polyphagia, and weight loss). Because of the increased incidence of concurrent diseases, it is imperative that the clinician spend ample time obtaining a careful history concerning all organ systems. Some diseases (e.g., pyometra, kidney failure, and hyperadrenocorticism) have historical signs resembling DKA and can initiate the metabolic derangements leading to DKA in a previously unidentified or insulin-regulated diabetic.

A complete and careful physical examination is critically important in any ketoacidotic animal. The initial physical examination should focus on an evaluation of the status of hydration, on the extent of central nervous system (CNS) depression, and on a careful search for any initiating cause for diabetic decompensation and ultimate ketoacidosis. Diabetic dogs and cats frequently suffer from concurrent infections, pancreatitis, cholangiohepatopathy, kidney disease, cardiac disease, or other insulin-antagonistic disorders (Bruskiewicz et al, 1997; Hume et al, 2006). A careful history, physical examination, and judicious use of laboratory tests can, in most circumstances, identify underlying concurrent disorders, lead to appropriate treatment, and increase the likelihood of a successful outcome.

Common physical examination findings suggestive of DKA include lethargy, dehydration, tachypnea, tachycardia, weakness, and sometimes a strong odor of acetone on the breath. Slow deep breathing (i.e., Kussmaul respiration) may be observed in animals with severe metabolic acidosis. Gastrointestinal tract signs (e.g., vomiting and abdominal pain) are common in dogs and cats with DKA; this is in part because of the common concurrent occurrence of pancreatitis. Other intraabdominal disorders should also be considered and diagnostic tests (e.g., abdominal ultrasound) performed to help identify the cause of the gastrointestinal signs. Additional physical examination findings associated with uncomplicated diabetes mellitus (e.g., hepatomegaly, cataracts, peripheral neuropathy) may also be identified (see Chapters 6 and 7).

ESTABLISHING THE DIAGNOSIS OF DIABETIC KETOSIS AND KETOACIDOSIS

A diagnosis of diabetes mellitus requires the presence of appropriate clinical signs (i.e., polyuria, polydipsia, polyphagia, and weight loss) and documentation of persistent fasting hyperglycemia and glycosuria. Measurement of the blood glucose concentration using a portable blood glucose monitoring device (see Protocol for Generating the Serial Blood Glucose Curve in the Hospital in Chapter 6) and testing for the presence of glycosuria using urine reagent test strips (e.g., Keto-Diastix)

allows the rapid confirmation of diabetes mellitus. The concurrent documentation of ketonuria establishes a diagnosis of DK or ketoacidosis. The subsequent documentation of metabolic acidosis differentiates DKA from DK. Commonly used nitroprusside reagent test strips for ketonuria (e.g., Keto-Diastix, Ketostix) measure only acetoacetate and its byproduct acetone. Beta-hydroxybutyrate has no ketone group and is therefore not detected by conventional nitroprusside tests. Beta-hydroxybutyrate is formed from acetoacetate in the presence of hydrogen ions; the more acidic the diabetic dog or cat is, the more β-hydroxybutyrate is formed. Urine ketone measurements do not reflect the severity of increase in blood β-hydroxybutyrate concentration, may not reflect the severity of the metabolic acidosis, and may be negative for ketones in dogs and cats in the early stages of DK and DKA. If ketonuria is not identified in a dog or cat with suspected DK or DKA, blood should be tested for the presence of β-hydroxybutyrate using a quantitative enzymatic assay or a portable blood glucose and ketone analyzer (e.g., Precision Xtra, Abbott Diagnostics; Fig. 8-6), or plasma from heparinized hematocrit tubes can be used to test for the presence of acetoacetate using urine reagent strips used to document ketonuria (Duarte et al, 2002; Brady et al, 2003; Hoenig et al, 2008; Di Tommaso et al, 2009; Zeugswetter and Pagitz, 2009).

In human diabetics, the predominate ketone body produced during DKA is β-hydroxybutyrate. The β-hydroxybutyrate-to-acetoacetate ratio can range from 3:1 to 20:1 depending on the severity of hypovolemia, tissue hypoxia, and lactic acidosis (Li et al, 1980; Goldstein, 1995). In the presence of circulatory collapse, an increase in lactic acid can shift the redox state to increase β-hydroxybutyrate at the expense of readily detectable acetoacetate. Severe hyperketonemia could be underestimated or even undetected if urine reagent test strips or blood tests that only measure acetoacetate and acetone are used to identify DK or DKA.

The predominate ketone body produced in diabetic dogs and cats is also believed to be β-hydroxybutyrate. Although serum β-hydroxybutyrate concentrations may be mildly increased in sick non-diabetic dogs and cats in a negative energy balance, documenting an increased serum β-hydroxybutyrate concentration in conjunction with hyperglycemia and glycosuria supports a diagnosis of DK or DKA, regardless of dipstick test

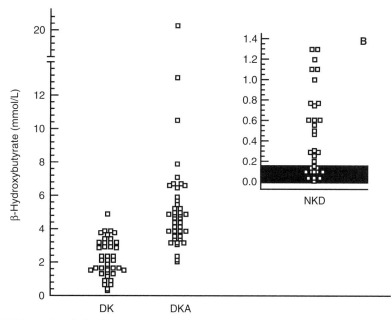

FIGURE 8-7 Serum beta-hydroxybutyrate (β-OHB) concentrations from dogs with diabetic ketoacidosis *(DKA)* and diabetic ketosis *(DK)*. The small plot *(B)* is a graphic depiction of serum β-OHB concentrations from dogs with non-ketotic diabetes mellitus *(NKD)* compared to the reference interval *(shaded area)*. (From Duarte R, et al.: Accuracy of serum β-hydroxybutyrate measurements for the diagnosis of diabetic ketoacidosis in 116 dogs. *J Vet Intern Med* 16:411, 2002.)

results for ketonuria (Di Tommaso et al, 2009; Zeugswetter et al, 2010; Aroch et al, 2012). The magnitude of increase in serum β-hydroxybutyrate concentration correlates with the severity of the metabolic acidosis with the highest concentrations identified in dogs with DKA (Duarte et al, 2002; Fig. 8-7). However, a recent study by Durocher, et al., (2008) suggested that acetoacetate may be the predominate ketone body in some dogs with DKA. Serum β-hydroxybutyrate and total ketone body concentrations were measured in 48 diabetic dogs. As expected, serum β-hydroxybutyrate concentrations were increased in the dogs, but when expressed as a percentage of total serum ketone concentration, serum β-hydroxybutyrate concentration decreased from approximately 60% to 20% as serum total ketone concentration (and presumably acetoacetate concentration) increased (Fig. 8-8). These findings suggest that the predominate ketone body (β-hydroxybutyrate versus acetoacetate) may differ between dogs. Regardless, measurement of β-hydroxybutyrate in blood is indicated whenever DK or DKA is suspected but ketonuria is absent.

In a recent study evaluating plasma and urine ketone measurements using dipstick methodology (Ketostix) in cats with DK and DKA based on increased plasma β-hydroxybutyrate concentrations, positive plasma and urine test results for acetoacetate were found in approximately 46% and 20% of the cats, respectively (Zeugswetter and Pagitz, 2009). The sensitivity of the plasma ketone dipstick test was 100%, and a negative plasma test result reliably excluded DKA, suggesting that the plasma ketone dipstick test may be a useful tool to rule out DKA in cats.

A subsequent study evaluating a hand-held glucose and ketone meter (Precision Xtra, Abbott) for measuring β-hydroxybutyrate in whole blood in diabetic cats showed a good linear correlation with a reference laboratory method at low to moderate β-hydroxybutyrate concentrations (Zeugswetter and Rebuzzi, 2012). Unfortunately, a significant negative bias was identified at high concentrations of β-hydroxybutyrate. Beta-hydroxybutyrate

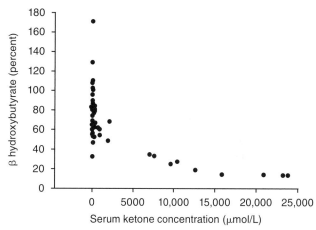

FIGURE 8-8 Scatterplot of serum β-hydroxybutyrate concentration, expressed as a percentage of serum ketone concentration, versus serum ketone concentration in 48 dogs with diabetes mellitus. (From Durocher LL, et al.: Acid-base and hormonal abnormalities in dogs with naturally occurring diabetes mellitus, *J Am Vet Med Assoc* 232:1310, 2008.)

concentrations greater than 2.55 mmol/L had a sensitivity of 94% but a specificity of 68% for diagnosing ketoacidemia. Many cats with high β-hydroxybutyrate concentrations and normal blood pH had an elevated chloride gap suggestive of superimposed hypochloremic metabolic alkalosis. The authors concluded that the ketone meter was a valid tool for excluding DKA in sick diabetic cats and for identifying resolution of ketonemia when treating a DKA cat.

The aggressiveness of the diagnostic evaluation and treatment of a dog or cat with DKA is dictated primarily by results of the history and physical examination. A diagnosis of severe DKA is indicated in dogs and cats with systemic signs of illness (i.e., lethargy, anorexia, and/or vomiting); a physical examination revealing dehydration, depression, weakness, and/or Kussmaul respiration; blood glucose concentration greater than 600 mg/dL (34 mmol/L); and severe metabolic acidosis as diagnosed by a total venous CO_2 or arterial bicarbonate concentration less than 12 mEq/L. History and physical examination findings are subjective, however, and a veterinarian may not be able to obtain quick acid-base information. Therefore, a diagnosis of severe DKA is often initially based on having an *ill* dog or cat with glucose and ketones in the urine. Dogs and cats with severe DKA require hospitalization and immediate initiation of fluid therapy (see Fluid Therapy). Additional diagnostic tests are necessary to care for these animals properly (see the next section), but therapy should proceed while remaining tests are pending.

A tentative diagnosis of DK is reserved for diabetic dogs and cats that are apparently healthy but have both glucose and ketones present in the urine. Systemic signs of illness are absent or mild, serious abnormalities are not readily identifiable on physical examination, and metabolic acidosis has not yet developed or is mild (i.e., total venous CO_2 or arterial bicarbonate concentration greater than 16 mEq/L). Dogs and cats with DK are not in need of immediate aggressive therapy and must be distinguished from the pet with a critical metabolic emergency. The apparently healthy ketotic diabetic can often be managed conservatively, usually without fluid therapy, whereas the animal with severe DKA requires a much more intensive therapeutic plan involving treatments with a variety of contingency alternatives based on numerous assessments of related parameters.

 ## IN-HOSPITAL DIAGNOSTIC EVALUATION

The laboratory evaluation of "healthy" ketotic diabetic dogs and cats is similar to that for non-ketotic diabetics (see Clinical Pathologic Abnormalities in Chapter 6 and Establishing the Diagnosis of Diabetes Mellitus in Chapter 7). The healthy ketotic diabetic can usually be managed conservatively, as contrasted with the needs of an extremely ill DKA pet. Critically important information for formulating the initial treatment protocol in the sick DKA pet include hematocrit and total plasma protein concentration; serum glucose, albumin, creatinine, and urea nitrogen concentrations; serum electrolytes; venous total CO_2 or arterial acid-base evaluation; and urine specific gravity. Abnormalities frequently associated with DKA are listed in Box 8-2. Once treatment for DKA is initiated, additional studies (e.g., a complete blood count [CBC], serum biochemistry panel, urinalysis, urine culture, thoracic radiographs, and abdominal ultrasound) or diagnostic tests for pancreatitis, diestrus in the female dog, and hyperthyroidism in the cat are usually warranted to identify underlying concurrent disorders (Box 8-3).

Urinalysis and Urine Culture

The urinalysis can serve several purposes simultaneously. The most obvious reason for obtaining a urine sample is to identify glycosuria and ketonuria. Urinary tract infection is a common and important contributing factor in DKA. The presence of bacteriuria, hematuria, and pyuria on urinalysis supports the presence of urinary tract infection and the need for culture of a urine sample. If possible, urine should be obtained by cystocentesis. Because of the high incidence of urinary tract infections in our cats and especially

---

BOX 8-2   Common Clinicopathologic Abnormalities Identified in Dogs and Cats with Diabetic Ketoacidosis

Neutrophilic leukocytosis, signs of toxicity if septic
Hemoconcentration
Hyperglycemia
Hypercholesterolemia, lipemia
Increased alkaline phosphatase activity
Increased alanine aminotransferase activity
Increased blood urea nitrogen (BUN) and serum creatinine concentrations
Hyponatremia
Hypochloremia
Hypokalemia
Metabolic acidosis
Hyperosmolality
Glycosuria
Ketonuria
Urinary tract infection

BOX 8-3   Diagnostic Tests for Insulin Resistance in Diabetic Dogs and Cats

Complete blood count (CBC), serum biochemistry panel, and urinalysis
Bacterial culture of the urine
Serum canine/feline pancreatic-specific lipase (SPEC cPL/fPL) (pancreatitis)
Serum trypsin-like immunoreactivity (TLI) (exocrine pancreatic insufficiency)
Adrenocortical function tests
    Urine cortisol-to-creatinine ratio (spontaneous hyperadrenocorticism)
    Low-dose dexamethasone suppression test (spontaneous hyperadrenocorticism)
    Adrenocorticotropic hormone (ACTH)-stimulation test (iatrogenic hyperadrenocorticism)
Thyroid function tests
    Baseline serum total and free thyroxine (hypothyroidism and hyperthyroidism)
    Serum thyroid-stimulating hormone (TSH; hypothyroidism)
Serum progesterone concentration (diestrus in intact female dog)
Fasting serum triglyceride concentration (hyperlipidemia)
Plasma growth hormone or serum insulin-like growth factor-1 (IGF-1) concentration (acromegaly)
Serum insulin concentration 24 hours after discontinuation of insulin therapy (insulin antibodies)
Abdominal ultrasonography (adrenomegaly, adrenal mass, pancreatitis, pancreatic mass, inflammatory bowel disease, neoplasia)
Thoracic radiography (cardiomegaly, neoplasia)
Computed tomography or magnetic resonance imaging (pituitary mass)

From Nelson RW, Couto CG: *Small animal internal medicine*, ed 5, St Louis, 2014, Elsevier/Mosby.

---

dogs with DKA, we routinely culture urine, regardless of findings on urinalysis (Bailiff et al, 2006). Proteinuria may be the result of urinary tract infection or glomerular damage secondary to disruption of the basement membrane. Evaluation of a urine protein-to-creatinine ratio performed on a urine sample void of infection or inflammation can help determine if the proteinuria is significant.

Azotemia is also common in DKA, and evaluation of urine specific gravity from a sample of urine obtained prior to initiation of fluid therapy is helpful in differentiating prerenal azotemia from primary kidney failure. Urine specific gravity must be assessed with the severity of glycosuria and the hydration status of the dog or cat kept in mind. If the animal is clinically dehydrated and has normal kidney function, its urine specific gravity should be greater than 1.030. Urine specific gravities that are less than 1.020 are suggestive of primary kidney disease or concurrent polyuria/polydipsia disorder (e.g., hyperadrenocorticism). Glycosuria will increase the urine specific gravity measured by refractometers and should be considered when interpreting urine specific gravity. As a general rule of thumb, 2% or 4+ glycosuria as measured on urine reagent test strips will increase the urine specific gravity 0.008 to 0.010 when urine specific gravity is measured by refractometry.

Oliguric and anuric kidney failure is an infrequent but grave complication of DKA. Severe hyperglycemia (> 600 mg/dL; 34 mmol/L) is not likely to occur without a significant reduction in the GFR due to primary kidney disease or severe dehydration and poor renal perfusion. It is critical that urine production be closely monitored in the severely ill DKA animal. Although diabetic dogs and cats are prone to develop infection, it is still strongly recommended that the animal with severe DKA and concurrent azotemia have an indwelling urinary catheter secured in the bladder and attached to a closed collection system. The urine volume produced over the initial 12 hours of therapy can be assessed and oliguric or anuric kidney failure quickly recognized. Rapid institution of appropriate measures to improve GFR and urine production can then be initiated. Urine production should increase once dehydration is corrected and normovolemia restored in the dog or cat with severe prerenal azotemia and decreased GFR. Once adequate urine production is confirmed, the indwelling urinary catheter can be removed.

The Minimum Data Base (Ketoacidosis Profile)

Blood Glucose

Although the average blood glucose concentration in dogs and cats with DKA is approximately 500 mg/dL (28 mmol/L), values can range from close to 200 mg/dL (11 mmol/L) to concentrations greater than 1000 mg/dL (56 mmol/L) (Fig. 8-9). Because hepatic production of glucose is excessive in dogs and cats with DKA and relative or absolute deficiencies of insulin always exist, it is likely that the degree of hyperglycemia is determined primarily by the severity of dehydration and corresponding decrease in GFR. Evidence suggests that blood glucose concentrations become extremely elevated (i.e., > 600 mg/dL; 34 mmol/L) only when the ECF volume has decreased to the point that urine flow and the capacity to excrete glucose are impaired. Studies have shown a marked reduction in the blood glucose concentration when humans with DKA were treated solely with fluids (i.e., no insulin) (Owen et al, 1981); these findings have also been seen clinically in diabetic dogs and cats (Fig. 8-10). An association has been made in diabetic humans between the maximum attainable blood glucose concentration and the severity of reduction in GFR (Kandel and Aberman, 1983). The initial blood glucose concentration also dictates, in part, how aggressive the initial fluid and insulin therapy should be. The higher the blood glucose concentration, the higher the plasma osmolality, and the more at-risk the animal is for developing cerebral edema

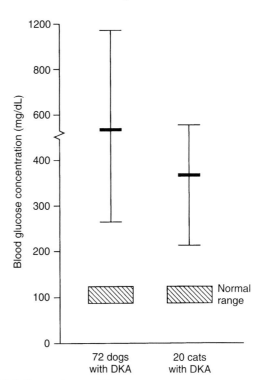

FIGURE 8-9 Mean and range of blood glucose concentration determined at the time diabetic ketoacidosis *(DKA)* was diagnosed in 72 dogs and 20 cats.

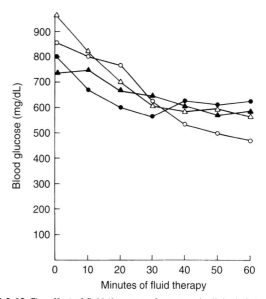

FIGURE 8-10 The effect of fluid therapy on four severely diabetic ketoacidotic dogs over a period of 1 hour, without insulin administration.

following a sudden decrease in plasma osmolality; therefore the rate of blood glucose decline needs to be slower during the initial hours of treatment.

Acid-Base Status

Metabolic acidosis is one of the hallmark clinical pathologic changes in DKA and is the direct result of an excess accumulation of ketone bodies in the blood. Excessive serum ketones can overwhelm the body's buffering system, causing an increase in arterial

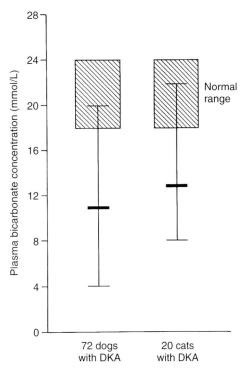

FIGURE 8-11 Mean and range of plasma bicarbonate concentration determined at the time diabetic ketoacidosis *(DKA)* was diagnosed in 72 dogs and 20 cats.

	TABLE 8-1		ARTERIAL pH, PCO_2, AND HCO_3^- IN SIMPLE ACUTE ACID-BASE DISORDERS

CONDITION	pH	ARTERIAL PCO_2	TOTAL VENOUS CO_2*
Acidosis			
Respiratory	↓	↑↑	↑
Metabolic	↓	↓	↓↓
Alkalosis			
Respiratory	↑	↓↓	↓
Metabolic	↑	↑	↑↑

Double arrows indicate primary change; HCO_3^-, bicarbonate ion; PCO_2, partial pressure of carbon dioxide.
*The total venous CO_2 concentration is equal to the arterial bicarbonate concentration.

hydrogen ion concentration, a decrease in serum bicarbonate, and a progressively worsening metabolic acidosis (Fig. 8-11).

Failure of the kidneys to compensate adequately for the acid load in DKA is partly the result of the physicochemical properties of β-hydroxybutyrate and acetoacetate. The renal threshold for these acids is low, and appreciable excretion occurs at plasma concentrations only slightly above normal. Thus, the renal tubules are easily overwhelmed when these acids are synthesized in excessive quantities by the liver. This creates a situation in which the amount of acid present surpasses the renal capacity for urine acidification. Furthermore, β-hydroxybutyrate and acetoacetate are relatively strong acids (pKa 4.70 and 3.58, respectively). Even at the lowest urinary pH, they are excreted mostly as sodium and potassium salts, resulting in the concomitant loss of bicarbonate.

Recognition of acidosis is usually straightforward with the use of arterial blood gas or venous total CO_2 determinations (Table 8-1). In DKA, the severity of changes in arterial blood gas or venous total CO_2 depends on the duration and severity of hyperketonemia at the time of presentation to the veterinarian. Arterial pH can range from 7.2 to as low as 6.6. Dogs and cats with arterial blood pH values less than 7.0 have life-threatening DKA and are often difficult to treat successfully (Hume et al, 2006). A tremendous amount of controversy surrounds therapy directed specifically at the acidosis component of DKA. A discussion on the pros and cons of bicarbonate therapy for animals with severe DKA is found in the Bicarbonate Therapy section later in this chapter.

Serum Sodium Concentration

The serum sodium concentration is a reflection of the relative amounts of water and sodium present in the body. With rare exception, dogs and cats with DKA have significant deficits in total body sodium, regardless of the measured serum concentration. In 72 dogs with DKA, 62% were hyponatremic and only 7% were hypernatremic (Fig. 8-12). Similarly, in 42 cats with

DKA, 80% were hyponatremic and only 5% were hypernatremic (Bruskiewicz et al, 1997).

Hyponatremia results from excessive urinary sodium loss caused by the osmotic diuresis induced by glycosuria and ketonuria. Because insulin enhances renal sodium reabsorption in the distal portion of the nephron, its absence results in sodium wasting. Hyperglucagonemia, vomiting, and diarrhea also contribute to the sodium loss in DKA (Foster and McGarry, 1983).

It is important to consider the severity of hyperglycemia when assessing the severity of hyponatremia in the dog or cat with DKA. Because glucose penetrates cells poorly in the absence of insulin, an increase in ECF glucose concentration creates a transcellular osmotic gradient that results in the movement of water out of the cells, a corresponding reduction in the plasma sodium concentration, and a falsely decreased measured sodium value. In general, for every 100 mg/dL of plasma glucose above the reference range, plasma sodium concentration decreases by approximately 1.6 mEq/L (DiBartola, 2012). Conversely, as insulin therapy drives glucose into the cells, water will follow and the plasma sodium concentration will increase. The measured sodium value should be corrected to a sodium value that accounts for hyperglycemia by using the following formula:

Corrected Na^+ = 1.6 × (measured glucose [mg/dL] − 100)/100 + measured Na^+

This reflects that the measured serum sodium value is decreased by approximately 1.6 mEq for every 100 mg/dL increase in glucose above 100 (Nugent, 2005).

Severe hypertriglyceridemia may occasionally cause factitious hyponatremia. Severe hypertriglyceridemia can be recognized by the presence of gross lipemia on visual inspection of serum or plasma or by the presence of lipemia retinalis on ophthalmoscopic examination and confirmed by measurement of triglyceride concentration in serum or plasma. Physiologic saline and Ringer's solutions have adequate sodium quantities for replacement of sodium deficiencies and are recommended as the initial fluids of choice for the treatment of severe DKA (see Fluid Therapy later in this chapter).

Serum Potassium Concentration

During DKA, intracellular dehydration occurs as hyperglycemia and water loss lead to increased plasma and ECF tonicity and a shift of water out of cells. This shift of water is also associated with a shift of potassium into the extracellular space (Kitabchi et al, 2001; Fig. 8-13). Potassium shifts are further enhanced by

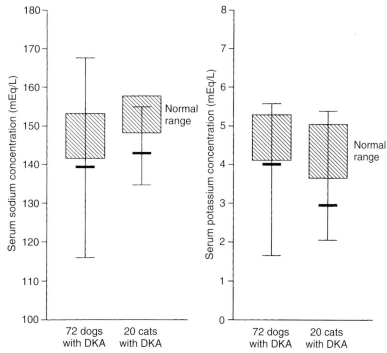

FIGURE 8-12 Mean and range of serum sodium and potassium concentrations determined at the time diabetic ketoacidosis *(DKA)* was diagnosed in 72 dogs and 20 cats.

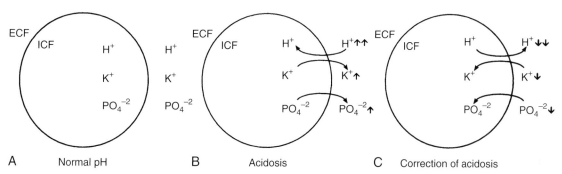

FIGURE 8-13 Redistribution of extracellular fluid *(ECF)* and intracellular fluid *(ICF)* hydrogen, potassium, and phosphate ions in response to a decrease in ECF pH (i.e., acidosis); an increase in ECF glucose and osmolality; and the translocation of water from the ICF to the ECF compartment and subsequent correction of acidosis and the intracellular shift of glucose and electrolytes with insulin treatment. **A,** Normal ECF pH. **B,** ECF H^+ concentration increases during acidosis, causing H^+ to move into cells and down its concentration gradient. Increase in ECF glucose and osmolality causes extracellular shift of water, K^+, and PO_4^{+2}. **C,** ECF H^+ concentration decreases during correction of acidosis, causing H^+ to move out of cells. Insulin administration and correction of acidemia cause an intracellular shift of glucose, K^+, and PO_4^{+2}, decreasing ECF K^+ and PO_4^{+2} concentration.

the presence of acidosis and the breakdown of intracellular protein secondary to insulin deficiency. Entry of potassium into cells is also impaired in the presence of insulinopenia. The osmotic diuresis induced by glycosuria and ketonuria causes marked urinary losses of potassium. Secondary hyperaldosteronism induced by plasma volume contraction, gastrointestinal losses, and decreased dietary intake augment the potassium deficiency (Kitabchi et al, 2001). As a consequence, most dogs and cats with DKA have a net deficit of total body potassium. Serum potassium concentrations can be decreased, normal, or increased, depending on the duration of illness, kidney function, and previous nutritional state of the dog or cat. Most dogs and cats with DKA have either normal or decreased serum potassium concentrations on pretreatment testing (see Fig. 8-12). In 72 dogs and 42 cats with DKA, 43% and 67% were hypokalemic and 10% and 7%

were hyperkalemic, respectively, at the time DKA was diagnosed (Bruskiewicz et al, 1997).

Knowing the serum potassium concentration and status of kidney function is critical when deciding on the aggressiveness of potassium supplementation in the intravenous (IV) fluids. Polyuric DKA animals are predisposed to *severe* hypokalemia, and oliguric/anuric animals are predisposed to *severe* hyperkalemia. Insulin treatment causes a marked translocation of potassium from the ECF to the intracellular fluid (ICF) compartment, which when combined with continuing kidney and gastrointestinal loss, can cause severe hypokalemia during the initial 24 to 48 hours of treatment. DKA dogs and cats that are hypokalemic on initial evaluation require aggressive potassium supplementation to their IV fluids to replace deficits and to prevent worsening hypokalemia (see Monitoring Fluid Therapy later in this chapter).

Blood Urea Nitrogen and Creatinine

The blood urea nitrogen (BUN) and serum creatinine concentrations are commonly elevated in DKA (Fig. 8-14) and are useful indicators of the severity of volume depletion. When evaluated in conjunction with the urine specific gravity and serum calcium and phosphorus concentrations, they can also help to identify concurrent primary kidney failure versus prerenal azotemia. In addition, the initial BUN or serum creatinine concentration can serve as a measure of the success of fluid therapy. A rapidly falling BUN and serum creatinine concentration in an azotemic dog or cat is consistent with proper fluid therapy, good urine output, and prerenal azotemia. The increased BUN and serum creatinine concentration that is slowly declining or static suggests inadequate fluid therapy or primary kidney failure. Serum creatinine concentrations may also be falsely increased due to interference from acetoacetate with some automated creatinine assays (Molitch et al, 1980; Nanji and Campbell, 1981).

Serum Osmolality

Hyperosmolality is a potentially serious development in DKA, one that can have profound effects on CNS function and consciousness. Of all the factors related to stupor or altered consciousness, including the serum levels of glucose, ketones, or arterial pH, the serum osmolality correlates best with the level of consciousness in humans with DKA. "Clouded consciousness" is an extremely subjective finding in humans, making recognition of such a problem guesswork in dogs or cats. Nevertheless, veterinarians and owners can usually recognize "depression" in the dog and cat, and, in our experience, the severity of this sign roughly correlates with the severity of hyperosmolality.

Fortunately, severe hyperosmolality (> 350 mOsm/kg of H_2O) occurs infrequently in dogs and cats with DKA, in part because of the concurrent prevalence of hyponatremia (see Fig. 8-12). Serum sodium concentration and, to a lesser extent, glucose are the primary determinants of *effective* serum osmolality. Cell membranes are permeable to potassium and urea and, as such, these solutes are *ineffective* osmoles. Hyperosmolality, if present, usually resolves with IV isotonic fluid and insulin therapy, albeit correction of the hyperosmolar state must be done slowly to minimize the shift of water from the extracellular to the intracellular compartment.

Many veterinary hospitals, especially those with a large emergency case load, have the necessary equipment to measure serum or plasma osmolality directly. One can calculate the approximate *effective* osmolality of serum or plasma using the following formula:

$$\textit{Effective ECF Osmolality (mOsm/kg)} = 2\,(Na^+) + 0.05\,(\text{glucose [mg/dL]})$$

or

$$= 2\,(Na^+) + \text{glucose (mmol/L)}$$

In an insulin deficient state, the intracellular movement of glucose in insulin-dependent tissues is impaired and the increase in extracellular glucose creates an osmotic gradient between the ECF and ICF compartments. For this reason, glucose is included in calculations of *effective* osmolality. In contrast, potassium and urea remain freely permeable across cell membranes regardless of insulin concentrations and therefore are not included in calculations of *effective* serum osmolality. The approximate normal range for *effective* serum osmolality in the dog and cat is 280 to 300 mOsm/kg.

Anion Gap

The metabolic acidosis stemming from hyperketonemia is an anion gap acidosis, which must be differentiated from other causes of anion gap acidosis (e.g., lactic acidosis, kidney failure, and/or ethylene glycol intoxication) and from hyperchloremic acidosis (Narins et al, 1994). The anion gap is calculated by subtracting the negatively charged anions, chloride and bicarbonate, from the most important positively charged cations, sodium and potassium. The normal anion gap for dogs and cats is 12 to 16 mEq/L (Feldman and Rosenberg, 1981). Anything greater than 16 mEq/L indicates the presence of an anion gap acidosis. The

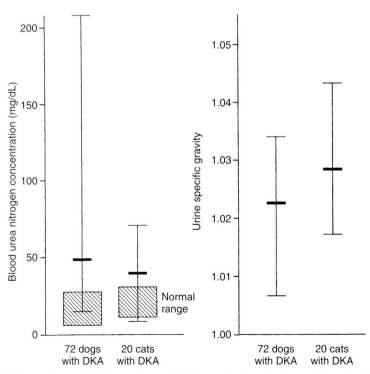

FIGURE 8-14 Mean and range of blood urea nitrogen (BUN) concentration and urine specific gravity determined at the time diabetic ketoacidosis *(DKA)* was diagnosed in 72 dogs and 20 cats.

unmeasured anions that comprise the normal anion gap include albumin and other circulating proteins, sulfate, phosphate, lactate, and a variety of organic acids.

The typical diabetic dog or cat in ketoacidosis has an anion gap that ranges from 20 to 35 mEq/L, and the increment in the anion gap above baseline approximates the decrement in serum bicarbonate concentration (Adrogué et al, 1982). A number of factors can disrupt the normal stoichiometry between acid retention, increment in the anion gap, and decrease in serum bicarbonate concentration (Box 8-4). Such disruption is common in DKA because urinary loss of ketoanions causes a disproportionately greater decrease in serum bicarbonate concentration compared with the increment in anion gap. In these cases, chloride replaces the missing ketoanion, and a component of hyperchloremic acidosis commonly accompanies the anion gap acidosis (Adrogué et al, 1982; 1984; Table 8-2). Dogs and cats that are volume contracted tend to have a pure anion gap acidosis, because the decrease in GFR and tubular avidity for sodium reabsorption limit the urinary loss of ketone bodies. Conversely, animals with DKA able to maintain salt and water intake avoid severe volume depletion. These animals have variable degrees of hyperchloremic acidosis due to the urinary excretion of ketone salts and a concomitant retention of chloride (see Table 8-2).

Completing the Data Base

Complete Blood Count

The CBC in uncomplicated DKA usually reveals a neutrophilic leukocytosis without evidence of toxic neutrophils (Bruskiewicz

---

BOX 8-4	Influences of Common Metabolic Disorders on the Calculated Anion Gap*

Increased Anion Gap
Diabetic ketoacidosis (DKA)
Lactic acidosis
    Tissue ischemia and/or hypoxemia
    Sepsis
    Malignancy
    Drugs
Uremic acidosis
Ethylene glycol intoxication
Salicylate intoxication

Normal Anion Gap
Diarrhea
Renal tubular acidosis
Hypoadrenocorticism
Hyperchloremic acidosis
Ammonium chloride
Carbonic anhydrase inhibitors

*These disorders are frequently associated with metabolic acidosis.

---

et al, 1997; Hume et al, 2006). The leukocytosis may occur secondary to the release of "stress" hormones or severe inflammation, especially if an underlying pancreatitis is present. White blood cell counts greater than 30,000/μL, the presence of toxic or degenerative neutrophils, or a significant left shift toward immaturity of the cells supports the presence of a severe inflammatory and/or infectious process as the cause of the leukocytosis. The red blood cell count and hematocrit should be consistent with hemoconcentration secondary to dehydration. A hematocrit below 35% in these typically volume-contracted animals should arouse suspicion that blood loss has occurred or that significant bone marrow suppression or another problem has resulted in anemia.

Liver Enzymes and Total Bilirubin

Clinical pathologic abnormalities associated with the liver are common in dogs and cats with DKA and are usually caused by hepatic lipidosis, pancreatitis, severe acidosis, hypovolemia, hypoxia, sepsis, and, less commonly, extrahepatic biliary obstruction caused by acute severe pancreatitis, acute and chronic hepatitis, and cholangiohepatitis. Serum alanine aminotransferase (ALT), aspartate aminotransferase (AST), and/or alkaline phosphatase (ALP) are usually increased, even in a non-ketotic diabetic animal. A more worrisome hepatopathy and/or acute severe pancreatitis should be suspected when icterus, a marked increase in serum liver enzyme activities (higher than expected with hepatic lipidosis), or abnormalities involving endogenous liver function tests (e.g., hypoalbuminemia, hypocholesterolemia, increased bile acids) are identified. Acute and chronic hepatitis and cholangiohepatitis should also be considered in diabetic dogs and cats with persistent lethargy and anorexia despite correction of the metabolic derangements associated with DKA. Hepatitis and cholangiohepatitis often occur in conjunction with pancreatitis. When appropriate, abdominal ultrasound and histologic evaluation of a liver biopsy specimen may be indicated to establish concurrent liver disease.

Pancreatic Enzymes

Because acute and chronic pancreatitis is so common in dogs and cats with DKA, a diagnostic evaluation for its existence is always warranted (Bruskiewicz et al, 1997; Hume et al, 2006). In our experience, abdominal ultrasound is the single best diagnostic test for identifying acute and chronic pancreatitis in the dog or cat with DKA (Fig. 8-15); however, results are equipment and operator dependent. Blood tests to assess for the presence of pancreatitis should also be considered in the newly-diagnosed diabetic dog or cat with DKA and in dogs or cats with recurring bouts of DKA, especially if abdominal ultrasound is not available. Measurement of canine and feline pancreatic-specific lipase (SPEC cPL and SPEC fPL) is currently the blood test of choice for identifying pancreatitis (Forman et al, 2004; Trivedi et al, 2011; McCord et al, 2012). Preliminary studies evaluating a less expensive novel catalytic assay for colorimetric determination of serum

---

TABLE 8-2	EXAMPLES OF SERUM ELECTROLYTE CONCENTRATIONS AND THEIR ASSOCIATED ANION GAPS IN ACIDOSIS

	SODIUM (mEq/L)	POTASSIUM (mEq/L)	CHLORIDE (mEq/L)	BICARBONATE (mEq/L)	ANION GAP* (mEq/L)
Normal	142	4	108	22	12
Hyperchloremic acidosis	142	4	118	12	12
Anion gap acidosis	142	4	108	12	22

*Anion gap = (Na + K) − (Cl + bicarbonate); the normal anion gap is 12 to 16 mEq/L.

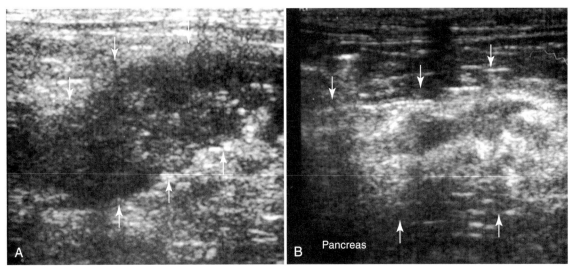

FIGURE 8-15 Abdominal ultrasound images of the pancreas *(arrows)* in a 10-year-old, spayed female Calico cat diagnosed with severe diabetic ketoacidosis (DKA) and acute pancreatitis. At presentation **(A)**, the pancreas was enlarged and diffusely hypoechoic. On the fifth day of treatment **(B)**, the pancreas was enlarged with a mixed echogenic pattern characterized by a hypoechoic center and a hyperechoic periphery, changes consistent with resolving pancreatitis. The cat underwent diabetic remission 5 weeks after discharge but was euthanized 2 years later because of reoccurring bouts of pancreatitis and insulin-requiring diabetes.

lipase activity in dogs and cats found substantial agreement with SPEC cPL and SPEC fPL results from the same blood samples, suggesting that the novel catalytic assay may offer a cost-effective alternative diagnostic test for pancreatitis in dogs and cats (Graca et al, 2005; Oppliger et al, 2013). Sensitivity and specificity of SPEC cPL and SPEC fPL varies between studies and is dependent on the severity of pancreatitis and the cutoff value (200 versus 400 μg/L in dogs; 6.8 versus 10 μg/L in cats) used to differentiate normal from pancreatitis (McCord et al, 2012; Bostrom et al, 2013). Serum SPEC cPL and SPEC fPL concentrations can be increased in dogs and cats with a histologically confirmed normal pancreas and normal in dogs and cats with histologically confirmed inflammation of the pancreas, especially when the inflammatory process is chronic and mild (Forman et al, 2004; McCord et al, 2012). Interpretation of serum SPEC cPL and SPEC fPL results should always be done in context with the history, physical examination, and additional findings on laboratory tests. Recognition of concurrent pancreatitis in the dog or cat with DKA has important implications regarding initial fluid therapy, subsequent dietary therapy, and prognosis. Fortunately, fluid therapy is the cornerstone of treatment for both DKA and pancreatitis.

Calcium and Phosphorus

The serum calcium and phosphorus concentrations are usually normal in the diabetic dog or cat with "uncomplicated" DKA. If concurrent primary kidney failure is present, the serum calcium concentration is typically normal, whereas the serum phosphorus concentration is increased. Hypocalcemia may occur in dogs and cats with concurrent pancreatitis, hypomagnesemia, or hypoproteinemia. The hypocalcemia is usually mild and does not require treatment per se. Hypercalcemia supports the existence of concurrent disease affiliated with the development of hypercalcemia (see Chapter 15).

Attention has been directed to serum phosphorus concentrations in dogs and cats with DKA, especially during the initial 24 hours of treatment. Phosphate, along with potassium, shifts from the intracellular to the extracellular compartment in response

to hyperglycemia and hyperosmolality (Kitabchi et al, 2001; see Fig. 8-13). Osmotic diuresis subsequently leads to enhanced urinary phosphate loss. Serum phosphorus concentrations can be decreased, normal, or increased, depending on the duration of illness and kidney function. Most dogs and cats with DKA have either normal or decreased serum phosphorus concentrations on pretreatment testing. Hypophosphatemia (< 3.0 mg/dL) was identified at initial presentation in 24% of 72 dogs and 48% of 42 cats with DKA (Bruskiewicz et al, 1997). In contrast, hyperphosphatemia (> 6.0 mg/dL) was identified in 14% and 26% of DKA dogs and cats, respectively, and usually occurred in conjunction with kidney failure.

Insulin treatment causes a marked translocation of phosphorus from the ECF to the ICF compartment. Within 24 hours of initiating treatment for DKA, serum phosphorus concentration can decline to severe levels (i.e., < 1 mg/dL) as a result of the dilutional effects of fluid therapy, the intracellular shift of phosphorus following the initiation of insulin therapy, and continuing kidney and gastrointestinal loss (Willard et al, 1987). Clinical signs usually do not develop until the serum phosphorus concentration is less than 1.5 mg/dL, and even at these low levels many dogs and cats remain asymptomatic. Hypophosphatemia primarily affects the hematologic and neuromuscular systems in the dog and cat (Forrester and Moreland, 1989). Hemolytic anemia is the most common and serious sequela to hypophosphatemia. Hypophosphatemia may decrease erythrocyte concentration of adenosine triphosphate (ATP) and/or alter red blood cell membrane lipids, which increases erythrocyte fragility, leading to hemolysis (Shilo et al, 1985; Adams et al, 1993). Hemolysis is usually not identified until the serum phosphorus concentration is 1 mg/dL or less. Hemolytic anemia can be life threatening if not recognized and treated. Neuromuscular signs include weakness, ataxia, and seizures, as well as anorexia and vomiting secondary to intestinal ileus. Phosphate therapy is indicated if clinical signs or hemolysis are identified or if the serum phosphorus concentration is less than 1.5 mg/dL, especially if a further decrease is possible (see Phosphate Supplementation).

Magnesium

The osmotic diuresis of DKA may cause significant urinary losses of magnesium and the development of hypomagnesemia (serum total magnesium concentration < 1.5 mg/dL; serum ionized magnesium concentration measured by ion-selective electrode < 1.0 mg/dL; Norris et al, 1999a; Fincham et al, 2004). In addition, the nature of the translocation of magnesium between the ICF and ECF compartments is similar to potassium in that factors that promote a shift of potassium into the ICF compartment (e.g., alkalosis, insulin, and/or glucose infusion) promote a similar shift in magnesium. During therapy for DKA, the serum total and ionized magnesium concentration can decline to severely low levels (i.e., less than 1 mg/dL and 0.5 mg/dL, respectively) as a result of the dilutional effects of fluid therapy and the intracellular shift of magnesium after the initiation of insulin therapy (Norris et al, 1999a; Hume et al, 2006). Clinical signs of hypomagnesemia do not usually occur until the serum total magnesium concentration is less than 1.0 mg/dL, and even at these low levels, many animals remain asymptomatic.

A magnesium deficiency can result in several nonspecific clinical signs, including lethargy, anorexia, muscle weakness (including dysphagia and dyspnea), muscle fasciculations, seizures, ataxia, and coma (Abbott and Rude, 1993; Martin et al, 1993; Dhupa and Proulx, 1998). Concurrent hypokalemia, hyponatremia, and hypocalcemia occur in animals with hypomagnesemia, although the prevalence of these electrolyte abnormalities may differ between species. These electrolyte abnormalities may also contribute to the development of clinical signs. Magnesium is a cofactor for all enzyme reactions that involve ATP, most notably the sodium-potassium ATPase pump. Deficiencies in magnesium may cause potassium-losing nephropathy and potassium wastage from the body and the resultant hypokalemia may be refractory to appropriate potassium replacement therapy. Magnesium deficiency may inhibit parathyroid hormone (PTH) secretion from the parathyroid gland, resulting in hypocalcemia (Bush et al, 2001). Magnesium deficiency causes the resting membrane potential of myocardial cells to be decreased and leads to increased Purkinje fiber excitability, with the consequent generation of arrhythmias (Abbott and Rude, 1993). Electrocardiographic changes include a prolonged PR interval, widened QRS complex, depressed ST segment, and peaked T waves. Cardiac arrhythmias associated with magnesium deficiency include atrial fibrillation, supraventricular tachycardia, ventricular tachycardia, and ventricular fibrillation. Hypomagnesemia also predisposes animals to digitalis-induced arrhythmias.

Unfortunately, assessing an animal's magnesium status is problematic because there is no simple, rapid, and accurate laboratory test to gauge total body magnesium status. Serum total magnesium represents 1% of the body's magnesium stores, and serum ionized magnesium represents 0.2% to 0.3% of total body magnesium stores. As a result, serum total and ionized magnesium concentrations do not always reflect total body magnesium status. A normal serum magnesium concentration may exist despite an intracellular magnesium deficiency. However, a low serum magnesium concentration would support the presence of a total body magnesium deficiency, especially when clinical signs or concurrent electrolyte abnormalities are consistent with hypomagnesemia. Magnesium exists in three distinct forms in serum: an ionized fraction, an anion-complexed fraction, and a protein-bound fraction. A serum ionized magnesium concentration determined using an ion-selective electrode more accurately assesses total body magnesium content than measurement of serum total magnesium and is recommended (Norris et al, 1999b). Fortunately, hypomagnesemia is not usually a clinically recognizable problem

---

BOX 8-5 Electrocardiographic Alterations Associated with Hypokalemia and Hyperkalemia in the Dog and Cat

Hypokalemia
Depressed T-wave amplitude
Depressed ST segment
Prolonged QT interval
Prominent U wave
Arrhythmias
  Supraventricular
  Ventricular

Hyperkalemia
Spiked T waves
Flattened P waves
Prolonged PR interval
Prolonged QRS interval
Decreased R-wave amplitude
Bradycardia
Complete heart block
Ventricular arrhythmias
Cardiac arrest

---

during management of DKA, and magnesium supplementation is not recommended unless hypomagnesemia is documented in dogs and cats with complications that have been associated with hypomagnesemia (e.g., persistent lethargy and anorexia; refractory hypokalemia, hypocalcemia, or both).

Diagnostic Imaging

Concurrent disorders (e.g., acute or chronic pancreatitis, pyometra, cholangiohepatitis, heart failure, bacterial pneumonia, and concurrent endocrinopathies) are common in dogs and cats with DKA. Many of these disorders actually perpetuate the metabolic derangements of DKA. Successful treatment of DKA requires recognition and treatment of these concurrent disorders. Abdominal and thoracic radiographs as well as abdominal ultrasonography are invaluable in confirming problems suspected after a review of the history and physical examination and in identifying problems previously unsuspected. In our hospital, thoracic radiography and abdominal ultrasonography are routine components of the diagnostic evaluation of any sick DKA dog or cat. However, radiographs and ultrasound scans are not usually obtained until more critical laboratory data (i.e., the *ketoacidotic profile*) have been analyzed and appropriate treatment for DKA initiated.

Electrocardiogram

The electrocardiogram (ECG) can be used to document and characterize suspected cardiac arrhythmias and for monitoring changes in serum potassium concentration during treatment of DKA. Use of the ECG is especially helpful for recognizing severe hypokalemia or hyperkalemia in hospitals where frequent monitoring of the serum potassium concentration is difficult because of lack of a point-of-care chemistry analyzer or because of economic constraints. The primary concern prior to and during treatment of DKA is hypokalemia. It must be emphasized that hypokalemia usually causes *subtle* changes in the ECG, especially when the serum potassium concentration is above 3.0 mEq/L (Box 8-5; Fig. 8-16). Changes in the ECG are more obvious when the serum potassium concentration is between 2.5 and 3.0 mEq/L, and alterations invariably occur with serum potassium levels below 2.5 mEq/L.

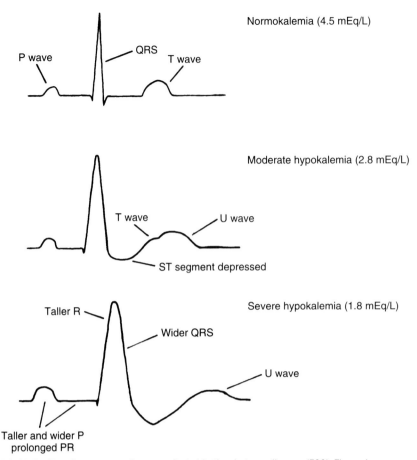

Normokalemia (4.5 mEq/L)

P wave   QRS   T wave

Moderate hypokalemia (2.8 mEq/L)

T wave   U wave

ST segment depressed

Severe hypokalemia (1.8 mEq/L)

Taller R   Wider QRS

U wave

Taller and wider P
prolonged PR

FIGURE 8-16 Profiles of serum potassium are reflected in the electrocardiogram (ECG). These changes are exaggerated here for illustration purposes. In practice, these changes can be quite subtle, indicating the necessity of a baseline ECG with simultaneous laboratory serum potassium.

The basic electrophysiologic alteration with hypokalemia is a gradual shift of the repolarization wave away from systole into diastole. The most consistent change on the ECG is prolongation of the QT interval. Additional findings include a progressive sagging of the ST segment, a decreased amplitude of the T wave, and a repolarization wave occurring after the T wave (U wave). In advanced hypokalemia, the amplitude and duration of the QRS complex are increased. It is believed that the QRS complex widens diffusely secondary to a generalized slowing of conduction in the ventricular myocardium or Purkinje fibers. The amplitude and the duration of the P wave increase, and the PR interval is slightly prolonged with hypokalemia. Atrial and ventricular premature contractions may also occur.

A complete description of the ECG findings in hyperkalemia is available in Chapter 12.

 ### TREATMENT OF "HEALTHY" DOGS AND CATS WITH DIABETIC KETOSIS

Diabetic dogs and cats that have ketonuria but not metabolic acidosis (i.e., DK) are often relatively healthy aside from the typical clinical signs of uncontrolled diabetes mellitus. DK may be identified in newly-diagnosed diabetic dogs and cats or in diabetic dogs and cats that are being treated with insulin. Identification of ketonuria in insulin-treated diabetic dogs and cats indicates that insulin treatment has become ineffective, usually because of a problem with the insulin treatment regimen, development of a concurrent disorder causing insulin resistance, or both. Critical evaluation of

the insulin treatment regimen and evaluation for concurrent disorders should be undertaken. If systemic signs of illness are absent or mild, inappetence is not present, serious abnormalities are not readily identifiable on physical examination, and metabolic acidosis is mild (i.e., total venous CO_2 or arterial bicarbonate concentration greater than 16 mEq/L), short-acting regular crystalline insulin can be administered subcutaneously three times daily until the ketonuria and ketonemia resolves. Fluid therapy and intensive care are usually not needed. Because regular crystalline insulin is potent insulin, the initial dosage (0.1 to 0.2 U/kg/injection) is lower than that recommended for longer-acting insulin preparations. To minimize hypoglycemia, the dog or cat should be fed one-third of its daily caloric intake at the time of each insulin injection. Subsequent adjustments in the insulin dose are based on clinical response and results of blood glucose measurements. Urine ketone concentrations should be monitored and, if available, blood glucose and β-hydroxybutyrate concentrations using a portable glucose and ketone meter (e.g., Precision Xtra, Abbott). A decrease in the blood glucose concentration implies a decrease in ketone production. This, in combination with metabolism of ketones and loss of ketones in urine, will usually correct ketosis within 48 to 96 hours of initiating insulin therapy. Prolonged ketonemia and ketonuria is suggestive of a significant concurrent illness (e.g., chronic pancreatitis) or inadequate blood insulin concentrations to suppress lipolysis and ketogenesis. Once the ketosis has resolved, insulin therapy may be initiated using longer-acting insulin preparations (see Chapters 6 and 7). As a general rule of thumb, the initial dosage of the longer-acting insulin preparation

---

BOX 8-6   Initial Management of the Dog or Cat with Severe Diabetic Ketoacidosis

Fluid Therapy

Type: 0.9% saline solution if hyponatremia is severe (< 130 mEq/L); isotonic crystalloid solution, such as Ringer's, lactated Ringer's solution, Plasma-Lyte 148¹ or Normosol-R if serum sodium concentration ≥ 130 mEq/L

Rate: 60 to 100 mL/kg/24 hours initially; adjust based on hydration status, urine output, persistence of fluid losses

Potassium supplement: Based on serum K⁺ concentration (see Table 8-4); if unknown, initially add 40 mEq KCl to each liter of fluids

Phosphate supplement: Administer if serum phosphorus concentration < 1.5 mg/dL; initial IV infusion rate is 0.01 to 0.03 mmol phosphate/kg/hour in calcium-free IV fluids

Dextrose supplement: Not indicated until blood glucose concentration is less than 250 mg/dL (14 mmol/L), then begin 5% dextrose infusion

Bicarbonate Therapy

Indication: Administer if plasma bicarbonate concentration is less than 12 mEq/L or total venous CO_2 concentration is less than 12 mmol/L; if not known, do not administer unless animal is severely ill and then only once

Amount: mEq HCO_3^- = body weight (kg) × 0.4 × (12 − animals HCO_3^-) × 0.5; if animal's HCO_3^- or total CO_2 concentration is unknown, use 10 in place of (12 − animal's HCO_3^-)

Administration: Add to IV fluids and give over 6 hours; do not give as bolus infusion

Retreatment: Only if plasma bicarbonate concentration remains less than 12 mEq/L after 6 hours of therapy

Insulin Therapy

Type: Regular crystalline insulin

Administration technique:

Intermittent IM technique: Initial dose, 0.1 to 0.2 U/kg IM; then 0.1 U/kg IM hourly until blood glucose concentration is less than 250 mg/dL (14 mmol/L), then switch to IM regular insulin every 4 to 6 hours or SC regular insulin every 6 to 8 hours

Low-dose IV infusion technique: To prepare infusion, add 2.2 U/kg (dogs) or 1.1 U/kg (cats) of regular insulin to 250 mL of 0.9% saline; run 50 mL through the drip set and discard; then administer via infusion or syringe pump through a line separate from that used for fluid therapy at an initial rate of 10 mL/hr; adjust infusion rate according to hourly blood glucose measurements; switch to SC regular insulin every 6 to 8 hours once blood glucose is less than 250 mg/dL or continue insulin infusion at a decreased rate to prevent hypoglycemia until the IV insulin preparation is exchanged for a longer-acting preparation

Goal: Gradual decline in blood glucose concentration, preferably around 50 mg/dL/hr (2.8 mmol/L/hr) until concentration is less than 250 mg/dL (14 mmol/L)

Ancillary Therapy

Concurrent pancreatitis is common in DKA; nothing by mouth and intensive fluid therapy usually indicated

Concurrent infections are common in DKA; use of broad-spectrum, parenteral antibiotics usually indicated

Additional therapy may be needed, depending on nature of concurrent disorders

Patient Monitoring

Blood glucose measurement every 1 to 2 hours initially; adjust insulin therapy and begin dextrose infusion when decreases below 250 mg/dL (14 mmol/L)

Hydration status, respiration, pulse every 2 to 4 hours; adjust fluids accordingly

Serum electrolyte and total venous CO_2 concentrations every 4 to 8 hours; adjust fluid and bicarbonate therapy accordingly

Urine output, glycosuria, urine and plasma ketones every 4 to 8 hours; adjust fluid therapy accordingly

Body weight, packed cell volume, temperature, and blood pressure every 6 to 8 hours

Additional monitoring, depending on concurrent disease

DKA, Diabetic ketoacidosis; *IM*, intramuscular; *IV*, intravenous; *SC*, subcutaneous.

---

is approximately the same as the dosage of regular crystalline insulin being administered at the time the switch in insulin is made with subsequent adjustments in the dosage based on the animal's response to the insulin.

 TREATMENT OF SICK DOGS AND CATS WITH DIABETIC KETOACIDOSIS

Intensive therapy is called for if the dog or cat has systemic signs of illness (e.g., lethargy, anorexia, and/or vomiting); physical examination reveals dehydration, depression, weakness, or a combination of these; or metabolic acidosis is severe (i.e., total venous CO_2 or arterial bicarbonate concentration less than 12 mEq/L). The five goals of treatment of a severely ill diabetic dog or cat with ketoacidosis are (1) to restore water and electrolyte losses; (2) to provide adequate amounts of insulin to suppress lipolysis, ketogenesis, and hepatic gluconeogenesis; (3) to correct acidosis; (4) to identify the factors precipitating the present illness; and (5) to provide a carbohydrate substrate (i.e., dextrose) when necessary to allow continued administration of insulin without causing hypoglycemia (Box 8-6). Proper therapy does not mean forcing a return to a normal state as rapidly as possible. Because osmotic and biochemical problems can arise as a result of overly aggressive therapy as well as from the disease itself, rapid changes in various vital parameters can be as harmful as, or more harmful than, no

change. If all abnormal parameters can be slowly returned toward normal over a period of 24 to 48 hours, therapy is more likely to be successful.

Fluid Therapy

Fig. 8-17 shows a flowchart for fluid therapy.

Composition and Rate of Administration

Initiation of appropriate fluid therapy should be the first step in the treatment of DKA, and in most cases it should precede the initiation of insulin therapy by 2 hours or longer to minimize the development of complications affiliated with insulin administration (see Monitoring and Complications of Therapy). Replacement of fluid deficiencies and maintenance of normal fluid balance are critical to ensure adequate cardiac output, blood pressure, and blood flow to all tissues. Improvement of renal blood flow is especially critical. In addition to the general beneficial aspects of fluid therapy in any dehydrated animal, fluid therapy can correct the deficiency in total body sodium and potassium, dampen the potassium-lowering effect of insulin treatment, and lower the blood glucose concentration in diabetics, even in the absence of insulin administration (see Fig. 8-10). Fluids enhance glucose excretion by increasing glomerular filtration and urine flow, and they decrease secretion of the diabetogenic hormones

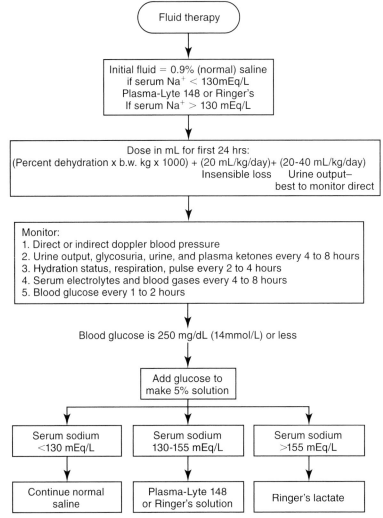

FIGURE 8-17 Intravenous (IV) fluid treatment plans for the dog or cat in diabetic ketoacidosis (DKA).

that stimulate hyperglycemia. The gradual decline in blood glucose combined with replacement of sodium for glucose in the ECF helps minimize the intracellular shift of water caused by a rapid decrease in ECF osmolality, thereby preventing cerebral edema (see Central Nervous System Signs [Cerebral Edema] under Monitoring and Complications of Therapy). Unfortunately, fluid therapy alone does not suppress ketogenesis (Foster and McGarry, 1983; Lebovitz, 1995). For this reason, insulin is always required to resolve the ketoacidotic state.

The type of parenteral fluid initially used depends on the animal's electrolyte status, blood glucose concentration, and osmolality. With rare exceptions, all dogs and cats with DKA have significant deficits in total body sodium, regardless of the measured serum concentration (see Serum Sodium Concentration earlier). Ringer's solution or Plasma-Lyte 148 (Baxter Healthcare Corp.) can be used for mild hyponatremia (serum sodium concentration of more than 130 mEq/L) and 0.9% (physiologic) saline solution for more severe hyponatremia (serum sodium concentration of less than 130 mEq/L) with appropriate potassium supplementation (see Fig. 8-17). Alternative isotonic crystalloid solutions that could be used include lactated Ringer's solution and Normosol-R (Abbott Laboratories). Each of these solutions has a slightly different electrolyte composition; none contain as much sodium as 0.9% saline (Table 8-3). Lactated Ringer's solution contains

lactate, and Plasma-Lyte 148 and Normosol-R contain acetate. Lactate and acetate are metabolized to bicarbonate. A theoretical contraindication for the use of crystalloid solutions that contain lactate centers on the increase in serum lactate concentration that could occur with use of these fluids. Lactate is metabolized in the liver in a similar manner as ketones, and hyperketonemia could reduce hepatic lactate metabolism. As such, administration of fluids containing lactate could increase lactate concentrations in the circulation and, because lactate is a negatively charged ion, promote further sodium and potassium loss in the urine as lactate is excreted (Macintire, 1995). However, in our experience, use of lactated Ringer's solution has not had a recognizable deleterious impact on development of complications or resolution of DKA in dogs and cats. Lactated Ringer's solution can be used in lieu of 0.9% saline to minimize the chloride load in animals that develop hyperchloremic acidosis during treatment of DKA.

Most dogs and cats with severe DKA usually are sodium depleted and therefore not suffering from dramatic hyperosmolality. Hypotonic fluids (e.g., 0.45% saline) are rarely indicated in dogs and cats with DKA, even when severe hyperosmolality is present. Hypotonic fluids do not provide adequate amounts of sodium to correct the sodium deficiency, restore normal fluid balance, or stabilize blood pressure. Rapid administration of hypotonic fluids can also cause a rapid decrease in the osmolality of

TABLE 8-3 ELECTROLYTE COMPOSITION OF COMMERCIALLY AVAILABLE FLUIDS

FLUID	NA+ (mEq/L)	CL− (mEq/L)	K+ (mEq/L)	GLUCOSE (g/L)	BUFFER* (mEq/L)	OSMOLARITY (mOsm/L)
0.9% saline†	154	154	0	0	0	308
0.45% saline†	77	77	0	0	0	154
Ringer's solution†	147	156	4	0	0	310
Lactated Ringer's solution†	130	109	4	0	28 (L)	272
Plasma-Lyte 148†	140	98	5	0	27 (A)	295
Normosol-R‡	140	98	5	0	27 (A)	296
Normosol-M‡	40	40	13	0	16 (A)	112
Plasma-Lyte 56†	40	40	13	0	16 (A)	110
5% dextrose in water†	0	0	0	50	0	252

*Buffers used: A, acetate; L, lactate.
†Baxter Healthcare Corp., Deerfield, IL.
‡Abbott Laboratories, Chicago, IL.

ECF, which may result in cerebral edema, deterioration in mentation, and eventually coma (see Monitoring and Complications of Therapy). Hyperosmolality is best treated with isotonic fluids and the judicious administration of insulin.

The initial volume and rate of fluid administration are determined by assessing the degree of shock, the dehydration deficit, the animal's maintenance requirements, plasma protein concentration, and presence or absence of cardiac disease. Fluid administration should be directed at gradually replacing hydration deficits over 24 hours while also supplying maintenance fluid needs and matching ongoing losses. Rapid replacement of fluids is rarely indicated unless the dog or cat is in shock. Once out of this critical phase, fluid replacement should be decreased in an effort to correct the fluid imbalance in a slow but steady manner. As a general rule of thumb, a fluid rate of 1.5 to 2 times maintenance (i.e., 60 to 100 ml/kg/24 hr) is typically chosen initially with subsequent adjustments based on frequent assessment of hydration status, urine output, severity of azotemia, and persistence of vomiting and diarrhea.

Monitoring Fluid Therapy

The rate of fluid administration and its effects on the animal must be monitored. Overzealous fluid therapy can lead to overhydration, pulmonary edema, and other "third-space" fluid loss with potentially serious consequences. Inadequate fluid administration can result in prolonged tissue underperfusion, hypoxia, continuing pancreatitis (if present), persistent prerenal azotemia, and the potential for development of primary kidney failure. Evaluation of fluid therapy should include subjective and objective assessments. Subjectively, the animal's alertness, heart rate, mucous membrane moisture, capillary refill time, pulse pressure, and skin turgor should be monitored and frequent pulmonary and cardiac auscultation performed. Objectively, serial evaluation of direct arterial or indirect Doppler blood pressure measurements, central venous pressure (CVP), urine output, body weight, and serum osmolality should be considered or completed.

Accurate assessment of urine output is extremely important in the sick ketoacidotic dog or cat, especially if azotemia is present. Diabetes-induced glomerular microangiopathy and/or the hemodynamic effects of ketoacidosis, concurrent necrotizing pancreatitis, or prolonged severe dehydration can lead to oliguric or anuric renal failure. Failure to produce urine within several hours of initiating fluid therapy is an alarming sign, and one that demands rapid recognition and an aggressive course of action. If urine production is in doubt, an indwelling urinary catheter should be secured in the bladder and attached to a closed collection system. Palpation of the bladder is not an accurate method for assessing urine output. A minimum of 1.0 to 2.0 mL of urine per kilogram of body weight per hour should be produced following the initial phase of fluid therapy. If urine production is minimal, the patency of the urinary catheter should be checked, the adequacy of fluid therapy evaluated (e.g., CVP, arterial blood pressure, subjective signs of excessive or inadequate fluids), and then attempts should be made to induce or increase the volume of urine produced with diuretics, mannitol, and/or dopamine.

Frequent assessment (ideally every 4 to 8 hours initially) of serum electrolytes and total venous CO_2 or arterial blood gases should be done and adjustments in fluid type and supplements made accordingly. Changes in serum electrolyte concentrations and blood gases are common and unpredictable during the initial 24 hours of treatment and the type of fluid (e.g., 0.9% saline, Plasma-Lyte 148, lactated Ringer's solution) and presence and amount of supplements (e.g., potassium, bicarbonate) in the fluids typically need to be adjusted several times during this period of time.

Potassium Supplementation

Fig. 8-18 shows a flow chart of potassium therapy.

Most dogs and cats with DKA have a net deficit of total body potassium due primarily to the marked urinary losses caused by the osmotic diuresis of glycosuria and ketonuria. Most dogs and cats with DKA initially have either normal or decreased serum potassium concentrations (see Fig. 8-12). During therapy for DKA, the serum potassium concentration decreases because of rehydration (dilution), insulin-mediated cellular uptake of potassium (with glucose), continued urinary losses, and correction of acidemia (translocation of potassium into the ICF compartment). Dogs and cats with hypokalemia require aggressive potassium replacement therapy to replace deficits and to prevent worsening, life-threatening hypokalemia after initiation of insulin therapy. The exception to potassium supplementation of fluids is hyperkalemia associated with oliguric kidney failure. Potassium supplementation should

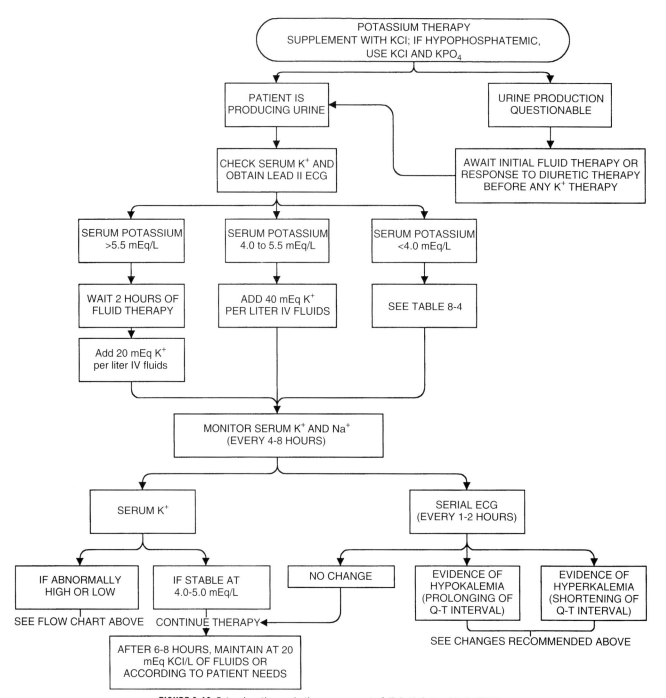

FIGURE 8-18 Potassium therapy in the management of diabetic ketoacidosis (DKA).

initially be withheld in these dogs and cats until glomerular filtration is restored, urine production increases, and hyperkalemia is resolving.

Ideally the amount of potassium required should be based on actual measurement of the serum potassium concentration (Table 8-4). If an accurate measurement of serum potassium is not available, potassium should be added to the liter of fluids to bring the potassium concentration to 40 mEq per liter. For example, 0.9% saline solution does not contain potassium, and Ringer's solution contains 4 mEq of potassium per liter; thus these fluids should be supplemented with 40 mEq and 36 mEq of potassium, respectively. Subsequent adjustments in potassium supplementation should be based on measurement of serum potassium, preferably every 4 to 8 hours until the dog or cat is stable and serum electrolytes are in the reference range.

Phosphate Supplementation

Serum phosphorus concentrations can be decreased, normal, or increased, depending on the duration of illness and kidney function. Most dogs and cats with DKA have either normal or decreased serum phosphorus concentrations on pretreatment testing. Within 24 hours of initiating treatment for DKA, serum phosphorus concentration can decline to severe levels (i.e., < 1 mg/dL) as a result of the dilutional effects of fluid therapy, the intracellular shift of phosphorus following the initiation of insulin therapy, and continuing kidney and gastrointestinal loss

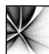

TABLE 8-4	GUIDELINES FOR POTASSIUM SUPPLEMENTATION IN INTRAVENOUS FLUIDS	
SERUM K+ (mEq/L)	**TYPICAL GUIDELINES** **K+ SUPPLEMENT/LITER OF FLUIDS**	**GUIDELINES FOR DIABETIC KETOACIDOSIS** **K+ SUPPLEMENT/LITER OF FLUIDS**
> 5.0	Wait	Wait
4.0-5.5	10	20 to 30
3.5-4.0	20	30 to 40
3.0-3.5	30	40 to 50
2.5-3.0	40	50 to 60
2.0-2.5	60	60 to 80
< 2.0	80	80

Total hourly potassium administration should not exceed 0.5 mEq/kg body weight.

(Willard et al, 1987). Hypophosphatemia affects primarily the hematologic and neuromuscular systems in dogs and cats (see Calcium and Phosphorus earlier in the chapter; Forrester and Moreland, 1989). Hemolytic anemia is the most common problem and can be life threatening if not recognized and treated. Severe hypophosphatemia may be clinically silent in many animals.

Phosphate therapy is indicated if clinical signs or hemolysis are identified or if the serum phosphorus concentration decreases to less than 1.5 mg/dL. Phosphate is supplemented by IV infusion. Potassium and sodium phosphate solutions contain 3 mmol of phosphate and either 4.4 mEq of potassium or 4 mEq of sodium per milliliter. The recommended dosage for phosphate supplementation is 0.01 to 0.03 mmol of phosphate per kilogram of body weight per hour, preferably administered in calcium-free IV fluids (e.g., 0.9% sodium chloride) (Willard, 1987). In dogs and cats with severe hypophosphatemia, the dosage may need to be increased to 0.03 to 0.12 mmol/kg/hr (Nichols and Crenshaw, 1995). Because the dose of phosphate necessary to replete an animal and the animal's response to therapy cannot be predicted, it is important to initially monitor the serum phosphorus concentration every 8 to 12 hours and adjust the phosphate infusion accordingly. Adverse effects from overzealous phosphate administration include iatrogenic hypocalcemia and its associated neuromuscular signs, hypernatremia, hypotension, and metastatic calcification (Forrester and Moreland, 1989). Serum total or preferably ionized calcium concentration should be measured at the same time as serum phosphorus concentration and the rate of phosphate infusion decreased if hypocalcemia is identified. Phosphorus supplementation is not indicated in dogs and cats with hypercalcemia, hyperphosphatemia, oliguria, or suspected tissue necrosis. If kidney function is in question, phosphorus supplementation should not be done until the status of kidney function and serum phosphorus concentration are known.

The routine supplementation of IV fluids with phosphorus during the initial 24 to 48 hours of treatment to prevent the development of severe hypophosphatemia, especially if the pretreatment serum phosphorus concentration is low, is controversial and varies with the experiences of the veterinarian queried. Routine phosphate supplementation is seldom recommended in treating DKA in humans, in part because several studies have failed to identify any apparent clinical benefit from

phosphate administration, and overzealous phosphate administration may cause hypocalcemia with tetany (Becker et al, 1983; Fisher and Kitabchi, 1983; Masharani and Karam, 2001). The use of low-dose insulin treatment regimens, as described in the Insulin Therapy section, helps reduce the intracellular shift of phosphate, and the frequent monitoring of serum phosphorus concentrations during therapy ensures early recognition of worrisome changes in the serum phosphorus concentration. Arguments for routine phosphate administration, especially if the pretreatment phosphorus concentration is low, center on concerns with hemolytic anemia and the desire to avoid this serious complication. Studies documenting the effect, if any, of prophylactic phosphate supplementation on the prevalence of hemolytic anemia have not been reported in dogs or cats with DKA. If the decision is made to prophylactically administer phosphate, it can be administered separately using the dosages discussed earlier or can be included as a component of potassium replacement in the fluids. When the latter approach is used, 5 to 10 mEq of the potassium supplement added to the liter of fluids should be potassium phosphate and the remainder of the potassium supplemented as potassium chloride. The serum phosphorus concentration should be monitored every 8 to 12 hours and the phosphate supplement adjusted accordingly.

Magnesium Supplementation

Hypomagnesemia is common in dogs and cats with DKA, and it often worsens during the initial treatment of DKA but resolves without treatment as the DKA resolves (Norris et al, 1999a). Clinical signs of hypomagnesemia do not usually occur until the serum total and ionized magnesium concentration is less than 1.0 and 0.4 mg/dL, respectively, and even at these low levels, many dogs and cats remain asymptomatic (see Magnesium under Completing the Data Base). What impact, if any, hypomagnesemia has on morbidity and response to treatment of DKA is not clear. To date there are no clinical studies that have yielded guidelines for magnesium replacement in dogs and cats; currently it is determined empirically. We do not routinely treat hypomagnesemia in dogs or cats with DKA unless problems with persistent lethargy, anorexia, weakness, or refractory hypokalemia or hypocalcemia are encountered after 24 to 48 hours of fluid and insulin therapy and another cause for the problem cannot be identified.

Parenteral solutions of magnesium sulfate (8.12 mEq of magnesium per gram) and magnesium chloride (9.25 mEq of magnesium per gram) salts are available. The IV doses for rapid and slow magnesium replacement are 0.5 to 1 mEq/kg/day and 0.3 to 0.5 mEq/kg/day, respectively, administered by constant-rate infusion in 5% dextrose in water or 0.9% sodium chloride (Dhupa and Shaffran, 1995; Hansen, 2000). Kidney function must be assessed before the administration of magnesium, and the magnesium dose must be reduced by 50% to 75% in azotemic animals. The administration of magnesium to animals being treated with digitalis cardioglycosides may cause serious conduction disturbances. Magnesium is incompatible with solutions containing sodium bicarbonate or calcium. Serum total or preferably ionized magnesium, calcium, and potassium concentrations should be monitored every 8 to 12 hours and adjustments in the rate of magnesium infusion made accordingly. The goal of therapy is the resolution of clinical signs or refractory hypokalemia or hypocalcemia. The parenteral administration of magnesium sulfate may cause significant hypocalcemia such that calcium infusion may be necessary. Other adverse effects of magnesium therapy include hypotension, atrioventricular and bundle-branch blocks, and in

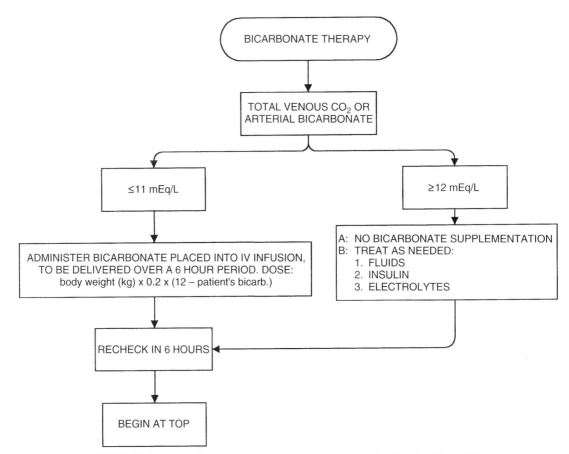

FIGURE 8-19 Bicarbonate treatment protocol for the management of diabetic ketoacidosis (DKA).

the event of overdose, respiratory depression and cardiac arrest. Overdoses are treated with IV calcium gluconate.

Bicarbonate Therapy

Fig. 8-19 shows a flow chart of bicarbonate therapy.

In humans with DKA, sodium bicarbonate treatment is reserved for patients with arterial pH of 7.0 or less and only with careful monitoring to prevent overcorrection. The primary concerns with sodium bicarbonate treatment are the potentially harmful consequences with overly aggressive bicarbonate administration, including exacerbation of hypokalemia from a rapid shift of potassium into cells, tissue anoxia from reduced dissociation of oxygen from hemoglobin when acidosis is rapidly reversed, and an exaggerated decrease in the cerebrospinal fluid (CSF) pH with resultant worsening of CNS function (Hale et al, 1984; Hood and Tannen, 1994; Kitabchi et al, 2001). The clinical presentation of the dog or cat, in conjunction with the plasma bicarbonate or total venous CO_2 concentration, should be used to determine the need for bicarbonate therapy. Bicarbonate supplementation is not recommended when plasma bicarbonate (or total venous CO_2) is 12 mEq/L or greater, especially if the animal is alert. An alert dog or cat probably has a normal or nearly normal pH in the CSF. The acidosis in these animals is corrected through insulin and fluid therapy. Improvement in renal perfusion enhances the urinary loss of ketoacid, and insulin therapy dramatically diminishes the production of ketoacid. Acetoacetate and β-hydroxybutyrate are also metabolically usable anions, and 1 mEq of bicarbonate is generated from each 1 mEq of ketoacid metabolized.

When the plasma bicarbonate concentration is 11 mEq/L or less (total venous CO_2 < 12 mEq/L), bicarbonate therapy should be initiated. Many of these animals have severe depression that may be a result of concurrent severe CNS acidosis. These can be difficult dogs and cats to treat, and the only safe therapeutic protocol involves correcting the metabolic acidosis slowly in the peripheral circulation via IV fluid supplementation, thereby avoiding major alterations in the pH of the CSF. As such, only a portion of the bicarbonate deficit is given initially over a 6-hour period of time.

The bicarbonate deficit (i.e., the milliequivalents of bicarbonate initially needed to correct acidosis to the critical level of 12 mEq/L over a period of 6 hours) is calculated as:

$$\text{mEq bicarbonate} = \text{body weight (kg)} \times 0.4 \times (12 - \text{animal's bicarbonate}) \times 0.5$$

or if the serum bicarbonate is not known:

$$\text{mEq bicarbonate} = \text{body weight (kg)} \times 2$$

The difference between the animal's serum bicarbonate concentration and the critical value of 12 mEq/L represents the treatable base deficit in DKA. If the animal's serum bicarbonate concentration is not known, the number 10 should be used for the treatable base deficit. The factor 0.4 corrects for the ECF space in which bicarbonate is distributed (40% of body weight). The factor 0.5 provides one-half of the required dose of bicarbonate in the IV infusion. In this manner, a conservative dose is given over a 6-hour period. Bicarbonate should not be given by bolus infusion (Ryder, 1984). After 6 hours of therapy, the acid-base status should be reevaluated and a new dosage calculated. Once the plasma bicarbonate level is greater than 12 mEq/L, further bicarbonate supplementation is not needed.

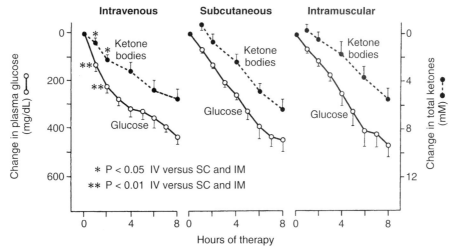

FIGURE 8-20 Effect of route of insulin therapy on reduction in plasma glucose and ketone concentrations in humans with diabetic ketoacidosis (DKA). Intravenous *(IV)* insulin was associated with a more rapid decline (initial 0 to 2 hours) in plasma glucose and ketone levels. Thereafter, no differences were noted between any of these groups. (Redrawn from Fisher JN, et al.: Diabetic ketoacidosis: low-dose insulin therapy by various routes, *N Engl J Med* 297:238-241, 1977. In DeFronzo RA, et al.: Diabetic ketoacidosis: a combined metabolic-nephrologic approach to therapy, *Diabetes Rev* 2:223, 1994; used with permission.) *IM,* Intramuscular; *SC,* subcutaneous.

Insulin Therapy

Insulin therapy is critical for the resolution of ketoacidosis. Insulin inhibits lipolysis and the mobilization of FFAs from triglycerides stored in adipose tissue, thereby decreasing the substrate necessary for ketone production; shifts hepatic metabolism from fat oxidation and ketogenesis to fat synthesis; suppresses hepatic gluconeogenesis; and promotes glucose and ketone metabolism by tissues (Hood and Tannen, 1994; DeFronzo et al, 1994). The net effect is decreased blood and urine glucose and ketone concentrations, decreased osmotic diuresis and electrolyte losses, and correction of metabolic acidosis. Overzealous insulin treatment can cause severe hypokalemia, hypophosphatemia, and hypoglycemia during the first 24 hours of treatment; these problems can be minimized by appropriate fluid therapy, frequent monitoring of serum electrolytes and blood glucose concentrations, and delaying the start of insulin treatment and modifying the initial insulin treatment protocol as indicated.

Initiating appropriate fluid therapy should always be the first step in the treatment of DKA. Delaying insulin therapy allows the benefits of fluid therapy to begin to be realized before the glucose, potassium, and phosphorus-lowering effects of insulin therapy commence. The question is how long to delay insulin therapy. We typically delay insulin therapy for a minimum of 2 hours after initiation of fluid therapy. Additional delays and decisions on the initial dosage of insulin administered are based on serum electrolyte results. If the serum potassium concentration is within the normal range after 2 hours of fluid therapy, insulin treatment should commence as described in the subsequent paragraphs. If hypokalemia persists, insulin therapy can be delayed an additional 2 hours to allow fluid therapy to replenish potassium, the initial insulin dose can be reduced to dampen the intracellular shift of potassium and phosphorus, or both can be done. The more severe the hypokalemia, the more inclined we are to delay insulin therapy and reduce the initial insulin dose. However, in our opinion, insulin therapy should be started within 4 hours of initiating fluid therapy.

Insulin therapy may not be as effective if a concurrent insulin-antagonistic disease is present, and it may be necessary to eliminate the disease while the animal is still ill to improve insulin effectiveness and resolve the ketoacidosis (e.g., a bitch in diestrus).

Regardless, insulin therapy is still indicated. The amount of insulin needed by an individual animal is difficult to predict. Therefore, an insulin preparation with a rapid onset of action and a brief duration of effect is ideal for making rapid adjustments in the dose and frequency of administration to meet the needs of that particular dog or cat. Rapid-acting regular crystalline insulin meets these criteria and is recommended for the treatment of DKA (Nelson et al, 1990). Rapid-acting insulin analogs (e.g., insulin lispro and insulin aspart) are also effective for treating DKA in humans, dogs, and presumably cats (Kitabchi et al, 2008; Sears et al, 2012).

Insulin protocols for the treatment of DKA include the hourly intramuscular (IM) technique (Chastain and Nichols, 1981), the constant low-dose IV infusion technique (Macintire, 1993; Claus et al, 2010), and the intermittent IM then subcutaneous (SC) technique (Feldman, 1980). All three routes (IV, IM, and SC) of insulin administration are effective in decreasing plasma glucose and ketone concentrations (Fig. 8-20). Arguments abound regarding the most appropriate route for initial insulin administration, arguments that are primarily based on personal experiences and preferences. Successful management of DKA does *not* depend on route of insulin administration. Rather, it depends on proper treatment of each disorder associated with DKA (see Box 8-6). All three protocols are effective.

Hourly Intramuscular Insulin Technique

Dogs and cats with severe DKA should receive an initial regular insulin loading dose of 0.1 to 0.2 U/kg followed by 0.1 U/kg every 1 to 2 hours thereafter (Fig. 8-21). The insulin dose can be reduced by 25% to 50% for the first two to three injections if hypokalemia is a concern. The insulin should be administered into the muscles of the rear legs to ensure that the injections are IM and do not go into fat or SC tissue where insulin absorption may be impaired in the dehydrated dog or cat. Diluting regular insulin 1:10 with sterile saline or special diluents available from the insulin manufacturer and using 0.3 mL U100 insulin syringes are helpful when small doses of insulin are required. By means of this insulin treatment regimen, the serum insulin concentration is typically increased to and maintained at approximately 100 μU/mL (700 pmol/L) (Fig. 8-22), which is an insulin concentration

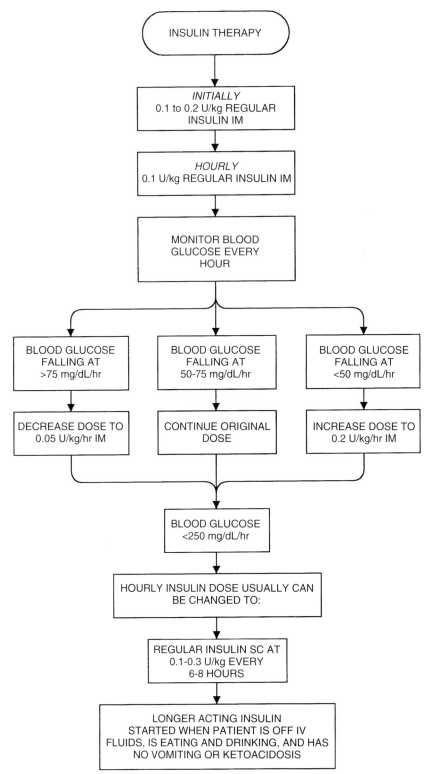

FIGURE 8-21 Hourly intramuscular (IM) insulin treatment protocol for the management of diabetic ketoacidosis (DKA). Similar principles for adjusting insulin therapy based on changes in the blood glucose concentration are used with the constant low-dose intravenous (IV) insulin infusion technique. *SC,* Subcutaneous.

that inhibits lipolysis, gluconeogenesis, and glycogenolysis and promotes utilization of glucose and ketones by tissues (Kitabchi et al, 2008).

The blood glucose concentration should initially be measured every hour using a point-of-care chemistry analyzer or portable blood glucose monitoring device and the insulin dosage adjusted accordingly (see Fig. 8-21). The goal of initial insulin therapy is to *slowly* lower the blood glucose concentration to the range of 200 to 250 mg/dL (11 to 14 mmol/L), preferably over a 6- to 10-hour time period. An hourly decline of 50 mg/dL (2.8 mmol/L) in the blood glucose concentration is ideal (Wagner et al, 1999). This provides a steady moderate decline, avoiding large shifts in osmolality.

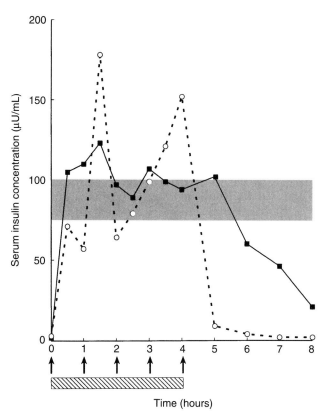

FIGURE 8-22 Mean serum insulin concentration in eight dogs with diabetic ketoacidosis (DKA) prior to and after the administration of regular crystalline insulin, 0.2 U/kg of body weight intramuscular (IM) (time 0) and then 0.1 U/kg IM hourly thereafter *(solid line)*, and in six dogs with DKA prior to and after continuous intravenous (IV) infusion of regular crystalline insulin *(dashed line)*, using a pediatric drip set. Insulin treatment was discontinued after the fourth hour in both groups of dogs. ↑, IM insulin administration; *hatched area,* IV insulin infusion; *shaded area,* ideal serum insulin concentration for treatment of DKA.

A declining blood glucose concentration also ensures that lipolysis and the supply of FFAs for ketone production have been effectively turned off. Glucose concentrations, however, decrease much more rapidly than ketone levels (Barrett and DeFronzo, 1984; Yeates and Blaufuss, 1990). In general, hyperglycemia is corrected within 12 hours, but ketosis often takes 48 to 72 hours to resolve.

Once the initial hourly insulin therapy brings the blood glucose concentration near 250 mg/dL (14 mmol/L), hourly administration of regular insulin should be discontinued and regular insulin given every 4 to 6 hours IM or, if hydration status is good, every 6 to 8 hours SC. The initial dose is usually 0.1 to 0.3 U/kg, with subsequent adjustments based on blood glucose concentrations. In addition, at this point, the IV infusion solution should have enough 50% dextrose added to create a 5% dextrose solution (100 mL of 50% dextrose added to each liter of fluids). The blood glucose concentration should be maintained between 150 and 300 mg/dL (8 to 17 mmol/L) until the dog or cat is stable and eating. Usually a 5% dextrose solution is adequate in maintaining the desired blood glucose concentration. If the blood glucose concentration dips below 150 mg/dL or increases above 300 mg/dL, the insulin dose can be decreased or increased accordingly. Dextrose helps minimize problems with hypoglycemia and allows insulin to be administered on schedule. Delaying the administration of insulin delays correction of the ketoacidotic state.

Marshall, et al., (2013) recently evaluated the efficacy of IM glargine with or without concurrent SC glargine administration in fifteen cats with DKA, adapting the protocol using regular insulin described earlier. All of the cats were initially administered 1 to 2 U of glargine IM, and for twelve cats 1 to 3 U of glargine SC. This was followed by intermittent IM glargine at intervals of 2 hours or more (range, 2 to 22 hours) and 1 to 3 U of glargine SC every 12 hours. Complications included hypoglycemia, hypokalemia, and hypophosphatemia. All fifteen cats survived and were discharged a median of 4 days after initiating treatment. The authors conclude that glargine may provide an alternative to regular insulin for the treatment of DKA in cats. Additional studies evaluating the safety and efficacy of glargine for treating DKA are needed before we would consider using basal insulin for the treatment of DKA.

Constant Low-Dose Intravenous Insulin Infusion Technique

Constant IV infusion of regular crystalline insulin is also effective in decreasing blood glucose concentrations. The decision to use the hourly IM technique versus constant IV insulin infusion is based primarily on clinician preference and availability of technical support and infusion pumps. To prepare the infusion, regular crystalline insulin (2.2 U/kg for dogs; 1.1 U/kg for cats) is added to 250 mL of 0.9% saline and initially administered at a rate of 10 mL/hr in a line separate from that used for fluid therapy (Church, 1983; Macintire, 1993). This provides an insulin infusion of 0.05 (cat) and 0.1 (dog) U/kg/hr, an infusion rate that has been shown to produce plasma insulin concentrations between 100 and 200 uU/mL (700 to 1400 pmol/L) in dogs (Macintire, 1993). Because insulin adheres to glass and plastic surfaces, approximately 50 mL of the insulin-containing fluid should be run through the drip set before it is administered to the animal. The rate of insulin infusion can be reduced for the initial 2 to 3 hours if hypokalemia is a concern. Two separate catheters are recommended for treatment: a peripheral catheter for insulin administration and a central catheter for fluid administration and blood sampling. An infusion or syringe pump should be used to ensure a constant rate of insulin infusion. Insulin infusions using pediatric drip sets may not provide a constant insulin infusion rate, especially if frequent monitoring of fluid administration is not possible (see Fig. 8-22). The goal of therapy is identical to that described for the hourly IM technique—to provide a continuous source of insulin at a dosage that causes a gradual decline in the blood glucose concentration. This goal is best attained with use of infusion or syringe pumps.

Adjustments in the infusion rate or the concentration of the insulin in the infusion (increased or decreased) are based on hourly measurements of blood glucose concentration; an hourly decline of 50 mg/dL (2.8 mmol/L) in the blood glucose concentration is ideal (Wagner et al, 1999). Once the blood glucose concentration approaches 250 mg/dL (14 mmol/L), the insulin infusion can be discontinued and regular insulin given every 4 to 6 hours IM or, if hydration status is good, every 6 to 8 hours SC, as discussed for the hourly IM protocol. Alternatively, the insulin infusion can be continued (at a decreased rate or decreased insulin concentration in the infusion to prevent hypoglycemia) until the insulin preparation is exchanged for a longer-acting product. Dextrose should be added to the IV fluids once the blood glucose concentration approaches 250 mg/dL, as discussed in the Hourly Intramuscular Insulin Technique section.

Claus, et al., (2010) recently compared the efficacy of three regular insulin doses (1.1 U/kg/d, 2.2 U/kg/d, and an escalating dosage from 1.1 to 2.2 U/kg during the course of the cat's stay) given by continuous IV infusion in 29 critically ill diabetic cats. There was no significant difference between groups regarding time required to reach a blood glucose of 250 mg/dL (14 mmol/L), change in serum potassium or phosphorus concentrations relative to baseline, length of time for resolution of ketonuria, or length of hospital stay. Sears, et al., (2012) evaluated the efficacy of the short-acting insulin analog lispro (Humalog, Eli Lilly) for the treatment of DKA using an IV constant rate infusion technique. Treatment with IV constant rate infusion of lispro was safe and as effective as treatment with regular crystalline insulin. Use of lispro insulin is a viable option for treating DKA, especially if the production of regular crystalline insulin is discontinued in the future.

Intermittent Intramuscular/Subcutaneous Insulin Technique

An intermittent IM followed by intermittent SC insulin technique has been described (Feldman, 1980). Although this technique was used successfully by us for years, it has been replaced with the hourly IM and constant IV insulin infusion techniques. The intermittent IM followed by intermittent SC insulin technique is less labor-intensive than the other techniques for insulin administration, but the decrease in blood glucose can be rapid and the risk of hypoglycemia is greater. The initial regular crystalline insulin dose is 0.25 U/kg, administered intramuscularly. Subsequent IM injections are repeated every 4 hours. Usually, insulin is administered intramuscularly only once or twice. Once the animal is rehydrated, the insulin is administered subcutaneously rather than intramuscularly every 6 to 8 hours. SC administration is not recommended initially because of problems with insulin absorption from SC sites of deposition in a dehydrated dog or cat. The dosage of IM or SC insulin is adjusted according to blood glucose concentrations, which initially should be measured hourly beginning with the first IM injection. An hourly decline of 50 mg/dL in the blood glucose concentration is ideal (Wagner et al, 1999). Subsequent insulin dosages should be decreased by 25% to 50% if this goal is exceeded. Dextrose should be added to the IV fluids once the blood glucose concentration approaches 250 mg/dL (14 mmol/L), as discussed in the Hourly Intramuscular Insulin Technique section.

Initiating Longer-Acting Insulin Therapy

Longer-acting insulin (e.g., Lente, protamine zinc insulin [PZI], glargine) are administered once the dog or cat is stable, eating, maintaining fluid balance without any IV infusions, and no longer acidotic, azotemic, or electrolyte-deficient. The initial dose of the longer-acting insulin is similar to the regular insulin dose being used just before switching to the longer-acting insulin. Subsequent adjustments in the longer-acting insulin dose should be based on clinical response and measurement of blood glucose concentrations, as described in Chapters 6 and 7.

Concurrent Illness

Therapy for DKA frequently involves the management of concurrent, often serious illness. Common concurrent illness in the dog and cat with DKA include pancreatitis, bacterial infection, congestive heart failure, chronic kidney disease, hepatobiliary disease, and insulin-antagonistic disorders, most notably hyperadrenocorticism (dog), hyperthyroidism (cat), and diestrus (intact female dog) (Bruskiewicz et al, 1997; Hume et al, 2006); It may be necessary in such animals to modify the therapy for DKA (e.g., fluid therapy with concurrent heart failure) or implement additional therapy (e.g., antibiotics), depending on the nature of the concurrent illness. Insulin therapy, however, should not be delayed or discontinued. Resolution of ketoacidosis can only be achieved through insulin therapy. If nothing is to be given per os, insulin therapy should be continued and the blood glucose concentration

maintained with IV dextrose infusions. If concurrent insulin-antagonistic disease is present, it may be necessary to treat the disease while the animal is still ill to improve the effectiveness of insulin and resolve the ketoacidosis (e.g., ovariohysterectomy in diestrual bitch).

Pancreatitis

Pancreatitis, acute or chronic, should always be assumed to be present in the dog or cat with DKA until proven otherwise. The diagnosis of pancreatitis should be based on a combination of presence of appropriate clinical signs; physical examination findings; abnormalities on the CBC, serum biochemistry panel, and urinalysis; results of serum pancreatic lipase immunoreactivity (see Pancreatic Enzymes earlier); radiographic evidence of a loss of detail in the right cranial abdomen accompanied by gas-filled duodenal ileus; and ultrasonographic evidence of enlargement of the pancreas and a hypoechoic to mixed echogenic pattern with or without mild to severe blockage of the bile duct (see Fig. 8-15). The presence of pancreatitis impacts fluid therapy and nutritional support during hospitalization, the duration of hospitalization, dietary recommendations, response to insulin treatment, the probability for recurrence of ketonuria and ketoacidosis following discharge from the hospital, and survival. Acute severe necrotizing pancreatitis is a common cause of death during the initial days of treatment of DKA, and the inability to prevent recurring bouts of chronic pancreatitis is one reason owners eventually elect euthanasia of their pet (Goossens et al, 1998). Avoidance of recurrent bouts of pancreatitis is critical to the long-term survival of the diabetic dog and cat. In the dog, this is primarily accomplished through appropriate dietary therapy. To date, inciting factors for development of pancreatitis in the cat have been poorly characterized, and the impact of diet, if any, on preventing recurrence of pancreatitis has yet to be clarified.

Bacterial Infections

The immunosuppressive effects of diabetes mellitus, in conjunction with the increased blood glucose concentration in body fluids, predisposes diabetic dogs and cats to bacterial infections (McMahon and Bistrian, 1995; Joshi et al, 1999). Urinary tract infections are most common, followed by infections of the oral cavity, skin, and pulmonary systems (Hess et al, 2000; Peikes et al, 2001). Life-threatening sepsis may develop in debilitated diabetics, those with severe concurrent illness (e.g., necrotizing pancreatitis), and those in which aseptic technique is not strictly followed during diagnostic and therapeutic procedures (e.g., placement of indwelling urinary or venous catheters). The clinician should always suspect infection in the DKA dog or cat. Urine cultures should be completed in all dogs and cats with DKA. Culture of blood and other fluids and tissues is usually dictated by the clinical signs and findings on the physical examination, routine blood tests, and diagnostic imaging. Whenever possible, the choice of antibiotic therapy should be based on results of culture and sensitivity testing.

Kidney Disease

Chronic and less commonly acute kidney disease may occur concurrently in dogs and cats with DKA. Abnormal kidney function may result from the deleterious effects of the diabetic state (i.e., diabetic nephropathy) or may be an independent problem that has developed in conjunction with diabetes in the geriatric dog or cat. Close monitoring of urine output and changes in BUN and serum creatinine concentration in response to fluid therapy are warranted whenever azotemia is identified in the dog or cat with newly diagnosed DKA. See the sections Urinalysis and Urine Culture, Blood Urea Nitrogen and Creatinine, and Monitoring Fluid Therapy for information on kidney function and DKA.

Hormonal Disorders Causing Insulin Resistance

Insulin resistance accompanies many of the concurrent disorders present in dogs and cats with DKA. The severity of insulin resistance is quite variable and depends on the underlying cause (see Table 6-11). Fortunately, most disorders cause mild insulin resistance; that is, the dog or cat remains responsive to insulin therapy even at the low insulin dosages often employed during the initial 24 to 72 hours of therapy, and ketoacidosis progressively resolves. Two major exceptions are diestrus-induced insulin resistance in the intact bitch and hyperadrenocorticism. Although acromegaly also causes severe insulin resistance in the cat, ketonuria is an infrequent finding and systemic illness from DKA is uncommon, despite an inability to establish any semblance of glycemic control with massive doses of insulin. Seemingly, insulin is able to inhibit lipolysis and the supply of FFAs for ketone production but unable to control hepatic glucose secretion and/or stimulate tissue glucose utilization to control hyperglycemia in these cats.

Diestrus. Increased progesterone secretion during the diestrual phase of the estrus cycle in the bitch directly antagonizes insulin action and stimulates growth hormone secretion which, in turn, causes severe insulin resistance and the potential for life-threatening DKA. Diestrus-induced insulin resistance can be difficult if not impossible to override, despite the administration of massive doses of regular crystalline insulin. As a consequence, the metabolic derangements associated with DKA progressively worsen—ultimately resulting in death of the bitch.

Intact bitches in DKA should always be assumed to be in diestrus and should be assumed to have a pyometra, regardless of owner statements regarding estrus activity or the lack thereof. Once initial therapy for DKA is initiated, abdominal ultrasound scans or radiographs should be evaluated for pyometra and a blood progesterone concentration should be determined. A blood progesterone concentration greater than 2 ng/mL is diagnostic for ovarian luteal activity and supports the diagnosis of diestrus. The bitch should undergo ovariohysterectomy as soon as safely possible. Timing of surgery depends on the severity of clinical signs. Severely ill bitches with DKA should be stabilized as best as possible with IV fluids, regular crystalline insulin, and if indicated, parenteral antibiotics for 6 to 24 hours prior to performing surgery. We rarely wait more than 24 hours from the time of diagnosis of pyometra or diestrus to ovariohysterectomy. Insulin resistance usually begins to resolve within a week of ovariohysterectomy. In some bitches, insulin-requiring diabetes mellitus may even resolve (see Chapter 6, Other Specific Types and Diabetic Remission).

Diestrus-induced insulin resistance and its effect on responsiveness of DKA to insulin therapy are not commonly encountered in cats, because essentially all female diabetic cats have been spayed at the time diabetes is diagnosed and progesterone does not stimulate growth hormone secretion in the cat (Peterson, 1987). Progesterone can cause insulin resistance, but the insulin resistance that develops during diestrus in the queen rarely causes significant problems, presumably because the insulin resistance is not severe and the increase in plasma progesterone is transient. In contrast, insulin resistance caused by chronic progesterone excess, as occurs with exogenous progestagen administration or a progesterone-secreting adrenocortical tumor, can cause diabetes mellitus and a clinical syndrome that mimics feline hyperadrenocorticism (Boord and Griffin, 1999; Rossmeisl et al, 2000; see Chapter 11).

Exogenous Glucocorticoids. Insulin resistance induced by exogenous glucocorticoid administration can antagonize treatment of DKA. In general, glucocorticoids should not be given to dogs and cats with DKA and should be discontinued in previously undiagnosed diabetic ketoacidotic dogs and cats. This includes oral, ocular, aural, and skin preparations. The exceptions are those situations in which glucocorticoids are necessary to control life-threatening disorders (e.g., immune-mediated disease). In these situations, the lowest dosage of glucocorticoid needed to control the disorder should be administered and alternatives to glucocorticoids (e.g., azathioprine or cyclosporine) should be sought. In addition, the clinician should be willing to compensate for the insulin-antagonistic effects of glucocorticoids by administering larger dosages of insulin than are typically required to control DKA.

Naturally-Acquired Hyperadrenocorticism. Hyperadrenocorticism is a well-recognized disorder in diabetic dogs and cats and is occasionally suspected in dogs and cats with newly diagnosed DK and DKA and insulin-treated dogs and cats with persistent ketonuria. For relatively healthy dogs and cats with DK, appropriate diagnostic tests should be undertaken and appropriate treatment initiated once the diagnosis of hyperadrenocorticism is confirmed (see Chapters 10 and 11). Despite its impaired efficacy, insulin should continue to be administered to inhibit lipolysis, suppress ketone production, and prevent deterioration of the ketoacidotic state. Ketosis typically resolves once hyperadrenocorticism is controlled.

Establishing a diagnosis of hyperadrenocorticism is more problematic in the ill ketoacidotic dog or cat, in part because of concerns regarding accuracy of results when the diagnostic tests used to diagnose hyperadrenocorticism are performed in dogs and cats with severe illness (Kaplan et al, 1995). Ideally, testing for hyperadrenocorticism should be postponed until DKA has resolved and the dog or cat is stable in the home environment. We rely on results of the urine cortisol-to-creatinine ratio, low dose dexamethasone suppression test, and ultrasonographic examination of the adrenal glands to help confirm the diagnosis of hyperadrenocorticism. Interpretation of results of the low dose dexamethasone suppression test and especially the urine cortisol-to-creatinine ratio should be done with care because of the increased potential for false positive test results in sick dogs and cats. Ideally, treatment for hyperadrenocorticism should not be initiated until the DKA has resolved with fluid and insulin therapy and the dog or cat is stable and eating.

Monitoring and Complications of Therapy

Complications induced by treatment of DKA are common and usually result from overly aggressive therapy, inadequate animal monitoring, and failure to reevaluate biochemical parameters in a timely manner (Box 8-7). DKA is a complex disorder that carries a high mortality rate if improperly managed. To minimize the occurrence of therapeutic complications and improve the chances of successful response to therapy, all abnormal parameters should be *slowly* returned toward normal (i.e., over a period of 24 to 48 hours), the physical and mental status of the animal must be evaluated frequently (at least three to four times daily), and fluid therapy, urine production, urine and plasma ketones, serum electrolytes, and blood gases every 4 to 8 hours. During the initial 24 hours, blood glucose concentrations should be measured every 1 to 2 hours. Fluid, insulin, and bicarbonate therapy typically require modification three or four times during the initial 24 hours of therapy. A CBC and serum biochemistry panel that

---

BOX 8-7 **Common Complications Caused by Treatment of Diabetic Ketoacidosis in Dogs and Cats**

- Hypoglycemia from excessive use of insulin or inadequate administration of glucose
- Hypokalemia from inadequate potassium supplementation
- Hypophosphatemia and hemolytic anemia from inadequate phosphorus supplementation
- Hypernatremia from excessive administration of physiologic saline or inadequate fluid intake
- Persistent oliguria from inadequate or inappropriately slow administration of fluids
- Persistent hypotension from inadequate or inappropriately slow administration of fluids
- Cerebral edema and neurologic signs from too rapid decrease in blood glucose and/or osmolality
- Paradoxical cerebral acidosis and neurologic signs from too rapid administration of bicarbonate

---

includes plasma proteins, creatinine, calcium, phosphorus, and magnesium should be evaluated every 24 hours until the dog or cat is stabilized and eating. Failure to recognize changes in the status of DKA and to respond accordingly invariably leads to potentially serious complications. The more common complications are discussed below.

Hypoglycemia

Hypoglycemia is a common problem during the initial days of treatment, especially when the dog or cat is anorectic and unable to ingest a dietary source of glucose to counter the glucose-lowering effects of insulin. The goal of initial insulin therapy, regardless of how the insulin is administered, is to *slowly* lower the blood glucose concentration to the range of 200 to 250 mg/dL (11 to 14 mmol/L), preferably over an 8- to 10-hour time period. Unfortunately, this goal can be quite difficult to attain, and the blood glucose concentration may drop precipitously. To avoid hypoglycemia, it is imperative that the blood glucose concentration initially be measured every hour using a point-of-care chemistry analyzer, or a portable blood glucose monitoring device, or a continuous glucose monitoring system (see Chapter 6, Fig. 6-23). Whenever the blood glucose concentration approaches 250 mg/dL, 50% dextrose should be added to the IV infusion solution to create a 5% dextrose solution. If hypoglycemia occurs (i.e., blood glucose less than 80 mg/dL; 4.5 mmol/L) or the dog or cat is symptomatic for hypoglycemia, 0.25 to 0.50 gm/kg body weight of 50% dextrose should be administered IV as needed until the 5% dextrose solution is able to maintain the blood glucose above 80 mg/dL. Insulin therapy should also be modified and, if necessary, discontinued but only for a few hours. Discontinuing insulin therapy interferes with resolution of the ketoacidosis.

Severe Hypokalemia

Dogs and cats with DKA are at risk for development of severe hypokalemia (< 2.0 mEq/L) during the initial 48 hours of therapy for reasons that are discussed in the Potassium Supplementation section earlier in the chapter. The most common clinical sign of hypokalemia is generalized skeletal muscle weakness. In cats, ventriflexion of the neck, forelimb hypermetria, and a broad-based hind limb stance may be observed. Cardiac consequences of hypokalemia include decreased myocardial contractility, decreased cardiac output, and disturbances in cardiac rhythm. Other metabolic

effects of hypokalemia include hypokalemic nephropathy, which is characterized by chronic tubulointerstitial nephritis, impaired kidney function, and azotemia and manifested clinically as polyuria, polydipsia, and impaired urine concentrating capability; hypokalemic polymyopathy, which is characterized by increased serum creatine kinase activity and electromyographic abnormalities; and paralytic ileus, manifested clinically as abdominal distention, anorexia, vomiting, and constipation (DiBartola and de Morais, 2012). Hypokalemic nephropathy and polymyopathy are most notable in cats. Cats seem more susceptible to the deleterious effects of hypokalemia than dogs. In dogs, signs may not be evident until the serum potassium concentration is less than 2.5 mEq/L, whereas in cats signs can be seen with serum potassium concentrations between 3 and 3.5 mEq/L. Clinical signs of hypokalemia can be mistakenly ascribed to other commonly encountered concurrent disorders (e.g., pancreatitis) and hypokalemia overlooked as a possible cause. Initial aggressive potassium replacement therapy, frequent monitoring of serum electrolytes, and subsequent adjustments in potassium replacement therapy are necessary to identify and prevent hypokalemia.

Central Nervous System Signs (Cerebral Edema)

Cerebral edema may result from excessive free water accumulation in the intravascular space during therapy for DKA. This typically results from a rapid decrease in the blood glucose concentration or after infusion of large quantities of hypotonic solutions (e.g., 0.45% saline). With insulin deficiency, the movement of glucose from the ECF to the ICF compartment is impaired. Glucose accumulation in the ECF causes a significant increase in ECF osmolality. A rapid increase in ECF glucose can result in cellular dehydration as water moves from the ICF to the ECF compartment in response to the increase in ECF osmolality. Neurologic signs develop as a consequence of neuronal dehydration in the CNS. Neurons in the CNS produce osmotically active substances including lactate, sorbitol, myoinositol, and idiogenic osmoles to compensate for the increasing osmolality of the ECF and prevent cellular dehydration. These intracellular substances can cause water to diffuse into the cell if the osmolality within the cell exceeds that within the ECF space. Idiogenic osmols within the neurons of a severely hyperglycemic animal is not associated with an osmotic gradient because of the equilibrium between the hyperosmotic ECF space (induced by glucose) and the hyperosmotic intracellular space (induced by idiogenic osmols). However, with aggressive fluid therapy and exogenous insulin administration, rapid reduction in blood glucose concentration and improved renal perfusion may cause a rapid reduction in ECF osmolality. A relative excess in free water accumulates in the ECF space. This water can then diffuse into the idiogenic osmol-induced hyperosmotic brain cells. A rapid decline in blood glucose concentration can thus result in cerebral edema and worsening CNS function. For these reasons, the veterinarian must be aware of the CNS status of the animal prior to initiation of therapy. If the animal becomes depressed or obtunded during treatment, it may be the result of the relatively rapidly decreasing blood glucose concentration leading to cerebral edema.

Mannitol is the most effective treatment for cerebral edema. Dexamethasone is usually recommended, but its efficacy has not been reported in diabetic dogs and cats. Passive hyperventilation to lower carbon dioxide pressure and diminish cerebral blood flow has also been recommended. Prophylactically avoiding cerebral edema through slow but progressive improvement in blood glucose concentration, serum electrolytes, and metabolic acidosis is the key.

Hemolytic Anemia

Life-threatening hemolytic anemia may develop during the initial 72 hours of therapy as a consequence of hypophosphatemia (see Phosphate Supplementation earlier in this chapter) (Willard et al, 1987; Adams et al, 1993; Bruskiewicz et al, 1997). The mechanism of hypophosphatemia-induced hemolysis is not known, but hemolysis may occur secondary to depletion of erythrocyte ATP, which is necessary for maintenance of cell membrane integrity; malfunction of the sodium-potassium pump secondary to erythrocyte ATP depletion and subsequent osmotic lysis; or alterations in red blood cell membrane lipids (Shilo et al, 1985; Adams et al, 1993).

Hypophosphatemia-induced hemolytic anemia can be serious, with hematocrits less than 15% reported in dogs and cats (Willard et al, 1987; Adams et al, 1993). Additional findings on a CBC include spherocytes, Heinz bodies, and hemoglobinemia. Treatment involves the IV administration of phosphate, and, if necessary, blood. Prevention of hypophosphatemia is the key to avoiding hemolytic anemia. Frequent monitoring of serum phosphorus concentration during the initial 24 to 48 hours of therapy for DKA and supplementation of the IV fluids with potassium or sodium phosphate when hypophosphatemia is identified is the cornerstone of prevention.

Severe Hypernatremia and Hyperchloremia

Occasionally, animals with DKA develop severe hypernatremia and hyperchloremia (see Fig. 8-12) as a result of water deprivation (i.e., inadequate fluid intake) in conjunction with urinary loss of large amounts of water in excess of electrolytes. Loss of water in excess of electrolytes creates hypertonic dehydration, a state of dehydration with few of the expected signs of severe fluid depletion (Edwards et al, 1983). Worsening hypernatremia, in combination with hyperglycemia, causes severe hyperosmolality (> 400 mOsm/kg) and CNS dysfunction. The initial critical signs of hypernatremia include irritability, weakness, and ataxia, but as the hypernatremia worsens, stupor progresses to coma and seizures. The progression and severity of these signs depend on the rate of onset, degree, and duration of hypernatremia. Therapy should be designed to replace fluid deficits, match continuing fluid losses, and decrease those losses when possible. (See Complications of the Modified Water Deprivation Test: Hypertonic Dehydration and Hypernatremia in Chapter 1 for details on the treatment of hypernatremic, hypertonic dehydration.)

It is important to consider factors that can result in artifactual changes in serum sodium concentrations. Severe lipemia can appear to *raise* the serum sodium concentration because lipemia displaces sodium into the non-lipemic volume of serum, making a normal serum sodium concentration appear increased. Hyperglycemia can also alter the serum sodium concentration. For each 100 mg/dL increment of serum glucose above the normal range, the serum sodium concentration *decreases* approximately 1.6 mEq/L (DiBartola, 2012).

PROGNOSIS

DKA remains one of the most difficult metabolic therapeutic challenges in veterinary medicine. One must remain aware of all the complicating factors in treatment and remember that fluid therapy, insulin, and potassium supplementation are the cornerstones of successful management. Added to these factors are close supervision and monitoring of the animal, without which failure rates are high, and identification and treatment of concurrent disease that is invariably present. Reported in-hospital mortality rates for DKA include 29% of 21 dogs (Macintire, 1993), 30% of 127 dogs (Hume et al, 2006), and 26% of 42 cats (Bruskiewicz et al, 1997), primarily as a result of severe concurrent illness. During the past decade in our hospital, the mortality rate has decreased to approximately 5%, and death has usually been attributed to underlying medical disorders (e.g., pancreatitis) that precipitated the DKA, client financial constraints, or both rather than to the metabolic complications of ketoacidosis (Claus et al, 2010). It is worth reiterating that a careful search should always be made, both at the time of initial history and physical examination and during therapy, for underlying problems that might have precipitated the episode of DKA or developed during treatment of DKA. In particular, pneumonia, sepsis, pancreatitis, and hormonal diseases causing insulin resistance are often silent at the time of presentation. Despite all precautions and diligent therapy, a fatal outcome cannot be avoided in some cases. Nevertheless, with logical therapy and careful monitoring, the goal of therapy for DKA (i.e., achieving a healthy diabetic dog or cat) is attainable. Diabetic remission is also possible in cats following resolution of DKA, especially in cats with concurrent pancreatic disease or cats being treated with glucocorticoids at the time DKA is diagnosed (Sieber-Ruckstuhl et al, 2008; Marshall et al, 2013).

HYPEROSMOLAR HYPERGLYCEMIC STATE

Diabetic hyperosmolar hyperglycemic state has historically been referred to by many terms, including *hyperosmolar non-ketotic syndrome, hyperosmolar coma, hyperglycemic hyperosmolar syndrome,* and *non-ketotic hyperosmolar syndrome.* Hyperosmolar hyperglycemic state (HHS) is the nomenclature recommended by the American Diabetes Association to emphasize the varying alterations in sensorium less than coma that are usually present in humans and that HHS may occur with mild ketosis and acidosis (Nugent, 2005). HHS is an uncommon complication of diabetes mellitus in the dog and cat. This syndrome is characterized by severe hyperglycemia (blood glucose concentration > 600 mg/dL; 34 mmol/L), hyperosmolality (> 350 mOsm/kg), and dehydration in the absence of significant ketosis. Progressively worsening lethargy ultimately leads to obtundation and coma as hyperosmolality becomes more severe. Concurrent disorders (e.g., kidney failure, congestive heart failure, infection, pulmonary disease and pancreatitis) are common, contribute to the progression of this syndrome, and negatively impact the prognosis. HHS is a diagnostic and therapeutic challenge that is associated with a high fatality rate (Koenig et al, 2004).

Pathogenesis

The pathogenesis of HHS is similar to that of DKA—a partial or relative insulin deficiency reduces glucose utilization by muscle, fat, and the liver while at the same time inducing hyperglucagonemia and increasing hepatic glucose output. Concurrent infection, inflammation, and organ system failure promote insulin resistance and secretion of counterregulatory hormones (e.g., catecholamines, cortisol) that exacerbate hyperglycemia. One theory for the lack of ketosis with HHS is the existence of a small population of functional beta-cells that are capable of secreting insulin, albeit in insufficient amounts to prevent hyperglycemia. However, the presence of small amounts of insulin is believed to prevent the development of ketosis by inhibiting lipolysis (see Role of Insulin Deficiency). Therefore, even though a low insulin-to-glucagon ratio promotes ketogenesis in the liver, the limited availability of precursor FFAs from the periphery restricts the rate at which ketones are formed (Ennis et al, 1994). Hepatic resistance to glucagon may also play a role in the lack of ketosis with HHS (Yen et al, 1980; Azain et al, 1985).

If a dog or cat is unable to maintain adequate fluid intake because of an associated acute or chronic illness (e.g., pancreatitis, gastroenteritis) or has suffered excessive fluid loss (e.g., diuretics for concurrent congestive heart failure), marked dehydration results. As plasma volume contracts, glomerular filtration is impaired, limiting renal glucose excretion and contributing markedly to the rise in blood glucose. The measured serum sodium concentration is usually decreased or within the reference range, but the "corrected" serum sodium concentration is typically in the reference range or increased and is contributing to the increase in plasma osmolality (see Serum Sodium Concentration earlier). As plasma osmolality increases, water is drawn out of cerebral neurons, resulting in mental obtundation and further impairment of water intake. A vicious cycle of worsening hyperosmolality, obtundation, inadequate fluid intake, dehydration, and prerenal azotemia ensues, ultimately resulting in coma and death.

The hyperglycemia of HHS (600 to 1600 mg/dL; 34 to 90 mmol/L) tends to be more severe than the hyperglycemia of DKA (300 to 600 mg/dL; 17 to 34 mmol/L). The increase in blood glucose concentration in HHS is, as in DKA, the result of increased production of glucose by the liver coupled with its diminished use by tissues. However, two additional factors in HHS allow the hyperglycemia to become more severe. First, impaired urine output in HHS diminishes excretion of glucose in urine (Foster and McGarry, 1989). Second, low or undetectable concentrations of ketoacid in the plasma and urine in HHS removes an important and early contributor to clinical signs. As a consequence, the hyperglycemia of HHS progresses for a longer period of time, and it is not until signs of severe hyperosmolality (i.e., lethargy, obtundation) or signs related to concurrent problems become evident to the owner that veterinary care is sought.

Some dogs and cats with HHS are acidotic despite low or undetectable concentrations of ketoacid in the plasma or urine. One cause for this disparity in expected versus real results is the fact that β-hydroxybutyrate (one of two major ketoacids) is not assayed by commonly used urine and plasma reagent strips or tablets (see Establishing the Diagnosis of Diabetic Ketosis and Ketoacidosis). Another cause for acidosis in non-ketotic diabetics is lactic acidosis. Lactic acid is the end product of anaerobic metabolism of glucose. The principal sources of this acid are erythrocytes (which lack the enzymes for aerobic oxidation), skeletal muscle, skin, and brain. Lactic acid is removed via hepatic, and to some degree renal, uptake with conversion first to pyruvate and eventually back to glucose, a process that requires oxygen. Lactic acidosis occurs when excess lactic acid accumulates in the blood. This can be the result of overproduction (tissue hypoxia), deficient removal (hepatic failure), or both (circulatory collapse). Like humans, dogs and cats with lactic acidosis are usually severely ill, with problems such as sepsis, hemorrhage, anemia, pulmonary disease, liver disease, and kidney failure.

Clinical Findings

Clinical Signs

The onset of HHS may be insidious, and it may be preceded for days or weeks by the classic signs of diabetes mellitus (polyuria, polydipsia, polyphagia, and weight loss). Progressive weakness, anorexia, and lethargy develop, usually in conjunction with a reduction in water intake. Additional clinical signs depend on the underlying precipitating disorder(s). Physical examination often reveals the presence of profound dehydration. These pets are typically lethargic, extremely depressed, or actually comatose. There is a direct relationship between the severity of the hyperosmolality and the severity of neurologic signs. Hypothermia and slow capillary refill time are common. Kussmaul respirations are absent unless severe metabolic (lactic) acidosis is present.

Laboratory Findings

Severe hyperglycemia is present, with blood glucose concentrations ranging from 600 to as high as 1600 mg/dL (34 to 90 mmol/L). Severe prerenal or renal azotemia is a common finding. These animals typically have depleted body potassium stores, despite the fact that serum potassium concentrations can be high, normal, or low. Serum sodium concentrations are also variable and may be low, normal, or elevated despite total body sodium depletion. Because glucose osmotically shifts water into the extracellular space, sodium is diluted and the measured value may be falsely decreased. The measured sodium value should be corrected to a sodium value that accounts for hyperglycemia by using the formula in Serum Sodium Concentration earlier in the chapter. The formula reflects that the measured serum sodium value is decreased by approximately 1.6 mEq for every 100 mg/dL increase in glucose above 100 (Nugent, 2005). A mild hyponatremia or a normal serum sodium concentration usually suggests moderate dehydration. Hypernatremia despite hyperglycemia suggests significant water loss has occurred and severe volume contraction and dehydration are present.

Hyperosmolality is a consistent finding in HHS and can exceed 400 mOsm/kg, especially in dogs and cats with hypernatremia and severe hyperglycemia. Plasma osmolality may be measured by determination of its freezing point with an osmometer or calculated using the formula given in Serum Osmolality earlier in the chapter.

Mild to moderate ketosis may occur with HHS in diabetic humans. HHS and DKA are two disorders believed to represent different points along a spectrum of emergencies caused by poorly-controlled diabetes (Kitabchi et al, 2006). Ketosis is usually absent in dogs and cats with HHS, although trace ketonuria may occur. Ketoacidosis is not a part of HHS but metabolic acidosis may be identified (usually in the form of lactic acidosis) owing to underlying disorders commonly affiliated with HHS in dogs and cats. Lactic acidosis depresses plasma bicarbonate concentrations and the arterial pH. An anion gap is present (see Anion Gap earlier in the chapter). Other causes of "anion gap" metabolic acidosis should be excluded (see Box 8-4). The diagnosis of lactic acidosis can be confirmed by measuring plasma lactate concentration.

Therapy

The goals of therapy for HHS are similar to DKA—that is, to correct severe dehydration and restore electrolyte losses, to provide adequate amounts of insulin to normalize intermediary metabolism, to correct the hyperosmolar state, and to identify and treat precipitating factors. Restoring intravascular volume and lost electrolytes using isotonic fluids has the highest priority. Osmolality is returned to normal by lowering the blood glucose concentration and by replacing water deficits. Initially, fluid therapy is used to lower the blood glucose concentration; insulin should not be administered until intravascular volume is restored, electrolyte derangements improved, and blood pressure stabilized. Careful and frequent monitoring of the dog's or cat's clinical and laboratory response to therapy is essential.

Fluid therapy is of paramount importance in treating HHS and is the primary mode of therapy for the initial 4 to 6 hours or longer. Derangements in total body water, sodium and potassium, hyperglycemia, and hyperosmolality are usually severe, in part because the lack of ketoacidosis and associated systemic signs of illness allows HHS to develop for a longer period of time before veterinary care is sought. Despite the severe hyperosmolality, the initial fluid of choice is isotonic (0.9%) saline with appropriate potassium supplementation. Isotonic saline will correct dehydration and improve blood flow to tissues, stabilize blood pressure, improve GFR and promote glycosuria, decrease blood glucose concentration, and replace sodium for glucose in the ECF space. The net effect is a slow reduction in ECF hyperosmolality, thereby minimizing development of cerebral edema. The initial goal of fluid therapy is correction of dehydration deficits. Half of the estimated dehydration deficit plus maintenance requirements should be replaced in the first 12 hours and the remainder in the next 12 to 24 hours.

The principles of potassium and phosphorus supplementation are similar to those discussed for DKA (see Potassium Supplementation and Phosphate Supplementation earlier in the chapter). Many dogs and cats with HHS are also in kidney failure (often oliguric) and may have hyperkalemia, hyperphosphatemia, and/or impaired ability to excrete a potassium load. As such, potassium and phosphorus supplementation should be based on measurement of serum concentrations and awareness of the status of kidney function and urine production. Usually, initial therapy consists of 20 mEq/L of potassium replacement (as potassium chloride) into the infusion fluids. Subsequent adjustments are based on measurements of serum electrolytes, which should be done frequently to quickly identify problems in serum electrolyte concentrations, should they arise.

Insulin therapy should be delayed (typically 4 to 6 hours or longer) until the positive benefits of fluid therapy are documented (i.e., correction of dehydration, stabilization of blood pressure, and improvement in urine production, hyperglycemia, hyperosmolality, and derangements in serum electrolyte concentrations). The need for insulin treatment is not as critical with HHS as with DKA; this is in part because ketone production and its metabolic consequences are minimal to nonexistent with HHS. Metabolic acidosis, if identified in HHS, is more likely caused by lactic acidosis, which can be improved with fluid therapy. In addition, insulin can cause a rapid decrease in the blood glucose concentration and ECF osmolality—changes that promote cerebral edema (see Central Nervous System Signs [Cerebral Edema]). The techniques for insulin administration are similar to those discussed for DKA (see Insulin Therapy). However, the insulin dosage used for the hourly IM technique or the insulin infusion rate used for the constant low-dose insulin infusion technique should be decreased by 50% initially to dampen the decrease in the blood glucose concentration and avoid a rapid decrease in ECF osmolality. Subsequent adjustments in the amount of insulin being administered are based on the rate of decline in the blood glucose concentration. The goal is a decrease of 50 mg/dL/hour (2.8 mmol/L/hour), although the rate of decrease is hard to predict or control, in part because of differences in insulin sensitivity between animals. Once the blood glucose concentration is less than 250 mg/dL (14 mmol/L), dextrose should be added to the IV fluids to make a 5% dextrose solution.

Monitoring urine output, blood pressure, blood glucose, serum electrolytes, creatinine, BUN, and urine glucose is imperative. As with ketoacidosis, the clinician must attempt to correct the hyperosmolality, hyperglycemia, and dehydration steadily (not precipitously) while stimulating diuresis to improve azotemia. These animals are critically ill and require close supervision.

The prognosis for recovery is guarded to poor. In a retrospective study of 17 diabetic cats with HHS, 65% did not survive the initial hospitalization, with most dying or being euthanized within 10 hours of presentation (Koenig et al, 2004). The long-term survival rate was low (12%). The most common concurrent disease affiliated with death or euthanasia in our animals with HHS is kidney failure.

REFERENCES

Abbott LG, Rude RK: Clinical manifestations of magnesium deficiency, *Miner Electrolyte Metab* 19:314, 1993.

Adams LG, et al.: Hypophosphatemia and hemolytic anemia associated with diabetes mellitus and hepatic lipidosis in cats, *J Vet Intern Med* 7:266, 1993.

Adrogué HJ, et al.: Plasma acid-base patterns in diabetic ketoacidosis, *N Engl J Med* 307:1603, 1982.

Adrogué HJ, et al.: Diabetic ketoacidosis: Role of the kidney in acid-base homeostasis reevaluated, *Kidney Int* 25:591, 1984.

Aroch I, et al.: A retrospective study of serum β-hydroxybutyric acid in 215 ill cats: clinical signs, laboratory findings and diagnoses, *Vet J* 191:240, 2012.

Azain MJ, et al.: Contributions of fatty acid and sterol synthesis to triglyceride and cholesterol secretion by the perfused rat liver in genetic hyperlipemia and obesity, *J Biol Chem* 260:174, 1985.

Bailiff NL, et al.: Frequency and risk factors for urinary tract infection in cats with diabetes mellitus, *J Vet Intern Med* 20:850, 2006.

Barrett EJ, DeFronzo RA: Diabetic ketoacidosis: diagnosis and treatment, *Hosp Pract* 19:89, 1984.

Becker DJ, et al.: Phosphate replacement during treatment of diabetic ketosis: effects on calcium and phosphorus homeostasis, *Am J Dis Child* 137:241, 1983.

Boord M, Griffin C: Progesterone secreting adrenal mass in a cat with clinical signs of hyperadrenocorticism, *J Am Vet Med Assoc* 214:666, 1999.

Bostrom BM, et al.: Chronic pancreatitis in dogs: a retrospective study of clinical, clinicopathological, and histopathological findings in 61 cases, *Vet J* 195:73, 2013.

Boyle PJ: Cushing's disease, glucocorticoid excess, glucocorticoid deficiency, and diabetes, *Diabetes Rev* 1:301, 1993.

Brady MA, et al.: Evaluating the use of plasma hematocrit samples to detect ketones utilizing urine dipstick colorimetric methodology in diabetic dogs and cats, *J Vet Emerg Crit Care* 13:1, 2003.

Bratusch-Marrain PR, et al.: The effect of growth hormone on glucose metabolism and insulin secretion in man, *J Clin Endocrinol Metab* 55:131, 1982.

Bruskiewicz KA, et al.: Diabetic ketosis and ketoacidosis in cats: 42 cases (1980-1995), *J Am Vet Med Assoc* 211:188, 1997.

Bush WW, et al.: Secondary hypoparathyroidism attributed to hypomagnesemia in a dog with protein-losing enteropathy, *J Am Vet Med Assoc* 219:1732, 2001.

Chastain CB, Nichols CS: Low-dose intramuscular insulin therapy for diabetic ketoacidosis in dogs, *J Am Vet Med Assoc* 178:561, 1981.

Cherrington AD, et al.: Insulin, glucagon, and glucose as regulators of hepatic glucose uptake and production in vivo, *Diabetes Metab Rev* 3:307, 1987.

Church DB: Diabetes mellitus. In Kirk RW, editor: *Current veterinary therapy VIII*, Philadelphia, 1983, WB Saunders, p 838.

Claus MA, et al.: Comparison of regular insulin infusion doses in critically ill diabetic cats: 29 cases (1999-2007), *J Vet Emerg Crit Care* 20:509, 2010.

Cryer PE: Catecholamines, pheochromocytoma, and diabetes, *Diabetes Rev* 1:309, 1993.

DeFronzo RA, et al.: Diabetic ketoacidosis: a combined metabolic-nephrologic approach to therapy, *Diabetes Rev* 2:209, 1994.

Dhupa N, Proulx J: Hypocalcemia and hypomagnesemia, *Vet Clin North Am Small Anim Pract* 28:587, 1998.

Dhupa N, Shaffran N: Continuous rate infusion formulas. In Ettinger SJ, Feldman EC, editors: *Textbook of veterinary internal medicine*, ed 4, Philadelphia, 1995, WB Saunders, p 2130.

DiBartola SP: Disorders of sodium and water: hypernatremia and hyponatremia. In DiBartola SP, editor: *Fluid, electrolyte, and acid-base disorders in small animal practice*, ed 4, St Louis, 2012, Elsevier Saunders, p 45.

DiBartola SP, de Morais HA: Disorders of potassium: hypokalemia and hyperkalemia. In DiBartola SP, editor: *Fluid, electrolyte, and acid-base disorders in small animal practice*, ed 4, St Louis, 2012, Elsevier Saunders, p 92.

Di Tommaso M, et al.: Evaluation of a portable meter to measure ketonemia and comparison of ketonuria for the diagnosis of canine diabetic ketoacidosis, *J Vet Intern Med* 23:466, 2009.

Duarte R, et al.: Accuracy of serum β-hydroxybutyrate measurements for the diagnosis of diabetic ketoacidosis in 116 dogs, *J Vet Intern Med* 16:411, 2002.

Durocher LL, et al.: Acid-base and hormonal abnormalities in dogs with naturally occurring diabetes mellitus, *J Am Vet Med Assoc* 232:1310, 2008.

Edwards DF, et al.: Hypernatremic, hypertonic dehydration in the dog with diabetes insipidus and gastric dilatation-volvulus, *J Am Vet Med Assoc* 182:973, 1983.

Ennis ED, et al.: The hyperosmolar hyperglycemic syndrome, *Diabetes Rev* 2:115, 1994.

Feldman BF, Rosenberg DP: Clinical use of anion and osmolal gaps in veterinary medicine, *J Am Vet Med Assoc* 178:396, 1981.

Feldman EC: Diabetic ketoacidosis in dogs, *Comp Cont Educ* 11:456, 1980.

Feldman EC, Nelson RW: *Canine and feline endocrinology and reproduction*, Philadelphia, 1987, WB Saunders.

Ferrannini E, et al.: Effect of free fatty acids on glucose production and utilization in man, *J Clin Invest* 72:1737, 1983.

Fincham SC, et al.: Evaluation of plasma-ionized magnesium concentration in 122 dogs with diabetes mellitus: a retrospective study, *J Vet Intern Med* 18:612, 2004.

Fisher JN, Kitabchi AE: A randomized study of phosphate therapy in the treatment of diabetic ketoacidosis, *J Clin Endocrinol Metab* 57:177, 1983.

Forman MA, et al.: Evaluation of serum pancreatic lipase immunoreactivity and helical computed tomography versus conventional testing for the diagnosis of feline pancreatitis, *J Vet Intern Med* 18:807, 2004.

Forrester SD, Moreland KJ: Hypophosphatemia: causes and clinical consequences, *J Vet Intern Med* 3:149, 1989.

Foster DW, McGarry JD: The metabolic derangements and treatment of diabetic ketoacidosis, *N Engl J Med* 309:159, 1983.

Foster DW, McGarry JD: Acute complications of diabetes: ketoacidosis, hyperosmolar coma, lactic acidosis. In DeGroot LJ, editor: *Endocrinology*, ed 2, Philadelphia, 1989, WB Saunders, p 1439.

Goldstein DE: Tests of glycemia in diabetes, *Diabetes Care* 18:896, 1995.

Goossens MM, et al.: Response to insulin treatment and survival in 104 cats with diabetes mellitus (1985-1995), *J Vet Intern Med* 12:1, 1998.

Graca R, et al.: Validation and diagnostic efficacy of a lipase assay using the substrate 1,2-o-dilauryl-rac-glycero-3-glutaric acid-(6'methylresorufin) ester for the diagnosis of acute pancreatitis in dogs, *Vet Clin Pathol* 34:39, 2005.

Groop LC, et al.: Effect of insulin on oxidative and non-oxidative pathways of glucose and FFA metabolism in NIDDM: evidence for multiple sites of insulin resistance, *J Clin Invest* 84:205, 1989.

Hale RJ, et al.: Metabolic effects of bicarbonate in the treatment of diabetic ketoacidosis, *Br Med J* 289:1035, 1984.

Hansen B: Disorders of magnesium. In DiBartola SP, editor: *Fluid therapy in small animal practice*, ed 2, Philadelphia, 2000, WB Saunders, p 175.

Hess RS, et al.: Concurrent disorders in dogs with diabetes mellitus: 221 cases (1993-1998), *J Am Vet Med Assoc* 217:1166, 2000.

Hoenig M, et al.: Use of a hand-held meter for the measurement of blood beta-hydroxybutyrate in dogs and cats, *J Vet Emerg Crit Care* 18:86, 2008.

Hood VL, Tannen RL: Maintenance of acid-base homeostasis during ketoacidosis and lactic acidosis: implications for therapy, *Diabetes Rev* 2:177, 1994.

Hume DZ, et al.: Outcome of dogs with diabetic ketoacidosis: 127 cases (1993-2003), *J Vet Intern Med* 20:547, 2006.

Joshi N, et al.: Infections in patients with diabetes mellitus, *N Engl J Med* 341:1906, 1999.

Kandel G, Aberman A: Selected developments in the understanding of diabetic ketoacidosis, *Can Med Assoc J* 128:392, 1983.

Kaplan AJ, et al.: Effects of disease on the results of diagnostic tests for use in detecting hyperadrenocorticism in dogs, *J Am Vet Med Assoc* 207:445, 1995.

Kitabchi AE, et al.: Management of hyperglycemic crises in patients with diabetes, *Diabetes Care* 24:131, 2001.

Kitabchi AE, et al.: Hyperglycemic crises in diabetes mellitus: diabetic ketoacidosis and hyperglycemic hyperosmolar state, *Endocrinol Metab Clin N Am* 35:725, 2006.

Kitabchi AE, et al.: Thirty years of personal experience in hyperglycemic crises: diabetic ketoacidosis and hyperglycemic hyperosmolar state, *J Clin Endocrinol Metab* 93:1541, 2008.

Koenig A, et al.: Hyperglycemic, hyperosmolar syndrome in feline diabetics: 17 cases (1995-2001), *J Vet Emerg Crit Care* 14:30, 2004.

Lebovitz HE: Diabetic ketoacidosis, *Lancet* 345:767, 1995.

Li PK, et al.: Direct, fixed time kinetic assays for β-hydroxybutyrate and acetoacetate with a centrifugal analyzer or a computer-baked spectrophotometer, *Clin Chem* 26:1713, 1980.

Luzi L, et al.: Metabolic effects of low-dose insulin therapy on glucose metabolism in diabetic ketoacidosis, *Diabetes* 37:1470, 1988.

Macintire DK: Treatment of diabetic ketoacidosis in dogs by continuous low-dose intravenous infusion of insulin, *J Am Vet Med Assoc* 202:1266, 1993.

Macintire DK: Emergency therapy of diabetic crises: Insulin overdose, diabetic ketoacidosis, and hyperosmolar coma, *Vet Clin North Am Small Anim Pract* 25:639, 1995.

Marshall RD, et al.: Intramuscular glargine with or without concurrent subcutaneous administration for treatment of feline diabetic ketoacidosis, *J Vet Emerg Crit Care* 23:286, 2013.

Martin L, et al.: Magnesium in the 1990's: Implications for veterinary critical care, *J Vet Emerg Crit Care* 3:105, 1993.

Masharani U, Karam JH: Pancreatic hormones and diabetes mellitus. In Greenspan FS, Gardner DG, editors: *Basic and clinical endocrinology*, ed 6, New York, 2001, McGraw-Hill, p 623.

McCord K, et al.: A multi-institutional study evaluating the diagnostic utility of the Spec cPL™ and SNAP® cPL™ in clinical acute pancreatitis in 84 dogs, *J Vet Intern Med* 26:888, 2012.

McGarry JD, et al.: Regulation of ketogenesis and the renaissance of carnitine palmitoyltransferase, *Diabetes Metab Rev* 5:271, 1989.

McMahon MM, Bistrian BR: Host defenses and susceptibility to infection in patients with diabetes mellitus, *Infect Dis Clin North Am* 9:1, 1995.

Molitch ME, et al.: Spurious serum creatinine elevations in ketoacidosis, *Ann Intern Med* 93:290, 1980.

Nanji AA, Campbell DJ: Falsely elevated serum creatinine values in diabetic ketoacidosis—clinical implications, *Clin Biochem* 14:91, 1981.

Narins RG, et al.: The metabolic acidoses. In Maxwell MH, Kleeman CR, editors: *Clinical disorders of fluid and electrolyte metabolism*, New York, 1994, McGraw-Hill, p 769.

Nelson RW, et al.: Absorption kinetics of regular insulin in dogs with alloxan-induced diabetes mellitus, *Am J Vet Res* 51:1671, 1990.

Nichols R, Crenshaw KL: Complications and concurrent disease associated with diabetic ketoacidosis and other severe forms of diabetes mellitus, *Vet Clin N Amer Small Anim Pract* 25:617, 1995.

Norris CR, et al.: Serum total and ionized magnesium concentrations and urinary fractional excretion of magnesium in cats with diabetes mellitus and diabetic ketoacidosis, *J Am Vet Med Assoc* 215:1455, 1999a.

Norris CR, et al.: Effect of a magnesium-deficient diet on serum and urine magnesium concentrations in healthy cats, *Am J Vet Res* 60:1159, 1999b.

Nugent BW: Hyperosmolar hyperglycemic state, *Emerg Med Clin N Am* 23:629, 2005.

Oppliger S, et al.: Agreement of the serum Spec fPL™ and 1,2-o-dilauryl-rac-glycero-3-glutaric acid-(6′-methylresorufin) ester lipase assay for determination of serum lipase in cats with suspicion of pancreatitis, *J Vet Intern Med* 13:27, 2013.

Owen OE, et al.: Renal function and effects of partial rehydration during diabetic ketoacidosis, *Diabetes* 30:510, 1981.

Peikes H, et al.: Dermatologic disorders in dogs with diabetes mellitus: 45 cases (1986-2000), *J Am Vet Med Assoc* 219:203, 2001.

Peterson ME: Effects of megestrol acetate on glucose tolerance and growth hormone secretion in the cat, *Res Vet Sci* 42:354, 1987.

Rossmeisl JH, et al.: Hyperadrenocorticism and hyperprogesteronemia in a cat with an adrenocortical adenocarcinoma, *J Am Anim Hosp Assoc* 36:512, 2000.

Ryder RE: Lactic acidosis: high-dose or low-dose bicarbonate therapy? *Diabetes Care* 7:99, 1984.

Sears KW, et al.: Use of lispro insulin for treatment of diabetic ketoacidosis in dogs, *J Vet Emerg Crit Care* 22:211, 2012.

Sherwin RS, et al.: Epinephrine and the regulation of glucose metabolism: effect of diabetes and hormonal interactions, *Metabolism* 29(Suppl 1):1146, 1980.

Shilo S, et al.: Acute hemolytic anemia caused by severe hypophosphatemia in diabetic ketoacidosis, *Acta Haematol* 73:55, 1985.

Sieber-Ruckstuhl S, et al.: Remission of diabetes mellitus in cats with diabetic ketoacidosis, *J Vet Intern Med* 22:1326, 2008.

Tessari P, et al.: Hyperaminoacidemia reduces insulin-mediated glucose disposal in healthy man, *Diabetologia* 28:870, 1985.

Thiebaud D, et al.: Effect of long chain triglyceride infusion on glucose metabolism in man, *Metabolism* 21:1128, 1982.

Tilg H, Moschen AR: Adipocytokines: mediators linking adipose tissue, inflammation and immunity, *Nat Rev Immunol* 6:772, 2006.

Trivedi S, et al.: Sensitivity and specificity of canine pancreas-specific lipase (cPL) and other markers for pancreatitis in 70 dogs with and without histopathologic evidence of pancreatitis, *J Vet Intern Med* 25:1241, 2011.

Wagner A, et al.: Therapy of severe diabetic ketoacidosis: zero-mortality under very-low-dose insulin application, *Diabetes Care* 22:674, 1999.

Willard MD, et al.: Severe hypophosphatemia associated with diabetes mellitus in six dogs and one cat, *J Am Vet Med Assoc* 190:1007, 1987.

Vick MM, et al.: Effects of systemic inflammation on insulin sensitivity in horses and inflammatory cytokine expression in adipose tissue, *Am J Vet Res* 69:130, 2008.

Yeates S, Blaufuss J: Managing the animal in diabetic ketoacidosis, *Focus Crit Care* 17:240, 1990.

Yen TT, et al.: Hepatic insensitivity to glucagon in ob/ob mice, *Res Commun Chem Pathol Pharmacol* 30:29, 1980.

Zammit VA: Regulation of ketone body metabolism: a cellular perspective, *Diabetes Rev* 2:132, 1994.

Zeugswetter F, Pagitz M: Ketone measurements using dipstick methodology in cats with diabetes mellitus, *J Sm Anim Pract* 50:4, 2009.

Zeugswetter F, Rebuzzi L: Point-of-care β-hydroxybutyrate measurement for the diagnosis of feline diabetic ketoacidaemia, *J Sm Anim Pract* 53:328, 2012.

Zeugswetter F, et al.: Efficacy of plasma β-hydroxybutyrate concentration as a marker for diabetes mellitus in acutely sick cats, *J Fel Med Surg* 12:300, 2010.

CHAPTER 9

Beta-Cell Neoplasia: Insulinoma

Richard W. Nelson

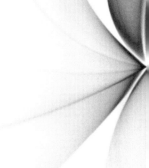

CHAPTER CONTENTS

Insulin-secreting beta-cell tumors (insulinomas) were first described in the dog by Slye and Wells in 1935. During the past seven decades, numerous publications have appeared in the veterinary literature addressing the clinical manifestations, diagnosis, treatment, and pathology of beta-cell tumors in dogs. Insulin-secreting beta-cell neoplasia is an uncommon diagnosis in dogs and a rare entity in cats. Despite excellent documentation of this disease, increased awareness of the clinical presentations, and well-established methods for establishing the diagnosis, treatment options remain limited and the prognosis remains guarded to poor. This chapter summarizes current concepts regarding the diagnosis and treatment of insulin-secreting beta-cell tumors in dogs and cats.

ETIOLOGY

Functional tumors arising from the beta cells of the pancreatic islets are malignant tumors that secrete insulin independent of the typically suppressive effects of hypoglycemia. Insulin is the most common product demonstrated in the neoplastic cells, and the clinical signs in such animals are primarily those that result from insulin-induced hypoglycemia. Beta-cell tumors, however, are not completely autonomous, and they respond to provocative stimuli, such as an increase in blood glucose by secreting insulin, often in excessive amounts. Immunohistochemical analysis of

beta-cell tumors has revealed a high incidence of multihormonal production, including pancreatic polypeptide, somatostatin, glucagon, serotonin, and gastrin (Hawkins et al, 1987; O'Brien et al, 1987; Minkus et al, 1997). Recently, using quantitative real-time polymerase chain reaction (PCR), significantly higher expression of genes encoding for growth hormone (GH) and insulin-like growth factor-1 (IGF-1) have been identified in metastases, compared to the primary beta-cell tumor and immunohistochemical examination of the beta-cell tumor and its metastases revealed expression of GH, IGF-1, and GH receptor in both primary beta-cell tumors and metastases (Buishand et al, 2012). The authors speculated that therapeutic intervention with agents that specifically antagonize the GH/IGF-1 axis or members of their signaling cascade may inhibit beta-cell tumor growth.

Malignant Versus Benign Potential

Beta-cell tumors are notorious for masking their malignant tendencies in the dog. Discrepancy is noted between the orderly arrangement of well-differentiated cells, the rarity of mitotic figures in most islet cell tumors, and the frequent metastasis of beta-cell tumors at the time of diagnosis (Kruth et al, 1982). Classifying beta-cell tumors as adenomas or adenocarcinomas based on their morphology often does not reflect their biologic behavior in humans and dogs (Mehlhaff, et al, 1985; Minkus et al, 1997). Differentiation of malignant from benign neoplasia is usually based on identification of metastasis at surgery or necropsy or the recurrence of hyperinsulinism and hypoglycemia days to months after surgical removal of a "solitary" pancreatic mass. Recent histopathologic evaluation of beta-cell tumors in 26 dogs revealed that 96% were highly cellular and exhibited nuclear atypia and 83% had an infiltrative growth pattern (Buishand et al, 2010). Vascular invasion was common, but the mitotic index was low in most tumors. Increased stromal fibrosis within the tumor was the only significant morphological prognostic marker identified in the study, a finding that illustrates the general lack of prognostic significance of histopathologic criteria in beta-cell tumors (Kruth et al, 1982; Mehlhaff et al, 1985; Caywood et al, 1988).

The malignant potential of beta-cell tumors is often underestimated in the dog. In our experience, virtually all beta-cell tumors in dogs are malignant, and most animals have microscopic or grossly visible metastatic lesions at the time of surgery. The most common sites of tumor spread are the regional lymphatics and lymph nodes (duodenal, mesenteric, hepatic, splenic), the liver, and the peripancreatic omentum. Pulmonary metastasis is typically not recognized until very late in the disease process. Identification of distant metastasis such as the gastrointestinal tract or bone marrow or gross invasion of the tumor into major blood vessels with tumor thrombus formation is uncommon (Pickens et al, 2005; Hambrook and Kudnig, 2012). In most dogs, hypoglycemia recurs days to weeks after surgical excision of the tumor. The high incidence of metastasis at the time afflicted dogs are initially examined results in part from the typically protracted time for worrisome clinical signs (e.g., collapsing episodes, seizures) to develop and become apparent to the owner and the interval between the time an owner initially observes signs and when assistance is sought from a veterinarian. Most dogs are symptomatic for 1 to 3 months before being brought to a veterinarian.

 ## PATHOPHYSIOLOGY

Maintenance of Euglycemia in the Healthy Dog

Glucose is essentially the sole metabolic fuel for the brain under normal physiologic conditions. Survival of the brain requires a continuous supply of glucose from the circulation which, in turn, requires maintenance of blood glucose concentration within or above the physiologic range. Glucose is derived from three sources: intestinal absorption that occurs after digestion of dietary carbohydrates; glycogenolysis, which is the breakdown of glycogen; and gluconeogenesis, which is the formation of glucose from precursors including lactate, amino acids (especially alanine and glutamine), and glycerol (Cryer, 2011). The liver is the major source of net endogenous glucose production through glycogenolysis and gluconeogenesis.

Exogenously derived energy, in the form of ingested carbohydrate, fat, and protein, provides enough fuel for 4 to 8 hours of cell metabolism. After this postprandial period, fuel for cellular metabolism must be derived from endogenous sources, primarily through production of glucose by the liver (Fig. 9-1). The liver initially provides glucose by the breakdown of stored hepatic glycogen (glycogenolysis). Liver glycogen stores are exhausted slowly in dogs, requiring 2 to 3 days of fasting, compared with only 24 hours of fasting in humans (de Bruijne et al, 1981). Hepatic glucose production is augmented by gluconeogenesis as the postprandial period increases and hepatic glycogen stores become depleted (Rothman et al, 1991). Gluconeogenesis is the formation of glucose from precursors (e.g., alanine, glutamine, lactate,

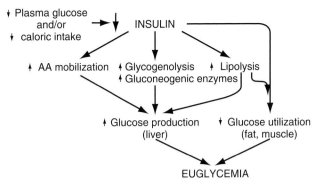

FIGURE 9-1 Hormonal and substrate changes by which euglycemia is maintained (and hypoglycemia is prevented) in normal subjects during a fast. The fall in the plasma insulin concentration is the key hormonal change resulting in increased glucose production and decreased glucose utilization. The decline in the plasma insulin concentration is, in turn, a result of a small decrease in the plasma glucose level (5 to 10 mg/dL) and/or a decrease in caloric intake. *AA,* Amino acid.

glycerol) delivered to the liver from peripheral stores. Muscle and other structural tissues supply amino acids, mainly alanine; blood cell elements supply lactate, the end product of glycolytic metabolism; and adipose tissue supplies glycerol from lipolysis of triglycerides (Karam, 2001). Oxidation of free fatty acids released from adipose cells during lipolysis supplies the energy required for gluconeogenesis and provides ketone bodies (i.e., acetoacetate, β-hydroxybutyrate), which can serve as alternative metabolic fuels for the brain during periods of prolonged fasting. Other requirements include a normal hepatic circulation, functioning hepatocytes capable of removing substrates from the circulation, and a complete complement of hepatic enzymes capable of converting these noncarbohydrate precursors into glucose.

The renal cortex also has the requisite enzymes for the production and release of glucose into the circulation, albeit the contribution is only about 5% during fasting (Stumvoll et al, 1995; Gerich et al, 2001). However, renal glucose production is regulated and under certain circumstances (e.g., glucose counterregulation, hepatic insufficiency) the contribution of glucose derived from renal gluconeogenesis can be as high as 40%. The kidney does not have glycogen stores and depends on gluconeogenesis as its only source of glucose production. Glutamine rather than alanine is the predominant amino acid substrate for renal gluconeogenesis. In addition to its contribution to glucose homeostasis during fasting, the kidney has been shown to be an important contributor to increasing blood glucose (i.e., glucose counterregulation) in the event of hypoglycemia. Although glucagon does not affect the kidney, the counterregulatory increase in epinephrine has been shown to stimulate gluconeogenesis in the renal cortex (Stumvoll et al, 1995; Gerich et al, 2001).

A normally functioning endocrine system is also necessary to maintain glucose homeostasis and prevent hypoglycemia. Rates of endogenous glucose influx into the circulation and glucose efflux out of the circulation into tissues other than the brain are regulated primarily by the blood glucose-lowering hormone insulin and the blood glucose-raising hormones, glucagon and epinephrine, such that systemic glucose balance is maintained, hypoglycemia and hyperglycemia are prevented, and a continuous supply of glucose to the brain is ensured (Cryer, 2011). In humans, when the blood glucose concentration exceeds approximately 110 mg/dL (6.2 mmol/L), insulin is secreted and the blood glucose concentration declines into the normal physiologic range (i.e., 70 to 110 mg/dL;

BOX 9-1   Autonomic Nervous System Response to Hypoglycemia

Alpha-Adrenergic Effects
Inhibition of endogenous insulin secretion
Stimulation of peripheral vasoconstriction causing increase in cerebral blood flow

Beta-Adrenergic Effects
Stimulation of hepatic and muscle glycogenolysis
Stimulation of plasma glucagon secretion
Stimulation of lipolysis generating free fatty acids
Impairment of glucose uptake by muscle
Increase in cardiac output causing increase in cerebral blood flow

Adrenomedullary Catecholamine Effects
Augmentation of alpha- and beta-adrenergic effects

Cholinergic Effects
Stimulation of pancreatic polypeptide secretion
Increase gastric motility
Produce hunger

Adapted from Karam JH: Hypoglycemic disorders. In Gardner DA, Shoback D, editors: *Greenspan's basic & clinical endocrinology,* ed 9, New York, 2011, McGraw-Hill, with permission.

BOX 9-2   Insulin and Counterregulatory Hormonal Response to Hypoglycemia

Insulin: Decreased Secretion
Reduced stimulation of beta cells by low glucose
Inhibition of insulin secretion by alpha-adrenergic nervous system and adrenomedullary catecholamines
Primary glucose regulatory factor, first defense against hypoglycemia

Glucagon: Increased Secretion
Direct stimulation of alpha cells by low glucose
Stimulation of glucagon secretion by beta-adrenergic nervous system and adrenomedullary catecholamines
Primary glucose counterregulatory factor, second defense against hypoglycemia

Catecholamines: Increased Secretion
Direct stimulation of sympathetic nervous system by low glucose
Direct secretion from the adrenal medulla in response to low glucose
Involved, third defense against hypoglycemia

Adrenocorticotropic Hormone and Cortisol: Increased Secretion
Direct stimulation of pituitary adrenocorticotropic hormone (ACTH) secretion in response to low glucose
Stimulation of pituitary-adrenocortical axis by the sympathetic nervous system
Involved but not critical

Growth Hormone: Increased Secretion
Direct stimulation of growth hormone (GH) in response to low glucose
Involved but not critical

3.9 to 6.2 mmol/L). When the blood glucose concentration decreases toward the lower limit of the normal physiologic range, insulin synthesis and secretion is inhibited, which limits tissue utilization of glucose and allows the blood glucose concentration to increase. If the blood glucose concentration decreases below the normal reference range, increased secretion of glucose counterregulatory hormones, most notably glucagon and epinephrine, increase the blood glucose concentration back into the normal physiologic range.

The signaling pathways in the pancreatic beta cell provide the mechanism whereby insulin secretion rates respond to changes in blood glucose concentration. Glucose enters the beta cell by facilitated diffusion mediated by glucose transporter 2 (GLUT-2) (see Origin of Clinical Signs). Intracellular glucose is phosphorylated to glucose-6-phospate by the enzyme glucokinase. Evidence suggests that glucokinase, by determining the rate of glycolysis, functions as the glucose sensor of the beta cell and is the primary mechanism by which the rate of insulin secretion adapts to changes in blood glucose (Buse et al, 2011). An increase in blood glucose levels results in an increase in the rate of glycolysis and a corresponding increase in the rate of insulin secretion by the beta cell, and vice versa. See the Insulin Synthesis, Structure, and Regulation section in Chapter 7 for more information on this topic.

Hypoglycemia and the Counterregulatory Response

The brain is wholly dependent on plasma glucose and counteracts declining plasma glucose concentrations with a carefully programmed neurogenic and hormonal response to mobilize storage depots of glycogen and fat and raise the plasma glucose concentration (Boxes 9-1 and 9-2). Hepatic glycogen reserves and gluconeogenesis in the liver and kidney directly supply the brain with glucose, and the mobilization of fatty acids from triglyceride depots provides energy for the large mass of skeletal and cardiac muscle, the renal cortex, the liver, and other tissues that use fatty acids as basic fuel; this spares glucose for use by tissues that remain dependent on glucose, including the central nervous system (CNS), erythrocytes, bone marrow, and renal medulla (Karam, 2001). The cascade of

events leading to endogenous glucose production is initiated by a blood glucose concentration that decreases below the normal physiologic range and the hormonal and neurogenic response to hypoglycemia intensifies as the hypoglycemia becomes more severe.

Insulin is the dominant glucose-lowering hormone. Hypoglycemia suppresses insulin secretion, which facilitates the mobilization of energy from existing energy stores (glycogenolysis, lipolysis), promotes hepatic gluconeogenesis and ketogenesis, promotes renal gluconeogenesis, and decreases glucose utilization by insulin-dependent tissues (Cryer and Polonsky, 1998; Karam, 2001). Glucose-raising or counterregulatory hormones include glucagon, epinephrine, GH, and cortisol (see Box 9-2). Insulin-induced hypoglycemia causes an increase in plasma glucagon, epinephrine, and norepinephrine concentrations at the onset of the glucose counterregulatory response, with increases in plasma GH and cortisol occurring later. Glucagon is the key counterregulatory hormone affecting recovery from acute hypoglycemia. In response to falling plasma glucose levels, glucagon is secreted by the alpha cells of the pancreatic islets into the hepatic portal circulation; it acts exclusively on the liver to activate glycogenolysis and gluconeogenesis (Cryer, 2011). Hepatic glucose production increases almost immediately.

The adrenergic-catecholamine response to hypoglycemia also plays a major role in recovery from hypoglycemia. Epinephrine has both direct and indirect effects, which stimulate hepatic glycogenolysis and hepatic and renal gluconeogenesis; provide muscle tissue with an alternative source of fuel by mobilizing muscle glycogen and stimulating lipolysis; mobilize gluconeogenic precursors (e.g., lactate, alanine, and glycerol); and inhibit glucose utilization by insulin-sensitive tissues (e.g., skeletal muscle) (Cryer, 1993; Karam, 2001). The role of cortisol and GH in the acute response to hypoglycemia is minimal but cortisol and GH may play roles in the defense against prolonged hypoglycemia (Boyle and Cryer, 1991). Cortisol facilitates lipolysis, promotes protein catabolism and the conversion of amino acids to glucose by the liver and kidney, and limits glucose utilization by insulin-dependent tissues. Similarly, GH promotes lipolysis and antagonizes the action of insulin on glucose utilization in muscle cells. However, the hyperglycemic effects of cortisol and GH do not appear for several hours after the hypoglycemic episode (Cryer and Polonsky, 1998).

The adrenergic neurogenic response to hypoglycemia acts directly to raise the blood glucose concentration and to stimulate hormonal responses that augment the adrenergic mobilization of energy stores (see Box 9-1). In dogs, hepatic glucose autoregulation is also an important glucose counterregulatory factor (Cryer and Polonsky, 1998). That is, the rate of hepatic glucose production is an inverse function of the blood glucose concentration independent of hormonal and neural regulatory factors.

Insulin Secretion in Dogs with Beta-Cell Neoplasia

In the dog or cat with an insulin-secreting tumor, neoplastic beta cells autonomously synthesize and release insulin despite hypoglycemia. As a result, tissue utilization of glucose continues, hypoglycemia progressively worsens, and clinical signs eventually appear. The onset of clinical signs is related to both the degree of hypoglycemia achieved and the rate at which it occurs. For example, a blood glucose concentration that gradually drops to 35 mg/dL (2 mmol/L) over an extended period (i.e., weeks) is much less likely to result in signs of hypoglycemia than is a blood glucose concentration of 35 mg/dL that develops rapidly over a few hours.

Failure of insulin secretion to decrease during periods of hypoglycemia predisposes a dog or cat with a beta-cell tumor to develop clinical signs of hypoglycemia during fasting and exercise. Insulin-secreting beta-cell tumors also remain responsive to many of the stimuli that promote insulin secretion in the healthy dog or cat, but the secretory response is often exaggerated, resulting in severe hypoglycemia. For example, clinical signs of hypoglycemia may occur after consumption of food that is easily digestible and rapidly absorbed or rapid intravenous (IV) administration of glucose to correct hypoglycemia.

Mechanism for Insulin-Induced Hypoglycemia

Insulin-secreting tumors and the associated hyperinsulinemia interfere with glucose homeostasis by decreasing the rate of glucose release from the liver and increasing the utilization of glucose by insulin-sensitive tissues (e.g., muscle, adipose tissue). Insulin interferes with mechanisms that promote hepatic glucose output by limiting circulating concentrations of substrates needed for gluconeogenesis. This effect is accomplished by inhibiting enzymes necessary for mobilizing amino acids from muscle and glycerol from adipose tissue. In addition, insulin decreases the activity of hepatic enzymes used in gluconeogenesis and glycogenolysis. Insulin also lowers blood glucose concentrations by stimulating glucose uptake and utilization in the liver, muscle, and adipose tissue. In essence, insulin increases tissue utilization of glucose already present in the extracellular space while interfering with hepatic production of glucose. The net effect is decreasing blood glucose concentrations because of increased tissue utilization of glucose.

Origin of Clinical Signs

Glucose is the primary fuel used by the CNS. Carbohydrate reserves in neural tissue are limited, and function of these cells depends on a continuous supply of glucose from sources outside the CNS. If the blood glucose concentration drops below a critical level, nervous system dysfunction occurs. In mammals the cerebral cortex is the first area to be affected by a shortage of glucose. The metabolically slower vegetative centers in the brainstem have less demand for blood glucose and are affected after the cerebral cortex.

The entrance of glucose into the neurons of the CNS occurs primarily by diffusion and is not insulin dependent. Because cell membranes are impermeable to hydrophilic molecules (e.g., glucose), all cells require carrier proteins to transport glucose across the lipid bilayers into the cytosol. All cells except those in the intestine and kidney have non–energy-dependent transporters that facilitate diffusion of glucose across cell membranes. To date, fourteen facilitative transporters have been identified in humans, and they include transporters for substrates other than glucose, including fructose, myoinositol, and urate (Thorens and Mueckler, 2010). The primary transporters involved in facilitative diffusion of glucose into cells are called *GLUT-1* through *GLUT-4*, with the numbers designating the order of their identity (Table 9-1). GLUT-1 is present in all tissues, has a very high affinity for glucose, and appears to mediate basal glucose uptake. GLUT-1 is an important component of the brain vascular system (blood brain barrier) that ensures adequate transport of plasma glucose into the CNS (Fig. 9-2). GLUT-2 has very high expression in pancreatic beta cells and the basolateral membranes of intestinal and renal epithelial cells and hepatocytes. GLUT-3 is the major glucose transporter on the neuronal surface, has a very high affinity for glucose, and is responsible for transferring glucose from the cerebrospinal fluid (CSF) into the neuronal cells. GLUT-4 is the major glucose transporter in adipocytes and skeletal muscle.

Blood insulin concentrations do not affect neuronal glucose transport or utilization. However, if hyperinsulinemia results in an inadequate glucose supply for intracellular oxidative processes in neurons, a resultant decline occurs in energy-rich phosphorylated compounds (adenosine triphosphate [ATP]) in neurons. This in turn results in cellular changes typical of hypoxia, increased vascular permeability, vasospasm, vascular dilation, and edema. Neuron death from anoxia follows. In acute hypoglycemia, histologic alterations are most marked in the cerebral cortex, basal ganglia, hippocampus, and vasomotor centers (see Feldman and Nelson [1987] for references). Although most of the damage from hypoglycemia occurs in the brain, peripheral nerve degeneration and

TABLE 9-1	GLUCOSE TRANSPORTERS IDENTIFIED IN HUMANS	
NAME	**MAJOR SITES OF EXPRESSION**	**AFFINITY FOR GLUCOSE***
GLUT-1	Brain vasculature, red blood cells, all tissues	High (Km = 1 mmol/L)
GLUT-2	Liver, pancreatic B cells, serosal surfaces of gut and kidney	Low (Km = 15-20 mmol/L)
GLUT-3	Brain neurons, also found in all tissues	High (Km < 1 mmol/L)
GLUT-4	Muscle, fat cells	Medium (Km = 2.5 to 5 mmol/L)

From Masharani U, Karam JH: Pancreatic hormones and diabetes mellitus. In Greenspan FS, Gardner DG, editors: *Basic and clinical endocrinology*, ed 6, New York, 2001, Lange Medical Books/McGraw-Hill, p. 630.
GLUT, Glucose transporter.
*Km represents the level of blood glucose at which the transporter has reached one-half of its maximum capacity to transport glucose. It is inversely proportional to the affinity.

demyelination are sometimes encountered (Braund et al, 1987). Other major organ systems, such as the heart, kidneys, and liver, also depend on glucose. However, an acute decrease in the blood glucose concentration results in clinical signs that involve the CNS before signs of any other major organ system dysfunction become apparent.

Prolonged, severe hypoglycemia may result in irreversible brain damage; however, it is uncommon for a dog to die during a hypoglycemic episode. Hypoglycemia is a potent stimulus for the release of the counterregulatory hormones that function to antagonize the effects of insulin and stimulate an increase in the blood glucose concentration (see Hypoglycemia and the Counterregulatory Response).

The clinical manifestations of hypoglycemia are believed to result from both a lack of glucose supply to the brain (neuroglycopenia) and stimulation of the sympathoadrenal system. The

neuroglycopenic signs common to dogs include lethargy, weakness, ataxia, disorientation, abnormal behavior, and seizures (Table 9-2). Clinical signs resulting from stimulation of the sympathoadrenal system include muscle tremors, shaking, nervousness, and restlessness. In humans, the symptoms related to release of catecholamines often precede those of neuroglycopenia and act as an early warning sign of an impending hypoglycemic attack (Karam, 2001). This illustrates the rapid response of catecholamine secretion to hypoglycemia and partly explains why canine patients with insulin-secreting tumors do not always progress to generalized seizure activity during a fast.

CLINICAL FEATURES

Signalment

Insulin-secreting tumors typically occur in middle-aged or older dogs. The mean age at the time of diagnosis of an insulin-secreting tumor in 123 dogs in our series at University of California, Davis (UC Davis), was 9 years, with a median age of 10 years and an age range of 3 to 14 years (Fig. 9-3). There is no gender predilection. A variety of breeds have been diagnosed with an insulin-secreting tumor at our hospital (Table 9-3). Labrador Retrievers and Golden Retrievers are the breeds most commonly diagnosed with this disease, which is probably a reflection of breed popularity in our region rather than a breed predisposition per se. In general, insulin-secreting

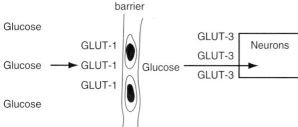

FIGURE 9-2 Glycemic regulation of glucose transporters. The center panel depicts the normal component of the high-affinity glucose transporter 1 (GLUT-1) on the vascular cells of the central nervous system (CNS) during euglycemia. An appropriate amount of glucose diffuses across the blood brain barrier and is transported into the neurons by another high-affinity glucose transporter, GLUT-3. The upper and lower panels, respectively, show adaptation by either downregulation of GLUT-1 in the face of chronic hyperglycemia (upper panel) or upregulation of GLUT-1 in the presence of chronic hypoglycemia. (From Karam JH: Hypoglycemic disorders. In Greenspan FS, Gardner DG, editors: *Basic and clinical endocrinology*, ed 6, New York, 2001, Lange Medical Books/McGraw-Hill, p. 701.)

TABLE 9-2	CLINICAL SIGNS ASSOCIATED WITH INSULIN-SECRETING TUMORS IN 117 DOGS	
CLINICAL SIGN	**NUMBER OF DOGS**	**PERCENT AGE**
Weakness	73	62
Seizures	61	52
Collapse	38	32
Tremors, shaking	25	21
Ataxia	22	19
Disoriented, abnormal behavior	22	19
Lethargy	21	15
Polyphagia	6	5
Weight gain	6	5

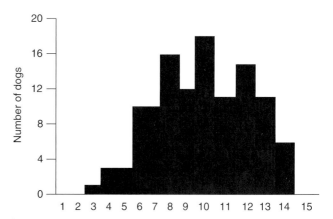

FIGURE 9-3 Age of 123 dogs at the time of initial diagnosis of an insulin-secreting islet cell tumor.

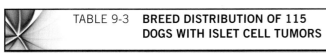

TABLE 9-3 BREED DISTRIBUTION OF 115 DOGS WITH ISLET CELL TUMORS

BREED	NUMBER OF DOGS	PERCENT
Labrador Retriever	17	15
Golden Retriever	11	10
Mixed-breeds	9	8
German Shepherd dog	7	6
Boxer	7	6
Terriers (Fox, Kerry Blue, West Highland White, Norwich)	7	6
Poodle	6	5
Irish Setter	6	5
Cocker Spaniel	6	5
Collie	5	4
Rottweiler	5	4
Border Collie	4	3
Doberman Pinscher	3	3
Samoyed	2	2
Staffordshire Terrier	2	2
Dachshund	2	2
Other breeds (one dog each)	16	10

tumors occur more commonly in large breeds of dogs. However, the size of the dog should never preclude an investigation for an insulin-secreting tumor in a hypoglycemic dog. We have diagnosed insulin-secreting tumors in dogs as small as a Pomeranian.

History

Clinical signs of an insulin-secreting tumor may have been observed for more than a year or as briefly as 1 day before veterinary care is sought. Most dogs, however, are symptomatic for 1 to 3 months before being brought to a veterinarian. In our most recent 30 dogs with an insulin-secreting tumor, clinical signs had been observed by the owners for an average of 5 weeks (range, 2 days to 4 months) before veterinary care was sought.

Clinical signs of an insulin-secreting tumor typically are caused by hypoglycemia and an increase in circulating catecholamine concentrations and include weakness, seizures, collapsing episodes, tremors, ataxia, and disorientation (see Table 9-2). One characteristic of hypoglycemic signs, regardless of the cause, is their episodic nature. Signs are generally observed intermittently for only a few seconds to minutes because of the compensatory counterregulatory mechanisms that usually increase the blood glucose concentration after the development of hypoglycemia. If these mechanisms are inadequate, seizures may occur as the blood glucose concentration continues to decrease. Seizures are usually self-limiting, typically lasting from 30 seconds to a few minutes. The seizure may stimulate further catecholamine secretion and activation of other counterregulatory mechanisms that increase the blood glucose concentration above critical levels (see Hypoglycemia and Counterregulatory Response).

The severity of clinical signs depends on the duration and severity of the hypoglycemia. Dogs with chronic fasting hypoglycemia or with recurring episodes appear to tolerate low blood glucose

concentrations (i.e., 20 to 30 mg/dL; 1.1 to 1.7 mmol/L) for prolonged periods without clinical signs, and only small additional changes in the blood glucose concentration are then required to produce symptomatic episodes. In these dogs, fasting, excitement, exercise, and eating may trigger the development of clinical signs. The "adaptation process" to chronic severe hypoglycemia is believed to involve "up-regulation" of the high-affinity glucose transporter, GLUT-1, on the vascular cells forming the blood brain barrier (see Fig. 9-2) (Karam, 2001).

In the healthy, exercising dog, a balance between increased glucose utilization by muscle, decreased glucose utilization by other tissues, and increased glucose production by the liver maintains the circulating blood glucose concentration in the normal range, allowing the brain to continue to function. The exercising dog with an insulin-secreting tumor has continuing glucose utilization not just by muscle but by all tissues, owing to the autonomous and continuing secretion of insulin. In addition, hepatic release of glucose is impaired. The potential for severe hypoglycemia is great, and this fact is supported by the number of owners who associate symptoms in their pets with jogging, play, or long walks. A similar pathophysiology is thought to explain the development of symptoms during periods of excitement. Insulin-secreting tumors are responsive to increases in the blood glucose concentration, and the insulin-secretory response can be exaggerated if the dog consumes food that is easily digestible and rapidly absorbed.

Physical Examination

Physical examination findings in dogs with an insulin-secreting tumor are often surprisingly unremarkable; dogs are usually free of visible or palpable abnormalities. Most abnormalities identified on the physical examination are nonspecific (Table 9-4). Weakness and lethargy, the most common findings, are identified in 29% and 17% of our cases, respectively. Episodes of collapse and seizures may occur during the examination but are uncommon. Afflicted dogs are usually free of palpable abnormalities, aside from findings commonly associated with aging. Weight gain is evident in some dogs and is a result of the anabolic effects of excess insulin in a dog with a normal or increased appetite. Failure to identify abnormalities on the physical examination, especially in an older, large-breed dog, is an important finding supportive of an insulin-secreting tumor.

Peripheral Neuropathy

Peripheral neuropathies have been reported in dogs with insulin-secreting tumors (Shahar et al, 1985; Braund et al, 1987; Van Ham et al, 1997). Clinical signs and physical examination findings range from paraparesis to tetraparesis, facial paresis to paralysis, sciatic hyporeflexia to areflexia, hypotonia, and muscle atrophy of the appendicular, masticatory and/or facial muscles. Sensory nerves may also be affected. A subclinical polyneuropathy has also been reported (Braund et al, 1987). The onset of clinical signs may be acute (days) or insidious (weeks to months). Abnormalities identified on electrodiagnostic testing include abnormal spontaneous potentials (e.g., positive sharp waves, fibrillation potentials) and slowed motor nerve conduction velocities (Braund et al, 1987). CSF analysis is usually unremarkable (Van Ham et al, 1997). Histopathologic findings in motor and sensory nerves include moderate to severe axonal necrosis, nerve fiber loss, and variable demyelination-remyelination (Braund et al, 1987; Schrauwen et al, 1996; Van Ham et al, 1997). Muscle changes reflect neurogenic atrophy. The pathogenesis of the polyneuropathy is not known. Proposed theories include metabolic derangements of the nerves induced by chronic and severe hypoglycemia or some

TABLE 9-4	PHYSICAL EXAMINATION FINDINGS ASSOCIATED WITH INSULIN-SECRETING TUMORS IN 78 DOGS	

PHYSICAL EXAMINATION FINDING	NUMBER OF DOGS	PERCENTAGE
Weakness	23	29
Lethargy	13	17
Collapsing	6	8
Tremors	5	6
Obtunded	5	6
Peripheral neuropathy	5	6
Seizures	4	5
No abnormalities identified	43	55

other tumor-induced metabolic deficiency, an immune-mediated paraneoplastic syndrome resulting from shared antigens between tumor and nerves, or toxic factors produced by the tumor that deleteriously affect the nerves (Kudo and Noguchi, 1985; Das and Hochberg, 1999; Heckmann et al, 2000). Treatment is aimed at surgical removal of the beta-cell tumor (Jeffery et al, 1994). Prednisone therapy (initially 0.5 mg/kg every 12 hours) may improve clinical signs (Van Ham et al, 1997). Correction of hypoglycemia, by itself, may or may not improve clinical signs caused by the peripheral neuropathy (Bergman et al, 1994). In our experience, the prognosis for improvement in clinical signs is guarded to poor, although the occasional dog shows remarkable improvement in ambulation following removal of the tumor and reestablishment of a normal blood glucose concentration.

CLINICAL PATHOLOGIC ABNORMALITIES

Virtually all dogs with insulin-secreting tumors remain undiagnosed and often unsuspected of having such tumors after completion of the history and physical examination. Most afflicted dogs have a history of episodic weakness or seizures—signs that encompass a wide variety of disorders (Box 9-3). The minimum diagnostic evaluation for dogs with these clinical signs should include a complete blood count (CBC), serum biochemical panel, and urinalysis in an effort to identify abnormalities supportive of one of the disorders outlined in Table 9-3. Therapy other than that required in an emergency situation should be withheld until a diagnosis has been made.

Results of the CBC and urinalysis in dogs with an insulin-secreting tumor are usually normal. Results of the serum biochemical profile, aside from the blood glucose concentration, are also usually normal. Hypoalbuminemia, hypophosphatemia, hypokalemia, and increased activity in alkaline phosphatase and alanine aminotransferase have been reported (Leifer et al, 1986), but these findings are considered nonspecific and not helpful in achieving a definitive diagnosis. A correlation has not been established between increased liver enzyme activity and obvious metastasis of beta-cell tumors to the liver.

The only consistent abnormality identified in serum biochemistry profiles is hypoglycemia. The mean initial blood glucose concentration in 123 of our dogs at UC Davis with an insulin-secreting tumor was 42 mg/dL, with a range of 15 to 78 mg/dL (0.84 to 4.4

BOX 9-3	A Partial Listing of the Numerous Disorders that may Result in Weakness

Neuromuscular Disorders
Infectious (e.g., canine distemper, bacterial, mycotic)
Inflammatory
Neoplasia
Cerebrovascular hemorrhage
Spinal disorders (e.g., type II disc disease; discospondylitis)
Degenerative myelopathy
Myasthenia gravis
Peripheral neuropathy
Polymyopathy/polymyositis

Polyarthritis
Immune-mediated
Infectious (e.g., rickettsial)
Degenerative

Cardiorespiratory
Congestive heart failure
Tachyarrhythmias/bradyarrhythmias
Heartworm disease
Bacterial endocarditis
Pneumonia (viral, bacterial, mycotic)
Pleural effusions

Hematologic Disorders
Anemia
Polycythemia
Hemangiosarcoma
Coagulopathy (e.g., warfarin-induced)

Metabolic Disorders
Hypoglycemia
Hypokalemia
Hyperkalemia
Hypercalcemia
Insulinoma
Hypothyroidism
Hypoadrenocorticism
Hyperadrenocorticism
Pheochromocytoma
Hepatic encephalopathy

mmol/L). The median blood glucose concentration was 38 mg/dL (2.1 mmol/L). One hundred and eleven of 123 dogs (90%) had a random blood glucose concentration less than 60 mg/dL (3.4 mmol/L). Dogs with insulin-secreting beta-cell tumors may occasionally have a blood glucose concentration between 60 and 70 mg/dL (3.4 and 3.9 mmol/L) on random testing. Such a finding does not eliminate hypoglycemia as a cause of episodic weakness or seizure activity. Fasting, with hourly evaluation of the blood glucose concentration, should be done to induce hypoglycemia in dogs with suspected insulin-secreting beta-cell tumor. The time required to induce hypoglycemia with fasting depends in part on the extent of disease at the time the dog is examined and ranges from a few hours to longer than 24 hours. Hypoglycemia (blood glucose < 60 mg/dL) will develop in most dogs with an insulin-secreting beta-cell tumor within 12 hours of withholding food. A fast of 8 or fewer hours was successful in demonstrating hypoglycemia in 33 of 35 trials in 31 dogs with insulin-secreting tumor (Kruth et al, 1982). We have had a few dogs require 12 to 24 hours of fasting before hypoglycemia became apparent and a couple of dogs that did not develop hypoglycemia after 30 hours of fasting. The clinical signs in these dogs were episodic and mild, and the diagnosis of beta-cell tumor was not established until 2 to 3 months after initial presentation.

DIFFERENTIAL DIAGNOSES FOR FASTING HYPOGLYCEMIA

Hypoglycemia is present if the blood glucose concentration is less than 60 mg/dL (3.4 mmol/L). It typically results from the excessive uptake of glucose by normal cells (e.g., during periods of hyperinsulinism, such as that which occurs with a beta-cell tumor or xylitol ingestion) or neoplastic cells, impaired hepatic gluconeogenesis and glycogenolysis (e.g., portal shunt, hepatic cirrhosis), a deficiency in diabetogenic hormones (e.g., hypocortisolism), an inadequate dietary intake of glucose and other substrates required for hepatic gluconeogenesis (e.g., anorexia in the neonate or toy breeds), or a combination of these mechanisms (e.g., sepsis; Box 9-4; Service, 1995). Iatrogenic hypoglycemia is a

common problem resulting from overzealous insulin administration in diabetic dogs and cats.

Congenital Hepatic Disease

Portovascular anomalies are the most common congenital cause of hepatic-induced hypoglycemia. Hypoglycemia develops despite an appropriate reduction in circulating insulin because of insufficient hepatic glycogen stores and inadequate hepatocellular function to support gluconeogenesis. Abnormalities suggestive of this disorder include microcytosis, hypoalbuminemia, hypocholesterolemia, decreased urea nitrogen, increased total bilirubin, ammonium biurate crystals in the urine, abnormal preprandial and postprandial bile acid concentrations, and small liver size on abdominal radiography or ultrasonography. Confirmatory tests include liver biopsy, angiography, nuclear scintigraphy, and identification of the shunt during abdominal ultrasound, computed tomography (CT) scanning or exploratory celiotomy.

Glycogen storage diseases (GSDs) are rare autosomal recessive disorders of glycogen metabolism that result from a congenital absolute or relative deficiency of one of the enzymes necessary to convert glycogen to glucose. In dogs, four breed-specific types of GSD have been described. Type Ia in Maltese terriers (von Gierke disease) is a deficiency in glucose-6-phosphatase caused by a mutated, defective glucose-6-phosphatase gene (Brix et al, 1995; Kishnani et al, 1997; 2001). Type II in Lapland dogs (Pompe disease) is a deficiency of lysosomal acid α-glucosidase (Walvoort et al, 1985). Type III in German Shepherd dogs and Curly-Coated Retrievers (Cori disease) is a deficiency of glycogen debranching enzyme (amylo-1,6-glucosidase; Fig. 9-4) (Hardy, 1989; Gregory et al, 2007). GSD in Curly-Coated Retrievers affects both liver and muscle (GSD type IIIa) and is caused by a mutation of the glycogen debranching enzyme gene *(AGL)* (Gregory et al, 2007). Type VII in English Springer Spaniels (Tarui disease) is a deficiency in phosphofructokinase (Giger et al, 1988; Smith et al, 1996). In cats, GSD type IV has been identified in Norwegian Forest cats, is caused by a deficiency in a glycogen branching enzyme (alpha-1,4 glucan 6 glycol transferase), and results in glycogen accumulation in skeletal and cardiac muscle and the nervous system (Fyfe et al, 1992).

Indicators for possible GSD in a juvenile dog include: clinical signs suggestive of hypoglycemia; progressive hepatomegaly characterized histologically by diffuse, marked hepatocellular vacuolation caused by glycogen accumulation; and hypoglycemia and increased hepatic enzyme activities identified on routine blood and urine tests. Serum glucose concentrations typically fail to increase after injection of glucagon in dogs with type Ia and type III GSDs. Confirmatory tests include histologic evaluation of hepatic biopsies and specific hepatic enzyme assays.

Acquired Hepatic Dysfunction

Hypoglycemia may result from progressive and severe destruction of the liver typically caused by primary or metastatic neoplasia or chronic inflammation leading to fibrosis, cirrhosis, and the development of acquired hepatic vascular shunts. There are numerous potential causes of chronic hepatic fibrosis in older dogs and cats. Hypoglycemia results from inadequate amounts of functional hepatic tissue for adequate storage of glycogen or for sufficient gluconeogenesis to sustain a normal blood glucose concentration during a fast. Serum insulin concentrations decline appropriately with worsening hypoglycemia, but this alone may be insufficient to prevent problems. Additional abnormalities suggestive of hepatic insufficiency include microcytosis, hypoalbuminemia,

---

BOX 9-4   Causes of Hypoglycemia in Dogs and Cats

Beta-cell tumor (insulinoma)*
Extra pancreatic neoplasia (see Box 9-5)
   Hepatocellular carcinoma, hepatoma*
   Leiomyosarcoma, leiomyoma*
Hepatobiliary disease*
   Portosystemic shunts
   Chronic fibrosis, cirrhosis
   Hepatic necrosis; toxins, infectious agents
   Primary and metastatic neoplasia
Sepsis*
   Severe canine babesiosis
   Septic peritonitis
Hypoadrenocorticism*
   Primary and secondary
Idiopathic hypoglycemia*
   Neonatal hypoglycemia
   Juvenile hypoglycemia (especially toy breeds)
   Hunting dog hypoglycemia
Exocrine pancreatic neoplasia
Pancreatitis
Glucagon deficiency (?)
Chronic kidney disease
Hypopituitarism
Severe polycythemia
Hepatic enzyme deficiencies
   Glycogen storage diseases (GSDs)
Severe malnutrition
Prolonged storage of whole blood*
Iatrogenic
   Insulin overdose*
   Sulfonylurea therapy
   Ethylene glycol ingestion
   Xylitol ingestion
   Alpha lipoic acid
   Dried chicken jerky treats
Artifact*
   Portable blood glucose monitoring (PBGM) devices
   Laboratory error

*Common cause.

hypocholesterolemia, decreased urea nitrogen, increased total bilirubin, ammonium biurate crystals in the urine, abnormal preprandial and postprandial bile acid concentrations, abnormal liver size on abdominal radiography, or abnormal echotexture or liver size on ultrasonography. Liver biopsy is helpful in confirming severe fibrosis or cirrhosis and may even identify a cause (e.g., neoplasia). The etiology of hepatic fibrosis and cirrhosis goes undiagnosed in most cases.

Adrenocortical Insufficiency (Addison's Disease)

Hypoglycemia in dogs with hypoadrenocorticism is caused by insufficient secretion of the glucocorticoids needed to stimulate hepatic mobilization and production of glucose (see Chapter 12). In this disorder, hypoglycemia occurs despite an appropriate reduction in the blood insulin concentration. Reduced insulin secretion must be accompanied by an increase in hepatic gluconeogenesis to correct hypoglycemia. Glucose synthesis is normally stimulated by gluconeogenic hormones. Without secretion of these hormones, as observed in hypoadrenocorticism, hypoglycemia is possible (Sherwin and Felig, 1981). Hypoadrenocorticism is most common in young and middle-aged dogs, and there is a gender predisposition for the female. Abnormalities on screening tests supportive of this diagnosis include a relative increase in the eosinophil and lymphocyte counts, mild nonregenerative anemia, mild to severe prerenal azotemia, hyperkalemia, hyponatremia, and hypercalcemia. Hypoglycemia may also develop with atypical hypoadrenocorticism, which is characterized by cortisol but not mineralocorticoid deficiency and normal serum electrolyte concentrations. The diagnosis of hypoadrenocorticism can be confirmed by abnormal results on adrenocorticotropic hormone (ACTH) stimulation test.

Glucagon Deficiency

Glucagon is the key counterregulatory hormone affecting recovery from acute hypoglycemia (Cryer and Gerich, 1985). In response to falling plasma glucose concentrations, glucagon is secreted by the alpha cells of the pancreatic islets into the hepatic portal circulation, and it acts exclusively on the liver to activate glycogenolysis and gluconeogenesis (Cryer and Polonsky, 1998). Hepatic glucose production is increased almost immediately. Abnormalities in the production or secretion of glucagon prevent a normal counterregulatory response to decreasing blood glucose concentrations and predispose the animal to hypoglycemia. A classic example is hypoglycemia unawareness in diabetic humans, which is a syndrome caused by deficient glucagon and catecholamine secretion, resulting in defective counterregulation, severe hypoglycemia, and diabetic coma (Gerich et al, 1991; Mokan et al, 1994; Meyer et al, 1998). Isolated glucagon deficiency that causes hypoglycemia has been reported in humans but is rare (Cryer and Polonsky, 1998). Typically, glucagon deficiency occurs in conjunction with excess insulin secretion, deficient catecholamine secretion, or increased tissue sensitivity to the actions of insulin; and this combination results in hypoglycemia. We have identified hypoglycemia in dogs and cats with severe pancreatitis and exocrine pancreatic adenocarcinoma, and we speculate that the destructive process associated with these disorders may alter the production and/or secretion of glucagon and insulin.

Hypopituitarism

GH and cortisol are glucose counterregulatory hormones involved in hepatic glucose synthesis and secretion. Failure of the pituitary gland to secrete ACTH, GH, or both may impact maintenance of glucose homeostasis and predispose the animal to hypoglycemia, especially in the fasting state. As in primary hypoadrenocorticism, insulin secretion diminishes appropriately for the degree of hypoglycemia, but this alone may not be sufficient to prevent clinical signs. GH deficiency is a rare cause of hypoglycemia and is usually diagnosed in young German Shepherd dogs as a congenital defect (see Chapter 2). Pituitary failure to secrete ACTH results in atrophy of the zona fasciculata of the adrenal cortex, impaired secretion of cortisol, and the development of secondary hypoadrenocorticism. No classic abnormalities are found on screening laboratory studies in animals with secondary hypoadrenocorticism. These dogs may have a mild nonregenerative anemia and fasting hypoglycemia, but serum electrolyte concentrations are

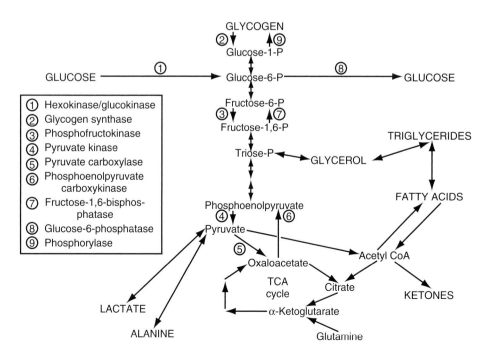

FIGURE 9-4 Schematic representation of glucose metabolism. (From Cryer PE, Polonsky KS: In Wilson JD, et al, editors: *Williams textbook of endocrinology,* ed 9, Philadelphia, 1998, WB Saunders, p. 940.) *Acetyl CoA,* Acetyl coenzyme A; *TCA,* tricarboxylic acid.

usually normal. An ACTH stimulation test and determination of a baseline endogenous ACTH concentration are used to establish the diagnosis of secondary hypoadrenocorticism (see Chapter 12).

Non–Beta-Cell Tumors

In humans, non–beta-cell tumors that cause hypoglycemia are usually of mesenchymal origin (e.g., leiomyosarcoma, fibrosarcoma). Hypoglycemia is caused less often by tumors of epithelial origin (e.g., hepatoma, carcinoid tumors) and hematopoietic origin (e.g., lymphoma, multiple myeloma) (Cryer and Polonsky, 1998). A variety of tumor types have also been reported to cause hypoglycemia in the dog (Box 9-5). In our hospital, hepatocellular carcinoma, hepatoma, leiomyoma, leiomyosarcoma, and tumors with extensive hepatic metastasis are most commonly associated with hypoglycemia (Cohen et al, 2003).

The pathogenesis of hypoglycemia associated with non–beta-cell tumors is undoubtedly multifactorial. Proposed mechanisms include excessive glucose utilization by the tumor, impaired hepatic glycogenolysis and gluconeogenesis as a result of tumor-induced hepatic destruction or inhibition of normal counterregulatory responses that prevent hypoglycemia, and secretion of an insulin-like molecule, specifically insulin-like growth factor-2 (IGF-2) that lowers the blood glucose concentration by enhancing glucose utilization by normal cells (Cryer and Polonsky, 1998). Although the major organ responsible for circulating insulin-like growth factors is the liver, it has been demonstrated that these factors are produced ubiquitously, particularly by mesenchymal cells (D'Ercole et al, 1984; Barreca et al, 1992). IGF-2 is structurally homologous to proinsulin, can bind to insulin receptors, and has direct insulin-like actions that result in hypoglycemia (de Groot et al, 2007). In addition, IGF-2 may suppress glucagon and GH secretion, which may also contribute to hypoglycemia (Cryer and Polonsky, 1998). Serum insulin concentrations are typically undetectable or in the lower end of the reference range with non–beta-cell tumors, in contrast to the high-normal to increased serum insulin concentrations seen with hypoglycemia induced by a beta-cell tumor (Beaudry et al, 1995; Bagley et al, 1996; Bellah and Ginn, 1996).

Paraneoplastic hypoglycemia affiliated with IGF-2 secretion has been reported in a dog with gastric leiomyoma, mammary carcinoma, hepatocellular carcinoma, and pancreatic neuroendocrine tumor (Boari et al, 1995; Zini et al, 2007; Finotello et al, 2009; Rossi et al, 2010). Blood glucose and serum insulin concentrations were low and serum IGF-2 concentrations were increased at presentation to the veterinary hospital in all dogs. Blood glucose and serum IGF-2 concentrations returned to the reference range in three dogs that underwent surgical removal of the tumor and results of immunohistochemical staining of tumor tissue were positive for IGF-2 in all four dogs. Interestingly, the dog with an IGF-2-secreting mammary carcinoma was an insulin-dependent diabetic dog prior to development of the mammary carcinoma; this dog developed problems with severe hypoglycemia as the tumor enlarged and became diabetic again after surgical removal of the tumor (Rossi et al, 2010).

In another study involving four dogs with hypoglycemia caused by smooth muscle tumors, the results of immunohistochemical staining for insulin were negative in the four tumors but positive for glucagon in three of the four tumors (Beaudry et al, 1995). The three smooth muscle tumors that stained positive for glucagon originated in either the stomach or jejunum, whereas the tumor that stained negative for glucagon originated in the spleen. Immunohistochemical staining for glucagon was negative in smooth muscle cells in normal adjacent tissue. The clinical relevance of this finding remains unclear, especially considering that glucagon should increase, not decrease, the blood glucose concentration.

Dogs with hypoglycemia caused by a non–beta-cell tumor may be brought to the veterinarian with clinical signs of hypoglycemia, or hypoglycemia may be a serendipitous finding on a serum biochemistry panel. In most dogs, non–beta-cell tumors that cause hypoglycemia are located in the liver or abdomen. Identification of a non–beta-cell tumor requires a thorough physical examination of the dog or cat, thoracic and abdominal radiography, abdominal ultrasonography, and histopathologic evaluation of biopsy specimens from identifiable masses. The association between a non–beta-cell tumor and hypoglycemia requires resolution of hypoglycemia after surgical excision of the tumor.

Neonatal and Juvenile Hypoglycemia

The fetus receives a continuous source of glucose via the placenta and does not depend on its own gluconeogenic capabilities to maintain an adequate blood glucose concentration. In contrast, the neonate depends on glycogenolysis and gluconeogenesis to maintain euglycemia during fasts, even if brief. Limited hepatic glycogen stores, small muscle mass, lack of adipose tissue, and decreased use of free fatty acids as an alternative energy source place the neonate at risk for developing hypoglycemia within hours of fasting (Chastain, 1990). Impaired gluconeogenesis as a result of delayed induction of one or more of the rate-limiting gluconeogenic enzymes is suspected in neonatal hypoglycemia of human infants (Cryer and Polonsky, 1998) and may play a role in neonatal hypoglycemia of puppies and kittens as well.

Hypoglycemia often occurs in conjunction with hypothermia, sepsis, starvation, toxic milk syndrome, or a combination of these problems. The ill neonate should always be evaluated for hypoglycemia. Orally administered glucose (e.g., 0.01 mL of 5% to 10% solution per gram of body weight) and frequent nursing or bottle feeding help correct and prevent hypoglycemia in the neonate.

Hypoglycemia of toy and miniature breed dogs younger than 6 months of age is common. Alanine deficiency has been implicated in this syndrome, as it has in young children (Chew et al, 1982). In humans, the rate of alanine release from muscle determines the rate of gluconeogenesis during starvation. Puppies with juvenile

---

| BOX 9-5 | **Histologic Classification of Non–Beta-Cell Tumors Associated with Hypoglycemia** |

Hepatocellular carcinoma, hepatoma
Leiomyosarcoma, leiomyoma
Hemangiosarcoma
Adenocarcinoma
    Mammary
    Nasal (horse)
    Pulmonary
    Salivary
    Gastric
    Small intestine
    Splenic
    Renal
Lymphoblastic leukemia
Plasmacytoma
Metastatic melanoma
Pancreatic neuroendocrine tumor

hypoglycemia are usually under extreme stress. They frequently have a history of recently being purchased, with an associated change in environment and diet. Gastrointestinal upset (vomiting, diarrhea, and/or anorexia) is typical and may or may not be associated with parasites. These puppies are quite fragile and are brought to veterinarians with signs that may include weakness, collapse, depression, ataxia, stupor, convulsions, hypothermia, and/or diarrhea. IV administration of glucose usually results in rapid clinical improvement. Frequent feedings prevent recurrences. This disorder virtually disappears with attainment of adult height and weight. If signs persist, a search for another disease that may be causing the hypoglycemia should be considered.

Endotoxic or Sepsis-Induced Hypoglycemia

Endotoxic or sepsis-induced hypoglycemia is a relatively uncommon cause of hypoglycemia in the dog and cat (Breitschwerdt et al, 1981). The pathogenesis of sepsis-induced hypoglycemia is not well characterized but is believed to result from increased tissue utilization of glucose in conjunction with decreased hepatic glucose production (Naylor and Kronfeld, 1985; Hargrove et al, 1988a; 1988b). Proposed mechanisms for increased glucose utilization include sepsis-induced production of insulin-like substances, interleukin-1–enhanced insulin secretion by beta cells, cytokine-enhanced increase in glucose transport into cells, and increased glucose utilization by bacteria and neutrophils (Commens et al, 1987; del Rey and Besedovsky, 1987). Increased glucose use by macrophage-rich tissues (e.g., the liver, spleen, and ileum) is responsible for most of the glucose utilization (Meszaros et al, 1988), with skeletal muscle accounting for an additional 25% (Meszaros et al, 1987). Decreased hepatic glucose production may result from impaired hepatic oxidative metabolism, increased anaerobic glycolysis of liver glucose, hypoxic injury to hepatic cells, or sepsis-induced interference with substrate delivery to the liver (see Feldman and Nelson [1987] for references). Endotoxin may also decrease glycogenolysis through depletion of hepatic and muscle glycogen stores and may impair hepatic gluconeogenesis.

In our hospital, sepsis-induced hypoglycemia is most commonly associated with parvovirus infection, abscesses, hemorrhagic gastroenteritis, pyothorax, pyometra, and gram-negative septicemia. Sepsis-induced hypoglycemia should be considered if a hypoglycemic animal is suffering from severe infection or significant leukocytosis (> 30,000 cells/μL). Artifactual hypoglycemia caused by delays in measuring the glucose concentration in a blood sample containing bacteria and marked leukocytosis may contribute to the low blood glucose measurement. A diagnosis of sepsis-induced hypoglycemia is based on identification of infection by means of a physical examination, CBC, radiography and ultrasonography, appropriate bacterial cultures, and resolution of hypoglycemia after initiation of appropriate antibiotic therapy. If severe infection is diagnosed in a dog or cat with hypoglycemia, pursuit of other causes of hypoglycemia is usually not warranted unless screening tests dictate otherwise or the hypoglycemia fails to resolve after initiation of appropriate antibiotic therapy.

Kidney Failure

The blood glucose concentration in dogs and cats with kidney failure is usually within the reference range. Occasionally dogs and cats develop hyperglycemia as a result of uremia-induced carbohydrate intolerance and insulin resistance or more commonly develop problems with glycemic control in a dog or cat with concurrent diabetes mellitus. Although critical illness caused by kidney failure

may cause hypoglycemia in humans, kidney failure-induced hypoglycemia is a very uncommon finding in dogs and cats (Edwards et al, 1987; Cryer, 2011). Proposed mechanisms for development of hypoglycemia in kidney failure include decreased renal gluconeogenesis in conjunction with impaired glucose production by the liver as a consequence of defective hepatic glycogenolysis and gluconeogenesis, limited availability of glucogenic substrates, inadequate glucose counterregulatory responses, decreased caloric intake, decreased renal degradation, and/or excretion of insulin (Fischer et al, 1986; Gerich et al, 2001).

Polycythemia

Severe polycythemia (hematocrit > 65%) may cause artifactual hypoglycemia secondary to increased glucose utilization by the markedly increased number of red blood cells in the blood sample. Polycythemia may be primary (i.e., polycythemia vera), or it may occur secondary to disorders that cause chronic systemic hypoxia (e.g., congenital right-to-left shunting of blood in the heart), to chronic renal hypoxia (e.g., renal neoplasia), or to erythropoietin-producing tumors.

Artifactual Hypoglycemia

Prolonged storage of blood before separation of serum or plasma causes the glucose concentration to decrease at a rate of approximately 7 mg/dL/h (0.4 mmol/L/h). Glycolysis by red and white blood cells becomes even more apparent in dogs and cats with erythrocytosis, leukocytosis, or sepsis. Therefore whole blood obtained for the measurement of the glucose concentration should be separated soon after collection (within 30 minutes), and the serum or plasma should be refrigerated or frozen until the assay is performed to minimize artifactual lowering of the blood glucose concentration. Glucose determinations from separated and refrigerated plasma or serum are reliable for as long as 48 hours after the separation and refrigeration of the specimen. Alternatively, plasma can be collected in sodium fluoride tubes; sodium fluoride inhibits glycolysis by erythrocytes, leukocytes, and platelets. Unfortunately, hemolysis is common in blood collected in sodium fluoride-treated tubes, which can result in slight decrements in glucose values owing to methodological problems in laboratory determinations.

Blood glucose values determined by many portable blood glucose monitoring (PBGM) devices designed for use by human diabetics are almost always lower than actual glucose values determined by bench-top methodologies (e.g., glucose oxidase and hexokinase methods). A notable exception is the AlphaTRAK glucometer designed for use in diabetic dogs and cats. Blood glucose values obtained with the AlphaTRAK can be high or low compared with actual glucose values (Cohen et al, 2009; Zini et al, 2009; Fig. 9-5). Failure to consider this "error" when using a PBGM device could result in an incorrect diagnosis of hypoglycemia. Fortunately, for most PBGM devices, the more severe the hypoglycemia, the more accurate the device becomes.

Laboratory error may also result in an incorrect value for any assay. Therefore it is wise to confirm a finding of hypoglycemia by means of evaluation of a second blood sample using bench-top methodology before more expensive studies are performed to identify the cause of hypoglycemia.

Iatrogenic Hypoglycemia (Toxicities)

Insulin and oral sulfonylurea drugs (e.g., glipizide, glyburide) are the only commonly available drugs that consistently lower the

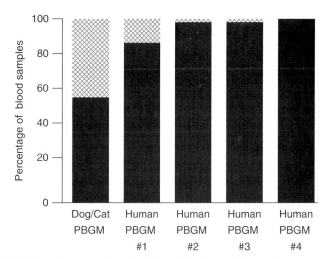

FIGURE 9-5 Frequency of low *(solid)* and high *(hatched)* blood glucose results measured in the same blood sample by five portable blood glucose monitoring *(PBGM)* meters designed for use in human diabetics and one meter (AlphaTRAK) designed for use in diabetic dogs and cats, compared with reference analyzer results. One hundred fifty-eight blood samples obtained from 49 dogs were evaluated. Blood glucose concentrations measured by the reference analyzer ranged from 41 to 639 mg/dL (2.3 to 35.8 mmol/L). (From Cohen TA, et al.: Evaluation of six portable blood glucose meters for measuring blood glucose concentration in dogs, *J Am Vet Med Assoc* 235:279, 2009.)

blood glucose concentration. In small animal practice, the most common cause of symptomatic hypoglycemia is an overdose of insulin in a diabetic dog and cat—a diagnosis that should always be suspected whenever a client reports signs resembling hypoglycemia in a diabetic pet.

Clinical hypoglycemia has been reported in dogs following the ingestion of alpha lipoic acid (Loftin and Herold, 2009), dried chicken jerky treats (Hooper and Roberts, 2011; Thompson et al, 2013), and xylitol (Murphy and Coleman, 2012). Alpha lipoic acid has antioxidant properties, is available as an over-the-counter supplement, and has been investigated as possible adjunctive treatment for various conditions, including diabetes mellitus and diabetic neuropathy. Ingestion of dried chicken jerky treats made in China caused Fanconi syndrome characterized by glucosuria and euglycemia or hypoglycemia in addition to lethargy, inappetence, and vomiting in dogs. Xylitol is a five-carbon sugar alcohol used as a sweetener and sugar substitute in many products including chewing gums, candies, baked goods, jellies, drink powders, vitamins, and nutritional supplements (Murphy and Coleman, 2012). Xylitol ingestion in dogs stimulates insulin secretion leading to potentially severe and life-threatening hypoglycemia, which may develop within 30 minutes to 12 hours after xylitol ingestion. Acute hepatic failure may develop 1 to 3 days later. Treatment for these toxicities included IV fluids with dextrose administration in addition to supportive care.

 ## DIAGNOSTIC APPROACH TO HYPOGLYCEMIA: PRIORITIZING THE DIFFERENTIALS

Hypoglycemia should always be confirmed in a second blood sample before initiating diagnostic studies to identify the cause. Careful evaluation of the animal's history, physical examination findings, and results of routine blood and urine tests (i.e., CBC, serum biochemistry panel, and urinalysis) usually provide clues to the underlying cause. Hypoglycemia in the puppy or kitten is

usually caused by idiopathic hypoglycemia, starvation, congenital portosystemic shunt, or sepsis. In young adult dogs or cats, hypoglycemia is usually caused by hepatobiliary disease, portosystemic shunt, hypoadrenocorticism, or sepsis. In older dogs or cats, hepatobiliary disease, beta-cell neoplasia, extrapancreatic neoplasia, hypoadrenocorticism, and sepsis are the most common causes.

The blood glucose concentration tends to be greater than 45 mg/dL (2.5 mmol/L) and is often an incidental finding in dogs and cats with hypoadrenocorticism or hepatobiliary disease, although severe hypoglycemia causing neurologic signs may occasionally occur. Additional clinical pathologic alterations are usually present (e.g., hyponatremia and hyperkalemia in animals with hypoadrenocorticism or increased liver enzyme activities, hypocholesterolemia, hypoalbuminemia, and a low blood urea nitrogen [BUN] concentration in animals with hepatobiliary disease). Normal serum electrolyte concentrations do not rule out a cortisol deficiency as the cause for hypoglycemia; atypical hypoadrenocorticism may be present. An ACTH stimulation test or liver function test (i.e., preprandial and postprandial bile acids) may be required to confirm the diagnosis. Severe hypoglycemia (less than 40 mg/dL; 2.2 mmol/L) may develop in neonates and juvenile kittens and puppies (especially toy breeds) and in animals with sepsis, beta-cell neoplasia, and extrapancreatic neoplasia—most notably hepatic adenocarcinoma and leiomyosarcoma. Sepsis is readily identified on the basis of physical examination findings and abnormal CBC findings, which include a neutrophilic leukocytosis (typically > 30,000/μL), a shift toward immaturity, and signs of toxicity. Extrapancreatic neoplasia can usually be identified on the basis of the physical examination, abdominal or thoracic radiography, and abdominal ultrasonography findings. Dogs with beta-cell neoplasia typically have normal physical examination findings aside from findings suggestive of hypoglycemia (e.g., weakness) and no abnormalities other than hypoglycemia identified on routine blood and urine tests. Measurement of baseline serum insulin concentration when the blood glucose is less than 60 mg/dL (3.4 mmol/L) is used to confirm the diagnosis of a beta-cell tumor.

 ## CONFIRMING THE DIAGNOSIS OF AN INSULIN-SECRETING BETA-CELL TUMOR: SERUM INSULIN DETERMINATION

The diagnosis of an insulin-secreting beta-cell tumor requires an initial confirmation of hypoglycemia followed by documentation of inappropriate insulin secretion and identification of a pancreatic mass using ultrasonography, CT, or exploratory celiotomy. Considering the potential differential diagnoses for hypoglycemia (see Box 9-4), a tentative diagnosis of insulin-secreting beta-cell tumor can often be made on the basis of the history, physical examination findings, and an absence of abnormalities other than hypoglycemia shown by routine blood tests.

Whipple's Triad

In 1935, the report that established insulin-secreting tumors of the pancreas as a clinical entity included a discussion of the three criteria to be used in confirming the diagnosis (Whipple and Grantz, 1935). These standards, now referred to as *Whipple's triad,* are: (1) the symptoms occur after fasting or exercise; (2) at the time of symptoms, the serum glucose concentration is less than 50 mg/dL (2.8 mmol/L); and (3) the symptoms are relieved by administration of glucose. Unfortunately, this triad can result from numerous causes of hypoglycemia and as such is nonspecific.

Determination of Baseline Insulin and Glucose Concentrations

Theory

The diagnosis of an insulin-secreting beta-cell tumor is established by evaluating the blood insulin concentration at a time when hypoglycemia is present. Hypoglycemia suppresses insulin secretion in normal animals, with the degree of suppression directly related to the severity of the hypoglycemia. Hypoglycemia fails to have this same suppressive effect on insulin secretion if the insulin is synthesized and secreted from autonomous neoplastic cells, because tumor cells that produce and secrete insulin are less responsive to hypoglycemia than normal beta cells. Invariably the dog with an insulin-secreting tumor will have an inappropriate excess of insulin relative to that needed for a particular blood glucose concentration. The relative excess of insulin is easiest to recognize when the blood glucose concentration is low, preferably less than 50 mg/dL (2.8 mmol/L). If the blood glucose concentration is low and the insulin concentration is in the upper half of the reference range or increased, the dog has a relative or absolute excess of insulin that can be explained by the presence of an insulin-secreting tumor that is insensitive to hypoglycemia. Confidence in identifying an inappropriate excess of insulin depends on the severity of the hypoglycemia; the lower the blood glucose concentration, the more confident the clinician can be in identifying inappropriate hyperinsulinemia, especially when the serum insulin concentration falls in the reference range.

Protocol

Most dogs with insulin-secreting neoplasia are persistently hypoglycemic. If the blood glucose concentration is less than 60 mg/dL (3.4 mmol/L) and preferably less than 50 mg/dL (2.8 mmol/L), serum should be submitted to a commercial veterinary endocrine laboratory for determination of the glucose and insulin concentrations. The insulin assay must be validated for use in dogs, and interpretation of insulin results should be based on the reference interval established by the laboratory utilized (Madarame et al, 2009; Öberg et al, 2011). If the dog's blood glucose concentration is greater than 60 mg/dL, fasting may be necessary to induce hypoglycemia. Blood glucose concentrations should be evaluated hourly during the fast and blood obtained for glucose and insulin determination when the blood glucose concentration is less than 60 mg/dL. It is important to remember that blood glucose results obtained from PBGM devices are often lower than results obtained using bench-top methodologies (Cohn et al, 2000; Wess and Reusch, 2000; Cohen et al, 2009; Zini et al, 2009). Ideally a blood sample for submission to a commercial laboratory for glucose and insulin determinations should not be obtained until the blood glucose measured on these devices is less than 50 mg/dL. Once fasting has induced hypoglycemia and the blood sample has been obtained for glucose and insulin determination, the dog can be fed several small meals over the next 2 to 3 hours to minimize overstimulation of the tumor and rebound hypoglycemia.

Interpretation

The serum insulin concentration must be evaluated from the same blood sample as and in relation to the blood glucose concentration (Box 9-6). A serum insulin concentration that exceeds the upper limit of the reference range in a dog with a corresponding blood glucose concentration of less than 60 mg/dL (3.4 mmol/L), in combination with appropriate clinical signs and clinical pathologic findings, strongly supports the diagnosis of an insulin-secreting tumor. An insulin-secreting tumor is also possible if the serum

BOX 9-6	Interpretation of Baseline Serum Insulin Concentration in Dogs with Hypoglycemia Believed to be Caused by Insulin-Secreting Beta-Cell Neoplasia

SERUM INSULIN CONCENTRATION	PROBABILITY OF BETA-CELL TUMOR*
Above reference range	High
Upper half of reference range	Possible
Lower half of reference range	Low
Below reference range	Ruled out

*Ideally, the blood glucose concentration determined by a bench-top methodology (i.e., glucose oxidase or hexokinase method) should be less than 50 mg/dL in the same blood sample submitted to the laboratory for insulin determination. Interpretation of serum insulin concentration is unreliable if the blood glucose concentration is greater than 60 mg/dL.

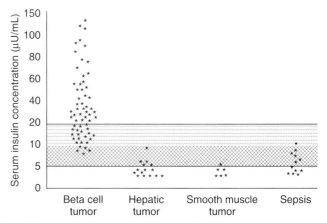

FIGURE 9-6 Serum insulin concentrations in dogs with hypoglycemia caused by an insulin-secreting beta-cell tumor, hepatoma or hepatocellular carcinoma, leiomyosarcoma, or sepsis. Although a serum insulin concentration in the high end of the normal range (i.e., > 10 μU/mL) is consistent with a beta-cell tumor, a serum insulin concentration in the low end of the normal range (i.e., 5 to 10 μU/mL) is not diagnostic for a beta-cell tumor. Shaded regions represent the high *(horizontal lines)* and low *(hatched area)* ends of the normal range.

insulin concentration is in the upper half of the reference range. Insulin values near the lower end of the reference range may be found in animals with other causes of hypoglycemia, as well as in those with insulin-secreting tumors (Fig. 9-6). Careful assessment of the history, physical examination findings, and diagnostic test results in relation to viable differentials for hypoglycemia in that dog and, if necessary, repeating serum glucose and insulin measurements when hypoglycemia is more severe will usually identify the cause of the hypoglycemia. In 101 of our dogs with a histologically confirmed beta-cell tumor and a blood glucose concentration less than 60 mg/dL, the serum insulin concentration was above the reference range in 74 dogs (73%); in the upper half of the reference range in 21 dogs (21%); and in the lower end of the reference range in 6 dogs (6%). No dog had a serum insulin concentration less than the reference range. Any serum insulin concentration below the reference range is consistent with insulinopenia and does not indicate the presence of an insulin-secreting tumor.

Insulin-to-Glucose Ratios

Several insulin-to-glucose ratios, including the insulin-to-glucose ratio, the glucose-to-insulin ratio, and the amended insulin-to-glucose ratio, have been recommended to evaluate the interrelationship between the blood glucose and insulin concentrations and to help establish the diagnosis of insulin-secreting tumor when the laboratory results are ambiguous (e.g., hypoglycemia is marginal and serum insulin concentrations remain in the reference range). Of these ratios, the amended insulin-to-glucose ratio is most commonly used. The amended insulin-to-glucose ratio is determined by entering the blood glucose and serum insulin concentrations in the following formula:

$$\frac{\text{serum insulin } (\mu U/mL) \times 10}{\text{blood glucose (mg/dL)} - 30}$$

The use of "- 30" in the formula is based on the theory that in normal humans, serum insulin concentrations are undetectable when the blood glucose concentration is less than 30 mg/dL (1.7 mmol/L). Whenever the blood glucose concentration is less than 30 mg/dL, the number 1 is used as the divisor. Extrapolating from the human literature, most authors have suggested that an amended insulin-to-glucose ratio greater than 30 is diagnostic of an insulin-secreting tumor. However, this test is not specific; that is, some dogs with other causes of hypoglycemia may have abnormal amended ratios (Leifer et al, 1986). The most common reason for lack of specificity is a detectable serum insulin concentration, albeit usually in the lower end of the reference range, despite hypoglycemia. This occurs most commonly with hepatic tumors and sepsis. We do not rely on insulin-to-glucose ratios for interpretation of blood insulin and glucose results. Rather, we interpret the absolute serum insulin concentration during hypoglycemia (see Box 9-6) in conjunction with the history, physical findings, and results of routine blood and urine tests.

Serum Fructosamine Concentration

Serum fructosamines are glycated proteins found in blood that are used to monitor control of glycemia in diabetic dogs and cats (see Chapters 6 and 7). Fructosamines result from an irreversible, nonenzymatic, insulin-independent binding of glucose to serum proteins and are a marker of the average blood glucose concentration during the circulating lifespan of the protein, which varies from 1 to 3 weeks depending on the protein. The extent of glycosylation of serum proteins is directly related to the blood glucose concentration; the lower the average blood glucose concentration during the preceding 2 to 3 weeks, the lower the serum fructosamine concentration, and vice versa. Serum fructosamine concentrations below the reference range support the existence of significant periods of hypoglycemia and an insulin secreting tumor, assuming the history and findings on physical examination and routine blood and urine test results are also consistent with the diagnosis. A serum fructosamine concentration below the reference interval may also occur with other disorders that cause prolonged periods of hypoglycemia or that interfere with the assay (see Table 6-8). Documenting a low serum fructosamine concentration in a dog with suspected insulinoma and blood glucose concentrations that remain greater than 60 mg/dL despite fasting provides support for additional diagnostics (e.g., diagnostic imaging) or exploratory surgery (Mellanby and Herrtage, 2002).

Provocative Testing

Several tests have been described that use agents that stimulate insulin secretion by normal and neoplastic beta cells; these include the glucagon tolerance test, the oral and IV glucose tolerance test, the tolbutamide tolerance test, and the epinephrine stimulation test. By evaluating the response of blood glucose and insulin concentrations for a period of time after administration of these agents, a differentiation between normal and neoplastic beta cells can potentially be made. We do not use any of these tests to establish the diagnosis of an insulin-secreting tumor, and they are not recommended. See the first edition of *Canine and Feline Endocrinology and Reproduction* (Feldman and Nelson, 1987) for more information on the use of provocative testing in dogs suspected of having beta-cell neoplasia.

 DIAGNOSTIC IMAGING

Diagnostic imaging is indicated to identify a pancreatic mass, to identify metastatic disease, and to localize the site of the mass in the pancreas (e.g., pancreatic body versus pancreatic limb); this information provides support for the diagnosis of a beta-cell tumor and a preliminary assessment of surgical resectability, likelihood of postoperative complications (e.g., pancreatitis), and prognosis. Abdominal ultrasound is widely available and is the initial imaging procedure used to assess the pancreas, peripancreatic tissues, and liver. Advanced diagnostic imaging, specifically dual-phase CT, is currently the most sensitive imaging procedure for identification of the primary mass and metastases and is recommended immediately prior to surgical exploration, if available.

Radiography

Abdominal radiographs are not helpful in establishing the diagnosis of an insulin-secreting tumor, partly because of the location of the pancreas and the small size of most insulin-secreting tumors. Insulin-secreting tumors are typically less than 3 cm in diameter at the time the diagnosis is established. Displacement of viscera or a visible mass in the right cranial quadrant of the abdominal cavity is extremely rare. Thoracic radiographs are of limited help in documenting metastatic disease, primarily because beta-cell tumors rarely metastasize to the lungs until late in the course of the disease. As such, thoracic radiographs are typically negative for metastatic disease when obtained at the time the diagnosis is established, and surgery is contemplated. The most common sites of early metastasis are the liver, regional lymph nodes, and peripancreatic omentum, which are regions where abdominal radiographs are also ineffective in identifying metastatic disease.

Ultrasonography

Abdominal ultrasonography can be used to identify a mass in the region of the pancreas and to look for evidence of potential metastatic disease in the liver and surrounding structures (Fig. 9-7). Because of the small size of most beta-cell tumors and similar echogenicity of the tumor and the adjacent normal pancreas, abdominal ultrasonographic findings are often interpreted as normal, although a pancreatic mass or metastatic lesion can be found at surgery. A normal abdominal ultrasonographic finding does not rule out the diagnosis of a beta-cell tumor.

Ultrasonic detection of a mass lesion in the region of the pancreas helps confirm the suspicion of beta-cell tumor in a dog with appropriate clinical signs and clinical pathologic abnormalities (Fig. 9-8). Identification of mass lesions in the hepatic parenchyma or peripancreatic tissue suggests metastatic disease. Occasionally only the metastatic sites are identified with ultrasound, and the tumor in the pancreas goes undetected. Failure to identify a mass lesion in the region of the pancreas or metastatic sites is common and does not rule out the presence of a beta-cell tumor.

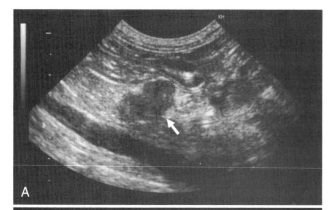

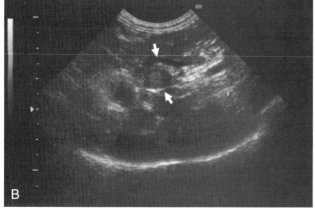

FIGURE 9-7 Ultrasonogram of the pancreas, showing an islet beta-cell tumor (*arrow;* **A**) and an enlarged hepatic lymph node (*arrows;* **B**) resulting from metastasis of the beta-cell tumor to the liver in a 9-year-old Cocker Spaniel. (From Nelson RW, Couto CG, editors: *Small animal internal medicine,* ed 5, St Louis, 2014, Elsevier, p. 817.)

In one study evaluating 13 dogs, the sensitivity of ultrasonography for detecting insulinomas was 69% and the sensitivity for detecting hepatic and lymph node metastasis was 44% (Lamb et al, 1995). In a more recent study evaluating 14 dogs, the sensitivity of ultrasonography for detecting insulinomas was 35% and ultrasonography was negative in all five dogs that had lymph node metastasis at surgery, and it was negative in two of four dogs with hepatic metastasis (Robben et al, 2005). Random evaluation of 58 dogs with surgically and histologically confirmed beta-cell neoplasia seen at UC Davis that underwent ultrasound evaluation of the abdomen prior to surgery identified a mass lesion in only 24 dogs (41%). Ultrasonography failed to identify diffuse infiltration of the pancreas by the tumor in two dogs and a mass that was not grossly visible at the time of surgery in two dogs. In one of these dogs, a 2.3 × 1.3 cm pancreatic mass was identified 1 year after the initial exploratory surgery. Tumors in the left limb of the pancreas were identified by ultrasound more often than those in the body or right limb. Similarly, larger tumors were more likely to be identified with ultrasonography although tumors greater than 2 cm × 2 cm were not identified.

The accuracy of ultrasound depends on the experience of the operator, quality of the ultrasound machine and sonogram images, size of the pancreatic mass, and presence of extraneous factors that affect results (e.g., bowel gas, obesity, movement of the dog). Failure to identify a pancreatic mass in a dog suspected of having a beta-cell tumor does not rule out the diagnosis or the presence of metastatic disease but is a further indication for exploratory surgery in the hopes of finding a small, excisable tumor.

Computed Tomography

Conventional pre- and postcontrast CT is reported to have better sensitivity than ultrasonography for the detection of beta-cell

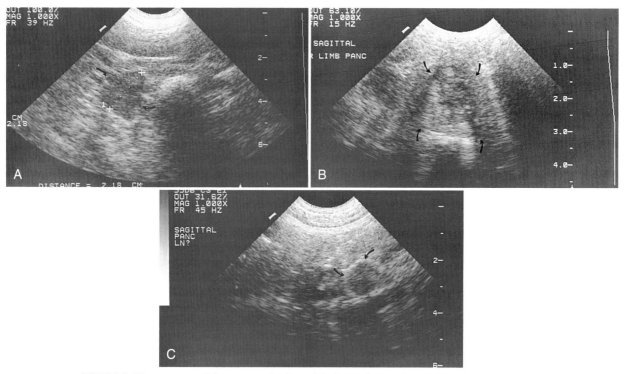

FIGURE 9-8 Ultrasonograms of the pancreas showing an islet beta-cell tumor *(arrows)* in a 13-year-old Borzoi **(A)** and a 14-year-old Miniature Poodle **(B). C,** Ultrasonogram of the peripancreatic tissue showing a metastatic beta-cell tumor *(arrows)* in a 5-year-old Golden Retriever.

tumors in dogs. In a series of 14 dogs with insulinoma, the sensitivity of conventional pre- and postcontrast CT for detection of insulinoma and lymph node metastasis was 71% and 40%, respectively (Robben et al, 2005). Unfortunately, CT also identified 28 false-positive lesions in lymph nodes. Conventional pre-and postcontrast CT has been replaced by dual-phase computed tomographic angiography (CTA) for the identification and localization of insulinomas and metastases in humans (Chatziioannou et al, 2001). Dual phase CTA techniques have been developed in dogs and preliminary studies in dogs with insulinoma have been promising (Caceres et al, 2006; Iseri et al, 2007; Mai and Caceres, 2008). During dual-phase CTA, images are acquired during the arterial and venous phases after IV injection of contrast medium. Most human insulinomas are histopathologically hypervascular, and the CT images obtained during the arterial phase may clearly delineate enhancing tumor lesions (Gritzmann et al, 2004). Insulinomas in dogs are also assumed to be hypervascular. A study evaluating dual-phase CTA of the pancreas in 10 healthy Beagle dogs identified an arterial phase peak at 15 ± 2 seconds after contrast medium injection followed by a venous phase peak where the pancreatic parenchyma was clearly delineated at 28 ± 9 seconds and appearance of the equilibrium phase approximately 70 seconds after injection (Fig. 9-9; Iseri et al, 2007). Caceres, et al., (2006) identified a purely arterial pancreatic window of 5 to 6 seconds after contrast administration in nine healthy Beagles. Evaluation of a dog with insulinoma revealed a hyperattenuating mass at the arterial phase of the dual-phase CTA, and the size and location of the tumor observed on the CT images were consistent with those seen at surgery (Iseri et al, 2007).

In a subsequent study involving three dogs with insulinoma, dual-phase CTA identified lesions not seen on ultrasonography, including the primary insulinoma in two dogs (Mai and Caceres, 2008). Findings with dual-phase CTA were in agreement with the surgical findings in all three dogs. In two dogs, the insulinomas had marked contrast enhancement during the arterial phase of the study with less enhancement during the venous phase and was isoattenuating to the rest of the pancreas during the delayed phase of the study. In the third dog, a metastasized lymph node but not the pancreatic insulinoma had strong enhancement at the arterial phase comparable to that seen in the primary insulinoma in the other two dogs. Lack of arterial enhancement of an insulinoma has been reported in humans with up to 45% of pancreatic insulinomas being hypo- to isoattenuating to the rest of the pancreas during the arterial phase (Van Hoe et al, 1995). Occasionally the tumor is hyperattenuating at the venous but not the arterial phase of the study. Evaluation of the arterial and venous phase of a contrast-enhanced CT is currently recommended immediately prior to surgery to identify the location of the primary insulinoma and its metastatic sites. The decision to either pursue surgery with medical treatment to follow, or cancel surgery and initiate medical treatment will be dependent, in part, on the findings of the CT study.

Scintigraphy

Somatostatin receptor scintigraphy using the radiopharmaceutical drug indium (In)-111 pentetreotide has been used to image pancreatic islet cell tumors in humans (Kvols et al, 1993; Lamberts et al, 1993). In humans, localization of beta-cell tumors with somatostatin receptor scintigraphy has been inconsistent and of limited value (Lamberts et al, 1991; Buetow et al, 1997). Positive and negative scan results have been correlated with the

presence or absence of somatostatin receptors in tumor biopsy samples. Five somatostatin receptor subtypes, designated sst1 to sst5, are recognized in human tissue (Reubi et al, 2001). One variable influencing the success of somatostatin receptor scintigraphy is the predominant somatostatin receptor subtype expressed by the insulinoma, which dictates its affinity for pentetreotide. Ligand binding studies on beta-cell tumors in humans have identified different subtypes of somatostatin receptors, with variable binding capacities for somatostatin and somatostatin analogs, which may explain the variability of results (Lamberts et al, 1991; Bruns et al, 1994).

In the dog, the predominant somatostatin receptor containing high-affinity binding sites for the somatostatin analog octreotide and the radiopharmaceutical In-111 pentetreotide in insulin-secreting tumors has been sst2 (Robben et al, 1997; Garden et al, 2005). Somatostatin receptor scintigraphy using radio-labeled

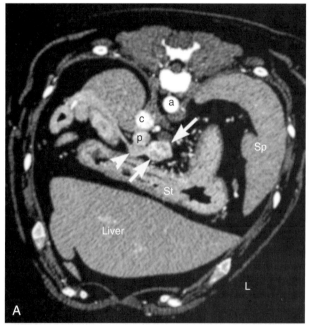
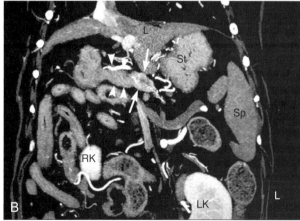

FIGURE 9-9 Transverse **(A)** computed tomography (CT) image and a maximum intensity projection CT image in the dorsal plane **(B)** of a pancreatic beta-cell tumor obtained during the arterial phase of dual-phase CT angiography in a dog that presented with severe hypoglycemia and inappropriate hyperinsulinemia. Note the marked distinction between the beta-cell tumor *(arrows)* and the remaining normal pancreas *(arrow heads)*. (Images courtesy of Dr. Eric Johnson.) *a,* aorta; *c,* caudal vena cava; *p,* portal vein; *St,* stomach, *Sp,* spleen; *RK* and *LK,* right and left kidney.

octreotide or In-111 pentetreotide was used to identify beta-cell neoplasia in seven dogs with inconclusive findings on abdominal ultrasonography (Robben et al, 1997; Lester et al, 1999). Somatostatin receptor scintigraphy was effective in identifying the primary insulin-secreting tumor in five of seven dogs and larger metastases in the regional lymph nodes and liver in three of three dogs and two of three dogs, respectively. Small metastases in the liver were not detected in one dog. In a subsequent study by Garden, et al., (2005) using In-111 pentetreotide, scintigraphic scans in four of five dogs with insulinoma showed that abnormal foci of In-111 pentetreotide activity attributed to the insulinoma but the anatomic location of the tumors was correctly predicted in only one of these dogs. The scan in the fifth dog was equivocal; a 1.5 cm insulinoma was identified in the distal left limb of the pancreas at surgery. In a series of 14 dogs with insulinoma, the sensitivity of single-photon emission CT using radiolabeled octreotide was 43% and lymph node metastasis was identified in none of five dogs (Robben et al, 2005). Negative scan results could reflect the expression of somatostatin receptors with low affinity for pentetreotide, low expression density of sst2 receptors, or small size of the tumor, rather than absence of the tumor itself (Garden et al, 2005).

Somatostatin receptor scintigraphy offers intriguing options for identifying insulin-secreting tumors and determining potential responsiveness of the tumor to octreotide therapy. Presumably, positive scintigraphic scans would also predict a positive response to treatment with the somatostatin analog octreotide (see Somatostatin Therapy).

 ## TREATMENT OF BETA-CELL NEOPLASIA

Surgical Versus Medical Therapy

Treatment options for a beta-cell tumor include surgical exploration, medical treatment for chronic hypoglycemia, or both. Surgery offers a chance to cure dogs with a resectable solitary mass. In dogs with nonresectable tumors or with obvious metastatic lesions, removal or "debulking" of as much abnormal tissue as possible frequently results in remission, or at least alleviation, of clinical signs and an improved response to medical treatment. Survival time is longer in dogs that undergo surgical exploration and tumor debulking followed by medical therapy, compared with dogs only treated medically (Tobin et al, 1999). Despite these benefits, surgery remains a relatively aggressive mode of diagnosis and treatment, in part because of the high prevalence of metastatic disease, the older age of many dogs at the time beta-cell neoplasia is diagnosed, the potential for postoperative pancreatitis, and the unpredictable response to surgery as it relates to improvement in hypoglycemia and clinical signs. As a general rule, we are less aggressive about recommending surgery in aged dogs (i.e., older than 12 years of age), dogs with extensive metastatic disease identified by diagnostic imaging, and dogs with concurrent disease that significantly enhances the anesthetic risk.

Medical management of chronic hypoglycemia should be initiated when an exploratory celiotomy is not performed or when metastatic or inoperable neoplasia results in recurrence of clinical signs. Medical therapy revolves around nonspecific antihormonal therapy designed to increase the blood glucose concentration and decrease the occurrence of clinical signs. Many dogs with metastatic disease can be managed medically for several months to more than a year. Medical therapy, however, has no potential for providing a "cure" or for preventing metastasis of malignant beta-cell neoplasia.

Perioperative Management of Dogs Undergoing Surgery

The intent of surgery should be to remove as much abnormal tissue as possible, including resectable sites of metastases. The success of surgery depends in part on providing appropriate fluid therapy, dextrose, and supportive care during the perioperative period to avoid severe hypoglycemia and postoperative pancreatitis and to improve the likelihood of an uneventful recovery. Euthanasia is not recommended regardless of the findings at surgery. Many dogs with metastatic disease can be managed medically for several months to more than a year.

Until surgery is performed, the dog should be protected from episodes of severe hypoglycemia. This can usually be accomplished through frequent feeding of small meals and administration of glucocorticoids (Box 9-7). A continuous IV infusion of a balanced

---

BOX 9-7   Long-Term Medical Therapy for Dogs with a Beta-Cell Tumor

Standard Treatments
1. Dietary therapy
   a. Feed canned or dry food in three to six small meals daily.
   b. Dietary fat, complex carbohydrates, and fiber help prolong postprandial glucose absorption.
   c. Avoid foods containing monosaccharides, disaccharides, propylene glycol, and corn syrup.
2. Limit exercise to walks; avoid strenuous exercise.
3. Glucocorticoid therapy
   a. Prednisone, 0.5 mg/kg divided into two doses initially.
   b. Gradually increase dose and frequency of administration, as needed.
   c. Goal is to control clinical signs, not to reestablish euglycemia.
   d. Consider alternative treatments if signs of iatrogenic hypercortisolism become severe or glucocorticoids become ineffective.

Additional Treatments
1. Diazoxide therapy
   a. Continue standard treatment; reduce glucocorticoid dose if polyuria and polydipsia is unacceptable.
   b. May initiate diazoxide early when glucocorticoid dose is low, or later when glucocorticoids become ineffective or polyuria and polydipsia becomes unacceptable.
   c. Diazoxide, 5 mg/kg every 12 hours initially.
   d. Gradually increase dose as needed, not to exceed 60 mg/kg/day.
   e. Goal is to control clinical signs, not to reestablish euglycemia.
2. Somatostatin therapy
   a. Continue standard treatment; reduce glucocorticoid dose if polyuria and polydipsia is unacceptable.
   b. Octreotide (Sandostatin), 10 to 40 μg/dog administered subcutaneously every 12 hours to every 8 hours.
3. Streptozotocin therapy
   a. Effectiveness in improving hypoglycemia, controlling clinical signs, and prolonging survival is variable and potentially severe adverse reactions are common (see Streptozotocin).
   b. Continue standard treatment; reduce glucocorticoid dose if polyuria and polydipsia is unacceptable.
   c. 0.9% saline diuresis for 3 hours, then streptozotocin, 500 mg/m^2, in 0.9% saline and administered intravenously over 2 hours, then 0.9% saline diuresis for 2 additional hours.
   d. Administer antiemetics immediately after streptozotocin administration to minimize vomiting.
   e. Repeat treatment every 3 weeks until hypoglycemia resolves or adverse reactions develop (e.g., pancreatitis, renal failure).

electrolyte solution containing 2.5% to 5% dextrose before, during, and immediately after surgery is important. Although this does not restore euglycemia, these solutions provide a substrate for CNS function, thereby minimizing CNS signs in most dogs. Concentrations of dextrose in excess of 5% should be avoided to prevent overstimulation of the pancreatic tumor and rebound, sometimes fatal, hypoglycemia. The IV dextrose infusion can be initiated the evening before surgery, at the time food and water are withheld, and continued throughout the perioperative period. Initiation of fluid therapy before surgery also helps ensure adequate circulation to the pancreas, thereby minimizing the risk of postoperative pancreatitis. The goal of the dextrose infusion is to prevent clinical signs of hypoglycemia and to maintain the blood glucose concentration at greater than 40 mg/dL (2.2 mmol/L), not to reestablish a normal blood glucose concentration. If the dextrose infusion is ineffective at preventing severe hypoglycemia during the perioperative period, a constant-rate infusion of glucagon should be considered (see Medical Therapy for an Acute Hypoglycemic Crisis). Glucagon is a potent stimulant of hepatic gluconeogenesis and is effective in maintaining normal blood glucose concentrations in dogs with an insulin-secreting tumor when administered by constant-rate infusion.

Intraoperative Considerations

Attention to the patient's blood glucose concentration and maintenance of adequate fluid therapy during surgery are imperative for the dog with beta-cell neoplasia. In a recent study, the addition of medetomidine (5 μg/kg IM) to the preanesthetic medication protocol significantly decreased plasma insulin concentrations, increased plasma glucose concentrations, and decreased the intraoperative glucose administration rate in 12 dogs undergoing surgery for beta-cell tumor, compared with 13 dogs that did not receive medetomidine prior to surgery (Guedes and Rude, 2013). These findings support the judicious use of medetomidine at low doses as an adjunct to the anesthetic management of dogs with beta-cell neoplasia.

Monitoring the blood glucose concentration every 30 to 60 minutes during surgery using a point-of-care or PBGM device allows objective assessment of the dog's blood glucose status. The goal is to maintain the blood glucose concentration greater than 40 mg/dL (2.2 mmol/L), not to establish a normal blood glucose concentration per se. Moderate changes in the blood glucose concentration can be monitored and adjustments made in the rate of IV dextrose administration, as needed, to prevent the

development of severe hypoglycemia (i.e., a blood glucose concentration < 40 mg/dL). Fortunately, it is uncommon for a dog in stable condition with a beta-cell tumor to require more than a 5% dextrose solution given intravenously during surgery. This infusion usually maintains the blood glucose concentration above 40 mg/dL. If a 5% dextrose infusion is ineffective in preventing severe hypoglycemia during surgery, a constant-rate infusion of glucagon should be considered (see Medical Therapy for an Acute Hypoglycemic Crisis).

Adequate fluid therapy just prior to, during, and immediately after surgery is extremely important for minimizing the development of pancreatitis. Digital manipulation and dissection of the pancreas cause inflammation. The severity of inflammation depends on the gentleness of the palpation, circulation to the pancreas, and surgical procedures performed. Providing adequate fluid therapy prior to and during surgery ensures that every means of maintaining circulation through the microvasculature of the pancreas has been used and helps minimize the development of pancreatitis. We routinely administer fluids at a rate of 60 to 100 mL/kg/24 hr during surgery and for 24 to 72 hours after the procedure, unless concurrent problems (e.g., heart failure, hypoproteinemia) are present that may affect the dog's ability to handle IV fluids.

During surgery, as much of the pancreas as possible should be examined visually. A complete, gentle digital inspection of this organ should then be undertaken. The importance of gentle handling of the pancreas cannot be overemphasized; failure to handle the organ gently may result in severe, potentially life-threatening pancreatitis. A thorough examination of the liver, surrounding lymph nodes, and omentum for metastatic sites should also be done.

Frequency of Tumor Identification. Most dogs with insulin-secreting tumors have masses that are easily visible to the surgeon inspecting the pancreas (Fig. 9-10). In a minority of dogs, the tumor is not visible but can be palpated during gentle but thorough digital examination of the pancreas. Multiple pancreatic masses may also occur. Ninety-nine (88%) of 111 dogs with insulin-secreting tumors at UC Davis had an obvious mass in the pancreas at the time of surgery.

Tumor Location. There is no predisposition for tumor location in the pancreas (Fig. 9-11). In our 99 dogs in which a mass was identified in the pancreas, the mass was located in the right (duodenal) limb of the pancreas in approximately 41%, in the left (splenic) limb of the pancreas in 40%, and in the central region

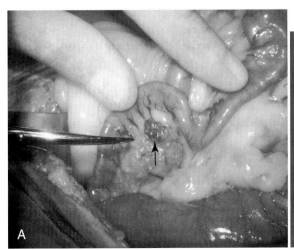
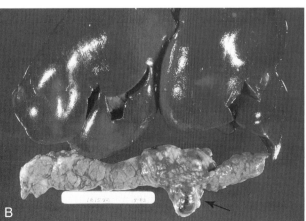

FIGURE 9-10 A and **B,** Photographs of pancreatic insulin-secreting islet beta-cell tumors *(arrows).*

(body) of the pancreas in 19%. In five of the remaining 12 dogs, a diffuse, microscopic islet cell carcinoma was recognized histologically in an arbitrarily resected portion of the right limb of the pancreas. Diffuse thickening of the pancreas was evident on digital palpation of the pancreas at the time of surgery in three of these five dogs; the pancreas was visually and digitally normal in two dogs. In three dogs, there was no visible mass and no metastatic sites, the pancreas was normal on digital palpation, and histologic examination of a portion of the right limb of the pancreas failed to identify an insulin-secreting tumor. One year later a pancreatic mass subsequently confirmed as an insulinoma was identified in one of the dogs. In two dogs, there was no visible mass and no metastatic sites, the pancreas was normal on digital palpation, and histologic examination of a portion of the right limb of the pancreas failed to identify an insulin-secreting tumor but subjectively there was marked increase in the number of islets and "islands" of beta cells scattered throughout the pancreas. Periodic evaluations of the dogs identified persistent hypoglycemia and hyperinsulinemia but failed to identify a pancreatic mass. One dog was lost to follow-up at 18 months after surgery and a necropsy was performed on the other dog approximately 5 years after surgery; histologic changes suggestive of "beta cell hyperplasia" were still evident, and a pancreatic mass was not identified. Enlargement of a mesenteric lymph node adjacent to the pancreas was evident in two dogs, but a mass was not identified in the pancreas per se. Histologic examination of the excised lymph node confirmed metastatic beta-cell tumor. Hyperinsulinism and hypoglycemia persisted in both dogs after surgery.

Tumor location has important ramifications for the success of surgery. In general, solitary tumors in the left or right limb of the pancreas are readily excisable with minimal damage to the pancreas and a low prevalence of postoperative pancreatitis. In contrast, tumors in the body of the pancreas are often intimately intertwined with the pancreatic ducts, blood vessels, and lymphatics. Surgical removal often requires extensive manipulation and dissection of the pancreas. Severe and potentially life-threatening pancreatitis that requires aggressive and often extended treatment is a common postoperative complication despite appropriate perioperative treatment aimed at preventing its development. In addition, complete excision of the tumor is almost impossible

and hypoglycemia typically recurs shortly after surgery. Prior to surgery we routinely discuss with the client the possible locations of the tumor and the implications that location has on attaining a successful outcome. We strongly recommend against tumor removal if the insulin-secreting tumor is located in the body of the pancreas because of the high probability of life-threatening postoperative complications. We inform the client that there is a one in five chance of the dog having inoperable disease and that if such disease is found, we advise closing the abdomen and treating the dog medically rather than risk the development of severe pancreatitis by trying to remove the tumor.

Failure to Identify a Mass: Use of Methylene Blue. IV methylene blue infusion has been advocated for intraoperative identification of a beta-cell tumor in the dog (Fingeroth and Smeak, 1988; Fingeroth et al, 1988). Methylene blue is an azo dye that, when administered intravenously, is concentrated in the parathyroid glands and endocrine pancreas. Methylene blue intensely stains hyperfunctional, adenomatous, or carcinomatous areas of these organs. Normal pancreatic endocrine tissue is stained a dusky slate blue, whereas hyperfunctioning tissue is stained more intensely, often a reddish blue. In one dog, methylene blue also successfully identified an ectopic islet cell tumor and differentiated metastatic from nonmetastatic nodules in surrounding tissue (Smeak et al, 1988).

Methylene blue is administered as an IV infusion by mixing appropriate volumes of methylene blue in 250 mL of normal isotonic saline solution to obtain a total dose of 3 mg methylene blue per kilogram of body weight (Fingeroth and Smeak, 1988). The entire solution is given over a period of 30 to 40 minutes. Maximal staining of the endocrine pancreas occurs approximately 30 minutes after initiation of the infusion. Complications with methylene blue infusion include Heinz body hemolytic anemia, acute kidney failure, pseudo-cyanosis (i.e., blue-appearing oral mucous membranes), green-tinged urine, and possibly pancreatitis. Hemolytic anemia is common, with the hematocrit declining to less than 25% 2 to 3 days after surgery.

We do not routinely use methylene blue because of its postoperative complications, the routine use of dual-phase CTA prior to surgery, and the ability to grossly identify abnormal tissue in the vast majority of our dogs with beta-cell neoplasia. If our surgeon fails to recognize a mass and the diagnosis has been confirmed by glucose and insulin measurements, the recommendation is to remove the right or left limb of the pancreas in the hope of removing the portion that contains the tumor. In theory, 90% of the pancreas could be removed without causing overt diabetes mellitus or exocrine pancreatic insufficiency.

Sites of Metastasis. Little correlation appears to exist between tumor size or shape and its malignant potential. A complete inspection of the abdominal contents is imperative to identify unsuspected abnormalities as well as sites of metastasis. The most common sites of tumor spread include the regional lymphatics and lymph nodes (duodenal, mesenteric, hepatic, splenic), the liver, and the peripancreatic omentum. Failure to identify metastatic disease is common during surgery. A solitary pancreatic mass is commonly removed in toto, with the belief that the dog has been "cured," only to have clinical signs of hyperinsulinism recur weeks to months later. In our experience, almost all beta-cell tumors in the dog are malignant. Unfortunately, initial clinical signs are often vague and not worrisome to the owner; weeks to months may elapse between the onset of clinical signs and establishment of the diagnosis, and as a result, the likelihood of metastasis at the time of exploratory surgery is high.

Recommendations if Metastasis Is Identified. Ideally, all abnormal-appearing tissue should be removed, if possible, and

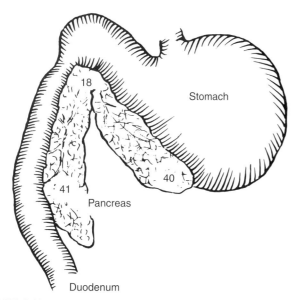

FIGURE 9-11 Diagram of tumor location in the pancreas in 99 dogs with an insulin-secreting islet beta-cell tumor.

submitted for histologic evaluation. When abnormal tissue cannot be entirely removed, debulking of the tumor mass may be beneficial. Biopsy of suspected tumor tissue is the least a surgeon should accomplish. The surgeon must always weigh the potential gains obtained with aggressive tumor removal and debulking against the potential complications that may develop as a result of the surgical procedure. This is especially important when dealing with the pancreas, because life-threatening pancreatitis can develop after extensive manipulation and dissection of the gland. Because medical treatment is a viable option after surgery, euthanasia at the time of surgery and heroic attempts to remove all abnormal tissue are not recommended in a dog with metastatic disease, especially if the latter course increases the risk of postoperative complications.

Postoperative Complications. The most common postoperative complications are pancreatitis, hyperglycemia, and hypoglycemia. The development of these complications is directly related to the expertise of the surgeon in handling the pancreas and excising these tumors, the location of the tumor in the pancreas (i.e., peripheral limb versus body), the presence or absence of functional metastases, and the adequacy of fluid therapy during the perioperative period.

Pancreatitis. IV administration of polyionic fluids with 2.5% to 5% dextrose (60 to 100 mL/kg/24 hr) and nothing by mouth prior to, during, and for 24 to 48 hours after surgery, followed by appropriate dietary therapy during the ensuing week, is helpful in minimizing the development of pancreatitis. We rely on physical examination findings in determining when to initiate oral water and a bland diet. Circulating pancreatic enzyme concentrations (e.g., canine pancreatic-specific lipase [cPL]) are usually not determined after surgery. Arbitrarily treating the dog for pancreatitis without determining the serum pancreatic enzyme concentrations beforehand has produced excellent results. Despite gentle handling of the pancreas during surgery, aggressive fluid therapy during the perioperative period, and appropriate dietary therapy during the postoperative period, nine (13%) of 70 dogs undergoing surgery for beta-cell tumor at UC Davis still developed clinical signs of acute pancreatitis. Three of the nine dogs died as a result of pancreatitis; the tumor was located in the body of the pancreas and was difficult to excise in all three dogs.

Diabetes Mellitus. Occasionally dogs develop transient diabetes mellitus after surgical removal of an insulin-secreting tumor. Diabetes mellitus is believed to result from inadequate insulin secretion by "atrophied" normal beta cells. Removal of all or a majority of the neoplastic cells acutely deprives the animal of insulin. Until the normal beta cells regain their secretory capability, the dog is hypoinsulinemic and may require exogenous insulin injections to maintain euglycemia. It was once thought that postsurgical hyperglycemia and glycosuria were excellent prognostic signs indicating total removal of insulin-secreting neoplastic cells. However, most of our dogs have required exogenous insulin only transiently after surgery and ultimately have required medical management for an exacerbation of an insulin-secreting tumor several weeks to months after their need for insulin therapy dissipates.

Postsurgical insulin therapy is initiated only when hyperglycemia and glycosuria persist for 1 to 2 days after discontinuation of all dextrose-containing IV fluids. Initial insulin therapy should be conservative—that is, 0.25 U of Lente or neutral protamine Hagedorn (NPH) insulin per kilogram of body weight given once daily. Subsequent adjustments in dosage or frequency of administration should be based on clinical response and blood glucose determinations (see Chapter 6).

The need for insulin treatment is usually transient, lasting from a few days to a few months. Most of these dogs still have neoplastic beta cells in the pancreas, liver, lymph nodes, or peripancreatic tissues that multiply and eventually reach a population density capable of secreting enough insulin to cause hypoglycemic signs to recur. For these dogs, resolution of diabetes is followed by a variable period of euglycemia, which eventually progresses to hypoglycemia. Owner evaluation of the pet's urine glucose is helpful in identifying when insulin therapy is no longer needed. Persistently negative urine glucose in conjunction with cessation of polyuria and polydipsia is an indication to discontinue insulin therapy. If hyperglycemia and glycosuria recur, insulin therapy can be reinstituted, but at a lower insulin dosage. The development of permanent insulin-requiring diabetes mellitus after surgical removal of a solitary insulin-secreting tumor is uncommon and implies additional abnormalities involving the beta cells (e.g., beta-cell degeneration, islet hypoplasia; see Chapter 6). Permanent diabetes mellitus has developed in only two of the dogs that underwent surgical removal of an insulin-secreting tumor at our hospital. Both dogs were lost to follow-up after 1 to 2 years, and at that time both dogs were still receiving insulin injections twice a day to control hyperglycemia.

Persistent Postoperative Hypoglycemia. Dogs that remain hypoglycemic after surgical removal of an insulin-secreting tumor have functional metastatic disease. Medical therapy should be initiated in dogs with persistent postoperative hypoglycemia. During the initial 48 to 72 postoperative hours, IV infusion of 2.5% to 5% dextrose should be continued. The goal is to prevent clinical signs of hypoglycemia (especially seizures), not to reestablish a normal blood glucose concentration. Additional therapy may be needed if hypoglycemic seizures occur (Box 9-8; also see Medical Therapy for an Acute Hypoglycemic Crisis). Small meals should be fed every 4 to 6 hours, beginning as soon after surgery as possible. A diet acceptable for the treatment of pancreatitis should be fed initially. Additional therapy may be needed, depending on the efficacy of the frequent feedings in maintaining remission of clinical hypoglycemia (see Medical Therapy for Chronic Hypoglycemia). If a dog becomes symptomatic despite the frequent feedings, medical therapy should be attempted before euthanasia is recommended.

BOX 9-8 **Medical Therapy for Hypoglycemic Seizures Caused by an Insulin-Secreting Beta-Cell Tumor**

Seizures at Home
Step 1: Rub sugar solution on pet's buccal mucosa.
Step 2: Once pet is sternal, feed a small meal.
Step 3: Call the veterinarian.

Seizures in Hospital
Step 1: Administer 1 to 5 mL (depending on dog size) of 50% dextrose (diluted) intravenously slowly over 1 to 2 minutes followed by continuous IV infusion of 5% dextrose in water (i.e., D5W).
Step 2: Once animal is sternal, feed a small meal.
Step 3: Initiate long-term medical therapy (see Box 9-7).

Intractable Seizures in Hospital
Step 1: Administer 2.5% to 5% dextrose in water intravenously at 1.5 to 2 times maintenance fluid rate.
Step 2: Add 0.5 to 1 mg of dexamethasone/kg to IV fluids and administer over 6 hours; repeat every 12 to 24 hours, as necessary.
Step 3: If above fails, administer glucagon USP (Eli Lilly) intravenously by constant rate infusion at an initial dosage of 5 to 10 ng/kg/min.
Step 4: If necessary, control seizure activity with diazepam or phenobarbital until medical treatment becomes effective in controlling hypoglycemia.

Evaluating the Long-Term Success of Surgery: Is the Dog Cured?

The long-term success of surgery can be difficult to predict in dogs with a "solitary" mass that is removed in toto and subsequent blood glucose concentration returns to normal. The most efficient and logical initial method for evaluating these patients for recurrence of beta-cell neoplasia is periodic measurement (i.e., every month initially) of a fasting blood glucose concentration. The fasting blood glucose concentration should be consistently greater than 70 mg/dL (3.9 mmol/L) if beta-cell neoplasia has not recurred. Recurrence of beta-cell neoplasia should be suspected if the blood glucose concentration is less than 70 mg/dL. Confirmation of recurrence requires measurement of the serum insulin concentration when the blood glucose concentration is less than 60 mg/dL (see Confirming the Diagnosis of an Insulin-Secreting Beta-Cell Tumor: Serum Insulin Determination).

Medical Therapy for an Acute Hypoglycemic Crisis

The acute onset of clinical signs caused by hypoglycemia typically occurs at home after exercise or consumption of food that is easily digestible and rapidly absorbed; during the immediate postoperative period in the dog with functioning metastases or inoperable neoplasia; or as a result of inadvertently aggressive IV dextrose administration at the time hypoglycemia is initially identified. Therapy depends on the severity of clinical signs and the location of the dog (i.e., home versus hospital) and initially involves administration of glucose, either as food or sugar solution by mouth or as an IV dextrose solution.

If an owner contacts a veterinarian by telephone and reports that the pet is having a hypoglycemic seizure, we do not recommend transporting the dog to a veterinary hospital. Rather, the owner should be instructed to rub a sugar solution on the pet's buccal mucosa. Hypoglycemic dogs usually respond in 1 to 2 minutes. The owner should be instructed to never place fingers in, or pour the sugar solution down, the pet's mouth. Once the dog or cat is sternal and cognizant of its surroundings, it should be fed a small meal and brought to the veterinarian.

At home subcutaneous administration of glucagon is used to treat severe hypoglycemia in human diabetics. Glucagon quickly increases blood glucose through stimulation of hepatic glycogenolysis and gluconeogenesis. In a recent study, subcutaneous administration of glucagon resulted in a rapid and significant increase in serum glucose concentrations in healthy Beagles but the effect was short-lived (Zeugswetter et al, 2012; Fig. 9-12). Although clinical trials are needed, at home glucagon emergency kits used to treat severe hypoglycemia in human diabetics may become a viable option for the short-term treatment of severe hypoglycemia in dogs or cats and provide the time needed to get the dog or cat to an emergency veterinary hospital for care (Niessen, 2012).

In the hospital, clinical signs of hypoglycemia can usually be alleviated initially with IV administration of 50% dextrose, diluted, followed by continuous IV infusion of 5% dextrose (i.e., dextrose 5% in water [D5W]). In dogs with beta cell neoplasia, dextrose should be administered in small amounts slowly (e.g., 1 to 5 mL increments depending on the size of the dog over a period of 1 to 2 minutes) to effect. Rapid administration of large boluses of glucose to a dog with suspected or proven beta cell neoplasia can result in severe rebound hypoglycemia caused by excessive insulin secretion by the tumor in response to the rapid increase in the blood glucose concentration. The goal of therapy is to control neurologic signs (primarily seizures), not correct hypoglycemia. Once neurologic signs have been controlled with judicious IV administration of dextrose, frequent feedings and glucocorticoids can be initiated (see Box 9-7).

If the dextrose infusion is ineffective in preventing severe hypoglycemia or breaking the cycle of hypoglycemia and hyperglycemia, a constant-rate infusion of glucagon should be considered. Glucagon is a potent stimulant of hepatic glycogenolysis and gluconeogenesis and is effective in maintaining normal blood glucose concentrations in dogs with beta-cell neoplasia when administered by constant-rate infusion (Fischer et al, 2000; Fig. 9-13). One milligram of lyophilized glucagon USP (Eli Lilly) is reconstituted with the diluent provided by the manufacturer, and the solution is added to 1 L of 0.9% saline, making a 1 µg/mL solution, which can be administered by syringe pump. The initial dosage is 5 to 10 ng per kilogram of body weight per minute. The dosage is adjusted as needed to maintain the blood glucose concentration between 60 and 100 mg/dL (3.4 and 5.6 mmol/L). When discontinuing

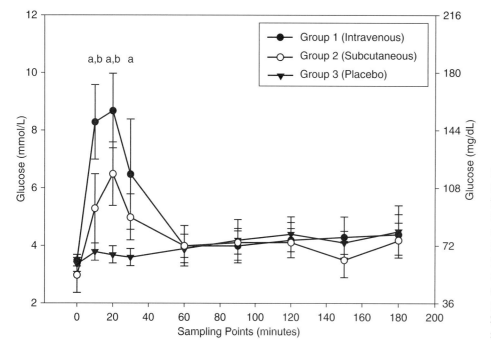

FIGURE 9-12 Mean glucose concentrations (mmol/L and mg/dL) over 180 minutes after the subcutaneous (SC) and intravenous (IV) injection of synthetic glucagon or 0.9% saline solution (placebo). (From Zeugswetter FK, et al.: Metabolic and hormonal responses to subcutaneous glucagon in healthy beagles, *J Vet Emer Crit Care* 22:558, 2012.) *Bars* indicate standard deviations. *a*, Significant difference of SC versus placebo injection; *b*, significant difference of SC versus IV injection; P < 0.05 is considered significant.

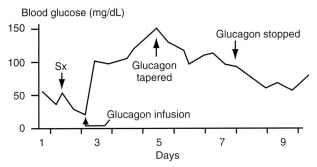

FIGURE 9-13 Blood glucose concentrations in a 13-year-old female spayed Pomeranian before and after surgical removal of an insulin-secreting islet beta-cell tumor. Pancreatitis and severe hypoglycemia developed postoperatively. The hypoglycemia resolved, and euglycemia was maintained after initiation of a constant-rate intravenous (IV) infusion of glucagon. The dosage of glucagon was gradually tapered beginning on day 5, feeding of small amounts of food was begun on day 7, and the IV glucagon infusion was stopped on day 8. Severe hypoglycemia did not recur. *Sx,* Surgery.

glucagon, the dose should be gradually decreased over 1 to 2 days and the blood glucose concentration monitored for recurrence of severe hypoglycemia.

Occasionally, a hypoglycemic dog with CNS signs fails to respond to glucose or glucagon administration. These signs could be the result of a disorder unrelated to hypoglycemia. However, irreversible cerebral lesions may result from long-term, severe hypoglycemia and the resultant cerebral hypoxia. Cerebral hypoxia predisposes the nervous tissue to edema, causing increased CSF pressure and cell death. These animals have a guarded to grave prognosis. Therapy is directed at providing a continuous supply of glucose as a 5% solution given intravenously or by stimulating hepatic glucose production with a constant-rate infusion of glucagon. Simultaneously, seizure activity is controlled with diazepam or stronger anticonvulsant medication (e.g., phenobarbital). Last, if cerebral edema is suspected, treatment with mannitol, furosemide, and/or dexamethasone should be considered (Fenner, 1995).

Medical Therapy for Chronic Hypoglycemia

See Box 9-7.

Background

Medical management for chronic hypoglycemia should be initiated when an exploratory celiotomy is not performed or when metastatic or inoperable neoplasia results in recurrence of clinical signs. The goals of medical therapy are to reduce the frequency and severity of clinical signs and to avoid an acute hypoglycemic crisis, not to establish euglycemia per se. Medical therapy typically involves nonspecific antihormonal therapy. Antihormonal therapy is palliative and should minimize hypoglycemia by providing a continuous source of glucose from the gastrointestinal tract (frequent feedings), increasing hepatic glycogenolysis and gluconeogenesis (glucocorticoids), or inhibiting the synthesis, secretion, or peripheral cellular actions of insulin (glucocorticoids, diazoxide, somatostatin). Antihormonal therapy consists primarily of frequent feedings and glucocorticoids (see Box 9-7). Surgical debulking of functional masses may enhance the effectiveness of medical therapy. The best results are obtained when surgical debulking is performed shortly after the diagnosis of an insulin-secreting tumor has been established, although we have had a few

dogs benefit from surgical debulking after medical treatment has become ineffective in controlling clinical signs of hypoglycemia. One of our dogs underwent surgical debulking on three separate occasions; the dog survived 3 years before succumbing to metastatic disease involving the lungs.

Alloxan and streptozotocin are drugs with specific toxicity directed at beta cells. The potential for serious adverse reactions has limited the use of these drugs for the treatment of insulin-secreting tumors in dogs. However, a viable treatment protocol using streptozotocin in dogs has been described, and studies to determine its value in the treatment of insulin-secreting tumors have been reported (Moore et al, 2002; Northrup et al, 2013).

Frequent Feedings

Dogs with insulin-secreting tumors have a persistent absolute or relative excess of circulating insulin. Frequent feedings provide a constant source of calories as a substrate for the excess insulin secreted by the tumor and help to reduce the frequency of hypoglycemic episodes. Diets high in fat, complex carbohydrates, and fiber delay gastric emptying, slow intestinal glucose absorption, and help minimize a rapid increase in the portal blood glucose concentration that could stimulate excessive pancreatic insulin secretion. Simple sugars are rapidly absorbed, have a potent stimulatory effect on insulin secretion by neoplastic beta cells, and should be avoided. A combination of canned and dry food, fed in three to six small meals daily, is recommended. Daily caloric intake should be controlled because hyperinsulinemia promotes obesity. Exercise should be limited to walks on a leash.

Glucocorticoid Therapy

Glucocorticoid therapy should be initiated when dietary manipulations are no longer effective in preventing clinical signs of hypoglycemia. Glucocorticoids antagonize the effects of insulin at the cellular level, stimulate hepatic glycogenolysis, and indirectly provide the necessary substrates for hepatic gluconeogenesis. Prednisone (dog) or prednisolone (cat) are the glucocorticoids most often used. The initial dosage is 0.25 mg/kg by mouth every 12 hours. Adjustments in the dose are based on clinical response. The dose of prednisone required to control clinical signs increases with time in response to growth of the tumor and its metastatic sites. Eventually, the adverse effects of prednisone, specifically polyuria and polydipsia, become unacceptable to clients. This typically occurs when the prednisone dosage approaches 1 mg/kg twice daily, although there is dog to dog variability in development of adverse effects and owner tolerance of the adverse effects. When adverse effects become intolerable, the dose of prednisone should be reduced by 25% to 50% (not stopped) and additional therapy considered.

Diazoxide Therapy

Diazoxide (Proglycem) is a benzothiadiazide diuretic that inhibits insulin secretion, stimulates hepatic gluconeogenesis and glycogenolysis, and inhibits tissue use of glucose. The net effect is the development of hyperglycemia. Diazoxide does not inhibit insulin synthesis and does not have cytotoxic (antineoplastic) effects. Diazoxide therapy can be initiated early in the medical treatment of a beta-cell tumor when the glucocorticoid dose is low and polyuria and polydipsia are acceptable to the client or can be initiated later when glucocorticoids are no longer effective in controlling clinical signs of hypoglycemia or the severity of polyuria and polydipsia has become unacceptable to the client. In the later situation, glucocorticoids should be continued but at a lower dose. The initial dosage of diazoxide is 5 mg/kg by mouth every 12 hours.

The dosage may gradually be increased as needed to control signs of hypoglycemia but should not exceed 60 mg/kg/day. Thiazide diuretics may potentiate the effects of diazoxide. The two drugs can be administered together to enhance hyperglycemic effects if diazoxide alone is not effective. The dosage of hydrochlorothiazide is 1 to 2 mg/kg by mouth every 12 hours.

The goal of diazoxide therapy is to establish a dosage at which hypoglycemia and its clinical signs are reduced or absent. In addition, the dosage should be low enough to avoid hyperglycemia (blood glucose concentrations > 180 mg/dL; 10 mmol/L) and its associated clinical signs. Reports of diazoxide use have appeared in the veterinary literature only sporadically (Leifer et al, 1986; Feldman and Nelson, 1987). Thirteen of 17 dogs with an insulin-secreting tumor in our series had a good clinical response, lasting 6 weeks to 20 months. In another report, nine of 14 dogs had a good response to diazoxide therapy (Leifer et al, 1986).

The most common adverse reactions to diazoxide administration are anorexia and vomiting. Administering diazoxide with a meal or decreasing the dosage, at least temporarily, is usually effective in controlling adverse gastrointestinal signs. Other potential complications include diarrhea, tachycardia, bone marrow suppression, aplastic anemia, thrombocytopenia, pancreatitis, diabetes mellitus, cataracts, and sodium and fluid retention (Feldman and Nelson, 1987). Diazoxide is metabolized in the liver, and the metabolites are excreted via the kidneys and biliary system. Adverse reactions or complications may develop more rapidly or at a lower dosage of diazoxide in a dog with concurrent hepatic dysfunction.

Somatostatin Therapy

Octreotide (Sandostatin) is an analog of somatostatin that inhibits the synthesis and secretion of insulin by normal and neoplastic beta cells. IV administration of octreotide can rapidly decrease the serum insulin concentration, causing a corresponding increase in the serum glucose concentration in dogs with insulin-secreting neoplasia (Robben et al, 1997; Fig. 9-14). The inhibitory actions of octreotide on insulin secretion can be maintained for several hours with subcutaneous administration (Fig. 9-15). The responsiveness of insulin-secreting tumors to the suppressive effects of octreotide varies and depends on the presence of membrane receptors on the tumor cells that bind somatostatin (Lamberts et al, 1990; Simpson et al, 1995). To date, five subtypes of somatostatin

receptors have been identified in humans (Patel, 1999). These subtypes show a tissue-specific distribution and differences in affinity for somatostatin and its analogs (Bruns et al, 1994). In humans, some insulin-secreting tumors have receptor subtypes that do not or only minimally bind octreotide, resulting in minimal to no effect by the analog on serum insulin and glucose concentrations (Lamberts et al, 1991; 1996). Autoradiography performed in dogs with insulin-secreting neoplasia suggests the presence of only one somatostatin receptor (sst2 receptors) in canine insulin-secreting tumors (Robben et al, 1997). The somatostatin receptor identified in canine insulin-secreting tumors contains high-affinity binding sites for octreotide and the radiopharmaceutical pentetreotide (see Scintigraphy). In that study, baseline plasma insulin concentrations, although varying widely, decreased significantly in all 10 dogs after octreotide administration. Unfortunately, octreotide is extremely expensive, must be administered by injection, has a relatively short (< 6 hours) suppressive effect on serum insulin concentrations in some dogs, clinical response to octreotide treatment is unpredictable, and some dogs that initially respond become refractory to octreotide treatment (Lothrop, 1989). Nevertheless, octreotide (10 to 40 μg SC twice or three times per day) is well tolerated and can be used for the management of both acute and chronic hypoglycemia in some dogs with insulin-secreting neoplasia. Adverse reactions have not been reported at these dosages.

Streptozotocin. Streptozotocin is a naturally occurring nitrosourea that is similar in structure to glucose and is taken up by the GLUT-2 transmembrane carrier protein but not by other glucose transporters (Schnedl et al, 1994). Because pancreatic beta cells have high concentrations of GLUT-2 transporters, streptozotocin selectively destroys pancreatic beta cells by depressing the pyridine nucleotides nicotinamide adenine dinucleotide (NAD) and reduced nicotinamide adenine dinucleotide (NADH). Two dogs with confirmed hyperinsulinism were treated with streptozotocin by Meyer in the 1970s. The first dog developed nephrotoxicosis and was euthanized 3 weeks after a single treatment with streptozotocin at a dosage of 1000 mg/kg body weight given intravenously over a 1-minute period. The second dog developed temporary remission of hypoglycemia that lasted approximately 50 days after two treatments with streptozotocin at a dosage of 500 mg/m² given intravenously over a 30-second period. The treatments were given 1 week apart, and mannitol was infused for 20 minutes before and after each streptozotocin treatment. The

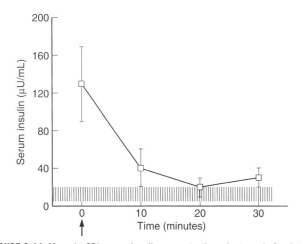

FIGURE 9-14 Mean (± SD) serum insulin concentration prior to and after intravenous (IV) administration of 100 μg of octreotide in six dogs with an insulin-secreting islet cell tumor. *Arrow,* Octreotide administration; *hatched area,* normal range for fasting serum insulin concentration.

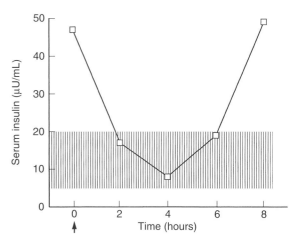

FIGURE 9-15 Serum insulin concentration prior to and after subcutaneous (SC) administration of 20 μg of octreotide to a dog with an insulin-secreting islet cell tumor. *Arrow,* Octreotide administration; *hatched area,* normal range for fasting serum insulin concentration.

dog developed a nephropathy and hepatopathy after a third treatment administered at day 97 and was euthanized shortly thereafter. As a result of these clinical reports, streptozotocin was not considered a viable treatment for insulin-secreting tumors in dogs.

In 2002, Moore and colleagues described a fluid diuresis protocol that allowed streptozotocin to be administered to dogs with insulin-secreting tumors with a minimum of adverse reactions. Fluid diuresis has been reported to ameliorate the renal toxicity of streptozotocin in humans, presumably as a result of less contact time between the drug and the renal tubular epithelium (Tobin et al, 1987; Kintzel, 2001). In Moore's study, diuresis with 0.9% sodium chloride at a rate of 18.3 mL/kg/hr administered through a peripherally located over-the-needle catheter was performed for 7 hours. Streptozotocin (Zanosar) was administered over a 2-hour period beginning 3 hours after initiation of the saline diuresis. The dose of streptozotocin (500 mg/m^2) was diluted in an appropriate volume of 0.9% saline to maintain the same rate of fluid administration for 2 hours. Saline diuresis was continued at the same fluid rate for an additional 2 hours after completion of the streptozotocin administration. Butorphanol (0.4 mg/kg IV) was given immediately after streptozotocin administration as an antiemetic. Streptozotocin treatments were repeated at 3-week intervals until there was evidence of tumor progression (i.e., increase in tumor size by greater than 50%), recurrence of hypoglycemia, or streptozotocin-induced toxicity that required supportive treatment.

Fifty-eight treatments were administered to 17 dogs with an insulin-secreting tumor at variable times after surgery (Moore et al, 2002). Sixteen of 17 dogs had metastatic disease. One dog developed azotemia, several dogs developed increases in serum alanine aminotransferase activity that appeared to resolve with cessation of treatment, and vomiting occurred in 18 (31%) of 58 streptozotocin treatments and was occasionally severe. Two dogs developed diabetes mellitus after receiving five treatments; two of three dogs had rapid resolution of paraneoplastic peripheral neuropathy; and two dogs had a measurable reduction in tumor size. Although the median survival time was longer in dogs treated with streptozotocin than in 15 control dogs with a similar stage of disease (163 versus 90 days, respectively), this difference was not statistically significant. The range for survival time was also similar between the two groups of dogs (streptozotocin-treated dogs, 16 to 309 days; control dogs, 0 to 426 days).

Because myelosuppression was not observed in the Moore study, Northrup, et al., (2013) investigated increasing dose intensity by decreasing the interval between streptozotocin dosing from 3 to 2 week intervals. Nineteen dogs with residual, local, metastatic, or recurrent insulinoma were treated with the streptozotocin and saline diuresis protocol described by Moore, et al., (2002) but administered biweekly rather than once every 3 weeks. Treatment was initiated after surgery for insulinoma or at the time of recurrence. The planned treatment protocol was five treatments per dog; however, 13 dogs received fewer than five treatments (median, 3; range, 1 to 4) primarily because of development of adverse events. Adverse events occurred in all dogs and included nausea, anorexia, acute emesis or regurgitation, diarrhea, increased liver enzyme activity, renal tubular injury, and hypoglycemic collapse or seizure during treatment. Mild to moderate gastrointestinal toxicity was the most common adverse event. Myelosuppression was not identified. Eight dogs developed diabetes mellitus and six of these dogs subsequently died or were euthanized. Median survival time for the 19 dogs was 308 days (range, 20 to 1404 days; Fig. 9-16). Median progression-free survival time, defined as the number of days from the first streptozotocin treatment until recurrence

of hypoglycemia, detection of local recurrence or metastasis, or death because of any cause, was 196 days (range, 20 to 840 days). Response rate to streptozotocin could not be determined from the results of this study because there was no control group of dogs with comparable metastatic or nonresectable insulinoma that were not treated, and survival times in the streptozotocin-treated dogs were confounded by concurrent symptomatic therapy, use of other cytotoxic therapies, and owner decision to euthanize. Bell, et al., (2005) reported on a Springer Spaniel treated with glucocorticoids and one treatment of streptozotocin for metastatic insulinoma that subsequently developed diabetes mellitus. The dog was euthanized 118 days after streptozotocin treatment because of cervical pain caused by metastasis of the tumor.

In our experience, the effectiveness of streptozotocin in improving hypoglycemia, controlling clinical signs, and prolonging survival time has been unpredictable and adverse events to streptozotocin (severe vomiting, acute pancreatitis, potentially severe kidney injury) are common and can be life-threatening. A thorough discussion of potential complications with streptozotocin treatment should always be undertaken with the owner prior to initiating treatment.

Phenytoin. Phenytoin is an anticonvulsant that inhibits the release of insulin by beta cells and may also directly impair the effects of insulin on peripheral tissues (Haemers and Rottiers, 1981). Unfortunately, phenytoin is not usually successful in controlling clinical signs of hypoglycemia. Only 30% of human patients with hyperinsulinism showed any beneficial effects after phenytoin administration (Haemers and Rottiers, 1981). Concurrent diazoxide administration is not recommended, because it results in a decrease in blood concentrations of phenytoin. Phenytoin has not been critically evaluated in dogs with beta-cell neoplasia.

Propranolol. Propranolol is a nonselective beta-adrenergic blocking drug that has no intrinsic sympathomimetic activity. Its potential usefulness in patients with beta-cell neoplasia probably involves its ability to block insulin secretion by beta cells. Insulin secretion is stimulated by the beta-adrenergic nervous system. However, propranolol may also induce hypoglycemia by impairing hepatic gluconeogenesis and glycogenolysis, normally induced by endogenous catecholamines. Propranolol has not been critically evaluated in dogs with beta cell neoplasia.

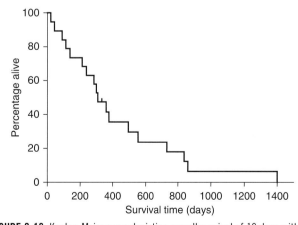

FIGURE 9-16 Kaplan-Meier curve depicting overall survival of 19 dogs with insulinoma treated with streptozotocin at 2-week intervals. The median survival time was 308 days (range, 20 to 1404 days). (From Northrup NC, et al.: Prospective evaluation of biweekly streptozotocin in 19 dogs with insulinoma, *J Vet Intern Med* 27:483, 2013.)

PROGNOSIS

Owing to the extremely high likelihood of malignancy in any dog with an insulin-secreting tumor (greater than 95%), the long-term prognosis is guarded to poor at best because beta-cell tumors almost always metastasize. The disease-free interval and survival time are difficult to predict. Survival time depends partly on the owner's willingness to treat the disease. Predictors of disease free interval and survival time in dogs with an insulin-secreting beta-cell tumor include tumor size, TNM (tumor, node, and metastasis) stage, stromal fibrosis within the tumor, and the Ki67 index (Caywood et al, 1988; Buishand et al, 2010). Ki67 is a proliferation marker expressed during the active phases of the cell cycle and absent in resting cells (Scholzen and Gerdes, 2000). The Ki67 index has been correlated with clinical outcome in humans with insulinoma (La Rosa et al, 2009).

Tobin and colleagues (1999) reported median survival time after diagnosis of 74 days (range, 8 to 508 days) and 381 days (range, 20 to 1758) in dogs treated medically versus dogs that initially underwent surgery followed by medical treatment, respectively. Polton and colleagues (2007) reported median survival time after diagnosis of 196 days (95% confidence interval [CI] 0 to 549 days) and 785 days (95% CI: 190 to 1380 days) in dogs treated medically versus dogs that initially underwent surgery followed by medical treatment, respectively. The shorter survival time for dogs treated medically in the Tobin study was partly due to a more severe stage of the disease at the time of diagnosis and the owners' feelings of hopelessness, which translated into early acceptance of euthanasia when clinical signs recurred. Polton, et al., (2007) reported a median disease free interval of 496 days (95% CI: 302 to 690 days) in 19 dogs that underwent partial pancreatectomy. The median disease free interval in 31 dogs that underwent partial pancreatectomy at Utrecht University was 244 days (range, 0 to 1116 days) and survival time was 258 days (range, 1 to 1146) (Tryfonidou et al, 1998).

The extent to which surgery can alter the prognosis depends on the clinical stage of the disease, most notably the extent of metastatic lesions. In one multi-university study, dogs with tumors confined to the pancreas (stage I) were normoglycemic for a median of 14 months after surgery, whereas dogs with metastasis to regional lymph nodes (stage II) or distant metastasis (stage III) were normoglycemic for a median of approximately 1 month (Caywood et al, 1988). Dogs with stage I or stage II disease had a median survival time of approximately 18 months, whereas those with stage III disease had a median survival time of less than 6 months. Approximately 50% of dogs with metastases to the liver were dead by 6 months, and all were dead by 18 months from the time of diagnosis.

In our experience, approximately 10% to 15% of dogs undergoing surgery for an insulin-secreting tumor die or are euthanized at the time of or within 1 month of surgery because of severe metastatic disease, uncontrollable postoperative hypoglycemia, or complications related to pancreatitis. An additional 20% to 25% of dogs die or are euthanized within 6 months of surgery because of severe metastatic disease and recurrence of clinical hypoglycemia. The remaining 60% to 70% live beyond 6 months postoperatively, many beyond 1 year after surgery, before uncontrollable hypoglycemia develops, resulting in death or necessitating euthanasia. Additional surgery to debulk metastatic lesions may improve the animal's responsiveness to medical therapy and prolong the survival time in some dogs that become nonresponsive to medical treatment after the initial surgery. Some dogs with metastatic disease do remarkably well (i.e., survive longer than 2 years) after aggressive surgical debulking of the tumor and its metastases.

INSULIN-SECRETING BETA-CELL TUMORS IN CATS

Insulin-secreting beta-cell tumors are rare in cats with only a few single cat case reports in the literature (McMillan, 1985; O'Brien et al, 1990; Hawks et al, 1992; Kraje, 2003; Greene and Bright, 2008) and one additional report in which the beta-cell tumor was an incidental finding at necropsy in a cat with ductal pancreatic adenocarcinoma (Carpenter et al, 1987). We have seen only two cats with beta-cell neoplasia during the past three decades, in contrast to more than 150 dogs with the disease during the same time interval.

The clinical characteristics of insulin-secreting beta-cell tumors in cats appear to be similar to those in dogs. To date, the disorder has affected aged cats, 12 to 17 years old. Interestingly, three cats have been Siamese. Immunohistochemical analysis of the beta-cell tumor in a few of these cats has revealed multihormonal productivity, with insulin and chromogranin A being the most common peptides demonstrated in the neoplastic cells (Kraje, 2003; Jackson et al, 2009). Clinical signs result from the effects of hyperinsulinism and included seizures, weakness, ataxia, lethargy, disorientation, and muscle twitching. Hypoglycemia (blood glucose concentration < 60 mg/dL; 3.4 mmol/L) was documented in each cat, and an inappropriately increased blood insulin concentration was documented in four cats in which insulin was measured. Abdominal ultrasound failed to identify a 1.5 to 2.0 cm pancreatic mass in one cat and a 0.4 cm pancreatic mass in another cat in which ultrasound was performed prior to surgery. A pancreatic mass was identified in five cats that underwent surgery, and hypoglycemia and clinical signs resolved in four of five cats after surgical excision of the mass. Four cats died or were euthanized 4 weeks, 5 weeks, 18 months, and 2 years after surgery, and three of these four cats were hypoglycemic at the time of death. Necropsy in one of these cats revealed metastasis to the liver and pancreatic lymph nodes. One cat was alive with no clinical signs suggestive of recurrence of the insulinoma 32 months after surgical removal of a solitary 0.4 cm pancreatic carcinoma (Greene and Bright, 2008).

Until more experience is gained with beta-cell neoplasia in cats, it seems prudent to approach this disorder in a manner similar to that used for dogs. Beta-cell neoplasia should be included in the list of differential diagnoses for persistent hypoglycemia in the older cat (see Box 9-4). The index of suspicion for beta-cell neoplasia should be heightened after a thorough review of the history, physical examination, and results of clinicopathologic tests and diagnostic imaging. However, as with the dog, failure to identify a pancreatic mass with abdominal ultrasound does not rule out a beta cell tumor. The diagnosis should be confirmed by documentation of an inappropriate serum insulin concentration despite the presence of hypoglycemia (see Confirming the Diagnosis of an Insulin-Secreting Beta-Cell Tumor: Serum Insulin Determination). Many commercially available radioimmunoassays for insulin work well in the dog but do not work in the cat (Lutz and Rand, 1993). It is imperative that the radioimmunoassay used to measure feline insulin is validated for cats and that species specific reference ranges are available.

Surgical exploration should be the initial treatment of choice for beta-cell neoplasia in the cat. However, the age of the cat, identification of metastatic disease using ultrasonography, or the existence of concurrent disease that increases the anesthetic risk may warrant a more conservative medical approach in some cats. Frequent feedings and prednisolone therapy have been effective in controlling clinical signs of hyperinsulinism and should be the mainstay of medical therapy for chronic hypoglycemia. The use of diazoxide has not been reported in the cat and is not recommended until its safety and dosing schedule have been investigated in cats. Similarly, the efficacy of octreotide for the treatment of feline beta-cell neoplasia remains to be reported.

REFERENCES

Bagley RS, et al.: Hypoglycemia associated with intraabdominal leiomyoma and leiomyosarcoma in six dogs, *J Am Vet Med Assoc* 208:69, 1996.

Barreca A, et al.: In vitro paracrine regulation of human keratinocyte growth by fibroblast-derived insulin-like growth factors, *J Cell Physiol* 151:262, 1992.

Beaudry D, et al.: Hypoglycemia in four dogs with smooth muscle tumors, *J Vet Intern Med* 9:415, 1995.

Bell R, et al.: Treatment of insulinoma in a springer spaniel with streptozotocin, *J Sm Anim Pract* 46:247, 2005.

Bellah JR, Ginn PE: Gastric leiomyosarcoma associated with hypoglycemia in a dog, *J Am Anim Hosp Assoc* 32:283, 1996.

Bergman PJ, et al.: Canine clinical peripheral neuropathy associated with pancreatic islet cell carcinoma, *Prog Vet Neurol* 5:57, 1994.

Boari A, et al.: Hypoglycemia in a dog with a leiomyoma of the gastric wall producing an insulin-like growth factor II–like peptide, *Eur J Endocrinol* 132:744, 1995.

Boyle PJ, Cryer PE: Growth hormone, cortisol, or both are involved in defense against but are not critical to recovery from prolonged hypoglycemia in humans, *Am J Physiol* 260:E395, 1991.

Braund KG, et al.: Insulinoma and subclinical peripheral neuropathy in two dogs, *J Vet Intern Med* 1:86, 1987.

Breitschwerdt EB, et al.: Hypoglycemia in four dogs with sepsis, *J Am Vet Med Assoc* 178:1072, 1981.

Brix A, et al.: Glycogen storage disease type Ia in two littermate Maltese puppies, *Vet Pathol* 32:460, 1995.

Bruns C, et al.: Molecular pharmacology of somatostatin receptor subtypes, *Ann N Y Acad Sci* 733:138, 1994.

Buetow PC, et al.: Islet cell tumors of the pancreas: clinical, radiological, and pathologic correlation in diagnosis and localization, *Radiographics* 17:453, 1997.

Buishand FO, et al.: Evaluation of clinicopathological criteria and the Ki67 index as prognostic indicators of canine insulinoma, *Vet J* 185:62, 2010.

Buishand FO, et al.: Expression of insulin-like growth factor-1 by canine insulinomas and their metastases, *Vet J* 191:334, 2012.

Buse JB, et al.: Type 2 diabetes mellitus. In Melmed S, Polonsky K, Larsen PR, Kronenberg HM, editors: *Williams textbook of endocrinology*, ed 12, Philadelphia, 2011, Elsevier, p 1371.

Caceres AV, et al.: Helical computed tomographic angiography of the normal canine pancreas, *Vet Radiol Ultrasound* 47:270, 2006.

Carpenter JL, et al.: Tumors and tumorlike lesions. In Holsworth J, editor: *Diseases of the cat: medicine and surgery*, Philadelphia, 1987, WB Saunders, p 406.

Caywood DD, et al.: Pancreatic insulin-secreting neoplasms: clinical, diagnostic, and prognostic features in 73 dogs, *J Am Anim Hosp Assoc* 24:577, 1988.

Chastain CB: Endocrine and metabolic systems. In Hoskins JD, editor: *Veterinary pediatrics*, Philadelphia, 1990, WB Saunders, p 249.

Chatziioannou A, et al.: Imaging and localization of pancreatic insulinomas, *Clin Imaging* 25:275, 2001.

Chew DJ, et al.: Hyperglycemia and hypoglycemia. In Klenner WR, editor: *Quick reference to veterinary medicine*, Philadelphia, 1982, JB Lippincott, p 432.

Cohen M, et al.: Gastrointestinal leiomyosarcoma in 14 dogs, *J Vet Intern Med* 17:107, 2003.

Cohen TA, et al.: Evaluation of six portable blood glucose meters for measuring blood glucose concentration in dogs, *J Am Vet Med Assoc* 235:276, 2009.

Cohn LA, et al.: Assessment of five portable blood glucose meters, a point-of-care analyzer, and color test strips for measuring blood glucose concentration in dogs, *J Am Vet Med Assoc* 216:198, 2000.

Commens PJ, et al.: Interleukin-1 is a potent modulator of insulin secretion from isolated rat islets of Langerhans, *Diabetes* 36:963, 1987.

Cryer PE: Catecholamines, pheochromocytoma and diabetes, *Diabetes Rev* 1:309, 1993.

Cryer PE: Hypoglycemia. In Melmed S, Polonsky K, Larsen PR, Kronenberg HM, editors: *Williams textbook of endocrinology*, ed 12, Philadelphia, 2011, Elsevier, p 1552.

Cryer PE, Gerich JE: Glucose counterregulation, hypoglycemia, and intensive insulin therapy in diabetes mellitus, *N Engl J Med* 313:232, 1985.

Cryer PE, Polonsky KS, et al.: Glucose homeostasis and hypoglycemia. In Wilson JD, editor: *Williams textbook of endocrinology*, ed 9, Philadelphia, 1998, WB Saunders, p 939.

Das H, Hochberg FH: Metastatic neoplasms and paraneoplastic syndromes. In Goetz CG, Pappert EJ, editors: *Textbook of clinical neurology*, Philadelphia, 1999, WB Saunders, p 957.

D'Ercole AJ, et al.: Tissue concentrations of somatomedin C: further evidence for multiple sites of synthesis and paracrine or autocrine mechanisms of action, *Proc Natl Acad Sci USA* 81:935, 1984.

de Bruijne JJ, et al.: Fat mobilization and plasma hormone levels in fasted dogs, *Metabolism* 30:190, 1981.

de Groot JW, et al.: Non-islet cell tumor-induced hypoglycaemia: a review of the literature including two new cases, *Endocr Relat Cancer* 14:979, 2007.

del Rey A, Besedovsky H: Interleukin 1 affects glucose homeostasis, *Am J Physiol* 253:R794, 1987.

Edwards DF, et al.: Hypoglycemia and chronic renal failure in a cat, *J Am Vet Med Assoc* 190:435, 1987.

Feldman EC, Nelson RW: *Canine and feline endocrinology and reproduction*, Philadelphia, 1987, WB Saunders.

Fenner WR: Diseases of the brain. In Ettinger SJ, Feldman EC, editors: *Textbook of veterinary internal medicine*, ed 4, Philadelphia, 1995, WB Saunders, p 578.

Fingeroth JM, Smeak DD: Intravenous methylene blue infusion for intraoperative identification of pancreatic islet cell tumors in dogs. II. Clinical trials and results in four dogs, *J Am Anim Hosp Assoc* 24:175, 1988.

Fingeroth JM, et al.: Intravenous methylene blue infusion for intraoperative identification of parathyroid gland and pancreatic islet cell tumors in dogs. I. Experimental determination of dose-related staining efficacy and toxicity, *J Am Anim Hosp Assoc* 24:165, 1988.

Finotello R, et al.: Pancreatic islet cell tumor secreting insulin-like growth factor type-II in a dog, *J Vet Intern Med* 23:1289, 2009.

Fischer JR, et al.: Glucagon constant-rate infusion: a novel strategy for the management of hyperinsulinemic-hypoglycemic crisis in the dog, *J Am Anim Hosp Assoc* 36:27, 2000.

Fischer KF, et al.: Hypoglycemia in hospitalized patients: causes and outcomes, *N Engl J Med* 315:1245, 1986.

Fyfe JC, et al.: Glycogen storage disease type IV: inherited deficiency of branching enzyme activity in cats, *Pediatr Res* 32:719, 1992.

Garden OA, et al.: Somatostatin receptor imaging in vivo by planar scintigraphy facilitates the diagnosis of canine insulinomas, *J Vet Intern Med* 19:168, 2005.

Gerich J, et al.: Hypoglycemia unawareness, *Endocr Rev* 12:356, 1991.

Gerich JE, et al.: Renal gluconeogenesis: its importance in human glucose homeostasis, *Diabetes Care* 24:382, 2001.

Giger U, et al.: Metabolic myopathy in canine muscle-type phosphofructokinase deficiency, *Muscle Nerve* 11:1260, 1988.

Greene SN, Bright RM: Insulinoma in a cat, *J Sm Anim Pract* 49:38, 2008.

Gregory BL, et al.: Glycogen storage disease type IIIa in curly-coated retrievers, *J Vet Intern Med* 21:40, 2007.

Gritzmann N, et al.: CT in the differentiation of pancreatic neoplasms-progress report, *Dig Dis* 22:6, 2004.

Guedes AG, Rude EP: Effects of pre-operative administration of medetomidine on plasma insulin and glucose concentrations in healthy dogs and dogs with insulinoma, *Vet Anaesth Analg* 40:472, 2013.

Haemers S, Rottiers R: Medical treatment of insulinoma, *Acta Clin Belg* 36:199, 1981.

Hambrook LY, Kudnig ST: Tumor thrombus formation in two dogs with insulinoma, *J Am Vet Med Assoc* 241:1065, 2012.

Hardy RM: Diseases of the liver and their treatment. In Ettinger SJ, editor: *Textbook of veterinary internal medicine*, ed 3, Philadelphia, 1989, WB Saunders, p 1479.

Hargrove DM, et al.: Adrenergic blockade does not abolish elevated glucose turnover during bacterial infection, *Am J Physiol* 254:E16, 1988a.

Hargrove DM, et al.: Adrenergic blockade prevents endotoxin-induced increases in glucose metabolism, *Am J Physiol* 255:E629, 1988b.

Hawkins KL, et al.: Immunocytochemistry of normal pancreatic islets and spontaneous islet cell tumors in dogs, *Vet Pathol* 24:170, 1987.

Hawks D, et al.: Insulin-secreting pancreatic (islet cell) carcinoma in a cat, *J Vet Intern Med* 6:193, 1992.

Heckmann JG, et al.: Hypoglycemic sensorimotor polyneuropathy associated with insulinoma, *Muscle Nerve* 23:1891, 2000.

Hooper AN, Roberts BK: Fanconi syndrome in four non-basenji dogs exposed to chicken jerky treats, *J Amer Anim Hosp Assoc* 47:178, 2011.

Iseri T, et al.: Dynamic computed tomography of the pancreas in normal dogs and in a dog with pancreatic insulinoma, *Vet Radiol Ultrasound* 48:328, 2007.

Jackson TC, et al.: Cellular and molecular characterization of a feline insulinoma, *J Vet Intern Med* 23:383, 2009.

Jeffery ND, et al.: Letter to the editor, *Prog Vet Neurol* 5:135, 1994.

Karam JH: Hypoglycemic disorders. In Greenspan FS, Gardner DG, editors: *Basic and clinical endocrinology*, ed 6, New York, 2001, Lange Medical Books/McGraw-Hill, p 699.

Kintzel PE: Anticancer drug–induced kidney disorders, *Drug Safety* 24:19, 2001.

Kishnani PS, et al.: Isolation and nucleotide sequence of canine glucose-6-phosphatase mRNA: identification of mutation in puppies with glycogen storage disease type Ia, *Biochem Mol Med* 61:168, 1997.

Kishnani PS, et al.: Canine model and genomic structural organization of glycogen storage disease type Ia (GSD Ia), *Vet Pathol* 38:83, 2001.

Kraje AC: Hypoglycemia and irreversible neurologic complications in a cat with insulinoma, *J Am Vet Med Assoc* 223:812, 2003.

Kruth SA, et al.: Insulin-secreting islet cell tumors: establishing a diagnosis and the clinical course of 25 dogs, *J Am Vet Med Assoc* 181:54, 1982.

Kudo M, Noguchi T: Immunoreactive myelin basic protein in tumor cells associated with carcinomatous neuropathy, *Am J Clin Pathol* 84:741, 1985.

Kvols LK, et al.: Evaluation of a radio-labeled somatostatin analog (I-123 octreotide) in the detection and localization of carcinoid and islet cell tumors, *Radiology* 197:129, 1993.

La Rosa S, et al.: Improved histologic and clinicopathologic criteria for prognostic evaluation of pancreatic endocrine tumors, *Human Path* 40:30, 2009.

Lamb CR, et al.: Ultrasonography of pancreatic neoplasia in the dog: a retrospective review of 16 cases, *Vet Rec* 137:65, 1995.

Lamberts S, et al.: Parallel in vivo and in vitro detection of functional somatostatin receptors in human endocrine pancreatic tumors: consequences with regard to diagnosis, localization and therapy, *J Clin Endocrinol Metab* 71:566, 1990.

Lamberts SJW, et al.: The role of somatostatin and its analogs in the diagnosis and treatment of tumors, *Endocrinol Rev* 12:450, 1991.

Lamberts SJW, et al.: Octreotide and related somatostatin analogs in the diagnosis and treatment of pituitary disease and somatostatin receptor scintigraphy, *Neuroendocrinology* 14:27, 1993.

Lamberts SWJ, et al.: Somatostatin analogs: future directions, *Metabolism* 45:104, 1996.

Leifer CE, et al.: Insulin-secreting tumor: diagnosis and medical and surgical management in 55 dogs, *J Am Vet Med Assoc* 188:60, 1986.

Lester NV, et al.: Scintigraphic diagnosis of insulinoma in a dog, *Vet Radiol Ultrasound* 40:174, 1999.

Loftin EG, Herold LV: Therapy and outcome of suspected alpha lipoic acid toxicity in two dogs, *J Vet Emerg Crit Care* 19:501, 2009.

Lothrop CD: Medical treatment of neuroendocrine tumors of the gastroenteropancreatic system with somatostatin. In Kirk RW, editor: *Current veterinary therapy X*, Philadelphia, 1989, WB Saunders, p 1020.

Lutz TA, Rand JS: Comparison of five commercial radioimmunoassay kits for the measurement of feline insulin, *Res Vet Sci* 55:64, 1993.

Madarame H, et al.: Retrospective study of canine insulinomas: eight cases (2005-2008), *J Vet Med Sci* 71:905, 2009.

Mai W, Caceres AV: Dual-phase computed tomographic angiography in three dogs with pancreatic insulinoma, *Vet Radiol Ultrasound* 49:141, 2008.

McMillan F: Functional pancreatic islet cell tumor in a cat, *J Am Anim Hosp Assoc* 21:741, 1985.

Mehlhaff CJ, et al.: Insulin-producing islet cell neoplasms: surgical considerations and general management in 35 dogs, *J Am Anim Hosp Assoc* 21:607, 1985.

Mellanby RJ, Herrtage ME: Insulinoma in a normoglycaemic dog with low serum fructosamine, *J Sm Anim Pract* 43:506, 2002.

Meszaros K, et al.: Increased uptake and phosphorylation of 2-deoxyglucose by skeletal muscles in endotoxin-treated rats, *Am J Physiol* 253:E33, 1987.

Meszaros K, et al.: In vivo glucose utilization by individual tissues during nonlethal hypermetabolic sepsis, *FASEB J* 2:3083, 1988.

Meyer C, et al.: Effects of autonomic neuropathy on counterregulation and awareness of hypoglycemia in type 1 diabetic patients, *Diabetes Care* 21:1960, 1998.

Minkus G, et al.: Canine neuroendocrine tumors of the pancreas: a study using image analysis techniques for the discrimination of metastatic versus nonmetastatic tumors, *Vet Pathol* 34:138, 1997.

Mokan M, et al.: Hypoglycemia unawareness in IDDM, *Diabetes Care* 17:1397, 1994.

Moore AS, et al.: Streptozotocin for treatment of pancreatic islet cell tumors in dogs: 17 cases (1989-1999), *J Am Vet Med Assoc* 221:811, 2002.

Murphy LA, Coleman AE: Xylitol toxicosis in dogs, *Vet Clin N Am Small Anim* 42:307, 2012.

Naylor JM, Kronfeld DS: In vivo studies of hypoglycemia and lactic acidosis in endotoxic shock, *Am J Physiol* 248:E309, 1985.

Niessen SJM: Glucagon: are we missing a (life-saving) trick? *J Vet Emerg Crit Care* 22:523, 2012.

Northrup NC, et al.: Prospective evaluation of biweekly streptozotocin in 19 dogs with insulinoma, *J Vet Intern Med* 27:483, 2013.

Öberg J, et al.: Validation of a species-optimized enzyme-linked immunosorbent assay for determination of serum concentrations of insulin in dogs, *Vet Clin Path* 40:66, 2011.

O'Brien TD, et al.: Canine pancreatic endocrine tumors: Immunohistochemical analysis of hormone content and amyloid, *Vet Pathol* 24:308, 1987.

O'Brien TD, et al.: Pancreatic endocrine tumor in a cat: clinical, pathological, and immunohistochemical evaluation, *J Am Anim Hosp Assoc* 26:453, 1990.

Patel YC: Somatostatin and its receptor family, *Front Neuroendocrinol* 20:157, 1999.

Pickens EH, et al.: Unique radiographic appearance of bone marrow metastasis of an insulin-secreting beta-cell carcinoma in a dog, *J Vet Intern Med* 19:350, 2005.

Polton GA, et al.: Improved survival in a retrospective cohort of 28 dogs with insulinoma, *J Sm Anim Pract* 48:151, 2007.

Reubi J, et al.: Somatostatin receptor sst1-sst5 expression in normal and neoplastic human tissues using receptor autoradiography with subtype-selective ligands, *Eur J Nucl Med* 28:836, 2001.

Robben JH, et al.: In vitro and in vivo detection of functional somatostatin receptors in canine insulinomas, *J Nucl Med* 38:1036, 1997.

Robben JH, et al.: Comparison of ultrasonography, computed tomography, and single-photon emission computed tomography for the detection and localization of canine insulinoma, *J Vet Intern Med* 19:15, 2005.

Rossi G, et al.: Paraneoplastic hypoglycemia in a diabetic dog with an insulin growth factor-2-producing mammary carcinoma, *Vet Clin Path* 39:480, 2010.

Rothman DL, et al.: Quantitation of hepatic glycogenolysis and gluconeogenesis in fasting humans with ^{13}C NMR, *Science* 254:573, 1991.

Schnedl WJ, et al.: STZ transport and cytotoxicity; specific enhancement of GLUT2-expressing cells, *Diabetes* 43:1326, 1994.

Scholzen T, Gerdes J: The Ki-67 protein: from the known and the unknown, *J Cell Physiol* 182:311, 2000.

Schrauwen E, et al.: Peripheral polyneuropathy associated with insulinoma in the dog: clinical, pathological, and electrodiagnostic features, *Prog Vet Neurol* 7:16, 1996.

Service FJ: Hypoglycemic disorders, *N Engl J Med* 332:1144, 1995.

Shahar R, et al.: Peripheral neuropathy in a dog with functional islet B-cell tumor and widespread metastasis, *J Am Vet Med Assoc* 187:175, 1985.

Sherwin RS, Felig P: Hypoglycemia. In Felig P, et al.: *Endocrinology and metabolism*, New York, 1981, McGraw-Hill, p 869.

Simpson KW, et al.: Evaluation of the long-acting somatostatin analogue octreotide in the management of insulinoma in three dogs, *J Small Anim Pract* 36:161, 1995.

Slye M, Wells HG: Tumor of islet tissue with hyperinsulinism in a dog, *Arch Pathol* 19:537, 1935.

Smeak DD, et al.: Intravenous methylene blue as a specific stain for primary and metastatic insulinoma in a dog, *J Am Anim Hosp Assoc* 24:478, 1988.

Smith BF, et al.: Molecular basis of canine muscle type phosphofructokinase deficiency, *J Biol Chem* 271:20070, 1996.

Stumvoll M, et al.: Uptake and release of glucose by the human kidney: postabsorptive rates and responses to epinephrine, *J Clin Invest* 96:2528, 1995.

Thompson MF, et al.: Acquired proximal renal tubulopathy in dogs exposed to a common dried chicken treat: retrospective study of 108 cases (2007-2009), *Aust Vet J* 91:368, 2013.

Thorens B, Mueckler M: Glucose transporters in the 21st century, *Am J Physiol Endocrinol Metab* 298:E141, 2010.

Tobin MV, et al.: Forced diuresis to reduce nephrotoxicity of streptozocin in the treatment of advanced metastatic insulinoma, *Br Med J* 294:1128, 1987.

Tobin RL, et al.: Outcome of surgical versus medical treatment of dogs with beta-cell neoplasia: 39 cases (1990-1997), *J Am Vet Med Assoc* 215:226, 1999.

Tryfonidou MA, et al.: A retrospective evaluation of 51 dogs with insulinoma, *Vet Quart* 20:114, 1998.

Van Ham L, et al.: Treatment of a dog with an insulinoma-related peripheral polyneuropathy with corticosteroids, *Vet Rec* 141:98, 1997.

Van Hoe L, et al.: Helical CT for the preoperative localization of islet cell tumors of the pancreas: value of arterial and parenchymal phase images, *Am J Roentgenol* 165:1437, 1995.

Walvoort HC, et al.: Comparative pathology of the canine model of glycogen storage disease type II (Pompe's disease), *J Inherit Metabl Dis* 8:38, 1985.

Wess G, Reusch C: Evaluation of five portable blood glucose meters for use in dogs, *J Am Vet Med Assoc* 216:203, 2000.

Whipple AO, Grantz VK: Adenoma of islet cells with hyperinsulinism: a review, *Ann Surg* 101:1299, 1935.

Zeugswetter FK, et al.: Metabolic and hormonal responses to subcutaneous glucagon in healthy beagles, *J Vet Emerg Crit Care* 22:558, 2012.

Zini E, et al.: Paraneoplastic hypoglycemia due to an insulin-like growth factor type-II secreting hepatocellular carcinoma, *J Vet Intern Med* 21:193, 2007.

Zini E, et al.: Evaluation of a new portable glucose meter designed for use in cats, *Schweiz Arch Tierheilkd* 151:448, 2009.

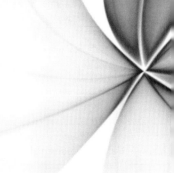

CHAPTER CONTENTS

In 1932, Dr. Harvey Cushing described eight humans with a disorder that he suggested was "the result of pituitary basophilism." Six of the eight humans had small, basophilic pituitary adenomas and clinical features of excess adrenocortical cortisol secretion. As other forms are now recognized for what was then considered a single condition, the eponym "Cushing's syndrome" is an umbrella term referring to the constellation of clinical and chemical abnormalities that result from chronic exposure to excessive concentrations of glucocorticoids (i.e., hyperadrenocorticism [HAC]). Specifically, the term "Cushing's disease" is applied to cases in which hypercortisolism occurs secondary to inappropriate excessive secretion of adrenocorticotropic hormone (ACTH; corticotropin) by the pituitary (i.e., pituitary-dependent hyperadrenocorticism [PDH]). Besides PDH, a pathophysiologic classification of HAC includes (1) autonomous secretion of cortisol by an adrenocortical carcinoma or adenoma, (2) iatrogenic resulting from exogenous glucocorticoid administration, (3) secretion of ACTH from an ectopic site (i.e., non-pituitary), (4) food-dependent cortisol secretion, and (5) pituitary hyperplasia caused by excess corticotropin-releasing hormone (CRH) secretion due to a hypothalamic disorder and, secondarily, adrenocortical hyperplasia (which is extremely rare in people and not yet reported in dogs or cats).

REGULATION OF GLUCOCORTICOID SECRETION

Corticotropin-Releasing Hormone

The hypothalamus, by secreting CRH into the hypophyseal portal system, exerts control over secretion of ACTH by the anterior pituitary (pars distalis). In turn, ACTH stimulates adrenocortical secretion of cortisol. Cortisol completes the circle by inhibiting secretion of hypothalamic and pituitary hormones (Fig. 10-1).

The CRH-secreting neurons are located in the anterior portion of the hypothalamic paraventricular nuclei. A polypeptide containing 41 amino acid residues, CRH has a long plasma half-life (approximately 60 minutes). In humans, both arginine vasopressin and angiotensin II potentiate CRH secretion and, in turn, ACTH; conversely, oxytocin inhibits CRH-mediated ACTH secretion. Roles for arginine vasopressin, oxytocin, and angiotensin II in regulating ACTH secretion have not been consistently demonstrated in dogs (Kemppainen and Sartin, 1987; Kemppainen et al, 1992).

Adrenocorticotropic Hormone

ACTH is a 39 amino acid peptide hormone with a half-life in blood of approximately 10 minutes. The amino terminal end of the ACTH molecule (amino acids 1 to 18) is responsible for its

biologic activity. Its primary function is to stimulate glucocorticoid secretion from the adrenal cortex. Stimulation of adrenocortical mineralocorticoid or sex hormone secretion is less important.

During synthesis, ACTH is derived from a large precursor molecule, pro-opiomelanocortin (POMC). In the pituitary cells responsible for ACTH secretion (corticotrophs), POMC is synthesized and processed into smaller, biologically active fragments including β-lipotropin (β-LPH), α–melanocyte-stimulating hormone (α-MSH), β-melanocyte-stimulating hormone (β-MSH), β-endorphin, and N-terminal fragment (Fig. 10-2). Two of the POMC fragments are contained within the structure of ACTH and, therefore, are byproducts of ACTH metabolism: α-MSH is the first 13 amino acids of ACTH and corticotropin-like intermediate lobe peptide (CLIP) is amino acids 18 to 39. Neither peptide is secreted as a separate hormone in humans.

In dogs, CRH controls ACTH release (Kemppainen and Sartin, 1987; Kemppainen et al, 1992). Both CRH and ACTH are secreted in a pulsatile manner with a diurnal rhythm in humans that results in a peak before awakening. Secretion of ACTH is episodic and pulsatile in healthy dogs and those with PDH (Kemppainen and Sartin, 1984a; Kooistra et al, 1997a). A circadian rhythm has not been convincingly demonstrated, although one study reported higher plasma ACTH concentrations in late afternoon than in the morning (Castillo et al, 2009). Many types of stress (e.g., pain, trauma, hypoxia, acute hypoglycemia, cold exposure, surgery, and inflammatory mediators) also stimulate ACTH secretion (Stewart, 2008).

The negative feedback effects of cortisol on the pituitary gland to diminish ACTH secretion occur within three time domains—fast, intermediate, and delayed. Fast feedback occurs within minutes in response to a rising cortisol concentration. Intermediate feedback occurs within 0.5 to 3 hours of cellular exposure to glucocorticoid and is present until delayed feedback begins approximately 9 hours after glucocorticoid exposure (Phillips and Tashjian, 1982; Dayanithi and Antoni, 1989; Antoni and Dayanithi, 1990). Delayed feedback appears to be mediated principally through suppression of the synthesis of both hypothalamic stimulatory peptides and pituitary ACTH. Type II glucocorticoid receptors (GRs) in the hypothalamus and pituitary likely interact with negative response elements in the gene for these peptides and decrease their transcription (Eberwine et al, 1987). Although negative feedback control of ACTH secretion at the pituitary corticotroph within the intermediate time domain is of fundamental biological (and potentially medical) importance, no one has yet ascertained how this process occurs. In addition to the negative feedback by adrenal steroid secretion, ACTH also exerts a negative feedback effect on (i.e., inhibits) its own secretion (short loop feedback), as depicted in Fig. 10-1.

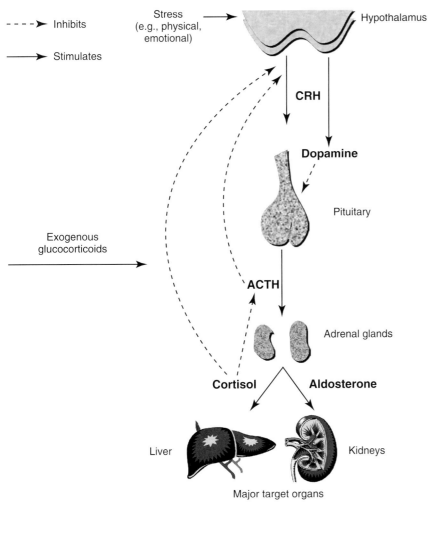

FIGURE 10-1 The hypothalamic-pituitary-adrenal axis, illustrating the various stimuli that enhance corticotropin-releasing hormone *(CRH)* secretion as well as negative feedback by cortisol at the hypothalamic and pituitary levels. *ACTH*, Adrenocorticotropic hormone.

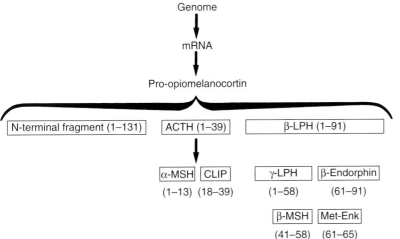

FIGURE 10-2 The processing of pro-opiomelanocortin (POMC) into its biologically active peptide hormones. *α-MSH*, α–melanocyte-stimulating hormone; *β-MSH*, β-melanocyte-stimulating hormone; *γ-LPH*, γ-lipotropin; *ACTH*, adrenocorticotropic hormone; *CLIP*, corticotropin-like intermediate lobe peptide; *mRNA*, messenger ribonucleic acid.

Dopamine

In humans and dogs, the pituitary gland is distinctly divided into an anterior section (pars distalis) and a posterior section (pars nervosa). However, dogs, unlike humans, also have a distinct area that separates the anterior and posterior lobes of the pituitary, the pars intermedia or intermediate lobe (Halmi et al, 1981). The pars intermedia has two distinct cell types. The predominant cells (A cells) immunostain intensely for α-MSH but weakly for

ACTH. The second population (B cells) stains strongly for ACTH and weakly for α-MSH. The intense ACTH staining of pars intermedia B cells is similar to the staining characteristics of ACTH-producing pars distalis cells (Halmi et al, 1981).

In comparison to regulation of the pars distalis, secretion of ACTH from the pars intermedia is under tonic negative regulation by dopamine secreted from the hypothalamic arcuate nucleus, as well as by serotonin and CRH. Compared to the pars

TABLE 10-1	NOMENCLATURE OF STEROIDOGENIC ENZYMES	
ENZYME	**GENE SYMBOL**	**TRIVIAL NAME**
P450scc	CYP11A1	Cholesterol side chain cleavage enzyme
3-β Hydroxysteroid dehydrogenase (3β-HSD)	HSD3B1 HSD3B2	3β-Hydroxysteroid dehydrogenase
P450c17	CYP17	17α-Hydroxylase; 17,20-lyase
P450c21	CYP21A2	21β-Hydroxylase
P450c11	CYP11B1	11β-Hydroxylase
P450c11AS	CYP11B2	P450aldo; aldosterone synthase; corticosterone methyloxidase

distalis, which is devoid of a nerve supply, the relatively avascular pars intermedia is innervated and controlled by dopaminergic and serotoninergic fibers from the brain (Peterson et al, 1982a).

Steroids

Zones of the Adrenal Cortex and Their Products

The main hormones secreted by the adrenal cortex are cortisol, corticosterone, and aldosterone. In dogs, cortisol and corticosterone are secreted in equal amounts. Histologically, the adrenal cortex is composed of three zones: the zonae glomerulosa, fasciculata, and reticularis. Most adrenal steroidogenic enzymes belong to the cytochrome P450 oxygenase family (Table 10-1). All zones can synthesize and secrete corticosterone. However, due to enzymatic differences between the zona glomerulosa and the inner two zones, the adrenal cortex functions as two separate units with differing regulation and secretory products.

The outer layer, the zona glomerulosa, produces aldosterone. It is deficient in 17α-hydroxylase activity (CYP17), rendering the zone incapable of making cortisol and sex hormones. In contrast, only cells in the zona glomerulosa contain the enzyme necessary for synthesizing aldosterone (i.e., aldosterone synthase) (Fig. 10-3).

The middle layer, the zona fasciculata, functions as a unit with the innermost layer, the zona reticularis. The zona fasciculata, however, secretes mostly glucocorticoids, and the zona reticularis secretes mainly sex hormones. Due to the presence of 17α-hydroxylase, both zones can synthesize 17 α-hydroxypregnenolone and 17α-hydroxyprogesterone, precursors of cortisol and sex hormones (Fig. 10-4).

Steroidogenesis

Cortisol, aldosterone, androgens, and estrogens are steroid hormones; the precursor for all is cholesterol. Low-density lipoprotein (LDL) particles account for approximately 80% of cholesterol delivered to the adrenal glands. A small pool of free cholesterol is available within the glands for rapid response to stimulation. When stimulation occurs, hydrolysis of stored cholesteryl esters to release cholesterol, cholesterol uptake from plasma lipoproteins, and cholesterol synthesis also occurs within the adrenal glands. The rate limiting-step in the production of adrenocortical steroid hormones is cholesterol transfer within mitochondria and is regulated by steroidogenic acute regulatory protein (StAR). Virtually no steroids are stored within the adrenal glands; thus, synthesis is constant and secretion requires activation of the biosynthetic pathway.

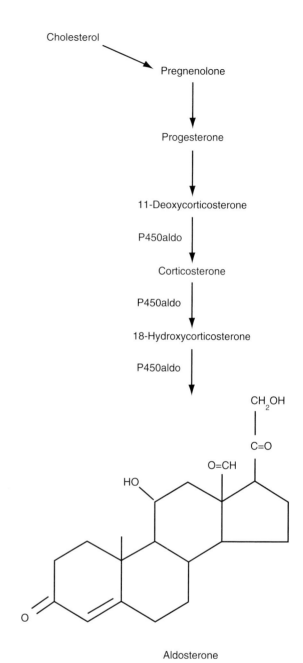

FIGURE 10-3 Steroid biosynthesis in the zona glomerulosa. The steps from cholesterol to 11-deoxycorticosterone are the same as in the zona fasciculata and zona reticularis. Only the zona glomerulosa contains aldosterone synthase, which catalyzes the conversion of 11-deoxycorticosterone to corticosterone and then to 18-hydroxycorticosterone and finally aldosterone.

Regulation of Cortisol Secretion

Besides being a secretory factor, ACTH is also a trophic hormone for the zonae fasciculata and reticularis. Delivery of ACTH to the adrenal cortex leads to rapid synthesis and secretion of cortisol and androgens. Plasma cortisol concentration increases within minutes of ACTH administration. Chronic adrenocortical stimulation by elevated ACTH concentrations leads to hyperplasia and hypertrophy; conversely, ACTH deficiency results in adrenocortical atrophy and decreased steroidogenesis, adrenal gland weight, and protein and nucleic acid content. Inflammatory mediators (e.g., interleukin-1, interleukin-6, and tumor necrosis factor-α) increase ACTH secretion either directly or by augmenting the effect of CRH (Stewart, 2008).

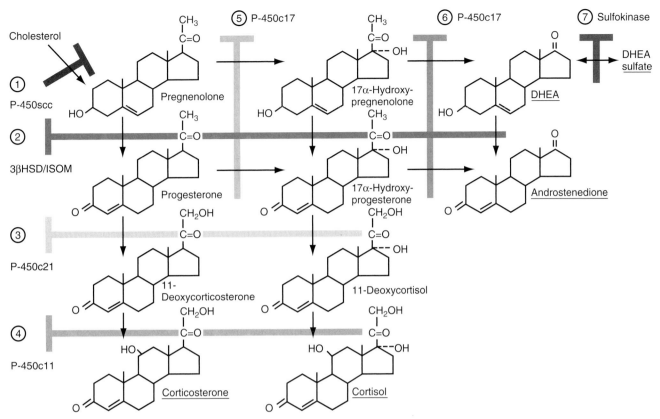

FIGURE 10-4 Steroid biosynthesis pathway in the adrenal cortex. The branching pathways for glucocorticoids, mineralocorticoids, and adrenal androgens and the structures of these steroids and their biosynthetic precursors are shown. Names of the biosynthetic enzymes are shown in Table 10-1. *DHEA,* Dehydroepiandrosterone.

Regulation of Aldosterone Secretion

Regulation of aldosterone synthesis is primarily by the renin-angiotensin system and serum potassium concentrations (see Chapter 12).

 PATHOLOGY AND PATHOPHYSIOLOGY

Pituitary-Dependent Hyperadrenocorticism

Pituitary Control, Feedback, and Cortisol Secretion

In normal dogs, ACTH secretion is episodic. In dogs with PDH, typically both the frequency and amplitude of ACTH secretory "bursts" are increased. Chronic ACTH oversecretion drives excess cortisol secretion and, eventually, adrenocortical hyperplasia. Dogs with HAC are exposed to more cortisol on a daily basis than healthy animals (Fig. 10-5), resulting in the clinical signs of HAC that are due to the effects of cortisol. Feedback inhibition of ACTH secreted from a pituitary adenoma by physiologic or excess levels of glucocorticoids is relatively ineffective (Fig. 10-6). If feedback inhibition of ACTH secretion by glucocorticoids functioned normally, PDH would not evolve.

Incidence of Pituitary Tumors

Eighty percent to 85% of dogs with naturally occurring HAC have PDH (Feldman, 1983a; 1983b). The reported incidence of histologically recognized pituitary tumors varies between 20% and 100% (Peterson et al, 1982a; Feldman, 1983a; 1983b; McNicol, 1987); the remainder of dogs reportedly has pituitary hyperplasia. The variation in reported incidence may be due in part to the persistence of the pathologist, as well as the microdissection

capabilities and staining capacities of the laboratory performing the histologic examination; some tumors can be quite small. In the author's experience, almost all dogs with PDH have a pituitary tumor. Functioning pituitary carcinomas occur rarely (Puente, 2003). Occasionally, more than one process may be present in the pituitary—for example, dogs with (1) two pituitary adenomas, each tumor apparently arising from a different pituitary lobe, or (2) both a tumor and hyperplasia of the pituitary.

Approximately 71% to 80% of pituitary tumors arise in the pars distalis. The remaining tumors originate in the pars intermedia (Peterson et al, 1982a; 1986a). Two types of pars intermedia tumors exist: dexamethasone non-suppressible with disproportionately elevated α-MSH levels and relatively dexamethasone-suppressible with normal to slightly elevated α-MSH concentrations (Peterson et al, 1986a). The two types appear to have identical clinical presentations; the cell type of origin has no known clinical significance.

Microadenoma Versus Macroadenoma

Pituitary tumors less than 10 mm in diameter are classified as microadenomas, whereas those more than 10 mm in diameter are classified as macroadenomas (Theon and Feldman, 1998). At the time of diagnosis of PDH, 31% to 48% of dogs have tumors less than 3 mm in diameter (Bertoy et al, 1995; Wood et al, 2007; Auriemma et al, 2009).

Pathology

Histologic classification of endocrine tissue is challenging. It is not unusual for pathologists to have difficulty distinguishing between normal and hyperplastic tissue. It may also be difficult to distinguish diffuse hyperplasia from adenomas as well as some

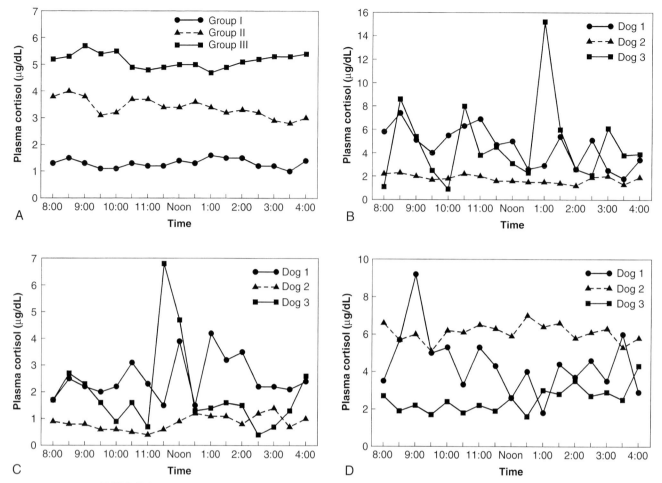

FIGURE 10-5 A, Mean plasma cortisol concentrations measured every 30 minutes for 8 hours in 15 normal dogs *(Group I),* 30 dogs with pituitary-dependent hyperadrenocorticism (PDH) *(Group II),* and 18 dogs with hyperadrenocorticism (HAC) secondary to an adrenocortical tumor (AT) *(Group III).* Demonstrating significant individual variation in plasma cortisol concentrations over time are values from three healthy dogs **(B),** three dogs with PDH **(C),** and three dogs with ATs **(D).**

adenomas from carcinomas. Thus, communication between clinician and pathologist, plus inclusion of laboratory and clinical impressions, may help the pathologist.

Grossly, larger adenomas often are attached to the base of the sella turcica but without invasion. As the diaphragma sellae is incomplete in dogs, pituitary growth occurs dorsad with invagination into the infundibular cavity and dilation of the infundibular recess and the third ventricle, with eventual compression or replacement of the hypothalamus. Larger neoplasms can have foci of hemorrhage, necrosis, mineralization, and liquefaction. Due to the ACTH secretion, bilateral adrenal gland enlargement is present. Nodules of yellow-orange cortical tissue can be found outside the adrenal capsule in the periadrenal fat and extending into the adrenal medulla. The corticomedullary junction is irregular and the medulla is compressed (Capen, 2007).

Histologically, pituitary corticotroph adenomas arising from the anterior pituitary are composed of well-differentiated chromophobic cells supported by fine connective tissue septa (see Chapter 2). Secretory cells are polyhedral to round. Secretory granules are not visible with standard light microscopy, but the cells will stain for ACTH and MSH; secretory granules can be demonstrated by electron microscopy. For tumors of the pars distalis, the demarcation between the neoplasm and pars distalis is often not distinct, and the pars distalis is either partly replaced by the neoplasm or severely compressed (Capen, 2007).

The histologic appearance of pars intermedia tumors is distinct from those of the pars distalis. Numerous colloid-filled follicles are present. Nests of cells between the follicles are primarily chromophobic, but occasional acidophilic or basophilic cells are present. Adenomas that secrete ACTH have prominent groups of large corticotrophs with abundant eosinophilic cytoplasm interspersed with variable numbers of smaller, more basophilic cells. Dense bands of fibrous connective tissue are occasionally interspersed between the follicles and chromophobic cells. Compression and invasion of the posterior pituitary is often present. If the tumor arises in the pars intermedia, the pars distalis is readily identifiable and sharply demarcated from the tumor. The pars distalis may have compression atrophy (Capen, 2007).

Etiology of Pituitary-Dependent Hyperadrenocorticism

Two main theories exist regarding the pathogenesis of pituitary tumors: (1) Excess stimulation by hypothalamic CRH secretion leading to corticotroph hyperplasia, and a somatic mutation of hyperplastic cells then leads to adenoma formation (i.e., the polyclonal theory), and (2) somatic mutation of a single corticotroph leading to clonal expansion (i.e., the monoclonal theory) (Castillo and Gallelli, 2010). The former is not widely believed; most pituitary tumors are monoclonal in humans, and hyperplastic areas are not detected surrounding adenomas. In addition, it would be difficult

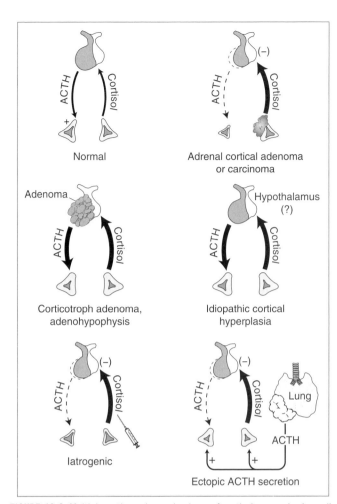

FIGURE 10-6 Multiple pathogenic mechanisms of cortisol excess in dogs. (In Maxie MG, editor: *Jubb, Kennedy and Palmer's pathology of domestic animals,* Philadelphia, 2007, Saunders, p. 339.) *ACTH,* Adrenocorticotropic hormone.

for one hypothalamic disorder to account for tumors arising in both the pars distalis and pars intermedia, because regulation of the two lobes is so different. Cerebrospinal fluid CRH concentrations are significantly lower in dogs with PDH than in healthy dogs (van Wijk et al, 1992). In addition, approximately 77% of dogs with PDH have no recurrence following hypophysectomy (Hanson et al, 2007); tumor regrowth should be common if the underlying problem were hypothalamic because the pituitary would continue to be stimulated.

Potential alterations in gene expression, oncogenes, and proliferation markers have been evaluated in canine corticotrophic tumors. Within 10 pars distalis adenomas, expression of the genes for POMC, CRH receptor 1 (CRHR1), glucocorticoid receptor, mineralocorticoid receptor (MR), and 11-β hydroxysteroid dehydrogenase (11β-HSD) type 1 and type 2 were determined. The messenger ribonucleic acid (mRNA) levels for POMC, CRHR1, and 11β-HSD2 were significantly increased approximately fourfold to fivefold, and for MR and 11β-HSD1 they were significantly decreased approximately twofold to threefold in adenomatous tissue compared with normal corticotrophic cells. The GR mRNA levels did not differ between adenomatous and normal corticotrophic cells (Teshima et al, 2009). The enzymes 11β-HSD1 and 11β-HSD2 are responsible for the conversion of inactive cortisone to active cortisol and vice versa, respectively, and help regulate glucocorticoid action. High expression of 11β-HSD2 with low 11β-HSD1 expression would lead to inactivation of cortisol within tumor cells, which could, at least in part,

explain resistance of corticotrophic adenomas to negative glucocorticoid feedback allowing continued ACTH secretion.

In humans and mice, the T-box transcription factor Tpit (Tbx19) is a marker of corticotrophs and melanotrophs and is necessary for POMC expression. Similarly, Tpit is expressed in normal and adenomatous canine pituitary tissue. Using adenomatous tissue from 14 dogs with PDH, the Tpit gene was screened for a tumor-specific mutation (e.g., a gain-of-function mutation), but none was identified. Interestingly, a missense polymorphism was discovered in the highly conserved DNA-binding domain for Tpit, the T-box, in one tumor sample, but the significance remains unknown (Hanson et al, 2008).

Leukemia inhibitor factor (LIF), a cytokine of the interleukin-6 family, activates the hypothalamic-pituitary axis and promotes corticotroph differentiation. Most cells of the canine pars distalis express LIF protein at low levels compared to rare cells in the pars intermedia; co-localization with ACTH is partial. Expression within 13 adenomas varied from high to almost undetectable. The LIF receptor (LIFR) is co-expressed with ACTH in cells of the pars intermedia and pars distalis. No mutations were identified in the LIFR gene of 14 corticotroph adenomas. Due to strong co-localization of LIFR and ACTH within adenomas, the possibility exists that LIFR pathway activation could play a role in tumor formation or progression (Hanson et al, 2010).

Activation of epithelial growth factor receptor (EGFR) occurs in a variety of human cancers, and epithelial growth factor (EGF) is a pituitary cell growth factor. Expression of EGFR is variable in canine pituitary corticotroph adenomas; however, for tumors expressing EGFR, treatment of cells in vitro with gefitinib, a tyrosine kinase inhibitor targeting the EGFR, decreased POMC expression. Thus, the EGFR may play a role in POMC overexpression in some corticotroph adenomas (Fukuoka et al, 2011).

In humans, KI-67 and proliferating cell nuclear antigen (PCNA) predict pituitary adenoma behavior and surgical outcome. The cell-cycle inhibitor p27kip1 is correlated with tumor recurrence after hypophysectomy. In one study in dogs, no significant differences in Ki-67, PCNA, and p27kip1 labeling indices were found between enlarged and non-enlarged pituitaries (van Rijn et al, 2010). Ishino and colleagues did find greater expression of Ki-67 in larger adenomas (Ishino et al, 2011). However, expression of minichromosome maintenance-7 (MCM-7) was significantly higher than that of Ki-67 in canine pituitary corticotroph adenomas. The MCM proteins are part of the DNA replication system and may be potential markers of neoplastic cell proliferation. Due to the higher expression of MCM-7, it may be a better proliferation marker than Ki-67 (Ishino et al, 2011).

Hyperadrenocorticism Due to Adrenal Tumor

Tumoral Secretion

Primary adrenocortical tumors (ATs), both adenomas and carcinomas, develop autonomously. Functioning, cortisol-secreting ATs secrete excessively, independent of pituitary control and in an episodic and random manner (see Fig. 10-5). Uncommonly, cortisol intermediates (e.g., desoxycorticosterone and corticosterone) are secreted (Reine et al, 1999; Behrend et al, 2004; Machida et al, 2007; Davies et al, 2008; Frankot et al, 2012). Due to negative feedback by cortisol or its intermediates, which can possess glucocorticoid activity, hypothalamic CRH and circulating ACTH concentrations are suppressed along with other POMC peptides (except α-MSH) (Peterson et al, 1986a). With low systemic ACTH concentrations, the contralateral adrenal cortex and the normal cells in the involved adrenal gland atrophy (see Fig. 10-6).

Pathology

Cortical adenomas are partially or completely surrounded by a fibrous connective tissue capsule, well-demarcated, and usually single. Larger adenomas are yellow to red, distort the gland's external surface, and are partially or completely encapsulated. Adjacent cortical tissue is compressed, and the medulla may be invaded. Small adenomas are more yellow and can be difficult to distinguish from areas of hyperplasia. Histologically, cortical adenomas are composed of well-differentiated cells resembling those of the normal zonae fasciculata or reticularis. The tumor cells are arranged in broad trabeculae or nests separated by small vascular spaces. The cells have abundant cytoplasm and are often vacuolated. Focal areas of hematopoiesis, calcification, or fat cell accumulation may be present (Capen, 2007).

Adrenal carcinomas are typically variegated, yellow-red, and friable. They are often fixed in location due to invasion of surrounding tissue, including the caudal vena cava. They are composed of highly pleomorphic secretory cells that are subdivided into small groups by fibrovascular stroma of variable thickness. Tumor cells are usually large and polyhedral with prominent nucleoli and densely eosinophilic or vacuolated cytoplasm. Areas of hemorrhage are common. The contralateral adrenal cortex is atrophied, consisting primarily of the adrenal capsule and zona glomerulosa. Atrophy may also be present in the remnants of the compressed adrenal cortex around the functional tumor (Capen, 2007).

Adenomas and carcinomas can be difficult to distinguish in some cases. Thorough evaluation of morphologic features combined with immunohistochemical assessment of the proliferation index may be useful. In one study, morphologic criteria significantly associated with carcinomas included being more than 2 cm in diameter, peripheral fibrosis, capsular invasion, a trabecular growth pattern, hemorrhage, and necrosis; hematopoiesis, fibrin thrombi, and cytoplasmic vacuolation were significantly associated with adenomas. A Ki-67 proliferation index was significantly higher in carcinomas. Mitotic index is low in adenomas and carcinomas (Labelle et al, 2004).

Bilateral Tumors

HAC caused by bilateral adenomas, carcinomas, or a combination of adenoma and carcinoma can occur (Ford et al, 1993; Hoerauf and Reusch, 1999; Anderson et al, 2001; Kyles et al, 2003; Stenske et al, 2005; Adissu et al, 2010). Although in a study of 15 dogs with HAC caused by functioning ATs, three (20%) had bilateral tumors (Hoerauf and Reusch, 1999), the author's experience is that the incidence of bilateral ATs is far lower. Pheochromocytomas and ATs may uncommonly occur simultaneously with one tumor per adrenal gland (Von Dehn et al, 1995; Thuroczy et al, 1998; Hylands, 2005). The presentation can be confusing, because ultrasonography may reveal bilateral adrenomegaly, and endocrine testing suggests an AT.

Etiology

Little is known about the pathogenesis of canine cortisol-secreting AT. In normal tissue, steroidogenesis is initiated by ACTH binding to its receptor (ACTH-R) on adrenocortical cells. Proteins involved in the second messenger system for the ACTH-R are protein kinase A (PKA) regulatory subunit 1 alpha (PRKAR1A) and the protein encoded by the stimulatory G protein alpha subunit gene (GNAS). The acute ultimate response to the binding of ACTH is mediated by StAR, which enhances cholesterol transport to the site of steroidogenesis. Alterations in expression of or mutations within genes for StAR, ACTH-R, steroidogenic enzymes, PRKAR1A, and GNAS could play a role in tumor pathogenesis. Expression of the genes for ACTH-R, StAR, cholesterol side-chain cleavage enzyme (CYPP11A), 17α-hydroxylase (CYP17), 3-β hydroxysteroid dehydrogenase (HSD3B2), 21-hydroxylase (CYP21), and

11β-hydroxylase (CYP11B1) was evaluated in cortisol-secreting adrenocortical adenomas and carcinomas. The expression of ACTH-R was significantly lower in carcinomas than in normal adrenal glands; thus, upregulation of steroidogenic enzymes is not responsible for hypercortisolemia, but significant downregulation of the ACTH-R might be associated with malignancy (Galac et al, 2010a). Functional mutations were not identified in genes for ACTH-R or PRKAR1A in tissue from 14 adenomas and 30 carcinomas. In comparison, 32% of tumors (four adenomas and 10 carcinomas) had missense mutations of GNAS; 11 were in codon 201, one in codon 203, and two in codon 227. Activating mutations would increase signaling from the receptor and, as a result, cortisol synthesis and secretion. Additional in vitro assays are necessary to establish a causal relationship between the mutations and tumor pathogenesis and whether the mutations are activating (Kool et al, 2013).

One case resembling human Carney complex, a familial human syndrome characterized by cardiac myxoma and extracardiac tumors associated with mutations in the PKA regulator gene PRKAR1A, has been reported. A 9-year-old female Golden Retriever had a left atrial ossifying myxosarcoma, bilateral adrenocortical adenomas, multiple areas of pituitary hyperplasia with expression of ACTH, and multiple pituitary Rathke cleft cysts. Genetic mutations were not detected in PRKAR1A (Adissu et al, 2010).

The presence of vasopressin receptors on canine cortisol-secreting AT has been theorized, because dogs with ACTH-independent hypercortisolism can secrete cortisol in response to lysine vasopressin (LVP) administration (van Wijk et al, 1994). Quantitative polymerase chain reaction (PCR) analysis of expression of receptors for luteinizing hormone (LH) and gastric inhibitory polypeptide (GIP) and the vasopressin receptors V_{1a}, V_{1b}, and V_2 in 23 cortisol-secreting AT did not find evidence of overexpression of any of the receptors as compared with normal adrenocortical tissue as a whole (i.e., all three adrenocortical zones were evaluated together). However, GIP and V_2 receptors were present in the zona fasciculata of approximately 50% of the tumors; neither receptor was present in the zona fasciculata of normal adrenal tissue. Thus, the presence of GIP and V_2 receptors in the zona fasciculata of an AT may play a role in the pathogenesis of a cortisol-secreting AT (Galac et al, 2010b).

Ectopic Adrenocorticotropic Hormone Syndrome

In humans, the ectopic ACTH syndrome comprises a varying group of tumors, including oat cell (small cell) carcinoma of the lung, thymoma, pancreatic islet cell tumors, carcinoid tumors, medullary carcinoma of the thyroid, and pheochromocytoma, which synthesize and secrete ACTH (Stewart, 2008). The tumors most commonly associated with ectopic ACTH syndrome arise from neuroendocrine tumors. Because ACTH production within the tumors is not typically sensitive to glucocorticoid-mediated negative feedback, high doses of dexamethasone do not typically effect cortisol concentrations (i.e., the tumors are dexamethasone-resistant). In addition, ectopic CRH secretion with or without ACTH can occur rarely (Stewart, 2008).

Ectopic ACTH syndrome has potentially been reported in three dogs (Churcher, 1999; Galac et al, 2005; Burgener et al, 2007). In one, ACTH was purportedly secreted from a primary hepatic carcinoid (Churcher, 1999), but both examination of pituitary function and morphology as well as proof of ectopic ACTH secretion were lacking. Second, HAC was diagnosed in a 5-year-old intact male Dachshund that had clinical signs consistent with HAC, a positive ACTH stimulation test, an elevated endogenous ACTH (eACTH) concentration, and bilateral adrenomegaly on ultrasound (Burgener et al, 2007). A low-dose dexamethasone suppression test (LDDST) was consistent with PDH. However, empty sella syndrome, a herniation of the subarachnoidal space into the sella turcica with invisible or reduced size of the pituitary gland, was diagnosed by magnetic resonance imaging (MRI). At necropsy, the pituitary was mainly fluid-filled. Although no non-pituitary tumor was found on necropsy, the lack of pituitary tumor tissue makes PDH unlikely. Given that partial suppression in response to dexamethasone was seen (which is not typical of ectopic ACTH syndrome), the possibility of false-positive test results for HAC must be considered.

The most convincing report is of an 8-year-old intact male German Shepherd (Galac et al, 2005). Cortisol secretion was not suppressed by high doses of dexamethasone, abdominal ultrasound revealed bilateral adrenomegaly, and eACTH concentrations were elevated; thus, dexamethasone-resistant PDH was believed to exist. Hypophysectomy was performed, but the clinical signs did not abate nor was a tumor found on histologic examination of the pituitary gland. Ten months after surgery, abdominal computed tomography (CT) revealed a mass in the area of the pancreas and liver nodules. Histologic examination of the mass, regional lymph nodes, and liver nodules allowed a diagnosis of metastatic neuroendocrine tumor. Although immunohistochemistry of the tumor was negative for ACTH, lack of staining does not rule out the possibility of ectopic ACTH production (Galac et al, 2005).

Adrenocortical Nodular Hyperplasia and Food-Dependent Hyperadrenocorticism

Macronodular, ACTH-dependent hyperplasia of the adrenals occurs in 10% to 40% of people with bilateral adrenocortical hyperplasia. One or more nodules are present and can be quite large. Some nodules may become autonomous from ACTH (Stewart, 2008). Macronodular hyperplasia also exists in dogs (Greco et al, 1999). In a retrospective study of dogs with HAC and concurrent pituitary and adrenal tumors, measurement of eACTH concentration was consistent with PDH in 11 dogs, with ATs in two, and was non-diagnostic in two. Four dogs had bilateral adrenal adenomas, potentially from transformation of macronodular hyperplasia to adenomas. The pathogenesis of macronodular hyperplasia in dogs is unclear, but, as in humans, it may represent a variant of PDH. However, why some dogs would develop diffuse adrenocortical hyperplasia and a minority develop nodular hyperplasia is unknown.

An ACTH-independent bilateral nodular adrenocortical hyperplasia occurs rarely in humans. Most cases are due to aberrant receptor expression within the adrenal cortex. Food-induced hypercortisolism due to enhanced adrenal responsiveness to GIP was the first type recognized, but aberrant expression of the vasopressin V_1, β-adrenergic, LH, serotonin, and angiotensin-1 receptors with resultant adrenal responsiveness have now been documented (Stewart, 2008).

Although not due to adrenocortical nodular changes, an ACTH-independent, food-dependent HAC has been described in one dog (Galac et al, 2007). The diagnosis was made due to a combination of (1) low plasma eACTH concentration in the absence of an AT, (2) at least a doubling in the urine cortisol-to-creatinine ratio (UC:CR) on two occasions in response to food, and (3) prevention of the meal-induced increase in cortisol concentration by octreotide, which is a diagnostic criteria for food-dependent HAC in humans. Because the dog of the case report had bilateral adrenomegaly on ultrasound, the low eACTH concentration was the means by which the etiology was determined to not be PDH. Potentially more cases of ACTH-independent HAC exist than are recognized because eACTH measurement is not always performed in the diagnosis of HAC.

Simultaneous Pituitary-Dependent and Adrenal-Dependent Hyperadrenocorticism

Rarely, dogs can have a functioning AT and a pituitary tumor (and bilateral adrenocortical hyperplasia) (Thuroczy et al, 1998; Greco et al, 1999). Endocrine evaluation of such dogs is diagnostic for HAC if the pituitary tumor is secreting ACTH and/or the adrenal tumor is secreting cortisol. However, tests to distinguish between pituitary-dependent and AT HAC provide confusing or contradictory results.

 ## SIGNALMENT

Age

HAC is a disease of middle-age and older dogs. The vast majority (≥ 89%) of dogs with PDH and those with functioning ATs are older than 6 years of age (Ling et al, 1979; Gallelli et al, 2010). More than 75% of dogs with PDH are older than 9 years of age, and the mean age is 8.6 to 11.7 years (Reusch and Feldman, 1991; Kipperman et al, 1992; Bertoy et al, 1995; Ortega et al, 1996; Wood et al, 2007; Gallelli et al, 2010; Lien et al, 2010: Bellumori et al, 2013). Dogs with HAC caused by functioning AT tend to be older than those with PDH. In one study, 92.5% of 41 dogs with ATs were 9 years of age or older (mean age 11.1 ± 2.3 years and 11.4 ± 2.1 years for dogs with adrenal carcinoma and adenoma, respectively) compared to 77% of 44 dogs with PDH (mean age 10.4 ± 3.2 years); however, no significant difference was detected between the two groups (Reusch and Feldman, 1991).

Gender

A gender predisposition has not been proven, but a female predisposition may exist. In multiple studies female dogs accounted for 63% to 76% of dogs (Reusch and Feldman, 1991; Bertoy et al, 1995; Ortega et al, 1996; Wood et al, 2007; Gallelli et al, 2010). However, no statistical comparisons were made to a control population to determine if females were truly overrepresented. In one study, a significant difference was not detected between the sex distribution of dogs with HAC and the general population (Ling et al, 1979); however, only 53% of dogs with HAC were female. In contrast, females are not the majority in all studies (Hess et al, 1998).

Breed/Body Weight

Overall, HAC occurs equally in purebred and mixed breed dogs (Bellumori et al, 2013). Although numerous breeds are commonly mentioned to be at increased risk, a statistical predisposition has been proven only for Poodles (likely Miniature Poodles only), Boxers, and Dachshunds (Ling et al, 1979). Various terrier breeds, especially Boston Terriers, Beagles, and German Shepherd dogs are often mentioned in studies. PDH and ATs have been diagnosed in virtually every breed (Tables 10-2 and 10-3) with PDH tending to occur more frequently in smaller dogs and ATs in larger dogs. Approximately 75% of dogs with PDH weigh less than 20 kg; in comparison, almost 50% of dogs with ATs, either adenoma or carcinoma, weigh more than 20 kg (Reusch and Feldman, 1991).

 ## HISTORY

Most articles outlining the clinical signs of HAC are at least 10 years old. Because of heightened awareness of HAC in the past 20 years, diagnosis is now likely made earlier in the course of the disease when clinical signs are fewer and subtler (Behrend

| | TABLE 10-2 | BREED DISTRIBUTION OF DOGS DIAGNOSED WITH PITUITARY-DEPENDENT HYPERADRENOCORTICISM (TOTAL: 750 DOGS)* |

PERCENTAGE	NUMBER	BREED
16%	119	Poodles (various breeds)
11%	84	Dachshunds
10%	76	Terriers (various breeds)
7%	54	Beagles
6%	48	German Shepherd dogs
5%	38	Labrador Retrievers
5%	36	Australian Shepherd
4%	30	Maltese
4%	28	Spaniel (various breeds)
3%	22	Schnauzer
3%	22	Lhasa Apso
2%	19	Chihuahua
2%	18	Boston terrier
2%	15	Golden Retrievers
2%	14	Shih Tzu
2%	12	Boxer
16%	115	Other breeds (38 breeds)

*Note: Data are observational; significant breed predisposition not assessed.

| | TABLE 10-3 | BREED DISTRIBUTION OF DOGS DIAGNOSED WITH FUNCTIONING ADRENOCORTICAL ADENOMA OR CARCINOMA CAUSING HYPERADRENOCORTICISM (TOTAL: 102 DOGS)* |

PERCENTAGE	BREED
15%	Poodles (various breeds)
12%	German Shepherd dogs
11%	Dachshunds
10%	Labrador Retrievers
8%	Terriers (various breeds)
5%	Cocker Spaniels
4%	Alaskan Malamute
4%	Boston terrier
4%	Shih Tzu
3%	Boxer
3%	Shetland Sheepdog
3%	English Springer Spaniel
3%	Australian Shepherd
15%	Other breeds (12 breeds)

*Note: Data are observational; significant breed predisposition not assessed.

| | TABLE 10-4 | CLINICAL MANIFESTATIONS OF CANINE HYPERADRENOCORTICISM* |

COMMON	LESS COMMON	UNCOMMON
Polyuria/polydipsia	Lethargy	Bruising
Polyphagia	Hyperpigmentation	Thromboemboli
Panting	Comedones	Ligament rupture
Abdominal distention	Pyoderma	Facial nerve palsy
Endocrine alopecia	Thin skin	Calcinosis cutis
Hepatomegaly	Poor hair regrowth	Pseudomyotonia
Muscle weakness	Urine dribbling	Testicular atrophy
Muscle wasting	Insulin-resistant diabetes mellitus	Persistent anestrus
Systemic hypertension		

Modified from Behrend EN, et al.: Diagnosis of spontaneous canine hyperadrenocorticism: 2012 ACVIM consensus statement (Small animal),*J Vet Int Med* 27:1292, 2013.
*Categorization of frequency is based on identification at the time of initial presentation.

et al, 2013). Accordingly, the current prevalence of clinical signs is likely less than published and not known.

Items of Importance *Not* in the History

Canine HAC is likely overdiagnosed due to the multitude of clinical signs and occurrence of false-positive results on screening tests. The primary indication for pursuing a diagnosis of HAC is the presence of one or more of the common clinical signs and physical examination findings (Behrend et al, 2013). Conversely, presence of clinical signs not associated with HAC is a reason to not pursue testing. Vomiting, diarrhea, coughing, sneezing, pain, or bleeding is not caused by HAC. Poor appetite and seizures are uncommon and, if related to HAC, are due to the presence of a pituitary macroadenoma.

General Review

Adult-Onset Hyperadrenocorticism

The clinical signs can be subtle or dramatic but usually progress slowly. Uncommonly, clinical signs may be intermittent with periods of remission (Peterson et al, 1982b). Not all dogs with HAC develop the same signs. Common signs include polydipsia, polyuria, polyphagia, abdominal enlargement, alopecia, panting, and muscle weakness (Table 10-4). Cutaneous changes may be the only clinical signs (Zur and White, 2011), so the presence of the common cutaneous manifestations of HAC, such as non-pruritic truncal alopecia and/or thin skin, without systemic signs warrants screening for the disease. The duration of clinical signs and the type of signs are similar between PDH and AT.

Hyperadrenocorticism in Young Dogs. Rarely, HAC has been diagnosed in dogs younger than 5 years of age (Figs. 10-7 and 10-8). Growth retardation was noted along with the typical clinical signs.

Polyuria and Polydipsia

Polyuria and polydipsia are extremely common signs associated with HAC. Polyuria may cause a loss of housebreaking or a need to urinate during the night. Polydipsia and polyuria previously

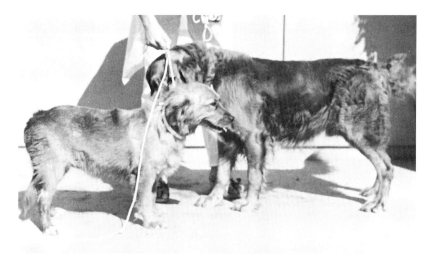

FIGURE 10-7 A 1-year-old dog with pituitary-dependent hyper-adrenocorticism (PDH) *(left)* and a normal adult. Note the short stature and immature hair coat in the young dog.

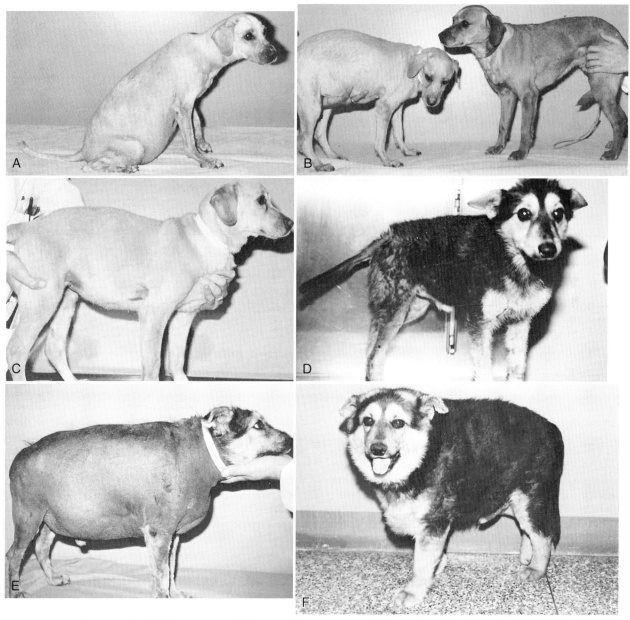

FIGURE 10-8 **A,** Mixed-breed 18-month-old dog with hyperadrenocorticism (HAC). **B,** Same dog *(left)* and a normal littermate. **C,** Same dog as in **A** 5 months after initiation of mitotane therapy. **D,** A 6-month-old German Shepherd dog with HAC. **E,** Same dog as in **D** after 4 years without therapy. **F,** Same dog as in **D** and **E** 4 months after initiation of therapy with mitotane.

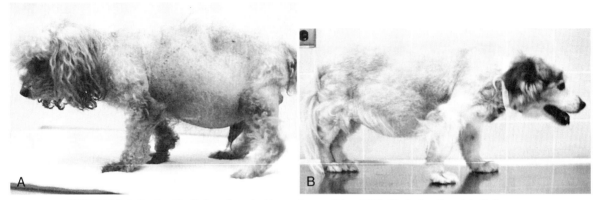

FIGURE 10-9 A, Poodle with pituitary-dependent hyperadrenocorticism (PDH), illustrating the pot-bellied appearance and diffuse alopecia sparing the head and distal extremities. **B,** A dog with PDH illustrating the pot-bellied appearance. The dog's hair was clipped 1 year previously; note the lack of regrowth.

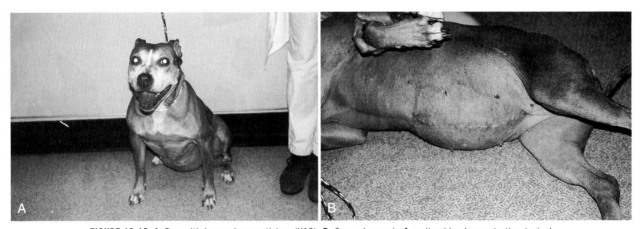

FIGURE 10-10 A, Dog with hyperadrenocorticism (HAC). **B,** Same dog as in **A** on its side, demonstrating typical pot-belly appearance.

has been documented in approximately 80% to 85% of dogs with HAC (Ling et al, 1979; Peterson, 1984). Owners often report the water intake to be two to 10 times normal.

The cause of the polyuria remains obscure. In dogs with HAC either due to PDH (*n* = 9) or AT (*n* = 6), the sensitivity and threshold of the osmoregulation of vasopressin secretion was abnormal in most (Biewenga et al, 1991). Direct effects of glucocorticoids on renal responsiveness to vasopressin may also exist (Biewenga et al, 1991) but are unproven. Although atrial natriuretic peptide concentrations are increased in the serum of humans with HAC (Yamaji et al, 1988) and could cause polyuria, it does not play a role in canine HAC (Vollmar et al, 1991). Direct compression of the posterior pituitary gland by an anterior pituitary tumor or compression of the hypothalamus or hypothalamic stalk can rarely cause concurrent diabetes insipidus (Ferguson and Biery, 1988; Goossens et al, 1995).

Appetite

Polyphagia may be troublesome, because affected dogs may resort to stealing food, eating garbage, begging continuously, and occasionally aggressively attacking or protecting food. It is assumed to be a direct effect of glucocorticoids, which is a unique effect in dogs. Polyphagia does not occur with cortisol excess in humans or cats.

Poor appetite can occur uncommonly in dogs with HAC. The most common reasons are the presence of a concurrent illness or

the dog could have a pituitary macroadenoma compressing adjacent structures and elevating cerebrospinal fluid pressure.

Abdominal Enlargement

The "potbellied" or pendulous abdominal profile is a classic clinical sign present in the majority of dogs with HAC (Figs. 10-9 and 10-10). It is believed to be the cumulative result of hepatomegaly filling out the cranial abdominal silhouette caudal to the rib cage, decreased strength of the abdominal muscles, fat accumulation within the abdomen, and, at times, an enlarged bladder due to polydipsia expanding the caudal abdomen.

Hepatomegaly is due to glycogen deposition (i.e., "steroid hepatopathy"). Muscle wasting is a direct result of protein catabolism due to excess cortisol. The mechanism responsible for fat redistribution is not understood.

Muscle Weakness and Lethargy

Dogs with HAC are usually capable of rising from a prone position and of going for short walks; however, exercise tolerance is often reduced. Muscle weakness may be demonstrated by an inability to climb stairs or to jump onto furniture or into a car. Owners may believe the problem is age-related. Muscle weakness is at least partly

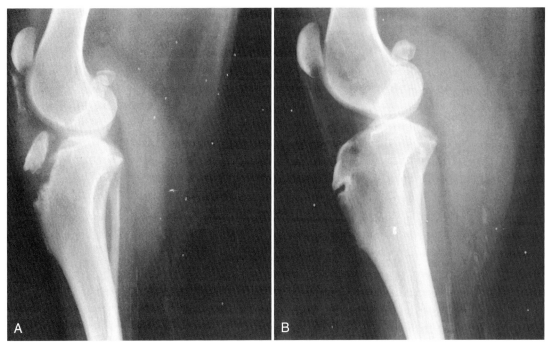

FIGURE 10-11 Radiographs of fracture of the tibial crest **(A)** in an 18-month-old dog with hyperadrenocorticism (HAC; see Fig. 10-10) with partially closed epiphyses. HAC delays epiphyseal closure in young dogs; note this dog's opposite stifle demonstrates delayed closure but no fracture **(B)**.

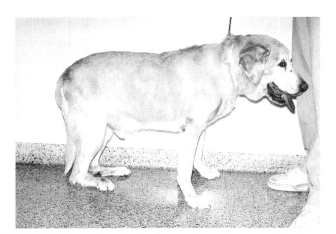

FIGURE 10-12 Dog with ruptured gastrocnemius muscles, a condition that may have occurred secondary to concurrent hyperadrenocorticism (HAC).

the result of muscle wasting caused by protein catabolism. Lethargy is probably an expression of muscle weakness and wasting.

Infrequently, affected dogs may not be capable of rising and may have difficulty standing for any length of time. A stress fracture across a tibial crest epiphysis, which had failed to close at a normal age, occurred in a juvenile dog with HAC (Fig. 10-11). Atraumatic rupture of both gastrocnemius muscles (Fig. 10-12) may have occurred in one dog secondary to spontaneous HAC; unilateral rupture has occurred secondary to glucocorticoid administration and iatrogenic HAC (Rewerts et al, 1997).

Cutaneous Markers

Cases seen by dermatologists may have a different constellation of findings than those seen by others. Cutaneous manifestations can occur without systemic signs (Zur and White, 2011). One report by dermatologists described cutaneous signs in 100% of 60 dogs with

HAC: 80% had some form of alopecia; 57% had pyoderma; 43% had hyperpigmentation; 25% were pruritic owing to seborrhea, calcinosis cutis, demodicosis, or pyoderma; 12% had thin skin; 5% had comedones; and 2% had calcinosis cutis (White et al, 1989). A recent study, although small, documented similar incidences of the common dermatologic signs (i.e., pyoderma, thin skin, hyperpigmentation, and comedones). Interestingly, although pruritus is not expected in dogs with HAC due to the anti-inflammatory effects of cortisol, it was a major clinical sign in four of 10 dogs (Zur and White, 2011). Conversely, some dogs with HAC have no apparent dermatologic signs (Peterson, 1984; Reusch and Feldman, 1991).

Alopecia and Pruritus

The hair loss associated with HAC is a common owner concern. It is slowly progressive and may begin at points of wear (e.g., bony prominences), eventually involving the flanks, perineum, and abdomen. Atrophy of hair follicles and the pilosebaceous apparatus with keratin accumulation in atrophic hair follicles is common; the follicular atrophy disrupts attachment of the hair shaft to the follicle, causing hair loss. Alopecia can be mild to severe (Figs. 10-13 and 10-14) with only the head and distal extremities retaining a coat.

Failure to Regrow Shaved Hair

If a dog with HAC is shaved, hair regrowth is poor or nonexistent (see Figs. 10-9, *B*, and 10-15), and any new hair is typically abnormal (e.g., brittle, sparse, or fine) (see Fig. 10-15). In the author's experience, poor hair regrowth after clipping is uncommonly due to HAC; if it is, other clinical signs of HAC are present. If poor hair regrowth is the only clinical sign, it is more likely due to "post clipping alopecia," which is an idiopathic syndrome in which hair can take up to 12 months to regrow and is normal in appearance (Rhodes and Beale, 2002).

Thin Skin, Pyoderma, Seborrhea, and Demodicosis

Thin skin, poor healing (Fig. 10-16), and pyoderma can occur in dogs with canine HAC. Piloglandular and epidermal atrophy

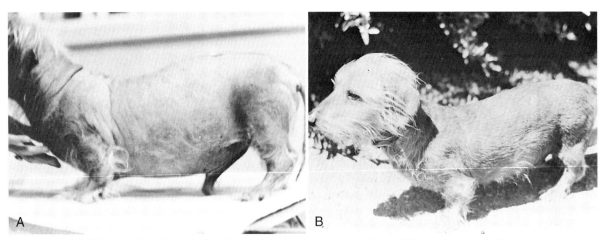

FIGURE 10-13 A, Dachshund with pituitary-dependent hyperadrenocorticism (PDH) showing severe, bilaterally symmetric alopecia. **B,** Same dog as in **A** 20 months after beginning therapy with mitotane.

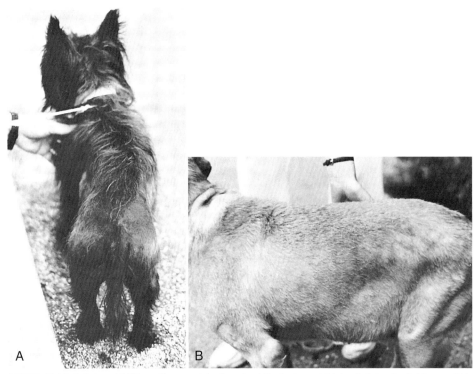

FIGURE 10-14 A, A dog with bilaterally symmetric alopecia of the flanks and thighs. **B,** Labrador Retriever, which had hyperadrenocorticism (HAC) caused by a functioning adrenal tumor, with alopecia and a poor hair coat secondary to HAC as well as a potbelly.

occur in 30% to 40% of dogs with HAC (White et al, 1989), which is likely due to the anti-proliferative effects of glucocorticoids on fibroblasts, with inhibition of collagen and mucopolysaccharide synthesis. Synthesis of collagen types I and III is decreased with topical glucocorticoid therapy in people (Valencia and Kerdel, 2012) and likely with HAC in dogs. In some dogs, the subcutaneous blood vessels are easily visualized. In addition, keratin-plugged follicles (comedones) can be found on the trunk, especially around the nipples and along the dorsal midline. Pyoderma is common, likely due to multiple local cutaneous changes as well as immunosuppression from excess cortisol, and may be poorly responsive to therapy (Zur and White, 2011). Adult-onset demodicosis has

been associated with naturally occurring HAC in approximately 10% of cases (White et al, 1989; Zur and White, 2011).

Bruising, Reduced Subcutaneous Fat, and Striae

The fragility observed with thin skin is also present in the blood vessels. Excessive bruising can follow venipuncture (Fig. 10-17) or other minor trauma. Rarely, bruising occurs secondary to the presence of metal staples in a surgical scar from years before (Fig. 10-18, *A* and *B*). Atrophy of subcutaneous tissue may predispose to bruising as well. Wounds heal more slowly, potentially with fragile, thin scar tissue (see Fig. 10-18, *C*). Healing skin lesions may undergo dehiscence because of the limited amount of fibrous tissue.

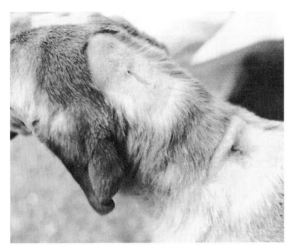

FIGURE 10-15 Close-up of the dog in Fig. 10-14, *B*. The areas shown had been shaved 8 months earlier prior to removal of small skin tumors. Note the failure of the hair to grow back, as well as the obvious surgical scars, which are the result of poor wound healing.

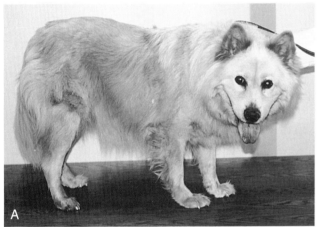

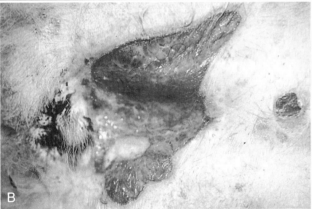

FIGURE 10-16 A, An 8-year-old mixed-breed dog that had been treated chronically with glucocorticoids. **B,** Open wounds on the ventral abdomen that were not healing, likely due to the effects of chronic glucocorticoid therapy.

Calcinosis Cutis and Cutaneous Metaplastic Ossification

Although previously stated to be pathognomonic of spontaneous or iatrogenic HAC, calcinosis cutis has also been reported as a consequence of fungal infection, treatment of hypoparathyroidism and renal failure, or as idiopathic. In general, large breed dogs

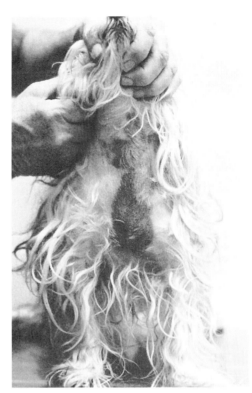

FIGURE 10-17 A dog with hyperadrenocorticism (HAC) that had two blood samples obtained from the jugular vein. The bruising was obvious 2 hours later.

appear to be predisposed. In one study, Rottweilers, Rottweiler/ Labrador retriever mixed breeds, Staffordshire Terriers, Boxers, Boxer mixed breeds, Akitas, and Pomeranians were significantly overrepresented, but the number of dogs in each breed was low (Doerr et al, 2013).

Calcinosis cutis is uncommon in dogs with HAC (White et al, 1989) but characteristic if it occurs. The pathophysiology is not known. On histopathology, calcinosis cutis is characterized by dermal, diffuse or multinodular, dystrophic calcium deposition. Subcutaneous involvement and osseous metaplasia may occur. Fibrosis and inflammation, mainly with histiocytes and lymphocytes, can be seen as well as other changes of HAC, such as epidermal atrophy (Doerr et al, 2013). Abnormal collagen fibrils due to the effects of glucocorticoids on collagen synthesis may attract ion deposition (Doerr et al, 2013), and secondary hyperparathyroidism may play a role (Ramsey et al, 2005). Affected dogs have firm, palpable erythematous papules to well-demarcated plaques that may feel mineralized. The most common location is the dorsum, followed by the head and inguinal area; other truncal locations may also be involved (Fig. 10-19), and the extremities are involved less frequently (Doerr et al, 2013). Calcinosis cutis does not always resolve with successful treatment of HAC.

Obesity

Owners of dogs with HAC usually comment on their pet's apparent weight gain. To the contrary, dogs with HAC do not usually gain a large amount of weight. Rather, most have fat redistribution and a potbellied appearance, which can be mistaken for weight gain. In dogs and humans, truncal obesity appears to occur at the expense of muscle and fat wasting from the extremities and subcutaneous stores.

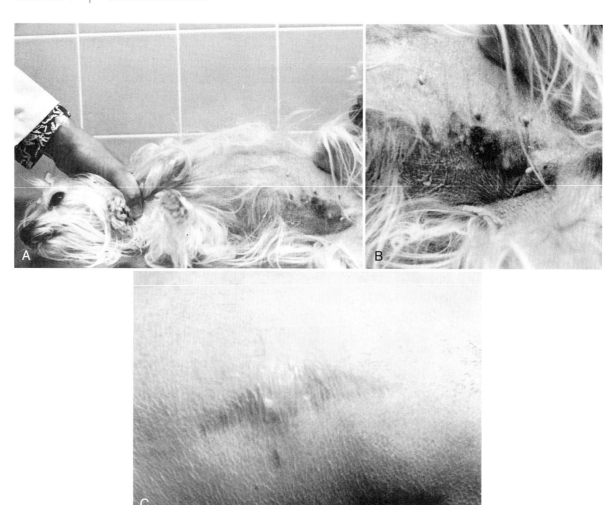

FIGURE 10-18 **A,** Bruising in the area of an ovariohysterectomy performed 8½ years earlier. **B,** Close-up of the bruising shown in **A** caused by metal sutures and a decrease in subcutaneous fat that normally "padded" the sutures. **C,** Thin, fragile, healed incision, typical of the poor healing in a dog with hyperadrenocorticism (HAC).

Respiratory Signs

Panting

Panting is common in dogs with HAC; dyspnea is possible due to thromboembolism (see later) but uncommon. Coughing is not associated with HAC.

Several possible reasons exist for panting. First, as with other muscles in the body, the respiratory muscles may be weak. Second, the increased pressure placed on the diaphragm from abdominal fat accumulation and hepatomegaly can accentuate disturbances in ventilatory mechanics. Third, pulmonary interstitial and bronchial mineralization can be present, leading to decreased lung compliance (Berry et al, 1994; 2000; Schwarz et al, 2000). Even if present, mineralization may not always be visible on plain radiographs. Last, minor pulmonary thromboemboli may cause panting or tachypnea. Any or all factors may be present in dogs with HAC. In one study, 33% of dogs with PDH were hypoxemic, and no thromboemboli were present (Berry et al, 2000). Concurrent disease (e.g., collapsing trachea) may exacerbate the respiratory issues of HAC.

Thromboembolism

Thromboembolism is a recognized problem in dogs with HAC (Keyes et al, 1993; Teshima et al, 2008; Sobel and Williams, 2009). Dogs with pulmonary thromboembolism (PTE) may have chronic, mild signs or may develop acute, severe respiratory distress.

Pneumothorax secondary to PTE has been reported (Sobel and Williams, 2009). The pathogenesis is described in more detail later (see Pulmonary Thromboembolism).

Reproductive Abnormalities

Owner concerns related to the reproductive tract in dogs with HAC are unusual, because most affected dogs are old, neutered, or both. No information exists in the literature regarding reproductive function specifically in dogs with HAC, nor sex hormone concentrations in female dogs with HAC or receiving exogenous glucocorticoids. Prednisone administration decreases basal testosterone concentrations in dogs (Kemppainen et al, 1983). Although decreased testosterone would be expected to lead to increased concentrations of LH from lack of negative feedback, in dogs with PDH, basal LH concentrations are not different from controls and, in fact, secretion was hyperresponsive to administration of gonadotropin-releasing hormone (GnRH). Thus, hypercortisolemia may affect LH secretion directly (Meij et al, 1997c).

Myotonia (Pseudomyotonia)

Quite rarely, dogs with HAC develop a distinct myopathy characterized by persistent, active muscle contraction after cessation of voluntary effort (Braund et al, 1980; Swinney et al, 1998; Cisneros

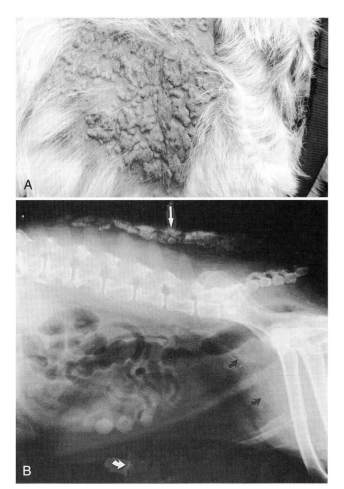

FIGURE 10-19 **A,** A 10-year-old female spayed Labrador Retriever with calcinosis cutis. Note the multifocal to coalescing, raised masses on the lateral aspect of the neck; the masses were palpably firm. Diffuse to patchy alopecia was present in the affected areas. **B,** Radiograph showing dorsal midline *(straight arrow)* and preputial *(curved white arrow)* calcinosis cutis, as well as calcified femoral arteries *(curved black arrows)*. (**A,** Photograph courtesy of Dr. Robert Kennis. In Rand J, editor: *Clinical endocrinology of companion animals,* Ames, IA, 2013, Wiley-Blackwell, p. 47.)

et al, 2011). Affected dogs develop a stilted gait, especially in the pelvic limbs, stiffness of the limbs, and enlarged muscles in the proximal limbs coincident with onset of other clinical signs of HAC (Cisneros et al, 2011). Inability to ambulate is possible (Fig. 10-20). Myotonic, bizarre, high-frequency discharges are noted on electromyography (Braund et al, 1980). Clinical response to resolution of HAC is not predictable (Swinney et al, 1998).

Myopathic changes in dogs with HAC-associated myotonia include fiber size variation, focal necrosis, internal nuclei, fiber splitting, subsarcolemmal aggregates, and fatty infiltration. Type 2 muscle fibers are preferentially involved. Mitochondrial changes are the most prominent ultrastructural feature. Evidence of demyelination suggests a chronic neuropathy may be present and underlie at least some of the muscular changes (Braund et al, 1980). However, histopathology may also be relatively unremarkable (Cisneros et al, 2011).

Facial Paralysis

Anecdotally, dogs with HAC are believed to rarely develop unilateral or bilateral facial nerve paralysis. An association has never been proven.

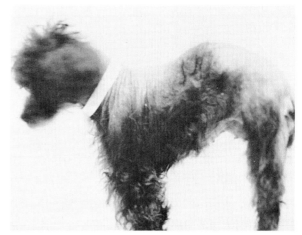

FIGURE 10-20 An 11-year-old dog with hyperadrenocorticism (HAC) and myotonia, resulting in extreme rigidity of the pelvic limbs and inability to walk.

PHYSICAL EXAMINATION

General Review

Common abnormalities include abdominal enlargement, panting, truncal obesity, bilaterally symmetric alopecia, hyperpigmentation, skin infections, comedones, and hepatomegaly (see Table 10-4). Remarkable variation exists in the number and severity of physical findings between patients.

Hyperpigmentation

Cutaneous hyperpigmentation may be diffuse or focal (see Fig. 10-8, *E*). Histologically, increased numbers of melanocytes are found in the stratum corneum, basal epidermis, and dermal tissues. The pathophysiology is not understood. Secretion of α-MSH from the pituitary may contribute to hyperpigmentation in dogs with PDH. However, as hyperpigmentation occurs as well in dogs with ATs, pituitary secretion is not the only cause.

Hepatomegaly

An enlarged liver, a classic sign with canine HAC, contributes to abdominal enlargement by filling out the cranial abdominal silhouette behind the rib cage. Hepatomegaly is easily palpated due to the weak abdominal muscles. If a dog thought to have HAC does not have hepatomegaly or if the liver is small, another condition or a serious concurrent disease should be suspected.

Grossly, the liver is typically large, pale, and friable. Histologic changes in dogs with naturally occurring HAC or exposure to exogenous glucocorticoid are the same and were previously referred to as *vacuolar hepatopathy* or *steroid hepatopathy.* The changes include increased hepatocyte size and centrilobular hepatocytic vacuolation with a few, often single, large vacuoles that displace the cell nucleus to the periphery. Glycogen accumulation is concentrated in periportal hepatocytes. Lipid deposits are not demonstrable with Sudan III stains. Hepatocellular necrosis, although present, is not a significant feature (Badylak and Van Vleet, 1981).

The term *vacuolar hepatopathy* is now recognized as a misnomer; the hepatic changes are not specific for HAC or glucocorticoid exposure. Of 336 dogs with vacuolar hepatopathy, only 55% were classified as having been exposed to glucocorticoids (Sepesy et al, 2006), and neoplasia and congenital or acquired hepatobiliary disease were common. The vacuolization was accompanied by elevated alkaline phosphatase (ALP) activity as well; the enzyme activity and vacuolar hepatopathy may be a marker of an illness-invoked physiologic stress.

Gonadal and Sex Hormone–Related Alterations

Due to low testosterone concentrations (see earlier), male dogs with HAC could have bilaterally small, soft, spongy testicles, and decreased libido. In females, in theory, decreased LH could suppress normal ovarian function and lead to prolonged anestrus (Meij et al, 1997c). Although dogs with PDH have hyperprolactinemia (Meij et al, 1997a; 1997c) independent of excesses in plasma cortisol, mammary development has not been reported in dogs with HAC.

In one case report, adrenal hypersecretion of androgens in a spayed female with HAC was hypothesized to have led to the development of recurrent perianal adenomas. However, the measured serum testosterone concentration was variable and did not correlate with development of the adenomas (Dow et al, 1988). Thus, no documentation exists of an adrenal source of androgens causing pathologic virilization in dogs (Johnson, 2013)

Ectopic Calcification

In addition to HAC causing calcinosis cutis, ectopic calcification may also involve the tracheal rings and bronchial walls, the kidneys, and (rarely) the major arteries and veins (see Fig. 10-19, *B*) (Berry et al, 2000; Schwarz et al, 2000). Because approximately 90% of dogs with HAC have elevated parathyroid hormone concentrations, soft tissue calcification has been speculated to be due, at least in part, to secondary hyperparathyroidism (Ramsey et al, 2005). Ectopic calcification may be noted only histologically in some dogs. Calcific band keratopathy, a syndrome characterized by a grey-white superficial corneal opacity horizontally oriented in the interpalpebral opening, was reported in two dogs with HAC (Ward et al, 1989).

Bruisability

Easy bruisability is common in people with HAC. It is not frequently observed in dogs, but it may be noted after venipuncture or trauma (see Figs. 10-17 and 10-18). Bruisability is likely due to cortisol-induced inhibition of collagen synthesis, leading to weaker blood vessel walls.

Sudden Acquired Retinal Degeneration Syndrome

Sudden acquired retinal degeneration syndrome (SARDS) is an idiopathic retinal disorder that produces sudden, permanent blindness in adult dogs. The syndrome is characterized by non-inflammatory degeneration and loss of retinal photoreceptors. An association has been suggested between SARDS and HAC because dogs with SARDS can have clinical signs suggestive of HAC (e.g., polyuria, polydipsia, polyphagia and weight gain) (van der Woerdt et al, 1991; Mattson et al, 1992; Montgomery et al, 2008; Stuckey et al, 2013). However, not all dogs with SARDS have signs consistent with HAC; indeed in one study only 33% of dogs with SARDS had systemic signs (Montgomery et al, 2008). Dogs with SARDS have had positive tests for HAC, but in others, negative or conflicting results were obtained (van der Woerdt et al, 1991; Mattson et al, 1992; Stuckey et al, 2013). The chance of a false-positive test result on a screening test for HAC due to the stress of acute blindness must be considered. Furthermore, the clinical signs suggestive of HAC, with the exception of polyphagia, typically resolve with time in dogs with SARDS (Mattson et al, 1992; Stuckey et al, 2013); no study has performed follow-up testing for HAC at 4 to 6 months after the initial diagnosis of SARDS. Thus, a link between SARDS and HAC is quite unsubstantiated.

Blindness

Blindness occurs rarely in dogs with PDH secondary to compression of the optic chiasm by a pituitary macroadenoma (Seruca et al, 2010). Blindness has also been reported in dogs with no optic chiasm compression, possibly due to changes in ophthalmic blood flow, interleukin-6, insulin, nitric oxide, triglycerides, and adiponectin (Cabrera Blatter et al, 2012a; 2012b). However, the proportion of blind dogs with HAC in the two studies by Cabrera Blatter and colleagues is much higher than reported elsewhere (14% and 43%), and the possibility exists that many dogs had SARDS and not HAC.

Acute Weakness Due to Non-Traumatic Rupture of an Adrenal Mass

Non-traumatic rupture of an AT is rare. In five dogs in which this occurred, severe lethargy, weakness, and pale mucous membranes developed acutely. Abdominal pain was detected on the physical examination. Each dog had acute intraabdominal or retroperitoneal hemorrhage, required immediate supportive therapy, and had emergency exploratory abdominal surgery (Vandenbergh et al, 1992; Whittemore et al, 2001). Both adenocarcinomas and adenomas have ruptured. Although this scenario is rare, it is one of the few situations (along with PTE) in which a dog with HAC may develop an acute, life-threatening illness.

Central Nervous System Signs

Central nervous system (CNS) signs can occur in dogs with PDH. Occasionally the CNS signs are present at the time of diagnosis of PDH; alternatively, small tumors can grow after diagnosis, and CNS signs develop within weeks to years (Nelson et al, 1989; Bertoy et al, 1996). Due to boney confines, pituitary masses expand dorsally and may compress or invade the hypothalamus and other suprasellar structures, may invaginate the pituitary stalk that connects the pituitary with the hypothalamus, or may dilate the infundibular recess and third ventricle. In addition, the second, third, and fourth cranial nerves may be affected (Capen, 2007).

When neurologic signs are first recognized in dogs with PDH, they can be nonspecific and subtle. Common initial signs include being dull, listlessness, and inappetence; they may progress to anorexia, restlessness, loss of interest in normal household activities, delayed response to stimuli, disorientation, and stupor. Other CNS signs reported in dogs with macrotumors include circling, pacing, head pressing, ataxia, behavioral alterations (i.e., aggression), blindness, adipsia, and seizures (Fig. 10-21 and Box 10-1; Nelson et al, 1989; Kipperman et al, 1992). A caveat exists, however, that neurologic signs can occur for other reasons in dogs with PDH (Wood et al, 2007). Thus, those reported in dogs with PDH may not have been due to the pituitary tumor itself. With severe hypothalamic compression, dysfunction of the autonomic nervous system develops rarely; clinical signs include adipsia, loss of temperature regulation, erratic heart rate, and stupor. These are considered terminal signs.

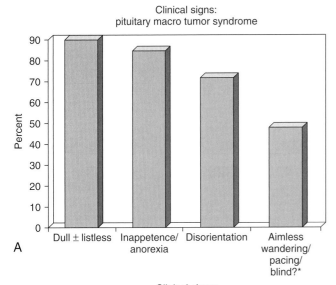

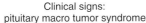

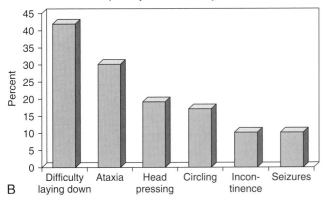

FIGURE 10-21 Bar graphs (**A** and **B**) illustrating the most common clinical signs observed in dogs with pituitary macroadenoma syndrome causing central nervous system (CNS) signs (note the difference in the vertical scale of the two graphs). *Note that it can be difficult in some cases to determine if a dog is truly blind or severely disoriented.

Predicting which pituitary tumor will grow is impossible. Although one study suggested macroadenomas (i.e., tumor >10 mm in height) were more likely in dogs weighing more than 20 kg (Duesberg et al, 1995), other studies found no relationship with weight (Nelson et al, 1989; Bertoy et al, 1995; Wood et al, 2007). In 21 dogs with PDH that did not have CNS signs at the time of diagnosis of HAC, 11 (52%) had a visible masses on MRI that ranged from 4 to 12 mm in height (Bertoy et al, 1995). Thirteen of the 21 dogs with PDH were followed over 1 year; five of the 13 had no mass visible originally, whereas eight dogs did. Over the year, six of the 13 dogs (46%) had tumor growth; two of the six did not have a visible mass on the initial MRI. In four dogs, a tumor was initially seen, and it increased in size over the year; two of the four dogs developed a macroadenoma with tumor height of 11 and 14 mm and had CNS signs (Bertoy et al, 1996).

Predicting which dogs will develop neurological signs is also impossible. Dogs can have neurological signs with tumors less than 10 mm diameter; conversely, dogs with a macroadenoma might not have detectable neurologic abnormalities (Nelson et al, 1989; Kipperman et al, 1992; Wood et al, 2007). No apparent relationship was detected in one study between the presence of a pituitary tumor regardless of size and the development of

BOX 10-1 Clinical Signs Caused by an Enlarging Pituitary Tumor in Dogs with Hyperadrenocorticism

Dullness, listlessness
Inappetence (poor appetite)/anorexia (no appetite)
Restlessness
Loss of interest in normal activities
Delayed response to various stimuli
Disorientation/aimless pacing
Altered mentation
Obtundation
Stupor
Ataxia
Circling
Head pressing
Behavior changes
Blindness
Seizures
Coma
Adipsia
Loss of temperature regulation

neurologic signs. In dogs with PDH, 71% of 84 dogs without neurologic abnormalities and 66% of 73 dogs with neurologic abnormalities had a pituitary macrotumor (Wood et al, 2007).

The diagnosis of a macroadenoma depends on imaging via CT or MRI. The possibility that the CNS abnormalities are an adverse effect of mitotane, if that is being administered, or due to a concurrent illness must be eliminated.

ROUTINE BLOOD AND URINE EVALUATION

General Approach

Any dog suspected of having HAC should be thoroughly evaluated before specific endocrine testing is done. Each dog should have a complete blood count (CBC), urinalysis with culture, and a complete serum chemistry profile performed. In addition, abdominal ultrasonography (preferred over radiography) should be considered. The initial results not only help ensure the correct diagnosis is being pursued; they also might identify concomitant medical problems.

Certain clinicopathologic changes are consistent with a diagnosis of HAC (Table 10-5), but none is pathognomonic. Laboratory test results must always be interpreted within the context of the history and physical examination. An absence of common clinical signs should strongly decrease the suspicion of HAC, and perhaps even stop pursuit of such a diagnosis. If consistent history and clinical signs are present, the greater the number of suggestive clinicopathologic abnormalities documented, the stronger the suspicion of HAC. Failure to identify clinicopathologic abnormalities should not, by itself, rule out HAC (Behrend et al, 2013).

Complete Blood Count

Neutrophilia and monocytosis are common due to steroid-enhanced capillary demargination of these cells and prevention of normal cellular egress from the circulation. Lymphopenia is most likely the result of steroid-induced lympholysis, and eosinopenia results from bone marrow sequestration of eosinophils. The constellation of changes

TABLE 10-5	HEMATOLOGIC, SERUM BIOCHEMICAL, URINE, AND RADIOGRAPHIC ABNORMALITIES THAT OCCUR WITH HYPERADRENOCORTICISM
TEST	**ABNORMALITY**
Complete blood count (CBC)	• Mature leukocytosis • Neutrophilia • Lymphopenia • Eosinopenia • Erythrocytosis; mild
Serum chemistries	• Increased alkaline phosphatase (ALP; sometimes extremely elevated) • Increased alanine aminotransferase (ALT) (usually mild) • Hypercholesterolemia • Hypertriglyceridemia • Hyperglycemia • Increased bile acids • Decreased blood urea nitrogen (BUN)
Urinalysis	• Urine specific gravity less than 1.015, often less than 1.008 • Proteinuria
Radiography/ultra sonography	• Hepatomegaly • Excellent abdominal contrast • Osteoporosis • Calcinosis cutis/dystrophic calcification • Adrenal calcification (usually adrenal tumor) • Pulmonary thromboembolism (PTE) (rare) • Calcified trachea and main stem bronchi • Pulmonary metastasis of adrenal carcinoma
Blood pressure	• Hypertension
Thyroid testing	• Low thyroxine (T_4) concentrations • Triiodothyronine (T_3) concentrations

in the white blood cell differential (i.e., overall leukocytosis with neutrophilia, monocytosis, eosinopenia, and lymphopenia) is called a "stress leukogram" and is common in dogs with HAC. A mild polycythemia can also occur. Approximately 75% to 80% of dogs with HAC have an increased platelet count (Pace et al, 2013; Rose et al, 2013). The significance of the thrombocytosis is unknown.

Serum Biochemical Profile

Alkaline Phosphatase

ALPs are a group of enzymes that catalyze the hydrolysis of phosphate esters. Their main source is the liver, with bone ALP contributing smaller amounts to the circulation; both forms have serum half-lives of approximately 3 days. Intestinal, placental, and renal ALPs are not detectable in serum, because their half-lives are only minutes.

A uniquely canine corticosteroid-induced alkaline phosphatase (CIALP) also can be measured in serum. The source is the bile canalicular membrane of hepatocytes (Sanecki et al, 1987). Exposure to exogenous and endogenous glucocorticoids increases synthesis of CIALP as well as other enzymes in the liver (liver ALP isoenzymes), kidneys, and intestines (Sanecki et al, 1987; Solter et al, 1993; Wiedmeyer et al, 2002a; 2002b).

Increased ALP activity is the most common routine abnormality on a serum biochemistry profile in dogs with HAC. Older literature

documented the presence of an elevated ALP activity in greater than 80% to 90% of dogs with HAC (Ling et al, 1979; Teske et al, 1989). Previously, approximately 15% of board-certified internists and dermatologists would not pursue a diagnosis of HAC if ALP activity was in the reference range (Behrend et al, 2002); however, given that dogs with HAC are likely currently diagnosed earlier in the course of disease, the percentage of dogs with HAC with an increased ALP activity may be lower. Thus, using an ALP activity within the reference range as a means to rule out HAC may not be a wise practice.

Alanine Aminotransferase

Alanine aminotransferase (ALT) activity is commonly increased in HAC, but the elevation is usually mild (i.e., < 400 IU/L). Elevations in serum ALP activity are relatively greater than that of ALT. Increases in ALT are not believed to be due to increased gene expression (Hadley et al, 1990) but secondary to damage caused by swollen hepatocytes, glycogen accumulation, or interference with hepatic blood flow.

Cholesterol and Triglycerides

Glucocorticoid stimulation of lipolysis causes an increase in blood lipid and cholesterol concentrations. Ninety percent of dogs with HAC have hypercholesterolemia. Approximately 10% of dogs with HAC have serum cholesterol concentrations less than 250 mg/dL; 15% have concentrations of 250 to 300 mg/dL; and 75% have concentrations greater than 300 mg/dL (Fig. 10-22; Ortega et al, 1995). Hypertriglyceridemia is also common (see Fig. 10-22). Lipid distribution within particles can also be altered (e.g., the amount of cholesterol in very–low-density, low-density, and high-density lipoprotein fractions) (Jerico et al, 2009).

Blood Glucose and Serum Insulin

Glucocorticoids antagonize the effects of insulin, leading to increased hepatic gluconeogenesis and decreased peripheral glucose utilization. Thus, dogs with HAC can have mild hyperglycemia (Peterson et al, 1984a; 1986b; Elliott et al, 1997). Insulin concentrations can be elevated (Wolfsheimer and Peterson, 1991; Montgomery et al, 1996; Cho et al, 2014). Binding of erythrocyte insulin receptors is decreased in dogs with HAC, but it may be the cause or effect of hyperinsulinemia (Wolfsheimer and Peterson, 1991). A small percentage of dogs with HAC have overt diabetes mellitus.

Blood Urea Nitrogen

The polyuria of HAC leads to continual urinary loss of blood urea nitrogen (BUN). Thus, BUN can be below the reference range (Behrend et al, 2013).

Phosphate

Hypophosphatemia had been reported to occur in approximately one-third of dogs with HAC (Peterson, 1984), potentially from a glucocorticoid-induced increase in urinary phosphate excretion. More recently, however, hyperphosphatemia was noted in most dogs with HAC in one study (Ramsey et al, 2005). The reason for the difference is not apparent. The finding of hyperphosphatemia was unexpected and was possibly an artifactual elevation due to lipemia (Ramsey et al, 2005).

Bile Acids

Pre- and post-prandial bile acid concentrations may be mildly increased in up to 30% of dogs with HAC (Reusch, 2005). Parameters of liver function such as bile acid concentration or bromosulfophthalein (BSP) retention have been inconsistently affected

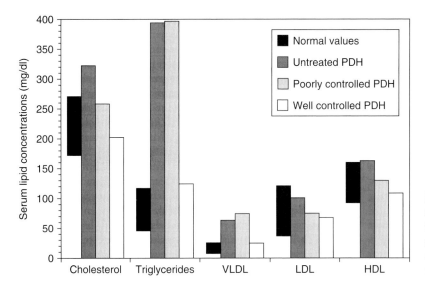

FIGURE 10-22 Serum cholesterol, triglyceride, and cholesterol content in very-low density lipoprotein (VLDL), low-density lipoprotein (LDL), and high-density lipoprotein (HDL) particles in normal dogs, dogs with untreated hyperadrenocorticism (HAC) and poorly controlled and well-controlled treated dogs with naturally occurring HAC.

by glucocorticoid administration (Badylak and Van Vleet, 1981; DeNovo and Prasee, 1983; Solter et al, 1994). Any change in liver function, however, is not considered to be clinically important.

Electrolytes

Although of little diagnostic or clinical significance, mild hypernatremia, hypochloremia, and hypokalemia can be seen in some dogs with HAC (Ling et al, 1979).

Amylase and Lipase

Pancreatitis is uncommon in dogs with HAC. Although a link between glucocorticoids and pancreatitis has previously been postulated, the concerns have largely been dismissed (see Chapter 14).

Urinalysis

Concentration

The most frequent urinalysis abnormality in dogs with HAC is dilute urine (specific gravity < 1.020). A large percentage of dogs with HAC have a specific gravity in a randomly obtained urine sample less than 1.015 (Smets et al, 2012). Owners of any dog suspected of having polyuria/polydipsia should obtain a urine sample by clean-catch prior to bringing their pet to the hospital. Hospitalization can alter drinking behavior, and a dog polyuric and polydipsic at home may drink less when hospitalized; dogs with HAC can concentrate their urine to some degree if water-deprived. It should also be noted that a single urine sample with a low specific gravity does not by itself prove the presence of polyuria/polydipsia.

Glucose

By itself, HAC should not cause glucosuria. The presence of glucose in the urine of a dog with HAC signifies the presence of another problem, most likely diabetes mellitus.

Proteinuria

Proteinuria occurs in more than half of dogs with HAC (Ortega et al, 1996; Hurley and Vaden, 1998; Lien et al, 2010; Smets et al, 2012); the exact percentage varies between studies and is not clearly stated in all of them. The proteinuria is typically mild to moderate (i.e., urine protein-to-creatinine ratio [UPCR] < 5). Hypoalbuminemia does not occur secondary to proteinuria due to HAC; thus, if hypoalbuminemia is present, another cause for proteinuria should be sought. In untreated dogs with HAC, median UPCR

was 0.70 (range, 0.03 to 4.2) in one study (Hurley and Vaden, 1998) and 1.66 in another (Smets et al, 2012). When comparing dogs with PDH and AT, the mean UPCR were 1.47 ± 1.69 and 2.74 ± 2.8, respectively (Ortega et al, 1996). The UPCR in dogs with ATs was significantly higher than that for dogs with PDH.

Microalbuminuria (urine albumin-to-creatinine ratio 0.03 to 0.3) and albuminuria (urine albumin-to-creatinine ratio > 0.3) were present in 38.6% and 48.5%, respectively, of dogs with HAC. Interestingly, the incidence of microalbuminuria was significantly higher in dogs with PDH versus ATs (52.5% versus 20%), whereas the incidence of albuminuria was significantly lower in dogs with PDH versus ATs (32.5% versus 70%) (Lien et al, 2010).

The etiology of the proteinuria is unclear. The underlying glomerular lesion is typically glomerulosclerosis (Ortega et al, 1996; Waters et al, 1997). In one study, the ACTH-stimulated cortisol concentration correlated with the UPCR (Ortega et al, 1996). Hypertension is common in dogs with HAC and could contribute. However, conflicting results have been obtained with regard to correlation between systemic blood pressure and degree of proteinuria (Ortega et al, 1996; Lien et al, 2010). Glucocorticoids may induce glomerular hypertension (Ortega et al, 1996).

Treatment of HAC typically improves the proteinuria, but it does not resolve in 20% to 40% (Ortega et al, 1996; Hurley and Vaden, 1998; Smets et al, 2012). After treatment and adequate cortisol suppression, the UPCR in five dogs with PDH remained high (1.2 to 6.5). In dogs in which the UPCR normalized, it required more than 4 to 12 weeks of control of the HAC (Hurley and Vaden, 1998). For 16 dogs with well-controlled PDH or four whose AT had been removed, the mean UPCR was 0.64 ± 0.98 and 1.1 ± 1.32.

Urinary Tract Infection

In two studies, approximately half the dogs with HAC had a urinary tract infection (UTI) at the time of initial examination. However, less than 5% had clinical signs of infection, and approximately 18% had pyuria and bacteriuria noted on urine sediment exam (Ling et al, 1979; Forrester et al, 1999). Whether the infection was in the lower or upper urinary tract (i.e., pyelonephritis) was not determined. Likely, increased urinary cortisol concentration suppresses inflammation and thus clinical signs. Therefore, a urine culture should be considered in the initial work-up of dogs with HAC. The bacteria isolated are common, and the sensitivities are typical of any UTI (Forrester et al, 1999). HAC may also cause persistent UTI or reinfection

(Seguin et al, 2003). The high incidence of UTI could be due to immunosuppression due to glucocorticoid excess. Also, dilute urine increases susceptibility to UTI (Lulich and Osborne, 1994). Whether dogs with HAC have a higher incidence of pyelonephritis is unknown.

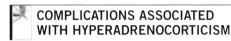

COMPLICATIONS ASSOCIATED WITH HYPERADRENOCORTICISM

Urinary Crystals and Calculi

Of 20 dogs with both HAC and urolithiasis, 16 had calcium-containing uroliths (13 with calcium oxalate and one each with calcium apatite, mixed calcium hydrogen phosphate, and dihydrate carbonate-apatite struvite), and four had struvite calculi. Dogs with HAC and urolithiasis were 10 times more likely to have calcium-containing stones than breed-matched controls with urolithiasis but not HAC (Hess et al, 1998). In humans, glucocorticoids increase urinary calcium excretion, which in turn may increase the risk of development of calcium-containing uroliths. The incidence of urinary calculi in dogs with HAC is unknown but seems to be quite low.

Hypertension

Moderate, sustained hypertension occurs in more than 90% of humans with HAC. Multiple factors have been implicated in its development, including excessive secretion of renin (the protein that acts to release angiotensin I), activation of the renin-angiotensin system via alternative stimulators, enhanced vascular sensitivity to pressors (e.g., catecholamines and adrenergic agonists), reduction of vasodilator prostaglandins, and increased secretion of non–zona glomerulosa mineralocorticoids (e.g., deoxycorticosterone) (Yamaji et al, 1988).

The reported incidence of hypertension in dogs with HAC is 31% to 86%. Comparison between studies is difficult because the methods of blood pressure measurement are not the same and the definition of hypertension varies slightly. Normal blood pressure can also vary between breeds (Bodey and Michell, 1996). The degree of hypertension is often mild to moderate, but reported mean systolic blood pressure ranges from approximately 160 mm Hg to 202 mm Hg (Ortega et al, 1996; Goy-Thollot et al, 2002; Lien et al, 2010; Smets et al, 2012; Arenas et al, 2014). In one study, mean blood pressure was higher in dogs with ATs (164.1 ± 36.7 mm Hg) versus dogs with PDH (142.2 ± 24.9) (Lien et al, 2010), but no difference was found in another (Ortega et al, 1996).

The etiology of the hypertension is unknown and likely multifactorial. Aldosterone concentrations are decreased in dogs with PDH (Golden and Lothrop, 1988; Goy-Thollot et al, 2002). Hypercortisolemia could contribute to hypertension because pressor sensitivity to norepinephrine infusion is increased in dogs with iatrogenic HAC (Martinez et al, 2005). Hypertension typically improves with control of HAC but does not resolve in all dogs (Ortega et al, 1996; Goy-Thollot et al, 2002; Smets et al, 2012), potentially suggesting that HAC causes chronic, irreversible changes in some patients.

Hypertension raises concern because of its sequelae such as left ventricular hypertrophy and renal damage and potential to exacerbate congestive heart failure if present due to cardiac disease. Blood pressure should be measured in dogs diagnosed with HAC especially because severe hypertension may occur. If the hypertension is mild (e.g., < 180 mm Hg systolic), therapy for HAC can be initiated and the blood pressure reevaluated after control is obtained; antihypertensive therapy can then be

initiated if needed. If systolic blood pressure is more than 180 mm Hg, which means the risk of target organ damage is considered to be high, antihypertensive therapy should be considered; once the HAC is controlled, the need for anti-hypertension medications should be reevaluated.

Hypothyroidism

Clinical signs and routine laboratory changes associated with hypothyroidism and HAC can overlap (e.g., lethargy, hypercholesterolemia, and bilaterally symmetric, non-pruritic alopecia). (It should be noted that polyuria/polydipsia is not a sign of hypothyroidism.) Determining which disease is present can be difficult because hypercortisolemia causes secondary hypothyroidism and may also alter thyroid hormone binding to plasma proteins, enhance the metabolism of thyroid hormone, or decrease peripheral deiodination of thyroxine (T_4) to triiodothyronine (T_3) (Ferguson and Peterson, 1992). Approximately 40% to 60% of dogs with HAC have decreased basal serum T_4 and/or T_3 concentrations, and 24% have decreased free T_4 concentrations (Peterson et al, 1984b; Ferguson and Peterson, 1992). Given that secondary hypothyroidism typically resolves with treatment of HAC (Ferguson and Peterson, 1992) and that concurrent spontaneous hypothyroidism and HAC occurs rarely (Blois et al, 2011), if a patient is suspected to have both hypothyroidism and HAC and if HAC is confirmed, it should be treated and thyroid replacement therapy should be postponed. Once the HAC is controlled, thyroid function should be reassessed.

Diabetes Mellitus

Diabetes mellitus and HAC can occur concurrently. Either can be diagnosed first, with the other disease following at variable lengths of time. How often they occur concurrently is not clear but is likely not often. Diagnosis of HAC in a diabetic can be exceedingly difficult (see later) clouding the issue; uncontrolled diabetes mellitus can cause false-positive results on screening tests for HAC and give the incorrect impression of a high rate of concurrence.

Gallbladder Mucocele

An association between HAC and gallbladder mucoceles has been postulated, but remains to be proven. In one study, 23% of 30 dogs with mucocele were reported to have HAC (Pike et al, 2004). Similarly, in 78 dogs with gallbladder mucocele, 21% had HAC, and the odds of a mucocele in dogs with HAC were 29 times that of age- and breed-matched dogs without HAC (Mesich et al, 2009). However, how the diagnosis of HAC was made was not described in the former study, and the diagnosis could not be confirmed by the authors in either study given the retrospective nature of the studies. In a third study, only two of 58 dogs with a mucocele had HAC (Kutsunai, 2014). Because hyperlipidemia may be a risk factor for mucocele formation (Kutsunai, 2014) and the majority of dogs with HAC are hyperlipidemic, the possibility exists that hypercortisolemia does not contribute directly to mucocele formation. In six dogs treated with hydrocortisone (8 mg/kg every 12 hours) for 3 months, all of them developed gallbladder sludge by day 56, but so had three of six control dogs; no significant differences were seen between groups at any sampling time. Solutes associated with gallbladder sludge in humans (i.e., bilirubin, cholesterol, and calcium) were decreased by hydrocortisone administration (Kook et al, 2011). However, the study by Kook and colleagues was small, and HAC could lead to mucocele formation by other mechanisms (e.g., changes in gallbladder motility or in glycoproteins, such as mucin) (Kook et al, 2011; Mesich et al, 2009).

Pulmonary Thromboembolism

PTE is a complication of hypercoagulability, blood stasis, and damage to the endothelial lining of blood vessels (LaRue and Murtaugh, 1990) and ranges in importance from incidental and clinically irrelevant thromboembolism to massive embolism with sudden death. Hypercoagulability leads to thrombi formation in the leg, pelvic, and arm veins of people with proximal extension as clots propagate. As thrombi form in the deep veins, they may dislodge and embolize to the pulmonary arteries. Pulmonary arterial obstruction and platelet release of vasoactive agents, such as serotonin, worsen pulmonary resistance. The resulting increase in alveolar dead space and redistribution of blood flow creates areas with ventilation to perfusion mismatch, impairs gas exchange, and stimulates alveolar hyperventilation. Reflex bronchoconstriction augments airway resistance. Lung edema (if present) decreases pulmonary compliance. As right ventricular afterload increases, right ventricular wall tension rises, possibly leading to right ventricular dilation, dysfunction, and ischemia (Goldhaber, 1998).

PTE is a potential complication of HAC (Keyes et al, 1993; Teshima et al, 2008; Sobel and Williams, 2009), as well as several other disorders (Box 10-2), and is due, at least in part, to HAC-induced hypercoagulability. Humans with HAC are four times more likely to suffer thromboembolic complications than the general population (Meaney et al, 1997). Patients who undergo surgery for HAC are specifically predisposed to thrombosis (Reitmeyer et al, 2002). Other factors present in dogs with HAC that may predispose patients for PTE are obesity, hypertension, increased hematocrit (resulting in vascular stasis), and prolonged periods of recumbency.

Although overall it appears that dogs with naturally occurring HAC have hypercoagulable tendencies, study results have been inconsistent. No evidence of hypercoagulability was found in one study, but it included only nine dogs with untreated HAC and may have been underpowered (Klose et al, 2011). Levels of procoagulation factors II, V, VII, IX, X, XII, and fibrinogen are significantly increased in dogs with HAC (Feldman et al, 1986; Jacoby et al, 2001). Antithrombin, an anti-thrombotic agent, was significantly decreased in one study, which could allow clot formation (Jacoby et al, 2001); however, other studies did not find the same (Feldman et al, 1986; Pace et al, 2013; Park et al, 2013). A marker of subclinical thrombosis, thrombin-antithrombin (TAT)

complexes, may be significantly increased in dogs with HAC, and inhibition of fibrinolytic activity is not associated with HAC (Jacoby et al, 2001; Pace et al, 2013). Changes in thromboelastography consistent with hypercoagulability can also occur in dogs with HAC (Pace et al, 2013; Park et al, 2013; Rose et al, 2013). However, not all dogs with HAC have changes consistent with hypercoagulability; for those that do, no specific, consistent pattern can be identified. Furthermore, evidence of hypercoagulability has not been shown to have a clinical correlation with PTE (i.e., many dogs have at least one marker of hypercoagulability, but PTE secondary to HAC is considered rare).

Severe PTE is one of the few complications of HAC that can be fatal. Occurrence of PTE should be considered in all dogs with HAC that acutely develop tachypnea, orthopnea, and/or dyspnea. Anecdotally, PTE is believed by some to be more common after adrenalectomy or after initiation of medical therapy for HAC. Thoracic radiography is an important component of the evaluation of any dyspneic animal. Radiographs of dogs with PTE may reveal pleural effusion, loss of the pulmonary artery, alveolar infiltrates, cardiomegaly, hyperlucent lung fields, enlargement of the main pulmonary artery, or no abnormalities (Johnson et al, 1999). Alternatively, increased diameter and blunting of the pulmonary arteries, lack of perfusion of the obstructed pulmonary vasculature, and overperfusion of the unobstructed pulmonary vasculature may be seen (Fig. 10-23). Normal thoracic radiographs in a dyspneic patient that lacks large airway obstruction may be consistent with PTE. Further discussion of PTE is beyond the scope of this chapter.

SPECIFIC EVALUATION OF THE PITUITARY-ADRENOCORTICAL AXIS

A suspicion of HAC should be established from the history, physical examination findings, results of routine laboratory tests (CBC, serum biochemistry profile, and urinalysis), radiographs, and/or ultrasonography. Confirmation of a diagnosis of HAC

BOX 10-2 Primary Clinical Disorders in 29 Dogs with Pulmonary Thromboembolism*

Immune mediated hemolytic anemia
Neoplasia
Systemic bacterial disease
  Sepsis
  Pneumonia
  Pyothorax
  Endocarditis
Hyperadrenocorticism (HAC)
Amyloidosis (protein-losing nephropathy)
Cardiomyopathy
Megaesophagus

*Modified from Johnson LR, et al.: Pulmonary thromboembolism in 29 dogs: 1985-1995, *J Vet Intern Med* 13:338, 1999.

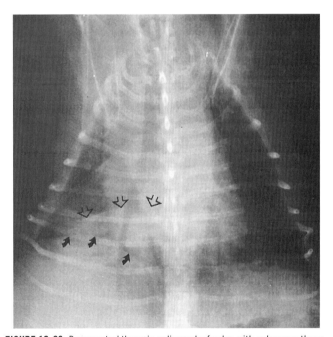

FIGURE 10-23 Dorsoventral thoracic radiograph of a dog with pulmonary thromboembolism (PTE) that resulted in a focal area of density, which is outlined by the *arrows.*

must be done with specific endocrine tests. The evaluation for HAC proceeds through two basic steps of screening and differentiating. Screening tests (e.g., LDDST, ACTH stimulation test, and UC:CR measurement) confirm or rule out the existence of HAC. If a diagnosis of HAC is confirmed, the second step is to perform a biochemical differentiating test or imaging to distinguish between PDH and AT.

The mainstay of diagnostic procedures is measurement of plasma, serum, or urine cortisol concentrations. Assays for cortisol include radioimmunoassay (RIA), enzyme-linked immunosorbent assay (ELISA), and chemiluminescence. To the author's knowledge, data regarding in-house cortisol measurements have not been reported in the peer-reviewed literature.

For measurement of cortisol in blood, serum or plasma can be used. The samples should be centrifuged within 2 hours of collection. Cortisol concentrations in plasma are stable, and cooling of the sample is not necessary; serum, however, should be shipped cold (Reimers et al, 1991; Behrend et al, 1998). However, to best ensure adequate sample integrity, after centrifugation, samples should either be refrigerated for up to 24 hours or frozen for longer at –20° C. Urine can be stored at 4° C for up to 4 days or at –20° C for more than 5 days. Samples should be sent to the laboratory overnight; sample type will not matter, and no special packaging is needed (Behrend et al, 2013).

The extent to which lipemia and hemolysis interfere with assay performance is assay-dependent. Exogenous glucocorticoids can interfere with measurement of cortisol in two ways. First, certain synthetic glucocorticoids (e.g., hydrocortisone, prednisone, prednisolone, and methylprednisolone) can cross-react in cortisol assays, falsely elevating the apparent cortisol concentration. The degree of cross-reactivity is assay-dependent. To avoid cross-reactivity, no synthetic glucocorticoid that cross-reacts should be given for at least 12 hours before a sample is drawn for measurement of cortisol; a 24-hour withdrawal can be observed for greater assurance that the synthetic glucocorticoid has been cleared. Second, exogenous glucocorticoids can exert negative feedback on the hypothalamic-pituitary-adrenal axis and cause adrenocortical atrophy, suppressing cortisol concentrations. The amount of time necessary for recovery of the hypothalamic-pituitary-adrenal axis after discontinuation of exogenous glucocorticoid therapy is unpredictable and variable depending on patient factors, the dose and form of glucocorticoid, and the duration of therapy (see Chapter 14).

In the following section, reference ranges will not be provided. Each laboratory must establish its own. Measured concentrations can vary between methods and even between laboratories using the same method (Behrend et al, 2013).

SCREENING TESTS: CONFIRMING A DIAGNOSIS OF HYPERADRENOCORTICISM

Screening tests for spontaneous HAC aid in distinguishing dogs with HAC from dogs that do not have HAC. Diagnosis of HAC depends on demonstration of either 1) increased cortisol production, or 2) decreased sensitivity of the hypothalamic-pituitary-adrenal axis to negative glucocorticoid feedback. Routinely used screening tests include the ACTH stimulation test, LDDST, and the UC:CR. No test has 100% diagnostic accuracy, and all can have false-positive results (i.e., a dog that does not have HAC has a test consistent with the diagnosis) and false-negative results (i.e., a dog with HAC has normal test results). In some cases, more than one test must be done to fully rule in or rule out a diagnosis of HAC. Positive and negative predictive values are dependent upon disease prevalence. In a population appropriately screened so that disease prevalence is high, diagnostic tests will be more accurate. No biochemical test

can predict the size of a pituitary tumor. In order to determine if a macroadenoma is present, imaging must be performed.

It must be emphasized that the decision to treat a dog for HAC should never be based solely on laboratory results. If a dog has no clinical signs, treatment is not recommended (see later).

Sensitivity and Specificity

In order to understand how good a test is, comprehension of the statistical terms sensitivity and specificity is helpful. Sensitivity is the percentage of individuals with the disease who are correctly identified by the test. It reflects the false-negative rate. For example, if the LDDST is 95% sensitive for diagnosing HAC, of all dogs with the disease, 95% have abnormal LDDST results consistent with HAC, and the other 5% do not (i.e., the test is false negative in 5% and the diagnosis would be missed). Specificity is the percentage of individuals without the disease who have a negative result. It reflects the false-positive rate. For example, if the ACTH stimulation test has a specificity of 86% for diagnosing HAC, of all dogs with a negative ACTH stimulation test result, 86% do not have the disease, and 14% have a false-positive result.

Sensitivity and specificity are never 100% for any test. Therefore, more than one screening test may be necessary for the diagnosis of HAC, especially in dogs without classic clinical signs of the disease or in those with known non-adrenal disease (e.g., diabetes mellitus). If a test is negative but suspicion for HAC remains, another test should be performed. If more than one test is negative, the possibility that the patient does not have HAC must be considered. Alternatively, the patient may have mild HAC and the tests have not yet become positive. It may be worthwhile to retest in 3 to 6 months if clinical signs progress.

Special Considerations

Phenobarbital Administration

Side effects of phenobarbital include polydipsia, polyuria, and polyphagia. In addition, phenobarbital administration can cause increases in serum ALP activity (Foster et al, 2000b; Muller et al, 2000b). Thus, suspicion of HAC can arise in dogs receiving phenobarbital therapy. Unfortunately, confirmation of HAC in phenobarbital-treated dogs is challenging. Although no effect of phenobarbital on LDDST results overall has been documented, occasional phenobarbital-treated dogs may not show suppression (Chauvet et al, 1995; Foster et al, 2000a; Muller et al, 2000b). No effect on the ACTH stimulation test was documented overall or individually in healthy dogs treated with phenobarbital for 8 weeks (n = 12) (Dyer et al, 1994) or 29 weeks (n = 12) (Muller et al, 2000a), or in epileptic dogs treated for 1 year (n = 5) (Chauvet et al, 1995) or more than 2 years (n = 5) (Dyer et al, 1994). Thus, if a dog on phenobarbital is suspected to have HAC, consideration should be given to switching to another anticonvulsant. If clinical and laboratory abnormalities persist, substantiating the suspicion of HAC, testing may then be performed. If discontinuation of phenobarbital is impossible, LDDST results should be interpreted cautiously (Behrend et al, 2013). An ACTH stimulation test may be better in dogs on phenobarbital, but the lower sensitivity of the test (see later) must be considered.

Dogs with Known Disease, Especially Diabetes Mellitus

Suspicion of HAC can arise in dogs known to have a non-adrenal illness (NAI) (e.g., diabetes mellitus). Many illnesses affect results of HAC screening tests (Chastain et al, 1986; Kaplan et al, 1995; Gieger et al, 2003; Boozer et al, 2006). The likelihood of a false-positive result on a screening test can increase with the severity of the non-adrenal disease (Kaplan et al, 1995). Some dogs with NAI can have positive test results on both the LDDST and ACTH stimulation test and still not have HAC (Chastain et al, 1986). The UC:CR measured on a single urine sample is the least specific test when NAI is present (Kaplan et al, 1995; Gieger et al, 2003).

Ideally, testing for HAC should be avoided if serious NAI exists. Testing for HAC is not mandatory at the time suspicion arises. Postponing testing until concurrent illnesses are resolved or controlled is recommended, but the severity of the concurrent illness must be considered. In addition, some diseases cannot be resolved (e.g., diabetes mellitus). At the least, the non-adrenal disease should be controlled as best as possible before testing for HAC.

The degree of suspicion for HAC must be considered. Certain diseases can have similar clinical signs. For example, diabetic patients will have polyuria/polydipsia and polyphagia, hepatomegaly, and increased serum ALP activity. A strong suspicion for HAC in a diabetic should be built on the presence of clinical signs that are typical of HAC but not diabetes mellitus (e.g., bilaterally symmetrical alopecia or calcinosis cutis). If solid suggestion of HAC exists, diagnostic testing can be pursued earlier. However, the effect of NAI on the results of screening tests should be kept in mind and results interpreted cautiously.

Urine Cortisol-to-Creatinine Ratio

The UC:CR can be used to screen for HAC as an assessment of adrenocortical reserve. The advantages are that the test is safe and easy, has a high sensitivity, and is relatively inexpensive. Measurement of the UC:CR can also be combined with dexamethasone suppression testing, providing a differentiation test as well (see later). The main disadvantage is that the specificity can be quite low, depending on the laboratory performing the testing. The UC:CR without dexamethasone suppression can never differentiate between PDH and AT.

Protocol

A single, midstream free-catch urine sample is used. The urine should be centrifuged and at least 1.0 mL of supernatant submitted. To avoid the influence of stress, urine for a UC:CR should be collected at home at least 2 days after a visit to a veterinary clinic (Fig. 10-24) (van Vonderen et al, 1998). Although a UC:CR

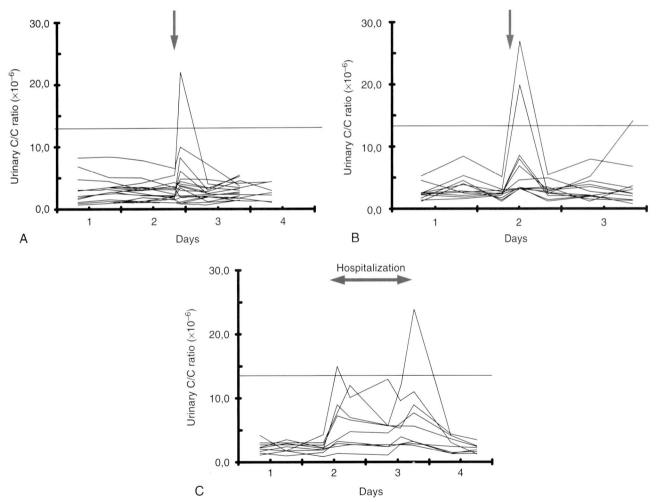

FIGURE 10-24 A, Urine cortisol-to-creatinine ratio (UC:CR) measured in 19 healthy pet dogs before and after a visit to a veterinary practice for yearly vaccination. The *arrow* indicates the time of the visit to the veterinary practice. The *line* indicates the upper reference limit of the assay. **B,** UC:CR measured in 12 pet dogs before and after a visit to a referral clinic for orthopedic examination. The *arrow* indicates the time of the visit to the referral clinic. The increase in the UC:CR on day 3 in one dog was most probably caused by an additional visit to a veterinary hospital. The *line* indicates the upper reference limit of the assay. **C,** UC:CR measured in nine healthy pet dogs before, during, and after a 1½-day hospitalization at a referral clinic. The *line* indicates the upper reference limit of the assay. (From van Vonderen IK, et al.: Influence of veterinary care on the urinary corticoid-to-creatinine ratio in dogs, *J Vet Intern Med* 12:431, 1998.)

sample can be collected at any time of day (Zeugswetter et al, 2010), morning urine may be preferred, because it usually represents several hours of urine production.

Interpretation

Urine cortisol excretion increases as a reflection of augmented adrenal secretion, adjusting for fluctuations in blood concentrations. Because creatinine excretion is relatively constant and kidney function is stable, dividing the urine cortisol concentration by the creatinine concentration negates the effect of urine volume in interpreting urine cortisol concentration.

Statistics

In one study of dogs with physical and biochemical changes consistent with HAC, the sensitivity of finding two basal UC:CRs above the cutoff level was 99%, and the specificity was 77% (Rijnberk et al, 1988a). In some dogs, considerable day-to-day variation exists in the UC:CR. In mild cases, a UC:CR may be just within the reference range 1 day and increased another day.

The assay used by Rijnberk and colleagues was proprietary and not available for use in the United States. In other studies, when a single, random urine sample was collected in veterinary hospitals, the reported sensitivity and specificity of the UC:CR for diagnosis of HAC ranges from 75% to 100% (Stolp et al, 1983; Smiley and Peterson, 1993; Kaplan et al, 1995; Jensen et al, 1997) and 20% to 25%, respectively (Stolp et al, 1983; Feldman and Mack, 1992; Smiley and Peterson, 1993; Kaplan et al, 1995; Fig. 10-25). Whether the assay used (Rijnberk et al, 1988a) or the collection of samples at home, or both, accounts for the higher specificity is unknown. Which assay is used can significantly affect results of UC:CR measurement (Kolevska and Svoboda, 2000).

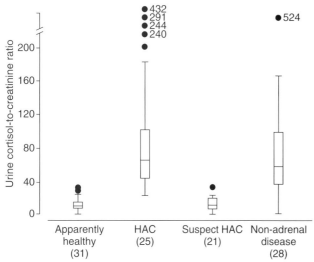

FIGURE 10-25 Box plots of urine cortisol-to-creatinine ratios (UC:CRs) found in apparently healthy dogs, dogs with hyperadrenocorticism *(HAC)*, dogs in which HAC was initially suspected but that did not have the disease *(suspect HAC)*, and dogs with a variety of severe, non-adrenal diseases. The number of dogs in each group is shown in parentheses. The box represents the interquartile range from the 25th to 75th percentiles (the middle half of the data). The horizontal bar through the box is the median. The upper whisker shows the 10th percentile and the lower whisker the 90th. Outlying data points are represented by the circles (exact value is given). (From Smiley LE, Peterson ME: Evaluation of a urine cortisol:creatinine ratio as a screening test for hyperadrenocorticism in dogs, *J Vet Intern Med* 7:163, 1993.)

Consequently, with assays currently available commercially, in the United States and Canada, a UC:CR is a good way to rule out the diagnosis of HAC but not to rule it in. With a sensitivity of more than 90%, it would be very unlikely that patients with a normal ratio would have HAC. However, because one study found the sensitivity of the UC:CR to be 75% (Kaplan et al, 1995), any dog with a normal UC:CR for which there is a high suspicion of HAC should be further evaluated by an LDDST or ACTH stimulation test. Due to the low specificity, an elevated UC:CR is not diagnostic for HAC. As a result, in patients with an elevated UC:CR, a diagnosis of HAC must always be confirmed with a LDDST or ACTH stimulation test.

Adrenocorticotropic Hormone Stimulation Test

The ACTH stimulation test assesses adrenocortical reserve. It is the gold standard for diagnosis of iatrogenic HAC, and it is the only test recommended for monitoring response to therapy for HAC. With regard to its use as a screening test for HAC, the advantages are that the test is safe, simple, and not time-consuming (lasting only 1 or 2 hours). The main disadvantage is a lower sensitivity than the LDDST, especially for dogs with an AT (see later). In addition, the ACTH stimulation test can never differentiate between PDH and AT. Although in one study the responses in dogs with adrenal carcinoma were higher than dogs with an adrenal adenoma (Peterson et al, 1982b), no consistent difference was noted in another (Feldman, 1983b).

Protocol

The test can begin at any time of day and without patient preparation. Numerous protocols have been published in healthy dogs and dogs with HAC. Synthetic polypeptides containing the biologically-active first 24 amino acids of ACTH are available (e.g., cosyntropin [Cortrosyn] or tetracosactide acetate [Synacthen]). Although in healthy dogs, doses as low as 0.5 μg/kg maximally stimulate cortisol secretion (Martin et al, 2007), only doses tested in dogs with HAC can be endorsed.

The currently recommended protocol is to administer 5 μg/kg cosyntropin or tetracosactrin intravenously with a maximum of 250 μg per dog; samples for cortisol measurement should be drawn before and 1 hour after administration (Kerl et al, 1999; Frank et al, 2000). Although cosyntropin can be administered intramuscularly in normal dogs with the same effect (Behrend et al, 2006), the intravenous (IV) route is preferred to avoid issues with drug absorption. Recently, a generic form, cosyntropin injection, was introduced for IV use only. No differences in cortisol concentrations were found in response to 250 μg Cortrosyn intramuscularly (IM) or cosyntropin injection IV in 18 healthy dogs (Cohen and Feldman, 2012). The study, however, included only healthy dogs, and the dose used (250 μg/dog) is higher than needed for the vast majority of dogs.

Using a dose of 5 μg/kg allows multiple uses of a single vial of cosyntropin. Cortrosyn can be reconstituted and frozen in aliquots at –20° C in plastic syringes for 6 months (Frank and Oliver, 1998). Because the effect of thawing and refreezing has not been investigated, the author recommends freezing in 50 μg aliquots, thawing only those needed for a test. Whether Synacthen or cosyntropin injection can be frozen has not been investigated.

In some countries, compounded ACTH preparations are available. In healthy dogs, after administration of four compounded products (2.2 U/kg IM), cortisol concentrations at 60 min were similar to each other as well as to concentrations after Cortrosyn (5 μg/kg IV). However, at later times cortisol concentrations varied considerably. Thus, if using compounded forms (2.2 U/kg IM), samples should be collected before and at 1 and 2 hours after injection

(Kemppainen et al, 2005). Certain caveats exist. First, dogs with HAC were not included in the study. Second, a single vial of ACTH from each compounding pharmacy was used. Whether gels obtained from any compounding pharmacy or even a different vial from the same compounding pharmacy would perform similarly is unknown.

A tetracosactrin depot product, (Synacthen depot), designed for protracted tetracosactrin release, has been evaluated in healthy dogs. Peak cortisol response occurred at 120 to 180 minutes after administration (250 µg/dog IM or 5 µg/kg IM). In comparison, the peak response to a non-depot cosyntropin occurred earlier (i.e., at 60 to 90 minutes) and was significantly higher (Ginel et al, 2012). Because the depot form has not been evaluated in dogs

with HAC in the peer-reviewed literature, its use cannot be recommended because the correct protocol in diseased dogs is unknown.

Interpretation

The absolute values for the pre- and post-ACTH cortisol concentrations must be assessed. Evaluation of ratios or relative changes is not recommended. Some laboratories include a borderline range for results of the post-ACTH cortisol concentration; if a dog's results falls within the range, HAC, unfortunately, cannot be ruled in or ruled out.

Dogs with PDH have bilateral adrenocortical hyperplasia with an increased capacity to synthesize and secrete excessive amounts of cortisol. Dogs with functioning ATs have a similar abnormal capacity to synthesize and secrete excess cortisol. Therefore, dogs with either PDH or AT have the potential for an exaggerated response to ACTH stimulation (Fig. 10-26). In dogs with iatrogenic HAC, the adrenal cortex is suppressed by exogenous glucocorticoid administration (see Chapter 14). Accordingly, endogenous cortisol concentrations are below the reference range, which is usually below the sensitivity of the assay (Fig. 10-27). Iatrogenic HAC is diagnosed on the basis of suppressed cortisol concentrations, the presence of clinical signs of HAC, and a history of exogenous glucocorticoid therapy by any route, including topical.

Test Statistics

The sensitivity of the ACTH stimulation test for canine HAC in general ranges from 57% to 95%. For dogs with HAC due to an AT, sensitivity is 57% to 63%; for dogs with PDH it is 80% to 83%. Specificity ranges from 59% to 93% (Reusch and Feldman, 1991; Kaplan et al, 1995; van Liew, et al, 1997; Gieger et al, 2003; Behrend et al, 2005; Monroe et al, 2012).

Influence of Drugs

Glucocorticoids of any form (see Chapter 14), progestagens (Selman et al, 1997), and ketoconazole (Willard et al, 1986) suppress cortisol secretion. Phenobarbital has no known effect on the ACTH stimulation test.

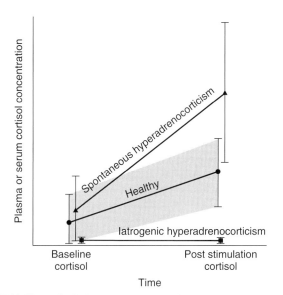

FIGURE 10-26 Idealized plasma or serum cortisol concentrations measured before and after administration of synthetic adrenocorticotropic hormone (ACTH) in healthy dogs, dogs with spontaneous hyperadrenocorticism (HAC), and those with iatrogenic HAC. The *gray area* denotes the reference range.

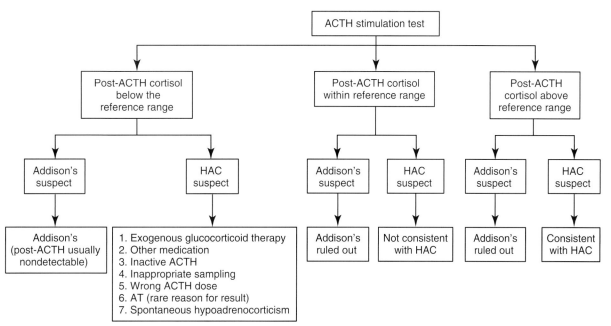

FIGURE 10-27 Algorithm for interpretation of adrenocorticotropic hormone *(ACTH)* stimulation test results for diagnosis of (screening for) hyperadrenocorticism *(HAC)*. (In Rand J, editor: *Clinical endocrinology of companion animals*, Ames, IA, 2013, Wiley-Blackwell, p. 51.)

Results below the Reference Range

Occasionally in dogs being screened for HAC, a less than normal ACTH response occurs. The most likely possibility is that the dog has received exogenous glucocorticoids, including topical. If glucocorticoid therapy has been carefully ruled out, other possibilities exist (see Fig. 10-27):

1. The patient has received progestagens or ketoconazole or any medication that suppresses cortisol secretion.
2. The ACTH used was inactive (e.g., the vial has expired, previously reconstituted cosyntropin was not stored correctly, or an ineffective compounded formulation was used).
3. The post-ACTH sample was collected at an inappropriate time. With compounded forms, the peak response can occur at 1 or 2 hours post-ACTH, even though most compounding pharmacies recommend only a 2-hour sample. If only a 2-hour post-ACTH sample is collected, the diagnostic cortisol concentration may be missed (Kemppainen et al, 2005).
4. The dose of ACTH was miscalculated and was too low.
5. Infrequently, a subnormal ACTH response is seen in dogs with ATs. The most likely explanation in such cases is that the AT is secreting either a progestin (Norman et al, 1999), or a cortisol intermediate, such as corticosterone (Behrend et al, 2004; Frankot et al, 2012). Progestins and some cortisol intermediates bind the glucocorticoid receptor, so they can cause the clinical signs of HAC and exert negative feedback on the pituitary, decreasing ACTH secretion. As a result, normal adrenocortical tissue atrophies and endogenous cortisol concentrations are below the reference range.
6. The patient has spontaneous hypoadrenocorticism. This would be unlikely because the clinical signs, for the most part, are not similar to those of HAC.

Low-Dose Dexamethasone Suppression Test

The LDDST demonstrates decreased hypothalamic-pituitary-adrenal axis sensitivity to negative glucocorticoid feedback, which is one of the two characteristics of HAC diagnosis. Additionally, dexamethasone may be metabolized quicker in dogs with HAC than in healthy dogs (Kemppainen and Peterson, 1993). Two large advantages of the LDDST are that the sensitivity for diagnosis of HAC is high, and the test differentiates between PDH and AT in approximately 40% of dogs with HAC. It is considered safe even though a single report exists of a dog that had a fatal anaphylactic reaction to dexamethasone (Schaer et al, 2005). The test is also relatively inexpensive. The disadvantages are that it has a lower specificity and it requires 8 hours to complete.

Protocol

To perform an LDDST, dexamethasone or dexamethasone sodium phosphate can be used as long as calculations are based on the concentration of the active ingredient. Dexamethasone (0.01 to 0.015 mg/kg) is administered intravenously, and blood should be drawn before and at 4 and 8 hours after injection (Behrend et al, 2013). Dexamethasone should be diluted in sterile saline, if necessary, for small dogs for accurate dosing. If part or all of the dexamethasone is given out of the vein, the test should be stopped, and a period of at least 48 hours should elapse before reinjection.

Interpretation

Lack of suppression on an LDDST is consistent with a diagnosis of HAC. Normally, dexamethasone feeds back onto the pituitary turning off ACTH secretion for up to 24 to 48 hours (Toutain et al, 1983). When systemic ACTH concentration falls, the secretory stimulus to the adrenal cortex diminishes, and cortisol release decreases. Thus, in normal dogs, plasma cortisol concentration 4 and 8 hours after dexamethasone is below the laboratory cutoff (e.g., < 1 to 1.5 µg/dL [30 to 45 nmol/L]). Conversely, a diagnosis of HAC is supported by an 8-hour post-dexamethasone plasma cortisol concentration above the laboratory cutoff (Fig. 10-28). With PDH, the pituitary tumor is relatively resistant to feedback. Thus, some ACTH secretion persists despite the dexamethasone injection and, in turn, cortisol release continues. For patients with an AT, endogenous ACTH (eACTH)

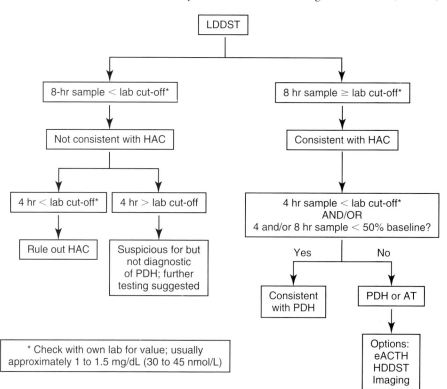

FIGURE 10-28 Algorithm for interpretation of low-dose dexamethasone suppression test *(LDDST)* results for diagnosis of (screening for) hyperadrenocorticism *(HAC)*. (Modified from Rand J, editor: *Clinical endocrinology of companion animals,* Ames, IA, 2013, Wiley-Blackwell, p. 50.) *AT,* Adrenocortical tumor; *eACTH,* endogenous ACTH; *HDDST,* high-dose dexamethasone suppression test; *PDH,* pituitary-dependent hyperadrenocorticism.

is already suppressed due to continuous, autonomous cortisol secretion from the tumor. Dexamethasone has no further effect on the pituitary, and adrenal cortisol secretion continues.

Statistics

The reported sensitivity and specificity of the LDDST ranges from 85% to 100% and from 44% to 73%, respectively (Feldman, 1983a; Chastain et al, 1986; Rijnberk et al, 1988a; Reusch and Feldman, 1991; Kaplan et al, 1995; Feldman et al, 1996; van Liew et al 1997; Mueller et al, 2006). By combining previous reports, it was determined that 640 tests were positive in 673 dogs for an overall sensitivity of 95.1% (Behrend and Kemppainen, 2001). In general, the more severe the NAI present, the more likely a false-positive test result (i.e., the lower the specificity) (Kaplan et al, 1995). Stress during a test may also potentially affect results (May et al, 2004).

Inverse Pattern

An "inverse" pattern, in which the cortisol concentration 8 hours after dexamethasone was within the reference range (i.e., suppressed) but the cortisol concentration 4 hours post-dexamethasone was increased, was described in five dogs with PDH (Mueller et al, 2006). Thus, although the inverse pattern is not diagnostic for HAC, it is highly suspicious. If the inverse pattern is obtained in a dog screened for HAC, further testing should be pursued.

Influence of Drugs

Dexamethasone is metabolized primarily by cytochrome P450 3A4. Agents that increase the enzyme's activity (e.g., carbamazepine, phenytoin, rifampicin, and barbiturates) accelerate dexamethasone clearance and could cause false-positive results on an LDDST. In veterinary medicine, only phenobarbital has been studied. Although no overall effect of phenobarbital on LDDST results has been found, occasional phenobarbital-treated dogs may not show suppression (Chauvet et al, 1995; Foster et al, 2000a; Muller et al, 2000a).

Combined Dexamethasone Suppression/Adrenocorticotropic Hormone Stimulation Test

The test combines a screening test (ACTH stimulation test) and a differentiating test (high-dose dexamethasone suppression test [HDDST]) with the aim of diagnosing and differentiating in one test. To perform the test, dexamethasone (0.1 mg/kg IV) is administered with a blood sample taken before and 2 to 6 hours later (Zerbe, 2000). Immediately after the second blood sample an ACTH stimulation test is performed. The arms of the test are interpreted as for the individual tests (i.e., HDDST and ACTH stimulation test) and with the same reference ranges. Test sensitivity has been estimated at 76% (Feldman, 1985), 86% (Feldman, 1986), and 93% (Zerbe, 2000). The author of the former two studies, therefore, concluded that due to the lower sensitivity, the test was not helpful and could not be advocated.

Part of the confusion may result in how the test is interpreted. If the test is evaluated as a whole (i.e., a diagnosis of HAC is made if a dog does not suppress in response to dexamethasone and has an elevated response to ACTH), then the sensitivity is relatively low. However, if the diagnosis is made on the basis of the ACTH stimulation portion alone, the sensitivity would be the same as performing an ACTH stimulation test without previous dexamethasone injection (as long as the ACTH is given within 8 hours of the dexamethasone [Kemppainen and Sartin, 1984b]). Thus, the combined test is subject to all of the caveats as the ACTH stimulation test alone. The dexamethasone suppression portion can then be viewed as a standalone differentiation test. However, the HDDST is not perfect either, and differentiation is not always achieved (see later section).

Tests Not Recommended as Screening Tests

Resting (Baseline) Cortisol Concentrations

Cortisol is secreted episodically; thus, values change throughout the day. Although mean daily cortisol concentration is increased in dogs with HAC, an individual, random measurement can be within the reference range. Conversely, dogs without HAC can have elevated baseline cortisol concentrations (Chastain et al, 1986; Church et al, 1994).

Serum Corticosteroid–Induced Alkaline Phosphatase Activity

As with total ALP activity, CIALP activity is elevated in most dogs with HAC or in dogs that have received exogenous glucocorticoids. Unfortunately, the specificity of CIALP activity measurement for the diagnosis of HAC is low (Fig. 10-29). In general, CIALP appears in a large number of samples when ALP is high for any reason (Eckersall et al, 1986) and can have CIALP accounting for at least 50% of the total (Eckersall et al, 1986; Kidney and Jackson, 1988; Wilson and Feldman, 1992; Solter et al, 1993). More importantly, dogs likely to be screened for HAC (e.g., those with diabetes mellitus or hypothyroidism or those given exogenous glucocorticoids or phenobarbital) can have elevated ALP levels with greater than 50% CIALP activity (Kidney and Jackson, 1988; Teske et al, 1989; Wilson and Feldman, 1992). Conversely, some dogs with HAC have little to no CIALP elevation (Kidney and Jackson, 1988; Teske et al, 1989). Overall, the sensitivity of elevated CIALP activity for glucocorticoid exposure (i.e., HAC or glucocorticoid therapy) is approximately 95%, but the specificity may be as low as 18% (Teske et al, 1989; Wilson and Feldman, 1992).

Abdominal Ultrasonography

Although dogs with HAC have adrenal gland measurements significantly greater than those of normal dogs (Barthez et al, 1995; Widmer and Guptill, 1995; Grooters et al, 1996; Hoerauf and Reusch, 1999; Choi et al, 2011), an overlap in the range of measurements occurs between dogs with HAC and normal dogs. Thickness (i.e., the dorsoventral dimension) has been suggested to be a better assessment of enlargement (Grooters et al, 1994; 1995; 1996), but overlap still exists between normal dogs and dogs with PDH (Grooters et al, 1996). In addition, the finding of an AT is not synonymous with HAC. Ultrasonography cannot distinguish a functional AT from a nonfunctional tumor, a pheochromocytoma, a metastatic lesion, or a granuloma.

DIFFERENTIATING PITUITARY-DEPENDENT HYPERADRENOCORTICISM AND ADRENOCORTICAL TUMOR

Differentiating tests should only be done after a screening test has confirmed the presence of HAC; differentiating tests cannot be interpreted if the diagnosis of HAC is in question. It is important to differentiate PDH and AT because treatment and prognosis differ. No clinical or routine biochemical features exist that aid in distinguishing dogs with functioning adrenal adenomas from those with adrenal carcinomas. Laboratory test options for differentiating include the HDDST and measurement of eACTH concentration. In some cases, the LDDST may provide the differentiation as well as the diagnosis. Imaging can also be performed to distinguish PDH and AT. As with the screening tests, no test is 100% accurate.

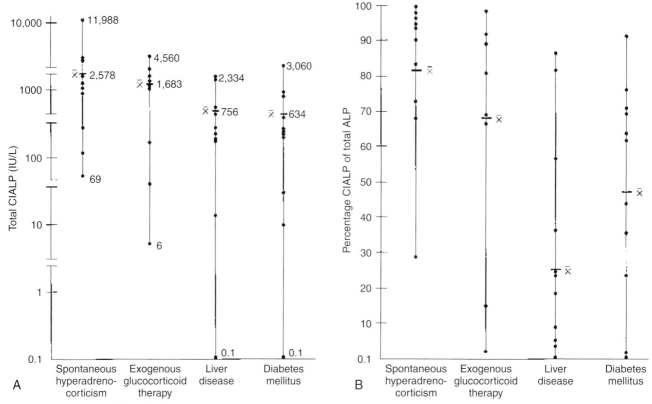

FIGURE 10-29 A, Mean and range of serum corticosteroid-induced alkaline phosphatase *(CIALP)* activity in dogs with naturally occurring hyperadrenocorticism (HAC), chronically treated with glucocorticoids, with liver disease, and with diabetes mellitus. **B,** The percentage of total serum alkaline phosphatase *(ALP)* activity accounted for by the CIALP fraction in the same four groups described in **A.** These graphs show that CIALP is a sensitive indicator of HAC (dogs with the disease usually have an elevated activity), but it is not a specific test (dogs with other conditions also can have a markedly elevated CIALP activity).

FIGURE 10-30 A, Of 178 dogs with naturally occurring hyperadrenocorticism (HAC) that were tested with both the low-dose and high-dose dexamethasone suppression tests (LDDST and HDDST), 111 dogs suppressed using one of the criteria defined in the text. Of the 111 dogs, 110 had pituitary-dependent hyperadrenocorticism *(PDH).* Twenty-nine of 30 dogs (97%) with adrenal tumors did not suppress using any of the criteria, and 38 of the 148 dogs with PDH (26%) did not suppress. **B,** Of the 109 dogs that suppressed on the HDDST, 86 (79%) had already shown suppression on the LDDST.

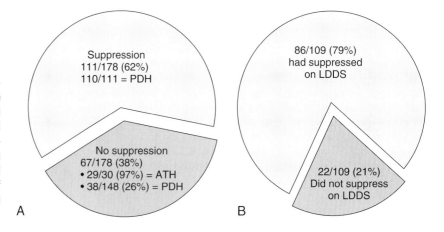

Suppression Tests

Low-Dose Dexamethasone Suppression Test

If the 8-hour post-dexamethasone concentration is greater than the laboratory cutoff (e.g., > 1 to 1.5 μg/dL [30 to 45 nmol/L]), results are consistent with HAC (see earlier; see Fig. 10-28). If, additionally, the 4-hour post-dexamethasone concentration is below the laboratory cutoff or if one or both post-dexamethasone concentrations is less than 50% of baseline, PDH is present (Feldman et al, 1996). If both post-dexamethasone concentrations are above the laboratory cutoff and neither is less than 50%

of baseline, either PDH or AT is possible. Approximately 60% of dogs with HAC can be determined to have PDH using an LDDST (Fig. 10-30). However, if the baseline cortisol is already less than the laboratory cutoff, these guidelines do not apply (Norman et al, 1999). In rare cases, dogs with an AT may meet one of these criteria for diagnosing PDH (Norman et al, 1999).

High-Dose Dexamethasone Suppression Test

Many of the advantages and disadvantages of the LDDST apply to the HDDST. One disadvantage of the HDDST is that it can never confirm the presence of an AT. If a dog does not suppress

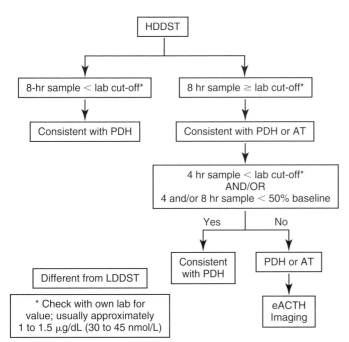

FIGURE 10-31 Algorithm for interpretation of high-dose dexamethasone suppression test *(HDDST)* results for differentiating between pituitary- and adrenal-dependent diseases. An HDDST should only be performed after a screening test has confirmed the presence of HAC. *AT,* Adrenocortical tumor; *eACTH,* endogenous adrenocorticotropic hormone; *LDDST,* low-dose dexamethasone suppression test; *PDH,* pituitary-dependent hyperadrenocorticism. (In Rand J, editor: *Clinical endocrinology of companion animals,* Ames IA, 2013, Wiley-Blackwell, p. 50.)

on the HDDST, there is approximately a fifty-fifty chance that it has PDH or AT, and another differentiation test must be done. In addition, if a diagnosis was made with the LDDST but a differentiation was not achieved, the HDDST is not likely to be able to differentiate either (Feldman et al, 1996), and another differentiation test should be pursued (see Fig. 10-30).

Protocol. The HDDST is performed similarly to the LDDST with respect to the timing of samples, but the dose used is tenfold higher (i.e., 0.1 mg/kg dexamethasone). The free alcohol form of dexamethasone should be avoided (Behrend et al, 2013). If any of the dexamethasone is given out of the vein, the test should be stopped and started again after at least 72 hours.

Interpretation. Even though the ability of cortisol to suppress ACTH secretion in dogs with PDH is abnormal, a large dose of dexamethasone may overcome the resistance to feedback. For dogs with an AT, a high dose of dexamethasone will have little to no effect on cortisol secretion, as for the low dose. Therefore, suppression to either below the laboratory cutoff or to less than 50% of baseline at either 4 or 8 hours post-dexamethasone is consistent with PDH (Fig. 10-31) (Feldman et al, 1996). Rarely dogs with an AT can have suppression to the borderline of the cutoff between PDH and AT (Feldman et al, 1996). Therefore, when baseline values are close to the laboratory cutoff for a suppressed value or when suppression is just at 50%, the results are suspect and warrant confirmation.

Statistics. In approximately 75% of dogs with PDH, cortisol concentrations meet the criteria for suppression on a HDDST. The remaining dogs with PDH do not demonstrate suppression even after receiving higher dexamethasone dosages (Feldman et al, 1996). In dogs with PDH that do not suppress, a large pituitary tumor is more likely (Kooistra et al, 1997b; Bosje et al, 2002). Additionally, lack of response may be due to the pituitary tumor having arisen from the intermediate lobe of the pituitary as compared with the anterior lobe (Peterson et al, 1986a; peterson, 1987). The intermediate lobe is not

normally under feedback control. Complete loss of feedback regulation in an anterior pituitary tumor is also possible.

Comparison of the Low-Dose and High-Dose Dexamethasone Suppression Test as Differentiating Tests

The largest study evaluating both suppression tests included 181 dogs with PDH and 35 with AT (Feldman et al, 1996). Some dogs with a mitotane-responsive AT may have been included in the PDH group. Approximately 75% of dogs with PDH met at least one criterion for suppression on either the LDDST or HDDST. Of dogs with PDH, 12% did not suppress on an LDDST but did on the HDDST. Dexamethasone resistance (i.e., no criteria were met on the LDDST) occurred in all dogs with ATs and the remainder of the dogs with PDH. However, two dogs with AT did meet the criteria for suppression on the HDDST. The criteria proposed in this study still are well accepted, although no follow-up studies have been performed for confirmation. In 41 dogs with ATs in another study, 28 LDDST and 30 HDDST were performed (Reusch and Feldman, 1991). No suppression was seen on any test.

Dexamethasone Suppression with Urine Cortisol-to-Creatinine Ratio

Decreased blood cortisol concentration after dexamethasone administration is reflected in a decreased UC:CR. The advantage of combining dexamethasone suppression with a UC:CR is that potentially screening and differentiating can be done with a single test that is safe and easy to perform.

Protocol. For the test, after collection of a morning urine sample on 2 consecutive days at home, three doses of dexamethasone should be administered (0.1 mg/kg by mouth at 6- to 8-hour intervals), and a third urine sample is collected the next morning.

Interpretation. The combination of dexamethasone suppression and UC:CR has been validated only using a proprietary assay (see Urine Cortisol-to-Creatinine Ratio). Using this assay, a decrease in the third UC:CR to less than 50% of the mean basal values is consistent with PDH (Galac et al, 1997). Lack of suppression does not confirm AT.

Statistics. In 160 dogs with HAC (49 with ATs and 111 with PDH), suppression to less than 50% of the basal UC:CR occurred in 72% of dogs with PDH (Galac et al, 2009). The remaining dogs with PDH were dexamethasone-resistant. In dogs with ATs, the maximum suppression was 44%.

Discordant Test Results

Discordance between results of suppression tests and other differentiating tests may occur. Changes in dexamethasone metabolism may also influence results of suppression tests (Behrend et al, 2013) (see the next section).

Endogenous Adrenocorticotropic Hormone Measurement

The advantages of measuring eACTH include the requirement of a single sample, and the test can definitively diagnose an AT. Measurement of eACTH is the most accurate standalone biochemical test for differentiating PDH from AT. On the other hand, eACTH is labile, and specific, strict guidelines for handling must be followed. Second, a grey zone exists in the results; if a measured concentration falls in the grey zone, a differentiation cannot be made. For example, at the Auburn University Endocrine Diagnostic Service an eACTH concentration less than 10 pg/mL is consistent with an AT, whereas more than 15 pg/mL is consistent with PDH. The area between is a "grey zone." Although other laboratories may have different cutoffs, a grey zone will exist. Concentrations of eACTH do not differ

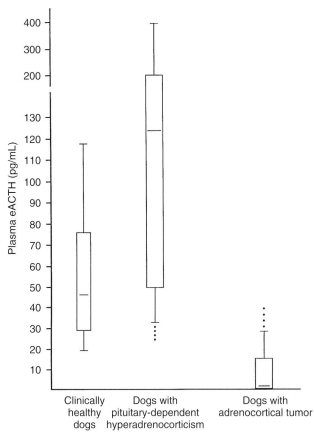

FIGURE 10-32 Endogenous plasma adrenocorticotropic hormone (*eACTH*) concentrations from clinically healthy dogs, dogs with pituitary-dependent hyperadrenocorticism (PDH) and dogs with cortisol-secreting adrenocortical carcinomas or adenomas. Each box represents the interquartile range from the 25th to 75th percentiles (the middle half of the data). The *horizontal bar* through the box is the median. The upper whisker indicates the 10th percentile, and the lower whisker indicates the 90th percentile. Outlying data points are represented by the *circles*.

between healthy dogs and those with PDH, so measurement is not useful to screen for HAC (Hanson et al, 2006).

RIA and chemiluminescent assays have been validated for eACTH measurement (Kemmpainen et al, 1994; Scott-Moncrieff et al, 2003; Rodriguez Pineiro et al, 2009; Zeugswetter et al, 2011). Measured concentrations are lower using chemiluminescent technology compared to RIA (Rodriguez Pineiro et al, 2009).

Protocol

Blood should be collected into chilled, silicon-coated glass or plastic tubes containing ethylenediaminetetraacetic acid (EDTA), centrifuged within 15 minutes (ideally in a cooled centrifuge), and the plasma transferred to plastic tubes and frozen immediately (Behrend et al, 2013). Samples must stay frozen until analysis; if a courier is used for quick transport to a reference laboratory, ice may be sufficient. If samples are shipped, they should be sent overnight packed in dry ice. Plasma proteases degrade eACTH rapidly if samples are not cooled appropriately. Addition of the protease inhibitor aprotinin (Trasylol) prevents eACTH degradation (Kemppainen et al, 1994). With the Immulite assay, aprotinin introduces an artifactual decrease (Scott-Moncrieff et al, 2003) and is not recommended.

No clear evidence exists that the specific time of sample collection affects the results or discriminatory power of the test. In healthy dogs, eACTH concentrations did not return to baseline until 24 hours after performance of an ACTH stimulation test and 12 hours after an LDDST (Bugbee et al, 2013).

Interpretation

In dogs with PDH, eACTH concentration is normal to elevated due to secretion from the pituitary tumor. In dogs with an AT, the autonomous tumoral secretion of cortisol turns off ACTH secretion; eACTH concentration should be below normal (Fig. 10-32).

Statistics

The accuracy for differentiating PDH from AT depends upon the analytical sensitivity and working range of the assay (Table 10-6). The most common problem with the eACTH assay is a poor working range at the lower end; some dogs with PDH have eACTH concentrations at or below what the assay can measure accurately,

---

 TABLE 10-6   RESULTS OF ENDOGENOUS ADRENOCORTICOTROPIC HORMONE ASSAYS FOR DOGS WITH HYPERADRENOCORTICISM*

STUDY	ASSAY	PITUITARY-DEPENDENT HYPERADRENOCORTICISM	ADRENOCORTICAL TUMOR	NUMBER INCORRECT
Zeugswetter et al, 2011	Immulite 1000	49 dogs	10 dogs	9/59
Rodriguez Pineiro et al, 2009	Immulite 2000	91 dogs (6 to 1250 pg/mL)	18 dogs (< 5 pg/mL)	0/109
Castillo et al, 2009	Nichols IRMA	5 dogs 9 to 30 pmol/L	NA	NA
Scott-Moncrieff et al, 2003	Immulite ACTH IRMA (Allegro)	11 dogs < 5 to 50 pg/mL 9 to 99 pg/mL	4 dogs < 10 pg/mL < 10 pg/mL	4/15 (Immulite) 3/15 (IRMA)
Gould et al, 2001	Nichols IRMA	21 dogs 28 to 1132 pg/mL 1 dog < 5 pg/mL	5 dogs < 5 pg/mL 1 dog 76 pg/mL	2/28

From Behrend et al.: Diagnosis of spontaneous canine hyperadrenocorticism: 2012 ACVIM consensus statement (Small animal), *J Vet Int Med* 27:1292, 2013.

ACTH, Adrenocorticotropic hormone; *IRMA*, immunoradiometric assay.

*Last 10 years with currently available assays only.

particularly with the Immulite 1000 analyzer. The largest study of eACTH in dogs with HAC used a two-site solid-phase chemiluminescent immunometric assay (Immulite ACTH kit and Immulite 2000 analyzer) and showed excellent discrimination between PDH and AT (Rodriguez Pineiro et al, 2009). No dogs with PDH had undetectable eACTH concentrations, which was likely due to the analytical sensitivity (5 pg/mL); however, the range of eACTH concentrations for dogs with PDH was 6 to 1250 pg/mL, with many dogs falling close to the lower end of the range. Thus, less sensitive assay systems (e.g., Immulite 1000) would likely have poorer discrimination. Intra-assay and inter-assay variability (increased at lower eACTH concentrations), pulsatile ACTH secretion, and inappropriate sample handling allowing ACTH degradation increase the likelihood of a falsely low value in dogs with PDH (Behrend et al, 2013).

When study results were combined, 240 (82%) of 292 tests in 245 dogs were diagnostic for PDH or AT. With repeat testing when the initial result was in the grey zone, 235 out of 245 dogs (96%) had a definitive differentiation (Behrend and Kemppainen, 2001). Unfortunately there is no way to predict when a blood concentration will be in the diagnostic range.

Discordant Test Results

Discordance between eACTH concentration and results of other differentiating tests sometimes occurs. Episodic eACTH secretion, poor assay sensitivity, and sample degradation are potential explanations. Stress and the presence of multiple adrenal disorders (e.g., PDH with pheochromocytoma or a cortisol-secreting AT with PDH) may also influence ACTH concentrations (Behrend et al, 2013). Ectopic ACTH secretion and food-stimulated cortisol secretion could also cause discordance (Galac et al, 2007; 2009).

Corticotropin-Releasing Hormone and Vasopressin Response Testing

Pituitary corticotropes respond to CRH and vasopressin. Accordingly, CRH and vasopressin stimulation tests have been evaluated as a differentiating test for HAC. Plasma ACTH and cortisol responses to CRH and lysine vasopressin (LVP) were assessed in healthy dogs and dogs with PDH or AT (van Wijk et al, 1994). Dogs with PDH had a greater response to vasopressin than to CRH, and AT cells acquired sensitivity to LVP independent of ACTH. In another study, the response to desmopressin, a synthetic form of vasopressin, was evaluated (Zeugswetter et al, 2008). Desmopressin was injected (4 μg IV) with samples collected before and after 30, 60, and 90 minutes. Desmopressin significantly stimulated cortisol secretion in dogs with PDH but not in dogs with ATs or other diseases. Using a cutoff value of a 10% increase over baseline, it was possible to exclude the presence of an AT in 75% of patients (Zeugswetter et al, 2008). However, because only seven dogs with ATs were included, further study is needed for verification. In addition, the test does not appear to provide much benefit over other biochemical differentiating tests.

DIAGNOSTIC IMAGING

Radiography

Screening

Diagnosis of HAC cannot be done solely with imaging and must rely on hormone tests. Moreover, finding normal-sized adrenal glands does not rule out HAC (Behrend et al, 2013).

Bronchial mineralization can be seen on thoracic radiographs and is consistent with a diagnosis of HAC. Changes consistent with PTE may be seen (see earlier section). If an AT is present, three-view thoracic radiographs should be taken for assessment; pulmonary metastases uncommonly occur with ATs (Anderson et al, 2001; Kyles et al, 2003; Schwartz et al, 2008; Arenas et al, 2014).

Changes associated with HAC that may be seen on abdominal radiographs include hepatomegaly, a pendulous abdomen, and dystrophic mineralization of structures, such as the renal pelvis, liver, gastric mucosa, and abdominal aorta (Penninck et al, 1988; Berry et al, 1994; Schwarz et al, 2000). Hepatomegaly is quite common (Penninck et al, 1988); conversely, finding a small liver makes HAC unlikely (Schwarz et al, 2000). Good contrast, due to abdominal (primarily omental) fat deposition, is usually observed (Fig. 10-33).

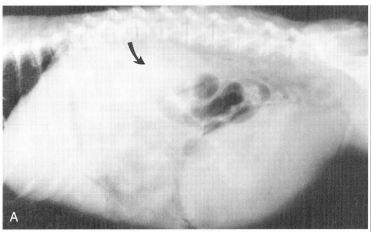
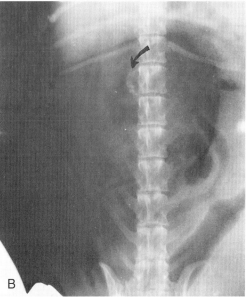

FIGURE 10-33 Lateral **(A)** and ventrodorsal **(B)** abdominal radiographs of a dog with a functioning adrenal tumor causing hyperadrenocorticism (HAC). Note the calcified adrenal tumor *(arrows)*, hepatomegaly, and excellent contrast due to fat mobilization.

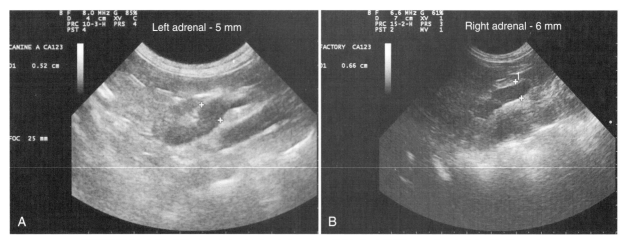

FIGURE 10-34 A, The left adrenal gland is located craniomedial to the left kidney and ventrolateral to the aorta between the caudal mesenteric and renal arteries. The typical shape is that of a peanut or dumbbell. The cursors are measuring the thickness of the caudal pole. **B,** The right adrenal gland has a variable shape including that of a "comma" or "boomerang." Because of the shape, it is difficult to image the entire gland in one plane. The extremities of the gland are often not symmetrical. The cursors are measuring the thickness of the caudal pole. The images were obtained in the sagittal plane with the dog in dorsal recumbency. The normal size of the adrenal glands is highly variable between dogs for both width and length. The most commonly cited value for the upper limit of normal is 7.4 mm in the dorsoventral dimension. (Images courtesy of Dr. Robert Cole.)

Osteopenia occurs with HAC from hypercalciuria, suppressed intestinal calcium absorption, and direct effects of cortisol on bone, but it is usually mild and clinically unimportant. Uncommonly, calcinosis cutis may be noted (see Fig. 10-19).

All thoracic and abdominal radiographic findings are not specific for HAC, and osteopenia can be easily misdiagnosed in any obese animal due to radiographic artifact (Schwarz et al, 2000). Therefore, these radiographic findings may increase the suspicion for HAC but would not aid in confirmation or differentiation. Abdominal radiography can be helpful in differentiation if an adrenal mass is found (see the following section).

Differentiation

Besides identifying nonspecific changes consistent with HAC, abdominal radiographs may be helpful for differentiation. In a compilation of 94 ATs in 88 dogs (six dogs had bilateral adenomas or carcinomas), 50 ATs (53.1%) were detected due to calcification within the tumor (40) and/or visualization of a mass (17) (Behrend and Kemppainen, 2001). Tumors less than 20 mm in diameter are not likely to be visualized (Voorhout et al, 1990). Both adenomas and carcinomas can contain mineral densities or appear as a mass cranial to the kidney. Although diffuse, ill-defined mineralization usually is associated with adrenal neoplasia discrete, well-marginated mineralization develops in clinically normal dogs and may be a dystrophic change (Widmer and Guptill, 1995). Mineralization also rarely occurs in the adrenals of dogs with PDH (Grooters et al, 1996). In dogs with bilateral tumors, only one may be visualized (Penninck et al, 1988; Reusch and Feldman, 1991; Ford et al, 1993). Consequently, finding one tumor does not rule out the presence of bilateral disease, but bilateral tumors are rare.

Abdominal Ultrasonography

Ultrasonography has more application as a differentiating tool than radiography because both adrenal glands are routinely visualized by experienced ultrasonographers. Small or non-calcified ATs can be detected, and bilateral adrenal enlargement can be documented in dogs with PDH. However, presence of gas in the gastric fundus or intestines, large body size, obesity, abdominal lymphadenopathy or masses, renal mineralization, or liver disease can prevent or complicate evaluation. Body size affects the ability to examine the right adrenal gland more than the left.

In healthy dogs, the left adrenal gland has a peanut or dumbbell shape when imaged in a sagittal plane, and the right adrenal gland has a V or comma shape when imaged in a mediolateral plane (Fig. 10-34). The contour of the glands should be smooth, and the parenchyma should be homogeneous and less echogenic than the adjacent renal cortex (Voorhout, 1990; Grooters et al, 1995; 1996). Because the adrenal glands' long axis is often misaligned with either the medial or dorsal plane of the body, cross-sectional images may lead to oblique views and miscalculation of glandular dimensions.

In dogs with PDH, bilateral adrenal enlargement may be found (Fig. 10-35). The adrenal margins appear more rounded, and the glands subjectively may appear thicker, giving them a "plump" appearance compared with adrenal glands of normal dogs (Grooters et al, 1996). Adrenal gland thickness (i.e., maximum dorsoventral dimension of the adrenal gland in a sagittal plane) is the most informative parameter for ultrasonographic assessment of the size of canine adrenal glands (Grooters et al, 1995; Barberet et al, 2010). The most accepted and commonly used measurement is a single cutoff value of 7.4 mm for normal maximum diameter of the larger of the cranial or the caudal pole in either a sagittal or transverse plane regardless of body weight. In studies, measurements greater than the cutoff had a sensitivity of 77% and a specificity of 80% for the diagnosis of PDH (Widmer and Guptill, 1995; Barthez et al, 1995), but breed and dog size was not taken into account. Body size may affect reference ranges (Barthez et al, 1995; Grooters et al, 1995; 1996; Douglass et al, 1997; Choi et al, 2011). The adrenal glands of dogs with PDH are often homogeneous and hypoechoic compared with adjacent renal cortices (Gould et al, 2001). Alternatively, variably sized focal areas of increased echogenicity may be seen. The areas represent either bilateral nodular cortical hyperplasia, an uncommon form of HAC (see Adrenocortical Nodular Hyperplasia and Food-Dependent Hyperadrenocorticism), or calcification of adrenal tissue (Grooters et al, 1996).

Asymmetry of shape within a single gland or of size between glands should not be interpreted as a tumor. Normal shape can vary (Fig. 10-36).

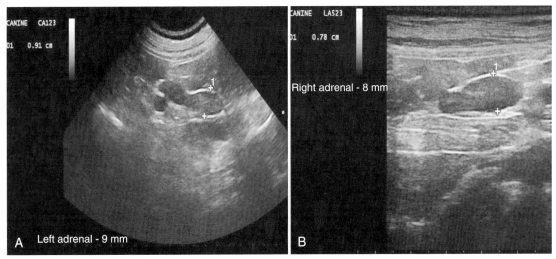

FIGURE 10-35 Bilateral adrenomegaly in a small breed dog with pituitary-dependent hyperadrenocorticism (PDH). The left adrenal gland **(A)** measures 9 mm and the right adrenal gland **(B)** measures 8 mm in dorsoventral dimensions. Both adrenal glands, although enlarged, maintain a typical shape. Both adrenal glands are slightly hypoechoic compared with normal; decreased echogenicity is often seen in patients with PDH. The images were obtained in the sagittal plane with the dog in dorsal recumbency. (Images courtesy of Dr. Robert Cole.)

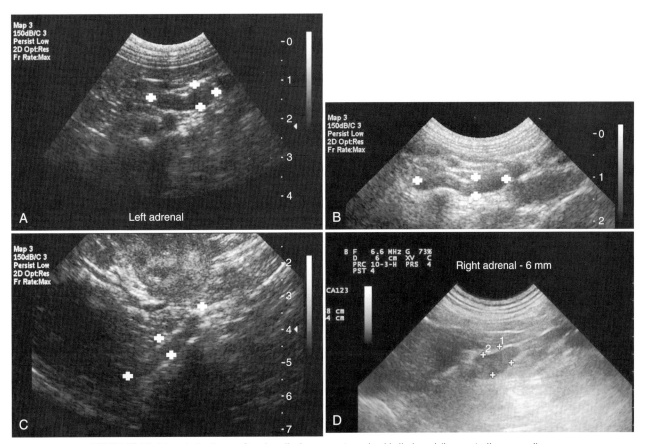

FIGURE 10-36 Adrenal glands are often described as peanut- or dumbbell-shaped (i.e., centrally narrowed), as shown in **A.** However, adrenal glands shapes are variable. Larger breed dogs often have adrenal glands that are more linear in shape without the central narrowing as shown in **B** and **C.** The right adrenal gland often has a "boomerang" or "comma" shape giving the cranial pole a widened appearance **(D).** The images were obtained in the sagittal plane with the dog in dorsal recumbency. (Images courtesy of Dr. Robert Cole.)

In some dogs, the cranial pole of the left adrenal is nearly twice as wide as the other regions. In the V-shaped right gland, the two sides may have different lengths (Grooters et al, 1995). The length of the two glands is typically not the same, and either the right or left gland may be the longer (Douglass et al, 1997). In dogs with PDH, mild asymmetry between the two glands may also occur (Benchekroun, 2010; Rodriguez Pineiro et al, 2011).

Ultrasonography defines location, size, and organ involvement of adrenal masses more precisely than radiography alone, but an AT is not always seen. In studies compiling 71 dogs, 68 of 79 (86%) tumors were found (eight had bilateral tumors) (Behrend and Kemppainen, 2001). When the tumor was missed, the affected adrenal gland appeared normal or was not visualized (Kantrowitz et al, 1986; Reusch and Feldman, 1991; Ford et al, 1993). The ultrasonographic appearance of an AT varies (Figs. 10-37 and 10-38). Moderate asymmetry, contralateral adrenocortical atrophy (adrenal width < 4 to 5 mm), and destruction of normal tissue architecture are consistent with a

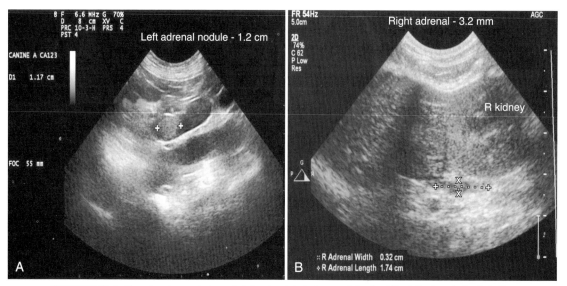

FIGURE 10-37 A, There is a hyperechoic, well-defined nodule in the cranial pole of the left adrenal gland. **B,** The contralateral gland is atrophied (3.2 mm), suggesting the nodule in the left adrenal is secreting cortisol. Most adrenal adenocarcinomas are larger and have a more variable echogenicity than what is displayed here. The images were obtained in the sagittal plane with the dog in dorsal recumbency. (Images courtesy of Dr. Robert Cole.)

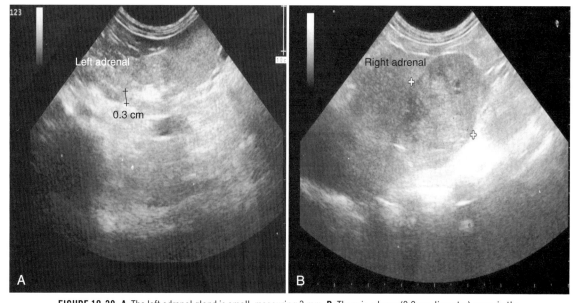

FIGURE 10-38 A, The left adrenal gland is small, measuring 3 mm. **B,** There is a large (2.2 cm diameter) mass in the area of the right adrenal gland. The mass has ill-defined borders, mixed echogenicity, and an abnormal shape; all changes are suggestive of malignancy. With most functional tumors, the contralateral adrenal gland will be smaller than normal, as in **A.** It is possible, however, for the contralateral adrenal gland to be within normal size limits. Most adrenal masses start as a small round to oval lesion, typically at one pole of the gland. As the mass continues to grow, the adrenal gland loses its normal shape and often takes a spherical/rounded shape with a variable echogenic appearance. It is very important to evaluate for local extension into the adjacent kidney or nearby vessels. The images were obtained in the sagittal plane with the dog in dorsal recumbency. (Images courtesy of Dr. Robert Cole.)

cortisol-secreting AT. The tumor may be hypoechoic, isoechoic, or hyperechoic compared to the renal cortex or have mixed echogenicity. Mineralization can be visualized as a hyperechoic area with acoustic shadowing (Kantrowitz et al, 1986; Voorhout et al, 1990; Besso et al, 1997; Hoerauf and Reusch, 1999). Areas of necrosis or hemorrhage can be anechoic, hypoechoic, or isoechoic. The adrenal gland may also simply appear enlarged (Ford et al, 1993). Distinguishing macronodular hyperplasia from an AT can be difficult with ultrasonography. A bilateral AT can be mistaken for bilateral adrenal hyperplasia, falsely providing a diagnosis of PDH.

Differentiation between an adrenal adenoma and carcinoma is unlikely with ultrasound because they can have a similar appearance. Neither echogenicity nor the presence of mineralization can be used. An adrenal gland width more than 4 cm correlates highly with malignancy. Lesions suggestive of metastasis may be found, especially in the liver (Reusch and Feldman, 1991). Evidence of invasion into the vena cava is suggestive of a carcinoma. Indication of invasion, however, can be missed (Besso et al, 1997; Voorhout et al, 1990). In one study of 34 dogs with 36 ATs, abdominal ultrasound was 100% sensitive and 96% specific for identifying the presence of a tumor thrombus within the caudal vena cava. However, when all forms of vascular invasion were evaluated, including patients with vascular wall invasion without a concurrent thrombus, sensitivity and specificity were 76% and 96%, respectively (Davis et al, 2012). With a cortisol-secreting AT, atrophy of the contralateral gland may not always be detectable by ultrasound. No significant difference exists between dimensions of normal adrenals and adrenals contralateral to an AT, and the normal two-layer appearance depicting the medulla and cortex may be seen in atrophied glands (Hoerauf and Reusch, 1999).

Computed Tomography and Magnetic Resonance Imaging

Pituitary

Pituitary imaging provides valuable information regarding treatment options and prognosis. With standard CT, pituitary tumors, if seen, are typically located in the sella turcica (Fig. 10-39) and extend dorsally and laterally along the base of the brain (Fig. 10-40). Of eight pituitary tumors, five were isodense on non-contrast scans, and the remainder were hyperdense. Bilaterally symmetric hydrocephalus, a mass effect, peritumoral edema, and mineralization may also be seen (Turrel et al, 1986; Nelson et al, 1989). Most tumors have minimal to marked contrast enhancement and well-defined margins (Turrel et al, 1986; Voorhout et al, 1990). Contrast enhancement can be homogenous or heterogenous; an area of hypoattenuation may also be seen (Turrel et al, 1986). Small pituitary tumors may not be visualized with or without contrast, so absence of a visualized mass does not rule out PDH. It is likely, however, that a tumor would be seen in all cases where a pituitary mass is causing neurological signs. In cases where neurological signs had developed, a mass was found (Nelson et al, 1989). In dogs with PDH with small pituitary lesions, contrast-enhanced CT may reveal a non-enlarged pituitary (Bertoy et al, 1995; Kooistra et al, 1997b; van der Vlugt-Meijer et al, 2004; Auriemma et al, 2009; Rodriguez Pineiro et al, 2011).

A variation of CT, dynamic contrast-enhanced CT, takes advantage of the difference in pituitary blood supply. Blood supply to the posterior pituitary is direct (arterial), whereas that of the anterior pituitary is mainly indirect via the pituitary portal system. In normal canine pituitaries, after IV administration of contrast medium, the posterior pituitary is identified first as an early intense enhancement of the central part of the gland. In later images, the anterior pituitary is

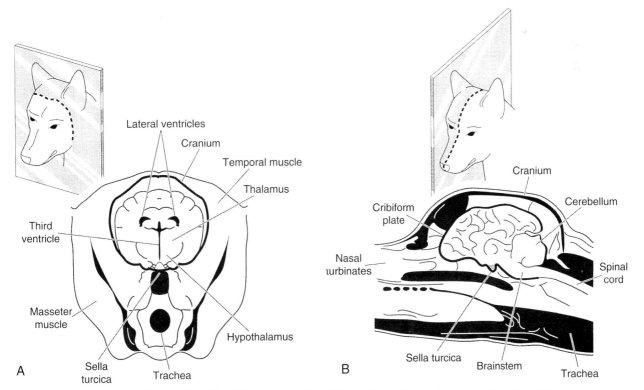

FIGURE 10-39 Orientation of the **(A)** transverse and **(B)** midline sagittal sections on brain scans. (From Bertoy EH, et al.: Magnetic resonance imaging of the brain in dogs with recently diagnosed but untreated pituitary-dependent hyperadrenocorticism, *J Am Vet Med Assoc* 206:651, 1995.)

visualized as a peripheral rim enhancement with a hypodense center (Love et al, 2000; van der Vlugt-Meijer et al, 2003). The initial phase has been termed the *pituitary flush.* The size of the pituitary relative to the brain (the P/B ratio) can also be assessed (Kooistra et al, 1997b). In dogs with PDH, small tumors can be visualized as an increase in P/B ratio or displacement or disruption of the pituitary flush, but the results may still be normal; thus, the sensitivity is not 100% (van der Vlugt-Meijer et al, 2004). If hypophysectomy is being considered, the greater sensitivity of dynamic CT for detecting a pituitary mass of any size may be helpful to ensure the correct treatment is being provided. In other cases, dynamic CT may not be warranted.

Treatment for a pituitary macroadenoma (i.e., an adenoma > 10 mm diameter) requires radiation therapy for local tumor control. Survival post-radiation depends on tumor size and the presence of neurological signs before treatment; the smaller the tumor and the milder the neurological signs (or absent), the better the response to therapy and the longer the survival (Goossens et al, 1998; Theon and Feldman, 1998). In dogs with PDH

followed for 1 year, six dogs (46%) had tumor growth. Of 13 with masses visible on MRI, four (36%) developed neurological signs within 1 year (Bertoy et al, 1995; 1996). Accordingly, CT or MRI should be considered in all dogs with PDH at the time of diagnosis. If no mass is seen, the dog should be treated medically with no follow-up imaging required. If a mass 3 to 7 mm in diameter is seen, medical treatment of the HAC should be administered and imaging should be repeated in 12 to 18 months. If the mass is more than 8 mm in diameter, radiation therapy should be pursued. Medical therapy can be added if clinical signs of HAC are still present after 3 to 6 months or if they recur (Feldman and Nelson, 2004). No benefit has been shown for irradiation of tumors smaller than 8 mm.

MRI has been utilized not as a differentiation test but to assess the size of a pituitary mass in known cases of PDH (Fig. 10-41). Using a 1.5-Tesla magnet for MRI, assessment of signal intensity on a T1-weighted image, as well as displacement of the posterior pituitary lobe, can be helpful in the diagnosis of PDH

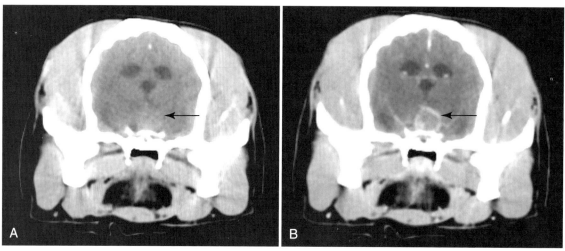

FIGURE 10-40 Pre- **(A)** and post- **(B)** contrast, transverse, 5-mm thick computed tomography (CT) images of the brain at the level of the pituitary fossa. Pre-contrast, mild hyperattenuation in the ventral calvarium dorsal to the pituitary fossa can be seen *(black arrow);* post-contrast, a ring enhancement of this area is visualized *(black arrow).* (Images courtesy of Dr. John Hathcock.)

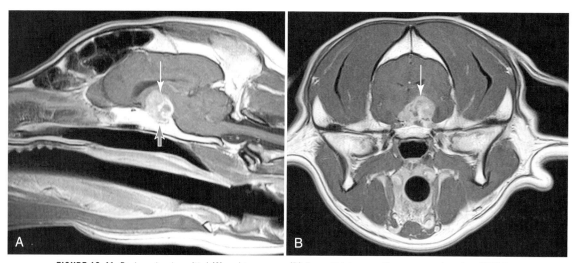

FIGURE 10-41 Post-contrast sagittal **(A)** and transverse **(B)** 5-mm thick magnetic resonance imaging (MRI) images at the level of the pituitary fossa. There is a large non-homogenous, markedly contrast-enhancing mass present in the ventral calvarium arising from the pituitary fossa. (Images courtesy of Dr. John Hathcock.)

(Taoda et al, 2011). However, low-field MRI (0.2-Tesla magnet) provides comparable information as dynamic CT on the presence of pituitary adenomas (Auriemma et al, 2009). In two studies of dogs with PDH that were showing neurologic signs not due to direct mitotane toxicity, a pituitary mass was seen in all. Typically masses causing neurological signs are more than 10 mm in diameter, but a Dachshund with a 5-mm mass had neurological signs. Most tumors are contrast-enhancing (Duesberg et al, 1995; Bertoy et al, 1996).

Although in one study the size of the pituitary tumor correlated with resistance to suppression by dexamethasone (Kooistra et al, 1997b), commercially available biochemical testing cannot reliably differentiate tumor size (Fig. 10-42) (Kipperman et al, 1992; Bertoy et al, 1995; Duesberg et al, 1995; Wood et al, 2007). The absence of neurological abnormalities does not exclude the presence of a pituitary macrotumor (Kipperman et al, 1992; Kooistra et al, 1997b). Measurement of POMC and a precursor to ACTH, pro-ACTH, may be helpful (Bosje et al, 2002; Granger et al, 2005) if the assays become commercially available.

In humans, an "empty sella" is a herniation of the subarachnoidal space into the sella turcica with invisible or reduced size of the pituitary gland; the empty sella syndrome may or may not be associated with endocrine disturbances (Konar et al, 2008). The MRI scans of 377 dogs were reviewed, and a partial or total empty sella was found in 11 (3.6%). Only one dog had a supposed endocrinopathy. The dog had elevations in serum ALP activity and cholesterol concentration, increased eACTH concentration, and bilaterally enlarged adrenal glands. Although an LDDST was supportive of PDH per the authors, the remnants of the pituitary gland found at post mortem were histologically normal (Konar et al, 2008). Thus, the diagnosis of HAC is questionable, and no evidence exists for a link between empty sella and endocrinopathies in general or HAC in particular in dogs.

Abdomen

Abdominal CT is a sensitive way of assessing adrenal gland structure (Fig. 10-43). Hyperplastic glands may appear slightly rounded in comparison to the normal adrenal glands, mineralization not apparent on radiography may be found, and hypoplasia of a gland contralateral to an AT can be seen (Bailey, 1986; Emms et al, 1986). However, enlargement is not always apparent in dogs with PDH (Emms et al, 1986). Unilateral nodular hyperplasia cannot be distinguished from an AT. Poor demarcation, irregular contrast enhancement, and a non-homogenous texture have been suggested to be evidence of malignancy (Voorhout et al, 1990). Contrast enhancement varies (Bailey, 1986; Emms et al, 1986). Although CT can be quite accurate for determining vascular invasion (Rodriguez Pineiro et al, 2011; Figs. 10-44 and 10-45), enlarged adrenal glands may adhere to or compress the vena cava suggesting invasion when it is not present (Emms et al, 1986; Voorhout et al, 1990).

TREATMENT—GENERAL APPROACH

Treatment options and protocols and prognosis vary depending on the form of HAC present. Therefore, differentiation between PDH and AT should be obtained before choosing a therapy. For PDH, the medical options are mainly trilostane and mitotane. In Europe and limited centers within the United States, hypophysectomy (i.e., complete pituitary removal) is available. For ATs, the treatment of choice is adrenalectomy. Surgery is not always possible, however, for numerous reasons. The main medical options are as for PDH. The protocol for mitotane use, however, may be different when treating AT (see Treatment—Medical Management Using Mitotane). Overall, therapy should be selected on the basis of the form of HAC as well as the veterinarian's experience.

Excellent rapport between veterinarian and owner is imperative during the long-term management of HAC. The surgical and medical options should be discussed in detail, including what is

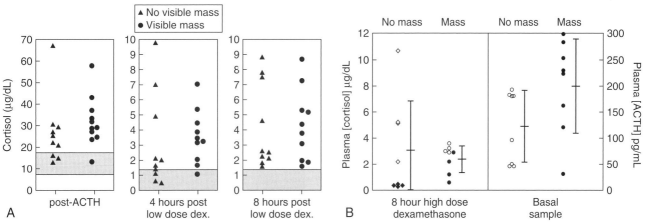

FIGURE 10-42 A, Plasma cortisol concentrations 1 hour after intramuscular (IM) administration of 0.25 mg of synthetic adrenocorticotropic hormone *(ACTH)* and 4 and 8 hours after intravenous (IV) administration of 0.01 mg/kg of dexamethasone in dogs with pituitary-dependent hyperadrenocorticism (PDH). *Triangles* denote dogs without a visible pituitary mass on magnetic resonance imaging (MRI) scan; *circles* denote dogs with a visible pituitary mass on MRI scan. *Shaded areas* indicate reference ranges. **B,** Plasma cortisol concentrations 8 hours after IV administration of 0.1 mg/kg of dexamethasone *(left),* and basal plasma endogenous ACTH (eACTH) concentrations *(right).* *Black diamonds* and *black circles* denote dogs with values less than 50% of baseline cortisol concentrations after dexamethasone administration; *open diamonds* and *open circles* denote dogs with values greater than 50% of baseline cortisol concentrations after dexamethasone administration. (From Bertoy EH, et al.: Magnetic resonance imaging of the brain in dogs with recently diagnosed but untreated pituitary-dependent hyperadrenocorticism, *J Am Vet Med Assoc* 206:651, 1995.)

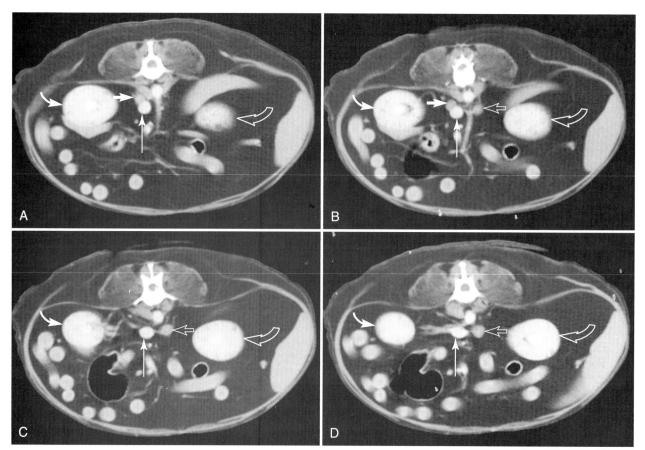

FIGURE 10-43 Series of post-contrast, transverse, 5-mm thick, computed tomography (CT) images demonstrating normal right and left adrenal glands and their relation to the caudal vena cava and right and left kidneys. The sequential scans (**A** through **D**) move progressively from cranial to caudal, showing the right adrenal *(short white arrow)* and right kidney *(curved white arrow)* first; the left adrenal *(short open arrow)* and left kidney *(curved open arrow)* are more caudal. Note also the round, caudal vena cava *(long white arrow)*. Vertebrae can be seen at the top. (Images courtesy of Dr. John Hathcock.)

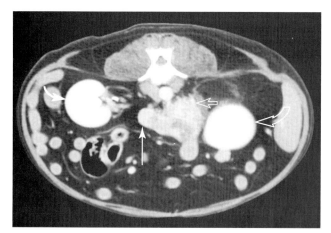

FIGURE 10-44 Post-contrast, transverse, 3-mm thick computed tomography (CT) image at the level of the cranial pole of left kidney. The left adrenal gland is enlarged and irregularly shaped with non-homogeneous, mild contrast enhancement *(short open arrow)*. The right adrenal gland is not visualized. The neoplastic mass extends into the lumen of the caudal vena cava *(long white arrow)*. The right *(curved white arrow)* and left *(curved open arrow)* kidneys can be seen. (Images courtesy of Dr. John Hathcock.)

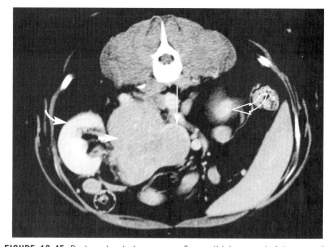

FIGURE 10-45 Post-contrast, transverse, 5-mm thick computed tomography (CT) image at the level of the right kidney *(curved white arrow)*. The right adrenal gland *(short white arrow)* is markedly enlarged and non-homogeneously, mildly contrast-enhancing. Invasion of the mass into the caudal vena cava is seen as a filling defect with a ring of contrast enhancement at the periphery of the caudal vena cava *(long white arrow)*. The cranial pole of the left kidney can be seen *(curved open arrow)*; the left adrenal gland is not visualized. (Image courtesy of Dr. John Hathcock.)

expected of the owner. Owners should understand the advantages and disadvantages of all therapies, including the fact that medical therapy will not cure the disease and therapy will be lifelong. In dogs with PDH, neither mitotane nor trilostane affect the pituitary tumor; therefore excessive ACTH secretion continues or becomes exaggerated (Nelson et al, 1985; Mantis et al, 2003; Witt and Neiger, 2004). Failure to continue therapy usually results in regrowth of the adrenal cortices and return of clinical signs.

To Treat or Not To Treat

An "urban legend" exists that survival is the same whether or not a dog with HAC is treated. That statement has never been scientifically evaluated. It may be true for some dogs, but likely not all. Importantly, treatment typically greatly improves quality of life for both the owner and dog.

On the other hand, not all dogs with positive tests for HAC need to be treated, and the decision should be made on a case-by-case basis. In deciding when to treat, consideration should be given to the dog, quality of life, the owner, and clinical signs. None of the drugs are cheap, and neither mitotane nor trilostane are benign; therefore, treatment is not to be taken lightly. If the only clinical sign is a benign clinicopathologic finding (e.g., elevated serum ALP activity) treatment is not warranted (neither is testing). If the issue is only cosmetic (e.g., poor hair) or very mild (e.g., slight increase in thirst and urination), a frank discussion should be had with the owner of the risks and benefits. In making the decision, further questioning of the owner on issues that might relate to clinical signs (e.g., the dog has stopped jumping on furniture—a sign of possible muscle weakness) can be helpful, as well as seeking evidence of clinical signs that the owner might not note (e.g., serial evaluation of urine samples collected at home for consistent suggestion of polyuria/polydipsia). It is also important to test for proteinuria by measurement of a UPCR and for hypertension by measurement of blood pressure. Both can damage the body; so if either or both are present and due to HAC, treatment may be more imperative. On the other hand, clinical signs may be recognized in retrospect; for example, an owner attributes decreased playing to old age, but when HAC is treated, the activity increases.

Treatment of HAC can unmask diseases that may be inapparent due to the anti-inflammatory effects of hypercortisolemia. For example, clinical signs of atopy or degenerative joint disease may develop with treatment of HAC as cortisol concentrations decrease.

Therapy Without Defining the Underlying Cause

At times, clear differentiation between PDH and AT is not possible due to such issues as owner financial constraints or inconclusive or conflicting results on differentiating tests. In such a situation, given that the vast majority of dogs have PDH, therapy can be initiated accordingly. However, the owners should understand that an accurate prognosis cannot be given and that attempting to differentiate between the forms once therapy is started is quite difficult, if not impossible.

 # TREATMENT—SURGERY

Adrenalectomy

Overview and Selection of Cases

Adrenalectomy is the treatment of choice for a cortisol-secreting AT. It is technically difficult, serious intra- and postoperative complications are common, and the reported mortality is variable but can exceed 25%. Thus, adrenalectomy should be undertaken only by experienced surgeons in a hospital with a well-equipped intensive care unit (ICU) and 24-hour observation and care.

Veterinarians should be realistic when recommending adrenalectomy. Medical treatment offers a viable alternative, especially for aged dogs or dogs at increased risk for anesthetic, surgical, or postsurgical problems and for dogs with documented metastatic disease or extensive major vein thrombosis. Dogs with tumors that are large (diameter > 5 cm), that have infiltrated the kidney or body wall, or that have extensive caudal vena caval invasion (especially thrombi that extend beyond the hepatic hilus) have a high probability of serious postoperative complications and a poor outcome. Similarly, so do dogs with metastatic lesions (typically in the liver and uncommonly in the lungs), with low antithrombin III concentrations, that are debilitated, or that have advanced clinical manifestations of HAC. In general, the probability of a successful outcome is lower, and the likelihood of perioperative complications is greater the larger the AT. Removal of an AT with a diameter of more than 5 cm can be difficult even when surgery is performed by an experienced surgeon. The larger the adrenal mass, the greater the probability it is a carcinoma and that metastasis has occurred, regardless of findings during the preoperative evaluation.

Several studies have evaluated prognostic factors for short-term survival after adrenalectomy (Schwartz et al, 2008; Lang et al, 2011; Massari et al, 2011; Barrera et al, 2013). All dogs undergoing adrenalectomy were included regardless of tumor type (i.e., ATs and pheochromocytomas), although 76% of 240 tumors were histologically classified as adrenocortical adenomas or carcinomas. The definition of short-term survival varied between studies, ranging from 6 to 14 days (i.e., dogs lived at least 6 to 14 days after adrenalectomy). Preoperative variables significantly associated with shorter survival times included size of the AT, presence and extent of vena caval invasion, concurrent azotemia, and presence of acute adrenal hemorrhage (Schwartz et al, 2008; Lang et al, 2011; Barrera et al, 2013). Intraoperative variables associated with shorter survival times included hemorrhage requiring a blood transfusion and concurrent nephrectomy (Schwartz et al, 2008; Barrera et al, 2013). Postoperative variables associated with shorter survival times included development of pancreatitis, PTE, acute renal failure, disseminated intravascular coagulation, hypotension, and hypoxemia (Schwartz et al, 2008; Barrera et al, 2013). In one study, extensive vena caval invasion was the most significant risk factor for poor short-term survival (Barrera et al, 2013).

Imaging provides valuable information about tumor size. In general, a "small" AT is arbitrarily defined as being 4 cm or less in maximum diameter and a "large" tumor is arbitrarily defined as 5 cm or more in maximum diameter. Small tumors are more likely to be adenomas, well-encapsulated, and somewhat easier to remove surgically than large tumors, which are usually carcinomas, not well-encapsulated, and can be difficult to excise surgically. However, adrenocortical carcinomas also may be "small." Histologic evaluation of any tumor is imperative in order to determine appropriate postoperative and long-term care.

Preoperative Evaluation and Management

Cortisol-secreting AT are challenging to manage following adrenalectomy, in part, because of concurrent immunosuppression, impaired wound healing, systemic hypertension, and a hypercoagulative state; frequent tumoral infiltration into surrounding blood vessels and soft tissues; potential postoperative development of pancreatitis (especially with a right-sided adrenal mass); and existence of hypoadrenocorticism following removal of the mass. The most worrisome complication of adrenalectomy is thromboembolism, which typically develops during or within 24 hours of surgery and carries a high mortality rate (see Postoperative Complications and Survival). Several steps may help minimize this complication. Medical control of the HAC prior to surgery for 3 to 4 weeks can reverse the metabolic derangements and minimize many of the complications associated with surgical removal of a cortisol-secreting AT. Because the treatment is expected to be short-term, trilostane may be preferred (Vetoryl, Dechra Veterinary Products; 1 mg/kg every 12 hours initially). An ACTH stimulation test should be performed and serum electrolytes should be measured prior to and 10 to 14 days after initiating treatment (see Treatment—Medical Management with Trilostane). The goals of therapy are improvement in clinical signs and a post-ACTH serum cortisol concentration between 2 and 6 µg/dL (55 to 170 nmol/L). The dosage of trilostane is adjusted as needed. Serum electrolytes are monitored for changes consistent with hypoaldosteronism. Adrenalectomy should be performed once the hypercortisolemia is controlled but no later than 30 days after initiating medical treatment, regardless of the state of control of the disease.

On the day prior to surgery, thoracic radiographs should be performed to ensure that metastatic disease is not present (Fig. 10-46) and an abdominal ultrasound—or better yet CT or MRI, if available—should be done to assess the size of the adrenal mass; presence of metastatic disease or invasion of the mass into the phrenicoabdominal vein, caudal vena cava, or surrounding tissues; and evidence of hemorrhage within the tumor or retroperitoneal space. Surgery may not be indicated if unexpected or previously unrecognized complications are identified, which significantly increase the risk for intra- or postoperative complications. Adrenal tumors typically metastasize to the liver or lungs, or both. Approximately 10% of dogs with HAC caused by an AT have obvious metastases at the time of initial examination.

Abdominal ultrasound is a good screening test for identification of metastases and vascular invasion (Davis et al, 2012). If metastasis is suspected, an ultrasound-guided biopsy of the lesions can be performed for confirmation. However, CT may be preferred, because significant and critical differences between findings on ultrasound versus CT regarding size of the tumor and presence and severity of vascular invasion and infiltration of surrounding soft tissues may occur. CT scans are a non-invasive and effective method for evaluating the size and shape of the adrenal glands and the presence and severity of invasion of the tumor into blood vessels, surrounding organs, and body wall. CT may also be used to identify metastatic disease (Voorhout et al, 1990; Widmer and Guptill, 1995; Hill and Scott-Moncrieff, 2001).

In addition to routine blood and urine tests, systemic blood pressure should be measured and hypertension treated accordingly. Cross-matching should be performed in anticipation of a blood transfusion during or after surgery. Assessment of a UPCR and serum antithrombin III concentrations is also recommended. If the UPCR is significantly increased, the antithrombin III concentration significantly decreased, or both, the dog may be at greater risk for thromboembolism than the typical dog with HAC (Ortega et al, 1995; Jacoby et al, 2001).

Surgical Approaches

The recommended surgical approach is either paracostal (flank), or ventral midline. In dogs, the ventral midline laparotomy is most commonly used; compared to other approaches, it provides the best

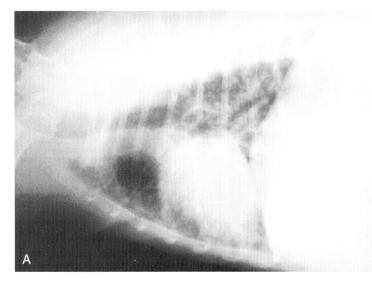
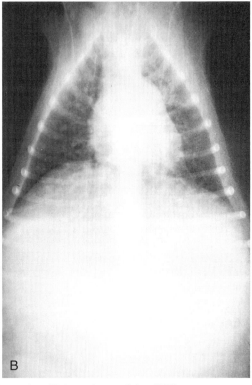

FIGURE 10-46 Lateral **(A)** and dorsoventral **(B)** thoracic radiographs from a dog with hyperadrenocorticism (HAC) caused by an adrenocortical tumor (AT) that has metastasized to the lungs.

opportunity for visualization of both adrenal glands as well as other abdominal structures for evidence of metastasis and provides better exposure of the vena cava if vascular occlusion is required during resection (Adin and Nelson, 2012). On the other hand, exposure of the dorsal retroperitoneal space can be challenging in deep-chested dogs and postoperative pancreatitis is a concern, especially with right-sided adrenal tumors (Fig. 10-47). For dogs with large masses and for tumors that are difficult to visualize, are invading vascular structures (most commonly the vena cava), or are infiltrating the kidney or abdominal wall, exposure can be improved by adding a flank (paracostal) incision to the ventral midline approach. Theoretically, the flank approach has the advantage of improved exposure to the dorsal abdomen, including the vena cava and aorta, and

it avoids the risk of abdominal herniation through a ventral midline incision in dogs with poor wound healing (see Fig. 10-47). It is best suited for unilateral, uncomplicated adrenal masses.

Laparoscopy

Laparoscopic adrenalectomy can be done in dogs with non-invasive adrenal masses. Advantages of minimally invasive laparoscopic adrenalectomy include better visualization of abdominal organs and the adrenal mass, limited manipulation of other abdominal organs, decreased surgical wound complications, improved postoperative comfort, faster recovery period, and a shorter hospital stay (Jiménez Peláez et al, 2008; Naan et al, 2013). Dogs are placed in a sternal or oblique lateral position, and three or four ports for

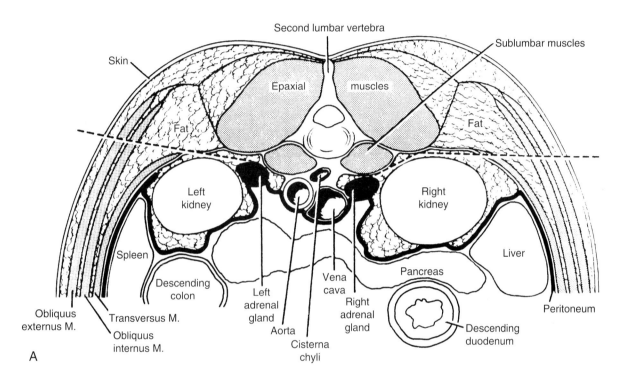

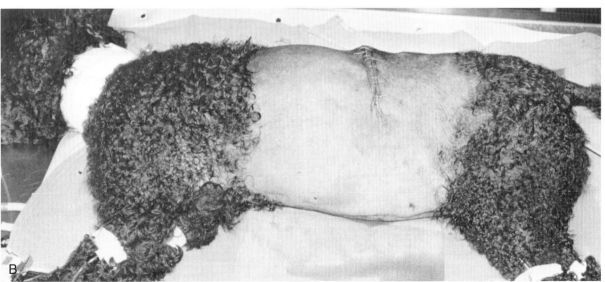

FIGURE 10-47 **A,** Anatomic diagram showing the location of the canine adrenal glands and the surgical approach *(dashed lines)* via paracostal incisions to each gland. **B,** Photograph of a dog with hyperadrenocorticism (HAC) caused by an adrenal tumor that was removed via the paracostal approach. (**A,** From Johnston D: Adrenalectomy via retroperitoneal approach in dogs, *J Am Vet Med Assoc* 170:1093, 1977.)

the camera, operative instruments, and a retractor are inserted into the abdominal cavity (Fig. 10-48). The abdominal viscera, including the pancreas, should move ventrally due to gravity, creating a working space for access to the adrenal mass while minimizing manipulation of other viscera (Fig. 10-49). Adrenal masses with a diameter up to 5 cm can be removed. In a preliminary evaluation, Mayhew and other soft tissue surgeons at the University of California, Davis (UC Davis) compared the perioperative morbidity and mortality in 23 dogs undergoing laparoscopic adrenalectomy to that of 25 dogs that underwent adrenalectomy using a ventral midline laparotomy. The ATs were similarly sized and non-invasive. Perioperative death did not occur in the laparoscopy group, but two dogs in the laparotomy group died. Surgery time and postoperative hospitalization time were significantly shorter in the laparoscopy group. In the UC Davis experience, with laparoscopy, recovery from surgery is quicker, postoperative discomfort

is noticeably less, most dogs are ambulatory a few hours post-anesthesia, and many are discharged the next day. Postoperative pancreatitis and PTE are very uncommon, especially if dogs are treated with trilostane for 3 to 4 weeks prior to surgery.

See *Small Animal Surgery* by Fossum (2012) and *Veterinary Surgery: Small Animal* by Tobias and Johnston (2012) for more detailed information on the surgical techniques for adrenalectomy.

Intra- and Postoperative Management

Autonomous cortisol secretion from an AT suppresses pituitary ACTH release via negative feedback, resulting in significant atrophy of normal cortisol-secreting cells in the contralateral adrenal gland. Therefore, acute hypocortisolism is expected after surgery. Suppression of eACTH by the tumor may also cause some atrophy of aldosterone-secreting cells.

Glucocorticoid therapy is not indicated before adrenalectomy, because it may worsen hypertension, cause overhydration, and increase the risk of thromboembolic episodes. Beginning with anesthesia, IV fluids should be administered at a surgical maintenance rate. In order to preemptively address the acute hypocortisolism that will occur, once the tumor is identified by the surgeon, dexamethasone (0.05 to 0.1 mg/kg) should be placed in the IV infusion bottle and given over 6 hours. A tapering dexamethasone dose (e.g., decreasing the dose by 0.02 mg/kg/24 hours but going no lower than 0.02 mg/kg) should continue to be administered IV at 12-hour intervals until the dog can safely be given oral medication without the danger of vomiting (typically 24 to 48 hours postoperatively). At that point, the glucocorticoid supplement should be switched to oral prednisone (0.25 to 0.5 mg/kg b.i.d. [bis in die; twice a day]). Once the dog is eating and drinking on its own, the frequency of prednisone administration should be decreased to once a day and given in the morning. The dosage is then gradually reduced in small increments at 2 to 4 week intervals during the ensuing 3 to 6 months, as long as the dog maintains an appetite and does not develop lethargy or vomiting, until the dosage is extremely low. If a unilateral adrenalectomy has been performed, prednisone supplementation can eventually be discontinued once the contralateral normal adrenocortical tissue becomes functional. ACTH stimulation tests can be used to guide prednisone therapy; if the dog has a normal ACTH stimulation test result, prednisone administration

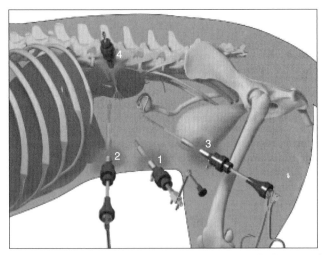

FIGURE 10-48 Schematic of portal placement in a dog undergoing laparoscopic adrenalectomy. The dog is placed in oblique lateral recumbency and four portals are placed for the camera *(1)*, operative instruments *(2 and 3)*, and a retractor *(4)*. (Illustration by Tim Vojt; from Adin CA. Nelson RW: Adrenal glands. In Tobias KM, Johnston SA, editors: *Veterinary surgery: small animal,* St Louis, 2012, Elsevier Saunders, p. 2040.)

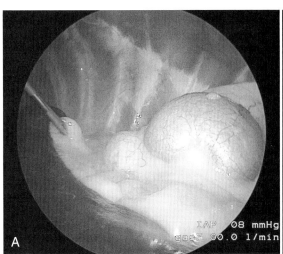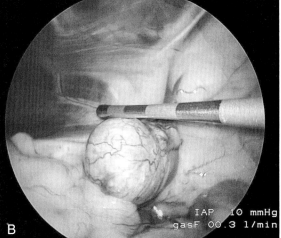

FIGURE 10-49 A, A cortisol-secreting adrenal mass *(left)* and laparoscopic images of the kidney *(right)* in a dog shortly after placement of the ports and insertion of the camera. The dog's head is to the left. **B,** Adrenal mass in **A** after dissection of the mass from surrounding structures and just prior to removal. (Images courtesy of Phil Mayhew.)

is no longer needed. An ACTH stimulation test can also be used to confirm a glucocorticoid deficiency and the need to increase the prednisone dosage if a dog becomes listless, anorectic, or ill during the tapering process. Lifelong prednisone at a dosage of 0.1 to 0.2 mg/kg administered once or twice daily is required for dogs that had a bilateral adrenalectomy.

Alternatively, rather than assuming that glucocorticoid supplementation is needed, an ACTH stimulation test may be completed 6 to 8 hours after surgery to assess the success of surgery and the need for glucocorticoid therapy. If results are low (pre-ACTH and post-ACTH serum cortisol concentrations < 1 μg/dL [30 nmol/L]), the surgery was likely a success, and this provides proof that glucocorticoid therapy is necessary; however, nonfunctional metastases are still a possibility. If the results are similar to those obtained prior to surgery, then remnant functional tumor tissue is still present and exogenous glucocorticoids are not necessary.

Serum electrolyte concentrations should be closely monitored postoperatively. Development of mild hyponatremia and hyperkalemia is common within 72 hours of surgery and usually resolves in 1 to 2 days as exogenous glucocorticoid doses are reduced and the dog begins to eat. Because short-term mineralocorticoid therapy is rather benign and because it is not possible to determine which dogs will have transient problems and which will have serious mineralocorticoid deficits, treatment is recommended if these abnormalities become worrisome (i.e., serum sodium < 135 mEq/L or serum potassium > 6.5 mEq/L) or if they persist longer than 72 hours. An injection of desoxycorticosterone pivalate (DOCP; Percorten-V, Novartis Pharmaceuticals) is recommended with measurement of serum electrolytes performed 14 and 25 days after the injection (see Chapter 12). If a unilateral adrenalectomy was done, the dog is healthy, and serum electrolytes are normal on day 25, the dog should be reevaluated 7 days later. If serum electrolytes are still normal, additional DOCP treatment is not needed. In the author's experience, a second dose has never been needed. If bilateral adrenalectomy is performed, DOCP therapy will be lifelong.

Alternatively, fludrocortisone acetate (0.02 mg/kg; see Chapter 12) can be used in place of DOCP. Oral mineralocorticoids can be given twice daily. If a unilateral adrenalectomy was performed, fludrocortisone administration can usually be tapered and discontinued within 1 to 2 weeks. Serum electrolyte concentrations can be measured during tapering and a few days after discontinuation to ensure that they are within reference ranges. If hyperkalemia or hyponatremia are present, the fludrocortisone dose should be increased or reinitiated, and tapering over 10 to 14 days should be attempted again.

Postoperative Complications and Survival

The most worrisome complication following removal of a cortisol-secreting AT is thromboembolism, which typically occurs during or within 24 hours of surgery and carries a high mortality rate. Several steps can help minimize this complication (see earlier). The first is to be realistic about case selection for adrenalectomy (see Overview and Selection of Cases). With proper case selection and management, anticoagulation therapy is no longer recommended unless PTE develops. Anesthetic drugs and pain medications should be administered at dosages that allow a dog to be ambulatory within 4 hours of surgery. Anesthesia time should be as short as possible; additional procedures "while the dog is under anesthesia" should not be done. If available, laparoscopic adrenalectomy should be performed whenever possible. Dogs should

have frequent, short walks (every 2 to 3 hours) to promote blood flow and minimize clot formation.

Postoperative complications following adrenalectomy are common with reported rates as high as 50%. Two recent retrospective studies reported postoperative complication rates of 30% and 35% for 60 and 41 dogs, respectively (Schwartz et al, 2008; Lang et al, 2011). Postoperative complications include pancreatitis, PTE, acute renal failure, septic peritonitis, hypoadrenocorticism, hypotension, cardiac arrhythmias, and cardiac arrest (Schwartz et al, 2008; Lang et al, 2011; Barrera et al, 2013).

In four recent studies, the reported postoperative mortality was 22% for 41 dogs with an adrenal tumor (Schwartz et al, 2008), 13% for 47 dogs with an AT (Lang et al, 2011), 15% for 52 dogs with an adrenal tumor (Massari et al, 2011), and 25.5% for 86 dogs with an adrenal tumor (Barrera et al, 2013). In total, post-adrenalectomy mortality was reported in 45 of 226 dogs (20%).

It is difficult to assess the severity of compromised wound healing in a dog with HAC. Thus, stitches should not be removed until regrowth of hair in the region of the incision is evident—no matter which surgical approach was used.

Median survival time for the dogs that survived the postoperative period and were discharged from the hospital was 690 days, 492 days, 953 days, and 48 months (Schwartz et al, 2008; Lang et al, 2011; Massari et al, 2011; Barrera et al, 2013). Long-term survival time was significantly shorter in dogs with adrenal adenocarcinomas, adrenal tumors with a diameter of 5 cm or more, metastases, and vena cava thrombosis (Massari et al, 2011). Survival time was also significantly shorter when adrenalectomy was combined with additional abdominal surgical intervention.

Hypophysectomy

For several decades, selective pituitary microsurgery using the transsphenoidal approach has been considered the treatment of choice for pituitary tumors causing HAC in humans (Melby, 1988; Rees et al, 2002). Initial studies in veterinary medicine developing the microsurgical technique, identifying postoperative complications and assessing postoperative pituitary function, or lack thereof, were done in healthy dogs approximately 25 years ago (Lantz et al, 1988; Niebauer and Evans, 1988; Niebauer et al, 1990). Since then, Meij and colleagues at Utrecht University, the Netherlands, have published several articles detailing their experiences with transsphenoidal hypophysectomy in dogs with PDH, beginning with a detailed description of their microsurgical technique and assessment of pituitary function after transsphenoidal hypophysectomy in healthy Beagle dogs (Meij et al, 1997a; 1997b) and followed by short-term (≤ 3 years) results of transsphenoidal hypophysectomy in 52 dogs with PDH (Meij et al, 1998).

In 2005, the Utrecht group reported on the long-term results of transsphenoidal hypophysectomy in 150 dogs with PDH (Hanson et al, 2005). Preoperatively, the pituitary glands, as measured by contrast-enhanced CT or MRI images, ranged in height from 2.1 to 15 mm (median, 5.1 mm), in width from 3.3 to 17 mm (median, 6.1 mm), and in length from 2 to 18 mm (median, 5.0 mm). The pituitary glands were not enlarged in 74 dogs, with a pituitary-to-brain ratio ranging from 0.15 to 0.31 and were enlarged in 76 dogs with pituitary-to-brain ratios ranging from 0.32 to 0.76.

Postoperative complications included central diabetes insipidus (CDI), hypernatremia, keratoconjunctivitis sicca (KCS), and secondary hypothyroidism (Meij et al, 1998; Hanson et al, 2005).

Postoperative hormonal replacement therapy included synthetic vasopressin (DDAVP), glucocorticoids, and levothyroxine. Postoperative CDI was transient in 78% of 127 dogs; DDAVP was discontinued 2 weeks after surgery in 47% and eventually discontinued in an additional 31% a median of 133 days (range, 28 to 1329 days) post-surgery (Hanson et al, 2005). CDI was present until death or until latest follow-up in 22% of the dogs. In another study, the incidence of postoperative permanent CDI in dogs undergoing transsphenoidal surgery for PDH was strongly influenced by the size of the pituitary tumor; the larger the tumor, the more likely for postoperative CDI to be permanent (Teshima et al, 2011).

Blepharospasm and KCS developed postoperatively in 31% of 150 dogs, occurred more frequently in the left eye, and required treatment for a median of 58 (right eye) and 70 days (left eye) (Hanson et al, 2005). Low tear production remained until death in approximately 7% of affected dogs. The KCS is believed to result from direct (trauma) or indirect (ischemia) neuropraxia of the major petrosal nerves during surgery (Meij et al, 1997a).

Twelve of the 150 dogs died within 4 weeks of surgery. One hundred twenty seven (92%) of 138 dogs that were alive after 4 weeks experienced remission within 8 weeks of surgery; remission was defined as resolution of clinical signs of HAC and UC:CR values in the reference range. Nine dogs had residual disease, one dog had suspected ectopic ACTH production, and one dog was lost to follow-up. HAC remained in remission in 95 of 127 dogs (75%). In 32 of 127 dogs (25%), signs of HAC and increased UC:CR values recurred at 6 weeks to 56 months (median, 18.3 months) after surgery. The 1-year, 2-year, 3-year, and 4-year estimated survival rate was approximately 84%, 76%, 72%, and 68%, respectively. The 1-year, 2-year, 3-year, and 4-year estimated relapse-free fraction was approximately 88%, 75%, 66%, and 59%, respectively. Survival and disease-free fractions of dogs with enlarged pituitaries (pituitary-to-brain ratios > 0.31) were significantly lower than in dogs with non-enlarged pituitaries.

Based on the experiences at Utrecht University, microsurgical transsphenoidal hypophysectomy is an effective long-term treatment of PDH in dogs. Early diagnosis of a corticotroph adenoma is important. Transsphenoidal hypophysectomy is most effective in dogs with non-enlarged or moderately enlarged pituitaries. Size of the pituitary tumor has a direct impact on survival, disease-free fractions, and incidence of permanent CDI in dogs. Unfortunately, the number of sites currently offering hypophysectomy as a treatment option for PDH is very limited in the United States.

TREATMENT—MEDICAL MANAGEMENT USING MITOTANE

Mitotane (o,p'-DDD [Lysodren]) was the mainstay of medical therapy of canine HAC for many years. A chlorinated hydrocarbon, mitotane is adrenocorticolytic, causing selective necrosis of the zona fasciculata and zona reticularis, which are the adrenocortical zones that secrete cortisol and sex hormones. Mitotane covalently binds to adrenal proteins following its metabolism in adrenocortical tissue to a reactive acyl chloride intermediate (Cai et al, 1995). The toxin is fairly specific for the adrenal glands (Kirk et al, 1974). However, in normal dogs, mitotane caused fatty degeneration and centrolobular atrophy of the liver, and hepatotoxicity secondary to mitotane therapy for HAC has occurred (Webb and Twedt, 2006).

The advantages of using mitotane are a high efficacy, especially for PDH, and the ability to monitor therapy objectively by use of an ACTH stimulation test. Disadvantages are a relatively high rate of adverse effects and the adrenocorticolytic effects may not be reversible. Although the zona glomerulosa is relatively resistant

to the effects of mitotane, aldosterone secretion can be decreased by mitotane (Golden and Lothrop, 1988; Goy-Thollot et al, 2002; Reid et al, 2014) and complete adrenocortical insufficiency can occur in 6% to 10% of dogs receiving mitotane (Kintzer and Peterson, 1991). Aldosterone deficiency can be life-threatening.

Interestingly, normal dogs appear relatively resistant to the adrenocorticolytic effects of mitotane. Four healthy dogs received 50 mg/kg of mitotane 5 days per week. Two of the four died after 20 and 21 months of therapy, respectively. The third dog was euthanized after 21 months of therapy, and the fourth dog was alive after 38 months of receiving the drug (Nelson and Woodard, 1949). An additional 10 dogs were treated at a dosage of 50 mg/kg/day. One dog died after 124 consecutive days of treatment, and a second died after 147 days. The remaining eight dogs were clinically healthy at the time of euthanasia, after 36 to 150 consecutive days of drug therapy. The dogs, however, had biochemical evidence of decreased adrenocortical reserve after 3 to 10 days of therapy (Kirk et al, 1974).

Therapy of HAC with mitotane occurs in two phases: induction (loading) and maintenance. Before initiation of therapy, the dog's attitude, activity, daily water intake, and appetite should be carefully observed. Awareness of these factors aids in assessment of treatment success or failure and in recognition of adverse reactions or the development of new problems, such as those associated with a growing pituitary tumor. The presence of a decreased appetite at any time is a contraindication to administration of mitotane without further assessment.

Loading is typically done with the patient at home. The loading phase can be long (see later). In addition, eating and drinking behavior are important to judgment of efficacy, and both can be diminished by hospitalization.

Pituitary-Dependent Hyperadrenocorticism

Loading Phase

General Protocol. Before dispensing the medication, the owner should receive thorough instructions on what should be monitored and when the drug should be discontinued. For treatment of PDH, a starting dose of 40 to 50 mg/kg divided twice daily (i.e., 20 to 25 mg/kg b.i.d.) by mouth should be used (Kintzer and Peterson, 1991). Mitotane should always be given with food, because this increases the bioavailability of intact tablets (Watson et al, 1987). In smaller dogs, division may be impossible due to a 500-mg pill size, and the drug can be given in one dose. Doses higher than 50 mg/kg/day increase the risk of complete cortisol deficiency (Kintzer and Peterson, 1991). Loading should end when appetite decreases, vomiting or diarrhea occurs, the patient becomes listless, water intake drops to less than 60 mL/kg/day (1 cup = 240 mL and 1 oz = 30 mL) or for a maximum of 8 days (Fig. 10-50). Feeding twice daily during loading allows better assessment of appetite. Appetite changes can be subtle, including eating slower than usual. In order to closely monitor the patient, best judge the endpoint, and impress on an owner the seriousness of overdosing, daily calls to the owner may be helpful. When signs suggest loading is complete or at the end of 8 days if no changes have occurred, adrenal reserve is assessed by ACTH stimulation testing. When performing ACTH stimulation tests for monitoring, a dose of 1 µg/kg cosyntropin can be used (Aldridge et al, 2014). If the signs of HAC have not changed, daily therapy can continue until the results of the ACTH stimulation test are known; otherwise, mitotane should be discontinued while awaiting the laboratory report.

Coadministration of glucocorticoids to ease loading or avoid signs of glucocorticoid deficiency if hypocortisolemia occurs is controversial. A concern is that coadministration of glucocorticoids

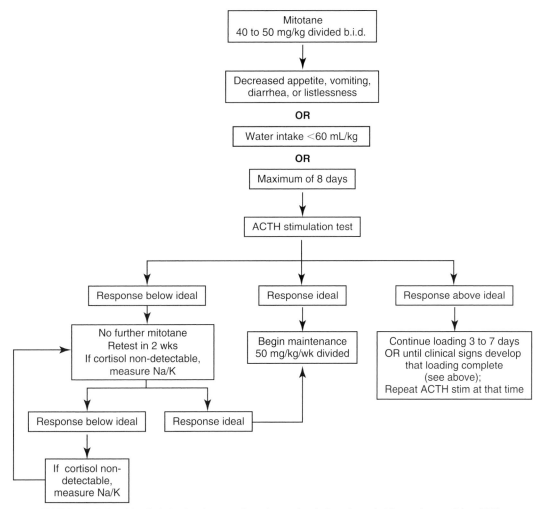

FIGURE 10-50 Algorithm for induction therapy using mitotane for pituitary-dependent hyperadrenocorticism (PDH). The ideal range for basal and adrenocorticotropic hormone *(ACTH)*-stimulated cortisol concentration is approximately 1 to 5 μg/dL (30 to 150 nmol/L) pre- and post-ACTH; readers should check with their laboratory for their recommended range. (In Rand J, editor: *Clinical endocrinology of companion animals,* Ames, IA, 2013, Wiley-Blackwell, p. 55.)

will obscure the endpoint leading to continued therapy and possible overdose; however, some authors do not believe that to be the case (Kintzer and Peterson, 1991). Prednisone can be dispensed (0.2 mg/kg) for an owner to give if moderate to severe vomiting and/or diarrhea occur. However, once prednisone is administered, an ACTH stimulation test should not be done for at least 12 hours due to cross reactivity of prednisone in cortisol assays.

The duration of loading cannot be predicted by severity of disease or pretreatment cortisol concentrations (Kintzer and Peterson, 1991). The success of mitotane therapy is judged mainly by performance of ACTH stimulation tests with the goal of the induction phase being serum cortisol concentrations pre- and post-ACTH stimulation in the lower part of the normal resting range (e.g., cortisol concentration of 1 to 5 μg/dL [30 to 150 nmol/L] pre- and post-ACTH). Clinical signs should be taken into account as well; for example, a post-ACTH cortisol concentration of approximately 5 to 8 μg/dL (150 to 220 nmol/L) is acceptable if the clinical signs have resolved and the dog is doing well. Dogs with PDH that continue to have responses to ACTH in the range for normal dogs (e.g., post-ACTH cortisol concentration of 8 to 20 μg/dL [220 to 560 nmol/L]) tend to have ongoing clinical signs. If pre- and post-ACTH cortisol concentrations are within the ideal range, maintenance therapy should begin. If cortisol concentrations are above the desired range, loading should continue for another 3 to

7 days depending on how close the concentrations are to the ideal or until clinical signs occur that suggest loading has been completed. Evaluation of the UC:CR is not a reliable monitoring tool (Angles et al, 1997; Guptill et al, 1997; Randolph et al, 1998).

The mean time required to achieve adequate control is 11 days, but up to 2 months is possible (Kintzer and Peterson, 1991). In general, smaller dogs (< 12.5 kg) and those receiving phenobarbital may require greater than average induction times. Approximately 33% of dogs will have a serum cortisol concentration less than ideal (e.g., post-ACTH cortisol concentration < 1 μg/dL [30 nmol/L]) after induction; mitotane therapy should be discontinued and an ACTH stimulation test performed after 2 weeks to assess adrenal function. Prednisone should be administered at physiological doses (0.2 mg/kg) during that time, but none should be given in the 12 to 24 hours before performing an ACTH stimulation test. In most dogs, serum cortisol concentrations will rise into the ideal range within 2 to 6 weeks, but up to 18 months may be needed (Kintzer and Peterson, 1991). When documentation of recovery of cortisol secretion occurs and the concentrations are in the ideal range, maintenance therapy can be initiated. If the cortisol concentrations are much greater than ideal when recovery is first recognized, loading will have to be performed again.

Adverse Effects. Adverse effects are generally gastrointestinal or neurological and include weakness, vomiting, anorexia, diarrhea, and/or ataxia. One or more adverse effects occur in approximately 25% of dogs with PDH during loading (Kintzer and Peterson, 1991). They develop as serum cortisol concentration falls rapidly and typically resolve quickly with appropriate therapy. If adverse effects occur, mitotane administration should be discontinued and prednisone administered (0.2 mg/kg) until the dog can be examined, an ACTH stimulation test performed, and serum electrolytes measured to assess possible aldosterone deficiency. Most dogs show a clinical response to glucocorticoid administration within 2 to 3 hours. Persistence of apparent adverse effects may signify the presence of another medical problem.

Gastrointestinal signs can be difficult to interpret because they could be due to direct drug toxicity, hypocortisolemia, or another problem (Fig. 10-51). It is the author's impression that during loading, dogs may develop a relative cortisol deficiency. Because they have been hypercortisolemic for a prolonged period, a sudden decrease in cortisol concentrations may cause signs of hypocortisolemia, even if the cortisol concentrations are within or slightly above the ideal range. It is further the author's impression that treatment with prednisone for 2 to 4 days suffices; the clinical signs abate and do not return after the prednisone is discontinued. If they do, another cause should be sought.

Resistance to Mitotane. If a dog does not respond to the induction protocol after 21 days, the following factors that could contribute to mitotane resistance should be considered:

1. The patient may have an AT, which is more resistant to mitotane.
2. The patient may be inherently resistant to mitotane; some dogs with PDH have required up to 60 days of daily therapy or doses of 100 to 150 mg/kg/day. Smaller dogs may require higher doses (Kintzer and Peterson, 1991).
3. The induction dose is too low. Dogs receiving less than 40 mg/kg/day are less likely to be adequately controlled after 10 days.
4. The drug is not being absorbed well. Ensure the medication is being given with food, preferably a fatty meal.
5. The diagnosis may be incorrect or the patient has iatrogenic HAC.
6. The drug may not be potent; replacing the owner's supply should be considered.
7. The dog is receiving another drug that is interfering with the actions of mitotane. In one study, the two dogs that required the highest weekly maintenance dosages of mitotane (330 and 318 mg/kg) were both receiving anticonvulsant drugs (Kintzer and Peterson, 1991).
8. The owner may not be giving the medication as directed.

Diabetic Patients. Special consideration should be given to patients with concomitant HAC and diabetes mellitus, although the combination is uncommon. Therapy for the diabetes mellitus should begin immediately upon diagnosis. If the two diseases are diagnosed simultaneously, a low dose of insulin should be initiated to prevent ketoacidosis (see Chapter 6). Attempts to control the diabetes mellitus are not recommended until the HAC is in remission because the insulin dose will diminish once cortisol concentrations decrease. Similarly, if a long-term diabetic has insulin resistance secondary to HAC and requires large doses of insulin for adequate glycemic control, treatment with mitotane usually removes the insulin resistance and can lead to a rapid decrease in insulin requirement. Consequently, insulin overdosage and hypoglycemia may occur if the insulin dose is not decreased. In eight out of 11 dogs with concurrent PDH and diabetes mellitus that were treated with mitotane, the mean insulin requirement decreased from 4.6 U/kg/day (range, 3.3 to 6.6) to 1.7 U/kg/day

(range, 0.7 to 2.2), usually within the first 3 weeks of therapy. In the other three dogs, the insulin requirement did not change despite control of the HAC (Peterson et al, 1981); another cause of insulin resistance was suspected.

To try to slow the return to insulin sensitivity and avoid hypoglycemia, the recommended induction dose for dogs with concurrent HAC and diabetes mellitus is 25 mg/kg once daily. Furthermore, although administration of prednisone during induction therapy for PDH is discouraged in general by some authors because it may obscure recognition of having achieved the endpoint of loading, prednisone (0.4 mg/kg once daily) should be given to diabetics receiving induction phase mitotane to help avoid hypoglycemia. Even with these precautions, diabetic patients should be monitored more closely than usual during induction. Because uncontrolled diabetes mellitus causes polyuria/polydipsia and polyphagia, decreases in water drinking, appetite, and urine production may not occur even if the HAC is controlled. If a dog is receiving insulin when mitotane therapy is initiated, the first recheck ACTH stimulation test should occur as usual (day 8 of loading), and the diabetic control should be checked as well.

Maintenance Therapy

General. Maintenance therapy will be necessary for the remainder of the dog's life, although the dose and frequency varies between patients and can vary in an individual patient over time (Fig. 10-52). In the absence of maintenance therapy, adrenal gland hyperplasia recurs in response to continued ACTH secretion. The maintenance phase uses a much lower mitotane dose of 50 mg/kg/week by mouth (Kintzer and Peterson, 1991) divided into as many days of treatment each week as is logical and convenient (e.g., if a dog is scheduled to receive one tablet weekly, one-quarter tablet can be given 4 days per week). Because approximately 60% of dogs with PDH on maintenance mitotane therapy, especially those receiving less than 50 mg/kg/week, relapse within 12 months of starting therapy (Kintzer and Peterson, 1991), an ACTH stimulation test should be performed 1, 3, and 6 months after initiating maintenance therapy and approximately every 3 months thereafter to ensure continued control. If the pre- and post-ACTH serum cortisol concentrations are in the ideal range, therapy can remain as is. If the post-ACTH cortisol concentration is mildly elevated (e.g., 5 to 9 µg/dL [150 to 250 nmol/L]), the maintenance dose should be increased 25% and the dog retested after 1 month to determine if adequate control has been achieved. If so, maintenance therapy should continue at the new dose. If serum cortisol concentrations are still above ideal, reinstitution of induction therapy should be considered. If the post-ACTH cortisol concentration is moderately to greatly increased (e.g., > 9 µg/dL [250 nmol/L]), loading therapy should be reinstituted. If induction therapy is reinitiated, the decision to end loading should be based on the same clinical signs as during the initial loading or it should be continued for a maximum of 7 days. Once serum cortisol concentrations are again within the ideal range, maintenance therapy should be reinstituted at a 50% higher mitotane dosage.

In 184 dogs with PDH treated with mitotane for a mean of 2 years, the final maintenance dosage required ranged from 27 to 330 mg/kg/week, with the two highest doses required by dogs also receiving phenobarbital. Median survival time was 1.7 years (range, 10 days to 8.2 years) with the response judged as excellent in 83%, fair in 16%, and poor in 0.6% (Kintzer and Peterson, 1991).

Adverse Effects. Approximately 33% of dogs on maintenance therapy develop adverse effects including anorexia, vomiting, weakness, diarrhea, and/or ataxia, typically shortly after initiation of a maintenance dosage or during periods of relapse when daily

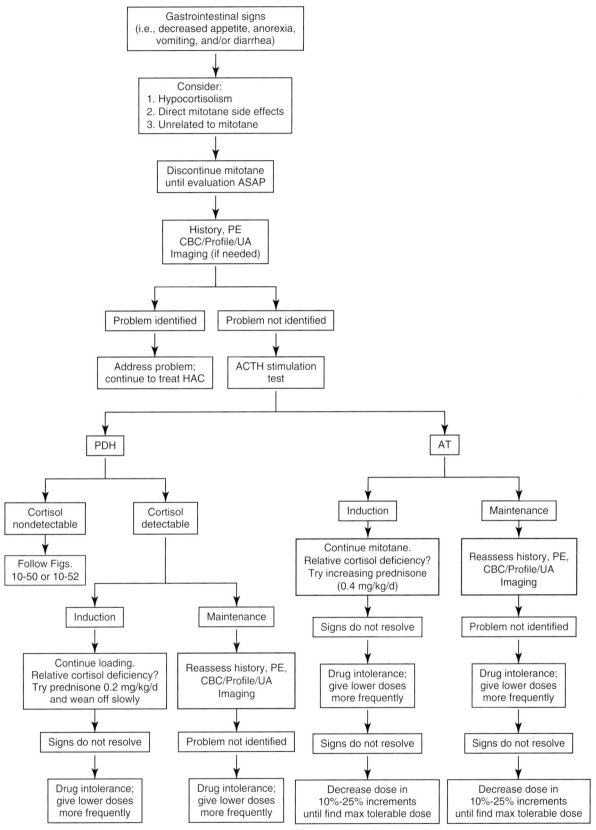

FIGURE 10-51 Algorithm for approach to gastrointestinal signs in a patient receiving mitotane. *ACTH,* Adreno-corticotropic hormone; *AT,* adrenocortical tumor; *CBC,* complete blood count; *HAC,* hyperadrenocorticism; *PDH,* pituitary-dependent hyperadrenocorticism; *PE,* physical examination; *profile,* complete serum biochemical profile; *UA,* urinalysis.

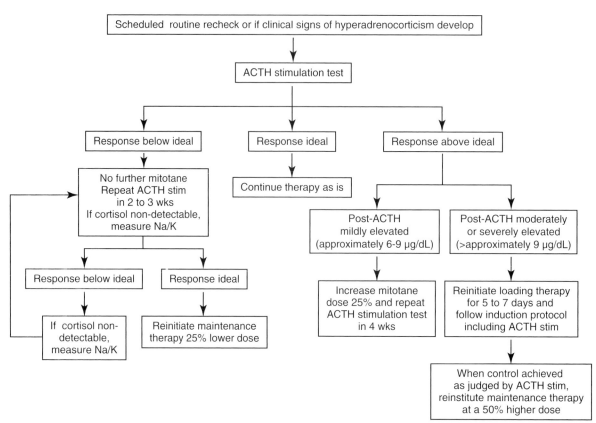

FIGURE 10-52 Algorithm for maintenance therapy using mitotane for pituitary-dependent hyperadrenocorticism (PDH). Ideal range for basal and adrenocorticotropic hormone *(ACTH)*-stimulated cortisol concentration is approximately 1 to 5 μg/dL (30 to 150 nmol/L) pre- and post-ACTH. (In Rand J, editor: *Clinical endocrinology of companion animals,* Ames, IA, 2013, Wiley-Blackwell, p. 56.) *AT,* Adrenocortical tumor; *CBC,* complete blood count; *PDH,* pituitary-dependent hyperadrenocorticism; *PE,* physical examination; *UA,* urinalysis.

therapy is reinstituted. If these develop, mitotane therapy should be discontinued, prednisone administered (0.2 mg/kg), an ACTH stimulation test performed, and serum electrolyte concentrations measured. Presence of glucocorticoid deficiency with or without mineralocorticoid deficiency can be documented and differentiated from direct drug toxicity. If the clinical signs are due to a hypoadrenal state, they should resolve quickly with prednisone administration. If the signs do not abate, presence of a non-adrenal illness should be suspected. Mitotane dose reduction may be necessary for dogs that develop adverse reactions or an alternate dosing scheme can be used (e.g., divide the dose into smaller amounts to be given more frequently during the course of the week).

If glucocorticoid deficiency is documented (e.g., pre- and post-ACTH serum cortisol concentration < 1.0 μg/dL [30 nmol/L]), mitotane therapy should be discontinued and physiological prednisone replacement therapy (0.2 mg/kg) continued until serum cortisol concentrations pre- and post-ACTH rise into the ideal range, which usually requires 2 to 6 weeks but can take months.

Decreased aldosterone secretion was previously thought to be uncommon and to occur only in dogs with cortisol deficiency. However, decreased aldosterone secretory reserve occurs in 79% of dogs with PDH treated with mitotane regardless of level of control of PDH and cannot be predicted by measurement of electrolyte concentrations (Reid et al, 2014). Although the zona glomerulosa is relatively resistant to the effects of mitotane, complete mineralocorticoid deficiency is seen in approximately 6% of dogs anywhere from 1 month to years after initiation of maintenance therapy and is often permanent (Kintzer and Peterson, 1991). The significance

of partial aldosterone deficiency is unclear. However, if a dog receiving mitotane is lethargic, weak, or hypotensive and cortisol deficiency or other disease is not present to explain the clinical signs, basal and ACTH-stimulated aldosterone concentrations should be measured. Aldosterone concentrations are best measured before and 30 minutes after ACTH if using cosyntropin for the ACTH stimulation test (Reid et al, 2014). If mineralocorticoid deficiency is present, the patient needs to be treated accordingly.

Neurological signs in a dog receiving mitotane (e.g., disorientation, dullness, or inappetence) may be due to direct drug toxicity or presence of a pituitary macroadenoma. If due to direct drug toxicity, signs occur the day the medication is given and usually resolve within a few hours. Imaging (i.e., CT or MRI) is required to confirm the presence of a large tumor. Of 173 dogs with PDH for which a cause of death or euthanasia was known, 6% developed a pituitary macroadenoma at 55 days to 5.6 years after initiation of mitotane therapy with a median of 9.7 months (Kintzer and Peterson, 1991).

Time Sequence for Improvement in Signs and Biochemical Abnormalities. If therapy is successful, the majority of clinical signs and complications of HAC resolve over time. Polyuria, polydipsia, and polyphagia should resolve when cortisol secretion is adequately controlled or shortly thereafter. Resolution of some clinical signs (e.g., muscle weakness, skin manifestations, non-healing wounds, and/or anestrus) may take 3 to 6 months or longer; calcinosis cutis may never fully clear. Dogs with cutaneous signs can have a period of severe seborrhea and a poor hair coat or worsening alopecia and pruritus, which may last 1 or 2 months, before a healthy hair coat

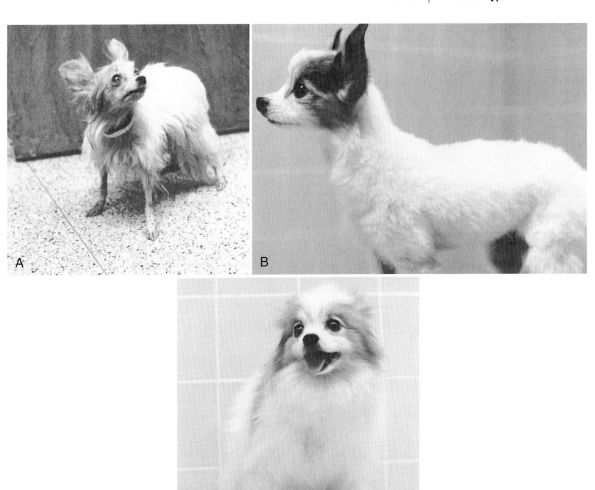

FIGURE 10-53 A Papillon with pituitary-dependent hyperadrenocorticism (PDH) **(A)** before therapy and 6 weeks after initiation of mitotane therapy **(B)**, which resulted in the appearance of a new, puppy-like hair coat. **C,** The same dog 10 weeks later, with a good, adult coat.

returns. Some dogs go through a phase of "puppy hair coat" before the normal adult coat returns (Fig. 10-53). A few dogs have dramatic changes in coat color after successful therapy (Fig. 10-54).

Liver enzyme activities may not normalize or improve. Serum cholesterol concentration may take months to decrease In humans, mitotane can increase serum lipid concentrations (Maher et al, 1992). Improvement in blood pressure can be detected within 3 to 6 months. Because hypertension may exist independent of the HAC, it does not dissipate in all treated dogs. Urine protein loss usually improves within 4 to 6 months of initiation of therapy, but proteinuria may not resolve (Ortega et al, 1996).

Stressful Situation. If a dog that is receiving mitotane undergoes any type of stress (e.g., illness, trauma, boarding, and/or elective surgery), glucocorticoid therapy should be initiated (≥ 0.2 mg/kg, adjusted or tapered as needed). An adequately treated dog with PDH has sufficient adrenal reserve for day-to-day living but may not have enough to handle major stress.

Development or Reemergence of Concurrent Problems during Therapy. The anti-inflammatory and immunosuppressive actions of cortisol can mask concurrent problems in dogs with HAC. Resolution of the HAC (due to mitotane or other therapy) may allow such problems (e.g., arthritis, atopy, and flea hypersensitivity) to become clinically obvious. Potentially, therapy with glucocorticoids may be indicated for treatment. Mitotane and glucocorticoids can be administered concomitantly. The patient will likely do better overall if the HAC is in remission, and a controlled dose of glucocorticoid is given as needed.

Planned Medical Adrenalectomy

An alternative protocol for treating PDH is aimed at non-selective adrenocorticolysis and complete destruction of adrenocortical tissue with substitution therapy for ensuing adrenocortical insufficiency. Mitotane is given for 25 days (50 to 75 mg/kg/day and up to 100 mg/kg daily for toy breeds), divided into 3 to 4 approximately equal and equally-spaced portions given with food. Lifelong glucocorticoid and mineralocorticoid therapy is begun on the third day of mitotane administration. Prednisone should be initiated at a temporarily high dose (1 mg/kg b.i.d.). Fludrocortisone (0.0125 mg/kg daily) and sodium chloride (0.1 mg/kg/day, divided over 2 to 3 meals) should also be administered (Rijnberk and Belshaw, 1988).

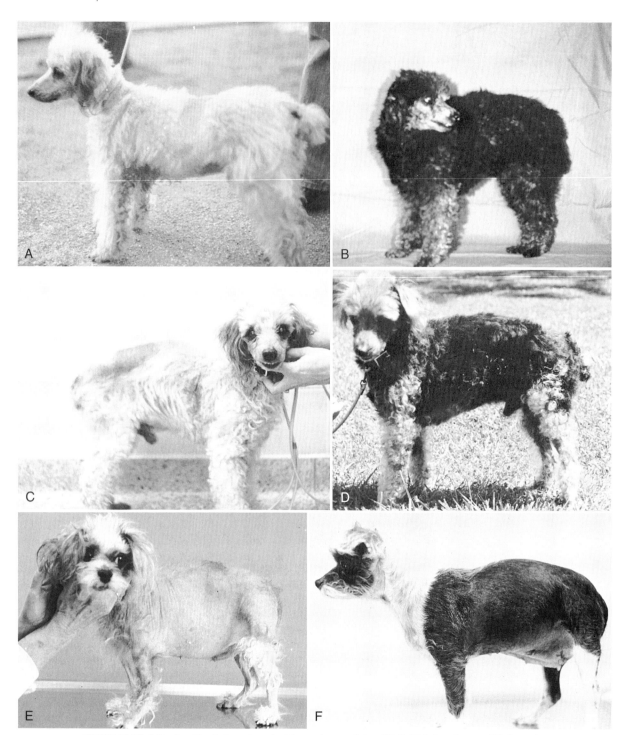

FIGURE 10-54 A Poodle with pituitary-dependent hyperadrenocorticism (PDH) **(A)** before therapy; **(B)** 2 months after institution of mitotane therapy, showing a dramatic change in the color of the hair coat; **(C)** after a relapse 4 years later; and **(D)** after reinstitution of mitotane therapy. **E,** A small, mixed-breed dog with PDH before mitotane therapy and **(F)** 2 months after starting therapy, showing a dramatic change in the coat color.

During the first month, owners should report by telephone at least weekly or as problems arise and should stop mitotane administration if any inappetence develops (Rijnberk and Belshaw, 1988). In this regimen, appetite change, if seen, is a direct toxic effect of the medication; cortisol deficiency is offset by the prednisone therapy. Glucocorticoid dosage may be increased temporarily if appetite diminishes. Usually mitotane can be resumed after 4 to 5 days when the appetite returns without further problem (Rijnberk and Belshaw, 1988). Fludrocortisone dose should be changed as needed to maintain normokalemia and normonatremia. Desoxycorticosterone pivalate (Percorten) may be used as an alternative to fludrocortisone (see Chapter 12 for more information).

The first follow-up visit should be 1 week after completion of mitotane administration. Serum electrolytes should be measured to ascertain if the fludrocortisone and salt doses are correct (Rijnberk and Belshaw, 1988). Performance of an ACTH stimulation test may be wise to ensure adequate control of the HAC. After the first follow-up visit, ACTH stimulation tests are performed only if clinical signs of HAC recur, but routine measurement of serum urea nitrogen and electrolyte concentrations is required to ensure adequate control of the hypoadrenocorticism.

The protocol was assessed in 129 dogs (den Hertog et al, 1999). The daily mitotane dose used was 31 to 125 mg/kg (median 59 mg/kg). Only 110 dogs received mitotane for 25 days. In four, administration was stopped due to adverse effects and not resumed; the other 15 dogs died in the first 25 days of treatment; seven died from hypoadrenocorticism. In 29% of the 110 dogs, mitotane administration was stopped temporarily due to development of anorexia, vomiting, weakness, depression, and/or diarrhea, but it was resumed within days (median 7 days; range, 1 to 63).

Convincing signs of partial or complete remission of the HAC such as hair regrowth and decreased water intake, appetite, and size were noted in 86%. Relapse occurred in 39% at a median of 402 days from the day therapy began (range, 84 to 1148). The dogs that were free of disease after 1, 2, and 3 years were 77%, 53%, and 44%, respectively. For all dogs, the survival fraction after 1, 2, and 3 years was 80%, 69%, and 61%, respectively. For the 110 dogs that received the full 25 days of therapy, the survival fraction after 1, 2, and 3 years was 87%, 77%, and 69%, respectively (den Hertog et al, 1999).

In another study that used a daily mitotane dose of 75 to 100 mg/kg/day in 46 dogs, median survival was approximately 2 years (Clemente et al, 2007). Although recurrence rate of HAC was only 29% (perhaps owing to a higher mitotane dose), 15 dogs suffered a hypoadrenal crisis during therapy. Overall incidence of side effects was 24%.

Although treatment of hypoadrenocorticism may appear easier than that of HAC, three main disadvantages exist for the alternative protocol, and its use is not recommended. First, mortality can be as high as 12% (den Hertog et al, 1999). Second, treatment of a hypoadrenal dog can be expensive. Third, and most importantly, failure to give medication to a hypoadrenal patient can be fatal, whereas missing a dose of mitotane will not put a patient in life-threatening danger.

Functioning Adrenocortical Tumors

In general, the preferred treatment for dogs with an AT causing HAC is adrenalectomy. However, surgery is not always possible. Some dogs have inoperable tumors or metastases at the time of diagnosis or are too debilitated for major surgery; some owners opt not to pursue surgery for a variety of reasons.

Two protocols have been advocated for treatment of an AT with mitotane. In general, dogs with AT are more resistant to the effects of mitotane than dogs with PDH (Kintzer and Peterson, 1994; Feldman et al, 1992). In the first, the ablative protocol, mitotane is used as a true chemotherapeutic drug; the goal is complete destruction of tumor tissue with serum cortisol concentrations pre- and post-ACTH below the normal resting range (e.g., < 0.3 μg/dL [< 10 nmol/L] on both samples) (Kintzer and Peterson, 1994). The other approach, the non-ablative protocol, uses mitotane with the same ideal ranges for cortisol concentrations as when treating PDH. The toxicity with the ablative protocol is likely higher. Destruction of all tumor tissue inherently makes sense, but which protocol provides a better prognosis is unknown.

Ablative Protocol

Loading. Mitotane induction dosage for treatment of an AT is 50 to 75 mg/kg/day. Although 20% of dogs with AT respond to the protocol for treating PDH, higher induction dosages and longer induction times are generally required for AT. The cumulative

induction dose of mitotane for PDH is usually 400 to 500 mg/kg, whereas that for dogs on the ablative protocol for AT is often up to 10 times higher. The goal is complete destruction of glucocorticoid-secreting tissue, so physiological doses of prednisone (0.2 mg/kg) should be administered concurrently (Kintzer and Peterson, 1994). The same clinical signs can be used to judge the endpoint of induction as when treating PDH with a maximum treatment span of 14 days. At the conclusion of a loading period, an ACTH stimulation should be performed (Fig. 10-55). When performing ACTH stimulation tests for monitoring, a dose of 1 μg/kg cosyntropin can be used (Aldridge et al, 2014).

If a partial response is seen but adequate control has not been achieved (i.e., pre- and post-ACTH cortisol concentration are lower than before treatment but not in the ideal range), mitotane should be continued at the same dosage and an ACTH stimulation test repeated every 10 to 14 days until serum cortisol concentrations fall within the ideal range. If after the initial loading dose the ACTH response is unaltered, the daily mitotane dosage should be increased in 50 mg/kg/day increments every 10 to 14 days as necessary, until an ACTH stimulation demonstrates a response to the medication or drug intolerance occurs. Therapy is then continued at the dosage at which a response was seen or at the highest tolerated dosage, and ACTH stimulation testing again performed every 10 to 14 days or if clinical signs suggest an endpoint has been reached. In 32 dogs with an AT, total induction time ranged from 10 days to 11 weeks with a mean of 24 days (Kintzer and Peterson, 1994).

Maintenance. Once cortisol concentrations pre- and post-ACTH are within the ideal range (i.e., < 1 μg/dL [30 nmol/L]) maintenance therapy should begin (75 to 100 mg mitotane/kg/week; Kintzer and Peterson, 1994). Daily prednisone administration should continue, because these dogs are cortisol deficient. An ACTH stimulation test should be performed after 1 month to assess control. If pre- or post-ACTH cortisol levels are within the normal resting range (i.e., 1 to 5 μg/dL [30-150 nmol/L]), the mitotane dose should be increased 50% and the dog should be retested in 1 month. If the cortisol levels are still above the resting range, induction therapy should be reinstituted; once ideal cortisol levels are again achieved, maintenance should be restarted at a 50% higher dosage than previously used. One month after a dose adjustment, ACTH stimulation should again be performed to assess control (Fig. 10-56). Once ongoing successful therapy is documented, an ACTH stimulation test should be done every 3 months or if clinical signs recur. Relapse occurs during maintenance in approximately 66% of dogs, usually due either to too low an initial maintenance dose or to tumor growth (Kintzer and Peterson, 1994).

As are induction doses, maintenance doses required for adequate control of an AT are higher than for PDH. In 32 dogs with an AT, the final mean maintenance dose required was 159 mg/kg/week, slightly more than double the average maintenance dose required to control PDH. Approximately 25% of dogs require maintenance doses greater than 150 mg/kg/week (Kintzer and Peterson, 1994).

Adverse Effects. Adverse effects, as described earlier, occur in approximately 60% of dogs. They can develop as long as 16 months after initiation of therapy, are more common during the maintenance rather than the induction phase, and are due either to direct mitotane toxicity or to adrenocortical insufficiency with the former being approximately twice as likely (Kintzer and Peterson, 1994).

If severe side effects occur, mitotane should be stopped, the prednisone dose increased to 0.4 mg/kg/day, and the dog reevaluated as soon as possible with an ACTH stimulation test and measurement of serum electrolyte concentrations to determine if complete

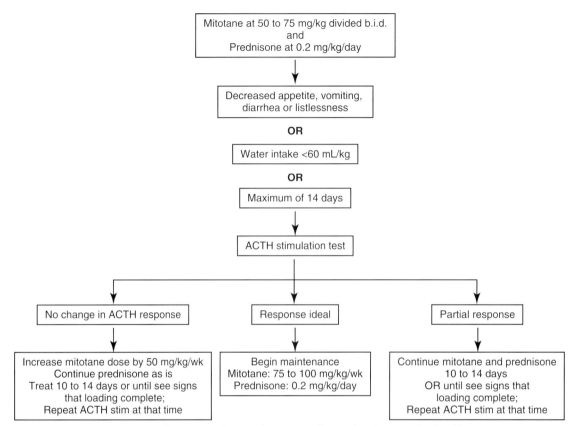

FIGURE 10-55 Algorithm for induction therapy using mitotane for an adrenal tumor using the ablative protocol. Ideal range for basal and adrenocorticotropic hormone *(ACTH)*-stimulated cortisol concentration is approximately less than 1 μg/dL (30 nmol/L) pre- and post-ACTH; normal resting range is approximately 1 to 5 μg/dL (30 to 150 nmol/L). (In Rand J, editor: *Clinical endocrinology of companion animals,* Ames, IA, 2013, Wiley-Blackwell, p. 57.)

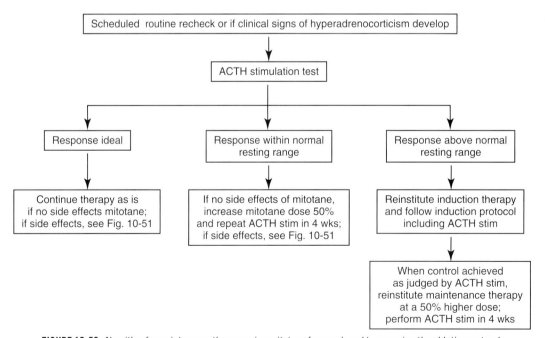

FIGURE 10-56 Algorithm for maintenance therapy using mitotane for an adrenal tumor using the ablative protocol. Ideal range for basal and adrenocorticotropic hormone *(ACTH)*-stimulated cortisol concentration is approximately less than 1μg/dL (30 nmol/L) pre- and post-ACTH; normal resting range is approximately 1 to 5 μg/dL (30 to 150 nmol/L). (In Rand J, editor: *Clinical endocrinology of companion animals,* Ames, IA, 2013, Wiley-Blackwell, p. 58.)

mineralocorticoid and glucocorticoid deficiency exists. If serum electrolytes are normal but pre- and post-ACTH serum cortisol concentrations are less than 1 µg/dL (30 nmol/L), aldosterone concentrations should be measured. If hypocortisolemia is present, mitotane therapy should be restarted and prednisone administration continued at a dosage of 0.4 mg/kg/day to exclude cortisol deficiency as the cause of the clinical signs. If adverse effects recur when mitotane is reinstituted despite an increased glucocorticoid dosage, direct drug toxicity or hypoaldosteronism are likely. If the adverse effects are direct mitotane toxicity, its administration can be temporarily discontinued and then reinstituted at a 25% to 50% lower dosage once signs of toxicosis have resolved. If hypocortisolemia, hypoaldosteronemia, hyponatremia, and hyperkalemia are present, the adrenocortical destruction may be permanent. Replacement therapy for both hormones should be instituted, and mitotane should not be administered until adrenal recovery can be documented via an ACTH stimulation test.

Prognosis. Of 32 dogs with an AT treated with mitotane, 66%, 28%, and 6% were judged by their owners to have a good to excellent, fair, and poor response, respectively. Mitotane does not appear to arrest metastatic tumor growth, and the response in dogs without evidence of metastatic disease is better than in dogs with metastases. Mean survival time of dogs with an AT treated with mitotane is 16 months (range, 20 days to 5.1 years) (Kintzer and Peterson, 1994).

Non-Ablative Protocol

Loading. The same treatment protocol is used as that for dogs with PDH with regard to dose and ideal cortisol concentrations pre- and post-ACTH. The initial dose is 50 mg/kg/day divided and given twice daily. When performing ACTH stimulation tests for monitoring, a dose of 1 µg/kg cosyntropin can be used (Aldridge et al, 2014). If at the first recheck after an initial 7 to 10 days of treatment the ACTH response test result demonstrates improvement but post-ACTH cortisol concentrations are not in the ideal range (i.e., 1 to 5 µg/dL [30-150 nmol/L]), loading should be continued with the same dose for up to an additional 10 days. If at the first recheck, the ACTH stimulation test result is similar to that obtained before therapy, the mitotane dose should be increased to 75 to 100 mg/kg/day divided and given twice daily for 7 to 10 days, and then another ACTH stimulation test performed. Lack of significant improvement in ACTH stimulation test results after the second loading phase indicates a need to continue the mitotane at the same or a higher dosage for an additional 7 to 10 days. The duration of the loading phase and the dosage required are then determined on an individual basis. In 13 dogs with AT treated with mitotane using the non-ablative protocol, only one dog had cortisol concentrations within the ideal range after 30 days of therapy (Feldman et al, 1992).

Maintenance. The same protocol is used as for PDH (see Fig. 10-52). Once induction is complete, maintenance therapy should begin at 50 mg/kg divided weekly into as many days of treatment each week as is logical and convenient (e.g., if a dog is scheduled to receive one tablet weekly, one-quarter tablet can be given 4 days per week). Dividing the dose into smaller portions can decrease adverse effects and make dose alteration easier if the need arises.

An ACTH stimulation test should be completed 1 and 3 months after the start of maintenance therapy. If the cortisol concentration after ACTH administration is approximately 5 to 10 µg/dL (150 to 275 nmol/L), the mitotane dosage should be increased by 25% weekly with ACTH stimulation testing done to guide further adjustments. If the post-ACTH cortisol concentration is more than 10 µg/dL (275 nmol/L), loading should be reinitiated. Once control is achieved, maintenance therapy should be resumed at a 50% higher dose than used previously. Some dogs remain stable for months or years on conservative dosages, whereas others receive mitotane daily at rather large doses. It is important to tailor treatment to the needs of each dog. Return of clinical signs suggestive of HAC should be managed by performing an ACTH stimulation test to confirm disease exacerbation and then, if indicated, increasing the dose of mitotane.

In one study, 13 dogs with PDH and 13 dogs with an AT were started on the non-ablative protocol with the same monitoring and dose adjustment protocol. Throughout the 6-month study, dogs with an AT were given at least four times the dose of mitotane as were dogs with PDH, yet the post-ACTH cortisol concentrations were at least three times higher in dogs with an AT. Clinical responses assessed by owners were consistently poorer in dogs with an AT. Only two of the 13 dogs (15%) with an AT were judged to have an excellent response (Feldman et al, 1992).

TREATMENT—MEDICAL MANAGEMENT WITH TRILOSTANE

Trilostane (Vetoryl) has been used to treat HAC for a number of years in Europe and is FDA-approved for treatment of canine HAC in the United States. A synthetic steroid analogue that inhibits the adrenal enzyme 3β-HSD, trilostane suppresses production of progesterone and its end-products, including cortisol and aldosterone. Additional enzymes such as 11β-hydroxylase and 11β-HSD may also be affected (Sieber-Ruckstuhl, 2006). The metabolite ketotrilostane is more potent than the parent compound (McGraw et al, 2010).

The advantages of using trilostane are a high efficacy and the ability to monitor therapy objectively by use of an ACTH stimulation test. Disadvantages are a relatively high rate of adverse effects, although potentially less than that of mitotane. Although as an enzyme inhibitor the effects of trilostane were expected to be fully reversible, adrenal necrosis can occur with resultant prolonged or permanent cortisol deficiency with or without aldosterone deficiency. Decreased aldosterone secretory reserve can occur (Wenger et al, 2004; Sieber-Ruckstuhl et al, 2006); it is common regardless of level of control of PDH and cannot be predicted by measurement of electrolyte concentrations (Reid et al, 2014). Aldosterone concentrations are best measured before and 30 minutes after ACTH if using cosyntropin for the ACTH stimulation test (Reid et al, 2014). Aldosterone deficiency can be life-threatening.

Trilostane is available as 10, 30, 60, and 120 mg capsules in the United States. Due to huge variations in trilostane content in capsules purchased from compounding pharmacies (Cook et al, 2012) and lack of knowledge regarding bioavailability and pharmacokinetics of the products supplied by compounding pharmacies, especially liquid formulations, use of brand name product (Vetoryl) only is recommended.

The protocol for trilostane use is the same whether treating PDH or an AT. As with mitotane, before initiation of therapy, the dog's mental status, activity, daily water intake, and appetite should be carefully observed. Awareness of these factors aids in assessment of treatment success or failure and in recognition of adverse reactions or the development of new problems, such as those associated with a growing pituitary tumor. The presence of a decreased appetite at any time is a contraindication to the administration of trilostane without further assessment.

General Protocol

The reported final dose required for control of HAC has varied greatly (Ruckstuhl et al, 2002; Braddock et al, 2003) with early studies finding effective dosages to be higher than currently recommended; the difference is likely due to initial inexperience.

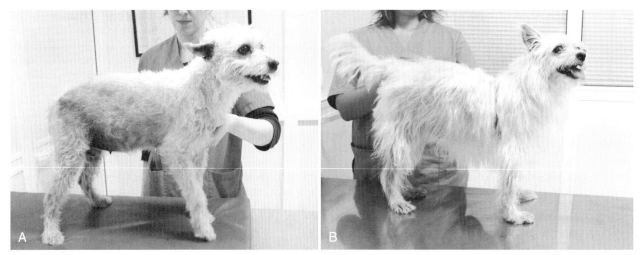

FIGURE 10-57 A, An 8-year-old mixed breed dog with pituitary-dependent hyperadrenocorticism (PDH) showing alopecia and a distended abdomen. **B,** Clinical signs of hyperadrenocorticism (HAC) resolved after treatment with trilostane. The dog is currently doing well after 33 months of treatment. (In Rand J, editor: *Clinical endocrinology of companion animals,* Ames, IA, 2013, Wiley-Blackwell, p. 61.)

The author uses a dose of 1 mg/kg twice daily or 2 mg/kg once daily, with the twice-daily dose being preferred (Fig. 10-57). Dosing to some extent will be based on the sizes of the capsules and the dog. Trilostane should be given with food to increase absorption from the gastrointestinal tract. Three times daily dosing may be needed in some dogs (Feldman, 2011). In any case, as with mitotane, dose adjustments will be required in most dogs and should be based on ACTH stimulation test results and clinical signs. In general, larger dogs (e.g., > 25 kg body weight) need lower doses on a per kilogram basis to control clinical signs (Alenza et al, 2006; Feldman and Kass, 2012).

If minor adverse effects are seen (see later), drug administration should be stopped for 3 to 5 days until they resolve and then restarted, giving trilostane less frequently for 1 week before continuing with the initial dosing scheme (i.e., every other day if dosing started once daily and give once daily if dosing was initiated twice daily). It is important to differentiate minor adverse effects from hypocortisolism; ACTH stimulation testing is needed.

The first ACTH stimulation test should be performed after 10 to 14 days or if decreased appetite, vomiting, diarrhea, or listlessness or normalization of water intake occurs. When performing ACTH stimulation tests for monitoring, a dose of 1 µg/kg cosyntropin can be used (Aldridge et al, 2014). Since trilostane absorption is affected by food, if the medication is usually given with food, the patient should not be fasted the morning of the test. Post-pill timing is crucial for dogs receiving trilostane. Some recommend initiating an ACTH stimulation test at 2 to 4 hours post-pill (Griebsch et al, 2014). However, insufficient data exist in the literature to determine the optimal time. The author recommends initiating the test at 4 to 6 hours post-pill. Keeping the timing of the test consistent for each patient may also be important (i.e., for an individual patient, always start the ACTH stimulation test at the same post-pill interval). The full effect of the drug may not be seen for approximately 30 days, so the first recheck is mainly to ensure that overdosing has not occurred. The dose should not be increased at the first recheck but should be decreased if serum cortisol concentrations are too low.

The ideal cortisol concentrations for a dog receiving trilostane therapy are approximately 1 to 5 µg/dL (30 to 150 nmol/L) pre- and post-ACTH; a cortisol concentration up to approximately 9 µg/dL (250 nmol/L) post-ACTH is considered acceptable if the patient is doing well and clinical signs of HAC are controlled

(Fig. 10-58). If the post-ACTH cortisol concentration is less than 1 µg/dL (30 nmol/L), the package insert states that trilostane administration should be suspended and restarted at a decreased dose after 3 to 7 days. In the authors' opinion, due to potential prolonged effects of trilostane, administration should be reinitiated only after recovery of adrenocortical function has been demonstrated by an ACTH stimulation test.

If the post-ACTH cortisol is 1 to 5 µg/dL (30 to 150 nmol/L), the dose should continue as is. If the post-ACTH cortisol is 5 to 9 µg/dL (150 to 250 nmol/L), the dose can be continued if the dog is doing well clinically and the clinical signs of HAC are controlled; if clinical signs are not controlled, twice-daily therapy should be used beginning with the same total dose. For example, if 60 mg was given once daily, the new dose should be 30 mg twice daily. Alternatively, a lower dose can be given in the evening (e.g., go from 60 mg once daily to 60 mg in the morning and 30 mg in the evening).

Except for the first recheck at 10 to 14 days after initiation of treatment, if the post-ACTH serum cortisol concentration is 5 to 9 µg/dL (150 to 250 nmol/L) and clinical signs of HAC are present, the trilostane dose should be increased. If after the first recheck, the post-ACTH cortisol concentration is more than 9 µg/dL (250 nmol/L), the trilostane dose should be increased whether or not clinical signs are present.

If the dog is already receiving twice-daily therapy and the cortisol concentrations are in the ideal range but the clinical signs are not controlled, two scenarios should be considered. One is that the dog needs to receive trilostane three times daily (Feldman, 2011). Alternatively, the clinical signs may not be due to HAC, and the diagnosis should be revisited.

An ACTH stimulation test should be performed 10 to 14 days after every dose adjustment. Once the clinical condition of the dog and the dose have stabilized, an ACTH stimulation test should be performed 30 and 90 days later and then every 3 months thereafter. The amount of dosage adjustment, either up or down, will likely be dictated by available capsule size, but it typically should be approximately 25%.

Twice-Daily Dosing

Trilostane may begin to lose effectiveness at 8 to 10 hours post-pill (Witt and Neiger, 2004; Bell et al, 2006; Vaughn et al, 2008). Although performing an ACTH stimulation test at 8 to 12 hours

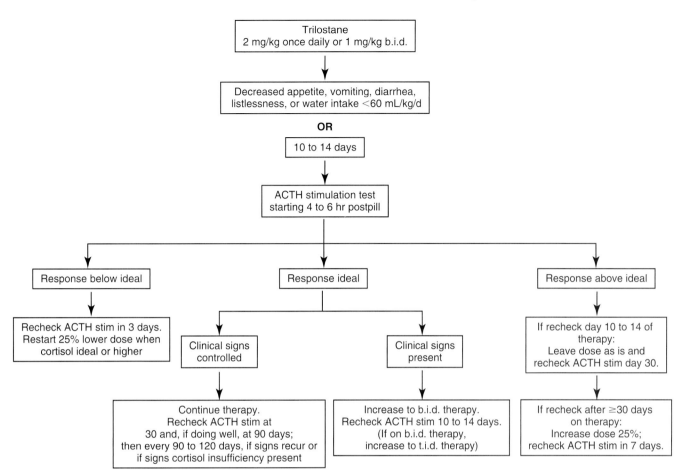

FIGURE 10-58 Algorithm for use of trilostane for treatment of hyperadrenocorticism (HAC). Ideal range for basal and adrenocorticotropic hormone *(ACTH)*-stimulated cortisol concentration is approximately 1 to 5 µg/dL (30 to 150 nmol/L) pre- and post-ACTH. Up to approximately 9 µg/dL (250 nmol/L) is considered acceptable if the clinical signs are controlled. *b.i.d.,* Twice-daily therapy; *t.i.d.,* three-times-daily therapy.

post-pill has been recommended for dogs on twice-daily trilostane therapy (Alenza et al, 2006), the optimal time has not been verified, and the author uses the same protocol as for once-daily therapy.

Twice-daily dosing might increase the likelihood of obtaining complete remission. At evaluation after 1 year of trilostane therapy for PDH, 12 of 12 dogs receiving trilostane twice daily had a complete clinical response. In comparison, of eight dogs receiving trilostane once daily, four had a complete clinical response, and two dogs each had partial or no clinical response, despite no dog having a post-ACTH cortisol concentration more than 9 µg/dL (250 nmol/L) (Arenas et al, 2013a).

Special consideration should be given to twice-daily dosing in dogs in which breaks in control of the HAC could be detrimental (e.g., dogs with concurrent diabetes mellitus or with proteinuria or PTE secondary to HAC). The duration of control of cortisol secretion afforded by trilostane varies between dogs and is not easily determined. Although clinical signs of HAC may be in remission, how long cortisol secretion must be controlled to improve or prevent the serious complications of HAC is unknown (for example: Is 12 hours of control out of 24 hours per day sufficient?).

Adequate control of HAC with mitotane significantly decreases blood pressure and proteinuria (Ortega et al, 1996). In dogs with PDH receiving trilostane therapy in one study, blood pressure was not significantly improved; UPCR decreased significantly, but approximately 38% remained proteinuric after 12 months (Smets et al, 2012). However, the study was small. Furthermore, some dogs received therapy twice daily and some once daily, and the effect of

dosing frequency was not evaluated. The consequences of control by either drug regarding development of recurrent infection or thromboembolic disease have not been evaluated.

Diabetic Patients

For dogs with diabetes mellitus and HAC, insulin doses are expected to decrease with treatment of HAC because hypercortisolemia causes insulin resistance. For dogs with both diseases receiving mitotane, the mean daily insulin requirement decreased from 4.6 U/kg/day to 1.7 U/kg/day in 8 of 11 dogs; the insulin requirement did not change in the other three dogs (Peterson et al, 1981). In a retrospective study of six dogs with concurrent diabetes mellitus and HAC treated for more than 2 months with trilostane, insulin requirements were not consistently reduced (McLauchlan et al, 2010). Three dogs received trilostane once daily.

Likely the same precautions apply when using trilostane in a dog with diabetes mellitus as when using mitotane (see Diabetic Patients). Attempts to control the diabetes mellitus are not recommended until the HAC is in remission because the insulin dose may diminish once cortisol concentrations decrease. Administration of prednisone (0.4 mg/kg once daily) to help avoid hypoglycemia should be considered during the early part of treatment when control is being achieved.

Alternate Monitoring

Given the expense of ACTH stimulation testing, alternate means for monitoring trilostane therapy have been evaluated. Although one paper suggested that basal cortisol concentrations within a specific range was highly suggestive that a patient was well controlled (Cook and Bond, 2010), a more recent study documented considerable overlap between excessively, adequately, and inadequately controlled dogs (Burkhardt et al, 2013). Similarly, an early paper suggested that measuring the UC:CR in a sample collected before administration of a trilostane dose could indicate duration of action (Braddock et al, 2003), but additional studies did not confirm use of UC:CR measurement either in samples collected before or 6 hours after trilostane administration (Vaughn et al, 2008; Galac et al, 2009). Thus, only ACTH stimulation testing can be used for monitoring trilostane therapy.

Adverse Effects

Reported adverse effects for the most part are relatively mild, including lethargy, weakness, decreased appetite, vomiting, and diarrhea. However, fatality has occurred. Reported rates of adverse effects vary from 25% to 40% (Neiger et al, 2002: Ruckstuhl et al, 2002; Alenza et al, 2006; Arenas et al, 2013a; 2014). One non–peer-reviewed report states mild, self-limiting side effects such as diarrhea, vomiting, and lethargy occur in 63% of dogs receiving trilostane (Neiger, 2004). Safety has not been evaluated in lactating dogs and males intended for breeding. Trilostane should not be given to pregnant females.

Excess adrenal gland suppression can occur and warrants discontinuing trilostane temporarily and lowering the dose (see earlier). Compared with mitotane, trilostane has fewer effects on aldosterone concentrations but hypoaldosteronism can occur regardless of level of control of PDH (Reid et al, 2014). Caution should be used in administering trilostane with an angiotensin converting enzyme (ACE) inhibitor or an aldosterone antagonist (e.g., spironolactone) because the suppressive effect on serum aldosterone concentration may be cumulative.

Prolonged Adrenal Suppression and Adrenal Necrosis

Although, in theory, as an enzyme inhibitor, the effects of trilostane should be reversible within 1 to 2 days, suppression can last weeks to years (Braddock et al, 2003; Alenza et al, 2006; Ramsey et al, 2008). After only three doses, one dog developed hypocortisolism that persisted for at least 1 year (Ramsey et al, 2008). Complete adrenal necrosis can occur secondary to trilostane administration as well (Chapman et al, 2004) and likely would be permanent. How often acute iatrogenic hypoadrenocorticism occurs in dogs treated with trilostane is unknown but is likely more common than originally believed. In one study, four of six dogs with PDH and one of one with an AT treated with trilostane had a degree of adrenal necrosis at necropsy. In two dogs, the damage was severe enough to potentially cause hypoadrenocorticism. Both dogs had received therapy with mitotane before trilostane but had been on trilostane for 15 and 22 months (Reusch et al, 2007). Thus, the contribution of each drug is unclear. Adrenal rupture, possibly secondary to adrenal necrosis, may have occurred (Vetoryl package insert). Interestingly, the necrosis is likely not a direct effect of trilostane but due to severely elevated ACTH concentrations that occur with trilostane use (Burkhardt et al, 2011); as cortisol concentrations decrease with trilostane therapy, negative feedback on the pituitary is diminished, and ACTH concentrations rise to very high concentrations (Witt and Neiger, 2004).

Efficacy for PDH

Trilostane is highly effective in suppressing cortisol secretion and controlling clinical signs in more than 90% of patients with PDH (Neiger et al, 2002; Ruckstuhl et al, 2002; Braddock et al, 2003; Alenza et al, 2006; Clemente et al, 2007; Vaughn et al, 2008; Galac et al, 2009). As with mitotane, many clinical signs

of HAC typically quickly resolve with control of cortisol concentrations, but certain ones such as dermatological abnormalities can take up to 3 months. Other abnormalities such as calcinosis cutis or myotonia may not fully resolve. A small proportion of dogs with PDH are not well controlled with trilostane (Ruckstuhl et al, 2002; Braddock et al, 2003; Vaughn et al, 2008).

Efficacy for Adrenocortical Tumor

Surgical removal of a cortisol-secreting AT is the recommended treatment, but if surgery is neither possible nor desired, trilostane can be used (Machida et al, 2007; Benchekroun et al, 2008; Helm et al, 2011; Arenas et al, 2014). Currently, the dose recommended is the same as for PDH. Clinical impressions are that the same dosage used for treatment of PDH is efficacious in dogs with AT at least in the short term. However, doses required for long-term control are unknown. One dog with an AT did receive a maximum dose of 17.2 mg/kg (Eastwood et al, 2003), which is higher than typical for PDH.

Prognosis

In 65 and 26 dogs with PDH treated with trilostane, median survival time was 662 days (range, 8 to 1,971) (Barker et al, 2005) and 549 days (Neiger et al, 2002), respectively. In 22 dogs treated with trilostane once daily for an AT, median survival time was 353 days (Helm et al, 2011). In eleven dogs with AT treated with twice-daily trilostane, the median survival time was 14 months (range, 3.3 to 55.0) (Arenas et al, 2014).

 ## TREATMENT—MEDICAL MANAGEMENT WITH KETOCONAZOLE

Ketoconazole, an imidazole derivative, is an orally active, broadspectrum antimycotic drug. It inhibits conversion of lanosterol to ergosterol and thus disturbs fungal membrane growth. At higher concentrations, ketoconazole affects steroid biosynthesis by interacting with the imidazole ring and the cytochrome P450 component of various mammalian steroidogenic enzyme systems. In normal dogs, ketoconazole administration decreases serum cortisol and testosterone, but not mineralocorticoid, concentrations (DeCoster et al, 1984; Willard et al, 1986). Ketoconazole is currently used rarely for treatment of canine HAC.

Protocol

Dosing of ketoconazole should be initiated at 5 mg/kg twice daily by mouth for 7 days, which is a low dosage to allow an evaluation period for development of side effects, such as gastroenteritis or hepatitis. Light feeding may help ameliorate gastritis. If no ill effects are observed during the first week, the dosage should be increased to 10 mg/kg b.i.d. by mouth for 14 days after which an ACTH stimulation test should be performed. The dosage requirement is determined from owner opinion and ACTH stimulation test monitoring. The ideal ranges for serum cortisol concentrations pre- and post-ACTH are approximately 1 to 5 µg/dL (30 to 150 nmol/L). If serum cortisol concentrations are above ideal, the ketoconazole dosage should be increased to 15 mg/kg b.i.d. by mouth and the dog monitored every 14 days (Feldman et al, 1990). Doses of at least 15 mg/kg b.i.d. are usually needed. Dosages equal to or greater than 20 mg/kg b.i.d. may be required (Feldman and Nelson, 1992; Behrend et al, 1999). At any time, if the cortisol concentrations are below ideal, ketoconazole administration should be stopped. Cortisol concentrations should return to pretreatment levels within 24 hours (Feldman et al, 1990); ketoconazole therapy can be reinitiated at a 25% dose reduction. If no response is seen or the disease progresses despite therapy, ketoconazole should be discontinued and alternative therapy begun.

Adverse Effects

Ketoconazole appears to be relatively safe with a low incidence of side effects. When seen, adverse effects may include anorexia, vomiting, elevated liver enzymes, diarrhea, and icterus (Behrend et al, 1999; Lien and Huang, 2008). Gastrointestinal adverse effects may be due to hypocortisolemia or direct drug toxicity. Uncommon side effects attributed to ketoconazole administration include depression, weakness, lethargy, trembling, liver failure, polyuria and polydipsia, thrombocytopenia, and dermatological changes, such as altered coat color, poor coat condition, and scaling (Behrend et al, 1999). Ketoconazole's effect on reproductive status has not been addressed, but it does decrease testosterone synthesis in healthy dogs (Willard et al, 1986) and should be used cautiously in male dogs intended for breeding.

Efficacy

The efficacy of ketoconazole for treating HAC is lower than that of mitotane and trilostane. After ketoconazole therapy, basal and post-ACTH cortisol concentrations may actually be higher than those pretreatment in some dogs (Feldman and Nelson, 2004). Of 132 veterinary internists and dermatologists surveyed, which are specialists likely to treat HAC, 52% considered ketoconazole to be effective in less than 25% of cases, 19% reported effectiveness in 25% to 49% of cases, and 14% each believed ketoconazole to be efficacious in 50% to 74% and 75% to 100% of cases (Behrend et al, 1999). A recent report suggested a higher efficacy of 70% in 48 dogs (Lien and Huang, 2008), but the follow-up on treated dogs was inconsistent and the ideal post-ACTH cortisol concentration used in the study was not as low as recommended by most authors. Thus, although ketoconazole may lower serum cortisol concentration in dogs with PDH and clinical improvement can be seen (Feldman et al, 1990; Lien and Huang, 2008), whether therapy is truly adequate in such a high percentage is unclear.

Three general indications previously existed for ketoconazole use. However, trilostane is now the first choice in such cases. First, ketoconazole was used when a patient could not tolerate mitotane. A second consideration was as a diagnostic aid in cases in which the diagnosis of HAC is unclear. If an ACTH stimulation test showed ketoconazole therapy had adequately controlled cortisol secretion, then any clinical signs present due to HAC should have resolved. If the disease was in remission, the diagnosis was confirmed. If no resolution of clinical signs was seen despite control of cortisol concentrations, HAC was ruled out as a diagnosis and ketoconazole discontinued. Ketoconazole provided a better alternative to trial therapy than mitotane, because mitotane's effects may be irreversible. It should be noted that although the effects of trilostane can be quickly reversible, they may not always be (see earlier). Third, because AT may be mitotane-resistant or the high doses of mitotane required to treat an AT may cause unacceptable side effects, ketoconazole was used for medical treatment of AT or pre-adrenalectomy to prepare the patient for surgery. No study has evaluated ketoconazole efficacy in a large number of dogs with AT.

 TREATMENT—OTHER MEDICATIONS

L-Deprenyl

Dopamine secretion from the hypothalamus tonically inhibits ACTH secretion from the intermediate lobe of the pituitary

(see Fig. 10-1). Thus, increasing dopamine concentrations or activity may inhibit ACTH oversecretion and be useful for treatment of PDH. Elevating dopamine can only be effective for PDH, however. Because ACTH secretion is suppressed in patients with an AT, dopamine agonism or increasing dopamine concentrations would have little, if any, further effect on ACTH release. Moreover, because ATs function autonomously of ACTH, lowering ACTH levels would not alter cortisol secretion.

Monoamine oxidase inhibitors, including selegiline (L-deprenyl, Anipryl), inhibit degradation of biogenic amines, most notably, dopamine. Unlike other monoamine oxidase inhibitors, selegiline is specific for cerebral monoamines (i.e., monoamine oxidase B). One study of 10 dogs suggested a 20% response rate (Reusch et al, 1999). The low rate is understandable because dopamine likely only inhibits intermediate lobe ACTH secretion and not secretion from the anterior pituitary; approximately 20% of canine PDH cases originate in the intermediate lobe. Unfortunately, only histopathology can differentiate anterior and intermediate lobe tumors. One study found selegiline to be ineffective for treatment of PDH (Braddock et al, 2004).

Use of selegiline to treat PDH is not recommended due to the low efficacy, but it could be tried in dogs with PDH that cannot tolerate mitotane and trilostane. Treatment should begin at 1 mg/kg orally once daily for 30 days. If no response is seen, the dose should be doubled for an additional 30 days. Failure to respond at that time indicates the need for an alternative therapy.

Selegiline therapy is relatively safe. Side effects are uncommon and usually mild, including vomiting, diarrhea, and ptyalism (Reusch et al, 1999; Braddock et al, 2003). Severe neurological disturbances and pancreatitis may have been caused by selegiline therapy (Reusch et al, 1999), but the neurological problems may also have been due to the presence of a large pituitary mass. Chronic selegiline therapy does not result in glucocorticoid insufficiency and, based on its mechanism of action, would not be expected to affect aldosterone secretion.

One disadvantage of selegiline is cost. Although the bioequivalency of generic preparations is the same among themselves, they are less bioavailable than the original product, L-deprenyl (Eldepryl); comparisons with the animal product Anipryl are not available. Thus, it may be wise to avoid the generic products. Another disadvantage of using selegiline for treating PDH is that monitoring of efficacy is based solely on subjective findings. The results of the ACTH stimulation test do not change in dogs receiving selegiline. Thus, other objective measures of effect, such as quantification of water intake or measurement of urine specific gravity should be utilized. L-deprenyl is degraded to amphetamine and methamphetamine. Thus, effects attributed to L-deprenyl administration, such as increased activity, may be due to the metabolic byproducts and not to an effect on the pituitary-adrenocortical axis.

Bromocriptine

Bromocriptine, a dopamine agonist, lowers plasma ACTH concentrations, but as with selegiline, likely only affects the pituitary intermediate lobe. Bromocriptine was administered to 47 dogs with PDH in total (Drucker and Peterson, 1980; Rijnberk et al, 1988b). Vomiting was a cause for treatment discontinuation in a large proportion, and only one of the 47 responded clinically. Thus, bromocriptine is not recommended for treatment of canine PDH.

Cyproheptadine

Increased CNS serotonin concentrations could theoretically increase pituitary ACTH secretion and, therefore, increased adrenal secretory activity. Cyproheptadine, a drug with antiserotonin, antihistamine, and anticholinergic effects, was used to treat nine dogs with PDH for 2 months—five at a dose of 0.3 mg/kg/day and four at a dose of 1 mg/kg/day; no dog improved (Stolp et al, 1984).

Retinoic Acid

Retinoic acid inhibits cell proliferation, growth, and invasion and induces apoptosis and differentiation in various tumors (Castillo and Gallelli, 2010). It decreases ACTH transcription and production in tumor cells in vitro and in experimental ACTH-producing tumors in vivo (Paez-Pereda et al, 2001). 9-*cis* retinoic acid was used to treat a total of 27 dogs with PDH in two studies at a dose of 2 mg/kg/day. Unfortunately, measurement of eACTH and α-MSH hormone concentrations and UC:CR were used to evaluate treatment, which makes the results difficult to interpret because these are not the typical tests used for therapeutic monitoring. Although the dogs treated with retinoic acid subjectively had greater resolution of clinical signs than the control group, the control therapy was ketoconazole, which is much less effective than trilostane or mitotane; thus, retinoic acid may have had an unfair advantage. Interestingly, pituitary tumor size decreased significantly in dogs that were treated for 180 days (Castillo et al, 2006; 2009). Although results were promising, more work needs to be done before retinoic acid therapy can be recommended, especially when proven therapies such as mitotane or trilostane are available. In addition, the retinoic acid used is not readily available and, at the doses used in the study, would likely be cost prohibitive to most owners.

Metyrapone and Aminoglutethimide

Metyrapone, an 11β-hydroxylase inhibitor, and aminoglutethimide, which inhibits conversion of cholesterol to pregnenolone, have both been used to reduce cortisol hypersecretion in people alone or in combination. Aminoglutethimide was administered to 10 dogs with PDH (5 mg/kg by mouth three times daily) for 1 month. A complete response was seen in only one dog and a partial response in three. Side effects including anorexia, vomiting, and weakness as well as elevations in liver enzymes were observed in the majority of dogs (Alenza et al, 2002). It is possible that longer treatment or use of other doses would have had greater efficacy. However, with the current data, its use cannot be recommended for treatment of PDH. To the author's knowledge, although metyrapone has been used to treat cats with PDH, no reports exist of metyrapone administration to dogs with HAC. Side effects in people are common. Furthermore, metyrapone is not consistently available.

TREATMENT—PITUITARY IRRADIATION

The normal pituitary gland in adult dogs is located in the hypophyseal fossa, which is an oval depression in the basisphenoid bone located ventral to the hypothalamus. The complex of boney structures around the pituitary gland has a saddle-like shape and is called the *sella turcica*. A normal pituitary gland remains within the sella turcica. The normal height of pituitary gland in dogs is 2.1 to 6.0 mm (Kooistra et al, 1997b). Pituitary tumors in dogs with PDH are variable in size; those that extend above the sella turcica are considered large (typically ≥ 10 mm in maximum height) and often referred to as *macrotumors,* either macroadenomas or macrocarcinomas. Large tumors may compress or invade the hypothalamus and thalamus and cause a spectrum of neurologic signs that include change in behavior, aggression, listlessness, obtundation, inappetence, pacing, circling, head pressing, and seizures (Theon and Feldman, 1998; Kent et al, 2007). Development of neurologic signs secondary to the compressive effects of a macrotumor is referred to as *pituitary macrotumor syndrome* (see Central Nervous System Signs). Development of pituitary macrotumor syndrome is associated with a shorter survival time, compared with dogs that do not develop it.

Radiation therapy can reduce tumor size and improve neurologic signs. It is the only effective treatment for pituitary macrotumors. Studies in dogs have used cobalt 60 teletherapy or 4, 5, and 6 MV photon teletherapy using a linear accelerator to deliver external beam megavoltage radiation. Total radiation doses have typically ranged from 35 to 50 Gy applied in 2.5- to 4-Gy fractions delivered 3 to 5 days per week over a period of 3 to 4 weeks. Fractionated treatment plans were developed to maximize tumor cell death while preserving normal tissue within the radiation field. As a late responding tissue, the CNS is most sensitive to the dose per fraction as well as the total radiation dose (Harris et al, 1997). Treatment plans that decrease the dose per fraction while increasing the number of doses have been recommended in an attempt to spare normal nervous tissue. Although this treatment approach is effective in reducing tumor volume and minimizing severity of neurologic signs and adverse effects of irradiation, it requires multiple anesthetic procedures and extended hospitalization time.

Stereotactic radiosurgery (SRS) is a relatively new procedure that delivers a single large radiation dose to a well-defined target while sparing surrounding tissue (Mariani et al, 2013). Several universities in the United States are utilizing SRS for the treatment of pituitary macrotumors in dogs with PDH and cats with acromegaly. At UC Davis, for example, a total dose of 24 Gy is administered in 8-Gy fractions on three consecutive days. Anesthetic procedures and hospitalization time are significantly reduced, the total radiation dose is minimized due to more accurate delivery of radiation to the tumor, and adverse effects have been minimal. Studies evaluating short- and long-term efficacy of SRS are currently in progress.

Adverse radiation effects are categorized as acute and late. Acute adverse effects occur in organs located within the treatment field that have rapidly dividing cells, most notably skin, pharyngeal mucosa, and the external auditory canal. Accordingly, acute adverse effects include alopecia involving the skin exposed to radiation, leukotrichia, mucositis, and transient lethargy and disorientation (Dow et al, 1990; Goossens et al, 1998; Kent et al, 2007). Concurrent treatment with low dose glucocorticoids (0.25 mg/kg prednisone once daily) during therapy may help decrease the occurrence of acute adverse effects. Late adverse effects develop months later, are irreversible, and occur in slowly-dividing tissues within the treatment field; they include infarction, demyelination and necrosis of the CNS, cranial nerve injury, pituitary-hypothalamic dysfunction, and neurologic impairment. Late adverse effects reported in dogs include deafness or partial hearing loss and vestibular and trigeminal nerve injury (Dow et al, 1990; Goossens et al, 1998; Theon and Feldman, 1998). The risk of late adverse effects depends on the volume of normal tissue treated, the daily radiation dose, and the total radiation dose administered. Higher total doses may improve local tumor control but increase the risk of late adverse effects, whereas with lower fractions, normal nerve tissue is more likely to be spared but reduction of tumor volume, improvement in neurologic signs, and survival time may be compromised (Gillette and Gillette, 1995; Brearley et al, 1999; de Fornel et al, 2007). Most studies to date have used a dosing protocol close to the limits of CNS tolerance (i.e., 40 to 48 Gy).

The goals of radiation therapy include shrinkage of the macrotumor, improvement or resolution of neurologic signs and the clinical manifestations of HAC, and prolonged survival with a good quality of life. All studies evaluating the effect of irradiation on pituitary tumor size, to date, have documented a significant decrease in almost all dogs treated (Dow et al, 1990; Goossens et al, 1998; Theon and Feldman, 1998; de Fornel et al, 2007; Kent et al, 2007). In some dogs the tumor was no longer detectable on subsequent CT imaging. The effects of radiation therapy on tumor size appeared quickly in some dogs (within 1 month after finishing treatment); the tumor continued to decrease in size over several months and could remain stable in size for up to 20 months (de Fornel et al, 2007). If neurologic signs were present, improvement or resolution occurred in most but not all dogs. Improvement in neurologic signs typically occurred within a month of beginning radiation therapy. Improvement or resolution of clinical signs of HAC did not occur in most dogs, suggesting that pituitary irradiation is more effective for controlling tumor growth than ACTH secretion. Pituitary ACTH hypersecretion usually persisted for months after radiation therapy, and most dogs required medical treatment of PDH to control clinical signs of HAC despite shrinkage of the pituitary tumor. A correlation between tumor size and ACTH secretion after radiation therapy was not identified in several studies (Dow et al, 1990; Goossens et al, 1998; Theon and Feldman, 1998).

Median overall survival time after irradiation has ranged from approximately 12 to 25 months (Dow et al, 1990; Theon and Feldman, 1998; Bley et al, 2005; de Fornel et al, 2007). In one study, the mean survival time was 1405 days (95% confidence interval [CI]: 1053 to 1757 days) for 19 dogs with pituitary masses (11 dogs had neurologic signs) irradiated with a total dose of 48 Gy (Kent et al, 2007). The 1-, 2-, and 3-year estimated survival was 93%, 87%, and 55%, respectively. In contrast, the mean survival time in 20 untreated control dogs with pituitary masses of comparable size (16 dogs had neurologic signs) was 551 days (95% CI: 271 to 829 days) and the 1-, 2-, and 3-year estimated survival was 45%, 32%, and 25%, respectively. Dogs treated with irradiation had significantly longer survival times, compared with untreated dogs with comparably sized pituitary masses (Fig. 10-59).

The ratio of pituitary tumor size to brain size has been used to correct for variations in dog size, including the ratios of pituitary gland height to brain area; of pituitary area to brain area; and of pituitary volume to brain volume (Kooistra et al, 1997b; Theon and Feldman, 1998). In the study by Kent and colleagues (2007), a pituitary-to-brain height ratio of more than 25% or a pituitary-to-brain area ratio of more than 5% was associated with decreased survival in dogs treated with irradiation. No dog with tumor heights less than 25% of brain height or with tumors less than 5% of the cross-sectional area of the brain died of their disease during the study period.

The severity of neurologic signs at presentation may also be a prognostic indicator for success of radiation therapy. In 24 dogs with PDH and neurologic signs, dogs with severe neurologic signs had a 6.6-fold higher risk of death due to their pituitary tumor than dogs with mild neurologic signs (Theon and Feldman, 1998). A significant correlation was detected between relative tumor size (i.e., pituitary tumor size relative to calvarium size) and severity of neurologic signs, remission of neurologic signs after radiation therapy, and duration of remission of clinical signs. Dogs with a relative tumor size of 12% or more had a fourfold higher risk of disease progression than dogs with a relative tumor size less than 12%.

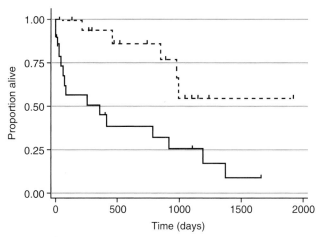

FIGURE 10-59 Survival distribution of dogs with pituitary masses that were treated with radiation therapy (RT) *(dashed line)* or that were not treated *(solid line)*. Nineteen dogs were treated with RT, and 20 dogs received no therapy. These curves were significantly different (log-rank test, P = 0.0039). Censored dogs are indicated by tick marks. (From Kent MS, et al.: Survival, neurologic response, and prognostic factors in dogs with pituitary masses treated with radiation therapy and untreated dogs, *J Vet Intern Med* 21:1027, 2007.)

The efficacy of irradiation of pituitary tumors of small relative size supports the importance of early diagnosis and treatment, preferably before neurologic signs develop. One year after irradiation of detectable pituitary masses measuring 3 to 14 mm in vertical height (median 6.5 mm) with a total dose of 44 Gy in six dogs with PDH and no neurologic signs, the size of the pituitary tumor had decreased by 25% in two dogs and was not detectable in four (Goossens et al, 1998). Clinical signs of PDH resolved in three dogs but recurred in two of them 6 and 9 months later. Clinical signs of PDH persisted in the remaining three dogs after radiation therapy. None of the dogs developed neurologic signs. Pituitary size did not correlate with the effects of radiation therapy.

Accordingly, routine pituitary imaging should be considered as part of the evaluation of a dog with newly-diagnosed PDH even if no clinical evidence of a large pituitary mass is present, especially if the client is willing to consider radiation therapy if a large pituitary mass is identified (see Treatment—Pituitary Irradiation). The preference is to perform CT imaging once clinical signs of HAC are controlled with medical treatment (i.e., trilostane or mitotane). For dogs treated medically for PDH, mean survival is approximately 30 months. While the rate of tumor growth is unpredictable, it may be safest for our patients to assume that a pituitary tumor will double or triple in size over a period of several years. If a dog has no visible pituitary mass (i.e., must be < 3 mm in greatest vertical height) at the first CT and the mass triples in size, the mass likely will never be large enough to be clinically significant. Hence, no follow-up with CT imaging is recommended. If a dog has a mass of 8 mm or more in greatest vertical height at the time of diagnosis of PDH, the mass would not even need to double in size before neurologic signs occur. Thus, radiation therapy is recommended. If a pituitary mass is 3 to 7 mm in greatest vertical height, doubling or tripling in size may or may not be problematic. Therefore, based on experience, the CT scan should be repeated in 12 months.

SPONTANEOUS REMISSION OF HYPERADRENOCORTICISM

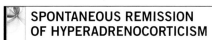

Spontaneous remission of HAC is a documented phenomenon in humans, either due to acute adrenal hemorrhage or pituitary infarction. One case report exists of a dog with presumed HAC, likely

PDH, which underwent spontaneous remission (Rockwell et al, 2005). In the dog, HAC was diagnosed by means of an ACTH stimulation test. Twelve days later, the dog had clinical signs and changes on routine biochemical tests consistent with spontaneous hypoadrenocorticism; cortisol and aldosterone concentrations were undetectable pre- and post-ACTH, and eACTH concentrations were elevated. Cytology of a fine needle aspirate of one of the adrenal glands was consistent with marked purulent inflammation. Thus, the spontaneous hypoadrenocorticism was believed to be due to adrenal necrosis. Because elevated eACTH concentrations can potentially cause adrenal necrosis (Burkhardt et al, 2011), the cause of the spontaneous remission was speculated to be the injection of exogenous ACTH given for the initial ACTH stimulation test. A similar occurrence has been documented in humans (Marcus et al, 1986).

Spontaneous remission has occurred in five dogs with histories, physical examination findings, and endocrine test results consistent with PDH (Feldman and Nelson, 2004). Treatment for HAC had not been pursued in any dog, because the owners believed they were improving. Subsequent evaluations demonstrated resolution of all evidence supporting a diagnosis of PDH. Given lack of development of hypoadrenocorticism, it is likely that remission of the HAC was caused by embolization of a pituitary tumor rather than adrenal necrosis.

PRIMARY MINERALOCORTICOID EXCESS: PRIMARY HYPERALDOSTERONISM

Primary hyperaldosteronism (Conn's syndrome) is an adrenocortical disorder characterized by excessive and autonomous secretion of the mineralocorticoid aldosterone. Primary hyperaldosteronism is typically caused by a unilateral solitary adenoma or carcinoma, although bilateral idiopathic adrenocortical hyperplasia has been identified (Breitschwerdt et al, 1985; Rijnberk et al, 2001; Behrend et al, 2005; Machida et al, 2007; Frankot et al, 2012). Primary hyperaldosteronism is perhaps the most common adrenal disease affecting cats but is rare in dogs. This disorder is covered briefly here, but see Chapter 11 for additional information on primary hyperaldosteronism.

The primary role of aldosterone is to maintain sodium and potassium balance and extracellular fluid volume. The primary regulators of aldosterone secretion include the renin-angiotensin-aldosterone system, plasma potassium and sodium concentrations, and ACTH. The primary target tissue for aldosterone is the kidneys where aldosterone promotes sodium absorption and potassium excretion. Excessive aldosterone secretion causes sodium retention and potassium depletion, which is manifested as a relatively mild increase in serum sodium concentration (typically 155 to 165 mEq/L) and a marked decrease in serum potassium concentration (typically < 3.0 mEq/L). Hypokalemia causes muscle weakness, which is the most common clinical sign of primary hyperaldosteronism. Hypernatremia and direct actions of aldosterone cause systemic hypertension, which, in turn, may cause ocular abnormalities, most notably retinal hemorrhage. Polyuria and polydipsia have been identified in dogs with primary hyperaldosteronism. The mechanism for polyuria and polydipsia is not clear, although mineralocorticoid-induced renal resistance to the actions of vasopressin and disturbed osmoregulation of vasopressin release has been documented (Rijnberk et al, 2001). Hyperaldosteronism-induced hypokalemia may also result in downregulation of aquaporin-2 water channels and urea transporters, thereby interfering with the ability to concentrate urine (see Chapter 1) (Robben et al, 2006; Sands and Bichet, 2006).

Primary hyperaldosteronism is a disease of middle-aged to older dogs presenting with owner complaints of lethargy, anorexia,

weakness, and polyuria/polydipsia. Tumors secreting both mineralocorticoids and glucocorticoids occur uncommonly (Behrend et al, 2005; Machida et al, 2007; Frankot et al, 2012), so clinical signs of and clinicopathologic changes consistent with glucocorticoid excess may also be present. The presence of severe hypokalemia and a serum sodium concentration at the upper end of or mildly above the reference range in combination with the finding of an adrenal mass on abdominal ultrasound should raise suspicion for primary hyperaldosteronism. However, aldosterone-secreting tumors can be quite small and normal ultrasound findings do not definitively rule out a mass or idiopathic adrenocortical hyperplasia.

Confirmation of an aldosterone-secreting tumor requires documenting markedly increased baseline plasma aldosterone concentrations (often > 3000 pmol/L) and suppressed plasma renin activity (i.e., increased aldosterone-to-renin ratio) in conjunction with exclusion of other causes of hypokalemia (see Chapters 11 and 12). Unfortunately, a canine plasma renin activity assay is not currently available. Other findings that help confirm a diagnosis of primary hyperaldosteronism include systemic hypertension and the presence of a metabolic alkalosis. The movement of potassium extracellularly results in a shift of hydrogen ions and an increased renal excretion of hydrogen ions leading to metabolic alkalosis. (Frankot et al, 2012).

The diagnostic value of increased urinary aldosterone-to-creatinine ratio and failure of the urinary aldosterone-to-creatinine ratio to suppress with administration of oral fludrocortisone acetate has been evaluated in cats (Djajadiningrat-Laanen et al, 2008; 2011). The major aldosterone forms present in human urine are aldosterone-18-glucuronide, tetrahydroaldosterone, and free aldosterone (Cartledge and Lawson, 2000). Commercially available kits for aldosterone measurement detect free aldosterone and aldosterone-18-glucuronide (after acid hydrolysis of the glucuronide). Syme and colleagues (2007) evaluated urine samples from eight normal dogs and found canine urine contained lower concentrations of aldosterone-18-glucuronide than human urine and, unlike feline or human urine, contained no detectable free aldosterone. Accordingly, urine tests may have limited to no diagnostic value for primary hyperaldosteronism in dogs, but they have not been evaluated.

Desoxycorticosterone-secreting tumors have been reported rarely (Reine et al, 1999; Davies et al, 2008). Clinical findings are the same as with primary hyperaldosteronism but aldosterone concentrations are low. As no assay for desoxycorticosterone measurement is commercially available, a diagnosis would be presumptive based on the constellation of diagnostic test results.

Unilateral adrenalectomy is the treatment of choice for a solitary adrenal mass, especially if no evidence of distant metastasis, vascular invasion, or infiltration of the mass into the kidney or body wall is found (see Adrenalectomy). Medical therapy involving the administration of oral potassium supplements, mineralocorticoid receptor blockers (e.g., spironolactone), and antihypertensive drugs (e.g., amlodipine) should be initiated until surgery can be performed (Sica, 2005). Medical therapy is also indicated for the long-term management of primary hyperaldosteronism when adrenalectomy is not performed and for dogs with suspected idiopathic adrenocortical hyperplasia.

In theory, autonomous aldosterone secretion from an AT should suppress normal zona glomerulosa cells within the contralateral adrenal gland. As such, hypoaldosteronism can occur postoperatively; serum electrolyte concentrations must be monitored frequently and IV fluid therapy adjusted accordingly to maintain serum potassium and sodium concentrations within or near reference intervals. If hypokalemia persists, oral potassium supplementation can be initiated once the dog tolerates oral medications. Serum ionized magnesium concentration should be monitored and hypomagnesemia treated, especially if hypokalemia is refractory to IV fluid therapy. Serum electrolyte derangements usually resolve within 24 to 72 hours of surgery, and mineralocorticoid replacement therapy is typically not needed. Mineralocorticoid treatment (i.e., oral fludrocortisone acetate or injectable desoxycorticosterone pivalate) is recommended if hyperkalemia and hyponatremia develop and persist for longer than 72 hours. Only one injection of desoxycorticosterone pivalate is required, and the daily dose of oral fludrocortisone acetate can be tapered and usually discontinued within a week. See Chapter 12 for more information on these medications.

Systemic hypertension usually improves or resolves within 48 to 72 hours after adrenalectomy. Antihypertensive medications should be initiated if hypertension persists. Attempts to wean off antihypertensive medications should be initiated during the ensuing month. Glucocorticoid replacement therapy is usually not indicated postoperatively, unless the tumor was secreting a glucocorticoid. An ACTH stimulation test can be performed 6 to 8 hours after adrenalectomy to assess the function of the zona fasciculata and reticularis of the remaining adrenal gland. If the tumor was known preoperatively to secrete a glucocorticoid, the same precautions and recommendations apply as when removing a cortisol-secreting tumor (see Adrenalectomy).

The prognosis for patients with primary hyperaldosteronism is similar to that for other AT. Surgical removal of an adenoma carries an excellent prognosis. The prognosis for a carcinoma is guarded. If metastatic sites exist, hyperaldosteronism, hypokalemia, and the associated clinical signs will recur. However, the tumor can be slow-growing with recurrence taking greater than a year following surgery. Management of recurrence with metastasectomy can be successful (Frankot et al, 2012). The prognosis for idiopathic adrenocortical hyperplasia is unknown and depends on the effectiveness of medical therapy. Bilateral adrenalectomy, in theory, should offer a cure, but the dog will require glucocorticoid and mineralocorticoid treatment for life.

UNEXPECTED DISCOVERY OF AN ADRENAL MASS

Ultrasonography has become a routine diagnostic tool for evaluation of soft tissue structures in the abdominal cavity. One consequence is the unexpected finding of a seemingly incidental adrenal mass (i.e., an "incidentaloma"). The incidence of finding an adrenal incidentaloma has been estimated at 4% overall but increases with age (Cook et al, 2014). Less commonly an AT is discovered during CT or MRI. Many factors determine the aggressiveness of the diagnostic and therapeutic approach to an adrenal incidentaloma, including the severity of concurrent problems, the original reason for performing abdominal ultrasound, the age of the dog, the likelihood that the mass is hormonally active, the probability that the mass is a malignant or benign tumor, the size and invasiveness of the mass, and the client's desires and willingness to pursue the problem. An adrenal mass may also be a metastasis from elsewhere. The first consideration is to be certain that an AT exists. Abdominal ultrasound should always be repeated to confirm the mass is a repeatable finding.

Bulbous enlargement or a "nodule" of the cranial or caudal pole of an otherwise normal-appearing adrenal gland is a common finding in older dogs and can be misinterpreted as an adrenal mass or tumor (Fig. 10-60). Bulbous enlargements or nodules have a maximum diameter typically less than 1.5 cm, and the

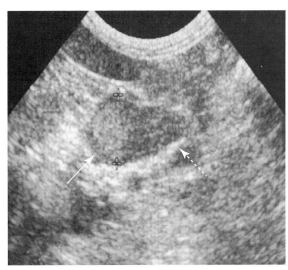

FIGURE 10-60 Abdominal ultrasound of a healthy dog revealed an incidental 1.2 cm-diameter "nodule" in the cranial pole of the adrenal gland *(solid arrow)*. The caudal pole of the adrenal gland appeared normal *(dashed arrow)*.

contralateral adrenal gland is usually normal in size and shape. A bulbous enlargement or nodule is usually not neoplastic or functional (i.e., autonomously secreting a hormone). Histologic examination often reveals normal tissue, inflammation, a granuloma, or a clinically irrelevant benign tumor (e.g., myelolipoma).

Less commonly, cortical tumors and pheochromocytomas in the early stages of development are identified. Of primary AT, approximately 75% are adrenocortical and the remainder are of neuroendocrine origin (Capen, 2007). A conservative approach centered on periodic monitoring with ultrasound, initially at monthly intervals, for changes in size of the nodule and appearance of the adrenal gland is recommended, especially if there are no clinical signs or findings on physical examination and routine blood and urine tests to support a functional adrenal tumor (Fig. 10-61). The chance of an incidentaloma being malignant may be between 14% and 30% (Cook et al, 2014). Of seven dogs with an incidentaloma of any type, three lesions were not found when ultrasound was performed again more than 4 months later. No growth was reported after more than 6 months in two dogs. In two dogs with initially larger tumors (16- and 25-mm in diameter), growth occurred. In the first, the mass grew to 25-mm diameter and invaded the vena cava within 10 months; in the second, the mass grew to 31-mm diameter within 8 months before the dog was lost to follow-up (Cook et al, 2014). In nine dogs with non–cortisol-secreting tumors followed for 12 months, no change was seen in seven (Arenas et al, 2013b).

An AT should be suspected when there is loss of the typical shape of the gland (i.e., the gland looks like a mass) regardless of size, there is asymmetry in shape and size between the affected and contralateral adrenal glands, or the mass has infiltrated the phrenicoabdominal vein, vena cava, or surrounding soft tissues (Fig. 10-62). If the mass is suspected to be malignant, adrenalectomy is the preferred treatment, but it may not be indicated if the mass is benign, small, hormonally inactive, and not infiltrating surrounding structures. Unfortunately, it can be difficult to determine whether an adrenal mass is neoplastic and malignant or benign before surgical removal and histopathologic evaluation. If the maximum diameter of the mass is 2 cm or more, chance of malignancy (Cook et al, 2014) and growth (Arenas et al, 2013b) may be high. Invasion into surrounding tissues and identification

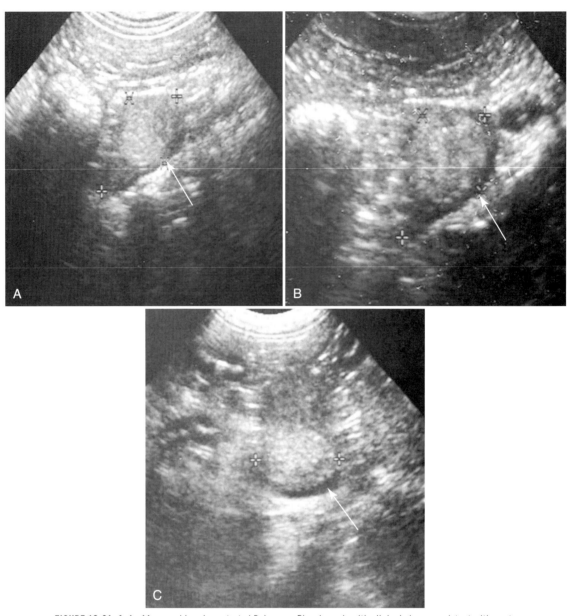

FIGURE 10-61 A, An 11-year-old male castrated Doberman Pinscher mix with clinical signs consistent with acute gastroenteritis. Abdominal ultrasound identified a 1.4 cm-diameter adrenal "nodule" *(arrow)* and a normal-size contralateral adrenal gland. The history, physical examination, and routine blood and urine tests were not supportive of adrenal disease, and the dog responded to symptomatic therapy for acute gastroenteritis. The adrenal nodule was periodically evaluated with ultrasound. Over the ensuing 2 years, the dog remained healthy, and minimal growth or change was noted in the echogenicity of the adrenal "nodule." **B,** The adrenal nodule 1 year after presentation; maximum diameter was 1.8 cm. **C,** The adrenal nodule 2 years after presentation; maximum diameter was 2.0 cm. (From Nelson RW, Couto CG: *Small animal internal medicine,* ed 5, St Louis, 2014, Elsevier Mosby, p. 859.)

of additional mass lesions with abdominal ultrasound and thoracic radiographs also suggest malignancy. The bigger the mass, the more likely it is malignant and the more likely metastasis has occurred, regardless of findings on abdominal ultrasound and thoracic radiographs. Cytological evaluation of specimens obtained by ultrasound-guided fine-needle aspiration of the adrenal mass may provide guidance regarding malignancy and origin of the mass (i.e., adrenal cortex versus medulla).

After confirming the existence of an unexpected adrenal mass, the clinician should review the history, physical examination, and results of routine blood and urine tests for evidence of hypercortisolism, hyperaldosteronism, or pheochromocytoma and should

perform appropriate tests to confirm the diagnosis, if indicated. An aggressive diagnostic and therapeutic approach is often not warranted for a small adrenal mass (< 2 cm in diameter), especially if the dog is healthy and there are no clinical signs related to adrenal dysfunction. In these cases, it may be preferable to determine the rate of growth of the mass by repeating abdominal ultrasound initially at monthly intervals. If the adrenal mass has not changed in size after 3 months, the time interval between ultrasound evaluations can be increased. However, if the adrenal mass is increasing in size, changing in appearance, or compressing or infiltrating surrounding blood vessels or soft tissues, or if clinical signs affiliated with an excess of cortisol, catecholamines, or aldosterone develop,

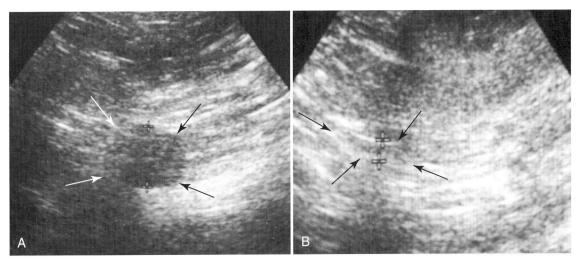

FIGURE 10-62 Ultrasound images of the adrenal gland in an 11-year-old castrated male Golden Retriever with adrenal-dependent hyperadrenocorticism (HAC). **A,** A cortisol-secreting tumor affecting the right adrenal gland *(arrows)* had a maximum diameter of 1.6 cm. Normal appearing adrenal tissue was not evident. **B,** The left adrenal gland had undergone marked atrophy *(arrows* and *crosses)* and had a maximum diameter less than 0.2 cm. (From Nelson RW, Couto CG: *Small animal internal medicine,* ed 5, St Louis, 2014, Elsevier Mosby, p. 831.)

adrenalectomy may be warranted. For non–cortisol-secreting tumors, median survival without surgery in 14 dogs was 29.8 ± 8.9 months (range, 1 to 96 months). Larger tumor size was associated with shorter survival (Arenas et al, 2013b).

See Chapter 13 for additional information.

 OCCULT HYPERADRENOCORTICISM

Due to the high incidence of HAC and relatively nonspecific clinical signs, older dogs are commonly screened for HAC. As discussed earlier, no screening test is perfect. Because HAC occurs in older dogs, patients tested for HAC often have concurrent disease. At the least, if they do not have HAC, they have a non-adrenal illnes (NAI) causing the clinical signs. In general, the more severe the NAI is the likelihood of a false-positive test result for HAC increases.

Due to the imprecision of diagnostic tests, HAC can be a difficult diagnosis to make. Clinicians are faced with a situation in which their clinical impressions are that patients have HAC, but the tests do not confirm the diagnosis and no alternative diagnosis is identified. Recently, in order to explain such circumstances, a syndrome termed *occult HAC* has been postulated. The 2012 American College of Veterinary Internal Medicine Small Animal Consensus Panel on the diagnosis of HAC defined the syndrome of atypical or occult HAC as, "[a] syndrome in which a dog appears to have HAC based on history, physical examination and clinicopathologic findings, but the LDDST, UC:CR *and* ACTH stimulation test fall into currently accepted reference ranges" (Behrend et al, 2013). Because the panel preferred the term *occult* over *atypical,* that is the name used here.

Occult HAC is supposedly caused by diversion of the normal adrenocortical pathways for cortisol and aldosterone synthesis into overproduction of sex hormones instead. The syndrome is diagnosed by performance of an ACTH stimulation test with measurement of serum sex hormone concentrations pre- and post-ACTH. However, conclusive evidence for the existence of occult HAC as a sex hormone-mediated condition is lacking. The Consensus Panel stated that sex hormones are not believed to be the cause of occult HAC (Behrend et al, 2013). Only 14 cases in

the veterinary literature meet the definition (Norman et al, 1999; Syme et al, 2001; Ristic et al, 2002; Benitah et al, 2005). No specific phenotype for occult HAC is apparent.

Although SARDS (Carter et al, 2009) and hyperphosphatasemia in Scottish Terriers (Zimmerman et al, 2010) have been linked with occult HAC, causative evidence is lacking. If only post-ACTH sex hormones are considered, no single sex hormone was elevated in more than 62% of dogs with retinal degeneration, and no hormone was consistently elevated. Similarly, in the Scottish Terriers, no single hormone was consistently elevated. More Scottish Terriers without hyperphosphatasemia had elevated sex hormones than did those with an enzyme elevation. Correlation is not causation.

Evidence for and Against the Existence of Occult Hyperadrenocorticism as a Sex Hormone–Mediated Disease

In evaluating adrenal hormone secretion, whether basal or ACTH-stimulated concentrations were measured in any study must be taken into account. For the diagnosis of standard HAC, determination of basal cortisol concentration is not reliable and never used by itself. No evidence exists that measurement of basal serum sex hormone concentrations are any more trustworthy for diagnosis of adrenal dysfunction; thus, the following discussion will focus on ACTH-stimulated concentrations.

Adrenal Sex Hormone and Cortisol Precursor Secretion as a Cause of Bilaterally Symmetrical Alopecia

Alopecia X is a condition most commonly affecting breeds, such as Poodles and plush-coated dogs (e.g., Pomeranians, Chow Chows, Samoyeds, and Keeshonds). It occurs in young adult dogs regardless of sex or neuter status. Clinical signs include loss of guard hairs, progressing to alopecia of the neck, tail, caudodorsum, perineum, caudal thighs, and ultimately trunk. In addition, the skin may become intensely hyperpigmented (Schmeitzel and Lothrop, 1995). With Alopecia X, no systemic signs are noted. Whether Alopecia X is a separate entity from occult HAC or represents dogs with occult HAC that only have cutaneous manifestations, as can occur with standard HAC (Zur and White, 2011), is unknown.

Evidence in Favor. Sex hormones can cause endocrine alopecia. Castration-responsive alopecia is recognized. Hyperestrogenism as well as hyperprogesteronism associated with Sertoli cell tumors, for example, can lead to bilaterally symmetrical alopecia. Estrogen administration for treatment of urinary incontinence has led to bilaterally symmetrical alopecia and histopathological changes consistent with endocrine alopecia (Watson, 1985)

The first report of Alopecia X described seven Pomeranians with bilaterally symmetrical alopecia and hyperpigmentation (Schmeitzel and Lothrop, 1990). Classic HAC was ruled out on the basis of normal ACTH stimulation test and LDDST results. Progesterone, 17-hydroxy-progesterone (17OHP), 11-deoxycortisol, dehydroepiandrosterone sulfate (DHEAS), androstenedione, testosterone, and estradiol were measured pre- and post-ACTH in the affected dogs, twelve unaffected Pomeranians, and nineteen non-Pomeranian control dogs. Only ACTH-stimulated 17OHP concentrations differed between affected and unaffected Pomeranians, but ACTH-stimulated progesterone and DHEAS concentrations were significantly higher in both groups of Pomeranians compared with controls. Given the constellation of abnormalities in affected and unaffected dogs, the alopecia was hypothesized to be due to a partial deficiency of 21-hydroxylase, an enzyme needed for cortisol synthesis.

In humans with 21-hydroxylase deficiency, cortisol is not synthesized and its precursors, most notably 17OHP and androgens, accumulate (Stewart, 2008). Because affected Pomeranians had normal cortisol concentrations, the enzyme deficiency was assumed to be partial (Schmeitzel and Lothrop, 1990). Family members of human patients have sex hormone elevations to a lesser magnitude and no clinical signs, thus explaining the findings (i.e., increased progesterone and DHEAS levels) in the unaffected Pomeranians (many of the affected and unaffected Pomeranians in the study were related). Subsequently, three Alaskan Malamutes with Alopecia X were reported to have ACTH-stimulated 17OHP concentrations above the reference range and that were significantly higher than those in three normal Alaskan Malamutes (Leone et al, 2005).

Evidence Against. Of six sex hormones assessed by Schmeitzel and Lothrop in the seven Pomeranians, only ACTH-stimulated serum 17OHP concentration was significantly different between affected and unaffected dogs. However, when affected males and females were assessed separately, the males did not have elevated serum 17OHP concentrations (Schmeitzel and Lothrop, 1990). In 276 dogs with Alopecia X, including 63 Pomeranians, only 73% had at least one basal or post-ACTH sex hormone concentration above the reference range (i.e., 27% had no elevations). Despite the preponderance of elevations in sex hormone concentrations, no consistent sex hormone abnormalities were identified. Of the ACTH-stimulated hormone concentrations, progesterone elevation was the most common abnormality, but it was found in only 36% of patients. Thus, it was concluded that Alopecia X should be referred to as alopecia associated with follicular arrest rather than an adrenal hormone imbalance (Frank et al, 2003).

Candidate genes in which mutations could cause the abnormalities, including 21-hydroxylase and enzymes in the cortisol synthesis pathway, have been cloned. No mutations affecting the primary structure of the enzyme or gene expression have been identified in the canine 21-hydroxylase gene (Takada et al, 2002).

17-Hydroxy-Progesterone, Other Sex Hormones, and Cortisol Precursors as Causes of Occult Hyperadrenocorticism

Evidence in Favor. Initially, a study of 24 dogs with clinical and routine laboratory findings suggestive of HAC was reported.

Eleven dogs with typical HAC with elevated cortisol responses to ACTH were assigned to Group 1. Of 13 dogs with normal ACTH stimulation test results, six had LDDST results consistent with HAC (Group 2A), four had negative LDDST results (Group 2B), and three had low plasma cortisol concentrations throughout testing, so the LDDST was not interpretable (Group 2C). Despite the variation in serum cortisol concentrations on the tests for standard HAC, all 24 dogs had elevated ACTH-stimulated 17OHP concentrations. Because ACTH-stimulated serum 17OHP concentration was elevated in dogs with both classic and occult HAC, it was concluded to be a marker of adrenal dysfunction (Ristic et al, 2002).

Numerous other studies have documented sex hormone concentration elevations in dogs with various forms of hypercortisolemia, either PDH or AT. Some studies were small, but elevations in DHEAS, testosterone, androstenedione, estradiol, progesterone, 17OHP, 21-deoxycortisol, 11-deoxycortisol, and corticosterone have been found in 40% to 100% (Frank et al, 2001; Behrend et al, 2005; Benitah et al, 2005; Hill et al, 2005; Sieber-Ruckstuhl et al, 2008).

In cases in which cortisol and sex hormones are both elevated, which hormone(s) is causing clinical signs of HAC is difficult or impossible to determine. However, sporadic reports exist of dogs with sex hormone-secreting AT and low serum cortisol concentrations but in which clinical signs of HAC were present, ostensibly due to the sex hormones. Two dogs with AT had clinical signs of HAC despite markedly suppressed ACTH-stimulated serum cortisol concentrations; one tumor secreted progesterone, 17OHP, testosterone, and DHEAS, whereas the other secreted androstenedione, estradiol, progesterone, and 17OHP (Syme et al, 2001). In a report of eight dogs with AT and signs of HAC, three had suppressed ACTH-stimulated serum cortisol concentrations and one had elevated 17OHP concentrations; no other sex hormones were measured in any dog nor in the other two with subnormal cortisol concentrations (Norman et al, 1999).

Evidence Against. It is difficult to understand how sex hormones cause clinical signs of HAC. The sex hormone most mentioned as a cause of occult HAC is progesterone. Due to its short half-life, however, little is known about the effects of elevated serum concentrations. Chronic progesterone excesses are not unique. In estrus and diestrus, serum progesterone concentration is elevated for 60 to 90 days and is higher than in dogs with HAC; yet no clinical signs of HAC develop (Bromel et al, 2010). In humans, clinically silent 17OHP-secreting ATs occur (Turton et al, 1992; Bondanelli et al, 1997). Massive elevations in serum 17OHP occur in humans with 21-hydroxylase deficiency (i.e., concentrations ranging from 3000 to 40,000 ng/dL [reference range, 20 to 600]) (Grumbach and Conte, 1998); yet clinically affected patients show signs either of aldosterone deficiency or androgen excess, such as virilization or loss of female cycling (Stewart, 2008), signs not reported in dogs with occult HAC. Lastly, a "cryptic" syndrome of 21-hydroxylase deficiency exists in which affected people lack 21-hydroxylase and have hormonal abnormalities but no clinical signs. The factors that impose the phenotypic variability on the genotypic abnormality are unknown (Grumbach and Conte, 1998), but abnormal sex hormone elevations by themselves are insufficient to cause clinical disease. Similarly, in dogs with Alopecia X, serum 17OHP concentrations can be quite elevated, similar to what is seen with dogs with purported occult HAC, yet none of the classical systemic clinical signs such as polyuria/polydipsia, polyphagia, pot belly, and panting are reported.

Two mechanisms have been proposed for progesterone's ability to cause signs of glucocorticoid excess. Synthetic progestins, compounds with progesterone-like actions, may either bind GRs

(Selman et al, 1997) or displace cortisol from its binding protein, elevating serum free cortisol concentrations (Juchem and Pollow, 1990). Indeed, progestins suppress eACTH secretion and cause adrenal atrophy, an action suggestive of glucocorticoid activity (Selman et al, 1997). Accordingly, progesterone may do the same. Examination of Pomeranians with Alopecia X, however, refutes the likelihood of either mechanism occurring. If elevated serum 17OHP concentration, as seen in the Pomeranians, is sufficient to cause clinical disease due to glucocorticoid actions of 17OHP, eACTH concentration should be suppressed due to negative feedback effects of glucocorticoids on the pituitary. Indeed, for dogs with proven sex hormone-secreting AT and signs of HAC despite hypocortisolemia, measured eACTH concentrations can be low (Syme et al, 2001). To the contrary, Pomeranians with elevated serum 17OHP concentrations had higher plasma ACTH concentrations than healthy dogs (Schmeitzel and Lothrop, 1990).

How AT could have a shift in hormone synthesis activity can be understood easily. Tumor cells are not normal and can undergo loss of differentiation, losing the ability to synthesize enzymes in the hormone synthesis pathways. In cases of pituitary-dependent occult HAC, how or why normal adrenocortical tissue should have altered steroid synthesis is unexplained.

Sex Hormone Panel Testing

Evidence in Favor. Measurement of serum sex hormone concentrations has been advocated as a means of diagnosing occult HAC. Use of a panel of hormones has been stated to increase sensitivity and specificity of the test over measurement of a single hormone alone. Elevations in concentrations of any hormone can be common, with estradiol elevations noted in approximately 40% of panels submitted to one reference laboratory (Oliver, 2007).

Evidence Against. It is reasonable to assume that dogs with NAI (e.g., a dog with diabetes mellitus) might not have the same ACTH response as healthy dogs because of adaptation of adrenocortical function to the stresses of chronic illness. Many stressed and sick dogs have increased cortisol concentrations and an exaggerated ACTH response, but they do not have HAC (Kaplan et al, 1995). In one study, post-ACTH serum cortisol and 17OHP concentrations were significantly correlated both in dogs with neoplasia and those suspected of having HAC, suggesting that as adrenal function is increased either by adrenal disease or nonspecifically by NAI, production of all hormones increases proportionately (Behrend et al, 2005).

For estradiol, a wide range of variability exists within and between dogs; random, basal estradiol concentrations in individual dogs often exceed the reference range (Frank et al, 2010). With regard to 17OHP, the specificity of measurement is 59% to 70% (i.e., the chance of a false-positive result is 30% to 41%) (Chapman et al, 2003; Behrend et al, 2005; Monroe et al, 2012). The specificity of progesterone measurement was determined to be 55% (Monroe et al, 2012). In six dogs with a pheochromocytoma or a nonfunctional AT, androstenedione, progesterone, 17OHP, testosterone, and/or estradiol concentrations were elevated (Hill et al, 2005). Therefore, dogs without adrenal disease clearly can have elevated sex hormones as well as cortisol concentrations, but sex hormones may be more likely to be falsely elevated by NAI as compared with cortisol.

Response to Treatment

Evidence in Favor. In dogs with either Alopecia X or purported occult HAC, treatment with agents that affect pituitary or adrenal function can resolve clinical signs. Melatonin, a neurohormone, controls seasonal reproductive and hair growth cycles

and alters sex hormone concentrations in intact dogs (Ashley et al, 1999). It was administered initially in 29 dogs with Alopecia X; 15 had partial hair regrowth at the first reevaluation (Frank et al, 2004). In three Alaskan Malamutes with Alopecia X, trilostane administration (3.0 to 3.6 mg/kg daily by mouth) resulted in complete hair regrowth within 6 months (Leone et al, 2005). Of 16 Pomeranians and eight Miniature Poodles with Alopecia X, 14 Pomeranians and all Poodles had hair regrowth in response to trilostane; the mean dose that caused hair regrowth was 11.8 mg/kg (range, 5 to 23.5) in Pomeranians and 9 mg/kg (range, 6.1 to 15.0) per day in Poodles (Cerundolo et al, 2004). In a study on occult HAC, nine dogs treated with trilostane or mitotane all had clinical improvement. Decreased ACTH-stimulated cortisol and/or 17OHP concentrations were documented in four of the nine (Ristic et al, 2002). Lastly, in one dog with clinical signs of HAC and normal post-ACTH-stimulated cortisol and LDDST results but an elevated ACTH-stimulated 17OHP concentration, clinical signs resolved with mitotane therapy (Benitah et al, 2005).

Evidence Against. The response to mitotane, melatonin, or trilostane is neither uniform nor predictable. In 15 Pomeranians with Alopecia X treated with melatonin (mean 1.3 mg/kg by mouth b.i.d.; range, 1.0 to 1.7) for 3 months, only six had mild to moderate hair regrowth (Frank et al, 2006). In the study evaluating 29 dogs diagnosed with Alopecia X treated with melatonin or mitotane, partial or complete hair regrowth was seen in only 62% overall. On mitotane, four of six dogs had partial to complete hair regrowth and two had none (Frank et al, 2004). More importantly, serum sex hormone concentrations did not change significantly in response to treatment nor correlate with whether response was seen. In dogs with partial or complete hair regrowth, 17OHP, androstenedione, and progesterone were still elevated in 36%, 21%, and 64%, respectively. In 16 Pomeranians and eight Miniature Poodles with Alopecia X (Cerundolo et al, 2004) and two dogs with occult HAC (Ristic et al, 2002) that responded to trilostane therapy, 17OHP concentrations were significantly elevated by therapy. Thus, hair coat and other clinical signs improve despite further increases in concentrations of the sex hormones purportedly underlying the clinical signs.

Indications for Diagnostic Testing

The author recognizes that cases that fulfill the criteria for occult HAC exist. However, sex hormones may simply be a marker of occult HAC, not the cause of it. At the current time, the recommended test is an ACTH stimulation test using the same protocol as with a standard test and measurement of cortisol, but the baseline and post-ACTH samples are used for measurement of sex hormones. Unfortunately, whether the protocol is optimal has not been evaluated.

Testing for occult HAC should not be undertaken if clinical indication for testing for classic HAC does not exist (Behrend et al, 2013). If the clinical picture fits, the primary indication for measuring adrenal sex hormones is when a dog is screened for HAC with an ACTH stimulation test or LDDST and all cortisol concentrations, including basal, are below the reference range. If administration of exogenous glucocorticoids of any form or administration of medications that alter cortisol synthesis (e.g., ketoconazole) are ruled out, a sex hormone-secreting AT may be present. Secretion of progesterone, 17OHP or a cortisol precursor (Reine et al, 1999; Syme et al, 2001) may suppress pituitary ACTH secretion and cause atrophy of normal adrenocortical tissue. The ultrasonographic finding of an AT in such patients would further support the diagnosis, but the lack of one does not rule it out.

If clinical signs are mild, waiting and retesting for classic HAC when progression is noted may be the best course of action. If clinical signs are moderate to severe, abdominal ultrasound should be performed. If the adrenal glands are normal, the differential diagnoses for the patient should be revisited. If bilateral adrenomegaly is present, pituitary imaging should be considered to identify a pituitary tumor causing early HAC. Lastly, food-stimulated HAC should be considered, because in these patients fasting cortisol concentration may be low (Behrend et al, 2013).

A few explanations exist for the existence of such cases (Behrend et al, 2013). First, the reference ranges and cutoff values for the LDDST need to be reestablished. The ACVIM Consensus Panel believed the cutoffs should be lower than they currently are; a decreased cutoff would result in some dogs diagnosed with occult HAC actually having typical HAC. Dogs with mild or early HAC that are "normal" on tests using current cutoff values may not be with revised (lower) values. Second, variable cortisol sensitivity exists in humans (Huizenga et al, 1998) and may occur in dogs. Dogs with high sensitivity may show clinical signs of HAC

at cortisol concentrations considered "normal" for the general population. Accordingly, the appropriate name for the syndrome may be *suspected HAC*. Third, dogs that meet the definition for occult HAC may have rare forms, such as food-dependent HAC. Other explanations may also exist.

Treatment

The treatment of occult HAC has not been widely studied, but it would depend on the form of the disease. If caused by an adrenal tumor, adrenalectomy would be preferred. If a tumor is not the etiology, melatonin, trilostane, and mitotane have all had some success (see earlier). The efficacy of trilostane would depend on which hormone is in excess. Because it is the author's opinion that the true mediator of occult HAC is unknown but may relate to adrenal function, mitotane may be preferred, because concentrations of all sex hormones and cortisol intermediates would be suppressed. Whether the protocol for using either drug for treating occult HAC should be different than when treating hypercortisolemia has never been evaluated.

REFERENCES

Adin CA, Nelson RW: Adrenal glands. In Tobias KM, Johnston SA, editors: *Veterinary surgery: small animal*, St Louis, 2012, Elsevier Saunders, p 2033.

Adissu HA, et al.: Cardiac myxosarcoma with adrenal adenoma and pituitary hyperplasia resembling Carney complex in a dog, *Vet Pathol* 47:354, 2010.

Aldridge C, et al.: Comparison of two doses for ACTH stimulation testing in dogs suspected of or treated for hyperadrenocorticism, *J Vet Int Med* 28:1025, 2014.

Alenza DP, et al.: Use of aminoglutethimide in the treatment of pituitary-dependent hyperadrenocorticism in the dog, *J Small Anim Pract* 43:104, 2002.

Alenza DP, et al.: Long-term efficacy of trilostane administered twice daily in dogs with pituitary-dependent hyperadrenocorticism, *J Am Anim Hosp Assoc* 42:269, 2006.

Anderson CR, et al.: Surgical treatment of adrenocortical tumors: 21 cases (1990-1996), *J Am Anim Hosp Assoc* 37:937, 2001.

Angles JM, et al.: Use of urine corticoid: creatinine ratio versus adrenocorticotropic hormone stimulation for monitoring mitotane treatment of pituitary-dependent hyperadrenocorticism in dogs, *J Am Vet Med Assoc* 211:1002, 1997.

Antoni FA, Dayanithi G: Evidence for distinct glucocorticoid and guanine 3',5'-monophosphate-effected inhibition of stimulated adrenocorticotropin release in vitro, *Endocrinology* 126:1355, 1990.

Arenas C, et al.: Evaluation of 2 trilostane protocols for the treatment of canine pituitary-dependent hyperadrenocorticism: twice daily versus once daily, *J Vet Intern Med* 27:1478, 2013a.

Arenas C, et al.: Clinical features, outcome and prognostic factors in dogs diagnosed with non-cortisol-secreting adrenal tumours without adrenalectomy: 20 cases (1994-2009), *Vet Record* 173:501, 2013b.

Arenas C, et al.: Long-term survival of dogs with adrenal-dependent hyperadrenocorticism: a comparison between mitotane and twice daily trilostane treatment, *J Vet Intern Med* 28:473, 2014.

Ashley PF, et al.: Effect of oral melatonin administration on sex hormone, prolactin and thyroid hormone concentrations in normal dogs, *J Am Vet Med Assoc* 215:1111, 1999.

Auriemma E, et al.: Computed tomography and low-magnetic resonance imaging of the pituitary gland in dogs with pituitary-dependent hyperadrenocorticism: 11 cases (2001-2003), *J Am Vet Med Assoc* 235:409, 2009.

Badylak SF, Van Vleet JF: Sequential morphologic and clinicopathologic alterations in dogs with experimentally induced glucocorticoid hepatopathy, *Am J Vet Res* 42:1310, 1981.

Bailey MQ: Use of x-ray-computed tomography as an aid in localization of adrenal masses in the dog, *J Am Vet Med Assoc* 188:1046, 1986.

Barberet V, et al.: Intra- and interobserver variability of ultrasonographic measurements of the adrenal glands in healthy beagles, *Vet Radiol Ultrasound* 51:656, 2010.

Barker EN, et al.: A comparison of the survival times of dogs treated with mitotane or trilostane for the pituitary-dependent hyperadrenocorticism, *J Vet Int Med* 19:810, 2005.

Barrera JS, et al.: Evaluation of risk factors for outcome associated with adrenal gland tumors with or without invasion of the caudal vena cava and treated via adrenalectomy in dogs: 86 cases (1993-2009), *J Am Vet Med Assoc* 242:1715, 2013.

Barthez P, et al.: Ultrasonographic evaluation of the adrenal glands in normal dogs and in dogs with hyperadrenocorticism, *J Am Vet Med Assoc* 207:1180, 1995.

Behrend EN, Kemppainen RJ: Diagnosis of canine hyperadrenocorticism, *Vet Clin North Am Sm Anim Pract* 31:985, 2001.

Behrend EN, et al.: Effect of storage conditions on cortisol, total thyroxine, and free thyroxine concentrations in serum and plasma of dogs, *J Am Vet Med Assoc* 212:1564, 1998.

Behrend EN, et al.: Treatment of hyperadrenocorticism in dogs: a survey of internists and dermatologists, *J Am Vet Med Assoc* 215:938, 1999.

Behrend EN, et al.: Diagnosis of hyperadrenocorticism in dogs: a survey of internists and dermatologists, *J Am Vet Med Assoc* 220:1643, 2002.

Behrend EN, et al.: Corticosterone- and aldosterone-secreting adrenocortical tumor in a dog, *J Am Vet Med Assoc* 226:1662, 2004.

Behrend EN, et al.: Serum 17-α-hydroxyprogesterone and corticosterone concentrations in dogs with non-adrenal neoplasia and dogs with suspected hyperadrenocorticism, *J Am Vet Med Assoc* 227:1762, 2005.

Behrend EN, et al.: Intramuscular administration of a low dose of ACTH for ACTH stimulation testing in dogs, *J Am Vet Med Assoc* 229:528, 2006.

Behrend EN, et al.: Diagnosis of spontaneous canine hyperadrenocorticism: 2012 ACVIM consensus statement (Small animal), *J Vet Int Med* 27:1292, 2013.

Bell R, et al.: Study of the effects of once daily doses trilostane on cortisol concentrations and responsiveness to adrenocorticotrophic hormone in hyperadrenocorticoid dogs, *Vet Rec* 159:277, 2006.

Bellumori TP, et al.: Prevalence of inherited disorders among mixed-breed and pure-bred dogs: 27,254 cases (1995-2010), *J Am Vet Med Assoc* 242:1549, 2013.

Benchekroun G: Ultrasonography criteria for differentiating ACTH dependency from ACTH independency in 47 dogs with hyperadrenocorticism and equivocal adrenal asymmetry, *J Vet Intern Med* 24:1077–1085, 2010.

Benchekroun G, et al.: Trilostane therapy for hyperadrenocorticism in three dogs with adrenocortical metastasis, *Vet Rec* 163:190, 2008.

Benitah N, et al.: Evaluation of serum 17-hydroxyprogesterone concentration after administration of ACTH in dogs with hyperadrenocorticism, *J Am Vet Med Assoc* 227:1095, 2005.

Berry CR, et al.: Pulmonary mineralization in four dogs with Cushing's syndrome, *Vet Radiol Ultrasound* 35:10, 1994.

Berry CR, et al.: Frequency of pulmonary mineralization and hypoxemia in 21 dogs with pituitary dependent hyperadrenocorticism, *J Vet Intern Med* 14:151, 2000.

Bertoy EH, et al.: Magnetic resonance imaging of the brain in dogs with recently diagnosed but untreated pituitary-dependent hyperadrenocorticism, *J Am Vet Med Assoc* 206:651, 1995.

Bertoy EH, et al.: One-year follow-up evaluation of magnetic resonance imaging of the brain in dogs with pituitary-dependent hyperadrenocorticism, *J Am Vet Med Assoc* 208:1268, 1996.

Besso JG, et al.: Retrospective ultrasonographic evaluation of adrenal lesions in 26 dogs, *Vet Radiol Ultrasound* 38:448, 1997.

Biewenga WJ, et al.: Osmoregulation of systemic vasopressin release during long-term glucocorticoid excess: a study in dogs with hyperadrenocorticism, *Acta Endocrinologica* 124:583, 1991.

Bley CR, et al.: Irradiation of brain tumors in dogs with neurologic disease, *J Vet Intern Med* 19:849, 2005.

Blois SL, et al.: Multiple endocrine diseases in dogs: 35 cases (1996-2009), *J Am Vet Med Assoc* 238:1616, 2011.

Bodey AR, Michell AR: Epidemiological study of blood pressure in domestic dogs, *J Small Anim Pract* 37:116, 1996.

Bondanelli M, et al.: Evaluation of hormonal function in a series on incidentally discovered adrenal masses, *Metabolism* 46:107, 1997.

Boozer AL, et al.: Pituitary-adrenal axis function in dogs with neoplasia, *Vet Comp Oncol* 3:194, 2006.

Bosje JT, et al.: Plasma concentrations of ACTH precursors correlate with pituitary size and resistance to dexamethasone in dogs with pituitary-dependent hyperadrenocorticism, *Domest Anim Endocrinol* 22:201, 2002.

Braddock JA, et al.: Trilostane treatment in dogs with pituitary-dependent hyperadrenocorticism, *Aust Vet J* 81:600, 2003.

Braddock JA, et al.: Inefficacy of selegiline in treatment of canine pituitary-dependent hyperadrenocorticism, *Aust Vet J* 82:272, 2004.

Braund KG, et al.: Subclinical myopathy associated with hyperadrenocorticism in the dog, *Vet Pathol* 17:134, 1980.

Brearley MJ, et al.: Hypofractionated RT of brain masses in dogs: a retrospective analysis of survival of 83 cases (1991-1996), *J Vet Intern Med* 13:408, 1999.

Breitschwerdt EB, et al.: Idiopathic hyperaldosteronism in a dog, *J Am Vet Med Assoc* 187:841, 1985.

Bromel C, et al.: Serum 17 α-hydroxyprogesterone concentrations during the reproductive cycle in healthy dogs and dogs with hyperadrenocorticism, *J Am Vet Med Assoc* 236:1208, 2010.

Bugbee AC, et al.: Effect of dexamethasone or synthetic ACTH administration on endogenous ACTH concentrations in healthy dogs, *Am J Vet Res* 74:1415, 2013.

Burgener IA, et al.: Empty sella syndrome, hyperadrenocorticism and megaesophagus in a dachshund, *J Small Anim Pract* 48:584, 2007.

Burkhardt WA, et al.: Adrenocorticotropic hormone, but not trilostane, causes severe adrenal hemorrhage, vacuolization, and apoptosis in rats, *Domest Anim Endocrinol* 40:155, 2011.

Burkhardt WA, et al.: Evaluation of baseline cortisol, endogenous ACTH and cortisol/ACTH ratio to monitor trilostane treatment in dogs with pituitary-dependent hyperadrenocorticism, *J Vet Intern Med* 27:919, 2013.

Cabrera Blatter MF, et al.: Blindness in dogs with pituitary dependent hyperadrenocorticism: relationship with glucose, cortisol and triglyceride concentration and with ophthalmic blood flow, *Res Vet Sci* 92:387, 2012a.

Cabrera Blatter MF, et al.: Interleukin-6 and insulin increase and nitric oxide and adiponectin decrease in blind dogs with pituitary-dependent hyperadrenocorticism, *Res Vet Sci* 93:1195, 2012b.

Cai W, et al.: Metabolic activation and binding of mitotane in adrenal cortex homogenates, *J Pharmaceut Sciences* 84:134, 1995.

Capen CC: Endocrine glands. In Maxie MG, editor: *Jubb, Kennedy and Palmer's pathology of domestic animals*, Philadelphia, 2007, Saunders/Elsevier, p 325.

Carter CT, et al.: Elevations in sex hormones in dogs with sudden acquired retinal degeneration syndrome (SARDS), *J Am Anim Hosp Assoc* 45:207, 2009.

Cartledge S, Lawson N: Aldosterone and renin measurements, *Annals Clin Biochem* 37:262, 2000.

Castillo V, Gallelli MF: Corticotroph adenoma in the dog: pathogenesis and new therapeutic possibilities, *Res Vet Sci* 88:26, 2010.

Castillo V, et al.: Retinoic acid as a novel medical therapy for Cushing's disease in dogs, *Endocrinology* 147:4438, 2006.

Castillo V, et al.: Diurnal ACTH and plasma cortisol variations in healthy dogs and in those with pituitary-dependent Cushing's syndrome before and after treatment with retinoic acid, *Res Vet Sci* 86:223, 2009.

Cerundolo R, et al.: Treatment of canine Alopecia X with trilostane, *Vet Dermatol* 15:2853, 2004.

Chapman PS, et al.: Evaluation of the basal and post-adrenocorticotrophic hormone serum concentrations of 17-hydroxyprogesterone for the diagnosis of hyperadrenocorticism in dogs, *Vet Rec* 153:771, 2003.

Chapman PS, et al.: Adrenal necrosis in a dog receiving trilostane for the treatment of hyperadrenocorticism, *J Small Anim Pract* 45:307, 2004.

Chastain CB, et al.: Evaluation of the hypothalamic pituitary-adrenal axis in clinically stressed dogs, *J Am Anim Hosp Assoc* 22:435, 1986.

Chauvet AE, et al.: Effects of phenobarbital administration on results of serum biochemical analyses and adrenocortical function tests in epileptic dogs, *J Am Vet Med Assoc* 207:1305, 1995.

Cho KD, et al.: Serum adipokine concentrations in dogs with naturally occurring pituitary-dependent hyperadrenocorticism, *J Vet Intern Med* 28:429, 2014.

Choi J, et al.: Ultrasonographic adrenal gland measurements in clinically normal small breed dogs and comparison with pituitary-dependent hyperadrenocorticism, *J Vet Med Sci* 73:985, 2011.

Church DB, et al.: Effect of nonadrenal illness, anaesthesia and surgery on plasma cortisol concentrations in dogs, *Res Vet Sci* 56:129, 1994.

Churcher RK: Hepatic carcinoid, hypercortisolism and hypokalaemia in a dog, *Aust Vet J* 77:641, 1999.

Cisneros LE, et al.: What is your neurologic diagnosis? Hyperadrenocorticism, *J Am Vet Med Assoc* 238:1247, 2011.

Clemente M, et al.: Comparison of non-selective adrenocorticolysis with mitotane or trilostane for the treatment of dogs with pituitary-dependent hyperadrenocorticism, *Vet Rec* 161:805, 2007.

Cohen TA, Feldman EC: Comparison of IV and IM formulations of synthetic ACTH for ACTH stimulation tests in healthy dogs, *J Vet Intern Med* 26:412, 2012.

Cook AK, Bond KG: Evaluation of the use of baseline cortisol concentration as a monitoring tool for dogs receiving trilostane as a treatment for hyperadrenocorticism, *J Am Vet Med Assoc* 237:801, 2010.

Cook AK, et al.: Pharmaceutical evaluation of compounded trilostane products, *J Am Anim Hosp Assoc* 48:228, 2012.

Cook AK, et al.: Clinical findings in dogs with incidental adrenal gland lesions determined by ultrasonography: 151 cases (2007-2010), *J Am Vet Med Assoc* 244:1181, 2014.

Davies DR, et al.: Hypokalaemic paresis, hypertension, alkalosis, and adrenal-dependent hyperadrenocorticism in a dog, *Aust Vet J* 86:139, 2008.

Davis MK, et al.: Ultrasonographic identification of vascular invasion by adrenal tumors in dogs, *Vet Radiol Ultrasound* 53:442, 2012.

Dayanithi G, Antoni FA: Rapid as well as delayed inhibitory effects of glucocorticoid hormones on pituitary adrenocorticotropic hormone release are mediated by type II glucocorticoid receptors and require newly synthesized messenger ribonucleic acid as well as protein, *Endocrinology* 125:308, 1989.

DeCoster R, et al.: Endocrinological effects of single daily ketoconazole administration in male beagle dogs, *Acta Endocrinologica* 107:275, 1984.

de Fornel P, et al.: Effects of radiotherapy on pituitary corticotroph macrotumors in dogs: a retrospective study of 12 cases, *Can Vet J* 48:481, 2007.

den Hertog E, et al.: Results of nonselective adrenocorticolysis by o,p'-DDD in 129 dogs with pituitary-dependent hyperadrenocorticism, *Vet Rec* 144:12, 1999.

DeNovo RC, Prasse KW: Comparison of serum biochemical and hepatic functional alterations in dogs treated with corticosteroids and hepatic duct ligation, *Am J Vet Res* 44:1703, 1983.

Djajadiningrat-Laanen SC, et al.: Urinary aldosterone to creatinine ratio in cats before and after suppression with salt or fludrocortisone acetate, *J Vet Intern Med* 22:1283, 2008.

Djajadiningrat-Laanen SC, et al.: Primary hyperaldosteronism: expanding the diagnostic net, *J Fel Med Surg* 13:651, 2011.

Doerr KA, et al.: Calcinosis cutis in dogs: histopathological and clinical analysis of 46 cases, *Vet Dermatol* 24:355, 2013.

Douglass JP, et al.: Ultrasonographic adrenal gland measurements in dogs without evidence of adrenal disease, *Vet Radiol Ultrasound* 38:124, 1997.

Dow SW, et al.: Perianal adenomas and hypertestosteronemia in a spayed bitch with pituitary-dependent hyperadrenocorticism, *J Am Vet Med Assoc* 192:1439, 1988.

Dow SW, et al.: Response of dogs with functional pituitary macroadenomas and macrocarcinomas to radiation, *J Small Anim Pract* 31:287, 1990.

Drucker WD, Peterson ME: Pharmacologic treatment of pituitary-dependent canine Cushing's disease, *Program of the Sixty-Second Annual Meeting of the Endocrine Society*, San Francisco, 1980, p 89.

Duesberg CA, et al.: Magnetic resonance imaging for diagnosis of pituitary macrotumors in dogs, *J Am Vet Med Assoc* 206:657, 1995.

Dyer KR, et al.: Effects of short- and long-term administration of phenobarbital on endogenous ACTH concentration and results of ACTH stimulation tests in dogs, *J Am Vet Med Assoc* 205:315, 1994.

Eastwood JM, et al.: Trilostane treatment of a dog with functional adrenocortical neoplasia, *J Small Anim Pract* 44:126, 2003.

Eberwine JH, et al.: Complex transcriptional regulation by glucocorticoids and corticotropin-releasing hormone of pro-opiomelanocortin gene expression in rat pituitary cultures, *DNA* 6:483, 1987.

Eckersall PD, et al.: The measurement of canine steroid-induced alkaline phosphatase by L-phenylalanine inhibition, *J Small Anim Pract* 27:411, 1986.

Elliott DA, et al.: Glycosylated hemoglobin concentrations in the blood of healthy dogs and dogs with naturally developing diabetes mellitus, pancreatic β-cell neoplasia, hyperadrenocorticism, and anemia, *J Am Vet Med Assoc* 211:723, 1997.

Emms SG, et al.: Evaluation of canine hyperadrenocorticism using computed tomography, *J Am Vet Med Assoc* 189:432, 1986.

Feldman BF, et al.: Hemostatic abnormalities in canine Cushing's syndrome, *Res Vet Sci* 41:228, 1986.

Feldman EC: Comparison of ACTH response and dexamethasone suppression as screening tests in canine hyperadrenocorticism, *J Am Vet Med Assoc* 182:505, 1983a.

Feldman EC: Distinguishing dogs with functioning adrenocortical tumors from dogs with pituitary-dependent hyperadrenocorticism, *J Am Vet Med Assoc* 183:195, 1983b.

Feldman EC: Evaluation of a combined dexamethasone suppression/ACTH stimulation test in dogs with hyperadrenocorticism, *J Am Vet Med Assoc* 187:49, 1985.

Feldman EC: Evaluation of a 6-hour combined dexamethasone suppression/ ACTH stimulation test in dogs with hyperadrenocorticism, *J Am Vet Med Assoc* 189:1562, 1986.

Feldman EC: Evaluation of twice-daily lower-dose trilostane treatment administered orally in dogs with naturally occurring hyperadrenocorticism, *J Am Vet Med Assoc* 238:1441, 2011.

Feldman EC, Kass PH: Trilostane dose versus body weight in the treatment of naturally occurring pituitary-dependent hyperadrenocorticism in dogs, *J Vet Intern Med* 26:1078, 2012.

Feldman EC, Mack RE: Urine cortisol:creatinine ratio as a screening test for hyperadrenocorticism in dogs, *J Am Vet Med Assoc* 200:1637, 1992.

Feldman EC, Nelson RW: Use of ketoconazole for control of canine hyperadrenocorticism. In Kirk RW, Bonagura JD, editors: *Current veterinary therapy XI*, Philadelphia, 1992, WB Saunders, p 349.

Feldman EC, Nelson RW: Canine hyperadrenocorticism (Cushing's syndrome). In Feldman EC, Nelson RW, editors: *Canine and feline endocrinology and reproduction*, St Louis, 2004, Saunders, p 252.

Feldman EC, et al.: Plasma cortisol response to ketoconazole administration in dogs with hyperadrenocorticism, *J Am Vet Med Assoc* 197:71, 1990.

Feldman EC, et al.: Comparison of mitotane treatment for adrenal tumor versus pituitary-dependent hyperadrenocorticism in dogs, *J Am Vet Med Assoc* 200:1642, 1992.

Feldman EC, et al.: Use of low- and high-dose dexamethasone tests for distinguishing pituitary dependent from adrenal tumor hyperadrenocorticism, *J Am Vet Med Assoc* 209:772, 1996.

Ferguson DC, Biery DN: Diabetes insipidus and hyperadrenocorticism associated with high plasma adrenocorticotropin concentration and a hypothalamic/pituitary mass in a dog, *J Am Vet Med Assoc* 193:835, 1988.

Ferguson DC, Peterson ME: Serum free and total iodothyronine concentrations in dogs with hyperadrenocorticism, *Am J Vet Res* 53:1636, 1992.

Ford SL, et al.: Hyperadrenocorticism caused by bilateral adrenocortical neoplasia in dogs: four cases (1983-1988), *J Am Vet Med Assoc* 202:789, 1993.

Forrester SD, et al.: Retrospective evaluation of urinary tract infection in 42 dogs with hyperadrenocorticism or diabetes mellitus or both, *J Vet Intern Med* 13:557, 1999.

Fossum TW: *Small animal surgery*, ed 4, St Louis, 2012, Mosby.

Foster SF, et al.: Effect of phenobarbitone on the low-dose dexamethasone suppression test and the urinary corticoid: creatinine ratio in dogs, *Aust Vet J* 78:19, 2000a.

Foster SF, et al.: Effects of phenobarbitone on serum biochemical tests in dogs, *Aust Vet J* 78:23, 2000b.

Frank LA, Oliver JW: Comparison of serum cortisol concentrations in clinically normal dogs after administration of freshly reconstituted versus reconstituted and stored frozen cosyntropin, *J Am Vet Med Assoc* 212:1569, 1998.

Frank LA, et al.: Cortisol concentrations following stimulation of healthy and adrenopathic dogs with two doses of tetracosactrin, *J Small Anim Pract* 41:308, 2000.

Frank LA, et al.: Steroidogenic response of adrenal tissues after administration of ACTH to dogs with hypercortisolemia, *J Am Vet Med Assoc* 218:214, 2001.

Frank LA, et al.: Retrospective evaluation of sex hormones and steroid hormone intermediates in dogs with alopecia, *Vet Dermatol* 14:91, 2003.

Frank LA, et al.: Adrenal steroid hormone concentrations in dogs with hair cycle arrest (Alopecia X) before and during treatment with melatonin and mitotane, *Vet Dermatol* 15:278, 2004.

Frank LA, et al.: Oestrogen receptor evaluation in Pomeranian dogs with hair cycle arrest (alopecia X) on melatonin supplementation, *Vet Dermatol* 17:252, 2006.

Frank LA, et al.: Variability of estradiol concentration in normal dogs, *Vet Dermat* 21:490, 2010.

Frankot JL, et al.: Adrenocortical carcinoma in a dog with incomplete excision managed long-term with metastasectomy alone, *J Am Anim Hosp Assoc* 48:417, 2012.

Fukuoka H, et al.: EGFR as a therapeutic target for human, canine, and mouse ACTH-secreting pituitary adenomas, *J Clin Invest* 121:4712, 2011.

Galac S, et al.: Urinary corticoid: creatinine ratios in the differentiation between pituitary dependent hyperadrenocorticism and hyperadrenocorticism due to adrenocortical tumour in the dog, *Vet Q* 19:17, 1997.

Galac S, et al.: Hyperadrenocorticism in a dog due to ectopic secretion of adrenocorticotropic hormone, *Domest Anim Endocrinol* 28:338, 2005.

Galac S, et al.: ACTH-independent hyperadrenocorticism due to food-dependent hypercortisolemia in a dog: a case report, *Vet J* 177:141, 2007.

Galac S, et al.: Urinary corticoid: creatinine ratios in dogs with pituitary-dependent hypercortisolism during trilostane treatment, *J Vet Int Med* 23:1214, 2009.

Galac S, et al.: Expression of the ACTH receptor, steroidogenic acute regulatory protein, and steroidogenic enzymes in canine cortisol-secreting adrenocortical tumors, *Domest Anim Endocrinol* 39:259, 2010a.

Galac S, et al.: Expression of receptors for luteinizing hormone, gastric-inhibitory polypeptide, and vasopressin in normal adrenal glands and cortisol-secreting adrenocortical tumors in dogs, *Domest Anim Endocrinol* 39:63, 2010b.

Gallelli MF, et al.: A comparative study by age and gender of the pituitary adenoma and ACTH and alpha-MSH secretion in dogs with pituitary-dependent hyperadrenocorticism, *Res Vet Sci* 88:33, 2010.

Gieger TL, et al.: Lymphoma as a model for chronic illness: effects on adrenocortical function testing, *J Vet Int Med* 17:154, 2003.

Gillette EL, Gillette SM: Principles of radiation therapy, *Semin Vet Med Surg (Small Animal)* 10:129, 1995.

Ginel PJ, et al.: Evaluation of serum concentrations of cortisol and sex hormones of adrenal gland origin after stimulation with two synthetic ACTH preparations in clinically normal dogs, *Am J Vet Res* 73:237, 2012.

Golden DL, Lothrop CD: A retrospective study of aldosterone secretion in normal and adrenopathic dogs, *J Vet Intern Med* 2:121, 1988.

Goldhaber SZ: Pulmonary embolism, *N Engl J Med* 339:93, 1998.

Goossens MMC, et al.: Central diabetes insipidus in a dog with a pro-opiomelanocortin-producing pituitary tumor not causing hyperadrenocorticism, *J Vet Int Med* 9:361, 1995.

Goossens MMC, et al.: Efficacy of cobalt 60 radiotherapy in dogs with pituitary-dependent hyperadrenocorticism, *J Am Vet Med Assoc* 212:374, 1998.

Gould SM: Use of endogenous ACTH concentration and adrenal ultrasonography to distinguish the cause of canine hyperadrenocorticism, *J Small Anim Pract* 42:113, 2001.

Goy-Thollot I, et al.: Investigation of the role of aldosterone in hypertension associated with spontaneous pituitary-dependent hyperadrenocorticism in dogs, *J Small Anim Pract* 43:489, 2002.

Granger N, et al.: Plasma pro-opiomelanocortin, pro-adrenocorticotropin hormone and pituitary adenoma size in dogs with Cushing's disease, *J Vet Int Med* 19:23, 2005.

Greco DS, et al.: Concurrent pituitary and adrenal tumors in dogs with hyperadrenocorticism: 17 cases (1978-1995), *J Am Vet Med Assoc* 214:1349, 1999.

Griebsch C, et al.: Effect of trilostane on hormone and serum electrolyte concentrations in dogs with pituitary-dependent hyperadrenocorticism, *J Vet Intern Med* 28:160, 2014.

Grooters AM, et al.: Evaluation of routine abdominal ultrasonography as a technique for imaging the canine adrenal glands, *J Am Anim Hosp Assoc* 30:457, 1994.

Grooters AM, et al.: Ultrasonographic parameters of normal canine adrenal glands: comparison to necropsy findings, *Vet Radiol Ultrasound* 36:126, 1995.

Grooters AM, et al.: Ultrasonographic characteristics of the adrenal glands in dogs with pituitary dependent hyperadrenocorticism: comparison with normal dogs, *J Vet Intern Med* 10:110, 1996.

Grumbach MM, Conte FA: Disorders of sex differentiation. In Wilson JD, Foster DW, Kronenberg HM, Larsen PR, editors: *Williams textbook of endocrinology*, Philadelphia, 1998, WB Saunders, p 1303.

Guptill L, et al.: Use of the urine cortisol:creatinine ratio to monitor treatment response in dogs with pituitary-dependent hyperadrenocorticism, *J Am Vet Med Assoc* 210:1158, 1997.

Hadley SP, et al.: Effect of glucocorticoids on alkaline phosphatase, alanine aminotransferase, and gamma-glutamyltransferase in cultured dog hepatocytes, *Enzyme* 43:89, 1990.

Halmi NS, et al.: Pituitary intermediate lobe in the dog: two cell types and high bioactive adrenocorticotropin content, *Science* 211:72, 1981.

Hanson JM, et al.: Efficacy of transsphenoidal hypophysectomy in treatment of dogs with pituitary-dependent hyperadrenocorticism, *J Vet Intern Med* 19:687, 2005.

Hanson JM, et al.: Plasma profiles of adrenocorticotropic hormone, cortisol, alpha-melanocyte-stimulating hormone, and growth hormone in dogs with pituitary-dependent hyperadrenocorticism before and after hypophysectomy, *J Endocrinol* 190:601, 2006.

Hanson JM, et al.: Prognostic factors for outcome after transsphenoidal hypophysectomy in dogs with pituitary-dependent hyperadrenocorticism, *J Neurosurg* 107:830, 2007.

Hanson JM, et al.: Expression and mutation analysis of Tpit in the canine pituitary gland and corticotroph adenomas, *Domest Anim Endocrinol* 34:217, 2008.

Hanson JM, et al.: Expression of leukemia inhibitory factor and leukemia inhibitory factor receptor in the canine pituitary gland and corticotrope adenomas, *Domest Anim Endocrinol* 38:260, 2010.

Harris D, et al.: Radiation therapy toxicities, *Vet Clin N Amer Sm Anim Pract* 27:37, 1997.

Helm JR, et al.: A comparison of factors that influence survival in dogs with adrenal-dependent hyperadrenocorticism treated with mitotane or trilostane, *J Vet Int Med* 25:251, 2011.

Hess RS, et al.: Association between hyperadrenocorticism and development of calcium containing uroliths in dogs with urolithiasis, *J Am Vet Med Assoc* 212:1889, 1998.

Hill K, Scott-Moncrieff JC: Tumors of the adrenal cortex causing hyperadrenocorticism, *Vet Med* 96:686, 2001.

Hill KE, et al.: Secretion of sex hormones in dogs with adrenal dysfunction, *J Am Vet Med Assoc* 226:556, 2005.

Hoerauf A, Reusch C: Ultrasonographic characteristics of both adrenal glands in 15 dogs with functional adrenocortical tumors, *J Am Anim Hosp Assoc* 35:193, 1999.

Huizenga NA, et al.: A polymorphism in the glucocorticoid receptor gene may be associated with an increased sensitivity to glucocorticoids in vivo, *J Clin Endocrinol Metab* 83:144, 1998.

Hurley KJ, Vaden SL: Evaluation of urine protein content in dogs with pituitary-dependent hyperadrenocorticism, *J Am Vet Med Assoc* 212:369, 1998.

Hylands R: Veterinary diagnostic imaging: malignant pheochromocytoma of the left adrenal gland invading the caudal vena cava, accompanied by a cortisol-secreting adrenocortical carcinoma of the right adrenal gland, *Can Vet J* 46:1156, 2005.

Ishino H, et al.: Ki-67 and minichromosome maintenance-7 (MCM7) expression in canine pituitary corticotroph adenomas, *Domest Anim Endocrinol* 41:207, 2011.

Jacoby RC, et al.: Biochemical basis for the hypercoagulable state seen in Cushing's syndrome, *Arch Surg* 139:1003, 2001.

Jensen AL, et al.: Evaluation of the urinary cortisol:creatinine ratio in the diagnosis of hyperadrenocorticism in dogs, *J Small Anim Pract* 38:99, 1997.

Jerico MM, et al.: Chromatographic analysis of lipid fractions in healthy dogs and dogs with obesity or hyperadrenocorticism, *J Vet Diagn Invest* 21:203, 2009.

Jiménez Peláez M, et al.: Laparoscopic adrenalectomy for treatment of unilateral adrenocortical carcinomas: technique, complications, and results in seven dogs, *Vet Surg* 37:444, 2008.

Johnson CA: Progesterone and prolactin-related disorders; adrenal dysfunction and sex hormones. In Rand J, editor: *Clinical endocrinology of companion animals*, Ames, IA, 2013, John Wiley and Sons, pp 487–503.

Johnson LR, et al.: Pulmonary thromboembolism in 29 dogs: 1985-1995, *J Vet Intern Med* 13:338, 1999.

Juchem M, Pollow K: Binding of oral contraceptive progestogens to serum proteins and cytoplasmic receptor, *Am J Obstet Gynecol* 163:2171, 1990.

Kantrowitz BM, et al.: Adrenal ultrasonography in the dog, *Vet Radiol* 27:15, 1986.

Kaplan AJ, et al.: Effects of disease on the results of diagnostic tests for use in detecting hyperadrenocorticism in dogs, *J Am Vet Med Assoc* 207:445, 1995.

Kemppainen RJ, Peterson ME: Circulating concentration of dexamethasone in healthy dogs, dogs with hyperadrenocorticism, and dogs with nonadrenal illness during dexamethasone suppression testing, *Am J Vet Res* 54:1765, 1993.

Kemppainen RJ, Sartin JL: Evidence for episodic but not circadian activity in plasma concentrations of adrenocorticotropin, cortisol and thyroxine in dogs, *J Endocrinol* 103:219, 1984a.

Kemppainen RJ, Sartin JL: Effects of single intravenous doses of dexamethasone on baseline plasma cortisol concentrations and response to synthetic ACTH in healthy dogs, *Am J Vet Res* 45:742, 1984b.

Kemppainen RJ, Sartin JL: Differential regulation of peptide release by the canine pars distalis and pars intermedia, *Front Horm Res* 17:18, 1987.

Kemppainen RJ, et al.: Effects of prednisone on thyroid and gonadal endocrine function in dogs, *J Endocr* 96:293, 1983.

Kemppainen RJ, et al.: Regulation of adrenocorticotropin secretion from cultured canine anterior pituitary cells, *Am J Vet Res* 53:2355, 1992.

Kemppainen RJ, et al.: Preservative effect of aprotinin on canine plasma immunoreactive adrenocorticotropin concentrations, *Dom Anim Endocr* 11:355, 1994.

Kemppainen RJ, et al.: Use of compounded adrenocorticotropic hormone (ACTH) for adrenal function testing in dogs, *J Am Anim Hosp Assoc* 41:368, 2005.

Kent MS, et al.: Survival, neurologic response, and prognostic factors in dogs with pituitary masses treated with radiation therapy and untreated dogs, *J Vet Intern Med* 21:1027, 2007.

Kerl ME, et al.: Evaluation of a low-dose synthetic adrenocorticotropic hormone stimulation test in clinically normal dogs and dogs with naturally developing hyperadrenocorticism, *J Am Vet Med Assoc* 214:1497, 1999.

Keyes ML, et al.: Pulmonary thromboembolism in dogs, *J Vet Emerg Crit Care* 3:23, 1993.

Kidney BA, Jackson ML: Diagnostic value of alkaline phosphatase isoenzyme separation by affinity electrophoresis in the dog, *Can Vet J* 52:106, 1988.

Kintzer PP, Peterson ME: Mitotane (o, p'DDD) treatment of 200 dogs with pituitary-dependent hyperadrenocorticism, *J Vet Intern Med* 5:182, 1991.

Kintzer PP, Peterson ME: Mitotane (o, p'-DDD) treatment of dogs with cortisol-secreting adrenocortical neoplasia: 32 cases (1980-1992), *J Am Vet Med Assoc* 205:54, 1994.

Kipperman BS, et al.: Pituitary tumor size, neurologic signs, and relation to endocrine test results in dogs with pituitary-dependent hyperadrenocorticism: 43 cases (1980-1990), *J Am Vet Med Assoc* 201:762, 1992.

Kirk GR, et al.: Effects of o,p'-DDD on plasma cortisol levels and histology of the adrenal gland in the normal dog, *J Am Anim Hosp Assoc* 10:179, 1974.

Klose TC, et al.: Evaluation of coagulation status in dogs with naturally occurring canine hyperadrenocorticism, *J Vet Emerg Crit Care* 21:625, 2011.

Kolevska F, Svoboda M: Immunoreactive cortisol measurement in canine urine and its validity in hyperadrenocorticism diagnosis, *Acta Vet Brno* 69:217, 2000.

Konar M, et al.: Magnetic resonance imaging features of empty sella in dogs, *Vet Radiol Ultrasound* 49:339, 2008.

Kooistra HS, et al.: Pulsatile secretion of alpha-MSH and the differential effects of dexamethasone and haloperidol on the secretion of alpha-MSH and ACTH in dogs, *J Endocrinol* 152:113, 1997a.

Kooistra HS, et al.: Correlation between impairment of glucocorticoid feedback and the size of the pituitary gland in dogs with pituitary-dependent hyperadrenocorticism, *J Endocrinol* 152:387, 1997b.

Kook PH, et al.: Effects of iatrogenic hypercortisolism on gallbladder sludge formation and biochemical bile constituents in dogs, *Vet J* 191:225, 2011.

Kool MM, et al.: Activating mutations of GNAS in canine cortisol-secreting adrenocortical tumors, *J Vet Intern Med* 27:1486, 2013.

Kutsunai M, et al.: The association between gall bladder mucoceles and hyperlipidaemia in dogs: a retrospective case control study, *Vet J* 199:76, 2014.

Kyles AE, et al.: Surgical management of adrenal gland tumors with and without associated tumor thrombi in dogs: 40 cases (1994-2001), *J Am Vet Med Assoc* 223:654, 2003.

Labelle P, et al.: Indicators of malignancy of canine adrenocortical tumors: histopathology and proliferation index, *Vet Pathol* 41:490, 2004.

Lang JM, et al.: Elective and emergency surgical management of adrenal gland tumors: 60 cases (1999-2006), *J Am Anim Hosp Assoc* 47:428, 2011.

Lantz GC, et al.: Transsphenoidal hypophysectomy in the clinically normal dog, *Am J Vet Res* 49:1134, 1988.

LaRue MJ, Murtaugh RJ: Pulmonary thromboembolism in dogs: 47 cases (1986-1987), *J Am Vet Med Assoc* 197:1368, 1990.

Leone F, et al.: The use of trilostane for the treatment of Alopecia X in Alaskan malamutes, *J Am Anim Hosp Assoc* 41:336, 2005.

Lien YH, et al.: Associations among systemic blood pressure, microalbuminuria and albuminuria in dogs affected with pituitary- and adrenal-dependent hyperadrenocorticism, *Acta Vet Scand* 52:61, 2010.

Lien YH, Huang H-P: Use of ketoconazole to treat dogs with pituitary-dependent hyperadrenocorticism: 48 cases (1994-2007), *J Am Vet Med Assoc* 233:1896, 2008.

Ling GV, et al.: Canine hyperadrenocorticism: pretreatment clinical and laboratory evaluation of 117 cases, *J Am Vet Med Assoc* 174:1211, 1979.

Love NE, et al.: The computed tomographic enhancement pattern of the normal canine pituitary gland, *Vet Radiol Ultrasound* 41:507, 2000.

Lulich JP, Osborne CA: Bacterial infections of the urinary tract. In Ettinger SJ, Feldman EC, editors: *Textbook of veterinary medicine*, Philadelphia, 1994, WB Saunders, p 1775.

Machida T, et al.: Aldosterone-, corticosterone- and cortisol-secreting adrenocortical carcinoma in a dog: case report, *J Vet Med Sci* 70:317, 2007.

Maher VMG, et al.: Possible mechanism and treatment of o, p' DDD-induced hypercholesterolemia, *Q J Med* 305:671, 1992.

Mantis P, et al.: Changes in ultrasonographic appearance of adrenal glands in dogs with pituitary-dependent hyperadrenocorticism treated with trilostane, *Vet Radiol Ultrasound* 44:682, 2003.

Marcus HI, et al.: Bilateral adrenal hemorrhage during ACTH treatment of ulcerative colitis, *Dis Colon Rectum* 29:130, 1986.

Mariani CL, et al.: Frameless stereotactic radiosurgery for the treatment of primary intracranial tumours in dogs, *Vet Comp Oncol*, 2013. [Epub ahead of print].

Martin LG, et al.: Effect of low doses of cosyntropin on serum cortisol concentrations in clinically normal dogs, *Am J Vet Res* 68:555, 2007.

Martinez NI, et al.: Evaluation of pressor sensitivity to norepinephrine infusion in dogs with iatrogenic hyperadrenocorticism. Pressor sensitivity in dogs with hyperadrenocorticism, *Res Vet Sci* 78:25, 2005.

Massari F, et al.: Adrenalectomy in dogs with adrenal gland tumors: 52 cases (2002-2008), *J Am Vet Med Assoc* 239:216, 2011.

Mattson A, et al.: Clinical features suggesting hyperadrenocorticism associated with sudden acquired retinal degeneration syndrome in a dog, *J Am Anim Hosp Assoc* 28:199, 1992.

May ER, et al.: Effects of a mock ultrasonographic procedure on cortisol concentrations during low-dose dexamethasone suppression testing in clinically normal adult dogs, *Am J Vet Res* 65:267, 2004.

McGraw AL, et al.: Determination of the concentrations of trilostane and keto-trilostane that inhibit ex vivo adrenal synthesis of cortisol, corticosterone and aldosterone, *Am J Vet Res* 72:661, 2010.

McLauchlan G, et al.: Retrospective evaluation of the effect of trilostane on insulin requirement and fructosamine concentration in eight diabetic dogs with hyperadrenocorticism, *J Small Anim Pract* 51:642, 2010.

McNicol AM: Pituitary morphology in canine pituitary-dependent hyperadrenocorticism, *Front Horm Res* 17:71, 1987.

Meaney JFM, et al.: Diagnosis of pulmonary embolism with magnetic resonance angiography, *N Engl J Med* 336:1422, 1997.

Meij BP, et al.: Residual pituitary function after transsphenoidal hypophysectomy in dogs with pituitary-dependent hyperadrenocorticism, *J Endocrinol* 155:531, 1997a.

Meij BP, et al.: Transsphenoidal hypophysectomy in Beagle dogs: evaluation of a microsurgical technique, *Vet Surg* 26:295, 1997b.

Meij BP, et al.: Alterations in anterior pituitary function of dogs with pituitary-dependent hyperadrenocorticism, *J Endocrinol* 154:505, 1997c.

Meij BP, et al.: Results of transsphenoidal hypophysectomy in 52 dogs with pituitary-dependent hyperadrenocorticism, *Vet Surg* 27:246, 1998.

Melby JC: Therapy for Cushing disease: a consensus for pituitary microsurgery, *Ann Intern Med* 109:445, 1988.

Mesich ML, et al.: Gall bladder mucoceles and their association with endocrinopathies in dogs: a retrospective case-control study, *J Small Anim Pract* 50:630, 2009.

Monroe WE, et al.: Concentrations of noncortisol adrenal steroids in response to ACTH in dogs with adrenal-dependent hyperadrenocorticism, pituitary-dependent hyperadrenocorticism, and nonadrenal illness, *J Vet Intern Med* 26:945, 2012.

Montgomery KW, et al.: Acute blindness in dogs: sudden acquired retinal degeneration syndrome versus neurological disease (140 cases, 2000-2006), *Vet Ophthalmol* 11:314, 2008.

Montgomery TM, et al.: Basal and glucagon-stimulated plasma C-peptide concentrations in healthy dogs, dogs with diabetes mellitus, and dogs with hyperadrenocorticism, *J Vet Intern Med* 10:116, 1996.

Mueller C, et al.: Low-dose dexamethasone test with "inverse" results: a possible new pattern of cortisol response, *Vet Rec* 159:489, 2006.

Muller PB, et al.: Effects of long-term phenobarbital treatment on the thyroid and adrenal axis and adrenal function tests in dogs, *J Vet Intern Med* 14:157, 2000a.

Muller PB, et al.: Effects of long-term phenobarbital treatment on the liver in dogs, *J Vet Intern Med* 14:165, 2000b.

Naan EC, et al.: Innovative approach to laparoscopic adrenalectomy for treatment of unilateral adrenal gland tumors in dogs, *Vet Surg* 42:710, 2013.

Neiger, R: Hyperadrenocorticism: the animal perspective—comparative efficacy and safety of trilostane, *Proceedings 22nd Ann Vet Med Forum,* p 699, 2004.

Neiger R, et al.: Trilostane treatment of 78 dogs with pituitary-dependent hyperadrenocorticism, *Vet Rec* 150:799, 2002.

Nelson AA, Woodard G: Severe adrenal cortical atrophy (cytotoxic) and hepatic damage produced in dogs by feeding 2, 2-bis (parachlorophenyl)-1, 1-trichloroethane (DDD or TDE), *Arch Pathol* 48:387, 1949.

Nelson RW, et al.: Effect of o, p'-DDD therapy on endogenous ACTH concentrations in dogs with hypophysis-dependent hyperadrenocorticism, *Am J Vet Res* 46:1534, 1985.

Nelson RW, et al.: Pituitary macroadenomas and macroadenocarcinomas in dogs treated with mitotane for pituitary-dependent hyperadrenocorticism: 13 cases (1981-1986), *J Am Vet Med Assoc* 194:1612, 1989.

Niebauer GW, Evans SM: Transsphenoidal hypophysectomy in the dog: a new technique, *Vet Surg* 17:296, 1988.

Niebauer GW, et al.: Study of long-term survival after transsphenoidal hypophysectomy in clinically normal dogs, *Am J Vet Res* 51:677, 1990.

Norman EJ, et al.: Dynamic adrenal function testing in eight dogs with hyperadrenocorticism associated with adrenocortical neoplasia, *Vet Rec* 144:551, 1999.

Oliver J: Steroid profiles in the diagnosis of canine adrenal disorders, Proc *25th Ann Vet Med Forum,* p 471, 2007.

Ortega T, et al.: Evaluation of fasting serum lipid profiles in dogs with Cushing's syndrome, *J Vet Intern Med* 9:182, 1995.

Ortega T, et al.: Systemic arterial blood pressure and urine protein/creatinine ratio in dogs with hyperadrenocorticism, *J Am Vet Med Assoc* 209:1724, 1996.

Pace SL, et al.: Assessment of coagulation and potential biochemical markers for hypercoagulability in canine hyperadrenocorticism, *J Vet Intern Med* 27:1113, 2013.

Paez-Pereda M, et al.: Retinoic acid prevents experimental Cushing's syndrome, *J Clin Invest* 108:1123, 2001.

Park FM, et al.: Hypercoagulability and ACTH-dependent hyperadrenocorticism in dogs, *J Vet Intern Med* 27:1136, 2013.

Penninck DG, et al.: Radiologic features of canine hyperadrenocorticism caused by autonomously functioning adrenocortical tumors: 23 cases (1978-1986), *J Am Vet Med Assoc* 192:1604, 1988.

Peterson ME: Hyperadrenocorticism, *Vet Clin North Am (Small Anim Pract)* 14:731, 1984.

Peterson ME: Pathophysiology of canine pituitary-dependent hyperadrenocorticism, *Front Horm Res* 17:37, 1987.

Peterson ME, et al.: Diagnosis and management of concurrent diabetes mellitus and hyperadrenocorticism in 30 dogs, *J Am Vet Med Assoc* 178:66, 1981.

Peterson ME, et al.: Immunocytochemical study of the hypophysis in 25 dogs with pituitary-dependent hyperadrenocorticism, *Acta Endocrinol* 101:15, 1982a.

Peterson ME, et al.: Plasma cortisol response to exogenous ACTH in 22 dogs with hyperadrenocorticism caused by an adrenocortical neoplasia, *J Am Vet Med Assoc* 180:542, 1982b.

Peterson ME, et al.: Decreased insulin sensitivity and glucose tolerance in spontaneous canine hyperadrenocorticism, *Res Vet Sci* 36:177, 1984a.

Peterson ME, et al.: Effects of spontaneous hyperadrenocorticism on serum thyroid hormone concentrations in the dog, *Am J Vet Res* 45:2034, 1984b.

Peterson ME, et al.: Plasma immunoreactive pro-opiomelanocortin peptides and cortisol in normal dogs and dogs with Addison's disease and Cushing's syndrome: basal concentrations, *Endocrinology* 119:720, 1986a.

Peterson ME, et al.: Effect of spontaneous hyperadrenocorticism on endogenous production and utilization of glucose in the dog, *Domest Anim Endocrinol* 3:117, 1986b.

Phillips M, Tashjian AH: Characterization of an early inhibitory effect of glucocorticoids on stimulated adrenocorticotropin and endorphin release from a clonal strain of mouse pituitary cells, *Endocrinology* 110:892, 1982.

Pike FS, et al.: Gallbladder mucocele in dogs: 30 cases (2000-2002), *J Am Vet Med Assoc* 224:1615, 2004.

Puente S: Pituitary carcinoma in an Airedale terrier, *Can Vet J* 44:240, 2003.

Ramsey IK, et al.: Hyperparathyroidism in dogs with hyperadrenocorticism, *J Small Anim Pract* 46:531, 2005.

Ramsey IK, et al.: Persistent isolated hypocortisolism following brief treatment with trilostane, *Aust Vet J* 86:491, 2008.

Randolph JF, et al.: Use of the urinary corticoid: creatinine ratio for monitoring dogs with pituitary-dependent hyperadrenocorticism during induction treatment with mitotane (o, p'-DDD), *Am J Vet Res* 59:258, 1998.

Rees DA, et al.: Long-term follow-up results of transsphenoidal surgery for Cushing's disease in a single centre using strict criteria for remission, *Clin Endocrinol (Oxf)* 56:541, 2002.

Reid LE, et al.: Effect of trilostane and mitotane on aldosterone secretory reserve in dogs with pituitary-dependent hyperadrenocorticism, *J Vet Intern Med* 28:443, 2014.

Reimers TJ, et al.: Effects of hemolysis and storage on quantification of hormones in blood samples from dogs, cattle, and horses, *Am J Vet Res* 52:1075, 1991.

Reine NJ, et al.: Deoxycorticosterone-secreting adrenocortical carcinoma in a dog, *J Vet Int Med* 13:386, 1999.

Reitmeyer M, et al.: The neurosurgical management of Cushing's disease, *Molec Cell Endocrinol* 197:73, 2002.

Reusch CE: Hyperadrenocorticism. In Ettinger SE, Feldman EC, editors: *Textbook of veterinary internal medicine*, ed 6, Philadelphia, 2005, Saunders/Elsevier.

Reusch CE, Feldman EC: Canine hyperadreno-corticism due to adrenocortical neoplasia, *J Vet Intern Med* 5:3, 1991.

Reusch CE, et al.: The efficacy of L-deprenyl in dogs with pituitary-dependent hyperadrenocorticism, *J Vet Intern Med* 13:291, 1999.

Reusch CE, et al.: Histological evaluation of the adrenal glands of seven dogs with hyperadrenocorticism treated with trilostane, *Vet Rec* 160:219, 2007.

Rewerts JM, et al.: Atraumatic rupture of the gastrocnemius muscle after corticosteroid administration in a dog, *J Am Vet Med Assoc* 210:655, 1997.

Rhodes KH, Beale KM: Alopecia, canine. In Rhodes KH, editor: *The 5-minute veterinary consult clinical companion: small animal dermatology*, Baltimore, 2002, Lippincott Williams and Wilkins, p 27.

Rijnberk A, Belshaw BE: An alternative protocol for the medical management of canine pituitary-dependent hyperadrenocorticism, *Vet Rec* 122:486, 1988.

Rijnberk A, et al.: Assessment of two tests for the diagnosis of canine hyperadrenocorticism, *Vet Rec* 122:178, 1988a.

Rijnberk A, et al.: Effects of bromocriptine on corticotropin, melanotropin, and corticosteroid secretion in dogs with pituitary-dependent hyperadrenocorticism, *J Endocrinol* 118:271, 1988b.

Rijnberk A, et al.: Aldosteronoma in a dog with polyuria as the leading symptom, *Domest Anim Endocrinol* 20:227, 2001.

Ristic JME, et al.: The use of 17-hydroxyprogesterone in the diagnosis of canine hyperadrenocorticism, *J Vet Intern Med* 16:433, 2002.

Robben JH, et al.: Cell biological aspects of the vasopressin type-2 receptor and aquaporin 2 channel in nephrogenic diabetes insipidus, *Am J Physiol Renal Physiol* 291:F257, 2006.

Rockwell JL, et al.: Spontaneous hypoadrenocorticism in a dog after a diagnosis of hyperadrenocorticism, *J Vet Int Med* 19:255, 2005.

Rodriguez Pineiro MI, et al.: Accuracy of an adrenocorticotropic hormone (ACTH) immunoluminometric assay for differentiating ACTH-dependent from ACTH-independent hyperadrenocorticism in dogs, *J Vet Intern Med* 23:850, 2009.

Rodriguez Pineiro MI, et al.: Use of computed tomography adrenal gland measurement for differentiating ACTH dependence from ACTH independence in 64 dogs with hyperadrenocorticism, *J Vet Intern Med* 25:1066, 2011.

Rose L, et al.: Effect of canine hyperadrenocorticism on coagulation parameters, *J Vet Intern Med* 27:207, 2013.

Ruckstuhl NS, et al.: Results of clinical examinations, laboratory tests, and ultrasonography in dogs with pituitary-dependent hyperadrenocorticism treated with trilostane, *Am J Vet Res* 63:506, 2002.

Sands JM, Bichet DG: Neprogenic diabetes insipidus, *Ann Intern Med* 144:186, 2006.

Sanecki RK, et al.: Subcellular location of corticosteroid-induced alkaline phosphatase in canine hepatocytes, *Vet Pathol* 24:296, 1987.

Schaer M, et al.: A case of fatal anaphylaxis in a dog associated with a dexamethasone suppression test, *J Vet Emerg Crit Care* 15:213, 2005.

Schmeitzel LP, Lothrop CD: Hormonal abnormalities in Pomeranians with normal coat and in Pomeranians with growth hormone-responsive dermatosis, *J Am Vet Med Assoc* 197:1333, 1990.

Schmeitzel LP, Lothrop CD: Congenital adrenal hyperplasia-like syndrome. In Bonagura JD, Kirk RW, editors: *Kirk's current veterinary therapy XII*, Philadelphia, 1995, WB Saunders/Elsevier, p 600.

Schwartz P, et al.: Evaluation of prognostic factors in the surgical treatment of adrenal gland tumors in dogs: 41 cases (1999-2005), *J Am Vet Med Assoc* 232:77, 2008.

Schwarz T, et al.: Osteopenia and other radiographic signs in canine hyperadrenocorticism, *J Small Anim Pract* 41:491, 2000.

Scott-Moncrieff JCR, et al.: Validation of chemiluminescent enzyme immunometric assay for plasma adrenocorticotropic hormone in the dog, *Vet Clin Pathol* 32:180, 2003.

Seguin MA, et al.: Persistent urinary tract infections and reinfections in 100 dogs (1989-1999), *J Vet Intern Med* 17:622, 2003.

Selman PJ, et al.: Effects of progestin administration on the hypothalamic-pituitary-adrenal axis and glucose homeostasis in dogs, *J Reprod Fertil Suppl* 51:345, 1997.

Sepesy LM, et al.: Vacuolar hepatopathy in dogs: 336 cases (1993-2005), *J Am Vet Med Assoc* 229:246, 2006.

Seruca C, et al.: Acute postretinal blindness: ophthalmologic, neurologic, and magnetic resonance imaging findings in dogs and cats (seven cases), *Vet Ophthalmol* 13:307, 2010.

Sica DA: Pharmacokinetics and pharmacodynamics of mineralocorticoid blocking agents and their effects on potassium homeostasis, *Heart Fail Rev* 10:23, 2005.

Sieber-Ruckstuhl NS, et al.: Cortisol, aldosterone, cortisol precursor, androgen and endogenous ACTH concentrations in dogs with pituitary-dependent hyperadrenocorticism treated with trilostane, *Domest Anim Endocrinol* 31:63, 2006.

Sieber-Ruckstuhl NS, et al.: Evaluation of cortisol precursors for the diagnosis of pituitary-dependent hypercortisolism in dogs, *Vet Rec* 162:673, 2008.

Smets PM, et al.: Long-term follow-up of renal function in dogs after treatment for ACTH-dependent hyperadrenocorticism, *J Vet Intern Med* 26:565, 2012.

Smiley LE, Peterson ME: Evaluation of a urine cortisol:creatinine ratio as a screening test for hyperadrenocorticism in dogs, *J Vet Intern Med* 7:163, 1993.

Sobel KE, Williams JE: Pneumothorax secondary to pulmonary thromboembolism in a dog, *J Vet Emerg Crit Care* 19:120, 2009.

Solter PF, et al.: Assessment of corticosteroid-induced isoenzyme as a screening test for hyperadrenocorticism in dogs, *J Am Vet Med Assoc* 203:534, 1993.

Solter PF, et al.: Hepatic total 3-alpha-hydroxy bile acid concentration and enzyme activities in prednisone-treated dogs, *Am J Vet Res* 55:1086, 1994.

Stenske KA, et al.: Acute polyarthritis and septicemia from mycoplasma edwardii after surgical removal of bilateral adrenal tumors in a dog, *J Vet Int Med* 19:768, 2005.

Stewart PM: The adrenal cortex. In Kronenberg HM, Melmed S, Polonsky KS, Larsen PR, editors: *William's textbook of endocrinology*, Philadelphia, 2008, Saunders/Elsevier, p 445.

Stolp R, et al.: Urinary corticoids in the diagnosis of canine hyperadrenocorticism, *Res Vet Sci* 34:141, 1983.

Stolp R, et al.: Results of cyproheptadine treatment in dogs with pituitary-dependent hyperadrenocorticism, *J Endocr* 101:311, 1984.

Stuckey JA, et al.: Long-term outcome of sudden acquired retinal degeneration syndrome in dogs, *J Am Vet Med Assoc* 243:1426, 2013.

Swinney GR, et al.: Myotonia associated with hyperadrenocorticism in two dogs, *Aust Vet J* 76:722, 1998.

Syme HM, et al.: Hyperadrenocorticism associated with excessive sex hormone production by an adrenocortical tumor in two dogs, *J Am Vet Med Assoc* 219:1725, 2001.

Syme HM, et al.: Measurement of aldosterone in feline, canine and human urine, *J Sm Anim Pract* 48:202, 2007.

Takada K, et al.: Cloning of canine 21-hydroxylase gene and its polymorphic analysis as a candidate gene for congenital adrenal hyperplasia-like syndrome in Pomeranians, *Res Vet Sci* 73:159, 2002.

Taoda T, et al.: Magnetic resonance imaging assessment of pituitary posterior lobe displacement in dogs with pituitary-dependent hyperadrenocorticism, *J Vet Med Sci* 73:725, 2011.

Teshima T, et al.: Cushing's disease complicated with thrombosis in a dog, *J Vet Med Sci* 70:487, 2008.

Teshima T, et al.: Expression of genes related to corticotropin production and glucocorticoid feedback in corticotroph adenomas of dogs with Cushing's disease, *Domest Anim Endocrinol* 36:3, 2009.

Teshima T, et al.: Central diabetes insipidus after transsphenoidal surgery in dogs with Cushing's disease, *J Vet Med Sci* 73:33, 2011.

Teske E, et al.: Corticosteroid-induced alkaline phosphatase isoenzyme in the diagnosis of canine hypercortism, *Vet Rec* 125:12, 1989.

Theon AP, Feldman EC: Megavoltage irradiation of pituitary macrotumors in dogs with neurologic signs, *J Am Vet Med Assoc* 213:225, 1998.

Thuroczy J, et al.: Multiple endocrine neoplasias in a dog: corticotrophic tumour, bilateral adrenocortical tumours and pheochromocytoma, *Vet Quart* 20:56, 1998.

Tobias KM, Johnston SA: *Veterinary surgery: small animal*, St Louis, 2012, Elsevier/Saunders.

Toutain PL, et al.: Pharmacokinetics of dexamethasone and its effect on adrenal gland function in the dog, *Am J Vet Res* 44:212, 1983.

Turrel JM, et al.: Computed tomographic characteristics of primary brain tumors in 50 dogs, *J Am Vet Med Assoc* 188:851, 1986.

Turton DB, et al.: Incidental adrenal nodules: association with exaggerated 17 hydroxy-progesterone response to adrenocorticotropic hormone, *J Endocrinol Invest* 15:789, 1992.

Valencia IC, Kerdel FA: Topical corticosteroids. In Goldsmith LA, Katz SI, Gilchrest BA, Paller AS, Leffell DJ, Wolff K, editors: *Fitzpatrick's dermatology in general medicine*, New York, 2012, McGraw Hill Medical, p 2659.

van der Vlugt-Meijer RH, et al.: Dynamic computed tomography of the pituitary gland in dogs with pituitary-dependent hyperadrenocorticism, *J Vet Int Med* 17:773, 2003.

van der Vlugt-Meijer RH, et al.: Dynamic computed tomographic evaluation of the pituitary gland in healthy dogs, *Am J Vet Res* 65:1518, 2004.

van der Woerdt A, et al.: Sudden acquired retinal degeneration in the dog: clinical and laboratory findings in 36 cases, *Prog Vet Comp Ophthalmol* 1:11, 1991.

Van Liew CH, et al.: Comparison of results of adrenocorticotropic hormone stimulation and low dose dexamethasone suppression tests with necropsy finding in dogs: 81 cases (1985-1995), *J Am Vet Med Assoc* 211:322, 1997.

van Rijn SJ, et al.: Expression of Ki-67, PCNA, and p27kip1 in canine pituitary corticotroph adenomas, *Domest Anim Endocrinol* 38:244, 2010.

van Vonderen IK, et al.: Influence of veterinary care on the urinary corticoid:creatinine ratio in dogs, *J Vet Intern Med* 12:431, 1998.

van Wijk PA, et al.: Corticotropin-releasing hormone and adrenocorticotropic hormone concentrations in cerebrospinal fluid of dogs with pituitary-dependent hyperadrenocorticism, *Endocrinology* 131:2659, 1992.

van Wijk PA, et al.: Responsiveness to corticotropin-releasing hormone and vasopressin in canine Cushing's syndrome, *Eur J Endocrinol* 130:410, 1994.

Vandenbergh AGGD, et al.: Haemorrhage from a canine adrenocortical tumour: a clinical emergency, *Vet Rec* 13:539, 1992.

Vaughn MA, et al.: Evaluation of twice-daily, low-dose trilostane treatment administered orally in dogs with naturally occurring hyperadrenocorticism, *J Am Vet Med Assoc* 232:1321, 2008.

Vollmar AM, et al.: Atrial natriuretic peptide concentration in dogs with congestive heart failure, chronic renal failure, and hyperadrenocorticism, *Am J Vet Res* 52:1831, 1991.

Von Dehn BJ, et al.: Pheochromocytoma in 6 dogs with naturally acquired hyperadrenocorticism: 1982-1992, *J Am Vet Med Assoc* 207:322, 1995.

Voorhout G, et al.: Computed tomography in the diagnosis of canine hyperadrenocorticism not suppressible by dexamethasone, *J Am Vet Med Assoc* 192:641, 1988

Voorhout G: X-ray-computed tomography, nephrotomography, and ultrasonography of the adrenal glands of healthy dogs, *Am J Vet Res* 51:625, 1990.

Voorhout G, et al.: Assessment of survey radiography and comparison with x-ray computed tomography for detection of hyperfunctioning adrenocortical tumors in dogs, *J Am Vet Med Assoc* 196:1799, 1990a.

Voorhout G, et al.: Nephrotomography and ultrasonography for the localization of hyperfunctioning adrenocortical tumors in dogs, *Am J Vet Res* 51:1280, 1990b.

Ward DA, et al.: Band keratopathy associated with hyperadrenocorticism in the dog, *J Am Anim Hosp Assoc* 25:583, 1989.

Waters CB, et al.: Effects of glucocorticoid therapy on urine protein-to-creatinine ratios and renal morphology in dogs, *J Vet Int Med* 11:172, 1997.

Watson ADJ: Oestrogen-induced alopecia in a bitch, *J Small Anim Pract* 26:17, 1985.

Watson ADJ, et al.: Systemic availability of o,p'-DDD in normal dogs, fasted and fed, and in dogs with hyperadrenocorticism, *Res Vet Sci* 43:160, 1987.

Webb CB, Twedt DC: Acute hepatopathy associated with mitotane administration in a dog, *J Am Anim Hosp Assoc* 42:298, 2006.

Wenger M, et al.: Effect of trilostane on serum concentrations of aldosterone, cortisol and potassium in dogs with pituitary-dependent hyperadrenocorticism, *Am J Vet Res* 65:1245, 2004.

White SD, et al.: Cutaneous markers of canine hyperadrenocorticism, *Compend Contin Educ* 11:446, 1989.

Whittemore JC, et al.: Nontraumatic rupture of an adrenal gland tumor causing intraabdominal or retroperitoneal hemorrhage in four dogs, *J Am Vet Med Assoc* 219:329, 2001.

Widmer WR, Guptill L: Imaging techniques for facilitating diagnosis of hyperadrenocorticism in dogs and cats, *J Am Vet Med Assoc* 206:1857, 1995.

Wiedmeyer CE, et al.: Alkaline phosphatase expression in tissues from glucocorticoid-treated dogs, *Am J Vet Res* 63:1083, 2002a.

Wiedmeyer CE, et al.: Kinetics of mRNA expression of alkaline phosphatase isoenzymes in hepatic tissues from glucocorticoid-treated dogs, *Am J Vet Res* 63:1089, 2002b.

Willard MD, et al.: Ketoconazole-induced changes in selected canine hormone concentrations, *Am J Vet Res* 47:2504, 1986.

Wilson SM, Feldman EC: Diagnostic value of the steroid-induced isoenzyme of alkaline phosphatase in the dog, *J Am Anim Hosp Assoc* 28:245, 1992.

Witt A, Neiger R: Adrenocorticotropic hormone levels in dogs with pituitary-dependent hyperadrenocorticism following trilostane therapy, *Vet Rec* 154:399, 2004.

Wolfsheimer KJ, Peterson ME: Erythrocyte insulin receptors in dogs with spontaneous hyperadrenocorticism, *Am J Vet Res* 52:917, 1991.

Wood FD, et al.: Diagnostic imaging findings and endocrine test results in dogs with pituitary-dependent hyperadrenocorticism that did or did not have neurologic abnormalities: 157 cases (1989-2005), *J Am Vet Med Assoc* 231:1081, 2007.

Yamaji T, et al.: Plasma levels of atrial natriuretic hormone in Cushing's syndrome, *J Clin Endocrinol Metab* 67:348, 1988.

Zerbe CA: Screening tests to diagnose hyperadrenocorticism in cats and dogs, *Compend Contin Educ* 22:17, 2000.

Zeugswetter F, et al.: The desmopressin stimulation test in dogs with Cushing's syndrome, *Domest Anim Endocrinol* 34:254, 2008.

Zeugswetter F, et al.: Tailored reference limits for urine corticoid: creatinine ratio in dogs to answer distinct clinical questions, *Vet Rec* 167:997, 2010.

Zeugswetter F, et al.: Diagnostic efficacy of plasma ACTH-measurement by a chemiluminometric assay in canine hyperadrenocorticism, *Schweiz Arch Tierheilkd* 153:111, 2011.

Zimmerman KL, et al.: Hyperphosphatasemia and concurrent adrenal gland dysfunction in apparently healthy Scottish terriers, *J Am Vet Med Assoc* 237:178, 2010.

Zur G, White SD: Hyperadrenocorticism in 10 dogs with skin lesions as the only presenting clinical signs, *J Am Anim Hosp Assoc* 47:419, 2011.

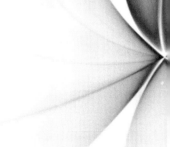

CHAPTER 11

Hyperadrenocorticism in Cats

Edward C. Feldman

CHAPTER CONTENTS

FELINE HYPERADRENOCORTICISM (FELINE CUSHING'S SYNDROME), HYPERALDOSTERONISM, SEX HORMONE SECRETING ADRENAL TUMORS

In 1932, long before the physiology of the adrenal cortex was understood and before identification of glucocorticoids, Dr. Harvey Cushing authored a report in which he described a group of people with a disorder that appeared to be "the result of pituitary basophilism." Subsequent study of the clinical, biochemical, and histologic features of these individuals are consistent with each having had a syndrome resulting from chronic exposure to excess circulating concentrations of glucocorticoids (cortisol). The eponym "Cushing's syndrome" is an umbrella term referring to all causes of "hyperadrenocorticism" in people and, more recently, in animals.

There are several causes for Cushing's syndrome. In addition to the common iatrogenic condition, one of the naturally occurring disorders is caused by an autonomously functioning, adrenocorticotropic hormone (ACTH)-secreting, pituitary tumor (usually an adenoma) resulting in excess cortisol synthesis/secretion and adrenocortical hyperplasia (pituitary dependent hyperadrenocorticism [PDH]). ACTH-secreting pituitary tumors have been demonstrated to be derived from a single aberrant cell line. A less common cause of naturally occurring hyperadrenocorticism (NOH) in animals is that caused by an autonomously functioning, cortisol-secreting, adrenocortical tumor (adenoma or carcinoma; adrenal tumor hyperadrenocorticism [ATH]). PDH is about five-to-six times more common in people, dogs, and cats than ATH. Both iatrogenic and NOH is being diagnosed with increasing frequency in cats. This rising number of cats diagnosed with hyperadrenocorticism is likely associated with feline medicine becoming more specialized, cats being better understood, owners requesting more sophisticated care, awareness of this condition increasing, veterinarians becoming more familiar with the many variations on the theme of glucocorticoid excess, and an expanding number of aging feline pets.

NOH is unusually common in dogs, resulting in veterinary clinicians becoming quite familiar with the condition and the inevitable comparisons of "dog hyperadrenocorticism" and hyperadrenocorticism in cats. There are both similarities and differences. The obvious clinical features of hyperadrenocorticism in dogs include polyuria, polydipsia, polyphagia, panting, muscle weakness, thin skin, potbelly, and symmetrical alopecia. These common and obvious signs in dogs are not noted with frequency in cats with hyperadrenocorticism unless they have diabetes mellitus which, in turn, causes polyuria and polydipsia (PU/PD). Confirming a diagnosis is more problematic in cats, in part because the disease is far less common. Most reports in the literature describe "obvious" diagnoses in cats with dramatic abnormalities, suggesting that confirming a diagnosis in subtle cases is difficult or that the subtle cases are not often recognized or reported. Most dogs with NOH respond quite well and live years after commencement of treatment. In cats, however, treatment is more frustrating and difficult.

Since the underlying physiologic causes for hyperadrenocorticism are similar in dogs, and cats, the reader interested in applied physiology and in mechanisms of disease is encouraged to review the appropriate sections in Chapter 10. The focus of this chapter is to review the current state of knowledge regarding the diagnosis and treatment of feline Cushing's syndrome (FCS) in cats. As will be discussed later in this chapter, some adrenocortical tumors in cats primarily secrete sex hormones and/or mineralocorticoids.

To aid in this discussion, information from the records of 56 cats diagnosed as having FCS at our hospital, including some reported in the literature (Duesberg et al, 1995) were added to the information from 31 cats described in the literature (Immink et al, 1992; Daley et al, 1993; Goossens et al, 1995; Schwedes, 1997; Watson and Herrtage, 1998; Moore et al, 2000a; Meij et al, 2001; Skelly et al, 2003; Neiger et al, 2004), for a total of 87 cats with naturally occurring FCS. This literature includes only those reports published since 1992, to have greater confidence that valid and currently available assays were used in the assessment of each cat and that current concepts in diagnosis and treatment were used. Before 1990, only a few cats with this disease were mentioned in the literature (Swift and Brown, 1976; Meijer et al, 1978; Peterson and Steele, 1986; Zerbe et al, 1987a; Nelson et al, 1988). Furthermore, in the reports that we arbitrarily chose to use, we set the following selection criteria: Each cat must have had clinical signs associated with FCS and each diagnosis must have been confirmed using an accepted screening test. Most cats had advanced imaging (computed tomography [CT] or magnetic

resonance imaging [MRI] scans) confirmation or histologic confirmation of the diagnosis.

 ## ETIOLOGY

Iatrogenic Cushing's Syndrome

Clinical signs of iatrogenic cortisol excess are relatively common in dogs. Clinical signs due to iatrogenic cortisol excess are much less dramatic or common in people and seem even less obvious in cats. This can be explained, in part, by what appears to be a relative insensitivity to the negative or deleterious side effects of chronic glucocorticoid administration in cats. In other words, owners of dogs being treated with glucocorticoids are far more likely to observe unwanted or worrisome side effects than are owners of similarly-treated cats, simply because cats do not often demonstrate such side effects.

In studies on cats experimentally treated with glucocorticoids, those treated for a 4-week period had few abnormalities on physical examination and no consistent hematologic or biochemical changes (Scott et al, 1979; 1982). When treated for 9 weeks or longer, most cats continued to have no or few clinical signs (Lowe et al, 2008). However, a minority of cats exhibited some of the following: polydipsia, polyuria, polyphagia, abdominal enlargement, lethargy, weakness, thin skin, and medial curling of their ear tips. Some cats with iatrogenic cortisol excess developed hepatomegaly, muscle wasting, ecchymoses, and skin fragility (Scott et al, 1979; 1982; Lowe et al, 2008). Many cortisol-treated cats tended to develop mild hyperglycemia, and a minority became overtly hyperglycemic due to diabetes mellitus. Less common abnormalities included increased white blood cell numbers, a "stress leukogram," increased liver enzyme activities, hypercholesterolemia, hypertriglyceridemia, glycogen accumulation in hepatocytes, and a vacuolar hepatopathy. Cataracts developed in some laboratory cats treated with topical glucocorticoids (Brightman, 1982; Zhan et al, 1992).

A small number of privately owned cats treated with exogenous glucocorticoids had "clinical iatrogenic FCS" and were reported (Green et al, 1995; Schaer and Ginn, 1999; Ferasin, 2001; Lien et al, 2006). Among the features likely due to chronic glucocorticoid exposure were abdominal enlargement, muscle wasting, poor hair coats, and skin fragility. The skin fragility in one report included thin skin, easy bruisability, and skin tears. Several cats had increased liver enzyme activities and hepatic vacuolar hepatopathy. In one report, four of twelve cats developed transient diabetes mellitus, and four of twelve had transient hypothyroidism (Lien et al, 2006). Diabetes mellitus in cats identified after initiation of glucocorticoid treatment may be transient. Some cats had PU/PD in one study, but urine specific gravities were more than 1.035 in all cats (Lien et al, 2006). Despite these observations, iatrogenic FCS usually does not cause owner-discernable concerns. Interestingly, some features of iatrogenic cortisol excess (e.g., ear curling) in cats are not commonly seen in cats with the naturally occurring condition.

Naturally Occurring Feline Hyperadrenocorticism

The causes of naturally occurring FCS are similar to those recognized in people and dogs. It has been suggested that resistance to glucocorticoid-induced side effects, likely in cats as compared with dogs, may help explain the relative low diagnosis rate of FCS in cats as compared with dogs. In other words, if excess glucocorticoids cause few clinical signs in cats, how would the diagnosis ever be suspected in the first place? Fewer than 100 cats have been reported in the veterinary literature that had been diagnosed with naturally occurring FCS. The incidence of the FCS in cats (assessed non-scientifically) does appear similar to the incidence of the syndrome in human beings. However, people seem more sensitive than cats (but less sensitive than dogs) to clinical side effects associated with glucocorticoid administration. Therefore, FCS may simply be less common in cats as compared with dogs and people.

The majority of cats with naturally occurring FCS (approximately 80%) have PDH. Cats with PDH have a pituitary tumor, adenomas far more common than carcinomas, that autonomously synthesize and secrete ACTH. The persistent excesses of ACTH, in turn, cause excess synthesis and secretion of glucocorticoid (cortisol) from the adrenal cortices. The excess circulating cortisol has effects on cells within organs throughout the body, including suppressive effects on healthy pituitary cells responsible for synthesis and secretion of ACTH, luteinizing hormone (LH), follicle-stimulating hormone (FSH), thyroid-stimulating hormone (also known as thyrotropin; TSH), and growth hormone (GH). Chronic exposure to excessive concentrations of circulating cortisol is also likely to have suppressive effects on the synthesis and secretion of antidiuretic hormone (ADH) from the posterior pituitary in dogs, but there is little evidence of this happening in cats. Over time, excesses in circulating ACTH cause adrenocortical hyperplasia and somewhat symmetrical adrenal gland enlargement.

At the time of PDH diagnosis in dogs, about 50% of their pituitary tumors are microscopic in size and about 50% are large enough to be visualized with CT or MRI scans (usually greater than 3 to 4 mm in greatest diameter). A similar number (approximately 50%) are grossly visible at surgery or necropsy. Approximately 20% to 30% of dogs with PDH, usually after successful management of the condition for a prolonged time period, develop pituitary tumors large enough to cause clinical signs secondary to the compressive or invasive effects of the mass. Although many of these clinical scenarios have been described in cats with FCS, their incidence is not as well established.

Approximately 20% of cats with FCS have an autonomously functioning adrenocortical tumor (adrenal tumor hyperadrenocortisolism, ATH). About 50% or more of adrenocortical tumors are adenomas and somewhat less than 50% are carcinomas. Regardless of their histologic classification, adrenocortical tumors that cause FCS do so via the autonomous and excessive synthesis and secretion of glucocorticoids (cortisol). Chronic and persistent exposure to excess cortisol, in turn, is responsible for the various problems (clinical, biochemical, and so on) that are conveniently placed under the umbrella "Cushing's syndrome." As mentioned, cortisol affects cells in every organ. As with PDH, the chronic and excessive amounts of circulating cortisol also cause chronic negative feedback to healthy cells within the hypothalamus and pituitary gland. In this condition, however, with both hypothalamus and pituitary suppressed, the chronic inhibition of synthesis and secretion of ACTH causes "normal" cortisol-secreting cells to atrophy within the zona fasciculata and zona reticularis of the adrenal cortices. Therefore, over time, the cortex of one adrenal gland contains a functioning tumor and atrophied non-tumorous cells, whereas the opposite adrenal cortex contains primarily atrophied cells and may appear small or thin on imaging studies or gross evaluation. Atrophy of the opposite (non-tumor containing) adrenal becomes clinically relevant not only on imaging studies, but when the adrenal containing the tumor is surgically removed as a treatment for FCS. In this scenario, the clinician must remember that the cells responsible for cortisol synthesis and secretion in the remaining adrenal cortex will likely be unable to immediately provide adequate hormone to sustain health. Therefore, such individuals are treated with tapering doses of exogenous glucocorticoids, allowing function to be regained over time.

	TABLE 11-1	AGE AT TIME OF FELINE CUSHING'S SYNDROME DIAGNOSIS IN 61 CATS*†
AGE (YEARS)	PITUITARY DEPENDENT NUMBER OF CATS	ADRENOCORTICAL TUMOR NUMBER OF CATS
5	1	—
6	5	—
7	2	—
8	3	1
9	4	2
10	4	1
11	5	2
12	6	3
13	4	2
14	6	2
15	2	2
16	3	—
17	1	—
Mean	11.0	11.9

*46 pituitary dependent hyperadrenocorticism; 15 adrenal tumor hyperadrenocorticism.
†Mean age of all 61 cats was 11.3 years

Later in this chapter, syndromes in cats with adrenocortical tumors synthesizing and secreting non-cortisol steroids will be reviewed.

 ## SIGNALMENT (AGE, SEX, BREED)

FCS is a disease of middle-aged and older cats. As can be seen in Table 11-1, both mean and median ages of 46 cats diagnosed as having PDH was 11 years (range, 5 to 17 years). The mean age of 15 cats, each with a functioning adrenocortical tumor, was 11.9 years (median 12 years), with a range of 8 to 15 years. The mean age for all 61 cats was just over 11 years. Among these 61 cats were 31 males and 29 females. All cats diagnosed as having naturally occurring FCS at our hospital had been neutered at an early age. The most commonly afflicted breed is the Domestic Short-Haired (DSH) cat (Table 11-2)—38 of 61 cats (62%), and if DSH and domestic long-haired cats are combined, the totals are 46 of 61 cats (75%). Cats representing various other breeds have been diagnosed with FCS.

 ## DURATION OF CLINICAL SIGNS, CHIEF COMPLAINT, AND GENERAL HISTORY

Duration of Clinical Signs

The duration of clinical signs or the duration of specific owner concerns were available for 53 cats diagnosed as having FCS (Table 11-3). The range in duration of signs was from as little as 1 month to greater than 12. Fifty-one of the 53 cats with either PDH or ATH had clinical signs for less than 1 year at the time of diagnosis.

Owner Chief Concern/Explanation for Being Referred

The "chief concern" is the primary reason or reasons that an owner seeks veterinary assistance, or in these cats, the primary reason(s) for seeing a specialist. The chief concern in 32 of 58 cats with FCS (55%) was "difficult to regulate diabetes mellitus." Most

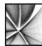

TABLE 11-2 BREEDS OF CATS WITH NATURALLY OCCURRING FELINE CUSHING'S SYNDROME (TOTAL OF 61 CATS)

BREED	Pituitary Dependent		Adrenocortical Tumor	
	NUMBER	PERCENTAGE	NUMBER	PERCENTAGE
Domestic Short-Hair	28	65	10	66
Domestic Long-Hair	7	13	1	7
Siamese	3	4	1	7
Persian	2	4	1	7
Abyssinian	2	4	—	—
European Short-Hair	2	4	—	—
Devon Rex	1	2	—	—
Japanese Bobtail	—	—	1	7
Russian Blue	1	2	1	—
Maine Coon	—	—	—	7
Total	46		15	

TABLE 11-3 DURATION OF CLINICAL SIGNS PRECEDING DIAGNOSIS OF FELINE CUSHING'S SYNDROME IN CATS (53 CATS)

DURATION (MONTHS)	NUMBER OF CATS WITH PITUITARY DEPENDENT DISEASE	NUMBER OF CATS WITH ADRENOCORTICAL TUMOR
1	2	—
2	6	1
3	5	1
4	3	3
5	4	2
6	4	1
7	1	3
8	2	—
9	2	1
10	3	—
11	—	—
12	4	3
> 12	2	—
Total	38	15

TABLE 11-4 CHIEF COMPLAINTS BY OWNERS OF CATS ULTIMATELY DIAGNOSED AS HAVING CUSHING'S SYNDROME

COMPLAINT	PITUITARY DEPENDENT (43 CATS)	ADRENOCORTICAL TUMOR (15 CATS)
Resistant diabetes mellitus (PD/PU/PP)[†]	28	4
Polyuria/polydipsia (of the eight non-diabetic)	6	2
Fragile (torn) skin	6	3
Weight loss	3	1
Lethargy	2	2
Alopecia/failure to regrow hair	2	2
Diarrhea	2	—
Weakness	1	—
Vomiting	1	—
Abdominal enlargement	1	1
Not grooming	1	—
Polyphagia	1	—
Referral for ultrasound	1	3
Referral for Cushing's syndrome	2	—

commonly, their diabetes mellitus was classified as difficult to regulate when owners felt that their pet had persistence of polyuria despite administration of insulin (Table 11-4). Other, less frequent observations that caused owners to believe their cats' diabetes mellitus was poorly controlled include continued weight loss, failure to gain weight, persistent lethargy, poor grooming habits, not consistently utilizing the litter box, and failing to be interactive with the family. Occasionally, "difficult to regulate diabetic" was designated by the referring veterinarian, rather than by the owner. Often, insulin dose and type had been altered numerous times by the primary care veterinarian in an effort to gain control of the diabetes mellitus prior to referral.

*Total of 58 cats; 50 of these 58 cats had diabetes mellitus, four had periodic diabetes mellitus, and four did not have diabetes mellitus.
[†]PD, Polydipsia; PP, polyphagia; PU, polyuria.

Owner chief concern was recorded in 58 cats. Forty-six of those 58 FCS cats had been previously diagnosed as having diabetes mellitus, four had been documented to have "episodic" diabetes mellitus prior to referral, and eight were not believed to be diabetic. Of the eight cats that did not have diabetes mellitus at the time of referral, six were believed to have PU/PD, and four of these six cats had diabetes when evaluated at our hospital. Thus, 50 of 58 FCS cats had

| TABLE 11-5 | OWNER OBSERVATIONS IN CATS WITH NATURALLY OCCURRING CUSHING'S SYNDROME (TOTAL OF 72 CATS) |

| OBSERVATION | Pituitary Dependent (57 Cats) | | Adrenocortical Tumor (15 Cats) | |
	NUMBER	PERCENTAGE	NUMBER	PERCENTAGE
Polyuria/polydipsia	46	80	11	73
Polyphagia	39	68	8	53
Weight loss	27	47	6	40
Lethargic/sleeps more	25	44	7	47
Weakness	20	35	4	27
Alopecia/failure to regrow hair	18	32	12	80
Stopped grooming	10	18	4	27
Coarse hair coat	9	16	2	13
Decreased appetite	4	7	2	13
Fragile (torn) skin	9	16	5	33
Weight gain/potbelly	5	9	4	27
Over grooming	2	4	1	6
Diarrhea	2	4	—	—
Periodic diabetes mellitus	4	7	—	—
Vomiting	1	2	—	—

diabetes mellitus when first seen at our hospital and four had had "episodes" of diabetes. Fourteen of the 46 diabetic cats were believed to be well controlled with insulin. Among the less common primary owner concerns were fragile (torn) skin in nine cats (16%), lethargy in four, weight loss in four, and alopecia or failure to regrow hair that had been previously shaved in four. Four cats were suspected as having FCS and were specifically referred for abdominal ultrasonography. Two cats were referred for "evaluation of Cushing's."

Owner Observations

Owner observations, other than their "chief concern," were available from 72 cats diagnosed as having FCS (57 cats with PDH; 15 cats with ATH; Table 11-5). The most common owner observation was PU/PD in 57 cats (79%), polyphagia in 47 (65%), weight loss or failure to gain weight in 33 (46%), and lethargy or reports of "sleeps more" in 32 cats (44%). Weakness, usually worse in the rear legs, was noted in 24 (33%) cats, 15 of whom had a plantigrade stance.

Concerns about skin problems were noted in a majority of the 62 cats; including the extremely worrisome fragile or torn skin noted in 14 cats (20%). Additionally, failure to grow hair after it had been shaved (usually for venipuncture or abdominal ultrasonography examination) was noted in 30 cats (42%), having "stopped grooming" was a concern in 14 cats (20%), and 11 owners thought their cat had abnormally coarse hair. Multiple skin problems were noted in some cats, whereas others had none. The owners of 21 cats with PDH (from the total of 57, or 37%) and the owners of three cats with ATH (from the total of 15, or 20%) did not mention any problem relative to the skin or hair coat. In general, owners of either PDH or ATH cats had similar observations, underscoring the final common denominator of chronic exposure to excess circulating cortisol. One exception was that 32% of PDH-cat owners noted alopecia or failure to regrow hair, whereas 80% of ATH cat owners mentioned this concern.

It has been suggested that clinical signs of FCS are not commonly detected by owners or veterinarians until these cats develop diabetes mellitus. Results of this review are in agreement with this concept for most afflicted cats. However, a few cats with FCS did not have diabetes mellitus and a few had signs that preceded development of diabetes mellitus. Thus, a suspicion of FCS may result from a history and physical examination in non-diabetic cats if thin skin, skin fragility, potbelly appearance, muscle atrophy, weakness (especially in the rear legs), or various hair coat disorders are noted. Any combination of these issues might lead to the suspicion of FCS in non-diabetic cats.

 PHYSICAL EXAMINATION ABNORMALITIES

The physical examination abnormalities from 72 cats with naturally occurring FCS are listed in Table 11-6. Many of the previously described owner concerns were obvious to the veterinarian performing the physical examination. The most common abnormalities observed included abdominal enlargement in 46 cats (66%; Fig. 11-1), muscle atrophy (44 cats; 61%), thin skin (43 cats; 60%), and an "unkempt" hair coat (35 cats; 49%). Less common abnormalities included hair loss, rear leg plantigrade stance, hepatomegaly, skin tears, bruising, and seborrhea. Two cats were noted to have abdominal masses, which were confirmed to be adrenal gland tumors (Immink et al, 1992). The finding of a palpable adrenal tumor is considered quite unusual.

 EXPLANATIONS FOR HISTORY AND PHYSICAL EXAMINATION ABNORMALITIES

Polyuria and Polydipsia

PU/PD are usually suspected after learning an owner's concerns of their pets' "inappropriate urination" and finding a urine specific gravity less than 1.020. These signs are, perhaps, the most common

| TABLE 11-6 | PHYSICAL EXAMINATION ABNORMALITIES IN 72 CATS WITH NATURALLY OCCURRING CUSHING'S SYNDROME | | | |

| | Pituitary Dependent (57 Cats) | | Adrenocortical Tumor (15 Cats) | |
OBSERVATION	NUMBER	PERCENTAGE	NUMBER	PERCENTAGE
Abdominal enlargement (potbelly)	35	61	11	73
Muscle atrophy	35	61	9	60
Thin skin	32	56	11	73
Unkempt hair coat	30	53	5	33
Hair loss	16	28	5	33
Hepatomegaly	11	19	3	20
Skin tears	11	19	2	13
Plantigrade stance	11	19	4	27
Bruising	7	12	3	20
Seborrhea	3	5	5	33
Palpable adrenal mass	—	—	2	13

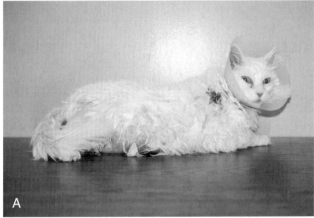

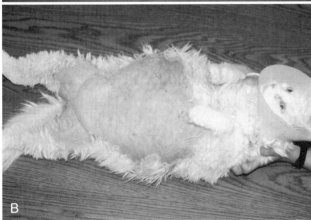

FIGURE 11-1 A, 12-year-old male cat with feline Cushing's syndrome (FCS). Note the unkempt appearance of the hair coat. **B,** Note the pot-bellied appearance and the thin skin. (The hair on the abdomen had been shaved for ultrasound evaluation.)

observations among owners of dogs with hyperadrenocorticism, yet only about 5% of those dogs have diabetes mellitus and glucosuria. This is a much lower percentage of diabetics than is seen in cats with FCS. It is thought that a majority of hypercortisolemic dogs have PU/PD due to central or nephrogenic diabetes insipidus which,

in turn, is secondary to their excess circulating cortisol concentrations. It is extremely unusual for such a dog to have concurrent chronic kidney disease (CKD). Cats with FCS, on the other hand, appear to develop PU/PD secondary to diabetes mellitus, CKD, or both. PU/PD occurs uncommonly in non-diabetic people or cats with naturally occurring or iatrogenic hyperadrenocorticism.

Polyuria, polydipsia, polyphagia, and weight loss are the classic signs of diabetes mellitus. For cats with FCS that also have diabetes mellitus (usually secondary to chronic excesses in systemic cortisol concentrations causing insulin resistance), the explanation for their PU/PD is the osmotic diuresis associated with glucosuria, especially if the diabetes is not well controlled. A small number of non-diabetic cats with FCS have been described with PU/PD, and most of them have had "episodes" of diabetes mellitus, CKD, or hyperthyroidism, which are all conditions associated with PU/PD. Although a huge majority of dogs with hyperadrenocorticism have low-to-low-normal blood urea nitrogen (BUN) and serum creatinine concentrations and randomly collected urine with specific gravities less than 1.020, only five urine samples from 52 cats with FCS (Table 11-7; 38 with PDH and 14 with ATH) had a specific gravity less than 1.020 (9%) and none was less than 1.008. Each of those five cats had an increase in their serum urea nitrogen, creatinine, or both (one was also hyperthyroid). Thus the observation of PU/PD in cats diagnosed as having FCS is noted almost exclusively in cats with glycosuria, CKD, or some additional cause of PU/PD (e.g., hyperthyroidism). Some "non-diabetic" FCS cats appear to have episodic insulin resistance with episodes of glycosuria and secondary PU/PD. This hyperglycemia and glycosuria may not be demonstrable at the time that in-hospital testing is carried out.

Polyphagia

Polyphagia is common in non-diabetic dogs with hyperadrenocorticism. This side effect is not a well-understood. Polyphagia is less common in cats with FCS, unless they are diabetic.

Weight Loss

A relative or absolute deficiency of insulin, definitive of diabetes mellitus, causes an inability to utilize glucose and a physiologic

TABLE 11-7	URINALYSIS RESULTS FROM 52 CATS WITH NATURALLY OCCURING CUSHING'S SYNDROME	
	Pituitary Dependent (38 Cats)	Adrenocortical Tumor (14 Cats)
URINALYSIS	NUMBER OF CATS	NUMBER OF CATS
Specific Gravity		
< 1.020	3	2
1.020 to 1.040	29	6
> 1.040	6	6
Protein		
Negative	19	6
Trace	11	3
> Trace	8	5
Bacterial Culture		
Negative	36	12
Positive	2	2
Ketones		
Negative	38	14
Positive	0	0

condition analogous to starvation. The physiologic response to starvation is hepatic synthesis of glucose and other sources of energy utilizing products derived from the breakdown of muscle and fat. This catabolism of muscle and fat is the explanation for weight loss. Since a majority of cats with FCS have diabetes mellitus, it is difficult for them to gain weight. This is certainly true of those cats whose diabetes is untreated. It is also true of those cats being treated with exogenous insulin but have resistance. Some cats are described as remaining thin (usually with a potbelly) and others have progressive weight loss despite insulin therapy. Nearly every cat with FCS that has an owner concern of weight loss (or failing to gain weight) has concurrent diabetes mellitus. Non-diabetic cats with FCS with CKD are also likely to lose weight. The third most common cause of weight loss among cats with FCS is concurrent hyperthyroidism. Weight loss or "remaining thin" is an important feature of FCS because acromegaly, a differential diagnosis for insulin resistance in cats, is a condition often associated with weight gain.

Weakness, Lethargy, Potbelly, and Bruising

Explanation for these clinical signs can be directly related to the physiologic effects of glucocorticoids. Cortisol causes protein catabolism and, thus, breakdown of muscle. Muscle breakdown leads to wasting and weakness, which is often obvious to owners (Robinson and Clamann, 1988). Alternatively, weakness may be interpreted by an owner to be "lethargy" or as an "increased amount of time spent sleeping." Furthermore, some cats with FCS have a plantigrade posture, which is most often related to the diabetic neuropathy seen in cats with diabetes mellitus and, in FCS, probably enhanced by steroid-induced muscle wasting.

Chronic cortisol excess is recognized to cause a redistribution of fat from areas throughout the body to the abdominal mesentery, increasing the weight of abdominal content. Abdominal distention is

the clinical consequence of this increased amount of abdominal content pressing down upon weakened abdominal musculature (see Fig. 11-1) and is a classic observation in people, dogs, and cats afflicted with hyperadrenocorticism. This type of abdominal distention is the "potbelly" appearance that is classic of Cushing's syndrome. Excess systemic glucocorticoids are associated with a relative decrease in the ability to heal due to blood vessel friability and a decrease in fibrous response to injury. Further, loss of subcutaneous fat (mobilized to the abdomen), blood vessels that are more superficial after losing their fat insulation, and decreases in normal healing properties increase the predisposition to bruising. In cats with FCS, bruising after venipuncture or clipping of hair can be dramatic.

Curled Ear Tips

As a component of the catabolic state associated with chronic glucocorticoid excesses, decreased strength of ligaments, tendons, and cartilaginous structures in general can be expected. Initial reports on iatrogenic FCS in cats included observations of "ear tip curling." However, this clinical sign has either not been mentioned or not observed in our experience nor in the cats comprising our review.

Dermatologic Abnormalities

Bilaterally symmetrical nonpruritic alopecia is common in hypercortisolemic dogs but not in cats. The alopecia that most FCS cat owners observe is due to a failure to regrow hair that has been clipped or hair that is lost as a result of normal or excessive grooming (Fig. 11-2). It is difficult to know whether "excessive" grooming truly exists. Are these cats grooming normally but causing hair loss, thereby also causing owner concern or are they grooming more than usual? In addition to hair loss, thin skin (Fig. 11-3), poor wound healing, skin fragility, and increased susceptibility to skin infections are typical sequelae to chronic excesses in circulating concentrations of cortisol. Chronic cortisol excess can result in atrophy of the epidermis, dermis, and hair follicles. This atrophy can be traced to glucocorticoid-induced suppression of dermal fibroblast and keratinocyte proliferation, as well as downregulation of collagen, hyaluronic acid, sulfated glycosaminoglycans, elastin, and tenascin-C expression (Schacke et al, 2002). Chronic skin infections are likely related to a combination of easily traumatized skin in individuals that lack the ability to heal normally and have glucocorticoid-induced suppression of their immune systems. Glucocorticoids have many immunosuppressive effects, including decreased macrophage expression of inflammatory cytokines, increased expression of some antiinflammatory cytokines, decreased function and maturation of dendritic cells, decreased T cell activation and proliferation in response to mitogens, decreased cell-mediated lysis of target cells, decreased mitogen-induced B cell proliferation, and decreased antibody production (Tuckermann et al, 2005; Lowe et al, 2008).

Skin fragility, not typical of dogs with NOH, and thin skin are well recognized concerns in cats with FCS (Fig. 11-4; see Tables 11-5 and 11-6). Some cats have wrinkling and folding of their skin due to the previously described dermal atrophy and decreased collagen expression. In some cats, their skin is so fragile as to be easily torn. These cats can create full-thickness, self-induced, dermal abrasions from simple grooming. It seems that the most common causes of skin tears are self-induced, associated with routine restraint, or they may be caused by owners pinching the skin to administer insulin. The combination of poor wound healing and increased susceptibility to infection can be serious and result in life-threatening sepsis.

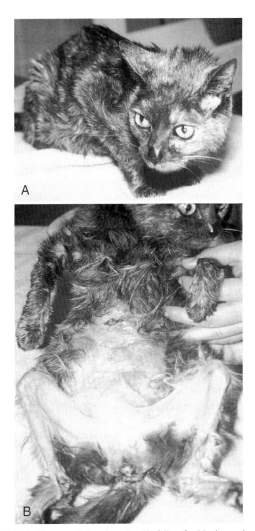

FIGURE 11-2 **A,** 10-year-old female cat with feline Cushing's syndrome (FCS). **B,** Note the hair loss sometimes associated with chronic exposure to excess cortisol.

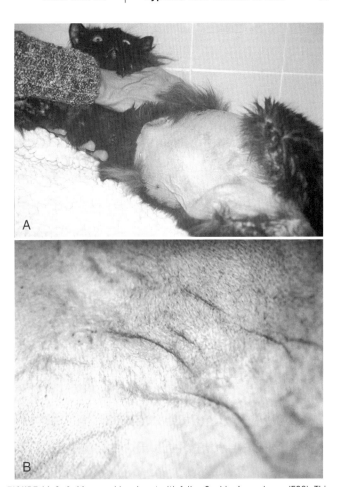

FIGURE 11-3 **A,** 11-year-old male cat with feline Cushing's syndrome (FCS). This cat had a progesterone-secreting tumor (see Excessive Sex-Hormone Secreting Adrenal Tumors in Cats). **B,** Note the thin skin sometimes associated with chronic exposure to excess cortisol.

ROUTINE CLINICAL PATHOLOGY (COMPLETE BLOOD COUNT, BIOCHEMISTRY, URINALYSIS)

Veterinarians working with dogs are familiar with the side effects associated with chronic excesses in circulating cortisone concentration (hyperadrenocorticism; "Cushing's syndrome") because glucocorticoids ("cortisols") are utilized in the management of many canine conditions, side effects are both common and obvious, and the naturally occurring condition is also frequently encountered. Veterinarians, hearing about side effects from almost every steroid-treated dog owner, are repeatedly reminded of "expected" steroid-induced clinical observations. Laboratory abnormalities are indistinguishable in both iatrogenic and naturally occurring conditions. Veterinary clinicians expect dogs with iatrogenic or naturally occurring Cushing's syndrome to have PU/PD, isosthenuria/hyposthenuria, low-normal or low BUN concentrations, increases in serum cholesterol concentration, and increases in alkaline phosphatase and alanine aminotransferase (ALT) activities. Keeping these alterations in mind, we can state once again with confidence, that "cats are not small dogs."

Complete Blood Count

Complete blood count (CBC) results from 53 cats with FCS can be reviewed in Table 11-8. The most important feature is the lack of consistency, in agreement with other investigators

(Gunn-Moore, 2005; Graves, 2010; Peterson, 2012). About half of 53 cats had a "stress leukogram" (neutrophilia and a relative reduction in both lymphocytes and eosinophils). Of their total white blood cell counts, 26 cats (49%) had a neutrophil percentage of more than 86%, 28 (53%) had a lymphocyte percentage of less than 5%, and 29 (55%) had an eosinophil percentage of less than 2%. Of the 53 cats, one was thrombocytopenic, one was leukopenic, and six were anemic. Of the anemic cats, only one had a hematocrit below 24% (that result was 16%), and five of the six had evidence of CKD, likely a contributing issue to their anemia.

Blood Glucose Concentrations and Diabetes Mellitus

Overview

Hyperglycemia represents the most common biochemistry abnormality in cats with FCS (Gunn-Moore, 2005; Lowe et al, 2007; Graves, 2010; Peterson, 2012). Fifty of 58 cats with FCS had diabetes mellitus when first seen at our hospital (four were diagnosed as diabetic at our hospital) and four had had "episodes" of diabetes. Fourteen of the 46 previously diagnosed diabetic cats were believed to be well controlled with insulin. Because a majority of cats with FCS were already being treated with insulin, it is not surprising that hypoglycemia would be identified on a few random blood glucose tests. On random blood glucose measurements in 52 FCS cats, 44 were hyperglycemic, six were hypoglycemic, and two were euglycemic. Both euglycemic and all six hypoglycemic cats were diabetic and

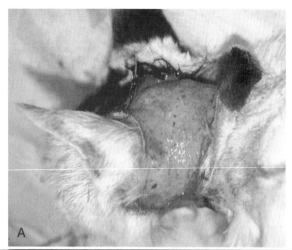

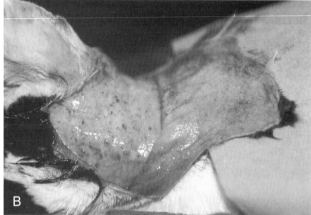

FIGURE 11-4 A, Skin tear in a 15-year-old male cat with feline Cushing's syndrome (FCS). **B,** Skin tear in a 10-year-old cat typical of the skin fragility sometimes associated with chronic exposure to excess cortisol.

had received insulin on the day of testing. The implication from these data is that virtually all the cats included in this review were hyperglycemic or had insulin-induced reduction in blood glucose. One fair question difficult to answer is: "Was stress-induced hyperglycemia a factor in these results?"

Hypoglycemia Versus Insulin Dose

Six of 52 cats with FCS evaluated with a randomly obtained biochemical profile in this review were found to be hypoglycemic, despite expected cortisol-induced insulin resistance. This incidence of hypoglycemia likely underestimates its frequency. Each was diabetic and each had received insulin the day of testing. Four of those six cats were described by their owners and referring veterinarians as "insulin-resistant." Insulin dose (per cat or per kg) among cats with FCS being treated for diabetes varies tremendously, but was often excessive (> 2.2 U/kg). Veterinarians are reminded that insulin can and frequently does induce hypoglycemia. It is also understood that veterinary clinicians occasionally need to manage cats with diabetes mellitus that appear to be "insulin resistant." One obvious response is to repeatedly increase insulin dose "as needed." However, increasing insulin dosage in an attempt to control "resistant" hyperglycemia in diabetic cats can become dangerous. An insulin dose in excess of 2.2 U/kg of body weight should be considered unsafe. Although we do not doubt that some cats appear responsive only to extremely high insulin doses after appearing resistant to lower doses, "resistance" is not a continuum. In other words, insulin resistance in cats with FCS seems to fluctuate or "wax and wane." If true, the

dose given when a cat appears resistant may be an overdose in the same cat at another time. Because some cats with FCS have had severe life-threatening hypoglycemic reactions to insulin, especially when insulin doses are in excess of 2.2 U/kg, it is recommended to maintain insulin doses below this admittedly arbitrary level.

Diabetes Mellitus and the Diagnosis of Feline Hyperadrenocorticism

Diabetes mellitus is among the more common conditions diagnosed in small animal practice and, along with hyperthyroidism, one of the two most frequently diagnosed endocrine disorders in cats. In contrast, FCS is considered uncommon-to-rare (Graves, 2010)—having been diagnosed in a few non-diabetic cats, a few cats with easily controlled diabetes mellitus, and many cats with apparent insulin resistance (Gunn-Moore, 2005). A large majority of cats with FCS are afflicted with concurrent diabetes mellitus (approximately 92% in our review) because it may be easier to suspect FCS in an insulin-resistant diabetic than in an older lethargic cat with a large abdomen. Thin skin, skin fragility, alopecia, failure to regrow hair after it has been clipped, muscle weakness, and PU/PD are potential owner concerns that may trigger testing and, ultimately, a diagnosis of FCS.

The Differential Diagnosis for "Difficult-to-Control" or "Insulin-Resistant" Diabetics

Progression of feline diabetes mellitus is notoriously difficult to predict, and the condition can be difficult to manage. Among the concerns to be addressed by the veterinary practitioner: Which "poorly controlled" diabetic cat is truly "insulin-resistant," and which of those truly insulin-resistant cats are candidates for FCS? We encourage veterinarians having difficulty controlling any diabetic cat to prioritize the potential explanations for "difficult control" with the least expensive and most likely explanations considered first. Topping this priority list should be the concept that in-hospital testing may not reflect what is happening in the home environment.

Owner opinion is the single most important monitoring tool in the long-term management of diabetes. If an owner is satisfied with their cat's response to therapy, decisions based on in-hospital test results should not supersede their opinion unless hypoglycemia is documented. In-hospital stress-induced hyperglycemia is common, and home glucose monitoring minimizes this concern. Veterinarians should also consider the possibility of an "error" in management when a diabetic cat fails to respond to insulin therapy as expected. Errors include, but are not restricted to, using the incorrect insulin, mixing the insulin improperly, drawing insulin into the syringe incorrectly, using incorrect syringes, using outdated insulin, and improper administration technique. Every time a diabetic cat is evaluated, owners should be assessed as they handle and administer insulin. Once these potential concerns have been dismissed, the veterinarian should consider the possibility that the insulin being used is being given at too low a dose, too high a dose, the insulin could be too weak, too potent, too short acting, or too long acting. Additionally, one should consider the possibility that a concurrent disorder exists that interferes with insulin sensitivity. This could include any infection (dental, urinary tract or skin, among others) or any source of non-septic inflammation (pancreatitis, among others). Additional conditions that could cause insulin resistance include CKD, neoplasia, heart disease, and trauma. Among the various endocrine causes for insulin resistance are acromegaly, sex hormone excess, and FCS.

Liver Enzyme Activities

A dramatic increase in serum alkaline phosphatase (SAP) activity (average > 1,000 IU/L) due to glucocorticoid-induction of an

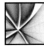

TABLE 11-8 COMPLETE BLOOD COUNT RESULTS FROM 53 CATS WITH NATURALLY OCCURRING CUSHING'S SYNDROME

	Pituitary Dependent (43 Cats)		Adrenocortical Tumor (10 Cats)	
	NUMBER	**PERCENTAGE**	**NUMBER**	**PERCENTAGE**
White Blood Cell Count				
< 6000	1	2	—	—
6000 to 17,000	26	60	6	60
17,000 to 25,000	10	23	3	30
> 25,000	6	14	1	10
% Neutrophils				
≤ 75	6	14	1	10
76 to 85	15	35	5	50
≥ 86	22	51	4	40
% Lymphocytes				
≤ 5	22	51	6	60
6 to 15	19	44	4	40
≥ 15	2	5	—	—
% Eosinophils				
≤ 2	24	56	5	50
3 to 6	13	30	4	40
≥ 7	6	14	1	10
Platelet Counts				
< 180,000	—	—	1	10
180,000 to 400,000	33	77	6	60
> 400,000	10	23	3	30
Hematocrit				
≤ 27	4	9	2	20
28 to 35	24	56	3	30
36 to 46	15	35	5	50
≥ 47	—	—	—	—

SAP isoenzyme is the most common serum biochemical abnormality (> 85%) recognized in dogs with NOH. By contrast, only five of 52 cats with FCS (9%) had an increased SAP. An important differential diagnosis for the increase in SAP in cats with diabetes mellitus is pancreatitis causing cholestasis. Further, the short half-life of SAP in cats as compared with dogs should increase concern regarding an increase. Although "steroid hepatopathy" has been observed in a few cats with iatrogenic hyperadrenocorticism, the changes are usually mild (Lowe et al, 2008; Graves, 2010). The cat has no corollary to the classic "steroid-induced-isoenzyme-of-SAP" known in dogs. In cats with FCS and diabetes mellitus, SAP activity may decrease into reference limits with insulin therapy alone, despite progression of the "Cushing's" (Peterson, 2012).

Another common biochemical abnormality in dogs with NOH (> 50%) is a mild to moderate increase in serum ALT activity. Increases in ALT were identified in 14 of 52 cats with FCS (27%). It is probable that increases in either or both liver enzyme activities in cats with FCS are secondary to hepatic changes associated with diabetes mellitus. Another cause for elderly cats to have increases in liver enzyme activities is

hyperthyroidism. However, of the 52 cats with FCS that had thyroid testing, hyperthyroidism was only diagnosed in two.

Serum Cholesterol and Thyroxine

Increase in serum cholesterol concentration is identified in more than 90% of dogs with diabetes mellitus and in more than 60% of dogs with NOH (less than 5% of dogs with hyperadrenocorticism have concurrent diabetes mellitus). Glucocorticoids inhibit lipoprotein lipase activity and increase activity of hormone-sensitive lipase, increasing both serum cholesterol and triglyceride concentrations. Increases in serum cholesterol concentration, however, are not common in cats with FCS, despite a majority having diabetes mellitus and, therefore, two physiologic stimuli for hypercholesterolemia. Serum cholesterol concentrations were increased in 13 of 52 (25%) cats with FCS in our review, each of whom had concurrent diabetes mellitus.

Chronic excesses in serum cortisol concentration feedback on the pituitary, decreasing TSH secretion and causing "secondary hypothyroidism." Hypothyroidism, primary or secondary, is a

TABLE 11-9	SERUM BIOCHEMICAL RESULTS FROM 52 CATS WITH NATURALLY OCCURRING CUSHING'S SYNDROME

Test and Reference Range		Pituitary Dependent (38 Cats)			Adrenocortical Tumor (14 Cats)		
SERUM		NUMBER WITHIN REFERENCE RANGE	NUMBER BELOW	NUMBER ABOVE	NUMBER WITHIN REFERENCE RANGE	NUMBER BELOW	NUMBER ABOVE
Alkaline phosphatase	(14 to 71 IU/L)	35	—	3	12	—	2
ALT	(28 to 106 IU/L)	24	—	14	12	2	—
Albumin	(2.7 to 3.9 g/dL)	33	5	—	9	3	2
Globulin	(2.9 to 4.3 g/dL)	17	—	21	9	—	5
Total protein	(5.6 to 8.4 g/dL)	31	—	7	12	—	2
BUN	(18 to 33 mg/dL)	17	—	21	8	—	6
Creatinine	(0.9 to 1.8 mg/dL)	26	1	11	10	—	4
Cholesterol	(89 to 258 mg/dL)	24	2	12	13	—	1
Glucose	(73 to 134 mg/dL)	0	4	34	2	2	10
Calcium	(9.4 to 11.4 mg/dL)	34	4	—	11	3	—
PO$_4$	(3.2 to 6.3 mg/dL)	34	2	2	11	—	3
TCO$_2$	(15 to 25 mm/L)	31	4	3	14	—	—
K	(3.6 to 5.3 mm/L)	37	1	—	12	2	—
Na	(145 to 156 mm/L)	36	2	—	12	—	2
T$_4$	(1.0 to 2.5 µg/dL)	33	5	—	12	—	2
Magnesium		3	0	3	2	0	1

ALT, Alanine aminotransferase; *BUN*, blood urea nitrogen; *PO$_4$*, phosphorus; *TCO$_2$*, total carbon dioxide; *K*, potassium; *Na*, sodium; *T$_4$*, thyroxine.

classic cause of hypercholesterolemia. Secondary hypothyroidism, together with the direct lipolytic actions of glucocorticoids are explanations for the increases in serum cholesterol concentration typically identified in non-diabetic dogs with hyperadrenocorticism. Of the 52 cats with FCS in our review, serum thyroxine (T$_4$) concentrations were lower than the reference range in five (9%), three of which had serum cholesterol concentrations within reference limits. Most cats with FCS are euthyroid. Histologically confirmed thyroid disease was only identified in the two cats with hyperthyroidism.

Blood (Serum) Urea Nitrogen, Serum Creatinine, Urinalysis

A consistent group of abnormalities seen in dogs that have hyperadrenocorticism are those related to PU/PD. A majority (> 90%) of hypercortisolemic dogs have urine specific gravities less than 1.020 (especially on samples obtained by owners from dogs in their home environment) and about 30% are less than 1.008. Polyuria in dogs represents one of the most frequent explanations for owners to seek veterinary care. In addition to PU/PD and isosthenuria/hyposthenuria in dogs with hyperadrenocorticism are their low-normal-to-low BUN and normal serum creatinine concentrations. These are classic features of canine hyperadrenocorticism. Increases in BUN are extremely uncommon in dogs with hypercortisolemia and represent a serious contraindication to treatment, because poor appetite and severity of CKD may be masked by hyperadrenocorticism. If the hyperadrenocorticism were to be treated, there is risk of "unmasking" and worsening CKD and its clinical signs.

A review of the serum biochemical and urinalysis data presented in Tables 11-7 and 11-9 from cats with naturally occurring FCS demonstrates several differences in results as compared with those from hypercortisolemic dogs. Not one of 52 cats with FCS had a BUN concentration below the reference range. Only five of 52 cats had a randomly obtained urine specific gravity less than 1.020. Each of those cats had isosthenuria secondary to CKD. Furthermore, 27 of 52 cats (52%) had an increased BUN concentration at the time of diagnosis. Fifteen of those 27 cats (29% of all 52) also had an increased serum creatinine concentration. It seems likely that the PU/PD recognized in some cats with FCS is secondary to CKD. Other polyuric conditions (e.g., hyperthyroidism) may need to be considered. There is little evidence to suggest that cats with FCS have a physiologic syndrome similar to the diabetes insipidus–like condition with dilute urine that occurs in hypercortisolemic dogs.

Serum Sodium, Serum Magnesium, Serum Potassium, and Muscle Weakness

Cats with FCS are often described by their owners as being weak, a condition most commonly related to "feline diabetic neuropathy" causing posterior paresis. Other possible contributors to weakness are the glucocorticoid-induced catabolic effects on muscle and hypokalemia, documented in three of the 52 cats with FCS (6%; see Primary Hyperaldosteronism in Cats). We recommend that serum electrolyte concentrations be evaluated in any weak patient. Assuming that these hypokalemic cats did not specifically have hyperaldosteronism, one may still hypothesize that circulating cortisol excess could act as weak mineralocorticoids and predispose cats to hypokalemia and muscle weakness. Serum sodium concentrations are usually within reference limits. Four of nine cats with FCS cats were hypermagnesemic, the significance of which is not yet fully appreciated.

Serum Calcium, Albumin, Globulins, and Total Protein

Perhaps related to the incidence of CKD in cats with FCS, seven of the 52 cats (13%) were mildly hypocalcemic (based on total serum calcium concentrations). However, each hypocalcemic cat also had a decreased serum albumin concentration. Eight of 52 cats had mild hypoalbuminemia. Hyperglobulinemia was observed on 26 of the 52 chemistry profiles (50%); this was perhaps simply a normal response to chronic antigen exposure, which occurs in any older individual. However, the degree of hyperglobulinemia was such that 11 of the 52 cats (21%) had hyperproteinemia.

Urinary Tract Infection

Urinary tract infection was confirmed in four of the 52 cats with FCS tested (8%; Table 11-9). Because many had been referred after being given antibiotics, perhaps this explains our failure to identify infection in more cats. In contrast, dogs with NOH have a high incidence of urinary tract infection and most are also referred after being treated with antibiotics.

Blood Pressure

Blood pressure assessments have not been commonly reported from cats with FCS, and there is little data regarding the incidence of hypertension among cats with iatrogenic or NOH. However, hypertension is quite common among human beings and dogs with NOH, presumably due to the weak but significant mineralocorticoid actions of glucocorticoids. Further, hypertension is often a component of CKD (common in cats with FCS) or of aldosteronism (unknown incidence).

"SCREENING TESTS" TO AID IN DIAGNOSING FELINE CUSHING'S SYNDROME

FCS is an uncommon condition, can be difficult to diagnose, and carries a guarded prognosis. Results from one of several endocrine tests may aid in discriminating cats that have naturally occurring FCS from cats that do not. The tests most commonly employed are the ACTH stimulation test, the low-dose dexamethasone suppression test (LDDST), and the urine cortisol-to-creatinine ratio (UC:CR); protocols for which can be seen in Table 11-10. Each of these tests has advantages, each has disadvantages, and no test is perfect. The diagnosis of FCS should be reserved for cats with clinical signs as well as endocrine test results consistent with the diagnosis.

Sensitivity and Specificity (A Simple Review)

Discussion on testing invariably includes the concepts of test sensitivity and specificity. Sensitivity, in simple terms, refers to the number of patients with a condition who test positive for that condition. An extremely sensitive test, for example, is glucosuria in dogs with diabetes mellitus. The test is 100% sensitive because diagnosis is restricted to dogs with glucosuria. Specificity refers to the number of patients who do not have a disease and do not test positive for that disease. Using glucosuria again, it is quite specific for diabetes mellitus because

"renal glucosuria" is uncommon. Although not perfect, glucosuria is a test that is strong in both sensitivity and specificity.

Urine Cortisol-to-Creatine Ratio (UC:CR)

Background in People and Dogs

One of the most sensitive and specific screening tests for a person suspected as having NOH is to measure the total amount of cortisol excreted in their urine over a 24-hour period as compared with healthy controls (repeating the test enhances result validity). Despite advances that have taken place since this 24-hour urine collection was introduced as a screening test for humans suspected as having hyperadrenocorticism more than 60 years ago, the test remains a "cornerstone" assessment (Molitch, 2012; Nieman, 2012). The amount of cortisol excreted in urine over a 24-hour period reliably reflects the total amount of cortisol synthesized and secreted over time. Assessing the 24-hour urine excretion of cortisol negates any concern of minute-to-minute pulsatile fluctuations in adrenocortical secretory patterns or any concern regarding diurnal patterns that could affect serum cortisol concentrations at any moment. The use of a randomly collected single urine sample, assessed for cortisol concentration and then compared via ratio with the urine creatinine (UC:CR) is a "short-cut" to the more cumbersome 24-hour collection of urine. See Chapter 10 for a thorough explanation.

Background in Cats

The UC:CR is readily available to veterinary clinicians. Its reference range is higher in cats than dogs, despite their relatively low urinary cortisol excretion rate. The higher UC:CR reference range in cats may be due to their higher glomerular filtration rates and/or lower renal free cortisol reabsorption rates (Goossens et al, 1995). As in dogs, UC:CR in cats is not affected by age, gender, or neuter status. Attributes of the UC:CR include its sensitivity, low expense, east of implementation, and straight-forward interpretation. About 70% to 90% of cats with FCS have an abnormal UC:CR. UC:CR reliability is enhanced if owners bring urine samples from home, usually using small quantities of litter or nonabsorbable litter to make urine easier to collect. Owners should be informed that at least two samples from separate days should be assessed and that a third sample may be necessary if the first results are contradictory. Home-collected urine negates concern of spurious results due to the stress associated with travel and in-hospital collection.

Those who do not recommend the UC:CR mention its lack of specificity. In evaluating the UC:CR from 16 ill cats in one study, three had test results consistent with FCS ($\geq 36 \times 10^{-6}$) and seven had results considered "borderline" (i.e., $10 - 36 \times 10^{-6}$). Thus 10 of 16 ill cats that did not have FCS had UC:CR results that could be considered consistent with that diagnosis (Henry et al, 1996). In a subsequent study, hyperthyroid cats were found to have increased UC:CR results (de Lange et al, 2004).

Test Interpretation

Two independent studies suggested similar reference ranges for feline UC:CR ($< 28 \times 10^{-6}$ and $< 36 \times 10^{-6}$) (Henry et al, 1996; Goossens et al, 1995, respectively). Both are higher than that for dogs ($\leq 16 \times 10^{-6}$). A UC:CR more than 36×10^{-6} is consistent with FCS in a cat with appropriate clinical signs and in-hospital test results. UC:CR values between 10 and 36×10^{-6} in cats with appropriate clinical signs should be considered "borderline," inconclusive, and worth repeating. It is possible for a cat with test results in this range to have FCS, as was true for

TABLE 11-10	A SUMMARY OF DIAGNOSTIC TEST PROTOCOLS USED IN CATS SUSPECTED OF HAVING CUSHING'S SYNDROME

SCREENING TESTS	TEST PROTOCOL
Urine cortisol-to-creatinine ratio (UC:CR)	1. Owner collects urine from the cat; urine is then taken to veterinary clinic. 2. Sensitivity and specificity improve if repeated on separate mornings.
Low-dose dexamethasone suppression test (LDDST)	1. Obtain blood for baseline control. 2. Administer 0.1 mg/kg dexamethasone, IV. 3. Obtain blood for cortisol 4 and 8 hours after dexamethasone.
Hair cortisol	Obtain appropriate samples for submission.
ACTH stimulation (ACTHST)	Not recommended.
Combination LDDST and ACTHST	Not recommended.

DISCRIMINATION TESTS	TEST PROTOCOL
High-dose dexamethasone suppression test (HDDST)	1. Owner collects two urine samples from the cat (on different days). 2. After second collection, give three doses of dexamethasone orally (0.1 mg/kg every 8 hours: 8 AM, 4 PM, and midnight). 3. Next morning, collect urine for HDDST portion of test.
Abdominal ultrasonography	Excellent ultrasonographer and equipment are quite important.
Plasma endogenous [ACTH] (ACTH precursors, as well)	1. Collect blood in chilled tube containing protease inhibitor. 2. Immediately separate plasma, freeze until assayed.
Low-dose dexamethasone suppression test (LDDST)	1. Protocol as described earlier and used as screening test. 2. Criteria as discrimination test are distinct (> 50% decrease from basal level); see text.
HDDST (in-hospital protocol)	1. Obtain blood for baseline cortisol. 2. Administer 1.0 mg/kg dexamethasone, IV. 3. Obtain blood for cortisol 4 and 8 hours after dexamethasone.
Abdominal radiographs	These are of limited value.

ACTH, Adrenocorticotropic hormone; *[ACTH],* ACTH concentration; *IV,* intravenous.

12 of the 48 cats in our review (Tables 11-11 and 11-12). The UC:CR has high negative predictive value, meaning that a reference range result makes the diagnosis of FCS much less likely (Graves, 2010).

Results

As can be seen from the data presented in Tables 11-11 and 11-12, UC:CR data was collated from a total of 48 cats with FCS (34 with PDH and 14 with ATH), including cats from the literature (Goossens et al, 1995 [six cats]; Schwedes, 1997 [one cat]; Skelly et al, 2003 [one cat]; Meij et al, 2001 [seven cats]; and Neiger et al, 2004 [five cats]). Thirty-five of the 48 cats (71%; 27 from the PDH group and 8 from the ATH group) had UC:CR results above the reference range, 12 cats (25%) had "borderline" (13 – 36 × 10⁻⁶) results (six from each group). One cat had a UC:CR result that was considered normal (that cat had PDH). Thus the UC:CR appears to be a sensitive test for confirming the diagnosis of FCS in cats; in that only 1/48 cats had a result within the reference range.

Conclusions

The UC:CR is a sensitive diagnostic aid for distinguishing cats that have FCS from cats that do not. Sensitivity of this test appears to be similar to that for dogs with NOH. Because specificity remains a concern, the negative predictive value of the UC:CR is emphasized (i.e., cats with a negative UC:CR are less likely to have FCS, especially if that result is repeatable). Veterinarians are encouraged to place a great deal of importance on the history, physical examination, and "routine" in-hospital test results when deciding whether to perform the UC:CR. Veterinarians are encouraged to consider having owners collect urine samples on two separate mornings from their cat as an excellent means of screening for FCS (please see the section, Urine Cortisol-to-Creatinine Ratio and High-Dose Dexamethasone Suppression Test).

ACTH Stimulation Test

Background

The adrenocorticotropic hormone stimulation test (ACTHST) has been recommended as an aid for confirming a diagnosis of NOH in dogs for about 50 years. More recently, the ACTHST has been recommended as an aid to confirm or refute the diagnosis of FCS, presumably as an extension of its use in dogs. A complete discussion on the physiologic basis for this test and its usefulness is provided in Chapter 10. In general, humans suspected of having hormone deficiency syndromes (e.g., hypoadrenocorticism [Addison's disease]), are typically evaluated with "provocative" or "stimulation" tests to aid in diagnosis, and those suspected of having hormone excess syndromes (e.g., NOH), are typically evaluated with suppression tests.

Background in Cats. Those who recommend using the ACTHST point out several attributes: the test requires little time (1 or 2 hours depending on the ACTH used), only two or three venipunctures are needed, results are easy to interpret, it is the only test useful for distinguishing iatrogenic from naturally occurring disease, and it is the only test used in the long-term monitoring of

TABLE 11-11 ENDOCRINE SCREENING TEST RESULTS FROM CATS WITH NATURALLY OCCURRING PITUITARY-DEPENDENT CUSHING'S SYNDROME

	Urine Cortisol-to-Creatinine Ratio	Serum Cortisol (μg/dL) Low-Dose Dexamethasone			Serum Cortisol (μg/dL) ACTH Stimulation		
		PRE	4 HOUR	8 HOUR	PRE	FIRST POST	SECOND OR FINAL POST
Reference range	$< 36 \times 10^{-6}$	1-5	< 1.4	< 1.4	0-5	5-15	5-15
Borderline range	$10 - 36 \times 10^{-6}$	—	0.9-1.3	0.9-1.3	—	15-19	15-19
Number of cats included	34	46	46	43	46	35	55
Number of results within reference range	1	—	4	0	23	24	33
Number of results in "borderline" range	6	—	0	0	—	3	5
Number of results consistent with Cushing's syndrome	27	—	42	43	—	8	17
Range of test results	$3 - 810 \times 10^{-6}$	1.5-20.2	0.3-14.9	1.5-14.7	1.5-27.3	5.4-32.7	5-36.0
Mean ± standard deviation	48.7 ± 31.6	6.8 ± 3.7	4.2 ± 2.9	4.9 ± 2.1	6.3 ± 3.8	12.2 ± 5.6	14.7 ± 10.1
Median	39	5.4	4.6	5.2	5.6	11.5	13.7

TABLE 11-12 ENDOCRINE SCREENING TEST RESULTS FROM 14 CATS WITH CUSHING'S SYNDROME CAUSED BY A FUNCTIONING ADRENOCORTICAL TUMOR

	Urine Cortisol-to-Creatinine Ratio	Plasma Cortisol (μg/dL) Low-Dose Dexamethasone			Plasma Cortisol (μg/dL) ACTH Stimulation		
		PRE	4 HOUR	8 HOUR	PRE	FIRST POST	SECOND OR FINAL POST
Reference range	$< 36 \times 10^{-6}$	0.5	< 1.4	< 1.4	0-5	5-15	5-15
"Borderline" range	$10 - 36 \times 10^{-6}$	—	0.9-1.3	0.9-1.3	—	15-19	15-19
Number of cats included	14	12	10	12	8	6	8
Number of results within reference range	0	—	0	0	5	4	4
Number of results in "borderline" range	6	—	—	—	—	1	—
Number of results consistent with Cushing's syndrome	8	—	10	12	—	1	4
Range of test results	$11 - 160 \times 10^{-6}$	1.5-11.0	1.5-11.6	1.8-10.2	2.6-11.8	2.7-50.0	3.3-52.8
Mean ± standard deviation	42 ± 81.4	4.9 ± 2.9	5.2 ± 3.5	4.9 ± 2.7	5.2 ± 3.4	17.3 ± 16.9	22.3 ± 18.2
Median	3.8	4.1	4.1	5.5	3.7	13.1	21.5

medically treated NOH dogs and cats. Detractors suggest that the test lacks sensitivity and specificity and is far more expensive than either the UC:CR or the LDDST.

A number of studies have evaluated the ACTHST in either laboratory or privately-owned cats. One of the earliest studies compared the use of two different doses of synthetic ACTH (cosyntropin) with the use of natural ACTH in stimulation tests conducted on privately-owned healthy cats. Synthetic ACTH was administered at doses of 125 and 250 μg per cat IM with blood samples obtained for cortisol analysis before administration and again at 15, 30, 60, 90, and 120 minutes after (Smith and Feldman, 1987). No significant difference was found between responses to the two doses of synthetic ACTH. Because two cats vomited and remained obtunded for several hours after receiving the higher dose, the lower dose was recommended. Peaks in plasma cortisol concentration were most often documented 30

and 60 minutes after starting the test, and therefore both post-ACTH sampling times were recommended. Using the mean ± standard deviation (SD) to establish the reference range for the post-ACTH plasma cortisol resulted in a range of about 6 to 19 μg/dL at 30 or 60 minutes after the intramuscular (IM) injection.

Response to intravenous (IV) synthetic tetracosactrin (another form of synthetic ACTH) was evaluated in laboratory cats given 125 μg/cat, IV. Cats demonstrated peak responses 180 minutes after injection (Sparkes et al, 1990). The longer duration of action and greater potency of IV versus IM administration was further supported in a subsequent study, again using 125 μg/cat. Peak cortisol response occurred between 60 and 90 minutes after starting the test (Peterson and Kemppainen, 1992a). No significant difference was noted in drug response after IV cosyntropin was compared with IV tetracosactrin in another study, and it was recommended that blood for cortisol be obtained

60, 90, 120, and 180 minutes after administration (Peterson and Kemppainen, 1992b). These two studies were followed by one in which 1.25, 12.5, and 125 µg of cosyntropin were administered to cats, demonstrating comparable peak cortisol responses after each dose but a more prolonged response with the highest dose (Peterson and Kemppainen, 1993). Another group demonstrated increases in hypothalamic-pituitary-adrenal activity as cats age (Goossens et al, 1995), although this phenomenon does not alter reference ranges. This study was then followed by one on overweight, older, privately-owned cats, using 125 or 250 µg of IV tetracosactrin/cat. Results complemented previous reports that had utilized young, relatively lean, laboratory cats. Peak cortisol concentrations after ACTH administration were similar to those reported in the other studies (Schoeman et al, 2000). Slight variations in post-ACTH cortisol concentration reference ranges may result from the use of cosyntropin versus tetracosactrin, various doses, or employing IV versus IM administration. The critical question, however, not addressed in any of these studies is simply whether or not the test should be employed in cats suspected of having FCS.

Test Interpretation. One generally agreed upon ACTHST protocol for cats is to administer 125 µg of synthetic ACTH, IV, with blood samples obtained 60, 90, 120, and 180 minutes after. (Veterinarians should use the protocol recommended by their laboratory.) Most laboratories suggest that post-ACTHST cortisol concentrations of 6 to 15 µg/dL are within their reference interval, 15 to 19 µg/dL are borderline and inconclusive, and results more than 19 µg/dL are consistent with FCS. Some laboratories may utilize slightly lower or higher reference intervals. Lower reference intervals could lose specificity, raising the risk that more cats without FCS are incorrectly diagnosed as having the condition. Higher reference intervals could lose sensitivity, potentially resulting in missing the diagnosis of FCS. As demonstrated in the study on privately owned, overweight cats that did not have FCS, baseline (pre-ACTH) cortisol concentrations were as high as 13 µg/dL and post-ACTH cortisol concentrations as high as 19.7 µgdL (Schoeman et al, 2000). Just the basal values, therefore, might include some cats in the FCS group if lower cortisol concentrations were considered "diagnostic," and others would have been described as "borderline." The ACTHST, regardless of dose, form of ACTH, timing, and so on has been demonstrated in most reports to have unacceptably poor sensitivity and specificity regarding its use as a screening for FCS.

Results. ACTHST results were available from 65 cats with FCS; 55 cats diagnosed with PDH and 10 with ATH. The results were from 51 cats in our series and 14 cats reported in the literature (Immink et al, 1992 [one cat]; Schwedes, 1997 [one cat]; Watson and Herrtage, 1998 [five cats]; Moore et al, 2000a [one cat]; Skelly et al, 2003 [one cat]; Neiger et al, 2004 [five cats]). All 65 cats had at least one post-ACTHST result, 56 had basal cortisol concentrations reported, and 41 had more than one post-ACTHST result. If only a solitary post-ACTH test result was available, it was arbitrarily considered the "final" result (see Tables 11-11 and 11-12). Thirty-eight of the 65 cats (58%) had post-ACTHST cortisol concentrations within the reference interval, five (8%) had "borderline" results, and 22 (34%) had abnormal results. Of the 55 cats with PDH, 33 (60%) had results within the reference interval, five (9%) had borderline results, and 17 (31%) had abnormal results. Of the 10 ATH cats, five had results within the reference interval and five were abnormal. Thus, the sensitivity (the number of cats that had FCS and tested positive) of the ACTHST for all the

cats was about 33%. Forty-one cats with FCS (35 with PDH, six with ATH) had two post-ACTH administration samples obtained, allowing assessment of the "middle" result (see Tables 11-11 and 11-12). Twenty eight cats (68%) had results within the reference interval, four (10%) had borderline results, and nine (22%) had abnormal results. There was little diagnostic value associated with adding the intermediate sample during ACTH stimulation testing.

Lack of ACTHST sensitivity as a screening test for FCS, demonstrated in our review, has also been noted by others (Gunn-Moore, 2005; Graves, 2010, Peterson, 2012). In a more recent study, 56% of cats with FCS had an abnormal ACTHST result (Valentin et al, 2014). Thus, the ACTHST is not sensitive as an aid in identifying cats with FCS, because so many of the results are normal. Evaluation of different blood sampling times and various doses of ACTH does not improve this index of diagnostic usefulness. Even a single basal serum cortisol measurement has a greater sensitivity (67%) for detecting cats with FCS than the ACTHST (Duesberg and Peterson, 1997; Graves, 2010). Specificity of the ACTHST has also been questioned (Graves, 2010; Peterson, 2012) because a variety of chronic illnesses not associated with FCS can influence results (Zerbe et al, 1987b). It has been suggested that "stress" associated with chronic illness could cause adrenocortical hyperplasia, accounting for an exaggerated cortisol response to ACTH (Peterson, 2012).

Conclusions. The attributes of ACTHST as a screening test for cats suspected as having FCS—the test is brief, easy to complete, and easy to interpret–all lose value when collated results indicate that it lacks sensitivity. Further, there are tests (UC:CR and LDDST) that are clearly superior. The ACTHST remains the best test to confirm iatrogenic hyperadrenocorticism, but this condition is rare in cats.

Low-Dose Dexamethasone Suppression Test (LDDST)

Background

A complete discussion on the physiologic basis for the LDDST and its usefulness is provided in Chapter 10. Use of the analogous "overnight LDDST" is a well-established test for confirming the diagnosis of NOH in people, with a sensitivity and specificity similar to that of the 24-hour urine cortisol excretion test. The basis of LDDST, as is true for the overnight test employed in people, assumes that administered dexamethasone circulates throughout the body, including to the hypothalamus and pituitary, in which it has potent suppressive effects. The "low" dose of dexamethasone is the minimum necessary to directly and completely suppress synthesis and secretion of both hypothalamic corticotrophin-releasing hormone (CRH) and pituitary ACTH in healthy individuals, which in turn decreases synthesis and secretion of adrenocortical glucocorticoids (Peterson and Graves, 1988). Effect of dexamethasone is profound within an hour and persists until the dexamethasone is metabolized, which is usually well beyond 8 to 10 hours (about 30 hours in dogs). Dexamethasone has been the traditional glucocorticoid for suppression testing because early cortisol assays cross-reacted with prednisone or prednisolone. Consistent hypothalamic-pituitary-adrenocortical axis suppression, in healthy individuals as well as those with non-adrenal illness, is the single most important criterion of a reliable LDDST.

Individuals with ATH have an autonomous, cortisol secreting, adrenal adenoma, or carcinoma. Secretion of glucocorticoids from these tumors is independent of hypothalamic-pituitary control. Glucocorticoids derived from adrenocortical tumors act the same as administered dexamethasone: it persistently and chronically suppresses hypothalamic and pituitary function. Therefore, administration of dexamethasone to a patient with ATH should have no suppressive effects on endogenous serum cortisol concentrations.

Individuals with PDH and secondary adrenocortical hyperplasia have a pituitary tumor less sensitive to glucocorticoid-associated negative feedback, otherwise hyperadrenocorticism would never develop. Administration of dexamethasone to an individual with PDH typically has one of two results: (1) the dexamethasone fails to cause lowering (suppression) of circulating cortisol concentrations because the pituitary tumor is resistant to negative feedback and results of this test are indistinguishable from that seen with ATH, or (2) hypothalamic, pituitary, and then adrenocortical cortisol secretion *is* suppressed and circulating cortisol concentrations do decrease, but this effect is far more transient than "normal" due to rapid metabolism of the administered drug. In this latter condition, dexamethasone causes a decrease in circulating cortisol concentrations, but rather than persisting for more than 8 hours, it lasts far less than 8 hours and circulating concentrations of cortisol "escape" from the suppression earlier in individuals with PDH than in healthy individuals.

Protocol

The LDDST dose and protocol established in dogs, 0.01 mg/kg of dexamethasone IV with cortisol concentrations determined before and 4 and 8 hours after administration, fails to cause suppression in 15% to 20% of healthy cats. Increasing the dose to 0.1 mg/kg was consistently effective in suppressing healthy cats but not cats with FCS (Smith and Feldman, 1987; Hoenig, 2002; Kley et al, 2007).

Test Interpretation

The established reference ranges for results 4 and 8 hours after administration of 0.1 mg/kg of dexamethasone in healthy cats is less than or equal to 0.8 µg/dL. A value greater than or equal to 1.4 µg/dL is consistent with a diagnosis of FCS due to PDH or ATH, in the context of a cat also having appropriate signs and supportive evidence. The "nondiagnostic" range of 0.9 to 1.3 µg/dL is meant improve both sensitivity and specificity by forcing additional testing.

Results

A total of 58 cats with FCS (46 with PDH and 12 with ATH) have their LDDST results included in Tables 11-11 and 11-12. Forty-seven cats were from our series, and data from 11 cats were obtained from the literature (Immink et al, 1992 [two cats]; Goossens et al, 1995 [three cats]; Meij et al, 2001 [three cats]; Neiger et al, 2004 [three cats]). Not all cats had both 4 and 8 hour post-LDDS results available. Forty-three out of 43 cats with PDH and 12 out of 12 cats with ATH cats (100%) had abnormal 8-hour LDDST results consistent with FCS (cortisol concentrations > 1.4 µg/dL), suggesting that this LDDST protocol is "highly sensitive" and more sensitive than either UC:CR or ACTHST. Although these results indicate 100% sensitivity, readers must understand that no test is perfect. In a related study, LDDST results were consistent with a diagnosis of FCS in 93% of afflicted cats (Valentin et al, 2014). Their conclusion was that the screening test of choice in the evaluation of a cat suspected as having FCS is the LDDST; however, there is no "gold standard."

Conclusions

The 0.1 mg/kg dexamethasone test is an excellent and extremely sensitive screening test in the evaluation of a cat suspected as having FCS. Specificity of the LDDST was not critically assessed here, although previous studies indicate that some cats with non-adrenal illness will have LDDST results consistent with FCS (Zerbe et al, 1987b; Duesberg and Peterson, 1997). The LDDST is the screening "test of choice" in evaluating a cat for FCS.

Hair Cortisol Concentrations

Hair cortisol concentrations were higher in dogs with NOH as compared with healthy dogs and ill dogs that did not have NOH (Corradini et al, 2013). This non-invasive laboratory aid could revolutionize the diagnosis of NOH in dogs and FCS in cats if results are both sensitive and specific.

Combined Dexamethasone Suppression Test/ Adrenocorticotropic Hormone Stimulation

This combination test can be completed in 1 day with collection of only three blood samples. An ACTHST is begun 3 to 5 hours after beginning the LDDST. However, the addition of the unacceptably insensitive ACTHST to the quite sensitive LDDST seems unnecessary while having the potential to provide misleading results. This test is *not* recommended (Peterson, 2012).

Combination "Screening" and "Discrimination" Tests

Urine Cortisol-to-Creatinine Ratio and High-Dose Dexamethasone Suppression Test

The Screening Portion of the Test. The UC:CR can be combined with a high-dose dexamethasone suppression test (HDDST) in a practical and cost-effective alternative to more "traditional" testing options (Goossens et al, 1995). This test is designed to be completed in the home environment, negating need for cats to be brought into the hospital with its attendant stress, time, and expense. Owners are instructed to collect urine from their cat on two separate mornings. It is not necessary for urine to be collected on consecutive days, but doing so shortens the process. There are a variety of methods for owners to obtain urine. Simply leaving their cat in a room with a box containing insufficient litter to absorb the urine produced overnight is easiest, allowing owners to pour urine into a clean container (alternatively, use nonabsorbable litter). Collected urine is then brought to the veterinarian for measurement of UC:CR. This portion of the test is the screening test to aid in separating cats with FCS (abnormally increased UC:CR) from cats that do not have the disease (UC:CR result within the reference range). The use of two separate samples is used to improve sensitivity and specificity by not relying on one result. If both samples suggest FCS, one may continue to the second phase of the test. If one result is within reference range and one is abnormal, additional samples (one or two) may be collected and evaluated.

The Discrimination Portion of the Test. Before interpreting this test, it is assumed that the previously obtained UC:CR results were abnormal and consistent with the strong clinical suspicion of FCS. In this second phase of the test, the owner should administer 0.1 mg/kg of dexamethasone orally every 8 hours beginning in the morning (i.e., dexamethasone is administered at about 8 AM, 4 PM, and midnight). That night, the cat should again be restricted to a location that allows urine to be collected on this third morning. The urine is delivered to the veterinarian and again assessed for UC:CR. Using the calculated mean from the first two samples, a result less than 50% of that mean (on average) would be consistent with PDH. A result more than 50% of that mean does not allow discrimination of PDH from ATH.

Conclusions. This test was suggested in the literature about two decades ago. It has not been critically evaluated, in part because FCS is an uncommon condition. The test may have a sensitivity and specificity as good as or better than other recommended protocols. It is not strongly recommended here only because we have little experience with this combination test. In people suspected as having NOH, a single overnight dexamethasone suppression test is a trusted and reliable screening test. Thus, the precedent for such a test in cats is solid (Molitch, 2012; Nieman, 2012).

 ## TESTS TO "DISCRIMINATE" PITUITARY FROM ADRENAL TUMOR CUSHING'S SYNDROME

After diagnosis of FCS has been confirmed, several tests can be used to help "discriminate" individuals with PDH from those with ATH. Four tests are commonly used to help "discriminate" ATH from PDH. These include the LDDST, the HDDST, plasma endogenous ACTH concentrations, and abdominal ultrasonography. Because of expense, need for specialized facilities and anesthesia, CT and MRI scans (although somewhat sensitive and quite specific) are not as widely used. The reason for discriminating ATH from PDH is their different therapeutic options. Ideally, adrenocortical tumors should be surgically removed. The most effective medical option for treating cats with ATH is trilostane. Pituitary tumors could also be surgically removed or treated with external radiation, but neither of these therapies is widely available. Trilostane is the medical alternative. If an owner is to refuse surgery in any scenario, it could be argued that discrimination testing is unnecessary.

Low-Dose Dexamethasone Suppression Test (LDDST)

Background

The LDDST, as discussed earlier, is extremely sensitive in helping to separate cats with FCS from cats that do not have the condition. Individuals with ATH typically demonstrate no response to administration of dexamethasone, whereas some with PDH do demonstrate suppression but for a shorter period of time than noted in healthy individuals. Three criteria define "suppression" on the LDDST in attempting to identify *dogs* likely to have PDH: a 4-hour cortisol less than a laboratory-determined absolute value (often < 1.4 µg/dL), a 4-hour cortisol less than 50% of the baseline value, and an 8-hour cortisol less than 50% of the baseline value. Approximately 65% of dogs with PDH demonstrate "suppression," because they meet one or more of these criteria.

Results

Forty-six cats with PDH in our review had their 4-hour cortisol concentrations assessed during LDDST, 42 had values more than 1.4 µg/dL (no suppression) and four had values less than or equal to 0.9 µg/dL. Ten cats with ATH had a 4-hour post LDDST blood sample assessed for cortisol, and all had both 4- and 8-hour results more than 1.4 µg/dL. Thus, use of the absolute value of less than 1.4 helped to identify only four of 56 cats (7%) with FCS as having PDH. All four results were correct, but sensitivity is poor. Use of more than 50% suppression from the

baseline cortisol concentration proved to be far more sensitive. Of 12 cats with FCS due to ATH, none demonstrated more than 50% suppression at either 4 or 8 hours. Of 46 cats with PDH, however, 24 cats (41% of all 58 cats; 52% of cats with PDH) demonstrated more than 50% suppression of serum cortisol concentrations at either 4 or 8 hours (seven cats at 4 hours, two cats at 8 hours, and 15 cats at both 4 and 8 hours). The LDDST does have sensitivity and specificity in discriminating ATH from PDH. In other words, a cat with FCS that meets any of the three established criteria for PDH on an LDDST, likely has PDH.

High-Dose Dexamethasone Suppression Test (HDDST)

Background

The HDDST is an aid for discriminating patients with PDH from those with ATH. Physiologic basis for this test, in part, is the same as for the LDDST: administration of dexamethasone decreases adrenocortical (endogenous) cortisol secretion via the suppression of hypothalamic synthesis and secretion of CRH, thereby decreasing pituitary ACTH synthesis and secretion. Dexamethasone also directly suppresses pituitary synthesis and secretion of ACTH. Without ACTH, adrenocortical cells cease synthesizing and secreting cortisol. As circulating cortisol is metabolized, plasma and urine cortisol concentrations decrease quickly after administration (within an hour) and remain suppressed throughout the period of dexamethasone activity (30 hours in healthy dogs).

Adrenocortical tumors function autonomously and are independent of hypothalamic and pituitary control. Negative feedback associated with chronic excesses in circulating glucocorticoids cause atrophy of pituitary ACTH-secreting cells in ATH patients. Therefore dexamethasone, regardless of dose administered, does not suppress cortisol secretion from an adrenocortical tumor. By contrast, although pituitary tumors in PDH function "somewhat" autonomously, secretion of ACTH by some (not all) pituitary tumors can be suppressed with "low" doses of dexamethasone. In dogs and cats with PDH, about 65% and 52%, respectively, demonstrate enough suppression on LDDST to indicate that ATH is not an explanation for their hyperadrenocorticism. Using a higher dose of dexamethasone is based on the concept that if some individuals with PDH demonstrate at least some suppression on LDDST, a higher dose will increase the number.

In-Hospital Protocol

Administer 10 times the dose of dexamethasone used for the LDDST. In cats, it is generally accepted to use a dexamethasone dose of 1.0 mg/kg, IV, with blood samples obtained for cortisol concentration before and 4 and 8 hours after administration. Remember, before employing this test, one should first confirm that the cat has FCS.

At-Home Protocol

An alternative method employs the UC:CR, and the entire test is carried out by the owner at home (described in previous section).

Interpretation of the In-Hospital HDDST

Four "criteria for suppression" can be utilized to aid in the interpretation of results: more than 50% decrease in cortisol concentration, from the basal value, at 4 or 8 hours; or cortisol concentrations less than 1.4 µg/dL at 4 hours or 8 hours. If any one of these four criteria for suppression is met, the result is most consistent with PDH. Failure to meet any of the criteria adds support for the diagnosis of FCS but is inconclusive regarding PDH versus ATH.

Interpretation of the At-Home Protocol. The interpretation of the at-home protocol is described in previous section.

Results

In-Hospital High-Dose Dexamethasone Suppression Test.

As seen in Table 11-13, HDDST results were available from 40 cats with confirmed FCS. Basal and 4- and 8-hour post-HDDST results were available from 24 cats with PDH and four with ATH. Only baseline and 8-hour samples were obtained from an additional 11 cats with PDH and one with ATH. There can only be two interpretations of HDDST results: (1) "consistent with PDH" can be applied to results demonstrating suppression, and (2) "inconclusive regarding PDH versus ATH discrimination" because none of the four criteria were met. Thirteen of 24 cats (54%) had "4-hour" HDDST results that demonstrated suppression; the results were consistent with PDH. All 13 cats had PDH. Thus suppression on the 4-hour test result was modestly sensitive but quite specific for PDH. The four cats with ATH and a 4-hour HDDST result failed to demonstrate suppression, as was expected. Also as expected, some cats (11 of 24; 46%) with PDH failed to respond to the HDDST at 4 hours. Thus failure to suppress plasma cortisol concentration at 4 hours was a nonspecific finding that included cats with ATH and PDH.

Fifteen of 40 cats (38%) had 8-hour HDDST results that demonstrated suppression; the results were consistent with PDH. All 15 of those cats did have PDH, correctly identifying 15 of 35 cats (43%) with PDH. Thus suppression on the 8-hour test result correctly identified cats with PDH. The five cats with ATH and an 8-hour HDDST result failed to demonstrate suppression, as was expected. Also as expected, some cats (20 of 35; 57%) with PDH failed to respond to the HDDST at 8 hours. Failure to suppress plasma cortisol concentration at 8 hours was a nonspecific finding that included cats with ATH and PDH. It is also of interest to note that the 8-hour test was available from all 24 PDH cats tested at 4 hours plus an additional 11 cats with PDH. However, only two additional cats with PDH demonstrated suppression at 8 hours. All 13 cats that met at least one of the two criteria for suppression at 4 hours met at least one of the two criteria for suppression at 8 hours. It seems reasonable to suggest only a 4-hour post-HDDST sample be obtained, because the 8-hour result has not offered significant new information.

Results

At-Home Urine High-Dose Dexamethasone Suppression Test.

As can be reviewed in Table 11-14, 13 cats were tested using the at-home protocol. All 13 cats had PDH (Goossens et al, 1995 [six cats]; Meij et al, 2001 [seven cats]). Ten of the 13 (77%) cats did demonstrate suppression on the UC:CR from the sample obtained post-dexamethasone, using the mean of two basal urine samples for the comparison. The entire test could be carried out by an owner, decreasing cost and stress.

TABLE 11-13 **HIGH-DOSE DEXAMETHASONE SUPPRESSION TEST AND PLASMA ENDOGENOUS ACTH RESULTS FROM CATS WITH CUSHING'S SYNDROME**

	Plasma Cortisol (µg/dL) High-Dose Dexamethasone Test			Plasma Endogenous ACTH
	PRE	**4 HOUR**	**8 HOUR**	**(pg/mL)**
Pituitary Dependent Hyperadrenocorticism (PDH)				
Reference range	0-5	< 1.4	< 1.4	10-60
Borderline range for PDH	—	—	—	10-45
Results consistent with PDH (definition)	—	< 1.4 or < 50% baseline	—	> 45
Number of cats	35	24	35	45
Number of results inconclusive (consistent with PDH or ATH)	—	11	20	3
Number of results consistent with PDH	—	13	15	42
Range of test results	2.4-39.0	0.2-15	0.1-25.8	38-3653
Mean (± standard deviation)	8.8 ± 8.8	3.0 ± 3.6	4.9 ± 6.2	457 ± 619
Median	5.3	0.9	2.4	221
Adrenocortical Tumor Hyperadrenocorticism (ATH)				
Reference range	0-5	< 1.4	< 1.4	10-60
Borderline range for ATH	—	—	—	10-45
Results consistent with ATH	—	> 1.4 or > 50% of baseline cortisol	—	Undetectable
Number of cats	5	4	5	6
Number of results inconclusive	—	0	0	0
Number of results consistent with ATH	—	4	5	6
Range of test results	3.0-7.1	3.7-6.1	4.4-6.1	All undetectable
Mean (± standard deviation)	5.1 ± 1.6	5.0 ± 0.8	5.0 ± 0.7	—
Median	4.9	4.7	4.7	—

ATH, Adrenal tumor hyperadrenocorticism; *PDH,* pituitary dependent hyperadrenocorticism.

TABLE 11-14	HIGH-DOSE DEXAMETHASONE SUPPRESSION TEST RESULTS FROM 13 CATS WITH PDH UTILIZING THE "AT-HOME" UC:CR PROTOCOL*				
CAT NUMBER	**FIRST BASAL UC:CR**	**SECOND BASAL UC.CR**	**MEAN UC:CR**	**POST-DEXAMETHASONE UC:CR**	**POSITIVE FOR PDH?**
1	139	145	142	13	Yes
2	37	64	51	5	Yes
3	75	82	78	92	No
4	125	155	140	41	Yes
5	104	103	104	26	Yes
6	228	316	272	18	Yes
7	—	—	272	18	Yes
8	—	—	80	117	No
9	—	—	119	5	Yes
10	—	—	73	17	Yes
11	—	—	72	27	Yes
12	—	—	105	119	No
13	—	—	77	7	Yes

All results compiled from Goossens MMC et al.: Urinary excretion of glucocorticoids in the diagnosis of hyperadrenocorticism in cats, *Domestic Anim Endocrinol* 12:355, 1995; and Meij BP, et al: Transsphenoidal hypophysectomy for treatment of pituitary-dependent hyperadrenocorticism in 7 cats, *Vet Surg* 30:72, 2001.
PDH, Pituitary dependent hyperadrenocorticism; *UC:CR,* urine cortisol-to-creatinine ratio.
*Suppression is defined as a post-dexamethasone UC:CR < 50% of the mean of two basal UC:CR. (All UC:CR results multiplied by 10^{-6}.)

Conclusions

The in-hospital HDDST is relatively easy to perform and interpret, not expensive, and not harmful. Suppression, after administering 1.0 mg/kg of dexamethasone IV, is consistent with PDH. Cats with ATH usually do not demonstrate suppression, whereas 52% of cats with PDH meet at least one criterion of suppression. The 0.1 mg/kg dexamethasone dose resulted in identification of only 22% of PDH cats. It is noted that the 1.0 mg/kg dexamethasone dose was most effective in identifying PDH at 4 hours. No cat with ATH demonstrated suppression at either 4 or 8 hours of the HDDST, but some cats with PDH also fail to suppress. Therefore, failure to demonstrate suppression should be considered an inconclusive result and is similar to results in human beings and dogs.

The at-home HDDST is easier to perform and interpret than the in-hospital protocol. In addition, at-home test results were superior to those utilizing the in-hospital tests in correctly discriminating PDH from ATH. Assuming an owner can administer dexamethasone, it seems reasonable to recommend the at-home protocol for both screening and discrimination testing, because this protocol is generally easier to perform, less expensive, easier to interpret, safer (less bruising and no chance of skin trauma), and as-good-as or more specific and sensitive.

Endogenous ACTH and ACTH Precursor Concentrations

Background

Circulating endogenous ACTH concentrations have been used to help discriminate people with PDH from those with ATH since the 1970s, and they have been used for the same purpose in dogs and cats since the 1980s. Individuals with ATH have autonomously functioning adrenocortical tumors that chronically suppress circulating concentrations of endogenous ACTH and its precursors. Those with PDH have an ACTH-secreting tumor associated with normal-to-increased concentrations.

The attributes of assessing endogenous ACTH include requiring only one blood sample, being easy to interpret and relatively reliable. However, it is important that blood samples for determination of endogenous ACTH concentration be handled as directed by your laboratory. ACTH is a labile protein that degrades quickly in plasma. Samples usually must be collected directly into a tube containing ethylenediaminetetraacetic acid (EDTA) anticoagulant, tubes must be made of plastic or silicone-coated glass (most glass EDTA collection tubes are siliconized); samples should be placed immediately on ice and centrifuged (ideally in a cold centrifuge). Harvested plasma must be placed in plastic tubing, frozen until assayed, and shipped on ice (Graves, 2010). Mishandled samples may falsely lower values suggesting an adrenal tumor (Peterson, 2012). Test results are not always definitive. Some people and dogs with hyperadrenocorticism due to either ATH or PDH have ACTH concentrations that overlap with the reference range. These drawbacks, together with the availability and diagnostic specificity of imaging studies (e.g., ultrasonography) have limited the use of endogenous ACTH assessment.

Some pituitary pars intermedia (PI) cells stain positively for ACTH as do virtually all pars distalis (PD) cells. In contrast, some PI cells cleave ACTH to α–melanocyte-stimulating hormone (MSH) and corticotropin-like intermediate lobe peptide (CLIP), suggesting that increases in plasma α-MSH concentrations could be expected in cats with PI adenomas. However, cats with the highest α-MSH concentrations were those with PD adenomas (Halmi and Krieger, 1983; Rijnberk, 1996; Meij et al, 2001). One explanation could be that the gene encoding the cleavage enzyme (proconvertase 2) may become "de-repressed" in the course of neoplastic transformation of PD corticotrophs (Low et al, 1993). Alternatively, as in people, some PD adenomas may originate from a sparse population of melanocyte cells (Coates et al, 1986). Cat PI and PD adenoma cells stain positively for both ACTH and α-MSH (Peterson et al, 1982).

TABLE 11-15 LENGTHS AND WIDTHS OF ADRENAL GLANDS MEASURED ULTRASONOGRAPHICALLY IN 20 HEALTHY AWAKE CATS

NUMBER OF CATS	PARAMETER	LENGTH OF RIGHT ADRENAL GLAND	WIDTH OF RIGHT ADRENAL GLAND	LENGTH OF LEFT ADRENAL GLAND	WIDTH OF LEFT ADRENAL GLAND
20	Range (cm)	0.7-1.4	0.3-0.45	0.45-1.3	0.3-0.5
	Median (cm)	1.0	0.4	0.9	0.4

From Zimmer C, et al.: Ultrasonographic examination of the adrenal gland and evaluation of the hypophyseal-adrenal axis in 20 cats, *J Small Anim Pract* 41:156, 2000.

Interpretation of Test Results

The reference range for endogenous ACTH concentrations in cats is slightly lower than for dogs (Feldman, 1981; Smith and Feldman, 1987). Most cats with PDH have endogenous ACTH concentrations from mid-reference range to several times higher than the upper limit of the assay. Cats with ATH (as well as cats with iatrogenic hyperadrenocorticism) have results that range from undetectable to the lower portion of most reference ranges. However, some cats with iatrogenic hyperadrenocorticism, ATH, or PDH have inconclusive results (Peterson et al, 1994; Duesberg and Peterson, 1997; Benchekroun et al, 2012).

Results

Plasma endogenous ACTH concentrations were available from 51 cats with FCS. Thirty-eight of these cats were from our series, and 13 were from the literature (Goossens et al, 1995 [six cats]; Meij et al, 2001 [seven cats]). All 13 cats from the literature had PDH, 32 cats from our series had PDH and six had ATH. As can be seen from Table 11-13, the results of endogenous ACTH testing were excellent. All six cats (100%) with ATH had undetectable concentrations, and 42 of 45 cats (93%) with PDH had concentrations more than 45 pg/mL. Nondiagnostic results from three cats with PDH (38, 40, and 41 pg/mL) were still distinct from the results obtained from cats with ATH. Twenty-five of 45 cats with PDH had results typical of those noted in dogs (45 to 450 pg/mL). However, 17 cats with PDH (38%) had plasma endogenous ACTH concentrations in excess of 450 pg/mL (range, 487 to 3850 pg/mL; mean, 1002 pg/mL ± a SD of 731). Why so many cats with PDH had extremely increased plasma endogenous ACTH concentrations (> 450 pg/mL) is not well understood. Is it that their pituitary tumors produce more ACTH, is the assay less reliable in cats, is the assay more reliable in cats, is the assay also measuring precursors in the cat, or is there some other explanation? The extremely high concentrations of ACTH, as noted in many cats from our series, were also noted by Meij and colleagues (2001). These authors pointed out that in one cat, the ACTH assay results as measured by an immunoradiometric assay (IRMA) was only about 20% of the value obtained with an assay employing a polyclonal antibody. It is possible, therefore, that the polyclonal antibody assay is suspect. Perhaps these pituitary tumors secreted precursor-molecule pro-opiomelanocortin (POMC) or POMC-derived peptides recognized as ACTH by the assay. Precursors of ACTH were above the reference range in eight of nine cats that had PDH (Benchekroun et al, 2012).

Conclusions

Measuring endogenous ACTH or its precursor concentrations in cats with confirmed FCS has value for discriminating PDH from ATH. However, since the diagnostic value, availability, and cost-effectiveness of imaging studies are excellent, use of endogenous ACTH testing is not common.

Abdominal Radiology

Changes noted on radiography of cats with FCS are similar to those seen in dogs. These changes include excellent contrast (due to fat deposition into the mesentery), hepatomegaly (which is usually secondary to diabetes mellitus in cats, as opposed to being more frequently secondary to steroid-induced hepatomegaly in dogs), and a pot-bellied appearance (caused by steroid-induced abdominal muscle weakness). Use of radiography has been replaced, for the most part, by abdominal ultrasonography as the key abdominal imaging study for cats known or suspected to have naturally occurring FCS. Ultrasonography is favored simply because adrenal glands are not routinely visualized via radiography unless the gland(s) is calcified or extremely enlarged (both situations are rare). By contrast, canine and feline adrenal glands can be routinely visualized on ultrasonography.

Abdominal Ultrasonography

Background

Knowledge regarding adrenal gland imaging in dogs developed sooner than cats (Barthez et al, 1995; Horauf and Reusch, 1995). A study on ultrasound appearance of adrenals in anesthetized healthy cats (Cartee and Finn-Bodner, 1993) was followed by a study on awake cats. In the latter report, both glands were visualized in each cat. Further, both left and right adrenal glands were virtually identical in size and shape, with both being oblong and oval-to-bean–shaped (Table 11-15; Zimmer et al, 2000). In general, the adrenal glands of cats are less echogenic than the surrounding tissues and the right adrenal may be technically more difficult to image. The central area of the adrenals were identified as more echogenic than the cortex in six of 20 cats. Readers are reminded that ultrasonography is a "subjective" diagnostic tool. In other words, results are dependent on skill and experience of the ultrasonographer, as well as on the equipment used.

Results

Results of abdominal ultrasonography in cats with FCS are summarized in Table 11-16. Forty-one cats were evaluated: Thirty-five cats from our series and six cats with results taken from the literature (Daley et al, 1993 [one cat]; Watson and Herrtage, 1998 [four cats]; Moore et al, 2000a [one cat]). Thirty-four of the 41 abdominal ultrasound results correctly identified either bilaterally symmetrical adrenals consistent with PDH or an adrenal nodule

TABLE 11-16	ABDOMINAL ULTRASOUND INTERPRETATIONS FROM 41 CATS WITH NATURALLY OCCURRING HYPERADRENOCORTICISM	
POSSIBLE FINDING		**NUMBER OF CATS**
Cats With Adrenal Tumor Hyperadrenocorticism (ATH) (9 Cats)		
R mass, L small		3
L mass, R small		0
R mass, L not seen		2
L mass, R not seen		2
Both adrenals enlarged		1
No adrenals seen		1
Cats with Pituitary Dependent Hyperadrenocorticism (PDH) (32 Cats)		
Both adrenals normal		5
Both adrenals enlarged		22
L normal or enlarged, R not seen		2
R normal or enlarged, L not seen		1
No adrenals seen		2

L, Left adrenal gland; R, right adrenal gland.

consistent with ATH. Three of the 41 cats (7%) had inconclusive studies, because no adrenal tissue was identified (two of these cats had PDH, and one had ATH). Four of the 41 cats (10%) had potentially misleading results: Three of 32 cats (9%) with PDH had one normal-to-increased-sized adrenal gland, with the other gland not visible, and one cat with ATH was thought to have enlargement of both glands. Twenty-seven of the 32 cats (84%) with PDH had both adrenal glands visualized and correctly described as being relatively equal-sized. A unilateral adrenal mass with the opposite gland being small or not visible was correctly observed in seven of nine cats (78%) with ATH. Thus, ultrasound results were correct in a total of 34 of 41 cats with FCS (83%). In a subsequent study of 32 FCS cats, the accuracy of ultrasound correctly discriminating PDH from ATH was 93% (Valentin et al, 2014).

Conclusions

Abdominal ultrasonography is not a screening test for separating cats with FCS from cats that do not have the condition. It is an excellent discrimination test for separating cats with ATH from those with PDH. Correct discrimination has been documented consistently in about 80% to 90% of cats with FCS (Duesberg and Peterson, 1997; Kley et al, 2007; Valentin et al, 2014). The reader is reminded that ultrasound examination results are subjective and success will vary.

Ultrasound-Guided Biopsy

Cats with FCS have undergone successful percutaneous biopsy of suspected adrenal masses. Although percutaneous biopsy can be completed with ultrasound guidance, one must weigh the benefit of obtaining a histologic description of adrenal tissue against risks of complication.

Computed Tomography (CT) and Magnetic Resonance Imaging (MRI) Scans

Background

It is recommended that the diagnosis of FCS due to PDH be confirmed before pursuing pituitary imaging using CT or MRI scanning. These imaging modalities provide a non-invasive means of visualizing some pituitary tumors; however, each technique requires specialized facilities and cats must be anesthetized. MRI scanning has been the imaging modality of choice for the pituitary gland area in people (Chakere et al, 1989; Stein et al, 1989). Compared with CT scans, MRI scans have superior anatomic resolution and soft tissue contrast. Also, MRI scans are less likely to create distracting artifacts when the middle and caudal fossae of the brain are imaged (Kaufman, 1984). MRI scanning allows acquisition of images oriented in any plane, which is an important feature when examining the pituitary fossa.

The purpose of considering a sophisticated diagnostic aid such as CT or MRI in a cat suspected of having FCS is to determine whether or not an obvious pituitary mass can be visualized prior to radiation therapy or surgery. In our experience, both CT and MRI scans consistently allow visualization of pituitary masses more than 3 mm in greatest diameter. Therefore, if only one modality is available, we would encourage using that tool. If both imaging modalities are available, we encourage veterinarians to choose whichever tool is less expensive or whichever tool requires the shortest duration of anesthesia.

In a study of healthy cats, the pituitary gland was measured using post-gadolinium (postcontrast) MRI studies in 17 cats. The cats were 1 to 15 years of age and weighed between 2.9 and 6.5 kg. Mean (± SD) pituitary length was 0.54 cm (± 0.06 cm) and the width was 0.5 cm (± 0.08 cm). Pituitary gland height measured on sagittal and transverse images was about 0.33 cm (± 0.05). Mean pituitary volume was about 0.05 cm^3. There were no significant correlations between weight, age, and pituitary volume. The pituitary gland appearance on the precontrast scan had "mixed signal intensity," whereas on postcontrast scans the pituitary appeared to have uniform enhancement (Wallack et al, 2003).

Abdominal imaging may be of interest prior to adrenalectomy. Specifically, imaging may identify vascular or local invasion. Assessment of the liver and other structures for evidence of metastatic disease or other concerns may be worthwhile.

Results

Pituitary imaging scan results were reviewed from 48 cats with confirmed PDH (Table 11-17). A visible mass (5 to 11 mm in greatest diameter) was identified in 34 cats (70%; Fig. 11-5). Thirteen of 22 cats (59%) from three different studies utilizing CT scans had a visible mass (Goossens et al, 1995; Meij et al, 2001; Benchekroun et al, 2012); in the UC Davis series, visible masses were identified in six of nine cats evaluated with CT and four of six evaluated with MRI. As veterinarians develop an ability to identify cats with PDH earlier in the course of disease progression, the "sensitivity" of CT and MRI scans for detecting pituitary tumors should decrease, because earlier diagnosis will be made in cats with smaller less detectable masses. Cats with confirmed PDH without a detectable mass should be assumed to have pituitary tumors simply too small to be seen.

Conclusions

Pituitary imaging serves several potential roles. Either CT or MRI scans could be used to help confirm a diagnosis of FCS (see Table

TABLE 11-17	COMPUTED TOMOGRAPHY (CT) AND MAGNETIC RESONANCE IMAGING (MRI) SCAN RESULTS FROM 48 CATS* WITH PDH		
RESULTS	CT SCAN	MRI SCAN	NOT SPECIFIED[†] CT/MRI
Normal study (no mass seen)	12 cats	2 cats	0 cats
Visible mass (5 to 11 mm in greatest diameter)	19 cats	6 cats	9 cats
Total	31 cats	8 cats	9 cats

*15 cats from UC Davis series; 9 cats from Benchekroun G, et al.: Plasma ACTH precursors in cats with pituitary-dependent hyperadrenocorticism, *J Vet Intern Med* 26:575, 2012; 9 cats from Valentin SY, et al.: Comparison of diagnostic tests and treatment options for feline hyperadrenocorticism: a retrospective review of 32 cases, *J Vet Intern Med* 28:481, 2014.
[†]7 cats from Meij BP, et al.: Transsphenoidal hypophysectomy for treatment of pituitary-dependent hyperadrenocorticism in 7 cats, *Vet Surg* 30:72, 2001; 6 cats from Goossens MMC, et al.: Urinary excretion of glucocorticoids in the diagnosis of hyperadrenocorticism in cats, *Domestic Anim Endocrinol* 12:355, 1995; 2 cats from Sellon RK, et al.: Linear-accelerator-based modified radiosurgical treatment of pituitary tumors in cats: 11 cases (1997-2008), *J Vet Intern Med* 23:1038, 2009.
CT, Computed tomography; *MRI,* magnetic resonance imaging.

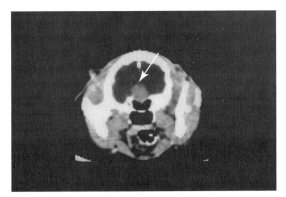

FIGURE 11-5 Computed tomography (CT) scan of the pituitary brain region from a cat with pituitary-dependent hyperadrenocorticism (PDH) demonstrating a pituitary mass.

11-17). This would be an expensive and insensitive approach, considering that UC:CR or LDDST results are much more sensitive, require no anesthesia, and are less expensive. Either CT or MRI scanning could be used as a discrimination test to help distinguish cats with PDH from those with ATH. This, too, is an expensive and insensitive approach because cats with ATH would have normal (unremarkable) scans along with those confirmed to have PDH but whose pituitary masses are too small for visualization. Thus a normal scan would yield virtually no information other than suggesting that a cat may have ATH or, if a cat has PDH, the tumor is small. The recommendation here is that CT or MRI scans be used to screen cats that might be scheduled to undergo hypophysectomy, pituitary radiation, or radiosurgery. Either CT or MRI scans could be used to evaluate a cat with central nervous system (CNS) signs to determine the likelihood of the macrotumor syndrome.

 MEDICAL TREATMENT

Introduction and the Options

Trilostane is the most efficacious medical treatment option effective in cats with PDH or ATH. Surgical management of FCS includes bilateral adrenalectomy or hypophysectomy for cats with PDH. Surgical removal of an adrenocortical tumor is the preferred treatment for cats with ATH. External beam radiation therapy can be utilized for cats with PDH, especially if the cat has a large (macro) pituitary tumor. No treatment modality has been employed in a large enough group of cats to allow solid recommendations, but experience with trilostane is promising.

Trilostane

Background

Trilostane is an orally active reversibly competitive 3-β hydroxysteroid dehydrogenase inhibitor of adrenocortical and gonadal steroid synthesis. (A full description of trilostane can be found in Chapter 10.) Trilostane inhibits synthesis of both glucocorticoids and mineralocorticoids. Although not efficacious for people with hyperadrenocorticism, trilostane therapy has successfully led to resolution of clinical and biochemical abnormalities associated with hyperadrenocorticism in dogs and cats. As an enzyme blocker, trilostane is effective only when administered consistently, usually once or twice daily. If medication is not given, the effect dissipates in hours. A small number of trilostane treated dogs have developed adrenal necrosis—an effect not described in cats. The number of cats treated with trilostane and reported in the literature (at least 30) is limited, but no other therapeutic modality has been used much more often and no other has had greater success (Skelly et al, 2003 [1 cat]; Neiger et al, 2004 [5 cats]; Mellett Keith et al, 2013 [15 cats]; Valentin et al, 2014 [9 cats]. Twenty-nine of these 30 cats had PDH. We have used trilostane for the treatment of 5 cats with FCS. Although trilostane is not recommended for dogs with pre-existing liver disease, kidney disease, or both, such parameters are often abnormal in cats with FCS, but influence of these conditions on response to therapy is not known.

Indications

The primary indication for using trilostane is for long-term treatment of PDH or ATH in cats. Among the reasons for using trilostane for a cat with ATH are owner refusal to consider surgery, presence of metastases, tumor size or location that negates surgery as an option, or one of many concurrent conditions making surgery an unacceptable risk (fragile skin, kidney disease, heart disease, and so on). Before surgery is performed on any cat with FCS, treatment with trilostane should be employed in an attempt to gain full control of the disease for a period of time (4 to 8 weeks). In this manner, many of the complications associated with surgery and the perioperative period can be minimized.

High Dose, Low Frequency Trilostane

The starting dose of trilostane, reported for 21 cats with FCS, varied from about 15 mg per cat once daily to 60 mg b.i.d. (twice a day; 120 mg/cat/day); 4.2 to 13.6 mg/kg, once or twice daily (Skelly et al, 2003; Neiger et al, 2004; Mellett Keith et al, 2013). Recommended starting doses are about 20 to 30 mg/cat orally per day, administered once daily or divided between feeding times (Peterson, 2012). The initial doses used in one study averaged 4.3 mg/kg, once daily (13 cats) and 3.3 mg/kg b.i.d. (2 cats) (Mellett Keith et al, 2013). Trilostane should always be administered during a meal or within 30 minutes of meal completion to enhance absorption of the drug.

Low-Dose, High-Frequency Trilostane

After experience with low-dose trilostane being effective in treating dogs with NOH (Vaughan et al, 2008), a similar approach was used in 4 FCS cats—3 with PDH and 1 with ATH (all managed by the author). Each cat was treated with about 1 mg/kg of body weight (rounded up to the next full kg of weight if needed), t.i.d. (three times a day). Purchased Vetoryl was compounded into appropriate-sized capsules, and good response in lowering cortisol concentrations and in resolving signs of FCS were achieved. In 3 cats, the dose was not changed, and in 1 cat, the dose was increased 20%. Trilostane should always be given during a meal or within 30 minutes of completion to enhance drug absorption.

Initial Home Treatment and Monitoring Recommendations

Medical therapy for cats with FCS is best carried out in their familiar home environment. Thus, treatment becomes the owner's responsibility. This is easy to discuss in a textbook but often quite difficult in reality. Remind owners that missing a dose occasionally should not be a problem. Assuming that an owner can consistently administer oral medication, treatment of FCS remains complicated. Therefore, prior to initiating therapy, the veterinarian is obligated to educate the owner as much as possible about FCS, the treatment plan, treatment goals, and potential complications. Treatment goals should never be a certain blood test result. Rather, the primary goal should be to have the owner see improvement in their pet's health and, therefore, therapy should be individualized to the needs of each cat. The patient should be thoroughly assessed before treatment with at least a body weight, history, physical examination, CBC, serum chemistry profile (including blood glucose and electrolytes), and urinalysis. Having this information from samples taken before treatment may be helpful when attempting to determine the explanation for predictable or unpredictable responses.

Cats with a Poor Appetite. No cat should be treated for FCS if inappetent or anorexic. Appetite issues should be understood and resolved prior to starting treatment because control of hyperadrenocorticism is always associated with a reduction in appetite. If appetite decreases with therapy, the veterinarian would want to know whether it is the result of treatment. In such a scenario, blood and urine tests become a valid means of detecting changes that likely took place after treatment began.

Conditions to Monitor. At a minimum, one must monitor the effects of trilostane on FCS, diabetes mellitus (if present), and kidney function. Veterinarians should also be aware of drug-induced side effects as well as changes in other concurrent conditions. Among the reported causes of death or euthanasia in treated FCS cats are kidney failure, worsening diabetes, or diabetes-related complications (ketoacidosis, hypoglycemic reactions, progressive weakness, and so on), overwhelming infection (especially of skin wounds), and perceived poor quality of life. FCS may mask concurrent conditions that become obvious as treatment progresses.

Feline Hyperadrenocorticism Cats with Diabetes Mellitus. Beginning with the first day of trilostane therapy, insulin dose in diabetic cats should be decreased by about 50% or to doses of 0.1 to 0.5 units per kg of body weight per dose, whichever is deemed appropriate. Reducing insulin dose anticipates the physiologic effect that decreases in circulating cortisol concentration

will reduce insulin antagonism and enhance insulin action. An attempt to avoid severe hypoglycemia is imperative, because such reactions are traumatic and dangerous for the patient as well as being frustrating, disappointing, and traumatic for owners.

Owners of cats with FCS and diabetes can provide their veterinarian with extremely valuable information. We encourage owners to monitor, as best they can, their cat's appetite, water intake, urine output, litter box usage, activity, muscle strength, interest in family members, grooming behavior, skin wound appearance (healing?), and any other pertinent information. If owners are willing and able, we recommend collection of an overnight urine sample (usually simply by removing most of the litter from the box or using nonabsorbable litter and restricting the cat to that room overnight). Urine should be obtained the morning of any planned in-hospital testing. This allows veterinary personnel to assess, at the least, specific gravity, glucosuria, and UC:CR. If owners are capable, we also recommend checking blood glucose concentrations, using the ear vein technique, every 2 hours over 10 hours every 5 to 7 days in the first month or so of trilostane treatment. Hyperglycemia is common. Euglycemia may be indicative of diabetes resolving or of the cat becoming more sensitive to insulin. Hypoglycemia always indicates insulin overdose. Some overdosed cats are no longer diabetic and others require an insulin dose reduction. Most cats with FCS and diabetes mellitus remain diabetic despite trilostane therapy. We are encouraged that using the low-dose trilostane protocol, two of three cats with PDH had resolution of both FCS and diabetes mellitus. Chapter 7 is dedicated to feline diabetes mellitus and should be consulted.

Feline Hyperadrenocorticism Cats with Chronic Kidney Disease (CKD). Valuable information can be gained from owners of a cat with FCS and CKD. As with owners of diabetic cats, we encourage these owners to monitor, as best they can, their cat's appetite, water intake, urine output, litter box usage, activity, muscle strength, interest in family members, grooming behavior, skin wound appearance (healing?), and any other pertinent information. Concerns regarding worsening kidney function will be raised if the appetite is abnormally poor, if weight loss is suspected, or if the cat has vomiting or worsening PU/PD. Resolution of NOH may be associated with unmasking severe CKD.

In-Hospital Monitoring

In-hospital rechecks should be planned 7 to 10 days after starting trilostane, again after a month, and then every 90 to 120 days. Schedules should be individualized. In the ideal situation, we ask owners to collect urine from their cat the morning of any scheduled recheck, as described. While repeatedly obtaining blood from FCS cats is problematic, it is difficult to avoid the ACTHST. While the ACTHST lacks sensitivity and is not recommended as a screening test for FCS, it remains the most informative and objective test used for monitoring response to trilostane administration. ACTHST should be started 2 to 3 hours after feeding and trilostane administration. Whatever the time period from trilostane administration, future ACTHST should begin using the same time interval.

Assessment of Trilostane Dose and Frequency. Together with the UC:CR result from owner collected urine, results of ACTHST will aid in determining if and what kind of adjustments in trilostane therapy are needed. A UC:CR result within the laboratory reference range indicates that a cat is receiving the correct dose or too much trilostane and that the frequency of administration is correct. The correctly dosed cat should be described by the owner as doing well, whereas the overdosed cat may be described as listless, inappetent, having diarrhea, and/or vomiting. The appropriately dosed cat should have a post-ACTHST cortisol concentration of about 2 to 6 µg/dL, whereas an over-dosed cat will have a cortisol concentration less than 2 µg/dL if the ACTHST is carried out at the correct time post-trilostane. If the UC:CR is above the reference limit, an increase in trilostane dose is indicated if the post-ACTHST cortisol concentration is more than 6 µg/dL. If the UC:CR is above the reference limit, an increase in the frequency of trilostane administration is indicated if the post-ACTHST result is in the desired range. This recommendation for repeatedly collecting urine is based on experience.

Assessment of Cats Not Doing Well. Ideally, if the trilostane dose is correct, the ACTHST result should be about 2 to 6 µg/dL. But these are not magic numbers with guaranteed results. Suggestions here are aids to achieving a positive response. Although ACTHST and UC:CR results are objective, owner opinion regarding response to therapy remains most important. If owner opinion and UC:CR or ACTHST results seem discordant, owner opinion should take precedence.

For example, an owner believes the cat is doing great but test results suggest underdose. In this scenario, no change in dose or frequency would be made. What if an owner believes the cat is doing great but test results suggest overdose? Here, we would recommend lowering the dose. Alternatively, an owner believes that the cat is doing poorly but UC:CR and ACTHST results look excellent. First, any cat described as being ill should have the trilostane discontinued because overdose is always a possibility and, even if not overdosed, continued treatment may negatively impact the cat's ability to respond to another condition. Our initial differential diagnoses would include worsening in diabetes control, pancreatitis, or CKD. Other problems may be encountered.

Results

In a study of five cats treated with trilostane, two died after 16 and 120 days of treatment, respectively. The remaining cats did improve and were alive at 6, 11, and 20 months (Neiger et al, 2004). In the study on 15 cats, survival ranged from 87 to 1280 days. The median survival was about 21 months. In this latter study, only cats treated for 60 days or longer were included, leaving the possibility that some trilostane treated cats failed to remain on the drug or survive 60 days (Mellett Keith et al, 2013). In both studies, cats with diabetes mellitus remained diabetic, although the condition was usually more responsive to treatment.

The four cats treated with low-dose trilostane included one with ATH that improved and had its adrenocortical tumor surgically removed with resolution of FCS. The three cats with PDH all improved clinically, no adverse side effects were noted, and two of the three experienced resolution of their diabetes mellitus. One cat whose diabetes resolved died from pancreatic adenocarcinoma 10 months after treatment started, and the other two are each alive after about 1 year.

Mitotane

A number of different protocols using mitotane (Lysodren; o,p'-DDD) for the medical management of cats with PDH have been used with varying levels of short-term success. Long-term results have been discouraging (Peterson, 1998). It is interesting to point out that human beings with PDH, like their feline counterparts, are not nearly as sensitive to o,p'-DDD as dogs. (See Chapter 10 for a complete discussion of o,p'-DDD.) When o,p'-DDD was given to clinically normal cats, only 50% demonstrated any adrenocortical suppression (Zerbe et al, 1987a). Adverse effects such as anorexia, vomiting, and lethargy have been described as common, even in cats that did not have discernable cortisol response

(Peterson et al, 1994; Duesberg and Peterson, 1997; Peterson, 2012). We have experience in using mitotane in four cats with FCS (Nelson et al, 1988). Mitotane does not effectively suppress adrenocortical function nor alleviate clinical signs of FCS, and its use is not recommended.

Ketoconazole

Ketoconazole, an imidazole derivative, is an orally active broad-spectrum antimycotic drug that has been used successfully in treating fungal disease in human beings and animals. At adequate doses, it inhibits both 11-β-hydroxylase and cholesterol side-chain cleavage enzymes, inhibiting mammalian steroid biosynthesis. Ketoconazole also has the potential to inhibit pituitary synthesis of ACTH by inhibiting adenyl cyclase activity in pituitary corticotrophs (Stalla et al, 1988). Doses used for mycotic infection can lead to significant reduction in serum androgen concentrations, and at higher doses, decreases in serum cortisol (Engelhardt et al, 1991). Ketoconazole is an efficacious oral medication for the treatment of human beings with PDH.

Ketoconazole does not seem to consistently suppress adrenocortical function in either normal cats or cats with FCS. A study of four healthy male cats given 30 mg/kg/day for 30 days failed to demonstrate significant changes in plasma testosterone or cortisol concentrations. Serum testosterone concentrations tended to decrease after the first 7 days of treatment, but in two of the four cats, values returned to near-pretreatment concentrations by day 30 (Willard et al, 1986). Our experience has been limited to using this drug in five cats with naturally occurring PDH. Three of the five cats responded moderately well but not completely. One cat demonstrated no response, and the fifth cat developed severe thrombocytopenia (which may or may not have been associated with the drug) several weeks after treatment was initiated. Use of ketoconazole for the treatment of cats with FCS is not recommended (Peterson, 2012).

Etomidate

Etomidate is a short-acting intravenously administered anesthetic agent used for anesthesia induction. Because it has been shown to have minimal deleterious effect on the cardiovascular system, this drug has been used to induce anesthesia in high-risk patients that are critically ill, hypovolemic, in shock, or have pre-existing cardiovascular disease. It has also been shown that administration of this drug suppresses adrenocortical function in people, dogs, and cats. One study on cats demonstrated profound suppression of adrenocortical function during 2 hours of anesthesia (Moon, 1997). Use of a sustained-release form of this drug could be an effective mode of therapy for cats with FCS.

Metyrapone

Metyrapone (Novartis; East Hanover, NJ) is an orally active drug that inhibits the enzymatic action of 11-β-hydroxylase, which is responsible for converting 11-deoxycortisol to cortisol. Because cortisol precursors have little or no biologic activity, inhibition of cortisol synthesis has the potential to resolve clinical signs and biochemical changes due to hyperadrenocorticism. In people, drugs like metyrapone have been recommended for short-term control prior to surgery, to resolve hyperadrenocorticism while waiting for radiation therapy to take effect, or to provide palliative treatment for metastatic disease (Verheist et al, 1991; Feelders et al, 2010).

Metyrapone has been documented to be effective in people with either PDH or ATH. Although adverse reactions are not common, transient hypocortisolemia has been reported. Chronic use of metyrapone has been demonstrated to result in a compensatory endogenous ACTH concentration increase and "override" of adrenal blockade of cortisol synthesis (Orth, 1978).

There are several reports of using metyrapone in cats with FCS. Clinical response without side effects (other than hypoglycemia) was achieved in two cats using 30 to 70 mg/kg orally, twice daily (Daley et al, 1993; Moore et al, 2000b). The lower end of the dose range should be used for the first 2 to 4 weeks, rechecking the cat and possibly completing an ACTHST. The dose can be increased, as needed, by small increments. Doses greater than 70 mg/kg, twice daily, are not recommended. Higher doses have been mentioned, although these higher doses have been associated with a strong suspicion of drug-induced vomiting and inappetence. Subjective clinical improvement was observed in three cats: One was lost to follow-up after 10 months of treatment, whereas two cats were treated for 21 days and 6 months, respectively, before each had successful bilateral adrenalectomy (Moore et al, 2000a). One of two additional cats was treated and reported to have had slight improvement (Peterson, 1988). Another cat demonstrated transient reduction in ACTHST cortisol concentrations, had resolution of clinical signs, and underwent subsequent successful adrenalectomy (Daley et al, 1993). Metyrapone is often difficult to obtain. There has not been a documented case of rising endogenous ACTH concentrations in cats, overriding adrenocortical blockade with either metyrapone or trilostane.

SURGERY AND LAPAROSCOPIC TREATMENT

Hypophysectomy

Background and Results

The treatment of choice for people with PDH is surgical removal of their pituitary tumor, thus eliminating the cause (Melby, 1988; Thorner et al, 1992). Pituitary tumors are primary and not caused by excessive hypothalamic stimulation. Their removal results in permanent resolution of PDH (Scholten-Sloof et al, 1992; Van Wijk et al, 1992). Hypophysectomy in cats has been used for both physiologic and pharmacologic studies (Reaves et al, 1981; Sallanon et al, 1988). In addition, transsphenoidal hypophysectomy in cats has been described in detail for advanced microsurgical training of physician neurosurgeons (Snyckers, 1975).

Microsurgical trans-sphenoidal hypophysectomy is an effective means of treating cats with PDH (Meij et al, 2001). However, this form of therapy requires CT or MRI imaging facilities to identify the mass, assess its size, establish location for the burr slot needed to perform the procedure, and determine if surgery is appropriate prior to the procedure. In addition to requiring an experienced surgeon, having facilities for perioperative care is imperative. Cats undergoing this procedure had both soft palate and mucoperiosteum incised to expose the sphenoid bone. Access to the pituitary fossa was completed using a burr and punches, the dura mater was incised, and the pituitary carefully extracted (Meij et al, 1997; 2001). The procedure is safest in cats with a small pituitary tumor. Regardless of tumor size, this procedure is associated with risk of surgical and medical problems. After the procedure, some cats develop transient or permanent hypopituitarism. This hypocortisolism, hypothyroidism, and diabetes insipidus requires at least short-term substitution therapy. Two of seven cats were alive 15 and 46 months after surgery, respectively,

at the time that the report was written and were in complete remission. Two of the five long-term survivors had resolution of diabetes mellitus (Meij et al, 2001).

Conclusions

The number of cats treated with hypophysectomy has been limited. However, as more experience is gained, there is no doubt that this could be the treatment of choice for cats with PDH, as it is for similarly afflicted human beings and dogs. Limiting factors include need for expertise and facilities to perform the surgery and the perioperative medical care. As expertise improves, it is anticipated that specific removal of ACTH-secreting tumors will be accomplished while preserving the healthy portion of the pituitary.

Adrenalectomy

Background

Pituitary surgery should provide a permanent cure. Bilateral adrenalectomy for PDH is another, rarely used means of permanently resolving FCS. Adrenal nodule or mass removal should be curative for ATH. Perhaps the most important questions to consider prior to surgery are whether the cat is a reasonable surgical and anesthesia risk and, after trilostane treatment for 4 to 12 weeks prior to surgery to control FCS, what would be gained from the surgery that has not been achieved with trilostane? One answer to this latter question is the cat would no longer need to be medicated, although diabetes mellitus and its need for therapy may not resolve. Again, consider risk versus reward, and be certain that the owner is well informed.

Managing Cats Pre- and Post-Adrenalectomy

Conservative volumes of IV fluids (2.5% dextrose if the cat is diabetic) should be started after withdrawal of food and water prior to surgery. During surgery and in the first days following, fluid therapy should be directed at maintaining hydration, being aggressive in the assumption that some of these cats will develop postsurgical pancreatitis, but not overloading a compromised cardiovascular system. General vague guidelines suggesting individualization of therapy is the only reasonable recommendation that can be made. Use of an antibiotic specific for an identified infection, based on culture and sensitivity results, may represent the best opportunity to avoid resistance. Insulin treated diabetics should be given 50% of the usual morning dose. Insulin dosing from this point until the cat is eating and drinking on its own will be challenging. When the surgeon begins removal of an adrenal tumor or the first of a bilateral adrenalectomy, dexamethasone should be administered (0.2 mg/kg, IV). That dose should be repeated IM when surgery is complete, and 0.1 mg/kg should be given between 10 PM and midnight. Some protocols utilize hydrocortisone. Those cats undergoing adrenocortical tumor removal will be predisposed to low cortisol concentrations because adrenocortical cells in the remaining gland will likely be atrophied. After bilateral adrenalectomy, no adrenal tissue remains.

The morning after surgery, an ACTHST should be completed. There should be an "Addisonian" result—both the basal and post-ACTHST cortisol concentration less than 2 μg/dL. If the result is as anticipated, surgery may have been a success. If results after surgery are similar to those obtained before, adrenal tissue or functioning metastatic sites remain.

After obtaining the ACTHST, begin giving 0.1 mg/kg of dexamethasone subcutaneous (SC), b.i.d. The switch to oral prednisolone replacement (Graham-Mize et al, 2004) should begin about 24 hours after the cat begins to eat without vomiting. Cats that had bilateral adrenalectomy are permanent Addisonians that will require glucocorticoid and mineralocorticoid replacement the remainder of their lives. They usually have their prednisolone replacement dose determined over a period of weeks to months. Those that had an adrenocortical tumor removed usually have their glucocorticoids tapered over a period of 2 to 4 months before discontinuing treatment.

After bilateral adrenalectomy, desoxycorticosterone pivalate (DOCP; Novartis, East Hanover, NJ) should be administered (2.2 mg/kg, IM). That dose should be repeated 21 to 25 days later, SC. Long-term dose and timing requirements should be individualized (see Chapter 12). It is not common for dogs or cats undergoing solitary adrenocortical tumor removal to need mineralocorticoid medication. If hyponatremia, hyperkalemia, or both are documented after surgery, DOCP should be given. ATH cats given DOCP, usually receive 50% of that dose when due in 25 days and then another 50% reduction is made for the final dose due at 50 days. From this time, it is quite uncommon for DOCP to be needed. During this entire period, monitoring serum electrolyte concentrations is important.

Serum renal parameters and electrolyte and glucose concentrations should continue to be assessed at the end of unilateral or bilateral adrenalectomy that evening, the next morning, and then daily until the cat is returned to the owner or until it is eating on its own without vomiting. The diabetes mellitus should be monitored and treated as if the cat were newly diagnosed, using conservative doses of insulin. The combination of resolved FCS, parenteral and then oral steroids, the stress of surgery and recovery, and a multitude of other factors make diabetes management challenging. Until the dose of oral glucocorticoids is discontinued in ATH cats or until the dose is stable after being tapered to that necessary for long-term health, insulin requirements are unpredictable.

Protocol: Surgery

If an obvious adrenal tumor is identified, it should be removed, especially if the opposite adrenal gland appears atrophied. If discrimination test results are definitive for PDH, both adrenal glands should be removed regardless of whether they appear normal or enlarged. If discrimination tests are not performed or inconclusive, the surgeon together with those managing the medical aspects should be prepared for intraoperative decisions. If the adrenals appear symmetrical in size and shape, they should be removed, whereas if one is obviously larger, that gland might be removed.

Protocol: Laparoscopy

Removal of adrenal masses via laparoscopy is becoming more common in veterinary practice (Smith et al, 2012). Mass size, location, presence of tumor thrombi, and invasion of local structures are all factors in deciding which animal is a candidate for this procedure as opposed to celiotomy. Laparoscopic adrenalectomy has the advantage of reducing perioperative complications.

Short-Term Complications

Complications are frequently encountered in cats undergoing surgery for FCS. Complications that are terminal or that lead a veterinarian to recommend euthanasia can be extremely disheartening to the owner and the entire veterinary team. Potential complications must be thoroughly explained to all decision makers before surgery. Some serious potential complications include sepsis, pancreatitis, thromboembolism, wound infection and/or dehiscence (surgical site or previous skin wounds due to fragility), and adrenocortical insufficiency (Duesberg et al, 1995). Sepsis is common because FCS predisposes to infection via immunosuppression and those with fragile skin can have seriously infected

wounds. Preoperative treatment with trilostane for a sufficient length of time to resolve as many FCS-related issues as possible should dramatically reduce complication rates.

Long-Term Complications, Including the Pituitary Macrotumor Syndrome

The consequences of a growing pituitary tumor are well described in dogs and information on cats is expanding. Questions exist regarding the effect of bilateral adrenalectomy or long-term inhibition of cortisol synthesis with drugs like trilostane on rate of pituitary tumor growth. Some believe that removal of cortisol negative feedback results in an increased rate of growth, a condition called *Nelson's syndrome* in people. Some believe that tumor growth rate is independent of physiologic influence. The possibility of enhanced pituitary tumor growth rate should be discussed with decision makers before surgery.

Experience

Experience with surgical management of FCS is limited and results have varied. Most cats survive surgery, and postsurgical complications are common. We have reviewed the experience of 21 cats that had PDH and bilateral adrenalectomy. These include 15 cats in our series and 6 cats from the literature (Watson and Herrtage, 1998 [4 cats]; Daley et al, 1993 [1 cat]; Moore et al, 2000a [1 cat]). Eight cats from our series have been reported (Duesberg et al, 1995). Thirteen of 21 cats survived surgery, had complete resolution of FCS, and lived for months or for more than 1 year (Daley et al, 1993; Watson and Herrtage, 1998; Moore et al, 2000). Five cats did not survive an appreciable period of time after surgery. One of the five died about 12 hours after surgery; no explanation was available. The second of five died from acute kidney failure 20 days after surgery (Watson and Herrtage, 1998). Two of the five cats died of sepsis within 1 month of surgery, both due to severely infected fragile skin. One of the five cats died of pulmonary thromboembolism about 3 weeks after surgery. Three additional cats from our series survived the surgery, had complete resolution of their FCS, but died within months of surgery. One died 4 months following surgery due to pancreatic carcinoma, and two died from apparent hypoadrenal crises 3 and 6 months after surgery, respectively.

Conclusions

Surgical resolution of FCS is difficult. Just the risk of exposing a cat with FCS to celiotomy is significant. Risk can be reduced with a combination of patient selection, preoperative trilostane therapy, minimal time for anesthesia and surgery, and thorough care after surgery. However, these remain older cats that often have serious problems involving other organ systems. Perhaps this is the reason that many cases of FCS are not treated. Bilateral adrenalectomy for PDH or tumor removal for ATH is an alternative to long-term oral trilostane therapy, hypophysectomy, or pituitary radiation.

PITUITARY RADIATION

Background

Ionizing radiation can be used in an attempt to destroy a benign or malignant tumor. This is a consultative discipline requiring a veterinary radiation oncologist and appropriate facilities. The objective of radiation therapy is tumor eradication with preservation of normal tissue structure and function (Theon, 2000). Facilities typically needed are a cobalt-60 photon irradiation unit or a linear accelerator photon unit. Treatment usually involves delivery of a predetermined total dose of radiation. Some protocols call for a large single dose, whereas others recommend smaller doses delivered in fractions over a period of several weeks. We are currently evaluating efficacy of a two-dose protocol, which still limits anesthesia, while possibly improving on disappointing experience with a single-dose approach.

Radiation therapy should always have potential benefit for the pet, even though outcome may not be entirely predictable. Because months may be required for effects of radiation therapy to be fully appreciated, many cats might benefit from prior trilostane control of FCS. Then, one can determine if the cat is a reasonable anesthesia risk. Trilostane should be continued for about 4 to 6 months after completion of radiation therapy. If a protocol calls for multiple treatment/anesthesia sessions, rapid anesthesia recovery is imperative. This provides cats with enough "conscious time" to eat prior to the obligatory cessation of food hours before the next scheduled anesthesia.

Experience

Radiation therapy has been used with partial success to treat a limited number of FCS cats with PDH (Peterson et al, 1994; Duesberg and Peterson, 1997; Feldman and Nelson, 2004; Mayer et al, 2006; Sellon et al, 2009). The most commonly noted benefit has been tumor shrinkage, prolonging survival in cats with large and/or invasive pituitary masses. Radiation offers a potential for cure, but resolution of FCS has only been reported in a minority of cats.

Our experience in treating PDH cats with pituitary radiation is limited to only seven cats with sufficient follow-up to determine response. Each had obvious clinical signs and five had insulin-resistant diabetes mellitus. Each cat had been evaluated either with a CT scan (3 cats) or an MRI scan (4 cats). Each of the seven cats had a visible pituitary mass (5 to 11 mm in greatest diameter). Four cats were treated with 15 fractions of radiation divided over a period of 3 weeks. One cat demonstrated no response and was euthanized 7 months after radiation because of continuing signs of diabetes mellitus and fragile skin. The two non-diabetic cats appeared to improve by losing weight, becoming more active, and demonstrating healthier skin. However, one of these two cats died of unknown reasons 3 months after completion of treatment, and the other died 14 months after completing radiation as a result of renal failure. The fourth and youngest cat (8 years old at the time of diagnosis) responded quite well to pituitary radiation with improvement in various parameters plus complete resolution of its diabetes mellitus. This cat has lived for 32 months. Each of three cats was treated with a single large dose of radiation. None of these cats had resolution of their FCS, and none had appreciable mass shrinkage. However, experience with seven cats is far too few to draw any conclusions. Pituitary radiation has potential to become a reasonable approach to management of PDH, but many more cats will need to be treated before opinions can be established.

PROGNOSIS

FCS is a serious condition that carries a guarded to grave prognosis. The deleterious effects of chronic hyperadrenocorticism on skin fragility, pancreatic endocrine function (diabetes mellitus), and the immune system are frequently responsible for morbidity and death of both treated as well as untreated cats. Treatment can be expensive, emotional (to the owner), and stressful (to the cat) without guarantee of success. Medical therapy with trilostane has great promise. Abdominal surgery has not been routinely successful because of the debilitated condition of most cats with FCS. This problem should be less of a concern if cats can be treated

with trilostane to resolve FCS before surgery. Pituitary radiation is limited by facilities required, expense, and the multiple anesthetic procedures that are part of some protocols. Hypophysectomy is limited by the few veterinarians who have this expertise. Again, there are the problems of expense and patient debilitation. Experience with "successful" therapies (adrenalectomy [unilateral or bilateral], radiation, hypophysectomy) has resulted in less than 50% of cats surviving well beyond 1 year. Remember, most cats that have FCS are not treated. Most of the treated cats are those considered most stable. Therefore, 50% survival at 1 year (an optimistic number) does not include those cats never treated. Also, as success improves in treating FCS, the incidence and severity of large pituitary tumors (macrotumor syndrome) is likely to increase.

PRIMARY HYPERALDOSTERONISM IN CATS

Background

The hormone aldosterone regulates both circulating concentrations of sodium and potassium and intravascular fluid volume homeostasis. It is the principle mineralocorticoid synthesized and secreted by the zona glomerulosa, the outermost zone of adrenal cortices, whose cells lack the capacity to synthesize cortisol. Increases in serum potassium directly stimulate release of aldosterone. Decreases in blood pressure, primarily sensed within the kidneys, stimulates synthesis and release of renin which, in turn, stimulates the angiotensins to stimulate secretion of aldosterone. After synthesis and secretion, aldosterone acts on the distal nephron to promote sodium reabsorption and excretion of potassium and hydrogen ions. In conserving sodium, aldosterone indirectly conserves water, raising blood volume and, in turn, blood pressure. Aldosterone directly increases blood pressure via enhancement of total peripheral resistance. This hormone is also synthesized in tissues within the heart, brain, and vasculature where it is thought to have paracrine or autocrine action (Djajadiningrat-Laanen et al, 2011).

Excess production of aldosterone can be primary or secondary. *Primary hyperaldosteronism (PHA)* is defined as the "autonomous secretion of the hormone by abnormal cells within the adrenal cortex." PHA is characterized by circulating aldosterone excess and renin suppression. For several decades after this condition was described by Conn (1955) it was considered rare. With better understanding, it is now thought to occur in about 6% of all people with arterial hypertension and about 11% of people with therapy-resistant hypertension (Fogari et al, 2007; Douma et al, 2008). Approximately two thirds of people with PHA have bilateral hyperplasia of the zona glomerulosa in whom plasma renin activity may be incompletely suppressed. About one-third of people with PHA have a solitary adenoma in which plasma renin activity is completely suppressed. Unilateral hyperplasia and aldosterone-producing carcinomas are uncommon-to-rare (White, 1994; Young, 2007). Afflicted patients typically have no abnormalities in cortisol production, plasma cortisol concentrations, or in cortisol metabolism. *Secondary hyperaldosteronism* is the result of a condition (e.g., heart failure and CKD) that stimulates renin secretion to begin the cascade of enzyme activity resulting in aldosterone synthesis and secretion. Thus, secondary hyperaldosteronism is associated with enhanced renin concentrations.

Sodium retention, associated with primary or secondary aldosteronism, increases extracellular fluid volume and blood pressure (hypertension). Despite increases in total body sodium content, serum sodium concentrations are usually normal. In cats, because glucocorticoids, estrogens, and progestagens are primarily excreted via bile into the intestines, it is likely that there are similar excretory pathways for aldosterone.

PHA has been described rather commonly in cats. Underdiagnosis, which seems likely, may be traced to the concept that progression of CKD can lead to hypertension, hypokalemia, or both. However, it appears that CKD may also be the result of PHA. Regardless, PHA may cause hypertension, hypokalemia, or both (Javadi et al, 2005; Djajadiningrat-Laanen et al, 2011). Hypertension and hypokalemia in cats with CKD are often treated symptomatically without further investigation of cause.

Etiology

Adrenocortical Neoplasia

Classically, PHA in cats is caused by a unilateral solitary adrenocortical adenoma or carcinoma. The incidence of malignant tumors (19 reported cases) exceeds that of solitary benign adenomas (11 reported cases). Feline PHA was first reported in 1983 by Eger and colleagues. In the past 15 years, cats with PHA have been reported more commonly (Flood et al, 1999; MacKay et al, 1999; Maggio et al, 2000; Moore et al, 2000b; Rijnberk et al, 2001; Reimer et al, 2005; Ash et al, 2005; DeClue et al, 2005; Rose et al, 2007; Briscoe et al, 2009; Renschler and Dean, 2009; Djajadiningrat-Laanen et al, 2011; 2013; Lo et al, 2014). Bilateral adrenal adenomas were identified in two cats. One cat with PHA also had an insulin secreting pancreatic tumor and a parathyroid hormone secreting adenoma. Some cats with PHA have had concurrent progestagen excess (DeClue et al, 2005; Briscoe et al, 2009), possibly due to enhanced production of intermediary products (Harvey and Refsal, 2012).

Adrenocortical Hyperplasia

Non–tumor-related PHA has been described in 13 cats (Javadi et al, 2005; Djajadiningrat-Laanen et al, 2013). Afflicted cats, at necropsy, were demonstrated to have bilateral adrenocortical hyperplasia, and most had evidence of CKD. Some cats had zona glomerulosa nodular hyperplasia, renal arteriolar sclerosis, glomerular sclerosis, tubular atrophy, and interstitial fibrosis (Javadi et al, 2005; Harvey and Refsal, 2012).

Clinical Features and In-Hospital Testing

Signalment and Signs

There does not appear to be a breed predisposition among cats diagnosed with PHA. The mean age at diagnosis is about 12 to 13 years and most are more than 10 years of age. Both genders have been represented, and most have been neutered. The most common clinical sign has been persistent and progressive weakness associated with hypokalemia, called *hypokalemic polymyopathy* (Harvey and Refsal, 2012). Usually seen at serum potassium concentrations less than 3 mg/dL, the most common owner observations have included cervical ventriflexion, hind limb weakness (sometimes plantigrade), difficulty jumping, listlessness, and ataxia. A few cats have had limb rigidity, dysphagia, or collapse. Some cats had episodic signs and a few had signs that were sudden in onset. Weakness was less worrisome in cats with adrenal hyperplasia (Javadi et al, 2005).

The second most common owner-perceived concern in cats with PHA has been associated with hypertension. Some hypertensive cats have had acute blindness and/or sudden change in eye color, usually due to intraocular hemorrhage or retinal detachments. Ocular signs are not as common in cats with adrenal tumors as they are in those with adrenal hyperplasia.

PU/PD have been described in less than 20% of cats with PHA. PU/PD may be due to a concurrent condition (e.g., diabetes mellitus, and/or CKD). Alternatively, hypokalemia can cause acquired and reversible nephrogenic diabetes insipidus (Harvey and Refsal, 2012). Systemic hypertension and hypokalemia have been associated with progressive loss of kidney function (Djajadiningrat-Laanen et al, 2013). About 20% of PHA cats have had decreases in appetite, about 10% have polyphagia, and a few have had worrisome weight loss. Other signs may be related to the insulin antagonistic effects of progestagen excess that also is seen in some cats with PHA.

Physical examination findings are usually related to hypokalemia or to hypertension. Hypertensive ocular signs include retinal detachment, hemorrhage, tortuous retinal vessels, and retinal edema. Weakness due to hypokalemia is consistent with owner observations. Some cats have had muscle atrophy, heart murmur, arrhythmias, palpable adrenal masses (three cats), and fragile skin (Djajadiningrat-Laanen et al, 2011).

In-Hospital Routine Testing

The one abnormality on laboratory testing typical for PHA is hypokalemia, documented in 42 of 50 cats with an adrenal tumor. Several of the remaining eight cats had serum potassium concentrations that were low-normal. Only a few differential diagnoses for low potassium are considered "common": CKD, diabetic ketoacidosis (the condition itself, under supplemented IV fluids, insulin, and bicarbonate all predispose to hypokalemia), acute gastrointestinal disease (vomiting, diarrhea, anorexia), and PHA. By contrast, about half of cats with adrenal hyperplasia have had normal serum potassium concentrations and the others have had mild hypokalemia (Javadi et al, 2005). Volume expansion due to sodium retention is "classic" for PHA, but serum sodium concentrations are usually within the reference range. About 85% of PHA cats are persistently hypertensive.

A number of cats described as having PHA secondary to adrenal hyperplasia have had CKD with abnormal increases in serum urea and creatinine concentrations. The combination of CKD and hypertension would tend to steer clinicians away from a separate investigation of the hypertension. Cats with adrenal tumors usually do not have evidence of CKD. Progressive renal damage associated with aldosterone excess has been implicated in some people due to a combination of increased intraglomerular capillary pressure, inflammation, and fibrosis. This may be associated with excesses in angiotensin II and the chronic hypokalemia of CKD. Hyperglycemia is not common, nor are abnormalities in serum phosphate.

Abdominal ultrasonography is a valuable diagnostic aid when assessing unexplained hypertension. Ultrasonography provides information regarding renal and adrenal anatomy, especially when searching for an adrenal nodule. Cats with an adrenocortical tumor evaluated with ultrasonography typically have had a 1 to 5 cm diameter adrenal mass (Harvey and Refsal, 2012). The contralateral adrenal is usually considered small. Bilateral adrenal tumors are not common (Quante et al, 2009). Adrenal masses that extend into or invade the vena cava or other vessels are called *tumor thrombi*. The liver, retroperitoneum, and other areas should be evaluated for evidence of metastases or unsuspected abnormalities. Abdominal CT or MRI examinations correctly detected a mass or hyperplasia in 32 of 38 cats with confirmed PHA (Flood et al, 1999; MacKay et al, 1999; Rijnberk et al, 2001; Ash et al, 2005; DeClue et al, 2005; Javadi et al, 2005; Rose et al, 2007; Renschler and Dean, 2009; Djajadiningrat-Laanen et al, 2013; Lo et al, 2014). Cats with non-tumor PHA do not have abnormal adrenals other than a few with subtle increases in adrenal echogenicity.

Confirming a Diagnosis: Plasma Aldosterone Concentrations and Abdominal Imaging

PHA should be strongly considered in any cat with an adrenal nodule identified on ultrasonography and unexplained hypokalemia or hypertension. The condition should also be suspected in hypertensive cats' refractory to therapy. Randomly obtained plasma aldosterone concentrations (PACs) have been above the reference range in 43 of 50 cats with a solitary adrenal mass (Djajadiningrat-Laanen et al, 2011; Lo et al, 2014). In this scenario, PHA is the most likely diagnosis, and a recommendation of surgery is supported. Aldosterone assays are widely available through commercial veterinary laboratories. Sample collection requirements are routine (Harvey and Refsal, 2012). Extremely high PACs have been reported in cats with PHA and in cats with CKD (Yu and Morris, 1998).

Diagnostic imaging with ultrasonography, MRI, and CT has been utilized to identify adrenal abnormalities, to evaluate for vascular invasion, and to attempt visualization of local or distant metastases. Absence of vascular invasion seen on imaging is not a guarantee that it does not exist. Although logic suggests that some adrenal masses may be too small to be detected, most have been easily visualized. Visualizing an adrenal mass does not indicate its function. In a study on people, 38% of CT/MRI scans did not accurately identify the source of aldosterone excess (Kempers et al, 2009). Thus, while extremely helpful, imaging is not a perfect screening test for PHA (Djajadiningrat-Laanen et al, 2011). Use of positron emission tomography (PET) or single photon emission computed tomography (SPECT) may prove valuable but have not yet been assessed.

Confirming a Diagnosis: Ratio of Urine Aldosterone to Creatinine

The urine aldosterone-to-creatinine ratio (UA:CR) theoretically provides a reflection of aldosterone concentrations over time. This test is not widely available. It has the advantages of urine not needing to be immediately frozen, and urine is easily collected. The UA:CR is often abnormal in cats with PHA, but sensitivity was less than with the random serum aldosterone assessment. The reference interval of the UA:CR is large and did not facilitate differentiation between healthy cats and those with PHA (Djajadiningrat-Laanen et al, 2008). A cat whose PAC is lower than anticipated may be in the early stages of this condition or may have simple minute-to-minute serum fluctuations.

Confirming a Diagnosis: Plasma Aldosterone and Renin Concentrations

Ideally, circulating aldosterone concentrations should be co-assessed with the renin concentration. Individuals with PHA (tumor) should have increases in plasma aldosterone and decreases in plasma renin concentrations, whereas both would be increased in CKD. The aldosterone-to-renin ratio (ARR) has been utilized to improve sensitivity and specificity, but reliable renin assays are not yet widely available, those results reported in PHA cats have been variable and not highly specific (Harvey and Refsal, 2012). In cats with adrenal tumors, the ARR can be quite increased, but in cats with idiopathic bilateral nodular hyperplasia, the ARR may be less impressive. Although the ARR is the gold standard for PHA screening, disadvantages of this test include the necessity for large blood samples, plasma must be instantly frozen, renin values may vary among laboratories, and repeat testing may be required because an unremarkable result does not rule out PHA (Javadi et al, 2004; 2005; Djajadiningrat-Laanen et al, 2011)

Provocative Mineralocorticoid Function Testing

The combination of owner-observed weakness, hypokalemia documented on routine blood chemistry, an adrenal nodule visualized on ultrasonography, and an increased randomly obtained circulating aldosterone concentration have proven quite sensitive and specific for diagnosing PHA. It is assumed that cats early in the course of their disease and those with a mild condition may not have all these abnormalities. Assessing aldosterone concentrations before and after ACTHST has not improved sensitivity and is not recommended. However, cats with PHA have been reported to have normal-to-low baseline serum cortisol concentrations with subnormal cortisol responses to ACTH (DeClue et al, 2011; Harvey and Refsal, 2012; Eiler et al, 2013). Excesses in aldosterone, its precursors, or other adrenocortical products may suppress endogenous ACTH synthesis and secretion sufficiently to account for the apparent decreases in cortisol. If true, this may help explain the poor appetite observed in some PHA cats.

Fludrocortisone (a synthetic mineralocorticoid described in Chapter 12) promotes sodium retention, water retention, and an increase in blood volume. In cats with a healthy renin-angiotensin-aldosterone system, fludrocortisone administration should suppress renin and aldosterone concentrations. Cats with PHA should be refractory to this effect. In studies of 23 healthy and one PHA cat, fludrocortisone given for 4 days at a dose of 0.05 mg/kg b.i.d. caused significant decreases in the healthy cats' UA:CR but not so for the cat with PHA (Djajadiningrat-Laanen et al, 2008; 2011; Matsuda et al, 2013). In a subsequent study of nine PHA cats and 10 non-PHA cats that were hypertensive and/or hypokalemic, results were not as sensitive as simply measuring the serum aldosterone concentration. PACs were abnormal in all PHA cats, whereas results were within or near the limit of the reference range in the non-PHA cats (Djajadiningrat-Laanen et al, 2013). Guidelines for provocative testing in people include assuring that serum potassium concentrations are normal before testing. Also, before testing, discontinuation of most medications for 2 to 4 weeks is recommended. Use of provocative testing may prove valuable as additional studies are completed. At this time, our recommended approach to a cat that may have PHA is to assess each adrenal via ultrasonography and to measure PAC if a nodule or mass is identified or suspected.

Treatment

Removal of an adrenal tumor is the treatment of choice for cats with PHA (Rose et al, 2007). Such masses can be removed via celiotomy or laparoscopy. Assessing each cat for tumor thrombi and for metastases is imperative before considering surgery. Preoperatively, hypokalemia should be treated with oral and/or parenteral potassium. After surgery, a high sodium diet has been recommended, although most PHA cats have not been so-treated (Djajadiningrat-Laanen et al, 2011). Temporary administration of oral fludrocortisone acetate or injectable DOCP could be administered post-surgically to manage hypoaldosteronism, but this has not usually been necessary (Lo et al, 2014). Perioperative complications have included hemorrhage, lethargy, anemia, anorexia, vomiting, dysphagia, hyperthermia, upper respiratory infection, and acute kidney failure (Djajadiningrat-Laanen et al, 2011; Lo et al, 2014). Hemorrhage was not predicted by tumor type, location, size, or vascular invasion. The cats that have survived the perioperative period have generally normalized and have an excellent long-term prognosis.

Cats with an unresectable mass, metastases, owners who choose not to have surgery on their cat, and cats with adrenal hyperplasia are managed medically via potassium supplementation and control of the hypertension. Spironolactone is the aldosterone receptor blocker most often employed at a dose of 2 mg/kg of body weight orally b.i.d. to help control the hypokalemia. Doses in excess of 4 mg/kg have been associated with anorexia, vomiting, and diarrhea. Hypertension may be treated with dihydropyridine calcium channel antagonists (e.g., amlodipine) either alone or in combination with a beta-adrenergic blocker or an angiotension-converting enzyme inhibitor (Brown et al, 2007). Cats with bilateral adrenal hyperplasia have more mild increases in PAC and can be maintained on medical therapy for extended time periods, but their prognosis is far more guarded (Djajadiningrat-Laanen et al, 2011; Harvey and Refsal, 2012; Lo et al, 2014).

EXCESSIVE SEX HORMONE–SECRETING ADRENAL TUMORS IN CATS

Background

Adrenocortical tumors have the potential for synthesizing and secreting a variety of steroid products other than cortisol and aldosterone. This physiologic process may be associated with neoplasia-related aberrant biosynthetic pathways and/or enzyme deficiencies. Specific precursors may accumulate due to one of these biosynthetic pathway blockages that would enhance alternative biochemical pathways to be followed, with synthesis of alternate products. Androgen, estrogen, and progestagen-secreting adrenocortical tumors have been diagnosed in people, dogs, and cats. Natural progesterone has a half-life in the blood of only a few minutes and serves as a precursor for androgens, estrogens, mineralocorticoids, and glucocorticoids in many mammals. Progesterone binds to albumin as well as cortisol-binding and sex-hormone-binding proteins. Theoretically, chronic excesses in progesterone results in excess "free" cortisol via their ability to competitively bind to cortisol-binding proteins in the circulation, simulating the actions of glucocorticoids. These physiologic processes, including insulin resistance, have been demonstrated in people, dogs, and cats (Selman et al, 1994; 1996; Syme et al, 2001). It has been suggested that adrenal tumors that synthesize steroids other than cortisol are usually carcinomas (Melian, 2012).

Clinical Features

Signalment and Signs

A relatively limited number of cats with increased secretion of progestagens or other sex hormones from adrenal gland tumors has been described (Boord and Griffin, 1999; Rossmeisl et al, 2000; Boag et al, 2004; DeClue et al, 2005; Millard et al, 2009; Blois et al, 2010; Meler et al, 2011). Some cats have had excesses in progestagens with typical signs of FCS. A few cats have had increased androgen concentrations (Rossmeisl et al, 2000; Boag et al, 2004; Millard et al, 2009). A cat with androgen excess may have facial enlargement, typical male territorial urine spraying behavior, produce urine with an unusually strong odor, and act aggressively. A castrated male cat developed penile spines (Millard et al, 2009).

Cats with excess progestagens are most likely to have clinical signs of FCS. To summarize, owners may be concerned about nonpruritic, progressive, symmetric alopecia; greasy and unkempt hair; or thin, easily bruised, fragile skin (see Fig. 11-3). Some owners may be concerned about their cat's diabetes mellitus or be frustrated with the difficulty in controlling the diabetes. Other owners have observed weakness, sudden blindness or changes in eye color (hypertension), polyphagia, unusual behavior, PU/PD, or abdominal distension.

In-Hospital Testing

The veterinarian, when learning any of these owner concerns or in attempting to treat a cat for diabetes or hypertension, for example, will attempt to find an explanation by conducting a logical, practical, and cost effective approach. This often begins with "routine" blood and urine testing. Other than persistent hyperglycemia and glycosuria in some cats, CBC or serum biochemistry abnormalities are not common in cats with sex-hormone-secreting adrenocortical tumors. Imaging studies are the next tests utilized. Thoracic radiographs as a health screen usually follow abdominal ultrasound. Ultrasound is preferred over radiographs because the concerns established for these cats involve potential pancreatic or adrenal abnormalities. Ultrasound is superior in evaluating these structures. Virtually every cat diagnosed with an adrenocortical tumor has had an adrenal mass visualized on abdominal ultrasonography. Once such a mass is identified, the logical next step is to rule out metastatic disease. The ultrasound examination should have included thorough evaluation of the area around the suspected mass for vascular or tissue invasion and the liver for possible spread. The lungs should be screened as well via radiographs. This allows thorough evaluation of the thorax for suspected or unsuspected issues. Assuming that an owner wishes to proceed and, ideally, if no evidence of metastasis is seen, hormone testing should be considered.

Most cats with a progestagen or androgen producing adrenal tumor have had low-normal or low basal and post-ACTHST plasma cortisol concentrations. Similar results have been noted for LDDST and UC:CR. Thus, if a cat appears to have FCS but does not have the expected abnormalities on screening test results, consideration of a sex hormone disorder is reasonable. Hormone concentrations that may be increased include 17α-hydroxyprogesterone, progesterone, estradiol, testosterone, and/or androstenedione (Melian, 2012). Most cats with a sex-hormone secreting adrenocortical tumor have had excessive basal concentrations of the hormone. Thus, for these adrenal tumors, basal hormone evaluations appear indicative of the underlying physiologic abnormalities. This should negate need for ACTHST. However, the test is recommended to further substantiate one of these unusual diagnoses (Millard et al, 2009; Melian, 2012).

Treatment and Prognosis

Surgical or laparoscopic removal of an adrenocortical tumor is the treatment of choice. Readers are encouraged to review that section earlier in the chapter regarding perioperative and long-term care. Whenever a cat has clinical evidence of FCS, preoperative treatment with trilostane may reduce morbidity and mortality. Readers are encouraged to review the sections on trilostane earlier in this chapter. Prognosis depends on presence of metastasis, successful removal of the tumor, how stable the cat is prior to treatment, and a myriad of other factors.

One male cat in our series was treated with aminoglutethimide (AGT; a drug we no longer recommend) for about 6 weeks in preparation for surgery. The cat did clinically improve dramatically with resolution of its thin fragile skin and diabetes mellitus. As the cat improved, it also developed dramatic mammary gland enlargement likely due to rapid decrease in plasma progesterone concentrations that stimulated, in turn, synthesis and secretion of prolactin. After AGT was discontinued, our surgeons were able to successfully remove the adrenal tumor. Successful surgery has also been reported in several other cats (Boord and Griffin, 1999).

REFERENCES

Ash RA, et al.: Primary hyperaldosteronism in the cat: a series of 13 cases, *J Feline Med Surg* 7:173, 2005.

Barthez PY, et al.: Ultrasonographic evaluation of the adrenal glands in dogs, *J Am Vet Med Assoc* 207:1180, 1995.

Benchekroun G, et al.: Plasma ACTH precursors in cats with pituitary-dependent hyperadrenocorticism, *J Vet Intern Med* 26:575, 2012.

Blois SL, et al.: Multiple endocrine diseases in cats: 15 cases (1997-2008), *J Feline Med Surg* 12:637, 2010.

Boag AK, et al.: Trilostane treatment of bilateral adrenal enlargement and excessive sex hormone production in a cat, *J Small Anim Pract* 45:263, 2004.

Boord M, Griffin C: Progesterone secreting adrenal mass in a cat with clinical signs of hyperadrenocorticism, *J Am Vet Med Assoc* 214:666, 1999.

Brightman AH: Ophthalmic use of glucocorticoids, *Vet Clin North Am Small Anim Pract* 12:33, 1982.

Briscoe K, et al.: Hyperaldosteronism and hyperprogesteronism in a cat, *J Feline Med Surg* 11:758, 2009.

Brown S, et al.: Guidelines for the identification, evaluation, and management of systemic hypertension in dogs and cats, *J Vet Intern Med* 21:542, 2007.

Cartee RE, Finn-Bodner ST: Ultrasound examination of the feline adrenal gland, *J Med Sonography* 9:327, 1993.

Chakere DW, et al.: Magnetic resonance imaging of pituitary and parasellar abnormalities, *Radio Clin North Am* 27:265, 1989.

Coates PJ, et al.: The distribution of immunoreactive-melanocyte-stimulating hormone cells in the adult human pituitary gland, *J Endocrinol* 111:335, 1986.

Conn JW: Primary hyperaldosteronism: a new clinical syndrome, *J Lab Clin Med* 45:3, 1955.

Corradini PA, et al.: Evaluation of hair cortisol in the diagnosis of hypercortisolism in dogs, *J Vet Intern Med* 27:1268, 2013.

Daley CA, et al.: Use of metyrapone to treat pituitary-dependent hyperadrenocorticism in a cat with large cutaneous wounds, *J Am Vet Med Assoc* 202:956, 1993.

DeClue AE, et al.: Hyperaldosteronism and hyperprogesteronism in a cat with an adrenal cortical carcinoma, *J Vet Intern Med* 19:355, 2005.

DeClue AE, et al.: Cortisol and aldosterone response to various doses of cosyntropin in healthy cats, *J Am Vet Med Assoc* 238:176, 2011.

de Lange MS, et al.: High urinary corticoid/creatinine ratios in cats with hyperthyroidism, *J Vet Intern Med* 18:152, 2004.

Djajadiningrat-Laanen SC, et al.: Urinary aldosterone to creatinine ratio in cats before and after suppression with salt or fludrocortisone acetate, *J Vet Intern Med* 22:1283, 2008.

Djajadiningrat-Laanen SC, et al.: Primary hyperaldosteronism: expanding the diagnostic net, *J Feline Med Surg* 13:641, 2011.

Djajadiningrat-Laanen SC, et al.: Evaluation of the oral fludrocortisone suppression test for diagnosing primary hyperaldosteronism in cats, *J Vet Intern Med* 27:1493, 2013.

Douma S, et al.: Prevalence of primary hyperaldosteronism in resistant hypertension: a retrospective observational study, *Lancet* 371:1921, 2008.

Duesberg CA, et al.: Adrenalectomy for treatment of hyperadrenocorticism in cats: 10 cases (1988-1992), *J Am Vet Med Assoc* 207:1066, 1995.

Duesberg CA, Peterson ME: Adrenal disorders in cats, *Vet Clin North Am Small Anim Pract* 27:321, 1997.

Eger CE, et al.: Primary aldosteronism (Conn's syndrome) in a cat: a case report and review of comparative aspects, *J Small Anim Pract* 24:293, 1983.

Eiler KC, et al.: Comparison of intravenous versus intramuscular administration of corticotropin-releasing hormone in healthy cats, *J Vet Intern Med* 27:516, 2013.

Engelhardt D, et al.: The influence of ketoconazole on human adrenal steroidogenesis: incubation studies with tissue slices, *Clin Endocrinol* 35:163, 1991.

Feelders RA, et al.: Medical treatment of Cushing's syndrome: adrenal-blocking drugs and ketoconazole, *Neuroendocrinology* 92(Suppl 1):111, 2010.

Feldman EC: The effect of functional adrenocortical tumors on plasma cortisol and corticotropin concentrations in dogs, *J Am Vet Med Assoc* 178:823, 1981.

Feldman EC, Nelson RW: Hyperadrenocorticism in cats (Cushing's syndrome). In Feldman EC, Nelson RW, editors: *Canine and feline endocrinology and reproduction*, ed 3, Philadelphia, 2004, Elsevier/Saunders, p 358.

Ferasin L: Iatrogenic hyperadrenocorticism in a cat following a short therapeutic course of methylprednisolone acetate, *J Feline Med Surg* 3:87, 2001.

Flood SM, et al.: Primary hyperaldosteronism in two cats, *J Am Anim Hosp Assoc* 35:411, 1999.

Fogari R, et al.: Prevalence of primary hyperaldosteronism among unselected hypertensive patients: a prospective study based on the use of an aldosterone/renin ratio above 25 as a screening test, *Hypertens Res* 30:111, 2007.

Goossens MMC, et al.: Urinary excretion of glucocorticoids in the diagnosis of hyperadrenocorticism in cats, *Domestic Anim Endocrinol* 12:355, 1995.

Graham-Mize CA, et al.: Absorption, bioavailability and activity of prednisone and prednisolone in cats. In Hillier A, Foster AP, Kwochka KW, editors: *Advances in veterinary dermatology*, vol 5. Vienna, 2004, Blackwell Publishing, p 152.

Graves TK: Hypercortisolism in cats (feline Cushing's syndrome). In Ettinger SJ, Feldman EC, editors: *Textbook of veterinary internal medicine*, ed 7, St Louis, 2010, Saunders/Elsevier, p 1840.

Green CE, et al.: Iatrogenic hyperadrenocorticism in a cat, *Feline Pract* 23:7, 1995.

Gunn-Moore D: Feline endocrinopathies, *Vet Clin Small Anim* 35:171, 2005.

Halmi NS, Krieger D: Immunocytochemistry of ACTH-related peptides in the hypophysis. In Bhatnagar AS, editor: *The anterior pituitary gland*, New York, 1983, Raven Press, pp 1–15.

Harvey AM, Refsal KR: Feline hyperaldosteronism. In Mooney CT, Peterson ME, editors: *Manual of small animal endocrinology*, ed 4, Cheltenham, 2012, British Small Animal Veterinary Association, p 204.

Henry CJ, et al.: Urine cortisol:creatinine ratio in healthy and sick cats, *J Vet Int Med* 10:123, 1996.

Hoenig M: Feline hyperadrenocorticism—where are we now? *J Feline Med Surg* 4:171, 2002.

Horauf A, Reusch C: Darstellung der nebennieren mittels ultraschall: untersuchungen bei gesunden hunden, hunden mit nicht endokrinen Erkrankungen sowie mit Cushing-Syndrom, *Kleintierpraxis* 40:337, 1995.

Immink WF, et al.: Hyperadrenocorticism in four cats, *Vet Q* 14:81, 1992.

Javadi S, et al.: Plasma renin activity and plasma concentrations of aldosterone, cortisol, adrenocorticotropic hormone, and alpha-melanocyte-stimulating hormone in healthy cats, *J Vet Intern Med* 18:625, 2004.

Javadi S, et al.: Primary hyperaldosteronism, a mediator of progressive renal disease in cats, *Domest Anim Endocrinol* 28:85, 2005.

Kaufman B: Magnetic resonance imaging of the pituitary gland, *Radio Clin North Am* 22:795, 1984.

Kempers MF, et al.: Systematic review: diagnostic procedures to differentiate unilateral from bilateral adrenal abnormality in primary aldosteronism, *Ann Intern Med* 151:329, 2009.

Kley S, et al.: Evaluation of the low-dose dexamethasone suppression test and ultrasonographic measurements of the adrenal glands in cats with diabetes mellitus, *Schweizer Archiv fur Tierheilkunde* 149:493, 2007.

Lien Y, et al.: Iatrogenic hyperadrenocorticism in 12 cats, *J Am Anim Hosp Assoc* 42:414, 2006.

Lo AJ, et al.: Treatment of aldosterone-secreting adrenocortical tumors in cats by unilateral adrenalectomy: 10 cases (2002-2012), *J Vet Int Med* 28:137, 2014.

Low MJ, et al.: Post-translational processing of pro-opiomelanocortin (POMC) in mouse pituitary melanotroph tumors induced by a POMC-Simian virus 40 large T antigen transgene, *J Biol Chem* 268:24967, 1993.

Lowe AD, et al.: A comparison of the diabetogenic effects of dexamethasone and prednisolone in cats, Twenty-second Proceedings of the North American Veterinary Dermatology Forum, *Kauai* 178, 2007.

Lowe AD, et al.: Clinical, clinicopathological and histological changes observed in 14 cats treated with glucocorticoids, *Vet Rec* 162:777, 2008.

MacKay AD, et al.: Successful surgical treatment of a cat with primary aldosteronism, *J Feline Med Surg* 1:117, 1999.

Maggio F, et al.: Ocular lesions associated with systemic hypertension in cats: 69 cases (1985-1998), *J Am Vet Med Assoc* 217:695, 2000.

Matsuda, et al.: Suppression of serum aldosterone following oral administration of fludrocortisone acetate in healthy cats (abstract), *J Vet Intern Med* 27:687, 2013.

Mayer NM, et al.: Outcomes of pituitary tumor irradiation in cats, *J Vet Intern Med* 20:1151, 2006.

Meij BP, et al.: Transsphenoidal hypophysectomy in beagle dogs: evaluation of a microsurgical technique, *Vet Surg* 26:295, 1997.

Meij BP, et al.: Transsphenoidal hypophysectomy for treatment of pituitary-dependent hyperadrenocorticism in 7 cats, *Vet Surg* 30:72, 2001.

Meijer JC, et al.: Cushing's syndrome due to adrenocortical adenoma in a cat, *Tijdschr Diergeneesk* 103:1048, 1978.

Melby JC: Therapy of Cushing's disease: a consensus for pituitary microsurgery, *Ann Int Med* 109:445, 1988.

Meler EN, et al.: Cyclic estrous-like behavior in a spayed cat associated with excessive sex-hormone production by an adrenocortical carcinoma, *J Feline Med Surg* 13:473, 2011.

Melian C: Investigation of adrenal masses. In Mooney CT, Peterson ME, editors: *BSAVA manual of canine and feline endocrinology*, ed 4, Gloucester, 2012, British Small Animal Veterinary Association, p 272.

Mellett Keith AM, et al.: Trilostane therapy for treatment of spontaneous hyperadrenocorticism in cats: 15 cases (2004-2012), *J Vet Intern Med* 27:1471, 2013.

Millard RP, et al.: Excessive production of sex hormones in a cat with an adrenocortical tumor, *J Am Vet Med Assoc* 234:505, 2009.

Molitch ME: Anterior Pituitary. In Goldman L, Schafer AI, editors: *Goldman's Cecil medicine*, ed 24, Philadelphia, 2012, Elsevier/Saunders, p 1431.

Moon PF: Cortisol suppression in cats after induction of anesthesia with etomidate, compared with ketamine-diazepam combination, *Am J Vet Res* 58:868, 1997.

Moore LE, et al.: Hyperadrenocorticism treated with metyrapone followed by bilateral adrenalectomy in a cat, *J Am Vet Med Assoc* 217:691, 2000a.

Moore LE, et al.: Use of abdominal ultrasonography in the diagnosis of primary hyperaldosteronism in a cat, *J Am Vet Med Assoc* 217:213, 2000b.

Neiger R, et al.: Trilostane therapy for treatment of pituitary-dependent hyperadrenocorticism in 5 cats, *J Vet Intern Med* 18:160, 2004.

Nelson RW, et al.: Hyperadrenocorticism in cats: seven cases (1978-1987), *J Am Vet Med Assoc* 193:245, 1988.

Nieman LK: Adrenal cortex. In Goldman L, Schafer AI, editors: *Goldman's Cecil medicine*, ed 24, Philadelphia, 2012, Elsevier/Saunders, p 1463.

Orth DN: Metyrapone is useful only as adjunctive therapy in Cushing's disease, *Ann Intern Med* 89:128, 1978.

Peterson ME: Endocrine disorders in cats: four emerging diseases, *Compend Contin Educ Pract Vet* 10:1353, 1988.

Peterson ME: Feline hyperadrenocorticism. In Torrance AG, Mooney CT, editors: *Manual of small animal endocrinology*, ed 2, Cheltenham, 1998, British Small Animal Veterinary Association, p 215.

Peterson ME: Feline hyperadrenocorticism. In Mooney CT, Peterson ME, editors: *Manual of small animal endocrinology*, ed 4, Cheltenham, 2012, British Small Animal Veterinary Association, p 190.

Peterson ME, Graves TK: Effects of low dosages of intravenous dexamethasone on serum cortisol concentrations in the normal cat, *Res Vet Sci* 44:38, 1988.

Peterson ME, Kemppainen RJ: Comparison of intravenous and intramuscular routes for administering cosyntropin for corticotropin stimulation testing in cats, *Am J Vet Res* 53:1392, 1992a.

Peterson ME, Kemppainen RJ: Comparison of the immunoreactive plasma corticotropin and cortisol responses to two synthetic corticotropin preparations (tetracosactrin and cosyntropin) in healthy cats, *Am J Vet Res* 53:1752, 1992b.

Peterson ME, Kemppainen RJ: Dose response relation between plasma concentrations of corticotropin and cortisol after administration of incremental doses cosyntropin for corticotropin stimulation testing in cats, *Am J Vet Res* 54:300, 1993.

Peterson ME, Steele P: Pituitary-dependent hyperadrenocorticism in a cat, *J Am Vet Med Assoc* 189:680, 1986.

Peterson ME, et al.: Immunocytochemical study of the hypophysis in 25 dogs with pituitary-dependent hyperadrenocorticism, *Acta Endocrinol (Copenh)* 101:15, 1982.

Peterson ME, et al.: Endocrine diseases. In Sherding RG, editors: *The cat: diagnosis and clinical management*, ed 2, New York, 1994, Churchill Livingstone, pp 1404.

Quante S, et al.: Hyperprogesteronism due to bilateral adrenal carcinomas in a cat with diabetes mellitus, *Schweizer Archiv fur Tierheilkunde* 151:437, 2009.

Reaves TA Jr, et al.: Vasopressin release by nicotine in the cat, *Peptides* 2:13, 1981.

Reimer SB, et al.: Multiple endocrine neoplasia type 1 in a cat, *J Am Vet Med Assoc* 227:101, 2005.

Renschler JS, Dean GA: What is your diagnosis? Abdominal mass aspirate in a cat with an increased Na:K ratio, *Vet Clin Pathol* 38:69, 2009.

Rijnberk A: Pituitary-dependent hyperadrenocorticism. In Rijnberk A, editor: *Clinical endocrinology of dogs and cats*, Dordrecht, The Netherlands, 1996, Kluwer Academic Publishers, pp 74–83.

Rijnberk A, et al.: Hyperaldosteronism in a cat with metastasised adrenocortical tumour, *Vet Q* 23:38, 2001.

Robinson AJ, Clamann HP: Effects of glucocorticoids on motor units in cat hindlimb muscles, *Muscle Nerve* 11:703, 1988.

Rose SA, et al.: Adrenalectomy and caval thrombectomy in a cat with primary hyperaldosteronism, *J Am Anim Hosp Assoc* 43:209, 2007.

Rossmeisl JH, et al.: Hyperadrenocorticism and hyperprogesteronemia in a cat with an adrenocortical adenocarcinoma, *J Am Anim Hosp Assoc* 36:512, 2000.

Sallanon M, et al.: Hypophysectomy does not disturb the sleep-waking cycle in the cat, *Neurosci Lett* 88:173, 1988.

Schacke H, et al.: Mechanisms involved in the side effects of glucocorticoids, *Pharmacol Ther* 96:23, 2002.

Schaer M, Ginn PE: Iatrogenic Cushing's syndrome and steroid hepatopathy in a cat, *J Am Anim Hosp Assoc* 35:48, 1999.

Schoeman JP, et al.: Cortisol response to two different doses of intravenous synthetic ACTH (tetracosactrin) in overweight cats, *J Small Anim Pract* 41:552, 2000.

Scholten-Sloof BE, et al.: Pituitary-dependent hyperadrenocorticism in a family of Dandie Dinmont terriers, *J Endocrinol* 135:535, 1992.

Schwedes CS: Mitotane (o,p'-DDD) treatment in a cat with hyperadrenocorticism, *J Small Anim Pract* 38:520, 1997.

Scott DW, et al.: Some effects of short-term methylprednisolone therapy in normal cats, *Cornell Vet* 69:104, 1979.

Scott DW, et al.: Iatrogenic Cushing's syndrome in the cat, *Fel Pract* 12:30, 1982.

Sellon RK, et al.: Linear-accelerator-based modified radiosurgical treatment of pituitary tumors in cats: 11 cases (1997-2008), *J Vet Intern Med* 23:1038, 2009.

Selman PJ, et al.: Progestin treatment in the dog, II: effects on the hypothalamic-pituitary-adrenocortical axis, *Eur J Endocrinol* 131:422, 1994.

Selman PJ, et al.: Binding specificity of medroxyprogesterone acetate and proligestone for the progesterone and glucocorticoid receptor in the dog, *Steroids* 61:133, 1996.

Skelly BJ, et al.: Use of trilostane for the treatment of pituitary-dependent hyperadrenocorticism in a cat, *J Small Anim Pract* 44:269, 2003.

Smith MC, Feldman EC: Plasma endogenous ACTH concentrations and plasma cortisol responses to synthetic ACTH and dexamethasone sodium phosphate in healthy cats, *Am J Vet Res* 48:1719, 1987.

Smith RR, et al.: Laparoscopic adrenalectomy for management of a functional adrenal tumor in a cat, *J Am Vet Med Assoc* 241:368, 2012.

Snyckers FD: Transsphenoidal selective anterior hypophysectomy in cats for microsurgical training: technical note, *J Neurosurgery* 43:774, 1975.

Sparkes AH, et al.: Assessment of adrenal function in cats: response to intravenous synthetic ACTH, *J Small Anim Pract* 31:2, 1990.

Stalla GK, et al.: Ketoconazole inhibits corticotropic cell function in vitro, *Endocrinology* 122:618, 1988.

Swift GA, Brown RH: Surgical treatment of Cushing's syndrome in the cat, *Vet Rec* 99:374, 1976.

Syme HM, et al.: Hyperadrenocorticism associated with excessive sex hormone production by an adrenocortical tumor in two dogs, *J Am Vet Med Assoc* 219:1725, 2001.

Stein AL, et al.: Computed tomography versus magnetic resonance imaging for the evaluation of suspected pituitary adenomas, *Obstet Gynecol* 73:996, 1989.

Theon A: Practical radiation therapy. In Ettinger SJ, Feldman EC, editors: *Textbook of veterinary internal medicine*, ed 5, Philadelphia, 2000, WB Saunders, p 489.

Thorner MO, et al.: Approach to pituitary disease. In Wilson JD, Foster DW, editors: *Williams textbook of endocrinology*, ed 8, Philadelphia, 1992, WB Saunders, p 246.

Tuckermann JP, et al.: Molecular mechanisms of glucocorticoids in the control of inflammation and lymphocyte apoptosis, *Crit Rev Clin Lab Sci* 42:71, 2005.

Valentin SY, et al.: Comparison of diagnostic tests and treatment options for feline hyperadrenocorticism: a retrospective review of 32 cases, *J Vet Intern Med* 28:481, 2014.

Van Wijk PA, et al.: Corticotropin-releasing hormone and adrenocorticotropic hormone concentrations in cerebrospinal fluid of dogs with pituitary-dependent hyperadrenocorticism, *Endocrinology* 131:2659, 1992.

Vaughan MA, et al.: Evaluation of twice daily, low-dose trilostane treatment administered orally in dogs with naturally occurring hyperadrenocorticism, *J Am Vet Med Assoc* 232:1321, 2008.

Verheist JA, et al.: Short and long-term responses to metyrapone in the medical management of 91 patients with Cushing's syndrome, *Clin Endocrinol* 35:169, 1991.

Wallack ST, et al.: Mensuration of the pituitary gland from magnetic resonance images in 17 cats, *Vet Radiol Ultrasound* 44:278, 2003.

Watson PJ, Herrtage ME: Hyperadrenocorticism in six cats, *J Small Anim Pract* 39:175, 1998.

White PC: Disorders of aldosterone biosynthesis and action, *N Engl J Med* 331:250, 1994.

Willard MD, et al.: Effect of long-term administration of ketoconazole in cats, *Am J Vet Res* 47:2510, 1986.

Young WF: Primary aldosteronism: renaissance of a syndrome, *Clin Endocrinol* 66:607, 2007.

Yu S, Morris JG: Plasma aldosterone concentration of cats, *Vet J* 155:63, 1998.

Zerbe CA, et al.: Hyperadrenocorticism in a cat, *J Am Vet Med Assoc* 190:559, 1987a.

Zerbe CA, et al.: Effect of nonadrenal illness on adrenal function in the cat, *Am J Vet Res* 48:451, 1987b.

Zhan GL, et al.: Steroid glaucoma: corticosteroid-induced ocular hypertension in cats, *Exp Eye Research* 54:211, 1992.

Zimmer C, et al.: Ultrasonographic examination of the adrenal gland and evaluation of the hypophyseal-adrenal axis in 20 cats, *J Small Anim Pract* 41:156, 2000.

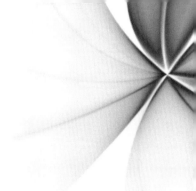

CHAPTER 12 | Hypoadrenocorticism

J. Catharine Scott-Moncrieff

BACKGROUND

The presence of the "suprarenal glands" was recognized by early anatomists, but their importance was not apparent until Thomas Addison described a clinical syndrome in humans that he associated with their dysfunction (Addison, 1855). Included in his description were "anemia, general languor, debility, remarkable feebleness of the heart's action, and irritability of the stomach." Autopsies usually revealed either tuberculous destruction or atrophy of the adrenal glands. At that time, no therapy was known, and patients who developed the disease died. About the same time that Thomas Addison described the clinical picture of adrenal insufficiency, In 1856, Brown-Sequard demonstrated that adrenalectomy resulted in death in experimental animals, thus documenting the necessity of the adrenal glands for maintaining life.

In 1930, crude lipid extracts from the adrenal cortex were demonstrated to contain substances that maintained the lives of adrenalectomized cats, and in 1933, sodium deficiency was demonstrated by Loeb to be a major component of Addison's disease. Cortisol and corticosterone were isolated from beef and porcine adrenal glands in 1937, and synthetic desoxycorticosterone acetate (DOCA) was shown to be of benefit in treatment of adrenal insufficiency by Thorn and his co-workers in 1942. By the mid-1950s, it was recognized that there were three major hormone types produced by the adrenal cortex: glucocorticoids (cortisol), mineralocorticoids (aldosterone), and androgens.

Naturally occurring adrenocortical insufficiency in a dog was initially reported as a clinical entity in 1953, and by the 1980s, brief accounts and then several series appeared in the veterinary literature (Willard et al, 1982). Since 1980, our knowledge of the pathogenesis, diagnosis, and treatment of canine Addison's disease has continued to expand. Feline hypoadrenocorticism was first described in the 1980s, and knowledge about the disease in this species is still limited.

 ## ADRENAL PHYSIOLOGY

The adrenal glands are made up of the adrenal medulla, which secretes catecholamines, and the adrenal cortex, which secretes glucocorticoids, mineralocorticoids, and androgens. Adrenal steroids are derived from cholesterol and all contain the cyclopentanoperhydrophenanthrene (CPPP) nucleus. Enzymes present in the adrenal cortex (P450scc, 17α-hydroxylase, 3β-hydroxysteroid dehydrogenase, 21β-hydroxylase, 11β-hydroxylase, and aldosterone synthase), catalyze formation of the different adrenal steroids (Fig. 12-1; Table 12-1). The major secretory products of the adrenal glands in dogs and cats are cortisol, aldosterone, and the androgens—dehydroepiandrosterone and androstenedione. Other hormones such as progesterone and 17α-hydroxyprogesterone are synthesized in the adrenal gland, but only small amounts are secreted into the systemic circulation in normal animals. Adrenal derived androgens serve as substrates for synthesis of estrogen and testosterone in peripheral tissues.

The adrenal cortex is composed of three histopathologic layers, the zona glomerulosa (ZG), the zona fasciculata (ZF), and the zona reticularis (ZR) (Fig. 12-2). The ZG is the outermost layer of the adrenal gland and is the only layer capable of synthesizing and secreting aldosterone, because it contains the aldosterone synthase enzyme (P450c11AS). The ZG does not contain the enzyme 17α-hydroxlase (P450 c17), so it is incapable of synthesizing cortisol or androgens. The ZF and ZR both synthesize androgens and cortisol.

Glucocorticoids

Regulation of Secretion

Synthesis and secretion of cortisol by the adrenal glands is regulated by the hypothalamic pituitary adrenal (HPA) axis (Fig. 12-3). Corticotrophin-releasing hormone (CRH) secreting neurons in the hypothalamus have axons that terminate in the anterior pituitary gland. CRH stimulates secretion of adrenocorticotropic hormone (ACTH) from the pituitary gland. ACTH is released into the blood, attaches to receptors in the adrenal cortex, and stimulates synthesis and secretion of cortisol. As the plasma cortisol concentration rises, cortisol inhibits CRH and ACTH release from the hypothalamus and pituitary by negative feedback. Increased ACTH concentration also inhibits CRH release from the hypothalamus. Although in people ACTH is secreted in a circadian rhythm with the highest concentrations of ACTH secreted in the early morning, a diurnal rhythm has not been documented in dogs and cats. Factors that stimulate CRH release include stress, hypoglycemia, and physical exercise. Other factors in addition to CRH that stimulate ACTH release include arginine vasopressin, angiotensin II, cholecystokinin, atrial natriuretic factor, and vasoactive peptides (Stewart, 2011).

Effects of Glucocorticoids

Glucocorticoids have a variety of effects throughout the body that make them crucial to normal homeostasis. Glucocorticoids stimulate hepatic gluconeogenesis and glycogenesis, and enhance protein and fat catabolism. They have a permissive action on many metabolic reactions (e.g., lipolysis and calorigenesis), and they are important in maintaining vascular reactivity to catecholamines. Glucocorticoids are also important in maintaining normal blood pressure, counteracting the effects of stress, and for maintaining normal function and maintenance of the gastrointestinal mucosa (Peterson et al, 1996). Glucocorticoids influence the digestion and intestinal absorption of nutrients and increase intestinal brush border and mitochondrial enzymes (Langlais-Burgess et al, 1995). Glucocorticoids also suppress vasopressin secretion due to negative feedback on vasopressin release by the periventricular nucleus. Cortisol binds to mineralocorticoid receptors as avidly as aldosterone but typically has only weak mineralocorticoid activity, because it is inactivated to cortisone by the aldosterone sensitive cells in the collecting tubules (Rose, 2001).

Consequences of Glucocorticoid Deficiency

Glucocorticoid deficiency results in hypotension, hypoglycemia, anorexia, vomiting, diarrhea, weight loss, decreased mobilization of protein and fat from tissues leading to muscular weakness, increased susceptibility to stress, and inability to maintain vascular tone and endothelial integrity. The pathogenesis of gastrointestinal signs in dogs with glucocorticoid deficiency is believed to be multifactorial. Factors that may play a role include decreased gastrointestinal motility, increased vascular permeability, poor tissue perfusion, hypovolemia, and vascular stasis, which can lead to mucosal hemorrhages, ulcers, and atrophy and inflammation of the gastric mucosa. Atrophy and mild inflammatory changes in the gastric mucosa have been documented both in humans with Addison's disease and in adrenalectomized animals (Peterson et al, 1996). Hyponatremia, although usually attributed to mineralocorticoid deficiency, may also occur with glucocorticoid deficiency secondary to stimulation of vasopressin secretion. Vasopressin secretion is stimulated both by hypovolemia and lack of negative feedback of cortisol on the paraventricular nucleus. Hyponatremia and loss of the renal medullary concentration gradient can lead to polyuria in isolated glucocorticoid deficiency (IGD).

Mineralocorticoids

Regulation of Secretion

Synthesis and secretion of aldosterone is regulated by the renin-angiotensin axis, the plasma potassium concentration, and, to a minor extent, the plasma sodium and ACTH concentrations (see Fig. 12-3). Increased plasma potassium concentrations and angiotensin II both markedly increase aldosterone release from the adrenal cortex. Increased angiotensin synthesis is stimulated by decreased extracellular fluid (ECF) volume, which results in increased renin secretion from the juxtaglomerular cells that surround the afferent arterioles as they enter the glomeruli. Renin acts on angiotensinogen to form angiotensin I, which is then converted to angiotensin II by angiotensin converting enzyme primarily in the lungs. Angiotensin II causes increased aldosterone synthesis and secretion by increasing conversion of cholesterol to pregnenolone and corticosterone to aldosterone. Increased plasma potassium also directly stimulates secretion of aldosterone by the adrenal gland. Total absence of ACTH decreases aldosterone secretion, but ACTH has little effect in controlling the rate of aldosterone secretion, and hypophysectomy does not result in mineralocorticoid deficiency (Meij et al, 1997).

Effects of Mineralocorticoids

Mineralocorticoids increase absorption of sodium and secretion of potassium in the kidney, sweat glands, salivary glands, and

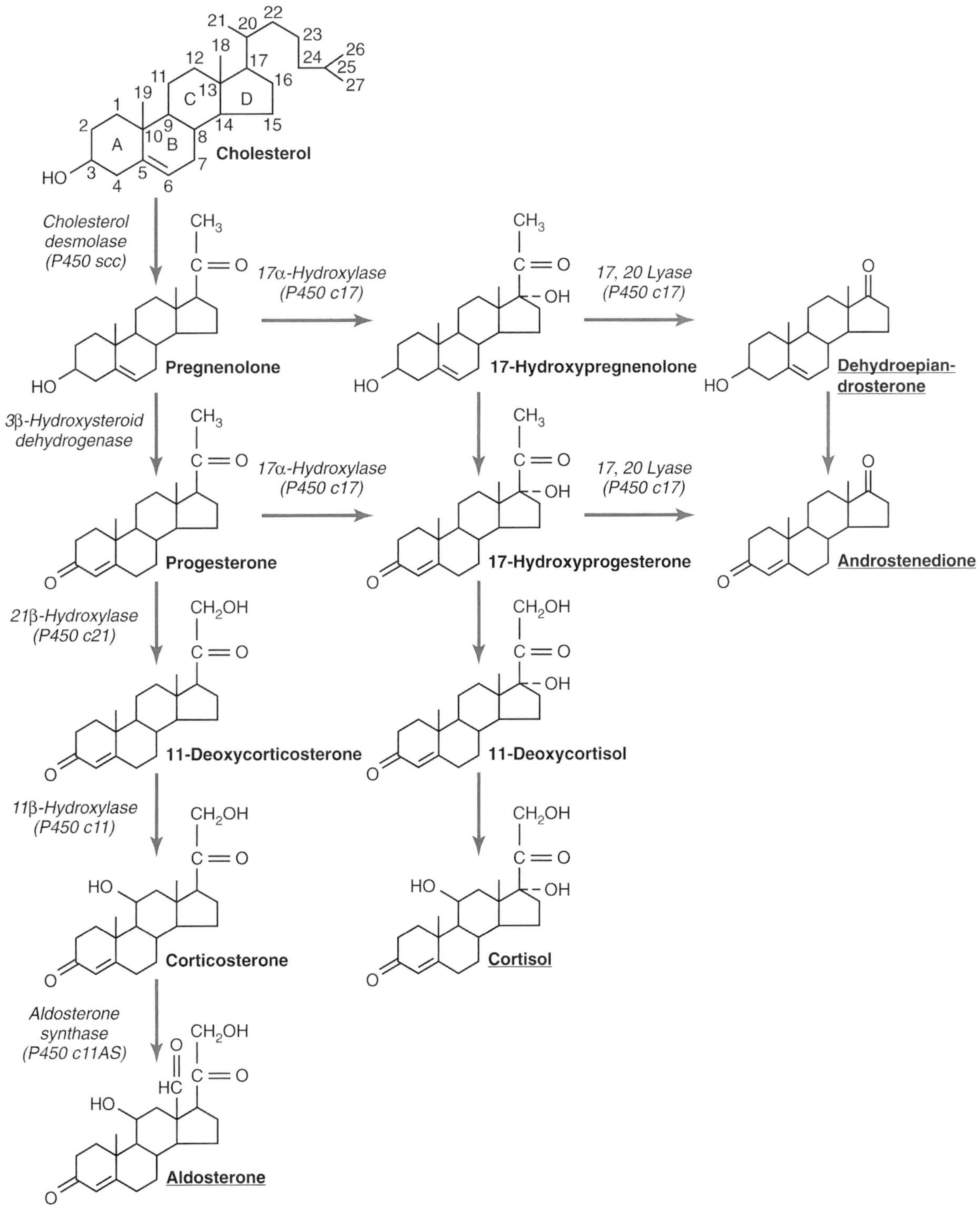

FIGURE 12-1 Major biosynthetic pathways of adrenocortical steroid biosynthesis. The major secretory products are underlined. Enzymes present in the adrenal cortex catalyze formation of the different adrenal steroids. (See Table 12-2 for nomenclature of adrenal steroid enzymes.) The zona glomerulosa (ZG), which produces aldosterone, lacks 17α-hydroxylase and therefore cannot synthesize 17α-hydroxypregnenolone and 17α-hydroxyprogesterone, which are the precursors of cortisol and the adrenal androgens. The zona fasciculata (ZF) and zona reticularis (ZR) produce cortisol, androgens, and small amounts of estrogens. These zones do not contain the aldosterone synthetase and therefore cannot convert 11-deoxycorticosterone to aldosterone. (From Ettinger SJ, Feldman EC: *Textbook of veterinary internal medicine,* ed 7, St Louis, 2010, Saunders/Elsevier.)

TABLE 12-1	NOMENCLATURE OF ADRENAL STEROID ENZYMES AND THEIR GENES	
ENZYME NAME	**ENZYME FAMILY**	**GENE**
P450 cholesterol side-chain cleavage (SCC) desmolase	Cytochrome P450 type I	*CYPIIA1*
3β-hydroxysteroid dehydrogenase (3β-HSD)	Short-chain alcohol dehydrogenase reductase superfamily	*HSDB32*
17α-hydroxylase /17, 20 lyase	Cytochrome P450 type II	*CYP17A1*
21β-hydroxylase	Cytochrome P450 type II	*CYP21A2*
11β-hydroxylase	Cytochrome P450 type I	*CYP11B1*
Aldosterone synthase	Cytochrome P450 type I	*CYP11B2*

Adapted from Melmed S, et al.: *Williams textbook for endocrinology,* ed 12, Philadelphia, 2011, Saunders/Elsevier.

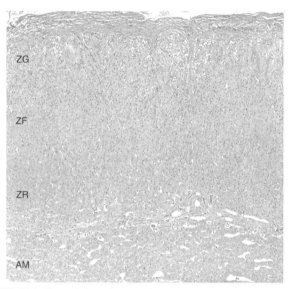

FIGURE 12-2 Histopathology of a normal adrenal gland showing the three layers of the adrenal cortex. Stain hematoxylin and eosin (H and E) 100× magnification. (Courtesy of Dr. M. Miller, Professor Department Comparative Pathobiology, Purdue University, West Lafayette, IN. In Ettinger SJ, Feldman EC: *Textbook of veterinary internal medicine,* ed 7, St Louis, 2010, Saunders/Elsevier.) *AM,* Adrenal medulla; *ZF,* zona fasciculate; *ZG,* zona glomerulosa; *ZR,* zona reticularis.

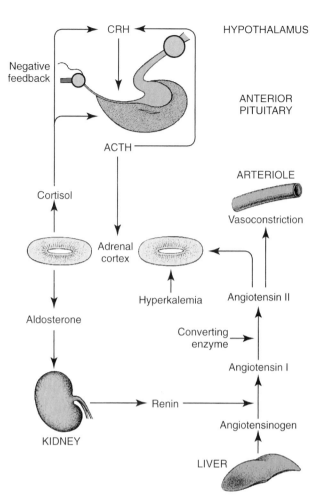

FIGURE 12-3 Regulation of cortisol and aldosterone secretion from the adrenal glands by the hypothalamic pituitary adrenal (HPA) axis and renin angiotensin system. (From Ettinger SJ, Feldman EC: *Textbook of veterinary internal medicine,* ed 7, St Louis, 2010, Saunders/Elsevier.)

intestinal epithelial cells. Thus aldosterone is critical in conserving body salt. The main site of action in the kidneys is the distal nephron (principal cells of the connecting segment and collecting tubules) where aldosterone promotes tubular resorption of sodium and chloride and excretion of potassium (Rose, 2001). In the connecting segment and cortical collecting tubule, aldosterone increases the number of sodium and potassium channels in the luminal membrane and increases the activity of the sodium-potassium adenosine triphosphatase (ATPase) pump in the basolateral membrane. Chloride is passively absorbed via the paracellular pathway. Potassium is exchanged for sodium by the sodium-potassium ATPase pump and then secreted from the cell into the lumen. Aldosterone also enhances sodium reabsorption but not potassium secretion in the papillary collecting tubules and causes secretion of hydrogen ions in exchange for sodium

in the intercalated cells of the cortical collecting tubules. Thus a deficiency of aldosterone causes a mild metabolic acidosis. Aldosterone also reduces the concentration of sodium and raises the concentration of potassium in sweat, saliva, and colonic secretions.

Consequences of Mineralocorticoid Deficiency

Hyponatremia and Hypochloremia. In adrenocortical insufficiency, lack of aldosterone secretion results in impaired ability to conserve sodium and chloride and to excrete potassium and hydrogen ions, leading to hyponatremia, hypochloremia, hyperkalemia, and metabolic acidosis. Loss of sodium and chloride lead to concurrent loss of water. Thus inability to retain sodium and chloride causes a reduced ECF volume that leads to progressive development of hypovolemia, hypotension, reduced cardiac output, and decreased glomerular filtration rate (GFR) leading to prerenal azotemia.

With an adequate sodium-chloride intake, mild aldosterone deficiency may be compensated for by increased sodium intake; however, if sodium intake diminishes due to anorexia or a change in diet or if sodium loss increases because of vomiting and/or diarrhea, continued loss of sodium and chloride through the gastrointestinal tract and kidneys leads to depletion of total body salt stores and severe volume depletion.

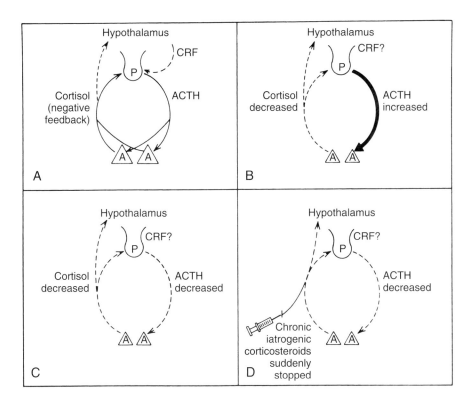

FIGURE 12-4 The pituitary-adrenal axis in normal dogs **(A)**; in dogs with loss of adrenocortical function and excess adrenocorticotropic hormone (ACTH) secretion due to a lack of negative feedback (the most common form of hypoadrenocorticism) **(B)**; in dogs with failure to secrete ACTH and secondary atrophy of the adrenal cortex, specifically the zona fasciculata (ZF) and zona reticularis (ZR) **(C)**; and in dogs that are chronically overtreated with exogenous glucocorticoids, causing insufficiency in pituitary ACTH secretion and secondary atrophy of the adrenal cortex **(D)**. (From Ettinger SJ: *Textbook of veterinary internal medicine*, ed 2, Philadelphia, 1983, WB Saunders.) *A,* Adrenal; *CRF,* corticotropin-releasing factor (hormone); *P,* pituitary.

Hyperkalemia. Mineralocorticoid deficiency results in progressively worsening hyperkalemia as a result of diminished renal perfusion, which reduces glomerular filtration and depresses cation exchange by the distal convoluted renal tubules. Hyperkalemia is worsened by metabolic acidosis, which promotes a shift of potassium ions from the intracellular to the extracellular space. The most prominent manifestation of hyperkalemia is the deleterious effect on cardiac function. Hyperkalemia causes decreased myocardial excitability, an increase in the myocardial refractory period, and slowed conduction. Hypoxia, secondary to hypovolemia and poor tissue perfusion, contributes to myocardial dysfunction. Ventricular fibrillation or cardiac standstill may eventually occur as the plasma potassium concentration exceeds 10 mEq/L.

Acidosis. Mild metabolic acidosis develops as a result of impaired ability to reabsorb bicarbonate and chloride ions in the renal tubules, as well as from failure of the poorly perfused kidneys to excrete metabolic waste products and hydrogen ions.

Polyuria/Polydipsia. Polyuria with compensatory polydipsia may result from aldosterone deficiency due to natriuresis and resultant loss of the renal medullary concentration gradient.

 PRIMARY VERSUS SECONDARY HYPOADRENOCORTICISM

Primary hypoadrenocorticism due to bilateral adrenal gland destruction accounts for the majority (more than 95%) of cases of canine hypoadrenocorticism. Loss of more than 90% of adrenocortical function is required before clinical signs of glucocorticoid and mineralocorticoid deficiency develop, so clinical hypoadrenocorticism only occurs when both adrenal cortices are destroyed (Fig. 12-4). Secondary hypoadrenocorticism due to reduced secretion of ACTH from the pituitary gland is a much rarer cause of adrenocortical failure. Loss of ACTH causes atrophy of the adrenal cortices (sparing the ZG) and impaired secretion of glucocorticoids but not mineralocorticoids.

GLUCOCORTICOID DEFICIENCY VERSUS MINERALOCORTICOID DEFICIENCY

In dogs, measurement of decreased cortisol concentration is used to confirm glucocorticoid deficiency; concurrent low aldosterone concentration is assumed if appropriate electrolyte abnormalities (hyponatremia and hyperkalemia) are present. In secondary hypoadrenocorticism, mineralocorticoid secretion is preserved because ACTH is only a minor player in control of aldosterone secretion, so electrolyte abnormalities are not expected, although mild hyponatramia can occur due to glucocorticoid deficiency alone. In most cases of primary hypoadrenocorticism, both cortisol and aldosterone secretion from the adrenal glands are impaired, resulting in hypocortisolemia and electrolyte abnormalities (e.g., hyponatremia and hyperkalemia); however up to 30% of dogs with primary hypoadrenocorticism have normal electrolyte concentrations at the time of initial diagnosis. This has been referred to in the literature as "atypical" or glucocorticoid deficient hypoadrenocorticism. It has been hypothesized that aldosterone concentrations in these dogs are normal due to sparing of the ZG; however, in most reported cases, the aldosterone concentration was not directly measured. In a recent study of aldosterone secretion in dogs with hypoadrenocorticism, four dogs that exhibited neither hyponatremia nor hyperkalemia had extremely low aldosterone concentrations, implying that maintenance of normal aldosterone concentrations cannot be the only reason by which normal electrolyte concentrations are maintained in dogs with atypical hypoadrenocorticism (Fig. 12-5; Baumstark et al, 2014). It is possible that increased dietary sodium intake compensates for increased natriuresis in some dogs with atypical hypoadrenocorticism. Increased renin concentrations indicating compensated failure of the ZG has been documented in humans with primary hypoadrenocorticism and normal electrolytes (Oelkers et al, 1992; Shiah, 1995). Isolated glucocorticoid deficiency (IGD) in people is a rare autosomal recessive disorder characterized by early onset of primary adrenocortical insufficiency without mineralocorticoid deficiency (Tsigos et al, 1995). Mutations of the ACTH receptor gene have been reported in several families

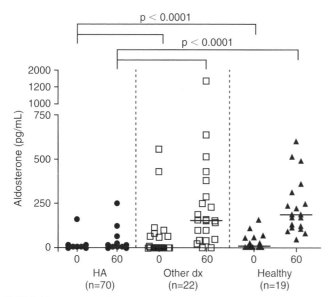

FIGURE 12-5 Baseline *(0)* and adrenocorticotropic hormone (ACTH) stimulated *(60)* serum aldosterone concentrations in dogs with hypoadrenocorticism *(HA; n = 70)*, dogs with diseases mimicking HA *(Other dx; n = 22)*, and healthy dogs *(Healthy; n = 19)*. (From Baumstark ME, et al.: Evaluation of aldosterone concentrations in dogs with hypoadrenocorticism, *J Vet Intern Med* 28:154, 2014.)

with IGD. Whether this syndrome is the cause of some cases of atypical hypoadrenocorticism in dogs is unknown. Pathology studies of dogs with lymphocytic plasmacytic adrenalitis have identified cases in which there is partial sparing of the ZG (Frank et al, 2013). Whether such cases have normal aldosterone concentrations has yet to be determined. Other proposed causes of normal electrolytes in dogs with primary hypoadrenocorticism include disparity in rate of destruction of glucocorticoid and mineralocorticoid secreting cells and influence of concurrent diseases such as hypothyroidism on the metabolic rate.

Deficiency of mineralocorticoid secretion but normal glucocorticoid secretion may also occur rarely in dogs. Isolated hypoaldosteronism is a rare syndrome in humans due either to inadequate secretion of renin by the kidneys (hyporeninemic hypoaldosteronism) or mutations in the biosynthetic cascade of aldosterone synthesis (hyperreninemic hypoaldosteronism) (White, 2004). The distinction between the two syndromes is based on measurement of renin concentrations. If the cause of hypoaldosteronism is primary adrenal dysfunction, renin concentrations should be high, whereas if it is due to kidney dysfunction, renin concentrations are low. Isolated case reports of hyporeninemic hypoaldosteronism in a dog with renal failure and hyperreninemic hypoaldosteronism in a dog that also had a heart base chemodectoma have been reported in the veterinary literature, but both syndromes are exceedingly rare (Lobetti, 1998; Kreissler and Langston, 2011). Mineralocorticoid deficiency occurring prior to development of glucocorticoid deficiency was reported in a dog with primary hypoadrenocorticism and hypothyroidism (McGonigle et al, 2013). Although renin was not measured, the progression from aldosterone deficiency to combined mineralocorticoid and glucocorticoid deficiency in the absence of renal disease suggested isolated hyperreninemic hypoaldosteronism.

PRIMARY ADRENOCORTICAL FAILURE

Development of the clinical syndrome associated with adrenocortical insufficiency is believed to require at least 90% destruction of adrenal cortices. Naturally occurring destruction of the adrenal

cortices is usually a gradual process, initially resulting in a "partial deficiency syndrome" characterized by inadequate adrenal reserve, with symptoms manifesting only during times of stress induced by surgery, trauma, infection, or changes of environment such as boarding. Basal hormone secretion in the unstressed state may be adequate to maintain near-normal plasma electrolyte concentrations and minimal clinical signs. For these dogs, the diagnosis can be confirmed only by measurement of adrenocortical reserve. As destruction of the adrenal cortices continues, hormone secretion becomes inadequate even under non-stressful conditions, and a metabolic crisis can result without any obvious inciting event.

The most common cause of primary adrenal failure in humans is immune mediated adrenalitis; however in some areas of the world, granulomatous adrenalitis due to tuberculosis is an important cause of hypoadrenocorticism (Box 12-1). In people, hypoadrenocorticism due to adrenalitis is 1.5 to 3.5 times more common in women than men (Mitchell and Pearce, 2012). Following the development of serum autoantibodies (usually to the steroidogenic enzyme 21-hydroxylase) there is a prolonged period of subclinical disease characterized by increased concentrations of ACTH and renin, before symptomatic adrenal failure develops (Mitchell and Pearce, 2012). Histologic examination of the adrenals reveals widespread infiltrates consisting of lymphocytes, plasma cells, and macrophages. In advanced stages, the cortex is replaced by fibrous tissue.

Large case series describing the underlying histopathologic abnormalities in dogs with hypoadrenocorticism have not been published, likely because most cases of hypoadrenocorticism are either successfully treated or the dog dies without a necropsy being performed. In most confirmed cases of hypoadrenocorticism the typical findings are of severe lymphoplasmacytic inflammation and adrenocortical atrophy involving all layers of the adrenal cortex (Fig. 12-6). In a study of 33 dogs with adrenalitis, inflammation was lymphoplasmacytic in 17 dogs, lymphocytic in four, lymphohistiocytic in one, granulomatous in three, and neutrophilic in eight dogs (Frank et al, 2013). Severe adrenocortical atrophy was observed predominantly in the dogs with lymphoplasmacytic inflammation. These dogs typically had nearly complete loss of cortical cells; however the ZG was partially spared in three dogs with lymphoplasmacytic adrenalitis and severe cortical atrophy. Non-lymphoid inflammation of the adrenal glands was usually multifocal, associated with systemic disease, and not associated with severe adrenocortical atrophy. Anti-adrenal antibodies have been detected in two dogs with primary hypoadrenocorticism, and it is believed that immune mediated adrenalitis is the most likely etiology for the majority of spontaneous cases of canine primary hypoadrenocorticism (Schaer et al, 1986); however, in most dogs with hypoadrenocorticism the cause is not proven and the etiology is classified as idiopathic. Although antibodies to adrenal cell antigens have been demonstrated by indirect immunofluorescence, no specific autoantibodies against a specific enzyme (e.g., the steroid 21-hydroxylase) have been identified in dogs with hypoadrenocorticism (Schaer et al, 1986). Dogs treated for hypoadrenocorticism for any length of time have complete loss of measurable cortical tissue with only mild residual mononuclear, lymphocytic, or lymphoplasmacytic inflammation and a thick fibrous capsule (Boujon et al, 1994; Frank et al, 2013). The pituitary gland is normal histologically in primary immune-mediated adrenocortical atrophy, but increased ACTH immunoreactivity has been identified in the anterior pituitary gland (Boujon et al, 1994).

Other rare causes of adrenalitis and primary hypoadrenocorticism in dogs include granulomatous destruction (e.g., blastomycosis, histoplasmosis, and cryptococcosis), amyloidosis,

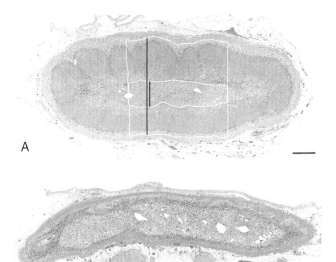

FIGURE 12-6 A, Histopathology of normal adrenal gland. **B,** Histopathology of adrenal gland with severe adrenocortical atrophy. Stained with H and E. The long black line marks the thickness of the entire gland, the short line the medullary thickness bar, 1 mm. (From Frank CB, et al.: Correlation of inflammation with adrenocortical atrophy in canine adrenalitis, *J Comp Pathol* 149:268, 2013.)

BOX 12-1 Etiology of Adrenocortical Insufficiency in Humans (Excluding Congenital Adrenal Hyperplasia)

Primary Causes: Addison's Disease

Autoimmune
   Sporadic
   Autoimmune polyendocrine syndrome type I (Addison's disease, chronic mucocutaneous candidiasis, hypoparathyroidism, dental enamel hypoplasia, alopecia, primary gonadal failure)
   Autoimmune polyendocrine syndrome type II (Schmidt syndrome) (Addison's disease, primary hypothyroidism, primary hypogonadism, insulin-dependent diabetes, pernicious anemia, vitiligo)
Infections
   Tuberculosis
   Fungal infections
   Cytomegalovirus
   HIV
Metastatic tumor
Infiltrations
   Amyloid
   Hemochromatosis
Intra-adrenal hemorrhage (Waterhouse-Friderichsen syndrome) after meningococcal septicemia
Adrenoleukodystrophies
Congenital adrenal hypoplasia
   DAX-1 *(NROB1)* mutations
   SF1 mutations
ACTH resistance syndromes
   MC2R gene mutations
   MRAP gene mutations
   AAAS (ALADIN) gene mutations (triple-A syndrome)
Bilateral adrenalectomy

Secondary Causes

Exogenous glucocorticoid therapy
Hypopituitarism
Selective removal of ACTH-secreting pituitary adenoma
Pituitary tumors and pituitary surgery, craniopharyngiomas
Pituitary apoplexy
Granulomatous disease (tuberculosis, sarcoid, eosinophilic granuloma)
Secondary tumor deposits (breast, bronchus)
Postpartum pituitary infarction (Sheehan syndrome)
Pituitary irradiation (effect usually delayed for several years)
Isolated ACTH deficiency
   Idiopathic
   Lymphocytic hypophysitis
   TPIT *(TBX19)* gene mutations
   PCSK1 gene mutation (POMC processing defect)
   POMC gene mutations
Multiple pituitary hormone deficiencies
   HESX1 gene mutations
   LHX4 gene mutations
   SOX3 gene mutations
   PROP1 gene mutations

From Melmed S, et al.: *Williams textbook for endocrinology,* ed 12, Philadelphia, 2011, Saunders/Elsevier.
ACTH, Adrenocorticotropic hormone; *HIV,* human immunodeficiency virus; *POMC,* pro-opiomelanocortin.

---

hemorrhagic infarction, and metastatic neoplasia (Labelle and De Cock, 2005; Rockwell et al, 2005; Reusch et al, 2007; Frank et al, 2013). The adrenal glands are a common site for tumor metastasis in dogs; 21% of dogs with disseminated neoplasia have adrenal metastases. The most common tumors that metastasize to the adrenal glands in dogs include pulmonary, mammary, prostatic, gastric, and pancreatic carcinomas and melanoma (Labelle and De Cock, 2005); however, only lymphoma and bilateral anaplastic neoplasia has been reported to cause adrenal gland failure in dogs (Labelle and De Cock, 2005; Kook et al, 2010). Hemorrhagic infarction of the adrenal gland (secondary to trauma, infection, necrosis, or coagulopathy) has been reported in dogs but is rare, and hypoadrenocorticism due to bilateral abscessing adrenalitis has been reported (Korth et al, 2008). Bilateral adrenal infarction secondary to a presumed increase in endogenous ACTH in a dog with previously diagnosed hyperadrenocorticism has also been described (Rockwell et al, 2005). Interestingly, in humans, intraadrenal hemorrhage with resultant necrosis is an important cause of adrenal gland failure, particularly in children with *Pseudomonas aeruginosa* infection and meningococcal septicemia (Stewart, 2011).

Iatrogenic primary hypoadrenocorticism may be caused by drugs such as mitotane, and trilostane (Reusch et al, 2007). Mitotane is cytotoxic to the adrenal gland and is well documented to cause adrenal gland necrosis in dogs. Although the glucocorticoid deficiency that occurs in many dogs during the induction phase of mitotane treatment for hyperadrenocorticism is usually transient once treatment is discontinued, 5% of dogs with hyperadrenocorticism treated with mitotane develop permanent mineralocorticoid deficient hypoadrenocorticism (Kintzer, 1991). Adrenal suppression caused by trilostane is usually reversible, but permanent primary hypoadrenocorticism due to adrenal necrosis and hemorrhage has also been reported in association with this drug (Reusch et al, 2007). Adrenal necrosis associated with trilostane treatment has been speculated to be caused by high circulating ACTH concentrations. This hypothesis is supported by studies in rats, showing that ACTH administration causes adrenal gland necrosis, vacuolization, and apoptosis of adrenocortical cells (Burkhardt et al, 2011). Primary hypoadrenocorticism has also been reported in Beagles exposed to aerosols of plutonium-238 (Weller et al, 1996).

POLYGLANDULAR AUTOIMMUNE SYNDROMES

Immune-mediated destruction of the adrenal glands in humans is commonly associated with other immune disorders. Two distinct immunoendocrinopathy syndromes have been described, autoimmune polyglandular disease type I and type II. Type I disease involves adrenal insufficiency, hypoparathyroidism, and chronic mucocutaneous candidiasis. Type II disease (also called *Schmidt syndrome*) involves adrenal insufficiency, thyroiditis, and insulin-dependent diabetes mellitus. Enzymes involved in steroidogenesis such as 17α-hydroxylase, 21α-hydroxylase, and the side-chain cleavage enzyme are target autoantigens in autoimmune Addison's disease in humans.

Polyglandular autoimmune disease is rare in dogs. Most canine reports resemble human type II autoimmune polyendocrine syndrome with hypoadrenocorticism and hypothyroidism being the most common concurrent disorders (Melendez, 1996; Blois, 2011). Two other diseases with possible immune mediated pathogenesis, diabetes mellitus, and hypoparathyroidism may also occur in dogs with hypoadrenocorticism (Bowen et al, 1986; Kooistra et al, 1995; Blois et al, 2011). Lymphocytic adenohypophysitis was documented in a dog with adrenalitis and primary thyroid atrophy (Adissu et al, 2010). In a study of 225 dogs with hypoadrenocorticism, a concomitant endocrinopathy was diagnosed in 5% of dogs (Peterson et al, 1996). In a case series of 10 dogs with concurrent hypoadrenocorticism and hypothyroidism, hypothyroidism was identified as a cause of poor response to treatment in dogs with hypoadrenocorticism (Melendez, 1996). Hypothyroidism should be considered in any dog with hypoadrenocorticism that has a poor clinical response to initial treatment for hypoadrenocorticism.

SECONDARY ADRENOCORTICAL FAILURE

Spontaneous Secondary Hypoadrenocorticism

Reduced secretion of ACTH by the pituitary gland results in decreased synthesis and secretion of adrenocortical hormones, especially glucocorticoids (see Fig. 12-4). Reduced secretion of CRH by the hypothalamus may also result in secondary adrenocortical failure. In humans destructive lesions in the pituitary or hypothalamus resulting in ACTH or CRH deficiency (or both) are usually caused by neoplasia; inflammation and trauma are less common causes (Velardo et al, 1992; Thodou et al, 1995; Platt et al, 1999; see Box 12-1). Pituitary hypopexy can result in an Addisonian crisis or spontaneous resolution of pituitary dependent hyperadrenocorticism. Pituitary hypopexy has been reported in dogs and resulted in acute neurologic signs and sudden death but adrenocortical function in these cases was not reported (Bertolini et al, 2007).

Iatrogenic Secondary Hypoadrenocorticism

Hypophysectomy for the treatment of pituitary dependent hyperadrenocorticism results in secondary hypoadrenocorticism, which is usually permanent unless there is disease relapse (Hanson, 2005).

More commonly, iatrogenic adrenal insufficiency is secondary to withdrawal of exogenous corticosteroid administration, although this only rarely results in clinical signs (see Fig. 12-4). Any dog chronically receiving amounts of corticosteroids sufficient

to suppress the hypothalamic-pituitary axis is susceptible to secondary adrenal atrophy. Adrenal suppression can occur within a few days of administration of ACTH-inhibiting doses of corticosteroids, although suppression is markedly variable among individuals. This individual variation is reflected in the fact that some dogs quickly develop clinical signs of iatrogenic Cushing's syndrome from relatively low doses of glucocorticoids, whereas others show no effect from higher doses. If adrenal suppression occurs, adrenal function usually recovers gradually (over a period of weeks) after hormone administration is stopped, usually taking more time if long-acting depot forms of glucocorticoids were used. Pituitary suppression has been documented not only with injectable and oral glucocorticoids but also with topical dermatologic, ophthalmic, and otic preparations (Roberts et al, 1984; Moriello et al, 1988; Murphy et al, 1990). Although estimates of the relative biologic effectiveness of synthetic steroids vary, studies have shown prednisone/prednisolone to be five times more potent than cortisol in suppressing ACTH secretion and dexamethasone to be 50 to 150 times more potent. Relatively small dosages of dexamethasone, therefore, may be sufficient to produce adrenal atrophy. The long-acting "depot" injectable corticosteroids (e.g., betamethasone) may suppress the pituitary-adrenocortical axis of dogs for as long as 5 weeks (Kemppainen et al, 1981; 1982). It is important to allow enough time for recovery of adrenal suppression after administration of glucocorticoids when planning testing of the pituitary adrenal axis. The length of time required depends upon the potency of the glucocorticoid product used, the dose, and the duration of administration. If only one dose of dexamethasone is administered, an ACTH stimulation test can be performed immediately because dexamethasone is not detected by assays for cortisol and because the amount of adrenal suppression that will result is mild enough that the response of a patient with spontaneous hypoadrenocorticism can be distinguished from the effects of glucocorticoid suppression. If other glucocorticoids are administered, time must be allowed for both metabolism and excretion of the administered glucocorticoid and recovery of adrenal gland atrophy. The waiting time necessary before being able to interpret the results of adrenal function testing ranges from as short as 48 hours in patients treated with one dose of prednisone or prednisolone to as long as 6 to 8 weeks in patients treated with a single dose of a depot preparation of glucocorticoid such as triamcinolone acetonide or methylprednisolone acetate (Behrend and Kemppainen, 1997). Oral administration of shorter acting or less potent glucocorticoids results in a quicker recovery of the adrenal axis. In one study of dogs treated with 5 weeks of prednisone at a dose of 0.55 mg/kg every 12 hours, complete HPA axis recovery was reported by 2 weeks after cessation of therapy (Moore and Hoenig, 1992). Suppression of the HPA axis in dogs treated with topical glucocorticoid therapy can last as long as 4 weeks depending upon the preparation. In some cases sequential stimulation tests may need to be performed to document full return of adrenal function.

SIGNALMENT

The prevalence of hypoadrenocorticism in dogs has been estimated at approximately 0.06% to 0.28% (Kelch et al, 1998). The disease is inherited as an autosomal recessive trait in the Standard Poodle, Portuguese Water dog, and Nova Scotia Duck Tolling Retriever and is also heritable in the Bearded Collie, although in this breed the mode of inheritance is not clear. In these four breeds, the estimated prevalence is higher than that in the general population although the reported rates may be artificially high because of biased sampling of dogs from concerned owners and breeders

| TABLE 12-2 | ESTIMATES OF HERITABILITY, ESTIMATED PREVALENCE OF HYPOADRENOCORTICISM, AND SEX PREDISPOSITION IN BREEDS WITH HERITABLE HYPOADRENOCORTICISM |

BREED	HERITABILITY	MODE OF INHERITANCE	ESTIMATED PREVALENCE	SEX PREDIS-POSITION
Standard Poodle	0.75	Autosomal recessive	8.6%	None
Portuguese Water dog	0.49	Autosomal recessive	1.5%	None
Nova Scotia Duck Tolling Retriever	0.98	Autosomal recessive	1.4%	None
Bearded Collie	0.76	Unknown	9.4%	None

From Ettinger SJ, Feldman EC: *Textbook of veterinary internal medicine,* ed 7, St Louis, 2010, Saunders/Elsevier.

(Tables 12-2 and 12-3; Shaker, 1988; Burton, 1997; Oberbauer et al, 2002; 2006; Famula et al, 2003; Hughes et al, 2007). Primary hypoadrenocorticism was also reported in a family of Leonbergers (Smallwood and Barsanti, 1995). Two disease associated loci on canine autosomes CFA 12 and 37, which are syntenic with the human DRB1 histocompatibility locus alleles HLA-DRB1*04 and DRB1*0301, have been identified in Portuguese Water dogs with hypoadrenocorticism (Chase et al, 2006). Dog leucocyte antigen (DLA) haplotypes are also associated with disease frequency in other dog breeds (Hughes 2010; 2011). For example in the Springer and Cocker Spaniel the DLA-DRB1*015:01—DQA1*006—DQB1*023:01 haplotype is significantly associated with disease risk (Massey et al, 2013). Markers on CFA 12 were associated with an increase in the frequency of the disease, whereas markers on CFA37 were associated with a decrease in frequency of the disease. Two markers on CFA12 FH2202 and FH2975 are within the canine DLA region, supporting the assumption that canine hypoadrenocorticism is an autoimmune disease (Chase et al, 2006). Many other breeds have been shown to have either an increased or decreased risk of hypoadrenocorticism (see Table 12-3; Peterson et al, 1996; Kelch et al, 1998; Adler, 2007; Thompson et al, 2007). Further genetic studies are necessary to establish the genetic cause of inherited hypoadrenocorticism in dogs. It has been proposed that canine hypoadrenocorticism may be a useful model for studying the mode of inheritance of human Addison's disease. Some of the same genes that are associated with susceptibility to Addison's disease in humans are also associated with canine hypoadrenocorticism (Short et al, 2013). There is a female predisposition for hypoadrenocorticism with approximately 70% of affected dogs being female; however, no sex predisposition has been demonstrated in the Standard Poodle, Portuguese water dog, Nova Scotia Duck Tolling Retriever, or Bearded Collie. In one study, neutered females and neutered males were each about three times more likely to develop the disease than their intact counterparts (Kelch et al, 1998). Median age of onset for all breeds is 4 years (range, 4 months to 14 years), and the majority are young to middle-aged dogs (Peterson et al, 1996). The disease has a younger age of onset in the Nova Scotia Duck Tolling Retriever, in which the median age of onset was 3 years (Hughes et al, 2007).

| TABLE 12-3 | BREEDS REPORTED TO BE EITHER AT INCREASED OR DECREASED RISK OF HYPOADRENOCORTICISM |

BREED	INCREASED RISK	DECREASED RISK
Airedale Terrier	X	
Basset Hound	X	
Bearded Collie	X	
Boxer		X
Chihuahua		X
Cocker Spaniel		X
Dalmatian		X
Golden Retriever		X
Great Dane	X	
Lhasa Apso		X
Nova Scotia Duck Tolling Retriever	X	
Pit Bull Terrier		X
Pomeranian		X
Portuguese Water Dog	X	
Rottweiler	X	
Saint Bernard	X	
Shetland Sheepdog		X
Shih Tzu		X
Springer Spaniel	X	
Standard Poodle	X	
West Highland White Terrier	X	
Wheaten Terrier	X	
Yorkshire Terrier		X

From Ettinger SJ, Feldman EC: *Textbook of veterinary internal medicine,* ed 7, St Louis, 2010, Saunders/Elsevier.

 HISTORY

Clinical signs in dogs with hypoadrenocorticism may be either acute or gradual in onset and commonly wax and wane. The clinical signs can be insidious in onset and owners may not realize the duration or severity of illness until treatment results in a dramatic improvement in activity level. Sometimes clinical illness is triggered by a stressful event. A history of episodic illness or gastrointestinal upset (lethargy, vomiting, diarrhea, and/or dehydration) that improves with supportive care (fluids, cage rest, and glucocorticoid administration) should alert the clinician to the possibility of hypoadrenocorticism, especially if clinical signs are recurrent. Clinical signs of hypoadrenocorticism are vague and none are pathognomonic for the disease. Anorexia, vomiting, lethargy/depression, weakness, weight loss, diarrhea, and shaking or shivering are all common; polyuria, polydipsia, and abdominal pain may also be observed. All of these clinical signs may be caused by glucocorticoid deficiency alone; however when mineralocorticoid deficiency is also present, polyuria, polydipsia, hypovolemic shock, collapse, and dehydration are more prominent, and the clinical signs tend to be more severe. Less common clinical manifestations of hypoadrenocorticism include seizures due to hypoglycemia, episodic muscle cramping, and gastrointestinal hemorrhage (Saito, 2002; Medinger et al, 1993; Levy, 1994; Syme and Scott-Moncrieff, 1998).

 PHYSICAL EXAMINATION

Abnormalities found on physical examination in dogs with hypoadrenocorticism are also vague and nonspecific. Poor body condition, lethargy, weakness, severe dehydration, abdominal pain, bradycardia, weak pulses, hypothermia, decreased capillary refill time, and other signs of hypovolemic shock may be evident on physical examination. The presence of bradycardia in a dog with other evidence for hypovolemic shock should be a red flag for the possibility of hypoadrenocorticism. Melena or hematochezia may occur and occasionally results in pale mucous membranes, weakness, and collapse due to anemia (Medinger et al, 1993). In some dogs with hypoadrenocorticism, especially those with glucocorticoid deficiency alone, the physical examination may be unremarkable (Peterson et al, 1996; Thompson et al, 2007).

Blood Pressure. Many dogs with hypoadrenocorticism have systolic hypotension at the time of initial evaluation. In one study of 53 dogs with hypoadrenocorticism, median systolic blood pressure was 90 mm Hg (range, 40 to 150 mm Hg), whereas in 110 dogs with other causes of illness, median blood pressure was 140 mm Hg (range, 50 to 210 mm Hg; Seth et al, 2011).

 CLINICAL PATHOLOGY

The classic clinicopathologic abnormalities of dogs with hypoadrenocorticism include hyponatremia, hyperkalemia, non-regenerative anemia, and lymphocytosis; however these changes are not present in all cases. Although diagnosis of a typical case of hypoadrenocorticism is usually straightforward, some dogs with hypoadrenocorticism have none of these classic clinicopathologic abnormalities. This less typical presentation can be a significant diagnostic challenge. Failure to consider hypoadrenocorticism as a differential diagnosis will result in a missed or incorrect diagnosis, leading to owner frustration or even death of the patient. It is therefore very important that the clinician considers hypoadrenocorticism as a possible differential diagnosis for any dog with vague clinical signs of illness. Although a low sodium-to-potassium ratio and a normal lymphocyte count in a sick dog increase the index of suspicion for hypoadrenocorticism, the diagnosis cannot be either confirmed or ruled out on this basis alone.

Abnormalities that may be observed on the complete blood count (CBC), biochemical panel, and urinalysis in dogs with hypoadrenocorticism are shown in Table 12-4 (Peterson et al, 1996; Feldman and Nelson, 2004). It is important to recognize that the clinicopathologic abnormalities seen in hypoadrenocorticism may mimic those observed in other diseases, such as hepatic failure (hypoglycemia, hypoalbuminemia, hypocholesterolemia, and increased alanine aminotransferase [ALT] and alkaline phosphatase [ALP]), renal failure (anemia, azotemia, hypercalcemia, hyperphosphatemia, and low urine specific gravity), insulinoma (hypoglycemia, increased ALT, and ALP), and protein losing enteropathy (hypoalbuminemia, hypocholesterolemia, and non-regenerative anemia); so unless the clinician maintains a high index of suspicion for a diagnosis of hypoadrenocorticism, the diagnosis may be missed.

Hematology

Typical hematologic abnormalities in dogs with hypoadrenocorticism include a nonregenerative, normocytic normochromic

TABLE 12-4	COMMON CLINICOPATHOLOGIC CHANGES OBSERVED IN DOGS SUFFERING FROM HYPOADRENOCORTICISM

CLINICOPATHOLOGIC CHANGES	PERCENTAGE AFFECTED
Complete Blood Count	
Eosinophilia	20
Lack of stress leukogram	92
Lymphocytosis	10
Neutrophilia	32
Nonregenerative anemia	27
Biochemical Panel	
Azotemia	88
Hypercalcemia	31
Hyperkalemia	95
Hyperphosphatemia	68
Hypoalbuminemia	6 to 39
Hypochloremia	42
Hypocholesterolemia	7
Hypoglycemia	17
Hyponatremia	81
Increased liver enzymes	30 to 50
Metabolic acidosis	40
Urine specific gravity < 1.030	**60**

From Ettinger SJ, Feldman EC: *Textbook of veterinary internal medicine,* ed 7, St Louis, 2010, Saunders/Elsevier.

anemia, eosinophilia, neutrophilia, and lymphocytosis; however, these changes are seen in only 10% to 30% of dogs (see Table 12-4). The anemia is typically of mild to moderate severity with hematocrits of 20% to 35% being typical. The anemia in hypoadrenocorticism is attributed to lack of red cell production due to cortisol deficiency in combination with gastrointestinal blood loss. Approximately 15% of dogs with hypoadrenocorticism have evidence of melena or hematochezia, and in approximately 5% of dogs, this can result in severe anemia (Medinger, 1993; Peterson et al, 1996). In some dogs, the mild anemia is initially masked by dehydration, and the anemia is only revealed after fluid rehydration. Dogs with hypoadrenocorticism that lack electrolyte changes (so called atypical Addison's disease or glucocorticoid deficient hypoadrenocorticism) are more likely to be anemic than those with evidence of concurrent mineralocorticoid deficiency (Thompson et al, 2007). This may relate to the longer duration of illness in these dogs and the fact that dehydration is less severe and less likely to mask anemia in this subgroup of dogs.

The most common abnormality on the leukogram in dogs with hypoadrenocorticism is the absence of a stress leukogram, which is an unexpected finding in the presence of systemic illness. The characteristics of a stress leukogram include lymphopenia, neutrophilia, and eosinopenia; dogs with Addison's disease may have lymphocytosis, eosinophilia (Box 12-2), or may have an unexpectedly normal neutrophil count or lymphocyte count. Cortisol causes lymphopenia due to redistribution of recirculating lymphocytes;

BOX 12-2	Potential Causes of Eosinophilia in Dogs and Cats

Parasitism
  Heartworm disease
  Gastrointestinal
  Dermatologic
  Other
Asthma
Nonparasitic dermatologic disease
Mast cell tumor, other neoplasia
Hypoadrenocorticism (Addison's disease)
Eosinophilic myositis
Eosinophilic pneumonitis/rhinitis/conjunctivitis
Eosinophilic enterocolitis (allergic colitis)
Eosinophilic leukemia
Eosinophilic granuloma complex
Eosinophilic vasculitis
Drug reaction

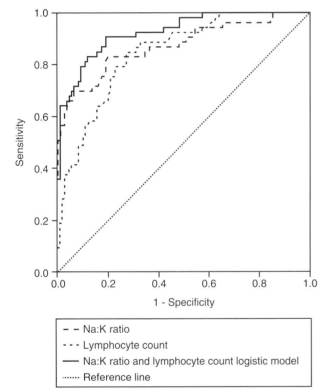

TABLE 12-5 SENSITIVITY AND SPECIFICITY OF THE SODIUM-TO-POTASSIUM RATIO OR LYMPHOCYTE COUNT FOR PREDICTING HYPOADRENOCORTICISM IN DOGS WITH A CLINICAL SUSPICION OF HYPOADRENOCORTICISM

	SENSITIVITY, % (95% CI)	SPECIFICITY, % (95% CI)
Sodium-to-Potassium Ratio		
< 40	100 (93-100)	15 (9-23)
< 35	94 (84-99)	35 (26-44)
< 28	74 (60-84)	84 (75-90)
< 27	70 (56-82)	94 (87-97)
< 24	62 (48-75)	96 (91-990)
< 20	51 (37-65)	100 (97-100)
Lymphocyte Count (cells × 10³/μL) (Reference Range: 0.9 to 5.5)		
> 0.75	100 (93-100)	35 (27-45)
> 1.0	92 (82-98)	46 (37-56)
> 1.2	89 (77-96)	56 (47-66)
> 1.4	87 (75-95)	69 (60-78)
> 1.6	79 (66-89)	77 (68-84)
> 1.8	64 (50-77)	83 (74-89)
> 2.0	58 (44-72)	85 (76-91)
> 2.2	57 (42-70)	89 (82-94)
> 2.4	49 (25-63)	92 (85-96)
> 5.0	19 (9-32)	99 (95-100)
> 6.0	9 (3-21)	100 (97-100)

From Seth M, et al.: White blood cell count and the sodium to potassium ration to screen for hypoadrenocorticism in dogs, *J Vet Intern Med* 25:1351, 2011.
CI, Confidence interval.

– – Na:K ratio
- - - Lymphocyte count
—— Na:K ratio and lymphocyte count logistic model
······ Reference line

FIGURE 12-7 Receiver operating characteristic (ROC) curves for the Na : K ratio *(coarse dashed line)*, absolute lymphocyte count *(fine dashed line)*, and a logistic regression model combining both of these variables *(solid bold line)* for discerning dogs with hypoadrenocorticism (HA) from dogs with a clinical suspicion of HA. The combined Na : K ROC curve is above and to the left of the other ROC curves at almost all values, indicating consistently superior sensitivity and specificity when compared to either variable alone. (From Seth M, et al.: White blood cell count and the sodium to potassium ration to screen for hypoadrenocorticism in dogs, *J Vet Intern Med* 25:1351, 2011.)

they remain transiently sequestered in the lymph nodes and bone marrow rather than entering the efferent lymph and blood. This does not occur in the absence of cortisol. In one study, only 8% of dogs with hypoadrenocorticism had lymphopenia on the CBC (Peterson et al, 1996). In another study, a lymphocyte count more

than 0.75 cells × 10³/μL had a sensitivity of 100%, meaning that all the dogs with hypoadrenocorticism had a lymphocyte count above this value (Fig. 12-7; Seth et al, 2011). Specificity of a lymphocyte count above 0.75 cells × 10³/μL was 35%, indicating that 35% of the dogs with lymphocyte counts more than 0.75 cells × 10³/μL were Addisonian (Table 12-5). Thus in this study the presence of lymphopenia excluded a diagnosis of hypoadrenocorticism (Seth et al, 2011). In the same study, dogs with hypoadrenocorticism had a higher eosinophil count and a lower neutrophil count, but these parameters were less useful in differentiating dogs with hypoadrenocorticism from dogs with other causes of systemic illness (Seth et al, 2011).

Serum Electrolyte Abnormalities

In a retrospective study of 225 dogs with hypoadrenocorticism, 96% of dogs were hyperkalemic and 81% were hyponatremic (Peterson et al, 1996). Other electrolyte abnormalities in dogs with hypoadrenocorticism may include hypochloremia, hyperphosphatemia, and hypercalcemia (see Table 12-4). Hypocalcemia occurs less commonly (9% of dogs) and is usually attributable to concurrent hypoalbuminemia (see Total Calcium/Ionized Calcium). Other serum biochemical abnormalities that have been reported in dogs with hypoadrenocorticism include azotemia, hypoalbuminemia, hypocholesterolemia, hypoglycemia, and increased liver enzymes. Appropriate treatment of hypoadrenocorticism results in complete resolution of these changes.

Hyponatremia and Hyperkalemia

Hyponatremia and hyperkalemia are caused by aldosterone deficiency with a resultant failure of the kidneys to conserve sodium (see Consequences of Mineralocorticoid Deficiency). Because sodium ions are exchanged for either potassium or hydrogen ions, impairment of renal tubular potassium and hydrogen secretion causes hyperkalemia and metabolic acidosis. Failure to conserve sodium results in profound fluid loss, shift of K+ ions to the extracellular compartment, prerenal azotemia due to decreased renal perfusion, and progressive hypovolemia. Glucocorticoid deficiency also contributes to hyponatremia due to increased secretion of vasopressin.

Sodium-to-Potassium Ratio. The normal Na:K ratio ranges from 27:1 to 40:1. Because of hyponatremia and hyperkalemia, the Na:K ratio is often low in dogs with hypoadrenocorticism, and this ratio can be used as a guide for planning emergency diagnosis and treatment while waiting for definitive test results. It is important to remember that electrolyte concentrations, and therefore the Na:K ratio, can be completely normal in dogs with both primary and secondary hypoadrenocorticism.

In a retrospective study of 76 dogs with hypoadrenocorticism and 200 control dogs, a Na:K ratio less than 24 was 100% specific for a diagnosis of hypoadrenocorticism (Adler et al, 2007); however, other studies have reported much lower specificity for the Na:K ratio. In two studies evaluating dogs with Na:K ratios less than 24 to 27, the proportion of dogs that had hypoadrenocorticism was 17% to 24%, suggesting that many other disorders can cause marked changes in the Na:K ratio (Roth and Tyler, 1999; Nielsen et al, 2008). Problems other than hypoadrenocorticism that were commonly associated with a low Na:K ratio included renal and urinary tract disease, gastrointestinal disease, cardiorespiratory disease, and sample contamination with potassium ethylenediaminetetraacetic acid (EDTA).

Normal Electrolytes in Hypoadrenocorticism. Although hyponatremia and hyperkalemia are the classic hallmarks of hypoadrenocorticism, it is now recognized that as many as 30% of dogs with hypoadrenocorticism lack these changes. This has been referred to as *atypical hypoadrenocorticism* or *glucocorticoid deficient hypoadrenocorticism.* In a study of 25 Nova Scotia Duck Tolling Retrievers with hypoadrenocorticism, 32% lacked both hyperkalemia and hyponatremia at the time of diagnosis (Hughes et al, 2007). In a retrospective study of 46 dogs with hypoadrenocorticism presented to a veterinary teaching hospital, 24% lacked hyponatremia and hyperkalemia (Thompson et al, 2007). Dogs without electrolyte changes tend to be older, have a longer duration of clinical signs, and are more likely to be anemic, hypoalbuminemic, and hypocholesterolemic. Reasons for normal electrolytes in dogs with hypoadrenocorticism include secondary hypoadrenocorticism, selective destruction of the ZF and reticularis, early stage disease in which destruction of the ZG is not complete, compensation for natriuresis by increased salt intake, or concurrent illnesses (e.g., hypothyroidism) that can mask electrolyte changes. In one report of dogs with hypoadrenocorticism that had symptoms of gastrointestinal hemorrhage, typical electrolyte changes were present initially, but by the time of referral the dogs were either normokalemic or even hypokalemic (Medinger et al, 1993). The decrease in serum potassium concentration by the

time of referral was attributed to anorexia, diarrhea, and administration of potassium-free fluids.

Concurrent diseases causing anorexia and decreased metabolic rate due to hypothyroidism can also mask the typical electrolyte changes of hypoadrenocorticism. Some dogs with primary adrenal failure will initially have normal electrolytes and later develop electrolyte abnormalities indicative of mineralocorticoid deficiency weeks to months later. In a retrospective study of eleven dogs with hypoadrenocorticism that lacked electrolyte changes at time of diagnosis, only one dog ultimately progressed to mineralocorticoid deficiency over a follow up time of 1 to 4½ years (Thompson et al, 2007). Other studies also suggest that only a small percentage of dogs with hypoadrenocorticism later progress to mineralocorticoid deficiency (Lifton et al, 1996; Sadek and Schaer, 1996; Baumstark et al, 2014). Most dogs that progress to develop evidence of mineralocorticoid deficiency do so within the first year after diagnosis. Because of the recognition of this less common presentation of hypoadrenocorticism, the absence of hyponatremia or hyperkalemia in a dog with suspected hypoadrenocorticism should not exclude the diagnosis; conversely reliance on measurement of electrolytes alone for diagnosis of hypoadrenocorticism is misleading, because there are many other causes of hyperkalemia and hyponatremia (Box 12-3). A suspicion of

---

BOX 12-3   Differential Diagnosis for Hyperkalemia and/or Hyponatremia in Dogs and Cats

  I. Hypoadrenocorticism
 II. Renal and urinary tract disease
   A. Primary acute renal failure
   B. Chronic severe oliguric or anuric renal failure
   C. Urethral obstruction longer than 24 hours duration
   D. Urine leakage into the peritoneal cavity
III. Severe liver failure
   A. Cirrhosis
   B. Neoplasia
IV. Severe gastrointestinal disease
   A. Parasitic infection
   B. Salmonellosis
   C. Viral enteritis (parvovirus)
   D. Gastric torsion
   E. Duodenal perforation
   F. Gastrointestinal malabsorption
  V. Severe metabolic or respiratory acidosis
   A. Diabetic ketoacidosis
   B. Pancreatitis
 VI. Pleural effusion
   A. Chylous effusion
   B. Repeated drainage of effusions
VII. Congestive heart failure (hyponatremia)
VIII. Massive tissue destruction
   A. Crush injury
   B. Extensive infection
   C. Hemolysis
 IX. Primary polydipsia (hyponatremia)
  X. Artifact
   A. Hyperkalemia
      1. Blood storage and hemolysis (especially from Akitas)
      2. Extreme leukocytosis or thrombocytosis
   B. Hyponatremia
      1. Lipemia

hypoadrenocorticism based on the presence of abnormal electrolytes should always be confirmed by an ACTH stimulation test.

Differential Diagnosis for Hyperkalemia and Hyponatremia. Dogs with hypoadrenocorticism must be distinguished from those with non-adrenal causes of hyperkalemia (see Box 12-3). Although the acute management of hyperkalemia is similar regardless of its cause (except for the need for specific treatment of urinary obstruction), the clinician must be certain of the diagnosis of hypoadrenocorticism because it requires lifelong therapy.

Renal and Urinary Tract Disorders. The most common non-adrenal causes of hyperkalemia are acute renal failure, urethral obstruction, and rupture of the bladder or ureter. Hyperkalemia is less common in chronic renal failure unless the dog or cat is terminally anuric or oliguric.

Gastrointestinal Disease. Gastrointestinal disorders may also result in serum electrolyte abnormalities consistent with Addison's disease. These electrolyte disturbances have been reported in dogs with intestinal parasitism (trichuriasis, ancylostomiasis), intestinal infection (salmonellosis), perforated duodenal ulcers, and gastric torsion (DiBartola et al, 1985; DiBartola, 1989; Roth and Tyler, 1999). Similar serum electrolyte abnormalities have been encountered in puppies with parvovirus infection or canine distemper. Severe malabsorption syndromes also occasionally cause hyperkalemia or hyponatremia or both. Hyponatremia in dogs with gastrointestinal disease is due to replacement of sodium lost from the gastrointestinal tract due to diarrhea by free water. Hyperkalemia is the result of hypovolemia, metabolic acidosis, and most importantly decreased renal distal tubular flow rate. Potassium secretion in the renal distal tubule depends on the serum potassium concentration, the cellular sodium-potassium ATPase activity induced by aldosterone, the electrochemical gradient that results from sodium reabsorption, and the luminal potassium concentration. Decreased distal tubular flow rate, especially in conjunction with hyponatremia, impairs potassium secretion because of poor sodium delivery (decreased electrochemical gradient) and potassium saturation of the luminal fluid (decreased concentration gradient) despite normal or increased concentration of aldosterone (Rose, 2001; Bissett et al, 2001). Dogs with trichuriasis, hyponatremia, and hyperkalemia do not have decreased serum concentrations of aldosterone (Graves et al, 1994).

Acidosis, Pancreatitis, and/or Trauma. Rapid cellular release of potassium and resultant hyperkalemia may occur as a result of severe acidosis or tissue destruction after surgery, crush injury, or inflammation. Although not common, examples of disorders that can cause hyperkalemia are pancreatitis, diabetic ketoacidosis, aortic thrombosis, and rhabdomyolysis secondary to heat stroke or prolonged exercise. These conditions may also be associated with impaired renal excretion of potassium.

Acidosis and insulin deficiency in diabetic ketoacidosis may lead to hyperkalemia, whereas hyperglycemia and hyperosmolality may result in concurrent hyponatremia (Roth and Tyler, 1999).

Pleural Effusions. Hyperkalemia and hyponatremia have been identified in some dogs with chylous pleural effusion after repeated pleural drainage procedures (Willard et al, 1991). Similar serum electrolyte abnormalities were identified in a dog with nonseptic, nonchylous effusion (Zenger, 1992). The incidence of these serum electrolyte abnormalities appears to be low, because only two of 17 dogs with experimentally induced chylothorax had hyperkalemia and hyponatremia (Fossum and Birchard, 1986; Willard et al, 1991). Hyperkalemia and hyponatremia may result from sodium loss in situations in which the effusion is drained, or from decreased effective circulating volume that causes activation of the renin-angiotensin-aldosterone axis and sodium and water

retention. Stimulation of thirst, impairment of free water excretion, and decreased renal distal tubular flow, combined with decreased sodium intake contribute to hyponatremia in this scenario (Willard et al, 1991).

Iatrogenic and/or Drug Therapy. Excess potassium intake is an uncommon cause of hyperkalemia except in patients with renal insufficiency. Hyperkalemia can develop with overzealous potassium supplementation in intravenous fluids, use of potassium containing salt substitutes, or administration of parenteral feeding solutions high in potassium. Potassium-sparing diuretics, angiotensin-converting enzyme inhibitors, and nonsteroidal anti-inflammatory drugs (NSAIDs) also have the potential to cause mild hyperkalemia (Willard, 1989). Renal excretion of potassium may also be decreased by drugs (e.g., trimethoprim), which block the luminal sodium ion channel in the cortical collecting tubule (Rubin et al, 1998).

Artifact. In vitro increases in the serum potassium concentration may occur due to sample contamination with potassium EDTA, or in some breeds if separation of red blood cells from plasma is delayed. The Akita breed appears to have unusually large concentrations of potassium in the red blood cells. In one study, six of eight Akitas had high erythrocyte potassium concentrations, and plasma from affected dogs displayed pseudohyperkalemia after being refrigerated in contact with red cells for longer than 4 hours (Rich et al, 1986). The rise in the plasma potassium concentration (pseudohyperkalemia) was progressive with prolonged red cell contact and was accompanied by a fall in plasma sodium. Extreme leukocytosis (> 100,000 mm³) or thrombocytosis (> 1,000,000 mm³) may allow sufficient amounts of potassium to be released into the serum during clotting to also falsely elevate the serum potassium value.

Lipemia. Lipemia may cause a false decrease in the plasma sodium concentration by displacing the aqueous plasma phase in which sodium ions are found. When the plasma sodium is measured, it is calculated based on the total volume of plasma including the lipid phase, which results in an artifactual hyponatremia.

Miscellaneous Disorders

Low sodium:potassium ratios have been described in dogs with pyometra, perhaps as a result of acidosis, gastrointestinal signs, and severe dehydration. Hyperkalemia and hyponatremia have also been described in three near-term pregnant Greyhounds (Schaer et al, 2000) and in dogs with disseminated neoplasia, congestive heart failure, and mushroom toxicity (Roth and Tyler, 1999).

Total Calcium/Ionized Calcium

An increase in total calcium concentration occurs in 30% to 40% of dogs with hypoadrenocorticism (Peterson and Feinman, 1982; Peterson et al, 1996; Adamantos and Boag, 2008), whereas 18% of dogs have ionized hypercalcemia (Adler et al, 2007). Increased total calcium may occur together with either increased or decreased ionized calcium (Adler et al, 2007; Adamantos and Boag, 2008). The mechanisms by which hypercalcemia occurs in Addison's disease are poorly understood, but volume contraction, decreased GFR, increased intestinal absorption of calcium, and decreased urinary excretion of calcium have been proposed. In eight dogs with concurrent hypoadrenocorticism and hypercalcemia, parathyroid hormone, parathyroid hormone related peptide, and 1,25 dihydroxyvitamin D concentrations were within their respective reference ranges in the majority of cases (Gow et al, 2009). An inverse relationship between venous pH and ionized calcium has been documented in dogs with hypoadrenocorticism, suggesting that acidosis may contribute to ionized hypercalcemia (Adler et al, 2007). Acidemia can lead to mild ionized hypercalcemia by decreasing protein binding of calcium. See Chapter 15 for more information regarding hypercalcemia.

Azotemia

Azotemia is common in hypoadrenocorticism due to hypovolemia, hypotension, and decreased renal perfusion (see Table 12-4). Delayed treatment of hypoadrenocorticism may result in secondary renal damage, although permanent renal failure is uncommon. In dogs with hypoadrenocorticism that are azotemic, serum creatinine concentrations are less likely to be increased than blood urea nitrogen (BUN) and sometimes are not increased to the same degree as BUN. One possible explanation for this disparity is hemorrhage into the gastrointestinal tract, which is common in Addison's disease. Gastrointestinal bleeding provides substrate for the production of ammonia, which is then absorbed into the portal circulation and converted to urea (BUN) by the liver. In such animals, BUN will be higher than predicted by the serum creatinine concentration.

Low Urine Specific Gravity

The urine specific gravity in a dog with normal renal function and prerenal uremia secondary to dehydration and decreased cardiac output should be greater than 1.030, whereas urine specific gravity in a dog with primary renal failure is within or near the isosthenuric range (1.008 to 1.020). Most dogs with hypoadrenocorticism have an impaired ability to concentrate urine because chronic urinary sodium loss causes a reduction in the renal medullary sodium content, loss of the normal medullary concentration gradient, and impaired capacity for water resorption by the renal collecting tubules. Hyponatremia also interferes with stimulation of vasopressin release by reducing serum osmolality. As a result, 60% of dogs with hypoadrenocorticism have urine specific gravity consistent with that expected in a dog with primary renal failure (see Table 12-4). Thus it may be difficult to distinguish hypoadrenocorticism from primary renal failure without measurement of serum cortisol concentrations (Box 12-4); hypoadrenocorticism should always be considered in an ill dog with azotemia and isosthenuria.

Hypoglycemia

Hypoglycemia occurs in up to 30% of dogs with hypoadrenocorticism and may be severe enough to cause seizures (Levy, 1994; Syme and Scott-Moncrieff, 1998; Lifton et al, 1996). Glucocorticoid deficiency causes decreased hepatic gluconeogenesis and increased peripheral sensitivity to insulin. Most, but not all dogs with hypoglycemia have other biochemical findings supportive of hypoadrenocorticism, such as hypocholesterolemia, hypoalbuminemia, and azotemia. Insulin concentrations in dogs with hypoadrenocorticism do not differ from those of dogs with nonadrenal illness (Gow et al, 2012). See Chapter 9 for more information regarding hypoglycemia.

Hypoalbuminemia and Hypocholesterolemia

Hypoalbuminemia and hypocholesterolemia are common in dogs with hypoadrenocorticism, and both abnormalities are more common in dogs with glucocorticoid deficient

---

BOX 12-4   Overlapping Clinical Manifestations of Hypoadrenocorticism Versus Other Diseases

I. Renal disease
   A. Weight loss, poor appetite, vomiting, and diarrhea
   B. Increased BUN, creatinine, acidosis; low albumin
   C. Urine specific gravity 1.008 to 1.020, when ill
   D. Responsive to IV fluids
II. Gastrointestinal disease
   A. Weight loss, poor appetite, vomiting, and diarrhea
   B. Decreased serum albumin and cholesterol
   C. Abnormal serum biochemistries correct with IV fluids
   D. Abnormal biopsies may be obtained
III. Hepatic disease
   A. Weight loss, poor appetite, vomiting, and diarrhea
   B. Decreased albumin, cholesterol, glucose ± BUN
   C. Microhepatia: Radiography or ultrasonography
   D. Abnormal liver enzyme activity ± liver function test results
   E. Abnormal liver biopsy results

BUN, Blood urea nitrogen; *IV*, intravenous.

---

hypoadrenocorticism (Langlais-Burgess et al, 1995; Thompson et al, 2007). This may be because dogs without electrolyte abnormalities are less likely to be hypovolemic and because these cases often have a longer duration of clinical signs prior to diagnosis (Thompson et al, 2007). Hypocholesterolemia in dogs with hypoadrenocorticism may be the result of either decreased fat absorption, or concurrent hepatopathy (Lifton et al, 1996). Glucocorticoids are believed to be important in fat absorption, and steatorrhea occurs in some people with hypoadrenocorticism. The cause of hypoalbuminemia in dogs with hypoadrenocorticism is unknown, but proposed mechanisms include anorexia, gastrointestinal blood loss due to mucosal ulceration, decreased synthesis due to hepatopathy, and protein losing enteropathy. Glucocorticoids have been reported to influence digestion and intestinal absorption of nutrients, especially amino acids. Increased vascular permeability has been documented in animals with glucocorticoid deficiency and could be the cause of protein losing enteropathy (Langlais-Burgess et al, 1995). Albumin is a negative acute phase protein, and thus hypoalbuminemia could also occur in dogs with hypoadrenocorticism and concurrent inflammation; however, most dogs with hypoadrenocorticism do not have evidence of concurrent inflammation.

Hepatic Dysfunction

Thirty percent of dogs with hypoadrenocorticism have mild increases in hepatic enzymes, and because these dogs may have concurrent hypoalbuminemia, hypocholesterolemia, and hypoglycemia, hypoadrenocorticism can mimic hepatic failure. Abnormalities in liver function tests (bile acids, ammonia tolerance test) have been reported in some dogs with hypoadrenocorticism (Feldman and Nelson, 2004). It has been speculated that immune mediated hepatitis may occur concurrently with hypoadrenocorticism in some dogs. Alternatively the liver could be secondarily affected due to hypotension and impaired tissue perfusion. Regardless, hepatic abnormalities detected in dogs with hypoadrenocorticism resolve with no specific treatment other than that for hypoadrenocorticism.

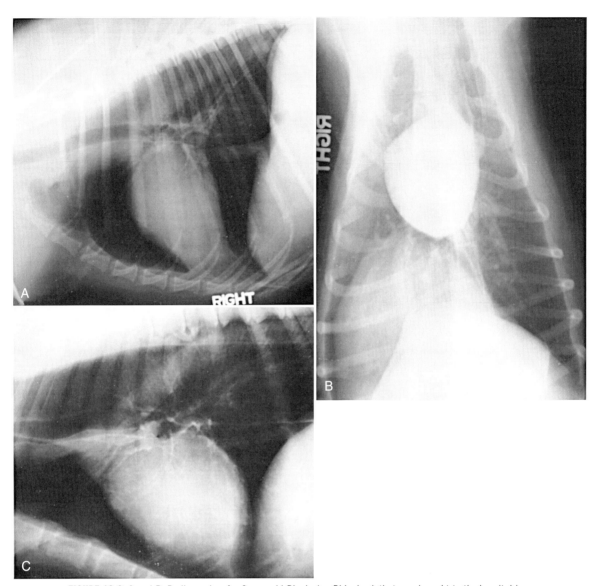

FIGURE 12-8 A and **B,** Radiographs of a 3-year-old Rhodesian Ridgeback that was brought to the hospital in a shock-like state secondary to hypoadrenocorticism. Note the small heart on both views and the small pulmonary vasculature due to poor cardiac output. **C,** Lateral thoracic view radiograph of a 5-year-old hypoadrenal dog with microcardia, a flattened caudal vena cava, and a dilated, air-filled esophagus. The esophageal dilation, which is seen occasionally in hypoadrenocorticism, is reversible with appropriate hormonal therapy for the primary disease.

Acid-Base Status

Hypoaldosteronism impairs renal tubular hydrogen ion secretion, which in conjunction with hypotension and poor perfusion of tissues, most likely accounts for the mild acidosis documented in many dogs suffering from hypoadrenocorticism. The metabolic acidosis is typically mild and rarely requires specific treatment. Adequate fluid and mineralocorticoid replacement therapy should restore renal perfusion, which in turn enhances urinary hydrogen ion excretion.

RADIOGRAPHY

Most untreated dogs with hypoadrenocorticism have one or more radiographic abnormalities on thoracic and abdominal radiographs, including microcardia, small cranial lobar pulmonary artery, narrow posterior vena cava, or microhepatia

(Fig. 12-8) (Melián et al, 1999). Changes occur as a result of hypovolemia; therefore they are more likely to be present in dogs with electrolyte abnormalities. Megaesophagus or esophageal dilation that is reversible with treatment of hypoadrenocorticism has been reported to occur in a small proportion of dogs with classic hypoadrenocorticism as well as those with glucocorticoid deficiency alone (Bartges and Nielson, 1992; Whitley, 1995; Lifton et al, 1996). In one study of 225 dogs with hypoadrenocorticism, one dog with megaesophagus was reported (Peterson et al, 1996); however, in a study of dogs with secondary hypoadrenocorticism, four of eleven dogs that had thoracic radiographs taken were diagnosed with megaesophagus (Lifton et al, 1996). Why some dogs with Addison's disease develop esophageal dilation is not clear. It has been proposed that the condition might be attributable to the effect of abnormal serum sodium and potassium concentrations on

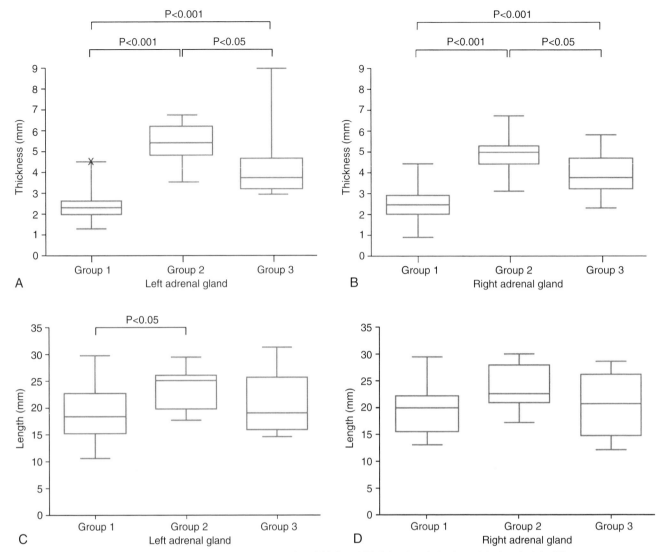

FIGURE 12-9 Measurements of the thickness of the **(A)** left and **(B)** right adrenal glands, and the length of the **(C)** left and **(D)** right adrenal glands for three groups of dogs. *Group 1,* Dogs with primary hypoadrenocorticism; *Group 2,* healthy control dogs; *Group 3.* dogs with diseases mimicking adrenal insufficiency. P values are indicated where differences between groups are significant. Note that in **A** the overlap between Groups 1 and 2 is limited to one dog indicated by X. (From Wenger M, et al.: Ultrasonographic evaluation of adrenal glands in dogs with primary hypoadrenocorticism and mimicking diseases, *Vet Rec* 167:207, 2010.)

membrane potential and neuromuscular function (Burrows, 1987); however, abnormal serum electrolyte concentrations are not always documented (Bartges and Nielson, 1992; Whitley, 1995). Cortisol deficiency and its associated muscle weakness may be the cause of megaesophagus because the condition typically resolves with treatment.

ABDOMINAL ULTRASOUND

Most dogs with hypoadrenocorticism have a measurable reduction in size of the adrenal glands on ultrasound examination, and sometimes the adrenal glands, particularly the right adrenal gland, cannot be identified by ultrasonography (Hoerauf, 1999). In a study of thirty dogs with hypoadrenocorticism, 14 healthy dogs, and 10 dogs with other causes of hyperkalemia and hyponatremia, the dogs with hypoadrenocorticism had significantly thinner adrenal glands than the other two groups and their left adrenal glands were also significantly shorter than

those of healthy dogs (Fig. 12-9; Wenger et al, 2010). The best discrimination between dogs with hypoadrenocorticism and those with normal adrenal function was obtained by measurement of the thickness of the left adrenal gland. Twenty eight of 29 dogs with hypoadrenocorticism had left adrenal gland thickness less than 3.2 mm, and there was minimal overlap between the groups. The right adrenal gland could not be visualized in eight dogs and was less than 3.2 mm in 18 of 22 dogs. Although there is some overlap, a left adrenal gland measuring less than 3.2 mm is strongly suggestive of hypoadrenocorticism. It is important to remember that identification of normal sized adrenal glands on ultrasound examination does not preclude a diagnosis of hypoadrenocorticism, and the presence of small adrenal glands, although supportive of a diagnosis of hypoadrenocorticism, is not adequate for confirmation. Normal adrenal gland size in Addisonian dogs may be the result of inflammation early in the disease process or more rarely may suggest granulomatous destruction, necrosis, or infiltrative disease, such as lymphoma or metastatic neoplasia (Parnell et al, 1999; Labelle and De Cock, 2005; Korth et al, 2008; Kook et al, 2010). Measurement of increased resistive index due to abnormal renal blood flow has been documented in a dog with hypoadrenocorticism (Koch et al, 1997). This presumably reflects renal vasoconstriction due to increased activity of the renin-angiotensin system.

ELECTROCARDIOGRAPHY

Potassium plays an important role in cell function and neuromuscular transmission and the effects of hyperkalemia in patients with hypoadrenocorticism can be life threatening. The most significant clinical effect of hyperkalemia is disturbed cardiac conduction, which can lead to bradycardia, ventricular fibrillation, or ventricular standstill, and can result in cardiac arrest. Plasma hyperkalemia decreases the ratio between intracellular potassium and plasma potassium resulting in a decrease in the resting membrane potential. Although this should increase membrane excitability, because persistent depolarization inactivates sodium channels in the cell membrane, there is actually a net decrease in excitability manifested clinically as muscle weakness and disturbed cardiac conduction (Rose, 2001).

Hyperkalemia results in a characteristic sequence of changes on the electrocardiogram (ECG) that reflect the effects of hyperkalemia on atrial and ventricular depolarization (P wave and QRS complex changes) and repolarization (represented by changes in the T wave for ventricular repolarization). Thus the ECG is a useful tool for rapid detection of hyperkalemia (Fig. 12-10). The earliest changes observed with mild hyperkalemia (potassium concentrations of 6.0 to 7.0 mEq/L) include "peaking" of T waves and a shortened QT interval. As the potassium rises above 7.0 mEq/L, there is prolongation of the PR interval and widening of the QRS complex and decreased amplitude, widening and eventual loss of the P wave when the potassium concentration exceeds 7.5 to 8.0 mEq/L. The final change that typically occurs as the potassium concentration increases greater than 10 to 11 mEq/L is a sine-wave pattern as the widened QRS complex merges with the T wave, followed by ventricular fibrillation or standstill.

It is important to remember that these potassium concentrations are only guidelines. Other factors such as hyponatremia, hypocalcemia, acidemia, and a rapid change in the potassium concentration enhance the effects of hyperkalemia, whereas hypercalcemia and hypernatremia counteract the membrane changes of hyperkalemia and decrease the cardiac effects of hyperkalemia; thus there is significant inter-patient variability in the cardiac effect of a certain potassium concentration. Regardless of its cause, marked hyperkalemia is an emergency situation that demands a quick therapeutic response. In addition to providing a tool for early recognition of hyperkalemia, the ECG also allows the clinician to easily, reliably, and inexpensively monitor therapy. As the hyperkalemia is treated, the various abnormalities present on an ECG resolve.

CONFIRMING THE DIAGNOSIS

Hormones that can be measured in the diagnostic approach to dogs with suspected hypoadrenocorticism include cortisol, aldosterone, endogenous ACTH, and renin concentrations. Although most dogs with hypoadrenocorticism have a deficiency of cortisol and aldosterone, routine diagnostic testing relies on measurement of cortisol concentrations. Aldosterone

concentrations are less commonly measured because the assay is not routinely run by commercial diagnostic laboratories. Aldosterone deficiency is presumed in dogs with hypocortisolemia that have hyponatremia and hyperkalemia. There are some weaknesses to this approach (see Glucocorticoid Deficiency Versus Mineralocorticoid Deficiency). Some dogs with hypoadrenocorticism that have normal electrolytes have low aldosterone concentrations, and some dogs with electrolyte abnormalities consistent with mineralocorticoid deficiency have normal or only slightly decreased aldosterone concentrations (Baumstark et al, 2014).

Basal Cortisol Concentrations

Plasma cortisol concentrations can be measured by radioimmunoassay, chemiluminescent assay, or enzyme-linked immunosorbent assay (ELISA; Russell et al, 2007). Reference ranges for plasma cortisol differ depending upon the specific assay. In-house cortisol assays are also available, but validation data have not been published in the peer reviewed literature; so results should be interpreted with caution. Cortisol is stable in plasma and urine at 4° C and 25° C for 5 days but decreases in serum at 4° C, 25° C, and 37° C (compared to 20° C; Behrend, 1995).

Measurement of a normal resting (basal) cortisol concentration is a useful test that can be used to exclude a diagnosis of hypoadrenocorticism. This approach is particularly helpful in dogs that have chronic clinical signs of illness. In a study of 123 dogs evaluated for suspicion of hypoadrenocorticism (110 with non-adrenal illness and 13 with hypoadrenocorticism), measurement of a basal cortisol less than 2 µg/dL was 100% sensitive for diagnosis of hypoadrenocorticism (Lennon et al, 2007; Fig. 12-11). In a study investigating 28 dogs with non-adrenal illness, pre-ACTH cortisol concentrations were less than 2.0 µg/dL in only 15 of 56 (27%) samples, suggesting that an ACTH stimulation test would have been unnecessary to rule out a diagnosis of hypoadrenocorticism in 73% of dogs (Fig. 12-12). Although a basal cortisol concentration more than 2.0 µg/dL is helpful in ruling out hypoadrenocorticism, it is important to understand that documentation of a low basal cortisol concentration is not adequate to confirm the diagnosis, because some normal dogs with a normal adrenal axis have a low basal cortisol concentration yet have a normal response to ACTH administration.

Adrenocorticotropic Hormone Stimulation Test

The ACTH stimulation test is a test of adrenal reserve and is considered the gold standard test for confirmation of a diagnosis of hypoadrenocorticism. Initial emergency treatment may need to be based on presence of characteristic clinical signs and electrolyte abnormalities; however the diagnosis should always be confirmed with an ACTH stimulation test prior to initiating long term treatment. Once treatment has been initiated, it is very difficult if not impossible to confirm the diagnosis without withdrawing treatment for several weeks. Synthetic polypeptides containing the biologically active first 24 amino acids of ACTH (Cortrosyn [cosyntropin] or Synacthen [tetracosactrin]) are the products of choice for performing an ACTH stimulation test (Behrend, 2013). Not all of these products have been directly compared in dogs but they are considered interchangeable. The lowest dose of ACTH that stimulates maximal secretion of cortisol in healthy dogs is 0.5 µg/kg (Martin, 2007). The lowest dose shown to result in maximal cortical stimulation in dogs with suspected adrenal

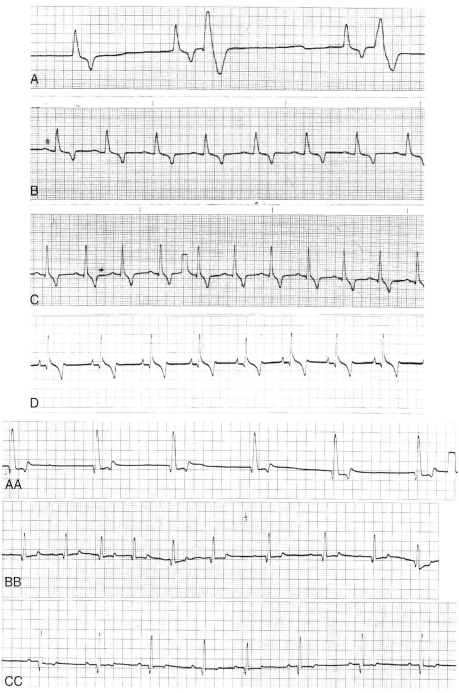

FIGURE 12-10 Serial electrocardiogram (ECG) segments obtained from two dogs with hypoadrenocorticism and hyperkalemia. **A** and **AA** both illustrate the effect of severe hyperkalemia, with the dog in **A** having a serum potassium concentration of 8.6 mEq/L and the dog in **AA** a measurement of 9.4 mEq/L. Note the lack of visible P waves, the short and wide QRS complexes, and the T waves, which are not of excessive amplitude. The ECG in **A** also reveals a bizarre-looking QRS complex following a more normal-appearing QRS complex. This bizarre wave represents a ventricular escape beat that could be the result of hypoxia or hyperkalemia or both. **B** and **BB** are ECGs from the same dogs as in **A** and **AA,** respectively. They were each obtained approximately 1 hour after institution of intravenous normal saline administration as the only treatment. The serum potassium concentrations had decreased to 7.6 mEq/L and 7.9 mEq/L, respectively. Two important factors to note: (1) improvement is seen in each case with the return of P waves, a more rapid heart rate, and disappearance of ventricular escape beats; and (2) abnormalities are still present, most obviously the prolonged P-R intervals (first-degree heart block), which alone suggest hyperkalemia, especially when associated with a widened QRS complex and a short Q-T interval. There are numerous other causes of P-R interval prolongation. In **C** and **CC,** the serum potassium concentrations are considerably lower, 6.2 mEq/L and 5.9 mEq/L, respectively. The P-R interval and P, QRS, and T waves are of shorter duration, and the R waves are taller. **D,** ECG from the dog in **A;** the serum potassium concentration is 5.6 mEq/L and a more spiked T wave is seen. (From Ettinger SJ: *Textbook of veterinary internal medicine,* ed 2, Philadelphia, 1983, WB Saunders.)

dysfunction is 5 μg/kg (Lathan, 2008). No differences in peak cortisol response between dosages of 5 μg/kg or 250 μg/dog have been documented in either healthy dogs or dogs with clinical signs of hypoadrenocorticism; therefore a dose of 5 μg/kg is recommended to decrease the cost of testing (Kerl, 1999; Frank et al, 2000; Behrend et al, 2006; Lathan et al, 2008; Fig. 12-13). Although

there are differences in peak concentration and duration of ACTH when administered intravenously versus intramuscularly, there is no difference in peak cortisol concentration in response to cosyntropin administered either intravenously or intramuscularly (Hansen et al, 1994; Cohen and Feldman, 2012). Blood samples for measurement of serum cortisol should be collected prior to and 60 to 90 minutes after administration of ACTH (Frank et al, 2000; Frank et al, 2004). Most protocols recommend that the second sample is collected at 60 minutes. Synthetic ACTH can be reconstituted and frozen at –20 ° C in plastic syringes for 6 months with no adverse effects on bioavailability (Frank and Oliver, 1998). Use of compounded ACTH gel is an alternative if synthetic ACTH is not available; however potential variability between compounding pharmacies makes this a less than ideal choice (Hill, 2004). In one study, cortisol concentrations at 60 minutes after administration were no different when compounded ACTH was administered at a dose of 2.2 U/kg IM compared to cosyntropin at 5 μg/kg IV, although there were differences at later time points (Kemppainen et al, 2005). Depot tetracosactide (250 μg intramuscularly [IM]) produced similar cortisol responses to cosyntropin at a dose of 5 μg/kg IV in healthy dogs, but it has not been evaluated in dogs with adrenal dysfunction (Ginel et al, 2012). Dogs do not exhibit a circadian rhythm in cortisol secretion, so the ACTH stimulation test can be performed at any time of day. In dogs with suspected hypoadrenocorticism, the ACTH stimulation test should be performed as soon as logistically possible. Fasting is not necessary unless the cortisol assay used is influenced by lipemia.

If it is clinically necessary to administer corticosteroids prior to performing the ACTH stimulation test, dexamethasone should be

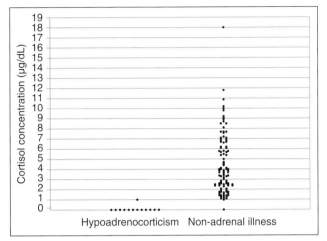

FIGURE 12-11 Basal serum or plasma cortisol concentrations in 13 dogs with hypoadrenocorticism and 110 dogs with non-adrenal gland illnesses. Samples with no detectable cortisol (< 1.0 μg/dL) were plotted with a value of 0. (From Lennon EM, et al.: Use of basal serum or plasma cortisol concentrations to rule out a diagnosis of hypoadrenocorticism in dogs: 123 cases (2000-2005), *J Am Vet Med Assoc* 231:413, 2007.)

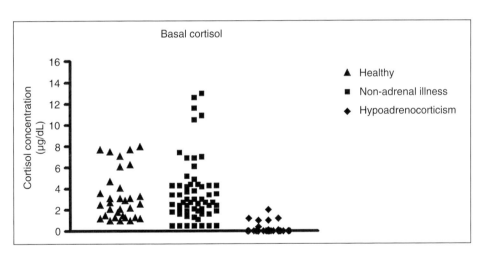

FIGURE 12-12 Basal cortisol concentrations in healthy dogs, dogs with hypoadrenocorticism, and dogs with non-adrenal illness.

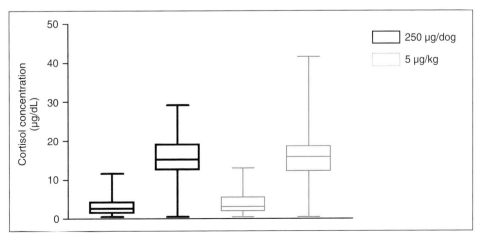

FIGURE 12-13 Plasma cortisol concentrations before and 1 hour following administration of cosyntropin at two different dosages in 28 dogs with suspected hypoadrenocorticism. The cortisol responses to adrenocorticotropic hormone (ACTH) were statistically equivalent.

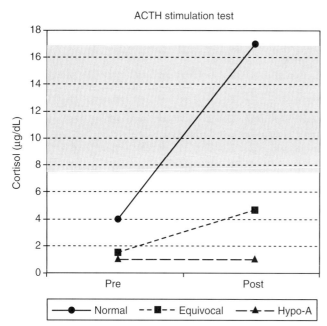

FIGURE 12-14 Response to adrenocorticotropic hormone (ACTH) showing a normal response, borderline response, and lack of suppression consistent with hypoadrenocorticism (post-cortisol < 2.0 µg/dL).

administered because of assay dependent cross reactivity among other steroids (prednisolone, prednisone, methylprednisolone, fludrocortisone, cortisone, and hydrocortisone). Even one dose of dexamethasone will suppress post ACTH cortisol concentration; however cortisol suppression after one dose of up to 5 mg/kg of dexamethasone did not exceed 35% of control, so it is unlikely that one dose would completely abolish the response to ACTH (Kemppainen et al, 1989).

The criteria for confirmation of the diagnosis of hypoadrenocorticism are a pre- and post-ACTH cortisol concentration less than the reference range for basal cortisol (usually 2 µg/dL). In most dogs with hypoadrenocorticism both the pre- and post-cortisol concentrations are less than 1 µg/dL. Although there is usually a clear distinction between the response to ACTH in a dog with hypoadrenocorticism and that of a dog with adequate adrenal reserve, sometimes borderline results occur (post ACTH cortisol concentrations between 2 and 8 µg/dL) (Fig. 12-14). Causes of inadequate response to ACTH stimulation other than hypoadrenocorticism, include prior glucocorticoid administration, treatment with mitotane, trilostane, or ketoconazole, poor potency of compounded ACTH gel, loss of potency of the ACTH product that was administered due to poor or extended storage, use of an inappropriate form or dose of ACTH, and errors in administration or sample collection (Box 12-5). Rarely, dogs with sex hormone secreting adrenal tumors have a suppressed response to ACTH; however, these dogs usually have overt signs of hyperadrenocorticism rather than signs of hypoadrenocorticism. In some cases, no other underlying cause of adrenal suppression can be identified. It is possible that dogs with progressive loss of adrenal function may initially have borderline results, but this is currently poorly documented. In secondary hypoadrenocorticism, the ACTH stimulation test shows no response because of adrenocortical atrophy due to lack of stimulation by ACTH. These cases may have more borderline cortisol concentrations after ACTH stimulation. Although individual data were not reported in a publication of 18 dogs with secondary hypoadrenocorticism, the mean post-ACTH plasma cortisol concentration was less than 2.0 µg/dL, and the highest value was 4.4 µg/dL (Lifton

---

BOX 12-5   Causes of an Inadequate Response in Adrenocorticotropic Hormone Stimulation Test

Primary hypoadrenocorticism
Secondary hypoadrenocorticism
Prior glucocorticoid administration*
Treatment with drugs that suppress adrenal gland function (trilostane, mitotane, ketoconazole)
Loss of potency of ACTH
Use of inappropriate dosage or form of ACTH
Errors in ACTH administration or sample collection
Sex hormone secreting adrenal tumors*
Critical illness related adrenal insufficiency*

ACTH, Adrenocorticotropic hormone.
*These animals may have clinical signs of hyperadrenocorticism.

et al, 1996). Critical illness related adrenal insufficiency (CIRCI, relative adrenal insufficiency) may decrease the relative change in cortisol concentration after ACTH administration, but in this situation the pre-cortisol is usually increased above the reference range (see Critical Illness Related Adrenal Insufficiency [Reactive Adrenal Insufficiency]; Martin et al, 2008). Whether dogs with CIRCI benefit from glucocorticoid supplementation is not yet known. In dogs in which no cause for a subnormal response can be established, the ACTH stimulation test should be repeated 1 to 4 weeks later to rule out whether there was a problem in performing the test and to identify possible progressive adrenal failure. Concurrent measurement of endogenous ACTH concentration in a sample collected prior to ACTH administration may be helpful in interpretation of the follow up ACTH stimulation test.

It is important to understand the limitations of the ACTH stimulation test. The results of ACTH stimulation testing do not distinguish between dogs with naturally occurring primary adrenocortical disease and those with secondary insufficiency due to pituitary failure, secondary insufficiency due to chronic iatrogenic corticosteroid administration, or dogs with primary adrenocortical destruction caused by o,p'-DDD (mitotane) or trilostane overdose. Therefore a detailed history is an important component of test interpretation. It should also be recognized that if hypoadrenocorticism is not present in a dog with systemic illness there may actually be an abnormally high response on the ACTH stimulation test. This should prompt investigation for other causes of systemic illness rather than pursuit of a diagnosis of hyperadrenocorticism.

Endogenous Adrenocorticotropic Hormone Concentration

Both a radioimmunoassay and a chemiluminescent assay have been validated for measurement of plasma ACTH in dogs (Scott-Moncrieff, 2003). Blood collected for measurement of ACTH must be handled with care because plasma ACTH is very labile. To avoid erroneously low values, blood specimens should not be allowed to stand at room temperature for even short periods. Contact with glass must be avoided during collection, separation, and storage, because the ACTH molecule adheres to glass causing erroneously low results. Blood samples should be collected in siliconized tubes containing EDTA as the anticoagulant. Plasma ACTH concentrations can be stored for later assay by freezing plasma samples in plastic containers and freezing (ideally at −20° C or lower). The protocol for sample collection and handling depends upon the assay utilized, and the individual laboratory should be consulted for handling recommendations and reference ranges.

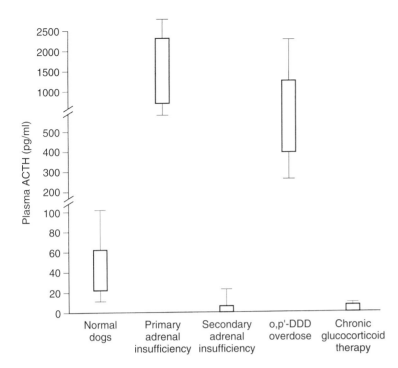

FIGURE 12-15 Plasma endogenous adrenocorticotropic hormone (ACTH) concentrations in normal dogs, dogs with primary adrenocortical failure causing lack of negative feedback to the pituitary, dogs with pituitary failure to secrete ACTH (secondary adrenal insufficiency) causing adrenocortical atrophy, dogs overdosed with the adrenocorticolytic agent o,p'-DDD (mitotane), and dogs chronically treated with glucocorticoids.

In dogs with confirmed hypoadrenocorticism that have normal electrolyte concentrations, measurement of an endogenous (basal) ACTH concentration is recommended to distinguish primary from secondary hypoadrenocorticism (Fig. 12-15). This allows the clinician to determine whether long-term monitoring of electrolyte concentrations is necessary. Measurement of an ACTH concentration above the reference range confirms a diagnosis of primary hypoadrenocorticism, whereas an ACTH concentration within or below the reference range is consistent with a diagnosis of secondary hypoadrenocorticism. In a study of 40 dogs with hypoadrenocorticism in which basal ACTH was measured, ACTH concentration in 35 dogs with primary hypoadrenocorticism ranged from 44 to 1254 pmol/L, and in five dogs with secondary hypoadrenocorticism it ranged from 1 to 2 pmol/L (reference range, 2.2 to 20 pmol/L; Peterson et al, 1996). Dogs with secondary hypoadrenocorticism would not be expected to ever require mineralocorticoid supplementation, whereas dogs with primary hypoadrenocorticism are at risk for progression to complete adrenal failure and ultimately may require mineralocorticoid as well as glucocorticoid supplementation. Interestingly, in one retrospective study that included 11 dogs with glucocorticoid deficient hypoadrenocorticism, only one dog ultimately developed mineralocorticoid deficiency, despite the fact that the majority of dogs (9 out of 11) were diagnosed as having primary hypoadrenocorticism based on measurement of ACTH concentrations greater than 25 pmol/L (Thompson et al, 2007). In another study of 18 dogs with hypoadrenocorticism that had normal electrolytes, two out of 18 dogs progressed to develop evidence of mineralocorticoid deficiency (Lifton et al, 1996). The number of dogs in this study that had primary versus secondary hypoadrenocorticism was not determined.

Cortisol-to-Adrenocorticotrophic Hormone Ratio

Measurement of cortisol-to-ACTH ratio (CAR) has been proposed as an alternative diagnostic test for primary hypoadrenocorticism in dogs (Javadi et al, 2006). In healthy dogs, cortisol increases in response to an increase in ACTH concentration. In primary hypoadrenocorticism, hypocortisolemia is present

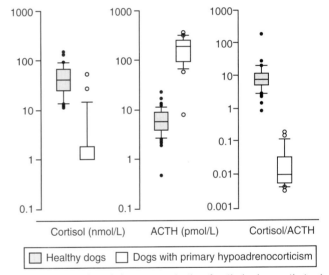

FIGURE 12-16 Box plots of plasma concentration of cortisol, adrenocorticotropic hormone (ACTH), and the cortisol-to-ACTH ratio (CAR) in 60 healthy dogs and 22 dogs with primary hypoadrenocorticism. Outlying data points are represented by *dots* and *open circles*. (From Javadi S, et al.: Aldosterone-to-renin and cortisol-to-adrenocorticotrophic hormone ratios in healthy dogs and dogs with primary hypoadrenocorticism, *J Vet Intern Med* 20:556, 2006.)

despite increased ACTH concentrations. In 22 dogs with primary hypoadrenocorticism and 60 healthy dogs in which cortisol and ACTH concentrations were measured, there was overlap between the groups for all basal hormone concentrations, however there was no overlap between the groups for the CAR (Javadi et al, 2006; Fig. 12-16). This finding was confirmed in another study evaluating healthy dogs, dogs with non-adrenal illness, and dogs with hypoadrenocorticism (Lathan, 2014; Fig. 12-17). These studies suggest that the CAR could potentially be used in place of the ACTH stimulation test for diagnosis of hypoadrenocorticism. The advantage of the CAR over the ACTH stimulation test is the need for collection of only one blood sample and

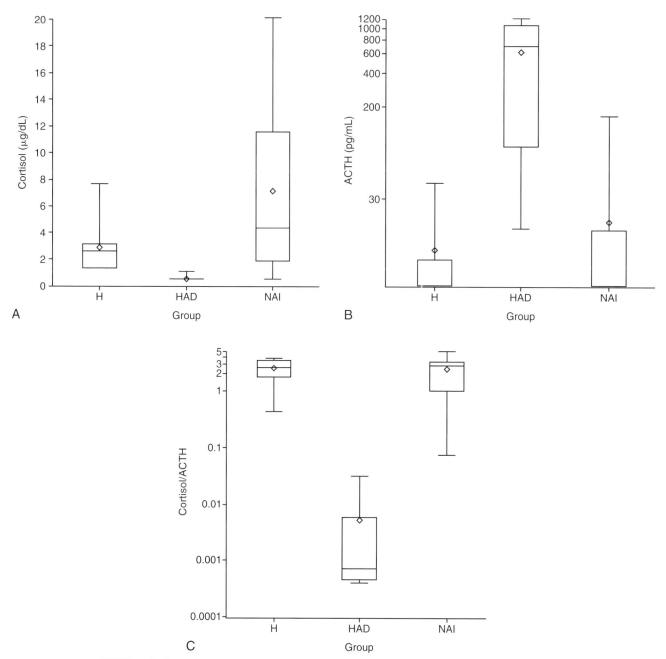

FIGURE 12-17 Box and whiskers plots comparing baseline cortisol **(A)**, adrenocorticotropic hormone (ACTH) concentrations **(B)**, and cortisol-to-ACTH ratio (CAR) **(C)** between three groups of dogs. *H,* Healthy, *HAD,* hypoadrenocorticism, *NAI,* non-adrenal illness. The *box* represents the interquartile range from the 25th to 75th percentile, the *horizontal bar through the box* represents the median, the *diamond in the box* represents the mean, and the *whiskers* represent the minimum and maximum values (range).

the cost savings that result from avoiding the ACTH stimulation test. Disadvantages include the special sample handling needed for samples submitted for measurement of endogenous ACTH and the higher cost of ACTH assays. Whether the CAR would be helpful in diagnosis of secondary hypoadrenocorticism requires further investigation.

Plasma Aldosterone Concentration

Diagnosis of hypoadrenocorticism has historically relied on cortisol concentration as an indicator of adrenal reserve, whereas plasma aldosterone concentrations (PACs) are more rarely

measured; this is primarily because plasma aldosterone assays are not as widely available as cortisol assays (Willard et al, 1987; Golden and Lothrop, 1988). Most studies investigating aldosterone concentrations in dogs have used a commercially available radioimmunoassay that has been validated for use in dogs (Coat-A-Count Aldosterone, Diagnostic Products Corp., Los Angeles, CA) (Sieber-Ruckstuhl, 2006). Samples may be stored refrigerated at 2° to 8° C for 7 days, or they may be stored frozen at –20° C for up to 2 months. Results are not affected by severe icterus, hemolysis, lipemia, or the serum protein concentration. In humans, a high sodium intake tends to suppress serum aldosterone, whereas a low sodium intake may increase values.

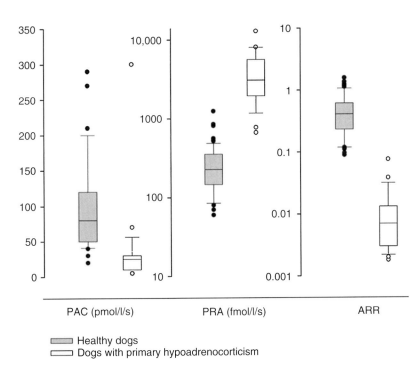

FIGURE 12-18 Box plots of plasma concentration of aldosterone *(PAC)*, plasma renin activity *(PRA)*, and the aldosterone-to-renin ratio *(ARR)* in 60 healthy dogs and 22 dogs with primary hypoadrenocorticism. Outlying data points are represented by *dots* and *open circles*. (From Javadi S, et al.: Aldosterone-to-renin and cortisol-to-adrenocorticotrophic hormone ratios in healthy dogs and dogs with primary hypoadrenocorticism, *J Vet Intern Med* 20:556, 2006.)

It is recommended that aldosterone concentrations are measured before, 30 minutes, and 60 minutes after administration of ACTH because aldosterone concentrations are higher at 30 minutes than 60 minutes in healthy dogs (Carlson, 2010). In dogs with pituitary hyperadrenocorticism treated with mitotane or trilostane, a significantly higher percentage of dogs had decreased aldosterone reserve detected at 30 minutes than at 60 minutes (Reid et al, 2014). However, in a study of seven dogs with hypoadrenocorticism and 22 dogs with non-adrenal illness, aldosterone concentrations were not different at 30, 45, or 60 minutes after ACTH administration, suggesting that earlier sampling times for measurement of aldosterone are not necessary in dogs with suspected hypoadrenocorticism (Baumstark et al, 2014).

In theory, measurement of PAC in dogs with hypoadrenocorticism should allow differentiation of secondary from primary hypoadrenocorticism and be useful in diagnosis of isolated hypoaldosteronism. In the majority of dogs with primary hypoadrenocorticism, aldosterone concentrations would be expected to be low, whereas in secondary hypoadrenocorticism PAC should be normal because ACTH has only a minor influence on aldosterone secretion. In most dogs with primary hypoadrenocorticism, basal and ACTH stimulated aldosterone concentrations are below the reference range (typically 7 to 105 pg/mL), although there is overlap with both healthy dogs and dogs with non-adrenal illness (Javadi et al, 2006; Baumstark et al, 2014). In a study of 70 dogs with hypoadrenocorticism, baseline and ACTH-stimulated aldosterone concentrations were undetectable in 64 out of 70 dogs and low in three dogs (Baumstark et al, 2014; see Fig. 12-5). In three dogs with hypoadrenocorticism, aldosterone concentrations were unexpectedly within the reference range despite the presence of hyperkalemia and hyponatremia. There was no correlation between sodium and aldosterone concentrations in dogs with hypoadrenocorticism in this study, and there was only a weak correlation between aldosterone and serum potassium concentrations (Baumstark et al, 2014). Additionally, in four dogs with primary hypoadrenocorticism that did not have characteristic electrolyte abnormalities, aldosterone concentrations were undetectable, suggesting that other mechanisms must have contributed

to maintenance of normal sodium and potassium in these dogs. There have been few studies investigating aldosterone concentrations in dogs with secondary hypoadrenocorticism. In 14 dogs with secondary hypoadrenocorticism, aldosterone concentrations ranged from normal to low (Feldman and Nelson, 2004). Further studies are necessary to evaluate the value of measurement of PAC concentration in dogs with hypoadrenocorticism. It is also important to recognize that circulating aldosterone concentrations in people are affected by sodium intake and whether the patient is standing or recumbent. These are factors that veterinarians cannot easily control, which makes evaluation of aldosterone concentrations potentially less reliable.

Aldosterone-to-Renin Ratio

Measurement of aldosterone-to-renin ratio (ARR) has been investigated in dogs with primary hypoadrenocorticism (Javadi et al, 2006). In dogs with primary hypoadrenocorticism and hypoaldosteronism, plasma renin activity should be high. In 22 dogs with primary hypoadrenocorticism and 60 normal dogs in which aldosterone and renin concentrations were measured, there was overlap between the groups for basal renin activity and aldosterone concentration; however, there was clear distinction between the groups when the ARR was calculated (Javadi et al, 2006; Fig. 12-18). Although measurement of the ARR has potential for diagnosis of hypoadrenocorticism, renin assays are not widely available and this test is rarely performed.

Cortisol-to-Creatinine Ratio

The cortisol-to-creatinine ratio has not been evaluated for diagnosis of spontaneous hypoadrenocorticism in dogs; however, it has been evaluated in dogs with mitotane and trilostane induced hypoadrenocorticism. Studies suggest that the cortisol-to-creatinine ratio is insensitive for detection of impending adrenocortical insufficiency in mitotane and trilostane treated dogs and is thus unlikely to be helpful in diagnosis of dogs with suspected adrenocortical insufficiency (Angles, 1997; Guptill, 1997; Randolph, 1998; Galac, 2009).

BOX 12-6 Emergency Management of Hypoadrenocorticism

- Place IV catheter in cephalic or jugular vein.
- If in hypovolemic shock, 0.9% saline as 90 mL/kg bolus (given as 20 to 30 mL/kg boluses).
- Continue fluid therapy with 0.9% saline IV, at 40 to 80 mL/kg/hour for next 1 to 2 hours, depending upon severity of hypotension and hyperkalemia. Then continue fluids at rate calculated based on maintenance requirements plus dehydration and ongoing losses. Take care to account for polyuria and polydipsia when considering maintenance requirements. Maintenance requirements may be higher than usual (90 to 120 mL/kg/day).
- If animal is hemodynamically unstable, administer one dose of dexamethasone (0.1 to 2.0 mg/kg IV).
- Collect blood and urine samples for CBC, biochemical profile (with electrolytes), urinalysis, and basal cortisol.
- Administer synthetic ACTH IV (5 μg/kg up to a maximum of 250 μg).
- Collect second blood sample for measurement of post ACTH cortisol 1 hour later.
- If glucocorticoids have not yet been administered, administer one dose of glucocorticoids after collection of the second blood sample:
  - Dexamethasone 0.1 to 2.0 mg/kg, or
  - Prednisolone sodium succinate 1 to 2 mg/kg IV, or
  - Hydrocortisone hemisuccinate or hydrocortisone phosphate 5 mg/kg or 0.3 mg/kg/hour IV.
- Continue dexamethasone every 12 hours (0.05 to 0.1 mg/kg) or prednisolone (0.5 mg/kg) every 6 hours or hydrocortisone 1 mg/kg every 6 hours until you can switch to oral glucocorticoids.
- If hyperkalemia is severe (> 6.5 mEq/L) or ECG changes (e.g., bradycardia, loss of P waves, or prolonged P-R interval) are present consider:
  - IV 10% calcium gluconate over 10 to 15 minutes (0.5 mL/kg or 2 to 10 mL/dog) to protect myocardium from effects of hyperkalemia.

- IV glucose (1 to 2 g/unit of insulin) and insulin (0.2 U/kg) to rapidly lower serum potassium followed by continued IV infusion of 5% dextrose in fluids.
- Correction acidosis (if serum bicarbonate < 10 mEq/L) or to aid in normalizing potassium concentration. Administer 25% to 50% of calculated dose IV over 6 hours. In most cases this is unnecessary because metabolic acidosis resolves rapidly with appropriate fluid therapy.
- Estimated deficit = 0.3 × BW (kg) × (24-patient HCO^3)
- Consider blood transfusion and synthetic colloids in dogs with anemia due to gastrointestinal blood loss.
- Administer IV dextrose in dogs with hypoglycemia as a diluted bolus (25%) or a 5% solution in fluids.
- Consider administration of one dose of an injectable mineralocorticoid (Percorten V; 2.2 mg/kg IM) while waiting for diagnosis to be confirmed if clinical suspicion of hypoadrenocorticism is high.

Monitor
- Serum electrolytes
- Blood glucose
- Acid-base status
- Blood pressure
- Urine output and central venous pressure (if severe azotemia)
- ECG (if hyperkalemia)

Follow-Up
- Continue IV fluids until oral intake begins.
- Continue injectable glucocorticoids until oral medications can be substituted.

ACTH, Adrenocorticotropic hormone; *BW*, body weight; *CBC*, complete blood count; *ECG*, electrocardiogram; *HCO³*, bicarbonate; *IV*, intravenous.

 ## CRITICAL ILLNESS INDUCED CORTICOSTEROID INSUFFICIENCY (RELATIVE ADRENAL INSUFFICIENCY)

Cortisol is an important part of the physiologic response to stress, and critical illness produces dramatic changes in the HPA axis due to increased ACTH and resultant cortisol concentrations due to the actions of circulating proinflammatory cytokines (Kaplan et al, 1995; Prittie et al, 2002; Martin, 2011). The increase in cortisol during critical illness is proportional to the severity of illness, and studies in both humans and dogs have shown a positive association between serum cortisol concentration and mortality (Schoeman et al, 2007; Martin, 2011). The syndrome of CIRCI, which was previously called *relative adrenal insufficiency,* is characterized by an inadequate production of cortisol in response to critical illness and has been most commonly described in human patients with sepsis (Martin, 2011). Possible underlying causes of CIRCI include decreased glucocorticoid synthesis caused by necrosis, thrombosis, or hemorrhage of the hypothalamus, pituitary gland, or adrenal glands, and effects of drugs on the HPA axis. Reduced access of glucocorticoids to target tissues and cells due to changes in pro-inflammatory cytokines, changes in concentration of binding proteins, and cortisol degradation at the tissue level may also contribute to changes in cellular cortisol concentrations. In patients with CIRCI, the basal cortisol concentration is usually normal or high, but there is a blunted cortisol response to ACTH administration. In veterinary patients, CIRCI is most commonly diagnosed on the basis of the absolute change in cortisol concentration (delta cortisol) after ACTH administration. In some but not all studies, a delta cortisol less than 3.0 μg/dL has been associated with

increased mortality (Burkitt et al, 2007; Martin et al, 2008). The most common clinical problem associated with CIRCI in human patients is hypotension refractory to fluid resuscitation, requiring vasopressor therapy. In a study of dogs with critical illness, those with a delta cortisol less than 3.0 were more likely to be receiving treatment with vasopressors (Martin et al, 2008). CIRCI is easily distinguished from true hypoadrenocorticism because basal cortisol concentrations are usually well within the reference range and the abnormality resolves once the illness resolves (Martin, 2011). Human patients with CIRCI given treatment with supplemental corticosteroids are more likely to be weaned off vasopressor and ventilator support, and there is a survival advantage for some groups of patients (Martin, 2011). Whether treatment of CIRCI with physiologic doses of glucocorticoids in dogs and cats with CIRCI improves outcome is currently unknown.

 ## TREATMENT OF HYPOADRENOCORTICISM

The approach to treatment of hypoadrenocorticism depends upon whether the patient is presented in an adrenal crisis or has more chronic clinical signs of illness.

 ## ACUTE MANAGEMENT

Prompt treatment of dogs with suspected Addison's disease that present in an adrenal crisis is vital for a good outcome, especially if profound electrolyte abnormalities are present. Hyperkalemia in particular can be life-threatening if not treated expeditiously. Aims of emergency treatment in dogs with suspected hypoadrenocorticism include correction of hypotension, hypovolemia, electrolyte imbalances, metabolic acidosis, hypoglycemia, and anemia if present. It is also important to confirm the diagnosis of hypoadrenocorticism at the time of initial presentation, because once replacement glucocorticoid therapy has been initiated, it is very difficult to retrospectively confirm the diagnosis. Although long term treatment of hypoadrenocorticism requires provision of adequate exogenous glucocorticoids and usually mineralocorticoids; in the short term, aggressive fluid therapy is the mainstay of treatment and will temporarily correct the majority of life-threatening electrolyte abnormalities.

The recommended approach to management of dogs with suspected hypoadrenocorticism that present with severe systemic signs of illness or hypovolemic shock is shown in Box 12-6. The goal should be to treat the manifestations of shock while at the same time confirming the diagnosis by performing an ACTH stimulation test. If the animal is assessed to be in hypovolemic shock, treatment of shock should take precedence over establishing an immediate diagnosis.

Fluid Therapy

Initial fluid support should be infusion of up to 90 mL/kg of a crystalloid solution given as 20 to 30 mL/kg boluses (each over approximately 20 minutes) until the patient is hemodynamically stable. An IV bolus of a synthetic colloid such as hetastarch (5 mL/kg over 30 minutes) should be considered in hypotensive patients that are hypoproteinemic (total protein < 4.5 g/dL). In patients with hypoadrenocorticism, 0.9% saline is traditionally recommended as the most appropriate fluid for emergency treatment because of hyponatremia and hyperkalemia; however disadvantages include the tendency for 0.9% saline to be acidifying and the potential concern of increasing the sodium concentration too rapidly, which can theoretically result in delayed central pontine myelinosis (O'Brien, 1994; Brady et al, 1999; see Chapter 1). Complications resulting from rapid correction of hyponatremia are believed to be more likely when hyponatremia has persisted for longer than 24 hours and fortunately are rare in dogs. It is recommended that sodium concentration should not increase by more than 10 to 12 mEq/L/day, and therefore treatment with hypertonic saline for fluid resuscitation should be avoided in patients with hyponatremia (Churcher et al, 1999).

Because of the potential disadvantages of 0.9% saline, some clinicians prefer using a buffered isotonic crystalloid solution containing low concentrations of potassium (4 to 5 mEq/L; e.g., lactated Ringer's solution or Normosol-R). These types of fluids still decrease the serum potassium by dilution and increased renal perfusion, as well as by improving metabolic acidosis, which will drive potassium intracellularly (Brown et al, 2008; Fig. 12-19).

Glucocorticoid Replacement

If immediate glucocorticoid supplementation is considered necessary prior to performing an ACTH stimulation test; because the patient is hemodynamically unstable, dexamethasone (0.1 to 2.0 mg/kg IV) should be the drug of choice because dexamethasone does not have cross reactivity with most cortisol assays. Although dexamethasone does decrease the cortisol response to ACTH by up to 35% for 1 to 3 days depending upon the dose administered, the results of dogs with non-adrenal illness can still be differentiated from the flat-line response of dogs with hypoadrenocorticism (Kemppainen et al, 1989). Ideally glucocorticoid supplementation should be delayed until after the ACTH stimulation test is complete, and at this point any rapid acting glucocorticoid such as hydrocortisone, dexamethasone, or prednisolone sodium succinate is appropriate. The recommended doses for glucocorticoid support in acute management of hypoadrenocortical crisis vary widely and are based upon clinical experience rather than prospective or retrospective studies of outcome (see Box 12-6). The recommended doses typically range from three to 10 times normal

physiologic requirements but even higher doses have been empirically recommended by some authors. Higher doses are typically recommended in dogs that are hemodynamically unstable. Our recommendations for glucocorticoid dosage are shown in Box 12-6.

Mineralocorticoid Replacement

Prior to confirmation of the diagnosis of hypoadrenocorticism, administration of one dose of an injectable mineralocorticoid (desoxycorticosterone pivalate [DOCP]) should be considered, depending upon the initial response of the patient to fluid therapy and the anticipated timeline for results of cortisol testing to be available. Point-of-care cortisol assays (e.g., SNAP Cortisol, IDEXX Laboratories) may be useful for initial confirmation of a diagnosis of hypoadrenocorticism, but the diagnosis should always be confirmed by results from a reference laboratory because validation of point-of-care assays has not been published in the peer reviewed literature. No clinically significant adverse effects have been demonstrated resulting from one dose of DOCP in dogs that do not have hypoadrenocorticism; the main disadvantage of treating with DOCP prior to confirmation of the diagnosis is the cost of the medication (Chow et al, 1993; Kaplan and Peterson, 1995).

Management of Hyperkalemia

In most dogs with hypoadrenocorticism, the serum potassium concentration rapidly decreases with fluid therapy. If severe hyperkalemia (potassium > 7.0 mEq/L) does not rapidly improve after institution of fluid therapy, or if bradyarrhythmias do not improve rapidly with fluid therapy, consideration should be given to emergency treatment of hyperkalemia (see Box 12-6). Treatment with 10% calcium gluconate (0.5 mL/kg) does not decrease the serum potassium but temporarily counteracts the impairment of myocardial excitability induced by hyperkalemia. This effect occurs rapidly but only lasts about 20 minutes. Intravenous administration of dextrose (1 to 2 g/unit of insulin) and insulin (0.2 U/kg) decreases the serum potassium concentration by driving potassium intracellularly. The effect lasts for 15 to 30 minutes, and the blood glucose must be monitored frequently (every 30 to 60 minutes) because of the risk of hypoglycemia especially in patients that are already predisposed to hypoglycemia. Correction of metabolic acidosis will also promote intracellular movement of potassium (Fig. 12-19). The ECG or point-of-care potassium assays should be used to monitor response during treatment of hyperkalemia.

Management of Metabolic Acidosis

In most dogs with hypoadrenocorticism, metabolic acidosis resolves with appropriate fluid therapy, and the authors rarely use sodium bicarbonate in dogs with hypoadrenocorticism. If hyperkalemia is severe and does not respond to the prior management strategies, or if severe acidosis (pH < 7.1 or Total CO_2 < 10 mEq/L) does not improve with fluid therapy, treatment with a conservative dose of sodium bicarbonate may be considered (see Box 12-6). Twenty-five percent to 50% of the calculated deficit should be administered over 4 to 6 hours. The bicarbonate deficit can be estimated based on the patient's bicarbonate concentration (see Box 12-6). Adverse effects of bicarbonate administration include metabolic alkalosis, paradoxical central nervous system (CNS) acidosis, and ionized hypocalcemia (Brown, 2008).

Other Supportive Care

Blood transfusion and colloidal support (plasma or synthetic colloid) is required in patients that have severe anemia due to gastrointestinal blood loss. Gastrointestinal protectants (sucralfate, H_2 blockers, and proton pump inhibitors), antiemetics

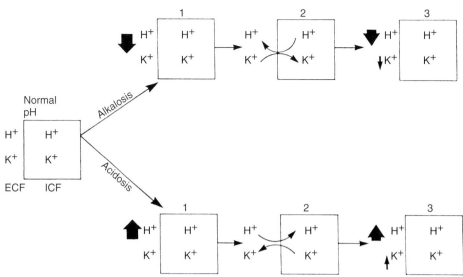

FIGURE 12-19 Redistribution of extracellular fluid *(ECF)* and intracellular fluid *(ICF)* potassium *(K+)* and hydrogen *(H+)* ions in response to changes in ECF pH. *Alkalosis: 1,* The H+ concentration decreases; *2,* H+ moves out of cells and down its concentration gradient and K+ moves into cells to maintain electrical neutrality; *3,* this contributes to the hypokalemia associated with alkalosis. *Acidosis: 1,* The H+ concentration increases; *2,* H+ moves into cells and down its concentration gradient, and K+ moves out of cells to maintain electrical neutrality; *3,* the result of electrolyte shifts, that is, the hyperkalemia associated with acidosis. The size of the arrow represents the degree of change from normal. (From Gabow P: Disorders of potassium metabolism. In Schrier RW, editor: *Renal and electrolyte disorders,* Boston, 1976, Little, Brown & Co.)

(metoclopramide, ondansetron, and maropitant citrate), and antibiotics may be indicated in individual patients with vomiting and diarrhea, gastrointestinal ulceration, or gastrointestinal ileus.

Complications of Hypoadrenal Crisis

Although most dogs with acute signs of hypoadrenocorticism respond rapidly to treatment within 24 to 48 hours of starting therapy, some dogs have a more prolonged recovery. Potential complications that may be encountered during treatment of a hypoadrenal crisis include severe gastrointestinal ulceration and hemorrhage, disseminated intravascular coagulation, sepsis due to bacterial translocation from the gastrointestinal tract, aspiration pneumonia secondary to megaesophagus, and disseminated intravascular coagulation (DIC). Patients with gastrointestinal ulceration and hemorrhage severe enough to require blood transfusion are rare but typically require much longer for recovery than other dogs with hypoadrenocorticism. Bleeding into the respiratory tract has occasionally been reported in dogs with severe hypoadrenal crisis. The cause is unknown but could potentially be caused by DIC. In dogs with hypoadrenocorticism that do not respond to treatment as expected, consideration should be given to investigation for more uncommon causes of hypoadrenocorticism, such as adrenal necrosis and granulomatous or neoplastic destruction of the adrenal glands.

LONG-TERM (MAINTENANCE) THERAPY

See Table 12-6.

Glucocorticoid Therapy

Once the diagnosis of hypoadrenocorticism has been confirmed and there has been a positive clinical response to parenteral treatment, long-term oral treatment with glucocorticoids should be initiated. Oral treatment should not begin until the patient is systemically well, is no longer vomiting, and has a good appetite.

TABLE 12-6	**LONG-TERM TREATMENT OF PRIMARY ADRENOCORTICAL INSUFFICIENCY***
Mineralocorticoid	DOCP injectable, approximately 2 mg/kg IM or SC every 14 to 35 days.
Glucocorticoid	Prednisone as needed, < 0.05 to 0.2 mg/kg daily or every other day.
or	
Mineralocorticoid	Fludrocortisone 0.02 mg/kg once a day or divided twice a day.
Glucocorticoid	Prednisone if needed, 0 to 0.2 mg/kg daily, or every other day.
Clinical follow-up	• Recheck monthly until dose stabilized then every 3 to 6 months. • Patients should maintain normal weight and activity. • Electrolytes and BUN should be normal.
Salt	No special addition if commercial diet.
Times of stress	Increase glucocorticoid therapy.

BUN, Blood urea nitrogen; *DOCP,* desoxycorticosterone pivalate; *IM,* intramuscular; *SC,* subcutaneous.
*Owner education is imperative.

Prednisone is the glucocorticoid supplement of choice in dogs. The starting dose is 0.1 to 0.22 mg/kg/day initially; the dose should then be gradually tapered over several weeks until the lowest dose that will control the clinical signs has been identified. Excessive prednisone supplementation should be avoided, because this will cause clinical signs of hyperadrenocorticism, which is the most common cause of polyuria and polydipsia in dogs treated for hypoadrenocorticism. In a study of 205 dogs with

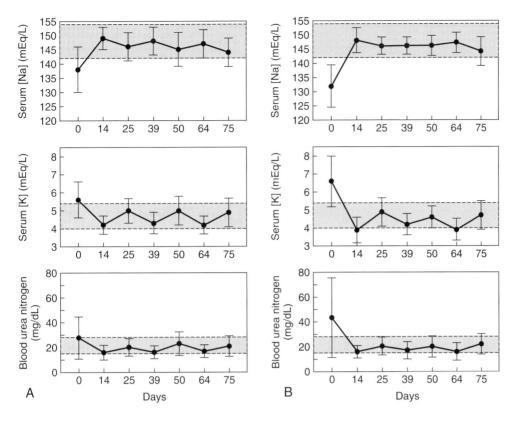

FIGURE 12-20 Serum biochemical values from 60 dogs given desoxycorticosterone pivalate (DOCP) intramuscularly for treatment of hypoadrenocorticism. **A,** *Top,* Serum sodium concentrations; *middle,* serum potassium concentrations; *bottom,* blood urea nitrogen (BUN) concentrations. **B,** Serum biochemical values (*top, middle,* and *bottom* same as for **A**) for nine dogs given DOCP for treatment of recently diagnosed hypoadrenocorticism. *Shaded areas* indicate reference ranges for each value. Results are reported as mean ± standard deviation (SD). (From Lynn RC, et al.: Efficacy of microcrystalline desoxycorticosterone pivalate for treatment of hypoadrenocorticism in dogs, *J Am Vet Med Assoc* 202:392, 1993.)

hypoadrenocorticism, the dose of prednisone used for long-term management ranged from less than 0.05 to 0.4 mg/kg/day (Kintzer and Peterson, 1997). Prednisone can be completely discontinued in as many as 50% of dogs being treated with fludrocortisone for mineralocorticoid replacement because of the intrinsic glucocorticoid activity of fludrocortisone. In contrast, because DOCP lacks glucocorticoid activity, dogs treated with DOCP should be treated with a low daily or every other day dose of prednisone.

Mineralocorticoid Therapy

Dogs with evidence of mineralocorticoid deficiency (hyperkalemia or hyponatremia) should also be treated with a mineralocorticoid, such as fludrocortisone or DOCP. The first dose of DOCP is either administered during the acute crisis when there is a high index of suspicion for hypoadrenocorticism or immediately after confirmation of the diagnosis once the results of an ACTH stimulation test are available.

Desoxycorticosterone Pivalate

DOCP (Percorten V, Novartis Corp.) is the only drug approved by the Food and Drug Administration (FDA) for treatment of hypoadrenocorticism in dogs, and is the treatment of choice in most dogs with hypoadrenocorticism. DOCP is a long-acting ester of DOCA, a synthetic mineralocorticoid that is no longer available in the United States. DOCP has no glucocorticoid activity and is formulated for veterinary use in a microcrystalline suspension for IM injection (Lynn and Feldman, 1991; Fig. 12-20). The drug may also be administered subcutaneously but should not be given intravenously (McCabe et al, 1995; Fig. 12-21). DOCP has a rapid onset of action and is effective within a few hours of injection, so no overlap is necessary when transitioning to DOCP from fludrocortisone. DOCP is administered at a starting dose of 2.2 mg/kg IM or subcutaneous (SC) every 25 days initially (Melián and Peterson, 1996). Serum electrolytes should be checked at 15 and 25 days after injection for the first 1 to 2 months

of treatment. The 15-day recheck allows titration of the dose, and the 25-day recheck allows adjustment of the frequency of administration required. If the electrolyte concentrations remain normal at 25 days, the interval between injections can be gradually increased to every 30 days; monthly injections are the most convenient for owners. In dogs that are well controlled on DOCP, electrolytes should remain within the reference range for the complete duration of the treatment period. Many dogs with hypoadrenocorticism require much lower doses than the recommended starting dose to achieve normal electrolyte concentrations. In one study, the dose of DOCP necessary for good control of hypoadrenocorticism, ranged from 0.8 to 3.4 mg/kg/dose administered at intervals ranging from 14 to 35 days (Kintzer and Peterson, 1997). Only six of 33 dogs ultimately required a dose more than 2.2 mg/kg. In a more recent study of 49 dogs with hypoadrenocorticism, 36 dogs were treated with an initial DOCP dose less than 2.2 mg/kg, and 19 of the dogs were treated with doses less than 1.0 mg/kg. No statistically significant relationship was found between initial DOCP dose and survival or posttreatment serum sodium or potassium concentrations and the authors concluded that initial doses less than 2.2 mg/kg may be effective in management of dogs with primary hypoadrenocorticism (Bates et al, 2013).

In our opinion it is not possible to predict which dogs can be effectively managed with lower doses of DOCP, so the most effective approach is to start at a dose of 2.2 mg/kg and then taper the dose by 10% a month while monitoring the sodium and potassium concentrations prior to each injection. Once the sodium and potassium concentrations start to trend outside the reference range prior to the next injection the next dose should be increased to the previous dose that resulted in normal electrolytes for the whole time period. A small minority of dogs require higher doses or a higher frequency of administration (every 14 to 24 days). Once the final dose of DOCP has been established, some owners are interested in learning how to administer DOCP at home and the frequency of veterinary reevaluation can be decreased to once every 3 to 6 months. It is important to note that especially

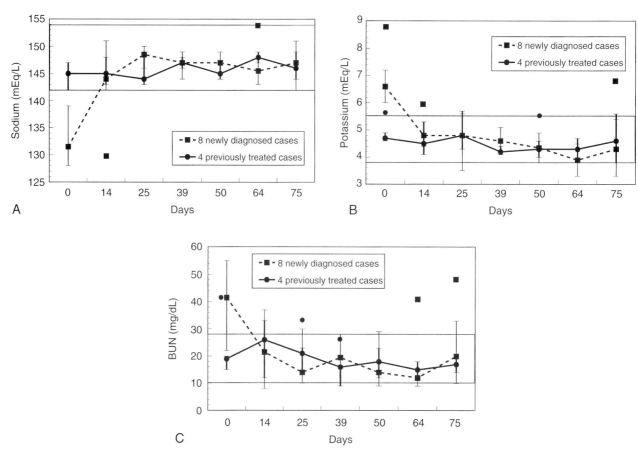

FIGURE 12-21 Serum biochemical values—sodium **(A)**, potassium **(B)**, blood urea nitrogen (BUN) **(C)**—from 12 dogs given desoxycorticosterone pivalate (DOCP) subcutaneously for treatment of hypoadrenocorticism. Mean values (± range) from newly diagnosed dogs *(dashed line)* and previously treated dogs *(solid line)* are separated; normal values are indicated by the *solid horizontal lines.* Outliers are indicated by *squares* (newly diagnosed dogs) or *dots* (previously diagnosed dogs) above or below the range lines. On day 75, one dog was hyperkalemic, and the same dog was azotemic on days 64 and 75. These abnormalities were resolved by administering the DOCP every 21 days rather than every 25 days.

in dogs maintained on lower doses of DOCP, the dose requirements of individual dogs may unexpectedly change over time, so it is important to reevaluate serum electrolyte concentrations on a regular basis (ideally every 3 months or if there is a change in body weight or clinical signs). Some clinicians recommend extending the dosing frequency of DOCP longer than 1 month rather than tapering the dose administered. We do not recommend this approach, because it can lead to problems with owner compliance and increase the risk of unexpected hypoadrenal crisis.

Some dogs treated with DOCP develop polyuria and polydipsia, which may be worse in the week after each injection. This can be due to either excessive glucocorticoid supplementation or excessive dosing of DOCP, resulting in excess circulating mineralocorticoids. In this situation the dose of glucocorticoids should be tapered first, and then the dose of DOCP should be tapered until the polyuria and polydipsia resolve.

Fludrocortisone Acetate

Fludrocortisone acetate (Florinef, Squibb) is an orally active synthetic mineralocorticoid that is an alternative option for mineralocorticoid supplementation if daily oral therapy is preferred. Fludrocortisone also possesses some intrinsic glucocorticoid activity, and additional glucocorticoid supplementation may not be required. The drug comes in 0.1 mg tablets, and the starting dose in dogs is 0.02 mg/kg by mouth either as a single dose or divided twice a day.

The dose of fludrocortisone required for control of clinical signs in a study of 190 dogs with hypoadrenocorticism ranged from 0.01 to 0.08 mg/kg/day, and the required dose typically increased over time (Kintzer and Peterson, 1997). Whether this reflects ongoing adrenal gland destruction, or is due to changes in metabolism or absorption of fludrocortisone is unknown. Interestingly, the average dose in a human with Addison's disease is 0.05 to 0.1 mg (one half to one tablet) daily. Because humans require a dramatically lower dose than dogs, it is presumed that dogs do not absorb the drug from the gastrointestinal tract as effectively or that they metabolize the drug more rapidly than humans. As with DOCP, the sodium and potassium concentration should be within the reference range in dogs that are well controlled on fludrocortisone. In some dogs, the dose required to achieve this either results in clinical signs due to the effects of excess glucocorticoid activity or becomes prohibitively expensive. In the past, salt supplementation has been recommended to decrease the dose required to maintain the sodium concentration within the reference range; however, this is not very effective and is no longer advocated. In one study, there was no difference in dose of fludrocortisone required between dogs that were treated with salt supplements and those that were not (Kintzer and Peterson, 1997). A change to treatment with DOCP is a more effective approach if the electrolyte concentrations are not effectively normalized with fludrocortisone.

Some dogs treated with fludrocortisone develop clinical signs of hyperadrenocorticism (e.g., polyuria and polydipsia) even at usual doses of fludrocortisone. The first step in this situation should be to withdraw any additional glucocorticoid supplementation. If the problem persists, it is possible that the clinical signs are due to the intrinsic glucocorticoid activity of fludrocortisone, and again consideration should be given to changing to treatment with DOCP.

Hydrocortisone Acetate

Treatment with hydrocortisone is often considered as an option for long term management of hypoadrenocorticism, because it is much cheaper than either fludrocortisone or DOCP. Unfortunately the ratio of glucocorticoid to mineralocorticoid activity of hydrocortisone is approximately 1:1, so an excessive glucocorticoid dose must be administered in order to achieve an adequate mineralocorticoid effect. This results in clinical signs of hyperadrenocorticism and this approach is therefore not recommended.

Treatment of Hypoadrenocorticism in the Absence of Electrolyte Abnormalities

Dogs without electrolyte abnormalities at the time of diagnosis initially only require glucocorticoid supplementation. These dogs either have secondary hypoadrenocorticism, or more commonly have atypical primary hypoadrenocorticism (see Glucocorticoid Deficiency Versus Mineralocorticoid Deficiency). Dogs with secondary hypoadrenocorticism can be identified by measurement of an endogenous ACTH concentration and identifying results either within or below the reference range for healthy dogs. These dogs do not develop electrolyte abnormalities because ACTH is not required for aldosterone secretion from the adrenal cortex, and these cases never require mineralocorticoid supplementation. Some dogs with atypical primary hypoadrenocorticism do later progress to complete adrenal failure and require mineralocorticoid supplementation, but the risk is difficult to predict in the individual patient. In one study, two dogs with glucocorticoid deficient hypoadrenocorticism died within a few days of discharge from the hospital due to progression to complete adrenal failure (Kintzer and Peterson, 1997); however, many other dogs do not progress over years of monitoring (Lifton et al., 1996; Hughes et al, 2007; Thompson et al, 2007; Baumstark et al, 2014). Because only a proportion of dogs later develop electrolyte abnormalities, mineralocorticoid treatment is not recommended as part of the initial treatment in dogs without electrolyte abnormalities at diagnosis; however, careful monitoring is recommended. Electrolyte concentrations should be monitored every 1 to 3 months for at least the first 12 months after diagnosis, and the owners should be educated about monitoring for clinical signs of mineralocorticoid deficiency. Most dogs that progress to complete adrenal failure do so within 1 year of diagnosis of glucocorticoid deficient hypoadrenocorticism (Lifton et al., 1996; Thompson et al, 2007). In human patients with hypoadrenocorticism, measurement of renin concentrations are used to guide need for mineralocorticoid treatment (Stewart, 2011), but measurement of renin concentration is not widely available in veterinary medicine.

 ## POOR RESPONSE TO THERAPY

Some dogs with confirmed hypoadrenocorticism do not respond well to treatment or have adverse effects associated with therapy. The most important cause of poor response to treatment is an inadequate mineralocorticoid dose. This is most commonly a problem in dogs treated with fludrocortisone. Other causes include incorrect diagnosis, failure to provide glucocorticoid supplementation in dogs treated with DOCP, or the presence of an undiagnosed concurrent illness, such as hypothyroidism, neoplasia, or fungal disease. One indication that a concurrent disease has been overlooked is the need for

glucocorticoid supplementation at a dose higher than the physiologic requirement. If a dog diagnosed with hypoadrenocorticism requires a prednisone dose of 0.5 mg/kg or greater to control clinical signs, this should be an indication to question the diagnosis and to investigate for the presence of other concurrent illness. The presence of megaesophagus or severe gastrointestinal hemorrhage can also complicate response to treatment and prolong recovery. The most common adverse effect of therapy is polyuria and polydipsia, which is most commonly associated with excessive glucocorticoid supplementation, an excessive dose of DOCP, or the intrinsic glucocorticoid activity of fludrocortisone. If polyuria and polydipsia are a problem, the glucocorticoid dose should be tapered or discontinued in dogs treated with fludrocortisone; and in dogs treated with DOCP, the dose should be gradually decreased. If the problem persists, consideration should be given to switching to an alternative mineralocorticoid treatment. If there is no improvement, further evaluation for other causes of polyuria and polydipsia should be considered.

 ## CONFIRMING THE DIAGNOSIS AFTER TREATMENT HAS ALREADY BEEN INITIATED

Unfortunately some dogs with suspected Addison's disease are treated based on suspicion rather than confirmation of the diagnosis. The expense of treatment may later prompt the owners to request that the diagnosis is confirmed. There are limited options in this situation because chronic glucocorticoid administration causes iatrogenic adrenocortical atrophy and a suppressed cortisol response to ACTH stimulation. The influence of mineralocorticoid treatment on the response to ACTH has not been investigated in dogs, but at least fludrocortisone would likely cause adrenocortical atrophy due to the intrinsic glucocorticoid activity of the drug. Thus the only way to confirm the diagnosis of hypoadrenocorticism is to withdraw therapy and monitor closely for clinical signs and electrolyte abnormalities. An ACTH stimulation test should be postponed if possible until at least 2 weeks after withdrawal of glucocorticoid supplementation. If clinical signs develop earlier, an ACTH stimulation test should be performed prior to reinstitution of therapy, but the test may be difficult to interpret depending upon the length of time that glucocorticoid treatment has been withheld. Alternatively the dose of mineralocorticoids can be gradually decreased, but this requires frequent monitoring of electrolytes each time that the dose is decreased.

 ## MANAGEMENT OF HYPOADRENOCORTICISM DURING STRESSFUL EVENTS

The dose of glucocorticoids required for normal maintenance may not be adequate during periods of stress. Examples of potentially stressful events include increased exercise or competition in working dogs or other unusual activities, such as boarding, veterinary visits, treatment of medical illness, or surgical interventions. It is recommended that the glucocorticoid dose is doubled in these situations to ensure that an adequate dose is provided.

PROGNOSIS

The prognosis for dogs with both primary and secondary hypoadrenocorticism is usually excellent, although the expense of mineralocorticoid supplementation especially in large breed dogs may cause some owners to consider euthanasia. In a study of 205 dogs treated for hypoadrenocorticism, the median survival time was 4.7 years (range, 7 days to 11.8 years) (Kintzer and Peterson, 1997). Factors such as age, breed, sex, and weight did not significantly influence survival time. The most important factor in the long-term response to therapy is owner education. The disease must be carefully described, and owners must be warned of the consequences of apparently mild illnesses. All owners should have glucocorticoids available to administer to their dogs in times of stress. The prognosis is more guarded in patients with underlying granulomatous or neoplastic causes of hypoadrenocorticism.

 IATROGENIC HYPOADRENOCORTICISM

Medical Treatment of Hyperadrenocorticism

Dogs treated medically for hyperadrenocorticism with either mitotane or trilostane sometimes develop hypoadrenocorticism. The diagnosis of hypoadrenocorticism must be confirmed by an ACTH stimulation test, because these drugs can also cause direct gastrointestinal toxicity. If clinical signs of cortisol deficiency (i.e., anorexia, vomiting, diarrhea, and/or weakness) are present but serum sodium and potassium concentrations are within reference ranges, only glucocorticoid treatment is required; this can then typically be tapered over a period of several weeks. If hyperkalemia and hyponatremia indicate concurrent mineralocorticoid deficiency, the treatment protocol is similar to that recommended for naturally occurring hypoadrenocorticism. Although mineralocorticoid deficiency induced by trilostane is usually reversible, mineralocorticoid deficiency induced by mitotane may be permanent and require life-long treatment (see Chapter 10).

Withdrawal of Chronic Glucocorticoid Therapy

Clinical signs due to iatrogenic hypocortisolism caused by chronic use of glucocorticoids that have been acutely discontinued are rare in dogs. Such cases should be treated by placing the dog back on a short-acting glucocorticoid (e.g., prednisone) and then slowly tapering the dose over a period of 1 to 2 months. We usually decrease glucocorticoid therapy to a physiologic dose (approximately 0.25 mg/kg/day) as quickly as possible (within a week). If that dose is tolerated for a week without recurrence of clinical signs, the dosage is reduced by administering the drug every other day rather than daily. After 2 weeks at this dose, the frequency is again reduced by giving the drug every 3 days. After 2 to 3 weeks at this dose, the prednisone can be discontinued. If signs recur after any dose reduction, the previous amount is usually reinstituted. If clinical signs continue to recur, complete reevaluation of the dog is recommended.

 FELINE HYPOADRENOCORTICISM

Etiology

Primary hypoadrenocorticism is a rare disease in cats. Since the first report in 1983, fewer than 40 cases have been described in the veterinary literature (Johnessee et al, 1983; Freudiger, 1986; Peterson et al, 1989; Berger and Reed, 1993; Parnell et al, 1999). An additional fifteen cases have been reported in book chapters (Hardy, 1995; Feldman and Nelson, 2004). The cause has been described as idiopathic adrenocortical atrophy in one cat with traumatically induced disease (Berger and Reed, 1993), and the condition occurred secondary to lymphoma of the adrenals in two cats (Parnell et al, 1999).

Signalment and Clinical Signs

The reported age of cats with Addison's disease has ranged from 1½ to 14 years. All have been Domestic Long-Haired or Domestic

CLINICAL FINDINGS	NUMBER OF CATS (%)
Historic Owner Complaints	
Lethargy/depression	10 (100)
Anorexia	10 (100)
Weight loss	9 (90)
Vomiting	4 (40)
Waxing-waning course of illness	4 (40)
Previous response to non-specific therapy	3 (30)
Polyuria/polydipsia	3 (30)
Physical Examination Findings	
Depression	10 (100)
Weakness	9 (90)
Dehydration	9 (90)
Hypothermia	8 (80)
Slow capillary refill time	5 (50)
Weak pulse	5 (50)
Collapse/unable to rise	3 (30)
Bradycardia	2 (20)
Painful abdomen	1 (10)

TABLE 12-7 CLINICAL FINDINGS IN 10 CATS WITH PRIMARY HYPOADRENOCORTICISM

From Peterson ME, et al.: Primary hyperadrenocorticism in ten cats, *J Vet Intern Med* 3:55, 1989.

Short-Haired cats. An equal number of males and females have been described, and all cats had been neutered.

The clinical signs and physical examination abnormalities are similar to those described for dogs (Table 12-7). The duration of signs noted by owners has been as short as a few days and as long as 3 to 4 months. The most common owner observations include lethargy, depression, anorexia, and weight loss. Less frequently noticed signs include vomiting, waxing-waning course of illness, polyuria, polydipsia, and previous response to nonspecific therapy, such as intravenous fluids or glucocorticoids. Diarrhea has not been reported (Peterson et al, 1989).

The most common physical examination abnormalities identified in these cats are depression, weakness, dehydration, hypothermia, slow capillary refill time, and weak femoral pulses. Less commonly observed examination findings included collapse, inability to rise, bradycardia, and painful abdomen (Peterson et al, 1989).

Laboratory, Radiographic, and Electrocardiogram Abnormalities

Hematologic abnormalities were not common but included mild anemia. Rarely, lymphocytosis, or eosinophilia has been noted. All of the cats have been hyponatremic, and all but one were hyperkalemic (Table 12-8). Hypochloremia, azotemia, and hyperphosphatemia were identified in almost all cats. Every cat had an abnormal sodium-to-potassium ratio (< 24:1). The hyperkalemia was not as severe as has been observed in dogs, with values of 5.4 to 7.6 mEq/L reported. Three of 10 cats were mildly acidotic, and one was hypercalcemic

TABLE 12-8	RESULTS OF LABORATORY TESTS IN 10 CATS WITH HYPOADRENOCORTICISM		
TEST	**MEAN STANDARD DEVIATION**	**RANGE**	**NORMAL RANGE**
Packed cell volume (%)	29.5 ± 5.8	21.2–39.2	25–38
Erythrocyte count ¥ 10^6/mm^3	6.4 ± 1.5	4.6–9.0	6–8.5
Hemoglobin (g/dL)	10.3 ± 1.7	7.3–12.6	8–15
Leukocytes/mm	11.656 ± 4335	7200–20,100	7000–15,000
Mature neutrophils	7586 ± 3514	4320–15,875	3500–11,250
Band neutrophils	144 ± 151	0–344	0–450
Lymphocytes	3348 ± 2233	1118–8410	1400–6000
Eosinophils	598 ± 935	145–3015	140–1400
Monocytes	178 ± 204	0–612	70–600
Serum glucose (mg/dL)	99.2 ± 24.9	71–139	70–150
Alanine aminotransferase (IU/L)	62.0 ± 21.0	43–100	10–80
Alkaline phosphatase (IU/L)	36.0 ± 29.7	10–108	10–80
Total bilirubin (mg/dL)	0.39 ± 0.23	0.1–0.8	0–0.5
Total protein (mg/dL)	6.5 ± 0.8	5.6–7.5	5.3–7.9
Albumin (mg/dL)	2.9 ± 0.5	2.3–3.5	2.3–3.8
Blood urea nitrogen (mg/dL)	55.6 ± 16.5	31–80	5–30
Creatinine (mg/dL)	3.2 ± 1.5	1.6–6.0	0.5–1.5
Total CO_2 (mEq/L)	18.6 ± 3.8	13–24	16–25
Inorganic phosphorus (mg/dL)	7.3 ± 0.94	6.1–9.1	3.0–6.0
Calcium (mg/dL)	10.7 ± 3.4	8.6–14.0	7.6–11.0
Sodium (mEq/L)	130.6 ± 8.1	111–138	140–155
Potassium (mEq/L)	6.2 ± 0.6	5.4–7.6	3.5–5.5
Chloride (mEq/L)	96.3 ± 9.7	74–108	100–120
Sodium-to-potassium ratio	21.0± 1.7	17.9–23.7	> 26
Urine specific gravity	1.028 ± 0.014	1.008–1.045	1.001–1.080
Serum cortisol (µg/dL)			
Basal	0.26 ± 0.28	0.1–0.8	0.5–5.0*
1-hour post-ACTH	0.29 ± 0.37	0.1–1.1	4.5–13.0*
2-hour post-ACTH	0.39 ± 0.44	0.1–1.3	4.0–14.5*
Plasma ACTH (pg/mL)	3767 ± 2667	500–8000	10–125†

From Peterson ME, et al.: Primary adrenocorticism in ten cats. *J Vet Intern Med* 3:55, 1989.

ACTH, Adrenocorticotropic hormone; *SD*, standard deviation.

*ACTH stimulation tests were performed in 33 clinically normal cats; mean ± SD: basal, 1-hour post-ACTH, and 2-hour post-ACTH cortisol concentrations were 2.1 ± 1.5 µg/dL, 7.9 ± 2.9 µg/dL, and 8.1 ± 2.7 µg/dL, respectively.

†Immunoreactive plasma ACTH concentrations were determined in 50 clinically normal cats; the mean (± SD) value was 36.7 ± 36.0 pg/mL.

(serum calcium concentration of 14 mg/dL). Hypoglycemia was reported in one cat.

The urine specific gravity was less than 1.030 in seven of 10 cats with naturally occurring Addison's disease. All 10 cats were dehydrated and azotemic. The BUN concentration ranged from 31 to 80 mg/dL with a mean of 55 mg/dL. As with dogs, similarities between the clinical descriptions, physical findings, and test results for cats with renal disease (which is common) and those with hypoadrenocorticism (which is rare) make diagnosis of the latter condition difficult.

Microcardia was identified on thoracic radiographs of five cats. This nonspecific finding supports the observed dehydration, hypovolemia, and hypotension thought to be present in these cats. Other cardiovascular abnormalities were not observed. Identified ECG abnormalities consisted of sinus bradycardia in two cats and atrial premature contractions in one cat. The characteristic changes in the T wave, P wave, P-R interval, and QRS complexes seen with hyperkalemia in dogs were not identified in these cats. The lack of these classic abnormalities on ECG is probably due to the relatively mild hyperkalemia documented in each of the cats.

Differential Diagnosis

The differential diagnosis for abnormal serum sodium and potassium concentrations should include gastrointestinal disease, renal disease, and ascites (Bissett et al, 2001). The differential diagnosis for low plasma cortisol concentrations with inadequate response to ACTH stimulation includes naturally occurring hypoadrenocorticism, chronic glucocorticoid administration, and chronic megestrol acetate administration, and failure to administer ACTH. The differential diagnosis of hypoadrenocorticism should include lymphoma, because this form of cancer is common in cats and adrenal involvement has been demonstrated (Parnell et al, 1999).

Confirming the Diagnosis

Adrenocorticotropic Hormone Stimulation Test

The ACTH stimulation test is the gold standard for diagnosis in cats, just as it is in dogs. However, the protocol in cats is slightly different. Half a vial (125 μg) of synthetic ACTH (Cortrosyn) should be administered intramuscularly with blood samples obtained immediately before and 30 and 60 minutes after injection.

The expected results in hypoadrenocorticism are similar to those in dogs: The pre-ACTH plasma cortisol concentration is usually undetectable or low-normal, and the post-ACTH plasma cortisol concentration is similar to the pre-ACTH value. As in dogs, both pre-ACTH and post-ACTH cortisol concentrations in Addisonian cats were less than 2.0 μg/dL (see Table 12-8). The basal plasma cortisol concentrations ranged from 0.1 to 0.8 μg/dL (reference range is 0.5 to 5.0 μg/dL). The 1- and 2-hour results were 0.1 to 1.1 μg/dL and 0.1 to 1.3 μg/dL, respectively (normal is 4.5 to 13.0 μg/dL) (see Table 12-8; Peterson et al, 1989).

Plasma Endogenous Adrenocorticotropic Hormone

Plasma ACTH concentrations were measured in seven of 10 cats with naturally occurring disease. Each cat had abnormally increased concentrations consistent with the diagnosis of primary adrenocortical disease. The values ranged from 500 to 8000 pg/mL with a mean of 3767 pg/mL (reference range for that assay is < 10 to 125 pg/mL; see Table 12-8).

 ## TREATMENT

Acute Management

The principles of therapy for cats are no different from those in dogs. Initial therapy includes aggressive intravenous administration of 0.9% normal saline over 2 to 4 hours to replace fluid deficits and restore blood pressure. After that has been accomplished, maintenance fluid therapy should be continued until the cat is eating and drinking with no vomiting or diarrhea. Glucocorticoid deficits should be replaced with dexamethasone (0.1 to 2 mg/kg IV or IM every 12 hours). Ideally, the ACTH stimulation test should be completed prior to administration of glucocorticoids. Mineralocorticoids can be administered in the form of DOCP prior to disease confirmation if appropriate (2.2 mg/kg IM every 25 days).

One feature of hypoadrenocorticism that is somewhat different in cats than in dogs is the slow response to therapy. Cats appear to remain weak, lethargic, and depressed for 3 to 5 days despite institution of appropriate therapy. Three of 10 cats were euthanized after only 2 to 5 days of treatment because of poor response. It is possible that they may have survived had they been treated for a longer period.

Long-Term (Maintenance) Therapy

As with acute management, long term treatment is no different from that recommended for dogs. Chronic mineralocorticoid therapy involves oral fludrocortisone acetate (0.05 to 0.10 mg b.i.d.) or injectable DOCP. Glucocorticoid replacement, as needed, is usually accomplished with prednisolone (starting dose 2.5 to 5 mg/day tapered to the minimal dose that controls clinical signs). Long-term oral administration of medication can be challenging in some cats, so other routes of administration (e.g., parenteral or transdermal) may need to be considered in some cats. Regular physical examinations (in addition to periodic monitoring of owner opinion regarding clinical response), serum electrolyte concentrations, and BUN levels are strongly recommended (just as for dogs) to ensure that treatment is appropriate.

Prognosis

The long-term prognosis for cats with hypoadrenocorticism is excellent unless underlying disease (e.g., lymphoma) is the cause of hypoadrenocorticism. As with dogs, committed cat owners who are well informed about the disease tend to have the best success. Frequent rechecks to ensure that glucocorticoid and mineralocorticoid supplementation is optimal is valuable. Six of seven cats that survived the hypoadrenal crisis were alive for a mean of 34 months (Peterson et al, 1989).

 ## CONGENITAL ADRENAL HYPERPLASIA

Congenital adrenal hyperplasia (CAH) is a group of inherited diseases that result from a deficiency of one or more of the enzymes required for cortisol and aldosterone synthesis in the adrenal cortex. CAH is the most common genetic endocrine disorder in humans, and the hormonal abnormalities and clinical manifestations depend upon the particular enzyme that is deficient. Clinical manifestations may include abnormal genital development, pseudohermaphroditism, virilization of females, salt wasting, and hypertension. Inheritance of all forms of CAH in humans is autosomal recessive, with an overall worldwide prevalence of 1 in 15,000 live births. Although mutations of any of the five adrenal enzymes required for cortisol biosynthesis can result in CAH, mutations of the genes encoding the 21β-hydroxylase enzyme and 11β-hydroxylase enzyme are the most common forms in people.

CAH is very rare in dogs and cats. Two cats with CAH due to 11β-hydroxylase deficiency and one dog with 17α-hydroxylase deficiency have been described (Breitschwert, 1989; Knighton, 2004; Owens, 2012). In one male and one female cat with 11β-hydroxylase deficiency, clinical signs included polyuria and polydipsia, foul smelling urine, presence of barbs on the penis of a castrated male cat and virilization of a female cat, hypertension and behavioral changes (Fig. 12-22). The diagnosis was made by demonstration of hypocortisolemia and hypoaldosteronemia and increases in plasma ACTH, desoxycorticosterone, dihydroepiandrosterone, 11-desoxycortisol, and pregnenolone (Knighton, 2004; Owens, 2012). Treatment with physiologic doses of prednisolone resolved the clinical signs and hormonal abnormalities. Congenital hyperplasia should be considered in the differential diagnosis for cats with unexplained hypertension, polyuria, polydipsia, presence of secondary sex characteristics after neutering, and behavioral abnormalities, such as inter-cat aggression.

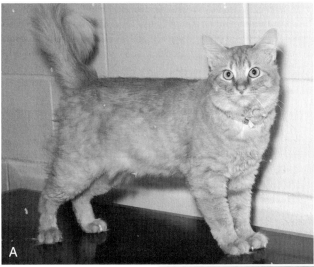
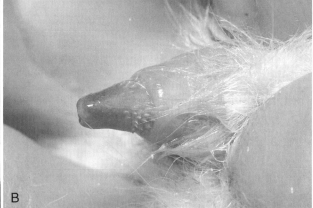
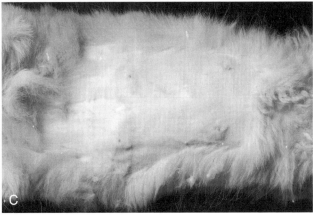

FIGURE 12-22 Three year old male cat with 11β-hydroxylase deficiency. **A,** The cat had a small body frame. **B,** Barbs were present on the penis despite evidence that the cat had previously been castrated. The barbs resolved with treatment. **C,** Gynecomastia was noted in this male castrated cat. This also resolved with treatment.

REFERENCES

Adamantos S, Boag A: Total and ionized calcium concentrations in dogs with hypoadrenocorticism, *Vet Rec* 163:25, 2008.

Addison T: *On the constitutional and local effects of disease of the suprarenal capsules*, London, 1855, Highley.

Adissu HA, et al.: Lymphocytic adenohypophysitis and adrenalitis in a dog with adrenal and thyroid atrophy, *Vet Pathol* 47:1082, 2010.

Adler JA, et al.: Abnormalities of serum electrolyte concentrations in dogs with hypoadrenocorticism, *J Vet Intern Med* 21:1168, 2007.

Angles JM, et al.: Use of the urine cortisol:creatinine ratio versus adrenocorticotrophic hormone stimulation testing for monitoring mitotane treatment of pituitary-dependent hyperadrenocorticism in dogs, *J Am Vet Med Assoc* 211:1002, 1997.

Bartges J, Nielson D: Reversible megaesophagus associated with atypical primary hypoadrenocorticism in a dog, *J Am Vet Med Assoc* 201:889, 1992.

Bates JA, et al.: Lower initial dose desoxycorticosterone pivalate for treatment of canine primary hypoadrenocorticism, *Aust Vet J* 91:77, 2013.

Baumstark ME, et al.: Evaluation of aldosterone concentrations in dogs with hypoadrenocorticism, *J Vet Intern Med* 28:154, 2014.

Behrend EN, Kemppainen RJ: Glucocorticoid therapy: pharmacology, indications, and complications, *Vet Clin Small Animal* 27:187, 1997.

Behrend EN, et al.: Effects of storage conditions on cortisol, total thyroxine and free thyroxine concentrations in serum and plasma of dogs, *J Am Vet Med Assoc* 212:1564–1568, 1995.

Behrend EN, et al.: Diagnosis of spontaneous canine hyperadrenocorticism: 2012 ACVIM Consensus Statement (Small Animal), *J Vet Intern Med* 27:1292, 2013.

Behrend EN, et al.: Intramuscular administration of a low dose of ACTH for ACTH stimulation testing in dogs, *J Am Vet Med Assoc* 229:528, 2006.

Berger SL, Reed J: Traumatically induced hypoadrenocorticism in a cat, *J Am Anim Hosp Assoc* 29:337, 1993.

Bertolini G, et al.: Pituitary apoplexy-like disease in 4 dogs, *J Vet Intern Med* 21:1251, 2007.

Bissett SA, et al.: Hyponatremia and hyperkalemia associated with peritoneal effusion in four cats, *J Am Vet Med Assoc* 218:1590, 2001.

Blois SL, et al.: Multiple endocrine diseases in dogs: 35 cases (1996-2009), *J Am Vet Med Assoc* 238:1616, 2011.

Boujon CE, et al.: Pituitary gland changes in canine hypoadrenocorticism: a functional and immunocytochemical study, *J Comp Pathol* 111:287, 1994.

Bowen D, et al.: Autoimmune polyglandular syndrome in a dog: a case report, *J Am Anim Hosp Assoc* 22:649, 1986.

Brady CA, et al.: Severe neurologic sequelae in a dog after treatment of hypoadrenal crisis, *J Am Vet Med Assoc* 215:222, 1999.

Breitschwert EB, et al.: Congenital adrenal hyperplasia in a dog because of 17-hydroxylase deficiency, in: Research abstract program of the 7th annual ACVIM Meeting, *J Vet Intern Med* 3:120, 1989 (abstract).

Brown AJ, et al.: Fluid therapy for vomiting and diarrhea, *Vet Clin Small Anim* 38:653, 2008.

Burkhardt WA, et al.: Adrenocorticotrophic hormone, but not trilostane, causes severe adrenal hemorrhage, vacuolization and apoptosis in rats, *Dom Anim Endocrinology* 40:155, 2011.

Burkitt JM, et al.: Relative adrenal insufficiency in dogs with sepsis, *J Vet Intern Med* 21:226, 2007.

Burrows C: Reversible megaesophagus in a dog with hypoadrenocorticism, *J Small Anim Pract* 28:1073, 1987.

Burton S, et al.: Hypoadrenocorticism in young related Nova Scotia duck tolling retrievers, *Can Vet J* 38:231, 1997.

Carlson KJ, et al.: Optimization of a test protocol to assess aldosterone secretory capacity in dogs, *J Vet Intern Med* 24:685, 2010 (abstract).

Chase K, et al.: Understanding the genetics of autoimmune disease: two loci that regulate late onset Addison's disease in Portuguese Water dogs, *Int J Immunogenet* 33:179, 2006.

Chow E, et al.: Toxicity of desoxycorticosterone pivalate given at high dosages to clinically normal Beagles for six months, *Am J Vet Res* 54:1954, 1993.

Churcher RK, et al.: Suspected myelinosis following rapid correction of hyponatremia in a dog, *J Am Anim Hosp Assoc* 35:493, 1999.

Cohen TA, Feldman EC: Comparison of IV and IM formulations of synthetic ACTH for ACTH stimulation tests in healthy dogs, *J Vet Intern Med* 26:412, 2012.

DiBartola SP: Hyponatremia, *Vet Clin North Am Small Anim Pract* 19:215, 1989.

DiBartola SP, et al.: Clinicopathologic findings resembling hypoadrenocorticism in dogs with primary gastrointestinal disease, *J Am Vet Med Assoc* 187:60, 1985.

Famula TR, et al.: Heritability and complex segregation analysis of hypoadrenocorticism in the standard poodle, *J Small Anim Pract* 44:8, 2003.

Feldman EC, Nelson RW: *Canine and feline endocrinology and reproduction*, ed 3, St Louis, 2004, Saunders/Elsevier.

Fossum TW, Birchard SJ: Lymphangiographic evaluation of experimentally induced chylothorax after ligation of the cranial vena cava in dogs, *Am J Vet Res* 47:976, 1986.

Frank CB, et al.: Correlation of inflammation with adrenocortical atrophy in canine adrenalitis, *J Comp Path* 149:268, 2013.

Frank LA, Oliver JW: Comparison of serum cortisol concentrations in clinically normal dogs after administration of freshly reconstituted versus reconstituted and stored frozen cosyntropin, *J Am Vet Med Assoc* 212:1569, 1998.

Frank LA, et al.: Cortisol concentrations following stimulation of healthy and adrenopathic dogs with two doses of tetracosactrin, *J Small Anim Pract* 41:308, 2000.

Frank LA, et al.: Serum concentrations of cortisol, sex hormones of adrenal origin, and adrenocortical steroid intermediates in healthy dogs following stimulation with two doses of cosyntropin, *Am J Vet Res* 65:1631, 2004.

Freudiger U: Literaturubersicht uber Nebennierenrinden—Erkrankungen der Katze und Beschreibung eines Falles von primarer Nebennierenrinden—Insuffizienz, *Schweiz Arch Tierheilk* 128:221, 1986.

Galac S, et al.: Urinary corticoid:creatinine ratios in dogs with pituitary-dependent hypercortisolism during trilostane treatment, *J Vet Intern Med* 23:1214, 2009.

Ginel PJ, et al.: Evaluation of serum concentrations of cortisol and sex hormones of adrenal gland origin after stimulation with two synthetic ACTH preparations in clinically normal dogs, *Am J Vet Res* 73:237, 2012.

Golden D, Lothrop CJ: A retrospective study of aldosterone secretion in normal and adrenopathic dogs, *J Vet Intern Med* 2:121, 1988.

Gow AG, et al.: Calcium metabolism in eight dogs with hypoadrenocorticism, *J Small Anim Pract* 50:426, 2009.

Gow AG, et al.: Insulin concentrations in dogs with hypoadrenocorticism, *Res Vet Sci* 93:97, 2012.

Graves TK, et al.: Basal and ACTH-stimulated plasma aldosterone concentrations are normal or increased in dogs with trichuriasis-pseudohypoadrenocorticism, *J Vet Intern Med* 8:287, 1994.

Guptill L, et al.: Use of the urine cortisol:creatinine ratio to monitor treatment response in dogs with pituitary-dependent hyperadrenocorticism, *J Am Vet Med Assoc* 210:1158, 1997.

Hardy RM: Hypoadrenocorticism. In Ettinger SJ, Feldman EC, editors: *Textbook of Veterinary Internal Medicine*, ed 4, Philadelphia, 1995, WB Saunders.

Hansen BL, et al.: Synthetic ACTH (Cosyntropin) stimulation tests in normal dogs: comparison of intravenous and intramuscular administration, *J Am Anim Hosp Assoc* 30:38, 1994.

Hill K, et al.: ACTH stimulation testing: a review and a study comparing synthetic and compounded products, *Vet Med February* 134, 2004.

Hoerauf A, Reusch C: Ultrasonographic evaluation of the adrenal glands in six dogs with hypoadrenocorticism, *J Am Anim Hosp Assoc* 35:214, 1999.

Hughes AM, et al.: Clinical features and heritability of hypoadrenocorticism in Nova Scotia Duck Tolling Retrievers: 25 cases (1994-2006), *J Am Vet Med Assoc* 231:407, 2007.

Hughes AM, et al.: Association of a dog leucocyte antigen class II haplotype with hypoadrenocorticism in Nova Scotia Duck Tolling Retrievers, *Tissue Antigens* 75:684, 2010.

Hughes AM, et al.: Examination of candidate genes for hypoadrenocorticism Nova Scotia Duck Tolling Retrievers, *Vet J* 187:212, 2011.

Javadi S, et al.: Aldosterone-to-renin and cortisol-to-adrenocorticotrophic hormone ratios in healthy dogs and dogs with primary hypoadrenocorticism, *J Vet Intern Med* 20:556, 2006.

Johnessee JS, et al.: Primary hypoadrenocorticism in a cat, *J Am Vet Med Assoc* 183:881, 1983.

Kaplan AJ, Peterson ME: Effects of desoxycorticosterone pivalate administration on blood pressure in dogs with primary hypoadrenocorticism, *J Am Vet Med Assoc* 206:327, 1995.

Kaplan AJ, et al.: Effects of disease on the results of diagnostic tests for use in detecting hyperadrenocorticism in dogs, *J Am Vet Med Assoc* 207:445, 1995.

Kelch WJ, et al.: Canine hypoadrenocorticism (Addison's disease), *Comp Small Anim Pract* 20:921, 1998.

Kemppainen RJ, et al.: Adrenocortical suppression in the dog after a single dose of methylprednisolone acetate, *Am J Vet Res* 42:822, 1981.

Kemppainen RJ, et al.: Adrenocortical suppression in the dog given a single intramuscular dose of prednisone or triamcinolone acetonide, *Am J Vet Res* 43:204, 1982.

Kemppainen RJ, et al.: Effects of a single intravenously administered dose of dexamethasone on response to the adrenocorticotrophic hormone stimulation test in dogs, *Am J Vet Res* 50:1914, 1989.

Kemppainen RJ, et al.: Use of compounded adrenocorticotrophic hormone (ACTH) for adrenal function testing in dogs, *J Am Anim Hosp Assoc* 30:41, 2005.

Kerl ME, et al.: Evaluation of a low-dose synthetic adrenocorticotropic hormone stimulation test in clinically normal dogs and dogs with naturally developing hyperadrenocorticism, *J Am Vet Med Assoc* 214:1497, 1999.

Kintzer PP, Peterson ME: Treatment and long-term follow-up of 205 dogs with hypoadrenocorticism, *J Vet Intern Med* 11:43, 1997.

Kintzer PP, Peterson ME: Mitotaine (op'-DDD) treatment of 200 dogs with pituitary-dependent hyperadrenocorticism, *J Vet Intern Med* 5:182, 1991.

Knighton EL: Congenital adrenal hyperplasia secondary to 11b-hydroxylase deficiency in a domestic cat, *J Am Vet Med Assoc* 225:238, 2004.

Koch J, et al.: Duplex Doppler measurements of renal blood flow in a dog with Addison's disease, *J Small Anim Pract* 38:124, 1997.

Kooistra HS, et al.: Polyglandular deficiency syndrome in a Boxer dog: thyroid hormone and glucocorticoid deficiency, *Vet Q* 17:59, 1995.

Kook PH, et al.: Addison's disease due to bilateral adrenal malignancy in a dog, *J Small Anim Pract* 51:333, 2010.

Korth R, et al.: Hypoadrenocorticism due to a bilateral abscessing inflammation of the adrenal cortex in a Rottweiler, *Kleinierpraxis* 53:479, 2008.

Kreissler JJ, Langston CE: A case of hyporeninemic hypoaldosteronism in the dog, *J Vet Intern Med* 25:944, 2011.

Labelle P, De Cock HE: Metastatic tumors to the adrenal glands in domestic animals, *Vet Pathol* 42:52, 2005.

Langlais-Burgess L, et al.: Concurrent hypoadrenocorticism and hypoalbuminemia in dogs: a retrospective study, *J Am Anim Hosp Assoc* 31:307, 1995.

Lathan P, et al.: Use of a low dose ACTH stimulation test for diagnosis of hypoadrenocorticism in dogs, *J Vet Intern Med* 22:1070, 2008.

Lathan P, et al.: Use of the cortisol-to-ACTH ratio for diagnosis of primary hypoadrenocorticism in dogs, *J Vet Intern Med* 28:1546, 2014.

Lennon EM, et al.: Use of basal serum or plasma cortisol concentrations to rule out a diagnosis of hypoadrenocorticism in dogs: 123 cases (2000-2005), *J Am Vet Med Assoc* 231:413, 2007.

Levy JK: Hypoglycemic seizures attributable to hypoadrenocorticism in a dog, *J Am Vet Med Assoc* 204:526, 1994.

Lifton SJ, et al.: Glucocorticoid-deficient hypoadrenocorticism in dogs: 18 cases (1986-1995), *J Am Vet Med Assoc* 209:2076, 1996.

Lobetti RG: Hyperreninemic hypoaldosteronism in a dog, *J S Afr Vet Assoc* 69:33, 1998.

Lynn R, Feldman EC: Treatment of hypoadrenocorticism with microcrystalline desoxycorticosterone pivalate, *Br Vet J* 147:478, 1991.

Lynn R, et al.: Efficacy of microcrystalline desoxycorticosterone pivalate for treatment of hypoadrenocorticism in dogs, *J Am Vet Med Assoc* 202:392, 1993.

Martin LG: Critical illness-related corticosteroid insufficiency in small animals, *Vet Clin Small Anim* 41:767, 2011.

Martin LG, et al.: Pituitary-adrenal function in dogs with acute critical illness, *J Am Vet Med Assoc* 233:87, 2008.

Martin LG, et al.: Effects of low doses of cosyntropin on serum cortisol concentrations in clinically normal dogs, *Am J Vet Res* 68:555, 2007.

Massey J, et al.: MHC class II association study in eight breeds of dog with hypoadrenocorticism, *Immunogenetics* 65:291, 2013.

McCabe M, et al.: Subcutaneous administration of desoxycorticosterone pivalate for the treatment of canine hypoadrenocorticism, *J Am Anim Hosp Assoc* 31:151, 1995.

McGonigle KM, et al.: Mineralocorticoid before glucocorticoid deficiency in a dog with primary hypoadrenocorticism and hypothyroidism, *J Am Anim Hosp Assoc* 49:54, 2013.

Medinger TL, et al.: Severe gastrointestinal tract hemorrhage in three dogs with hypoadrenocorticism, *J Am Vet Med Assoc* 202:1869, 1993.

Meij BP, et al.: Residual pituitary function after transsphenoidal hypophysectomy in dogs with pituitary dependent hyperadrenocorticism, *J Endocrinology* 155:531, 1997.

Melendez LD, et al.: Concurrent hypoadrenocorticism and hypothyroidism in 10 dogs, *J Vet Intern Med* 10:182, 1996 (abstract).

Melián C, Peterson ME: Diagnosis and treatment of naturally occurring hypoadrenocorticism in 42 dogs, *J Am Anim Pract* 37:268, 1996.

Melián C, et al.: Radiographic findings in dogs with naturally-occurring primary hypoadrenocorticism, *J Am Anim Hosp Assoc* 35:208, 1999.

Mitchell AL, Pearce SHS: Autoimmune Addison disease: pathophysiology and genetic complexity, *Nat Rev Endocrinol* 8:306, 2012.

Moore G, Hoenig M: Duration of pituitary and adrenocortical suppression after long-term administration of antiinflammatory doses of prednisone to dogs, *Am J Vet Res* 53:716, 1992.

Moriello K, et al.: Adrenocortical suppression associated with topical administration of glucocorticoids in dogs, *J Am Vet Med Assoc* 193:329, 1988.

Murphy CJ, et al.: Iatrogenic Cushing's syndrome in a dog caused by topical ophthalmic medications, *J Am Anim Hosp Assoc* 26:640, 1990.

Nielsen L, et al.: Low ratios of sodium to potassium in the serum of 238 dogs, *Vet Rec* 162:431, 2008.

Oberbauer AM, et al.: Inheritance of hypoadrenocorticism in Bearded Collies, *Am J Vet Res* 63:643, 2002.

Oberbauer AM, et al.: Genetic evaluation of Addison's disease in the Portuguese Water dog, *BMC Vet Res* 2:15, 2006.

O'Brien DP, et al.: Myelinolysis after correction of hyponatremia in two dogs, *J Vet Intern Med* 8:40, 1994.

Oelkers W, et al.: Diagnosis and therapy surveillance in Addison's disease: rapid adrenocorticotrophin (ACTH) test and measurement of plasma ACTH, renin activity, and aldosterone, *J Clin Endocrinol Metab* 75:259, 1992.

Olson PN, et al.: Effects of storage on concentration of hydrocortisone (cortisol) in canine serum and plasma, *Am J Vet Res* 42:1618, 1981.

Owens SL, et al.: Congenital adrenal hyperplasia associated with mutation in an 11beta-hydroxylase-like gene in a cat, *J Vet Intern Med* 26:1221, 2012.

Parnell NK, et al.: Hypoadrenocorticism as the primary manifestation of lymphoma in two cats, *J Am Vet Med Assoc* 214:1208, 1999.

Peterson ME, Feinman JM: Hypercalcemia associated with hypoadrenocorticism in 16 dogs, *J Am Vet Med Assoc* 181:802, 1982.

Peterson ME, et al.: Primary hypoadrenocorticism in ten cats, *J Vet Intern Med* 3:55, 1989.

Peterson ME, et al.: Pretreatment clinical and laboratory findings in dogs with hypoadrenocorticism: 225 cases (1979-1993), *J Am Vet Med Assoc* 208:85, 1996.

Platt SR, et al.: Secondary hypoadrenocorticism associated with craniocerebral trauma in a dog, *J Am Anim Hosp Assoc* 35:117, 1999.

Prittie JE, et al.: Pituitary ACTH and adrenocortical secretion in critically ill dogs, *J Am Vet Med Assoc* 220:615, 2002.

Randolph JF, et al.: Use of the urine cortisol-to-creatinine ratio for monitoring dogs with pituitary-dependent hyperadrenocorticism during induction treatment with mitotane (op'-DDD), *Am J Vet Res* 59:258, 1998.

Reid LE, et al.: Effect of trilostane and mitotane on aldosterone secretory reserve in dogs with pituitary-dependent hyperadrenocorticism, *J Vet Intern Med* 28:443, 2014.

Reusch CE, et al.: Histological evaluation of the adrenal glands of seven dogs treated with trilostane, *Vet Rec* 160:219, 2007.

Rich LJ, et al.: Elevated serum potassium associated with delayed separation of serum from clotted blood in dogs of the Akita breed, *Vet Clin Pathol* 15:12, 1986.

Roberts S, et al.: Effect of ophthalmic prednisolone acetate on the canine adrenal gland and hepatic function, *Am J Vet Res* 45:1711, 1984.

Rockwell JL, et al.: Spontaneous hypoadrenocorticism in a dog after a diagnosis of hyperadrenocorticism, *J Vet Intern Med* 19:255, 2005.

Rose BD, Post TW: *Clinical physiology of acid-base disorders*, ed 5., New York, 2001, McGraw-Hill. p. 178.

Roth L, Tyler RD: Evaluation of low sodium:potassium ratios in dogs, *J Vet Diag Invest* 11:60, 1999.

Rubin SI, et al.: Trimethoprim-induced exacerbation of hyperkalemia in a dog with hypoadrenocorticism, *J Vet Intern Med* 12:186, 1998.

Russell NJ, et al.: Comparison of radioimmunoassay and chemiluminescent assay methods to estimate canine blood cortisol concentrations, *Aust Vet J* 85:487, 2007.

Sadek D, Schaer M: Atypical Addison's disease in the dog: a retrospective survey of 14 cases, *J Am Anim Hosp Assoc* 32:159, 1996.

Saito M, et al.: Muscle cramps in two standard poodles with hypoadrenocorticism, *J Am Anim Hosp Assoc* 38:437, 2002.

Schaer M, et al.: Autoimmunity and Addison's disease in the dog, *J Am Anim Hosp Assoc* 22:789, 1986.

Schaer M, et al.: Combined hyponatremia and hyperkalemia mimicking an addisonian crisis in three near-term pregnant Greyhounds, *J Vet Intern Med* 14:121, 2000.

Schoeman JP, et al.: Serum cortisol and thyroxine concentrations as predictors of death in critically ill puppies with parvoviral diarrhea, *J Am Vet Med Assoc* 231:1534, 2007.

Scott-Moncrieff JCR, et al.: Validation of chemiluminescent enzyme immunometric assay for plasma adrenocorticotropic hormone in the dog, *Vet Clin Pathol* 32, 2003.

Seth M, et al.: White blood cell count and the sodium to potassium ratio to screen for hypoadrenocorticism in dogs, *J Vet Intern Med* 25:1351, 2011.

Shaker E, et al.: Hypoadrenocorticism in a family of Standard Poodles, *J Am Vet Med Assoc* 192:1091, 1988.

Shiah CJ, et al.: Diagnostic value of plasma aldosterone/potassium ratio in hypoaldosteronism, *J Formos Med Assoc* 94:248–254, 1995

Sieber-Ruckstuhl NS, et al.: Cortisol, aldosterone, cortisol precursor, androgen, andendogenous ACTH concentrations in dogs with pituitary-dependent hyperadrenocorticism treated with trilostane, *Domest Anim Endocrinol* 31:63, 2006.

Short AD, et al.: A candidate gene analysis of canine hypoadrenocorticism in 3 dog breeds, *J Heredity* 104:807, 2013.

Smallwood LJ, Barsanti J: Hypoadrenocorticism in a family of Leonbergers, *J Am Anim Hosp Assoc* 31:301, 1995.

Stewart PM, Krone NP: The adrenal cortex. In Melmed S, et al.: *Williams textbook for endocrinology*, ed 12, Philadelphia, 2011, Saunders/Elsevier.

Syme HM, Scott-Moncrieff JC: Chronic hypoglycemia in a hunting dog due to secondary hypoadrenocorticism, *J Small Anim Pract* 39:348, 1998.

Thodou E, et al.: Lymphocytic hypophysitis: clinicopathological findings, *J Clin Endocrinol Metab* 80:2302, 1995.

Thompson AL, et al.: Comparison of classic hypoadrenocorticism with glucocorticoid-deficient hypoadrenocorticism in dogs: 46 cases (1985-2005), *J Am Vet Med Assoc* 230:1190, 2007.

Tsigos C, et al.: A novel mutation of the adrenocorticotropin receptor (ACTH-R) gene in a family with the syndrome of isolated glucocorticoid deficiency, but no ACTH-R abnormalities in two families with the triple A syndrome, *J Clin Endocrinol Metab* 80:2186, 1995.

Velardo A, et al.: Isolated adrenocorticotropic hormone deficiency secondary to hypothalamic deficit of corticotropin-releasing hormone, *J Endocrinol Invest* 15:53, 1992.

Weller RE, et al.: Hypoadrenocorticism in beagles exposed to aerosols of plutonium-238 dioxide by inhalation, *Radiat Res* 146:688, 1996.

Wenger M, et al.: Ultrasonographic evaluation of adrenal glands in dogs with primary hypoadrenocorticism and mimicking diseases, *Vet Rec* 167:207, 2010.

White PC: Aldosterone synthase deficiency and related disorders, *Mol Cell Endocrinol* 217:81, 2004.

Whitley NT: Megaesophagus and glucocorticoid-deficient hypoadrenocorticism in a dog, *J Am Anim Pract* 36:132, 1995.

Willard MD: Disorders of potassium homeostasis, *Vet Clin North Am Small Anim Pract* 19:241, 1989.

Willard MD, et al.: Canine hypoadrenocorticism: report of 37 cases and review of 39 previously reported cases, *J Am Vet Med Assoc* 180:59, 1982.

Willard MD, et al.: Evaluation of plasma aldosterone concentrations before and after ACTH administration in clinically normal dogs and dogs with various diseases, *Am J Vet Res* 48:713, 1987.

Willard MD, et al.: Hyponatremia and hyperkalemia associated with idiopathic or experimentally induced chylothorax in four dogs, *J Am Vet Med Assoc* 199:353, 1991.

Zenger E: Persistent hyperkalemia associated with nonchylous pleural effusion in a dog, *J Am Anim Hosp Assoc* 28:411, 1992.

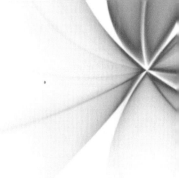

| CHAPTER 13 | Pheochromocytoma and Multiple Endocrine Neoplasia |

Claudia E. Reusch

CHAPTER CONTENTS

 ## HISTORY AND BACKGROUND

In 1884, an 18-year-old woman died at the University Hospital of Freiburg, a town in southern Germany. She had been suffering of recurrent episodes of palpitations, headaches, vomiting, pallor accompanied by a strong pulse, and retinitis (Manger, 2006). At autopsy, bilateral adrenal tumors were found in addition to myocardial hypertrophy and arterial changes in the kidneys. The pathologists diagnosed sarcoma for one adrenal tumor and angiosarcoma for the other. Felix Fränkel, a physician at the same hospital in which the woman had died, published the case in 1886 and suggested, which was different to the opinion of the pathologists, that the tumors were of the same type and that they had induced a generalized vasoactive disease (Fränkel, 1886). He did, however, not yet use the term *pheochromocytoma*. The original article of Fränkel was written in German; in 1984, it was translated into English as a Classic in Oncology (Classics in oncology, 1984). The case of the young woman was reconsidered by a research group of the same hospital in Freiburg 120 years after its publication (Neumann et al, 2007). The group hypothesized that the patient's pheochromocytoma had been an inherited condition because of her young age and the presence of bilateral disease. Because Fränkel had given the name and hometown of his patient in his paper (a fact which would be incompatible with today's regulations on data protection), they were able to start an extensive search for potential relatives. After contacting church offices, telephone directories, and the European-American Pheochromocytoma Registry, several descendants were identified who had developed pheochromocytomas between the age of 36 and 44 years. By molecular genetic testing, Neumann and colleagues were able to demonstrate germ-line RET mutations and hence provided evidence that the pheochromocytomas of the original patient and her family were in fact inherited as part of the multiple endocrine neoplasia type 2 (MEN-2) complex (Neumann et al, 2007).

The term *pheochromocytoma* was first proposed in 1912 by Ludwig Pick, a pathologist from Berlin, Germany. It comes from the Greek words *phaios* (dark), *chroma* (color), and *cytoma* (tumor), indicating the dark staining reaction caused by the oxidation of catecholamines when exposed to chromium salts (Manger, 2006; Young, 2011). In 1926, the first pheochromocytomas were successfully surgically removed by César Roux in Switzerland and Charles Mayo in the United States. In the following decades, epinephrine (in 1939) and norepinephrine (in 1949) were isolated from pheochromocytoma tissue; and in 1950, it was shown that patients with pheochromocytomas have elevated epinephrine and norepinephrine in plasma and urine (Manger, 2006; Young, 2011).

Approximately 80 years after Fränkel's publication, the first two cases of pheochromocytoma in dogs were described, interestingly also in Germany (Mueller et al, 1955; Tamaschke, 1955). The first pheochromocytoma in a cat was reported not until 1993 (Henry et al, 1993).

For many years pheochromocytoma in dogs and cats were usually identified as an incidental finding at necropsy, and ante mortem diagnoses were extremely rare. This was due to several reasons: low index of suspicion by veterinarians; the fact that clinical signs are highly variable, nonspecific, and often episodic; and lack of appropriate screening tests. During the past decade, awareness of the potential presence of pheochromocytomas in sick animals has increased, which is mainly due to the routine use of abdominal ultrasonography and the frequent identification of adrenal masses. Recently, biochemical testing (i.e., measurement of catecholamines and their metabolites in urine or plasma) has been introduced into veterinary medicine allowing specific diagnostic work-up.

 ## DEFINITION, EMBRYOLOGY, ANATOMY, AND ETIOLOGY

The World Health Organization (WHO) classification of endocrine tumors defines a pheochromocytoma as a tumor arising from catecholamine-producing chromaffin cells in the adrenal medulla. Tumors of the extra-adrenal sympathetic and parasympathetic paraganglia are classified as paragangliomas (Pacak et al, 2007). This definition will also be followed in this chapter. Pheochromocytoma (tumor of the adrenal medulla) is discussed in the following sections, and paraganglioma will be covered thereafter. The adrenal medulla, which comprises approximately one-fourth of the adrenal mass, develops during fetal life as part of the sympathetic nervous system. The latter arises from the primitive cells of the neural crest; groups of these cells migrate along the central vein and enter the adrenal cortex to form the adrenal medulla (Galac et al, 2010; Sjaastad et al, 2010; Fitzgerald, 2011). The cells of the adrenal medulla, called *pheochromocytes* or *chromaffin cells*, can be looked at as modified postganglionic sympathetic neurons lacking axons. They are stimulated by sympathetic preganglionic nerve fibers and secrete hormones into the bloodstream.

The adrenal medulla receives most of its blood through a portal vascular system from the adrenal cortex; consequently, it receives high concentrations of glucocorticoids. Cortisol induces the enzyme, phenylethanolamine-N-methyltransferase (PNMT), which is responsible for the conversion of norepinephrine to epinephrine (Fig. 13-1). Cells of the adrenal medulla, which synthesize epinephrine, are exposed to higher concentrations of glucocorticoids than cells that produce norepinephrine. The latter (i.e., cells that synthesize mostly norepinephrine) receive their blood supply by arteries that bypass the adrenal cortex (Fitzgerald, 2011).

In humans, pheochromocytoma is considered to be a rare tumor. The incidence has long been estimated to be as low as 2 to 8 cases per million people annually (Beard et al, 1983; Stenström and Svärdsudd, 1986). More recent autopsy studies, however, suggest that the incidence may be higher and that many cases remain undetected (McNeil et al, 2000). Many of the pheochromocytomas in humans develop sporadically, and their etiology is not understood. Recently, genetic screening revealed that a substantial percentage (20% to 30%) of patients with pheochromocytoma or paraganglioma have germline mutations in genes associated with genetic disease. So far, 10 genes have been identified, the three genes known best are: RET for MEN-2, VHL for von Hippel-Lindau disease, and NF1 for neurofibromatosis type 1 (Marini et al, 2006a; Maher et al, 2011; Fishbein and Nathanson, 2012; Table 13-1). It is assumed that the majority of human pheochromocytomas are benign; malignancy rates vary between 5% and 35% depending on the study. However, the biological behavior of pheochromocytoma is unpredictable, and reliable differentiation between benign and malignant tumors is difficult. The traditional position of the WHO is to base the diagnosis of malignancy on the presence of metastasis (and not on local invasion; Tischler et al, 2006; Carlsen et al, 2009). Because this approach requires life-long follow-up of patients, various techniques and markers, including the multiparameter scoring system Pheochromocytoma of the Adrenal Scaled Score (PASS), have been evaluated for their usefulness to predict malignancy. Results of the various studies differ; it seems, however, that none of the methods is 100% reliable (Carlsen et al, 2009; Agarwal et al, 2010; de Wailly et al, 2012; Eisenhofer et al, 2012). It may be interesting to follow future discussions on the criteria of malignancy. Although the WHO approach is clear, some pathologists challenge the definition because local invasion may also be potentially lethal (Tischler et al, 2006).

As in humans, pheochromocytoma is considered to be a rare tumor in dogs. According to currently available information they account for 0.01% to 0.1% of all canine tumors (Bailey and Page, 2007). However, due to the fact that comprehensive systemic evaluation has not been performed, it is possible that the true prevalence is higher. In cats, pheochromocytomas are extremely rare, and knowledge is limited to a few case reports (Henry et al, 1993; Chun et al, 1997; Calsyn et al, 2010). Growth rate of

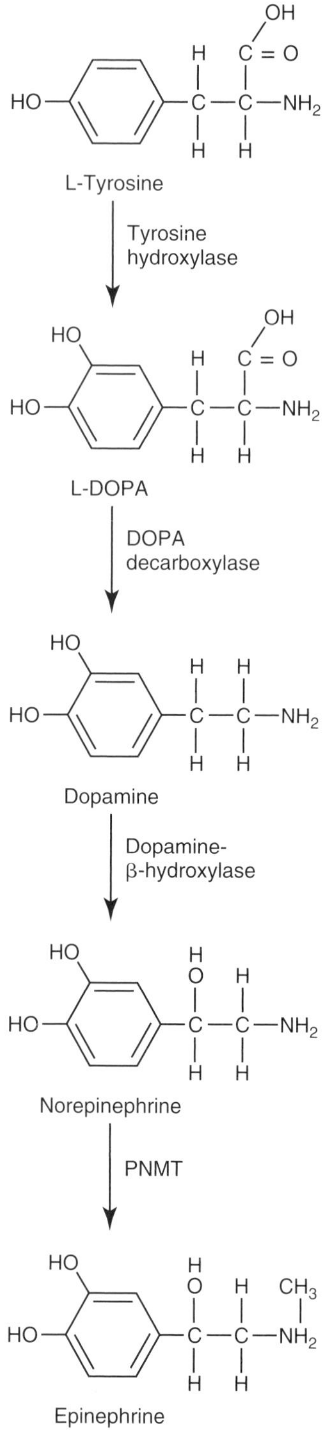

FIGURE 13-1 Biosynthetic pathway of catecholamines. (Redrawn from Fitzgerald PA: Adrenal medulla and paraganglia. In Gardner DA, Shoback D, editors: *Greenspan's Basic and Clinical Endocrinology,* ed 9, New York, 2011, McGraw-Hill, p. 351.) *L-DOPA,* L-dihydroxyphenylalanine; *PNMT,* phenylethanolamine-N-methyltransferase.

pheochromocytomas is unpredictable and may range from slow to quite rapid. The rate of malignant tumors seems to be much higher than in humans; however, those comparisons depend on how malignancy is perceived. As mentioned earlier, in human pheochromocytoma malignancy is currently defined by the presence of metastasis, not local invasion. In dogs, however, either local invasion or distant metastasis usually qualifies for the definition of malignancy. Information concerning the matter of malignancy

				OCCURRENCE OF
GENETIC SYNDROME	**INHERITANCE**	**GENE**	**CLINICAL FEATURES**	**PHEOCHROMOCYTOMA**
Multiple Endocrine Neoplasia Type 2				
Subtype 2A	Autosomal dominant	RET	• MTC • Hyperparathyroidism • Pheochromocytoma (often bilateral) • Cutaneous lichen amyloidosis • Hirschsprung disease	≈50%
Subtype 2B	Autosomal dominant	RET	• MTC • Pheochromocytoma (often bilateral) • Mucocutaneous neuromas • Skeletal deformities, joint laxity • Marfanoid habitus • Myelinated corneal nerves • Intestinal ganglioneuromas	≈50%
von Hippel-Lindau disease various subtypes	Autosomal dominant	VHL	• CNS hemangioblastoma • Renal angioma • Renal cell carcinoma • Pheochromocytoma (often bilateral) • Paraganglioma • Pancreatic NETs • Renal and pancreatic cysts • Endolymphatic sac tumors • Epididymal cystadenomas	≈10% to 20%
Neurofibromatosis type 1 (von Recklinghausen disease)	Autosomal dominant	NF1	• Cutaneous neurofibromas • Multiple café-au-lait spots • Axillary and inguinal freckling • Iris hamartomas • Pheochromocytoma (mostly unilateral) • Paraganglioma	≈5% to 7%

TABLE 13-1 **THE THREE BEST-KNOWN GENETIC SYNDROMES ASSOCIATED WITH PHEOCHROMOCYTOMA IN HUMANS***

Modified from Mackenzie IS, Brown MJ: Phaeochromocytomas, paragangliomas and neuroblastomas. In Wass JA, Stewart PM, Amiel SA, Davies MJ, editors: *Oxford Textbook of Endocrinology and Diabetes*, ed 2, Oxford, 2011, Oxford University Press, p. 798.
CNS, Central nervous system; *MTC*, medullary thyroid carcinoma; *NET*, neuroendocrine tumor.
*Please note that the occurrence rate of the disorders within the syndromes varies between patients, and only the approximate occurrence rate of pheochromocytoma is given. The syndromes (in particular, neurofibromatosis type 1) may also occur with various additional diseases.

in dogs is based mainly on the three largest case series published so far, including 123 dogs with pheochromocytoma (Bouayad et al, 1987; Gilson et al, 1994; Barthez et al, 1997). In 34% of the dogs, local invasion of adjacent vessels, such as vena phrenicoabdominales, vena cava caudalis, renal vessels, adrenal vessels, hepatic veins, and aorta or other tissue was found. Additionally, 20% of dogs had metastasis in regional lymph nodes, liver, spleen, kidneys, pancreas, lung, heart, bone, and central nervous system (CNS). In sum, more than 50% of canine pheochromocytomas were considered malignant, a number often quoted today. It may, however, be that small and potentially benign pheochromocytomas go undetected, and therefore the overall malignancy may be overestimated. In the three pheochromocytomas described in cats, so far invasion or metastasis was absent (Henry et al, 1993; Chun et al, 1997; Calsyn et al, 2010).

The size of pheochromocytomas is extremely variable, and their diameter ranges between a few millimeters and more than 15 centimeters. Most pheochromocytomas in dogs are unilateral, less than 10% are bilateral. Dogs with pheochromocytoma may have one or several additional endocrine neoplasias, such as glucocorticoid-producing adrenocortical adenoma or carcinoma,

adrenocorticotropic hormone (ACTH)-producing pituitary tumors, parathyroid tumor or hyperplasia, thyroid adenoma, or carcinoma and insulinoma (Peterson et al, 1982; Gilson et al, 1994; Wright et al, 1995; Barthez et al, 1997; Thuróczy et al, 1998). These patients may be considered to suffer a multiple endocrine neoplasia (MEN)-like disorder. However, inherited MEN syndromes, as they occur in humans, have thus far not been identified in dogs (see later). Coexistence of non-endocrine tumors is also common. In two case series, 50% and 54% of dogs with pheochromocytoma had additional endocrine or non-endocrine neoplasias (Gilson et al, 1994; Barthez et al, 1997).

PHYSIOLOGY AND PATHOPHYSIOLOGY

Catecholamines are molecules that contain a catechol structure (ortho-dihydroxybenzene) and a side chain with an amino group. Catecholamines include epinephrine (adrenaline), norepinephrine (noradrenaline), and dopamine (Young, 2011). They are synthesized from the amino acid tyrosine, which is derived from food or formed from phenylalanine in the liver (see Fig. 13-1). Tyrosine enters neurons and chromaffin cells and is converted to L-dihydroxyphenylalanine (L-DOPA) by the enzyme tyrosine hydroxylase. This conversion is the rate-limiting step in the catecholamine synthesis pathway; intracellular catecholamine depletion rapidly increases the enzyme activity, whereas increased catecholamine levels lead to its down-regulation. Dopa is decarboxylated to dopamine, which is the final product in some neurons. In the adrenal medulla and most sympathetic postganglionic neurons, dopamine is hydroxylated to norepinephrine. In most sympathetic postganglionic neurons, norepinephrine is the final product. Hydroxylation of dopamine to norepinephrine takes place after its active transport into granulated vesicles. In the adrenal medulla, norepinephrine is released from the vesicles into the cytoplasms of the chromaffin cells where the enzyme PNMT (see earlier) transforms it to epinephrine. Epinephrine is then transported into another vesicle (Cryer, 2001; Fitzgerald, 2011; Young, 2011). The expression of PNMT is enhanced by cortisol, which is present in high concentrations in the adrenal medulla due to the blood supply from the adrenal cortex. Although the enzyme PNMT is also found in other tissues than the adrenal medulla, the amount of epinephrine from extra-adrenal sources is small. This means that under physiological conditions, nearly all of the epinephrine in the circulation comes from the adrenal medulla, whereas circulating norepinephrine is mostly derived from postganglionic sympathetic neurons (Fitzgerald, 2011; Young, 2011). Within the adrenal medulla, the amount of stored epinephrine to norepinephrine varies between species. In the normal human medulla, 80% of catecholamines are epinephrine and 20% are norepinephrine. In dogs, 70% is epinephrine and 30% is norepinephrine; in cats, the percentages are 60% and 40% (Fitzgerald and Goldfien, 2004). Epinephrine and norepinephrine are stored in intracellular vesicles together with many other substances, such as chromogranins, adrenomedullin, neuropeptide Y, vasoactive intestinal peptide (VIP), enkephalins, pituitary adenylate cyclase activating polypeptide, and ACTH (Thouennon et al, 2010; Fitzgerald, 2011). The question of the physiological relevance of those peptides is an area of intensive research. Chromogranin A (CGA) for instance, which is widely used as diagnostic marker for tumors of neuroendocrine origin, seems to have an important role for storage and release of catecholamines (Loh et al, 2004; Elias et al, 2010).

Secretion of catecholamines takes place by exocytosis of the intracellular vesicles as part of the activation of the sympathetic nervous system. Catecholamine secretion increases with exercise, perceived danger, surgery, hypovolemia, hypotension, hypoglycemia, and many other stressful events (Galac et al, 2010; Fitzgerald, 2011). The plasma half-life of catecholamines is extremely short (1 to 3 minutes). Metabolism of secreted catecholamines occurs mostly in the liver and kidney; they may also be inactivated by conjugation, which happens mainly in the gastrointestinal tract. Metabolites of catecholamines, conjugates, and free catecholamines are excreted in the urine; free catecholamines account for only a small amount (Fitzgerald, 2011). Two enzyme systems are involved in the catecholamine metabolism: catechol-O-methyltransferase (COMT) and monoamine oxidase (MAO). In the normal adrenal medulla and in pheochromocytoma, membrane-bound COMT metabolizes epinephrine to metanephrine and norepinephrine to normetanephrine (Fig. 13-2). It is important to understand that most metabolism of catecholamines happens in the same cells in which they are produced (Eisenhofer et al, 2004a). In contrast to the catecholamines that are released only intermittently (by means of exocytosis of storage vesicles), their metabolites are constantly leaking into the circulation. This difference explains why the measurement of metanephrines (which equals the sum of metanephrine and normetanephrine) is superior to the measurement of catecholamines in the diagnosis of pheochromocytoma (Eisenhofer, 2001).

Catecholamines act by binding to receptors located in the cell membrane of the target cells. From there, signal transduction to intracellular sites takes place via G-proteins (i.e., adrenergic receptors are so-called G-protein coupled receptors). They are present in most cells of the body and are responsible to mediate the body's reaction to stress. The two broad categories of α- and β-receptors have further expanded into nine receptor subtypes: three α_1 (α_{1a}, α_{1b}, and α_{1d}), three α_2 (α_{2A}, α_{2B}, and α_{2C}), and three β (β_1, β_2, and β_3) (Cotecchia, 2010). Epinephrine and norepinephrine both act on α- and β-adrenergic receptors. They have approximately the same potency to stimulate α- and β_1-receptors. Epinephrine is much more potent to stimulate β_2, and norepinephrine is more potent to stimulate β_3-receptors (Fitzgerald, 2011). The effects of catecholamines depend on the density of the different receptors and their subtypes on specific organs and the relative concentrations of epinephrine and norepinephrine. Additionally, the effects may be modulated by receptor dynamics (e.g., phenomena known as receptor desensitization and resensitization; Tsujimoto et al, 1984; García-Sáinz et al, 2011; Vasudevan et al, 2011). Norepinephrine causes vasoconstriction (α_1) and increase in cardiac contractility and rate (β_1). The effects are modulated by reflex mechanism (e.g., an increase in heart rate is limited by simultaneous vagal stimulation). Epinephrine, through activation of α_1 and β_1 receptors, has the same effects as norepinephrine. However, epinephrine also stimulates β_2 receptors, which causes vasodilation in skeletal muscles. The effect of epinephrine on blood pressure is therefore variable and depends on its plasma concentration: At low concentrations epinephrine mainly stimulates β_2 receptors leading to vasodilation, and at higher concentrations the effect on α_1 receptors dominates causing vasoconstriction (Sjaastad et al, 2010; Fitzgerald, 2011). Table 13-2 gives an overview over the physiologic effects of catecholamines. In short, those effects support the organisms in stressful events and mediate the "fright, flight, fight" response—increase in heart rate and contractility, increase in blood pressure, increase in respiration rate, decrease in gastrointestinal motility, increase in blood glucose and fatty acids, and increased alertness.

The clinical signs in patients with a pheochromocytoma can be explained by the known actions of catecholamines or less frequently by tumor size and invasiveness. Catecholamine secretion from pheochromocytomas is highly variable with regard to relative amounts and types of catecholamines as well as to time of release (i.e., episodic versus continuous). In humans, these differences have been shown to be due to differences in expression of genes responsible for the regulation of the catecholamine synthesis pathway and differences in genes encoding the components of the complex secretory processes (Eisenhofer et al, 2011). Different to the normal medulla, the majority of pheochromocytomas in humans produce more norepinephrine than epinephrine, and many pheochromocytomas produce both catecholamines. Some tumors produce predominantly epinephrine (Fitzgerald, 2011). Recent studies have categorized human pheochromocytomas as with either noradrenergic or adrenergic phenotypes. The adrenergic phenotype represents a situation in which the enzyme PNMT (the enzyme that converts norepinephrine to epinephrine) is expressed, and the tumor secretes norepinephrine and epinephrine in various proportions. In the noradrenergic phenotype, PNMT is lacking and tumors produce

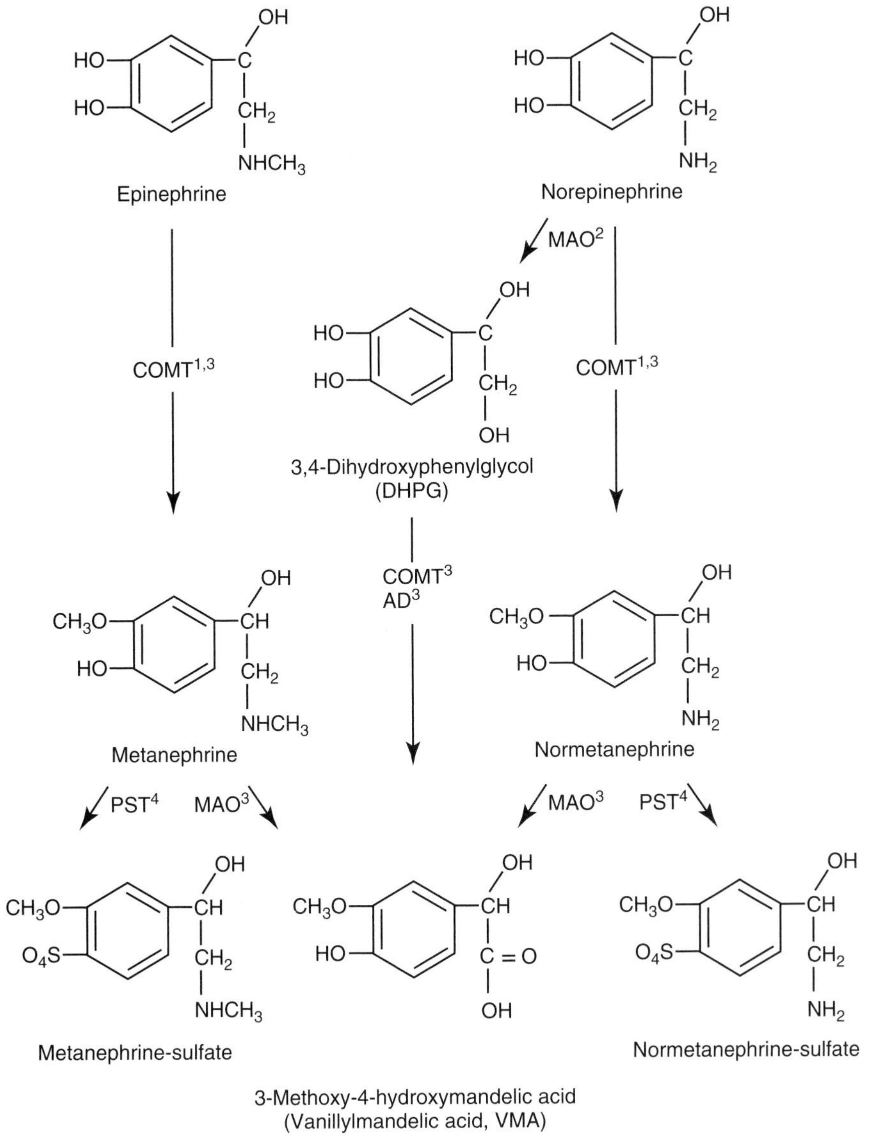

FIGURE 13-2 Metabolism of catecholamines by catechol-O-methyltransferase (COMT), monoamine oxidase (MAO), aldehyde dehydrogenase (AD), and phenol-sulfotransferase (PST). *1,* adrenal medulla or pheochromocytoma; *2,* sympathetic nerves; *3,* liver and kidneys; *4,* gastrointestinal tract, platelets, and lungs. (Modified from Fitzgerald PA: Adrenal medulla and paraganglia. In Gardner DA, Shoback D, editors: *Greenspan's Basic and Clinical Endocrinology,* ed 9, New York, 2011, McGraw-Hill, p. 351, with permission.)

predominantly norepinephrine (Eisenhofer et al, 2004b; 2008a; 2011; Pacak, 2011). In tumors with an adrenergic phenotype, the epinephrine content may vary between 11% and 90% of the combined epinephrine and norepinephrine content; in noradrenergic phenotype tumors, epinephrine content is less than 10% (Eisenhofer et al, 2005a). It was shown that the kind of mutation determines the phenotype: tumors due to RET, NF1, and the newly discovered TMEM127 mutations have an adrenergic phenotype, whereas tumors due to *VHL* mutations have a noradrenergic phenotype (Mannelli et al, 2012a). Metastasis of pheochromocytoma usually produces predominantly norepinephrine (Pacak, 2011). On very rare occasions pheochromocytomas may only produce dopamine (dopaminergic phenotype). Those tumors are caused by a lack of expression of the enzyme dopamine β-hydroxylase, which converts dopamine to norepinephrine; typically they are not associated with hypertension (Feldman et al, 1979; Mannelli et al, 2012a).

In general, tumor size in humans is positively correlated with the amount of catecholamines and metanephrines released into the circulation (i.e., small tumors secrete less than large tumors). The relationship between size and released concentration is stronger for metanephrines than for catecholamines (Eisenhofer et al, 2005a). This is most likely due to the fact that metanephrines are released continuously, whereas catecholamines are usually secreted episodically.

Catecholamine release from pheochromocytoma happens spontaneously and may be induced by various factors and drugs. The latter is a particular problematic issue in patients with an unrecognized tumor (Eisenhofer et al, 2007; Mannelli et al, 2012a; Box 13-1).

In addition to catecholamines and metanephrines, pheochromocytomas may secrete a multitude of other peptides. Those may add abnormalities to the clinical picture (e.g., hypercalcemia in case of parathyroid hormone–related peptide [PTHrp] secretion) and/or may counterbalance catecholamine effects (Box 13-2). Human pheochromocytomas may also produce inflammatory cytokines, and several cases of systemic inflammatory syndrome have been described (Tokuda et al, 2009).

Some human pheochromocytomas may present as clinically silent, termed *subclinical* pheochromocytomas. However, true nonsecretory pheochromocytomas are very rare; they may sometimes be associated with certain mutations. Apparently subclinical pheochromocytomas may cause sudden hypertensive crisis and even death. There are various reasons why those tumors may

TABLE 13-2 CATECHOLAMINE RECEPTORS SUBTYPES, TISSUE LOCATIONS, AND ACTIONS

CATECHOLAMINE RECEPTOR	TISSUE LOCATION	ACTION FOLLOWING RECEPTOR ACTIVATION
α_1	• Vascular smooth muscle • Liver • Eye • Skin • Prostate • Uterus • Intestines • Spleen capsule	• Increases vasoconstriction (increases blood pressure) • Increases glycogenolysis and gluconeogenesis • Increases ciliary muscle contraction (pupil dilation) • Increases pilomotor smooth muscle contraction (erects hairs) • Increases contraction and ejaculation • Increases gravid uterus contraction • Increases sphincter tone and relaxes smooth muscle • Contracts spleen volume, expelling blood
α_2	• Preganglionic nerves • Vascular smooth muscle • Pancreatic islet cells • Blood platelets • Adipose cells • Brain	• Decreases release of neurotransmitter • Increases vasoconstriction (increases blood pressure) • Decreases release of insulin and glucagon • Increases platelet aggregation • Decreases lipolysis • Decreases norepinephrine release
β_1	• Myocardium • Kidney (juxtaglomerular apparatus) • Adipose cells • Most tissues • Nerves	• Increases force and rate of contraction • Increases secretion of renin • Increases lipolysis • Increases calorigenesis • Increases conduction velocity
β_2	• Vascular smooth muscle • Bronchiolar smooth muscle • Liver • Intestinal smooth muscle • Pancreatic islet cells • Adipose tissue • Muscles • Liver and kidney • Uterus smooth muscle	• Decreases vasoconstriction (increases blood flow) • Decreases contraction (bronchial dilation) • Increases glycogenolysis and gluconeogenesis • Decreases intestinal motility; increases sphincter tone • Increases release of insulin and glucagon • Increases lipolysis • Increases muscle contraction speed and glycogenolysis • Increases peripheral conversion of T_4 to T_3 • Decreases nongravid uterine contraction (uterine relaxation)
β_3	• Adipose cells • Intestinal smooth muscle	• Increases lipolysis • Increases intestinal motility
Dopamine$_1$	• Vascular smooth muscle • Renal tubule	• Decreases vasoconstriction (vasodilation) • Enhances natriuresis
Dopamine$_2$	• Sympathetic nerves • Pituitary lactotrophs • Gastrointestinal tract	• Inhibits synaptic release of norepinephrine • Inhibits prolactin release • Paracrine functions

Modified from Fitzgerald PA: Adrenal medulla and paraganglia. In Gardner DA, Shoback D, editors: *Greenspan's basic and clinical endocrinology*, ed 9, New York, 2011, McGraw-Hill, p. 353, with permission.
Dopamine$_1$, Dopamine$_1$-like family of receptors; *dopamine$_2$*, dopamine$_2$-like family of receptors; T_3, triiodothyronine; T_4, thyroxine.

appear silent, such as small tumor size in the early stages of development, large tumors with extensive tissue loss due to necrosis and hemorrhage, paroxysmal symptoms with long asymptomatic periods and low medical awareness, and counteraction of the effects of catecholamines by co-secreted peptides (Mannelli et al, 2012a).

Information on pathophysiological aspects of pheochromocytoma in dogs is scarce. However, many of the findings in dogs appear to be similar to those in humans. As in humans, clinical signs including hypertension occur paroxysmal in most dogs with pheochromocytoma pointing to sporadic (and unpredictable) catecholamine secretion. Some dogs reveal more constant clinical signs, which is most likely associated with continuous catecholamine release at a lower rate. There are also dogs that are clinically asymptomatic (or have extremely mild signs), and the pheochromocytoma is an incidental finding. As in humans, there seems to be a correlation between severity and presence of clinical signs and tumor size. Very small pheochromocytomas are more

often an incidental finding than large tumors, and very serious clinical signs are more often associated with large than with small tumors (Feldman and Nelson, 2004a). Investigation of catecholamines and metanephrines in urine and plasma has only recently been started, and secretion patterns have not yet been established. According to our preliminary results, norepinephrine concentrations are increased in most dogs with pheochromocytoma, whereas a minority of dogs also reveals an increase in epinephrine (Kook et al, 2007; 2010; Quante et al, 2010; Salesov et al, 2012). Therefore, it is likely that also in canine pheochromocytoma, norepinephrine is the predominant catecholamine. By means of immunohistochemical stainings, it has been shown that neoplastic cells also contain various peptides (e.g., somatostatin, CGA, substance P, VIP, synaptophysin, galanin, leu-enkephalin, met-enkephalin, and S 100 protein) (Wilson et al, 1986; Cuervo et al, 1994; Sako et al, 2001). It is likely that those peptides contribute to the clinical picture.

BOX 13-1   Factors that have been Reported to Induce Hypertensive Crisis in Human Patients with Pheochromocytoma

Mechanical/Physical Influences
- Palpation of abdomen
- Physical exercise
- Change of posture
- Cough or sneezing
- Defecation
- Sexual intercourse
- Delivery
- Surgery
- Invasive diagnostic procedures

Drugs
- Monoamine oxidase (MAO) inhibitors
- Tricyclic antidepressants
- β-blockers
- Metoclopramide
- Sympathomimetics
- Decongestants
- Glucagon
- Glucocorticoids
- Adrenocorticotropic hormone (ACTH)
- Opiates
- Histamine
- Tyramine
- Alcohol
- Nicotine
- Chlorpromazine
- Chemotherapy

Others
- Pain
- Emotional stress
- Cold exposure
- Food and drinks containing tyramine (e.g., aged cheese, meats, fish, chocolate, bananas, beer, and wine)

Modified from Fitzgerald PA: Adrenal medulla and paraganglia. In Gardner DA, Shoback D, editors: *Greenspan's basic and clinical endocrinology*, ed 9, New York, 2011, McGraw-Hill; Mannelli M, et al.: Subclinical phaeochromocytoma, *Best Pract Res Clin Endocrinol Metab* 26:507, 2012a, with permission.

BOX 13-2   Substances that may be Co-Secreted with Catecholamines and Metanephrines in Human Patients with Pheochromocytoma

Peptide	Correlated Signs
Vasoactive intestinal peptide (VIP)	Diarrhea, flushes
Substance P	Flushes
Somatostatin	Constipation
Enkephalin	Constipation
Motilin	Diarrhea
Neuropeptide Y	Vasoconstriction
Renin	Hypertension
Corticotropin-releasing factor (CRF)	Hypercortisolism
Adrenocorticotrophic hormone (ACTH)	Hypercortisolism
Melanocyte-stimulating hormone (MSH)	Melanodermia
Parathyroid hormone (PTH)	Hypercalcemia
PTH-related peptide (PTHrp)	Hypercalcemia
Endothelin	Vasoconstriction
Erythropoietin	Polycythemia
Angiotensin converting enzyme (ACE)	Hypertension
Growth hormone-releasing hormone (GHRH)	Acromegaly
Interleukin-6 (IL-6)	Fever
Neuron-specific enolase (NSE)	
Chromogranin A (CGA)	
Insulin-like growth factor-2 (IGF-2)	Hypoglycemia
Atrial natriuretic peptide (ANP)	Polyuria, hypotension
Calcitonin	
Calcitonin-related peptide (CGRP)	Vasodilation
Pituitary adenylate-cyclase activating peptide	Vasodilation
Adrenomedullin	Vasodilation

Modified from Mannelli M, et al.: Subclinical phaeochromocytoma, *Best Pract Res Clin Endocrinol Metab* 26:507, 2012a, with permission; amended by Fukuda I, et al.: Clinical features of insulin-like growth factor-II producing non-islet-cell tumor hypoglycemia, *Growth Horm IGF Res* 16:211, 2006.

(e.g., Golden Retriever, Labrador Retriever, Boxer, Doberman, German Shepherd, poodle, and terrier breeds) may just reflect their popularity.

The three cats described with pheochromocytoma so far were 7, 11, and 15 years old, two were castrated males, and one was a spayed female. All three were Domestic Short-Hair cats (Henry et al, 1993; Chun et al, 1997; Calsyn et al, 2010).

Clinical Manifestations

Clinical signs are most often the result of the secretion of excessive amounts of catecholamines by the pheochromocytoma. Less commonly, they are due to the space-occupying or invasive nature of the tumor or metastasis (Box 13-3). Pheochromocytoma should be considered a potentially life-threatening disease that may result in collapse and sudden death due to massive catecholamine release or tumor rupture.

Hormone secretion from the tumors is highly variable, and consequently, the clinical picture varies considerably. The triggers for catecholamine secretion are usually unknown. Dogs may have some clinical signs at all times (e.g., lethargy, polydipsia/polyuria) with paroxysmal episodes of additional signs (e.g., panting, tachycardia), and other dogs may be clinically unremarkable between episodes. The episodes may occur frequently, such as several times per day or several times per week, or they may only recur after

Signalment

Since the first description of pheochromocytoma in dogs in 1955 (Mueller et al, 1955; Tamaschke, 1955), a little more than 200 cases have been published. Of those, 123 are part of three large case series (Bouayad et al, 1987; Gilson et al, 1994; Barthez et al, 1997); the others have been described either as single case reports or small case series comprising fewer than 10 cases.

Pheochromocytoma may be seen at any age; however, it occurs most commonly in older dogs. In the three case series, age ranged between 1 and 18 years with means between 11 and 12 years. In the other case reports and small case series, most dogs were 7 years and older, only approximately 5% of dogs were younger. There is no sex predilection because the relation between male and female dogs is approximately 1:1. Neutering also does not seem to have an obvious influence, because neutered as well as intact male and female dogs are affected. There also does not seem to be a breed predilection: pheochromocytomas have been described in more than 40 breeds. The somewhat higher frequency in some breeds

---

BOX 13-3   Categories of Clinical Signs in Dogs with Pheochromocytoma

CLINICAL SIGNS	SYMPTOMS
Clinical signs and findings caused by catecholamine excess	
Nonspecific	Anorexia, weight loss, lethargy
Related to cardiorespiratory system and/or hypertension	Tachypnea, dyspnea, panting, tachycardia, arrhythmias, collapse, pale mucus membranes, hemorrhages, acute blindness
Related to neuromuscular system	Weakness, anxiety, pacing, disorientation, muscle tremor, seizures
Miscellaneous	Polyuria/polydipsia, vomiting, diarrhea, abdominal enlargement, abdominal pain
Clinical signs caused by large, invasive tumor	Abdominal enlargement, ascites, abdominal pain, hind limb edema
Clinical signs caused by tumor rupture	Acute severe lethargy, painful abdomen, tachypnea, weakness, collapse, tachycardia, pale mucus membranes, prolonged capillary refill time
Clinical signs caused by metastasis	To brain: Seizures and other central nervous system (CNS) signs. To vertebral canal or bone: Tetraparesis, paraparesis, lameness, swelling, local pain

---

weeks to months. Their severity may range from very mild to life-threatening; severity of episodes may be similar each time or may progress over time (the latter is seen more often). The duration of symptoms before presentation of the patient to the veterinarian ranges from a few hours to several years. Many of the clinical signs may be explained by more common diseases and therefore the possibility of a pheochromocytoma may not be considered by the clinician. Additional difficulties occur if the time intervals between episodes are rather long and no link is made between them. Furthermore, the tumors often occur in conjunction with other serious diseases that are often more obvious and draw away the attention from a concurrent pheochromocytoma. In the three large case series, the percentage of dogs in which the presence of a pheochromocytoma was not considered and was an incidental finding (mostly at necropsy) ranged between 24% and 57% (Bouayad et al, 1987; Gilson et al, 1994; Barthez et al, 1997).

The clinical manifestations related to excessive catecholamine secretion may be categorized as follows (see Box 13-3):

- Nonspecific: Anorexia, weight loss, and/or lethargy
- Related to the cardiorespiratory system and/or hypertension: Tachypnea, dyspnea, panting, tachycardia, arrhythmias (mostly tachyarrhythmias), collapse, pale mucus membranes, nasal hemorrhage, gingival hemorrhage, ocular hemorrhage, and/or acute blindness
- Related to the neuromuscular system: Weakness, anxiety, pacing, disorientation, muscle tremor, and/or seizures
- Miscellaneous: Polyuria/polydipsia, vomiting, diarrhea, abdominal enlargement, and/or abdominal pain

Those categories reflect the enormous variability of clinical signs associated with pheochromocytoma, and it may be helpful to memorize them. Theoretically, a pheochromocytoma may be considered several times per day, because most sick dogs presented to the veterinarian have one or several of the problems mentioned earlier. Of course, pheochromocytoma is still a rare disease; nevertheless, one should remember that many pheochromocytomas are still overlooked due to a low level of medical awareness.

The most frequent clinical signs are weakness, lethargy, tachypnea/panting, and collapse. Those signs often occur as intermittent episodes associated with intermittent catecholamine release. They may, however, also present as acute events (e.g., associated with tumor rupture, bleeding, and potential catecholamine surge). Other frequent signs seen by owners or found by the veterinarian during physical examinations are anorexia, weight loss, cardiac arrhythmias, tachycardia, polyuria/polydipsia, vomiting, and abdominal pain.

Cardiac arrhythmias are usually tachyarrhythmias (mostly supraventricular tachycardias, but ventricular premature complexes and ventricular tachycardia are also seen); so far only one case of pheochromocytoma-associated bradyarrhythmia (Mobitz type II atrioventricular [AV] block) has been described (Brown et al, 2007a).

Box 13-4 gives an overview over clinical signs and findings in 105 dogs with pheochromocytoma that have been described during the past decades. The box only includes those dogs in which the clinical signs were specified. Because not all authors may have listed all clinical signs and some of the signs may have been due to concurrent diseases, there may be some overestimations or underestimations. The signs and approximate percentages correspond relatively well with a compilation of clinical signs and findings in 40 dogs with pheochromocytoma with no other concurrent disorder. Those dogs had been seen at the University of California, Davis, and were included in the previous edition of this textbook (Tables 13-3 and 13-4). The pathophysiological mechanisms for some of the clinical signs are difficult to explain and may be multifactorial. For instance, polyuria/polydipsia may be due to excessive catecholamine release, release of other peptides from the tumor, or may represent a form of tumor-induced, secondary nephrogenic diabetes insipidus. The presence of polyuria/polydipsia is particularly challenging if it is the predominant sign. Together with the finding of an adrenal mass during work-up, it may be mistaken as evidence for adrenal-dependent hyperadrenocorticism, and the possibility of a pheochromocytoma may not be considered. It is also important to be aware that seizures in a dog with pheochromocytoma may be due to different causes. They may be caused by catecholamine-induced vasospasms, catecholamine/hypertension associated bleeding into the CNS, and also by brain metastasis from the pheochromocytoma. It is therefore advisable to perform brain imaging in any dog with (suspected) pheochromocytoma and seizures. Interestingly, the percentage of dogs presented with nasal bleeding, retinal bleeding, retinal detachment, and blindness is rather low. The reason is unclear. It may be that the presence of pheochromocytoma goes unnoticed in some dogs with retinal detachment and blindness because no complete work-up is performed. Alternatively, the catecholamine release and hypertensive episodes may not be frequent enough to cause these kinds of damage.

Clinical signs may also be caused by large tumor size, invasiveness into surrounding structures, and by metastasis. Invasion of adjacent structures most often affects the vena cava caudalis. Occlusion of the vena cava caudalis (partial or complete) is either by tumor thrombosis within the lumen or by large tumor size—both may cause ascites, hind limb edema, and distention of the caudal epigastric veins. However, clinical signs may also be absent although the vena cava is occluded, which is most likely due to

BOX 13-4	Frequency of Clinical Signs and Findings in Dogs with Pheochromocytoma*
Clinical sign	**Percentage of Dogs**
Weakness	40%
Tachypnea/panting	30%
Lethargy	24%
Collapse	21%
Anorexia	19%
Weight loss	19%
Cardiac arrhythmias	19%
Polyuria/polydipsia	15%
Pale mucus membranes	14%
Tachycardia	13%
Abdominal pain	13%
Abdominal distension (ascites and/or mass)	12%
Dyspnea	12%
Vomiting	12%
Hind limb lameness or paraparesis	10%
Cough	9%
Palpable abdominal mass	8%
Seizures	7%
Ataxia	6%
Weak pulse	4%
Cyanosis	3%
Front leg lameness	3%
Nasal/ocular bleeding	3%
Congestive heart failure/cardiac arrest	3%
Fever	2%
Injected mucus membranes	2%
Restlessness/pacing	1%
Muscle tremor	1%
Diarrhea	1%
Dilated pupils	1%
Jugular distension	1%
Regurgitation	1%
Quadriparesis	1%
Distension of caudal epigastric veins	1%

*The data are compiled from 105 dogs with pheochromocytoma that have been described during the past decades in three larger case series and 25 case reports or small case series. Only dogs that had shown clinical signs were used (i.e., asymptomatic dogs were excluded). Dogs with additional other endocrine tumors were also excluded. The given percentages should be considered as approximate numbers, because history taking and physical examination were of course not standardized between the studies. Some of the dogs had concurrent diseases, which may have contributed to the clinical signs. For comparison see Tables 13-3 and 13-4.

TABLE 13-3	FREQUENCY OF CLINICAL SIGNS IN 40 DOGS WITH PHEOCHROMOCYTOMA AND IDENTIFICATION OF NO OTHER CONCURRENT DISEASE*	
CLINICAL SIGN	**NUMBER OF DOGS**	**PERCENTAGE OF DOGS**
Collapsing episodes[†]	13	33%
Weakness[†]	12	30%
Panting/tachypnea[†]	12	30%
Polyuria/polydipsia	10	25%
Lethargy	10	25%
Vomiting	9	23%
Inappetence	8	20%
Anxiety/agitation/pacing[†]	6	15%
Diarrhea	4	10%
Abdominal distention	4	10%
Hemorrhage (nasal, ocular, gingival)	4	10%
Acute blindness	3	8%
Tremors[†]	3	8%
Weight loss	3	8%
Tachycardia/ "pounding" heart[†]	2	5%
Rear limb edema	2	5%
Tender or painful abdomen	2	5%
Adipsia	1	3%
No clinical signs	4	10%

*Those dogs had been seen at the University of California, Davis.
[†]Usually reported to be intermittent by the owner.

presented with acute onset of lethargy, tachypnea, weakness or collapse, tachycardia, pale mucus membranes, prolonged capillary refill time, and painful abdomen (Whittemore et al, 2001; Williams and Hackner, 2001). Emergency work-up including ultrasonography, clinical pathology, and emergency treatment is required in those cases.

Pheochromocytoma may metastasize into many organs, including regional lymph nodes, liver, spleen, kidneys, pancreas, lung, heart, bone, and CNS. Metastasis into the brain may lead to seizures and other CNS signs (Gilson et al, 1994). Metastasis to the vertebral canal, causing tetraparesis or paraparesis depending on the localization, and metastasis to bone (scapula, humerus, femur, and/or tibia), causing lameness, swelling, and pain have been reported several times (White and Cheyne, 1977; Stowater, 1979; Berzon, 1981; Platt et al, 1998; Head and Daniel, 2004; Boes et al, 2009; Spall et al, 2011).

As mentioned earlier, there seems to be a correlation between tumor size and severity of clinical signs. Small tumors are often an incidental finding or associated with relatively mild signs. Large tumors are often found in patients with serious clinical signs, invasion into the vena cava, and/or tumor rupture.

Physical examination findings are variable and depend on the secretory activity of the tumor at the time of the examination, and they depend on tumor size and the presence or absence of clinically relevant metastasis or if the tumor has ruptured. In a substantial

the development of collateral circulation (Bouayad et al, 1987; Santamarina et al, 2003). Aortic thromboembolism with painful and weak hind limbs, paraparesis, absence of femoral pulse, and cold distal extremities may occur in rare cases (Gilson et al, 1994; Santamarina et al, 2003). Dorsal extension of a pheochromocytoma into the vertebral canal with paresis has been described (Platt et al, 1998).

Spontaneous tumor rupture with retroperitoneal hemorrhage may occur as a rare event, either as the only and first presentation or in association with other clinical signs of pheochromocytoma during the course of the disease. This risk needs to be explained to owners of dogs with relatively large tumors who are reluctant to proceed to surgery. Dogs with tumor rupture are

TABLE 13-4	FREQUENCY OF ABNORMAL FINDINGS ON PHYSICAL EXAMINATION IN 40 DOGS WITH PHEOCHROMOCYTOMA AND IDENTIFICATION OF NO OTHER CONCURRENT DISEASE*	
PHYSICAL FINDING	**NUMBER OF DOGS**	**PERCENTAGE OF DOGS**
Panting, tachypnea	15	38%
Weakness	9	23%
Tachycardia	7	18%
Thin, muscle wasting	6	15%
Cardiac arrhythmias	6	15%
Hemorrhage (nasal, gingival, and/or ocular)	6	15%
Weak pulses	4	10%
Pale mucous membranes	4	10%
Abdominal pain	4	10%
Ascites	4	10%
Lethargy	3	8%
Palpable abdominal mass	2	5%
Shocky	2	5%
Blindness, retinal detachment	2	5%
Rear limb edema	1	3%
Shaking, muscle tremors	1	3%
Lateral recumbency	1	3%
Anterior uveitis	1	3%
Unremarkable	15	38%

*Those dogs had been seen at the University of California, Davis.
Common geriatric findings, such as lipomas, dental disease, and incidental cardiac murmurs are excluded.

proportion of dogs, the physical examination is unremarkable with regard to the pheochromocytoma. However, because the dogs usually are older, concurrent diseases are frequently present (in approximately 50% of cases). Because those diseases may have an impact on further work-up and prognosis, careful clinical evaluation of the patients is warranted.

Of the three cats with pheochromocytoma described so far, one had no clinical signs (Chun et al, 1997). One of the two symptomatic cats just had polyuria/polydipsia; the other one had polyuria/polydipsia, polyphagia, aggression, weight gain, and an unkempt hair coat with areas of alopecia. Because the latter cat had a glucocorticoid-producing adrenocortical adenoma in addition to the pheochromocytoma, the clinical signs were thought to be caused by the hypercortisolemia (Henry et al, 1993; Calsyn et al, 2010).

CLINICAL PATHOLOGY

There are no consistent changes in the complete blood count (CBC), serum biochemistry panel, and urinalysis, which would support the suspicion of a pheochromocytoma. Dogs with pheochromocytoma may show one or several abnormalities; they may also have normal laboratory results. A compilation of laboratory results of dogs with pheochromocytoma that have been published during the last decades is given later. A little more than 100 dogs were included; dogs with concurrent endocrine neoplasia were not used. The reader should be aware that the percentages are approximate numbers, because not all authors may have listed all abnormalities, in particular if they were minor.

- CBC: Mild to moderate anemia (45%), leucocytosis or stress leukogram (37%), thrombocytopenia (8%), thrombocytosis (6%). The anemia usually is nonregenerative and may be an anemia associated with chronic disease; the latter may either be the pheochromocytoma or another concurrent disease. Polycythemia may also be seen in a few cases, possibly due to hemoconcentration, release of erythropoietin from the kidneys associated with catecholamine-induced ischemia, or it may result from erythropoietin release from the pheochromocytoma (Mannelli et al, 2012a). Thrombocytosis has been associated with chronically bleeding pheochromocytomas, whereas no association was found between bleeding from the tumor and thrombocytopenia (Gilson et al, 1994; Feldman and Nelson, 2004a).
- Biochemistry panel: Increased alkaline phosphatase (ALP; 44%), increased alanine aminotransferase (ALT; 33%), increased aspartate aminotransferase (AST; 27%), increased blood urea nitrogen (BUN; 25%), increased creatinine (21%), hypercholesterolemia (23%), hypoalbuminemia (21%), hyperglycemia (8%), hyperphosphatemia (8%), hypokalemia (7%), and hyponatremia (7%). Increase in liver enzymes is the most frequent biochemical abnormality. There is no obvious correlation of an increase in liver enzymes and the presence of metastasis or tumor stage (Gilson et al, 1994; Feldman and Nelson, 2004a). Potential explanations are hypertension-induced hepatopathy or concurrent disease (Barthez et al, 1997). In humans, it is known that pheochromocytomas may release inflammatory cytokines (Kang et al, 2005); this would be another potential explanation for the increase in liver enzymes in dogs. Azotemia may be prerenal or renal due to volume-depletion and/or catecholamine induced vasoconstriction and renal ischemia.
- Hypercholesterolemia is most likely due to catecholamine-induced lipolysis and the conversion of excess fatty acids to cholesterol and other lipids in the liver. Increased cholesterol levels have been seen most often in advanced-stage tumors (Gilson et al, 1994). Hyperglycemia is usually mild or moderate and most often does not require therapeutic intervention. Overt diabetes and diabetic ketoacidosis have been described in a small number of dogs with pheochromocytoma; however, it was not clear if the diabetes was caused by the catecholamine excess (Feldman and Nelson, 2004a). Catecholamines have various effects on carbohydrate metabolism and insulin secretion. They stimulate gluconeogenesis and glycogenolysis and limit peripheral glucose utilization. They both suppress (α_2) and stimulate (β_2) insulin secretion, whereby the suppressive effect generally predominates (Cryer, 2001).

Information on urinalysis is scarce in the literature. In our own population of dogs with pheochromocytoma, urine specific gravity ranged from 1.006 to 1.044 and was in the hyposthenuric or isosthenuric range in about half of the dogs. Catecholamines, in particular norepinephrine, suppress the release of antidiuretic hormone (ADH; Berl et al, 1974), which may, at least in part, explain low urine specific gravity and the polyuria and polydipsia seen in some of the dogs. Proteinuria may be present in approximately 30% of patients and may be caused by hypertension-induced kidney damage or concurrent diseases.

Blood Pressure Measurement

In humans, hypertension is one of the key features of pheochromocytoma, which affects 80% to 90% of patients (Prejbisz et al, 2011). Hypertension in humans is defined as systolic/diastolic blood pressure greater than or equal to 140/90 mm Hg; blood pressure less than 120/80 mm Hg is considered normal. According to the latest (seventh) report of the Joint National Committee on Prevention, Detection, Evaluation and Treatment of High Blood Pressure, values in between the two are allocated to the newly introduced category of prehypertension (Chobanian et al, 2003). Contrary to previous assumptions that an increase in diastolic blood pressure is more worrisome than in systolic pressure, it has been shown that hypertension-associated risks are more accurately attributed to systolic pressure (Black, 2004).

In dogs and cats, the importance of hypertension began to be recognized 20 to 25 years ago. Similar to the guidelines for humans, the American College of Veterinary Internal Medicine provides a consensus statement for dogs and cats (Brown et al, 2007b). There is some controversy with regard to the threshold values that should be considered as hypertension. The guidelines classify blood pressure in dogs and cats with regard to risk of target-organ damage into four categories. Minimal risk is present if systolic blood pressure is less than 150 mm Hg and diastolic pressure is less than 95 mm Hg, and one may roughly say that these numbers represent normal blood pressure. Although studies have not determined if an increase in systolic pressure is more damaging than an increase in diastolic pressure, there has been emphasis in addressing systolic hypertension in dogs and cats (Reusch et al, 2010). Major causes of inaccurate blood pressure results are technical errors associated with personnel inexperience. Therefore, to obtain reliable results, the person making the measurement should be patient and skilled in the handling of animals, clients, and equipment (Brown et al, 2007b). Although direct blood pressure measurement (by catheterizing a peripheral artery) is considered the gold standard, veterinarians usually rely on indirect methods, including Doppler flow detection, oscillometry, or high definition oscillometry. Blood pressure is influenced by many physiological factors (e.g., age, sex, and breed), and it decreases during rest and sleep and increases during exercise. It can also increase due to stress and anxiety; this so-called white coat effect may lead to the false assumption of hypertension. To minimize this risk and to avoid mistakes, the veterinarian or the technician should follow a standardized protocol. Among various other issues, it is important that the dog or cat is not subjected to any manipulation before blood pressure is measured, that the patient is allowed to acclimatize in a quiet room, that several measurements are taken (in the author's hospital the mean of 10 measurements is used), and that the first readings are discarded (Reusch et al, 2010). The reader is referred to the detailed protocol on how to organize a blood pressure measurement session of the Consensus Statement of the American College of Veterinary Internal Medicine (ACVIM; Brown et al, 2007b).

Hypertension is classified as idiopathic (primary or essential) or secondary. Primary hypertension is thought to be rare in dogs and may account for up to 20% of cases in cats. Secondary hypertension is subclassified into renal and endocrine hypertension. Primary hyperaldosteronism, hyperadrenocorticism, pheochromocytoma, hyperthyroidism, and diabetes mellitus are causes for endocrine hypertension in dogs and cats. In humans, other endocrine disorders (e.g., hypothyroidism, hyperparathyroidism, and acromegaly) have been associated with hypertension; there are no reports in dogs or cats.

In human pheochromocytoma, hypertension occurs primarily from the secretion of norepinephrine, whereas epinephrine has a more variable influence on blood pressure. Additional factors that might contribute to hypertension are the co-secretion of neuropeptide Y, a potent vasoconstrictor, or a compromised blood flow in the renal artery due to compression by a large tumor, causing increased renin production (Fitzgerald, 2011). Various blood pressure patterns are known to exist: (1) sustained but variable hypertension with paroxysmal severe hypertensive peaks (approximately 50% of human patients), (2) normotension between paroxysmal hypertensive peaks, (3) sustained stable hypertension, and (4) normotension. Interestingly, in pheochromocytomas that exclusively produce epinephrine, hypotension is possible and even shock may occur. Other peptides, co-secreted with catecholamines, such as adrenomedullin, may also play a role in the induction of hypotension. Tumors that predominantly produce dopamine are rare; they are usually associated with normotension or hypotension (Fitzgerald, 2011; Kitamura et al, 2012). Although pheochromocytoma is an uncommon cause for hypertension because it affects approximately one in 1000 people with hypertension, it is associated with potentially fatal cardiovascular complications. Lethal outcome is particularly common if the tumor is undiagnosed, because a multitude of factors and drugs may provoke catecholamine release (Galetta et al, 2010; Prejbisz et al, 2011; see Box 13-1).

In dogs with pheochromocytoma, lesions attributed to hypertension were described decades ago. Main histological changes were thickening and hyalinization of the Bowman capsule; medial hypertrophy and sclerosis of pulmonary, splenic, and renal arteries; and hyaline degeneration of arterioles in the brain (Howard and Nielsen, 1965). Unfortunately, in many dogs with pheochromocytoma, blood pressure was not measured, and up until now no studies with regard to correlation between the type of catecholamine released and any blood pressure pattern have been performed. Blood pressure measurements are available in fewer than 50 dogs with pheochromocytoma; a little more than 50% had hypertension (Table 13-5). Similar to the situation in humans, the increase in blood pressure in dogs may range from mild to severe; the maximum systolic pressure reported was 325 mm Hg. Hypotension was seen in one dog (Reusch et al, 2010). As already mentioned, it is currently not possible to determine blood pressure patterns as in humans. However, repeated measurements in a small group of dogs with pheochromocytomas in our hospital suggest that there may be similar patterns as in humans. Two of five dogs had multiple systolic blood pressure measurements constantly below 160 mm Hg. One dog had variable paroxysmal hypertensive peaks with maximal systolic values of 270 mm Hg, one dog had marked fluctuations between 55 and 175 mm Hg, and another dog had a single episode of an increased systolic pressure with 180 mm Hg (Kook et al, 2010).

It is important to remember that hypertension is not pathognomonic for pheochromocytoma and is also frequently found in hyperadrenocorticism, which is one of the most important differential diagnoses.

Diagnostic Imaging

Abdominal and Thoracic Radiographs

Survey abdominal radiographs play a limited role in the diagnostic work-up of dogs with pheochromocytoma.

In a recent study on surgical outcome, 13% of canine pheochromocytomas were small with a diameter less than 2.5 cm, 42%

TABLE 13-5   BLOOD PRESSURE MEASUREMENTS IN DOGS WITH PHEOCHROMOCYTOMA

STUDY*	NUMBER OF DOGS WITH PHEOCHRO-MOCYTOMA	NUMBER OF DOGS WITH BLOOD PRES-SURE MEASUREMENT	NUMBER OF DOGS CLASSIFIED AS BE-ING HYPERTENSIVE	DEFINITION OF SYS-TOLIC HYPERTENSION (mm Hg)	RANGE OF SYSTOLIC BLOOD PRESSURE IN ALL DOGS (mm Hg)	MEASURING TECHNIQUE
Gilson et al, 1994	50	7	6	>160	164 to 325	Indirect, Doppler
Barthez et al, 1997	61	23	10	>160	135 to 214	Indirect, oscillometric
Williams and Hackner, 2001	1	1	1	Not given	200 to 240, continuous monitoring	Indirect, oscillometric
Brown et al, 2007a	1	1	1	Not given	240, several measurements	Indirect, Doppler
Kook et al, 2007	7	5	3	>160	55 to 270 (see text)	Indirect, Doppler, and oscillometric
Bommarito et al, 2011	1	1	0	Not given	Not given	Indirect, oscillometric
Guillaumot et al, 2012	1	1	1	Not given	160	Indirect, oscillometric

*In some studies diastolic and mean pressures were recorded in addition to systolic pressures. To facilitate comparison, only systolic blood pressure results are given here.

were of moderate size with diameters between 2.6 and 4.9 cm, and 45% were found to be large with diameters greater than or equal to 5.0 cm. Sixty-two percent of the tumors were located in the right adrenal gland (Herrera et al, 2008). The study was not meant to investigate the role of radiology and does not give details on radiological findings; it is mentioned here to give the reader an impression on distribution of tumor sizes. By means of plain radiographs, small and moderate sized tumors may not be visible—in particular if located in the right adrenal gland. Detectable tumors display as a mass of soft tissue opacity adjacent to the kidney, possibly with displacement of the kidney and other abdominal organs. Mineralization is rare in pheochromocytoma, further hampering their radiological visibility. Other potential findings are distortion of renal shape or poor visualization of kidneys, reduced serosal detail due to ascites, enlargement of the vena cava caudalis, and hepatomegaly; the latter may or may not be associated with pheochromocytoma. In case of tumor rupture, diffuse retroperitoneal soft tissue opacity, reflecting retroperitoneal hemorrhage may be seen (Fig. 13-3). Thoracic radiography currently still plays a role to search for pulmonary metastasis and is therefore of particular importance if adrenalectomy is planned. Pulmonary nodules (reflecting metastasis) have previously been reported in approximately 10% of dogs with pheochromocytoma (Gilson et al, 1994; Barthez et al, 1997). They may be missed by radiology, and it has been shown that computed tomography (CT) is more sensitive for their detection (Armbrust et al, 2012). Most likely, thoracic radiographs will soon be replaced by CT to search for metastasis—at least in larger institutions. Other radiological abnormalities, which have been reported in dogs with pheochromocytoma, include generalized cardiomegaly, right or left ventricular enlargement, and pulmonary edema. Those changes may be caused by the pheochromocytoma, although a cause and effect relationship has not been proven. In humans, left ventricular hypertrophy, hypertensive cardiomyopathy, myocarditis, and dilated cardiomyopathy (including the relatively new phenomenon of takotsubo cardiomyopathy) are known to occur either as a consequence of systemic hypertension and/or high levels of catecholamines (Prejbisz et al, 2011).

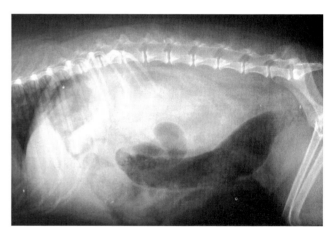

FIGURE 13-3 Abdominal radiograph of a Papillon (spayed, 10-year-old female). The dog was diagnosed with pheochromocytoma and invasion into the vena cava caudalis. The owner opted for medical treatment with phenoxybenzamine. Fourteen months after the diagnosis, the dog was presented to the referring veterinarian with acute collapse, pale mucus membranes, prolonged capillary refill time (CRT), tachycardia, abdominal pain, and a packed cell volume (PCV) of 28%. Diffuse retroperitoneal soft tissue opacity is seen, reflecting retroperitoneal hemorrhage due to rupture of the tumor. (Courtesy of Dr. Markus Haller, Boniswil, Switzerland.)

Abdominal Ultrasonography

Abdominal ultrasonography has major advantages over radiography for the imaging of the adrenal glands, such as higher resolution to visualize small masses, potential to detect retroperitoneal effusion and invasion of the tumor into surrounding vessels and tissues, and assessment of other abdominal organs for distant metastasis (Figs. 13-4, 13-5, and 13-6). Often, a pheochromocytoma is only considered after detection of an abnormal adrenal gland on abdominal ultrasonography. Careful consideration of the patient's history and physical examination is required. Areas of heterogenous or hyperechoic parenchyma within the adrenal gland, adrenal nodules, or masses are frequent findings and are not always

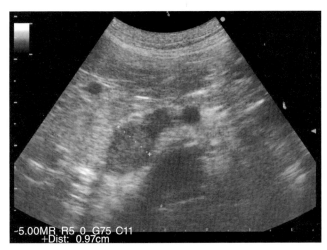

FIGURE 13-4 Ultrasonographic image of a small pheochromocytoma in a 12-year-old, spayed female Fox Terrier. The tumor presented as hyperechoic nodular enlargement of the cranial pole of the left adrenal gland (sagittal plane). The maximum diameter of the tumor was 0.97 cm. (Courtesy of Dr. Matthias Dennler and Prof. Patrick Kircher, Division of Diagnostic Imaging, Vetsuisse Faculty, University of Zurich, Zurich, Switzerland.)

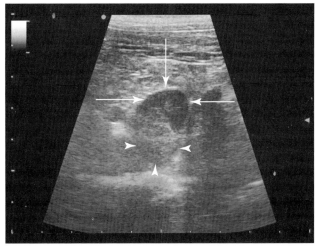

FIGURE 13-6 Ultrasonographic image of a tumor thrombus in the caudal vena cava (transverse plane) in an 11-year-old, castrated male Jack Russel Terrier. The thrombus originated from a pheochromocytoma in the right adrenal gland. Invasion of the tumor into the vena cava was confirmed by computed tomography (CT) (see Fig. 13-8). *Arrows,* non-occluded lumen of caudal vena cava; *arrowheads,* tumor thrombus in lumen of caudal vena cava. (Courtesy of Dr. Matthias Dennler and Prof. Patrick Kircher, Division of Diagnostic Imaging, Vetsuisse Faculty, University of Zurich, Zurich, Switzerland.)

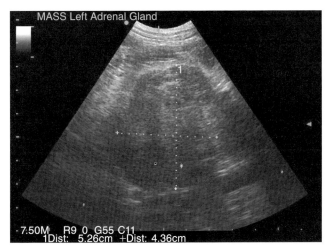

FIGURE 13-5 Ultrasonographic image (dorsal plane) of a large pheochromocytoma in a 13-year-old, spayed female Standard Schnauzer. The dog was admitted to the hospital as an emergency because of sudden onset of abdominal pain. Ultrasonographic evaluation of the abdomen revealed a large heterogenous mass with irregular margins (maximum diameter of 5.3 cm) in the area of the left adrenal gland. However, there was no evidence of tumor rupture or hemorrhage. Because transducer pressure in the area of the mass aggravated abdominal pain, further evaluation by computed tomography (CT) was performed (see Fig. 13-7). The mass was confirmed to be a pheochromocytoma by histopathology after successful adrenalectomy. (Courtesy of Dr. Matthias Dennler and Prof. Patrick Kircher, Division of Diagnostic Imaging, Vetsuisse Faculty, University of Zurich, Zurich, Switzerland.)

---

associated with disease. This is due to the fact that nowadays most sick animals undergo ultrasonography at some point during the work-up; today, most sonographers are able to visualize the adrenal glands, and the high-quality equipment allows detection of even small lesions. Finding an adrenal mass can create a diagnostic challenge due to the many differential diagnosis (see Incidental Discovered Adrenal Mass (Incidentaloma) later; Box 13-5).

The normal adrenal glands are hypoechoic to the surrounding fat. The left adrenal gland resembles a dumbbell; the right

BOX 13-5	**Main Important Differential Diagnosis of an Incidentally Discovered Adrenal Mass**

Hormonally Active Adrenal Nodule/Mass
- Aldosterone-producing adenoma, carcinoma, or hyperplasia
- Glucocorticoid-producing adenoma or carcinoma
- Adrenocortical hyperplasia (ACTH-dependent or ACTH-independent)
- Sex-hormone producing adenoma or carcinoma
- Pheochromocytoma

Hormonally Inactive Adrenal Nodule/Mass
- Hormonally silent adenoma, carcinoma, or hyperplasia
- Metastasis
- Miscellaneous: Myelolipoma, lipoma, cyst. abscess hematoma, or granuloma

ACTH, Adrenocorticotropic hormone.

adrenal gland looks similar to a comma. The phrenicoabdominal vein bisects the ventral surface of each gland and may serve as a marker (i.e., to differentiate the adrenal gland from a lymph node, which may look alike). Occasionally, a thin hyperechoic line, which is considered to be the corticomedullary junction, can be seen. The adrenal glands are usually evaluated with 7.5 to 10.0 MHz transducers. There are a number of techniques for locating the adrenal glands either in dorsal or lateral recumbency, which is mainly a question of personal preference. Pheochromocytomas may present as nodules (focal increase in thickness with normal global shape of the adrenal gland) or as a mass (diffuse increase in thickness and/or length with distortion of normal shape) (Besso et al, 1997). They may range in size between a few millimeters to more than 10 centimeters in diameter. The smallest pheochromocytoma seen by the author was 2 mm in diameter in a dog with recurrent diarrhea. Echogenicity is highly variable; nodules and masses may be hypo-, iso-, or hyperechoic (compared to the kidney); and echogenicity may be homo- or heterogenous. Masses may have a multicystic or multilobular architecture. Anechoic, non-far enhancing areas may represent foci of necrosis and hemorrhage. No pattern of echogenicity or architecture is specific for pheochromocytomas, and other adrenal masses (e.g., cortisol-producing tumors) may look alike (Besso et al, 1997; Rosenstein, 2000). The only difference is that mineralization is rare in pheochromocytoma and is relatively common in cortisol-producing tumors. However, this fact is not helpful to differentiate between the two tumor types in an individual dog.

Ultrasonography is also helpful to detect metastasis into abdominal organs and local invasion into surrounding structures, such as veins and kidneys. *Tumor thrombus* is a term for a mass formed by the extension of a nonvascular tumor into a blood vessel. In dogs with pheochromocytoma, tumor thrombi are common and may affect any of the surrounding vessels. Most commonly, tumor thrombi involve the caudal vena cava, which has been reported to occur in up to 56% of cases. They may originate from thrombi that first invade the phrenicoabdominal vein and then extend further into the vena cava. Tumor thrombi confined to the phrenicoabdominal vein may represent early stages of thrombus formation (Kyles et al, 2003). Invasion of the vena cava has been seen more often with right-sided pheochromocytoma; however, they also occur with left-sided pheochromocytoma. By means of ultrasonography (including Doppler) it may be difficult to differentiate compression of a vessel from vascular invasion (tumor thrombus) and a blood clot ("true" thrombus). In a study on 40 dogs with various adrenal tumors, abdominal ultrasonography had a sensitivity of 80% and specificity of 90% for the diagnosis of a thrombus in the vena cava (Kyles et al, 2003). Due to the small size of the vessel, detection of thrombi in the phrenicoabdominal vein is generally difficult. The question on a potential correlation between tumor size and invasiveness has not been addressed in a large number of dogs. It is, however, likely that invasion is rare as long as the pheochromocytoma is small (maximum diameter less than 2 cm).

Most pheochromocytomas are unilateral; in this case, the contralateral adrenal has a normal shape and size. However, bilateral pheochromocytoma may occur, and pheochromocytoma may also coexist with other types of nodule/mass in the contralateral adrenal gland. In those cases, interpretation of ultrasonographic (and clinical) findings is particularly difficult. The biggest challenge often is to differentiate between a cortisol-producing adrenal tumor and a pheochromocytoma. Unfortunately, this is not possible by means of ultrasonography. In theory, the contralateral gland of a cortisol-producing mass should be small due to atrophy, whereas it is normal in the case of a pheochromocytoma. However, the atrophy of the contralateral gland may not be apparent ultrasonographically (Hoerauf and Reusch, 1999).

Computed Tomography and Magnetic Resonance Imaging

CT has several advantages over ultrasonography. It may be particularly useful in patients where the adrenal gland is difficult to visualize (e.g., in large breed or obese dogs) (Morandi, 2011). It also allows a more precise and complete evaluation of tumor size, shape, and architecture. Most importantly, contrast-enhanced CT is superior to ultrasonography to detect vascular invasion (Figs. 13-7 and 13-8). In many cases, it enables reliable differentiation between vascular invasion and mural compression of veins from the tumor, and also between a tumor thrombus and a blood clot. On CT, pheochromocytomas appear as soft-tissue masses in the mid-dorsal abdomen;

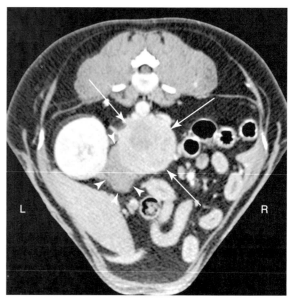

FIGURE 13-7 Transverse computed tomography (CT) image of the adrenal tumor in the equilibrium phase after intravenous (IV) administration of iodinated contrast medium in the 13-year-old Standard Schnauzer (see Fig. 13-5). The left adrenal gland is markedly enlarged and demonstrates heterogenous, moderate contrast enhancement *(arrows)*. The irregular defined, large area between left adrenal and kidney without contrast enhancement was interpreted as hemorrhage from the tumor *(arrowheads)*. Adrenalectomy confirmed the CT findings, and the tumor was classified as pheochromocytoma by histopathology. This case nicely demonstrates the superior performance of CT compared to ultrasonography with regard to a more precise and complete evaluation of tumor size, shape, and architecture. CT is also superior to detect hemorrhage—in particular if the amount of blood is only small to moderate. (Courtesy of Dr. Matthias Dennler and Prof. Patrick Kircher, Division of Diagnostic Imaging, Vetsuisse Faculty, University of Zurich, Zurich, Switzerland.)

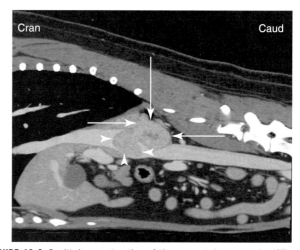

FIGURE 13-8 Sagittal reconstruction of the computed tomography (CT) angiography of the 11-year-old Jack Russell Terrier shown in Fig. 13-6 in the venous phase after intravenous (IV) administration of iodinated contrast medium. The tumor thrombus originated from a pheochromocytoma in the right adrenal gland and expanded into the lumen of the caudal vena cava. CT is superior to ultrasonography to detect vascular invasion of an adrenal tumor and also enables a precise determination of the exact extent of the thrombus. The arrows point to the tumor and the arrowheads show the tumor invasion into caudal vena cava. (Courtesy of Dr. Matthias Dennler and Prof. Patrick Kircher, Division of Diagnostic Imaging, Vetsuisse Faculty, University of Zurich, Zurich, Switzerland.)

further findings include irregular margins, heterogenous contrast-enhancement with regions of highly vascular parenchyma, and foci of low attenuation (Rosenstein, 2000). In one study, vascular invasion into the phrenicoabdominal vein, vena cava, and renal vein was correctly identified in 11 of 12 cases. Invasion into the phrenicoabdominal vein was missed in only one case, which was thought to be due to relatively thick image collimation. Mural compression was also correctly differentiated from vascular invasion. The sensitivity and specificity of contrast-enhanced CT for vascular invasion compared to surgery or pathology was 92% and 100%, respectively. CT also correctly identified invasion into hypaxial and epaxial musculature (Schultz et al, 2009).

In humans, it is known that ionic (high osmolar) contrast media used for contrast-enhanced CT may stimulate catecholamine release from a pheochromocytoma and may induce a hypertensive crisis. Non-ionic (low osmolar) contrast media do not have this side effect and are therefore considered to be much safer (Baid et al, 2009; Chew, 2010). Although there are no reports on this side effect in dogs, it seems appropriate to use non-ionic contrast media.

Magnetic resonance imaging (MRI) may be superior to CT to ascertain vascular invasion due to superior resolution and contrast (Gavin and Holmes, 2009). It may also be more accurate to determine the exact extent of a tumor thrombus in the vena cava, as has been demonstrated in humans (Goldfarb et al, 1990; Rosenstein, 2000). However, availability of MRI is currently more limited than that of CT; other disadvantages are longer scanning time and higher costs.

For appropriate surgical planning (e.g., decision between midline coeliotomy or laparoscopy) knowledge on invasion into vasculature is important. Invasion into other tissue, such as hypaxial and epaxial musculature, has a profound impact on the feasibility of tumor excision. Therefore, contrast-enhanced CT or MRI prior to surgery is indicated in any patient in whom invasiveness of the tumor is a concern.

In human medicine, attempts have been made to differentiate between the various tumor types of the adrenal gland and also to differentiate primary adrenal tumors from metastasis. Findings previously considered to be characteristic included the following: lower unenhanced CT density in adenomas compared to malignant tumors, very high contrast-enhanced CT density in pheochromocytoma, slower wash-out of contrast in malignant tumors including pheochromocytoma, and high signal intensity on T2-weighted MRI images, a feature described as light-bulb signs in pheochromocytoma. However, recent studies revealed large overlap between pheochromocytoma and other adrenal tumors, and therefore, CT and MRI cannot definitively identify an adrenal mass as a pheochromocytoma (Blake et al, 2010; Fitzgerald, 2011; Leung et al, 2013).

In dogs, there are no studies so far on CT and MRI characteristics of the various adrenal tumors. It is likely, however, that the situation is similar to humans (i.e., diagnosis of a pheochromocytoma is most likely not possible by means of those two modalities).

Functional Medical Imaging

Functional medical imaging provides information about the functional characteristics of a tumor. Nuclear medicine scanning techniques used for functional imaging are scintigraphy, single photon emission computed tomography (SPECT) and positron emission tomography (PET). These modalities involve the application of radiotracers, which are taken up by the tumor cells (Timmers et al, 2012). In human medicine, functional imaging is considered complimentary to anatomic imaging (CT, MRI) and usually used after

a mass has been identified by the latter. It is now well accepted in humans, however, that the presence of a pheochromocytoma/paraganglioma has to be proven by biochemical tests first. The purpose of functional imaging is to localize the primary tumor, to search for multiple primary tumors (which often occur in some genetic disorders in humans), and to search for metastasis. The isotope most often used is [123]iodine-metaiodobenzylguanidine (^{123}I-MIBG). ^{123}I-MIBG is a norepinephrine analog that localizes first to presynaptic adrenergic nerves and sympathomedullary tissue and then into cytoplasmic storage vesicles. Its uptake is proportional to the number of neurosecretory granules within the tumor (Leung et al, 2013). ^{123}I-MIBG SPECT is preferred over ^{123}I-MIBG scintigraphy due to higher sensitivity. Sensitivity and specificity have been reported to be 77% to 90% and 95% to 100% respectively (Leung et al, 2013). Combining SPECT scanning with CT, which is now possible on hybrid SPECT/CT machines, has the advantage of simultaneous delivery of morphological and functional data and has enhanced sensitivity (Fitzgerald, 2011; Timmers et al, 2012; Leung et al, 2013). Because the sensitivity and resolution of PET is superior to SPECT, PET imaging has grown rapidly together with the development of new tracers (e.g., ^{18}F-FDA, ^{18}F-DOPA, and ^{18}F-FDG). Similar to SPECT/CT, PET is combined with CT to produce very sensitive and accurate three-dimensional images (Fitzgerald, 2011; Timmers et al, 2012). Functional imaging is considered to be a very promising tool in human medicine, and further development in this area will certainly allow an even more exact tumor characterization.

In dogs, knowledge on functional imaging is scarce. ^{123}I-MIBG scintigraphy has been successfully used in one dog to demonstrate an area of focal intense uptake in the area of the right adrenal gland. After surgical excision, the mass was confirmed to be a pheochromocytoma (Berry et al, 1993). PET scanning with ^{18}F-fluorobenzylguanidine (^{18}F-PFBG) has been investigated in three dogs with adrenal masses. PET images showed increased uptake in the right adrenal gland in two dogs in which histology confirmed pheochromocytoma. In the third dog, no increased uptake was found, and exploratory laparotomy confirmed the absence of an adrenal mass (Berry et al, 2002). As in humans, functional imaging in dogs may have great potential in the future for characterization of adrenal masses. Currently, costs and availability are limiting factors.

Percutaneous Fine-Needle Aspiration and Biopsy of the Adrenal Glands

In human medicine, the question of whether adrenal masses should be biopsied has been discussed in a large number of publications. According to the North American Neuroendocrine Tumor Society (NANETS) guidelines, diagnosis of pheochromocytoma (and paraganglioma) relies on biochemical evidence of catecholamine production by the tumor. Biochemical testing should be performed in symptomatic patients, patients with known hereditary risk for developing pheochromocytoma/paraganglioma, and patients with an incidentaloma (Chen et al, 2010). Those guidelines do not even mention biopsy as a diagnostic tool. Other guidelines specifically state that fine-needle aspiration of an incidentaloma is contraindicated if a pheochromocytoma has not been excluded by biochemical testing (National Institutes of Health, 2002; Terzolo et al, 2011). A high rate of biopsy related complications including death have been reported in human patients with pheochromocytoma. A study from the Mayo Clinic revealed problems in 70% of patients, including hematoma, severe hypertension, severe pain, delay in surgical treatment, error in diagnosis, and difficulty in resecting the mass during surgery due to inflammation and retroperitoneal fixation (Vanderveen et al, 2009).

In veterinary medicine, fine-needle aspiration of pheochromocytomas has been reported in a few dogs and a cat (Chun et al, 1997; Rosenstein, 2000; Spall et al, 2011). In most cases, cytological evaluation suggested the tumor to be of endocrine or neuroendocrine origin. However, large studies would be needed to evaluate the diagnostic accuracy of fine-needle aspiration of adrenal masses. So far, no complications have been reported. There is, however, no reason to believe, that complication rates would be less in dogs and cats than in humans. Therefore, before fine-needle aspiration or core biopsy of adrenal masses in dogs and cats are performed, the risks should be weighed carefully against benefits.

Biochemical Testing

Biochemical testing has been performed in humans for many years and various tests have been developed. In dogs, the same tests are used; however, their evaluation has only recently been initiated. Some important details of the tests routinely used in humans today are discussed in the following section.

Human Medicine

Catecholamines and Metanephrines. In human medicine, there is consensus that all patients with suspected pheochromocytoma should undergo biochemical testing and that the diagnosis relies on the demonstration of excessive production of catecholamines (Lenders et al, 2005; Pacak et al, 2007; Chen et al, 2010). Many products of the catecholamine pathway have been assessed as potential markers for the disease, including urine catecholamines, urine metanephrines, urine vanillylmandelic acid (VMA), plasma catecholamines, and plasma metanephrines.

In order to understand the various tests that are offered by the laboratories, knowledge of the current terminology is essential. The term *catecholamines* includes dopamine, norepinephrine, and epinephrine. The term *metanephrines* in the plural form refers to the sum of normetanephrine and metanephrine, which are the major metabolites of norepinephrine and epinephrine. The term does not include methoxytyramine, the metabolite of dopamine. Previously, measuring techniques were only able to analyze the two metabolites together (i.e., measurement of metanephrines). Today, high-performance liquid chromatography (HPLC) assays allow separate analysis of normetanephrine and metanephrine, which is termed *fractionated* metanephrines (Eisenhofer, 2001). Catecholamines as well as their metabolites (except VMA) are converted to sulfate conjugates, mainly in gastrointestinal tissues. The term *total* is used to describe the sum of free (unconjugated) and conjugated parameters (Eisenhofer, 2001; Eisenhofer et al, 2001; 2008b; Grouzmann et al, 2010).

In plasma and urine, sulfate-conjugated metanephrines are present in much higher concentrations than the free forms. Total metanephrines are determined after samples are subjected to a deconjugation step so that both previously conjugated and free forms are measured. This is sometimes termed *deconjugated* metanephrines, which largely reflect the sulfate-conjugated forms, due to their abundance. The measurement of total metanephrines is analytically easier than the measurement of the free forms (Grouzmann et al, 2010). In urine, total (deconjugated) metanephrines are measured; in plasma, measurement of both free and total as separate tests is available. The standard procedure for the urine test in humans is collecting urine over a 24-hour period; rarely measurement is performed in spot urine samples, relating the concentrations to urinary creatinine.

Reference laboratories usually perform analyses of catecholamines and metanephrines either by means of high-performance liquid chromatography with electrochemical detection (HPLC-ECD) or tandem mass spectroscopy (LC/MS/MS).

Understanding the biochemical tests also requires some knowledge on the pathways for synthesis and metabolism of catecholamines. Comprehensive reviews of this complex matter have been published by Eisenhofer, et al. (2001b; 2008b), Pacak (2011), and others. The reader is also referred to the Physiology and Pathophysiology section at the beginning of this chapter and to Figs. 13-1 and 13-2.

In humans, most pheochromocytomas are hormonally active and produce catecholamines; however, there is large variation depending on the expression of the biosynthetic pathway and differences in the secretory processes (Eisenhofer et al, 2011). The activities of the enzymes tyrosine hydroxylase, L-amino acid decarboxylase and dopamine β-hydroxylase are usually very high in pheochromocytomas, which is the basis of the overproduction of catecholamines (Pacak, 2011). Most human pheochromocytomas produce more norepinephrine than epinephrine, and many produce both catecholamines. A few tumors produce predominantly epinephrine, and very rarely, pheochromocytomas only produce dopamine.

Pheochromocytomas (like normal chromaffin cells) express COMT, which is responsible for catecholamine metabolism. It converts norepinephrine to normetanephrine and epinephrine to metanephrine. Within the chromaffin cells, catecholamines permanently leak from storage vesicles into the cytoplasm where they are continuously metabolized to metanephrines. The release of the parent catecholamines into the circulation is highly variable, and it often occurs only intermittently or at low rates. In contrast, metanephrines are continuously released into the circulation (Eisenhofer et al, 2004a; 2008b; Lenders et al, 2005; Pacak, 2011; Fig. 13-9). In humans with pheochromocytoma, more than 94% of plasma metanephrines are derived from the metabolism

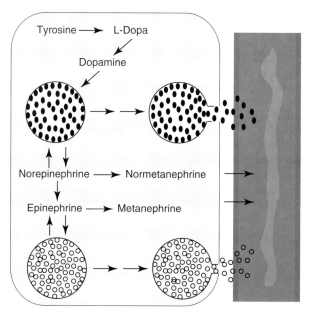

FIGURE 13-9 Main pathways of catecholamine synthesis, metabolism, and secretion in pheochromocytoma. (Graph redrawn and modified from Pacak, K: Pheochromocytoma: a catecholamine and oxidative stress disorder, *Endocr Regul* 45:65, 2011.)

of catecholamines by COMT within the tumor and not by the action of extra-adrenal COMT on catecholamines released into the circulation (Eisenhofer et al, 2004a). Therefore, there is consensus in human medicine that measurement of metanephrines is superior to measurement of catecholamines for the diagnosis of pheochromocytoma (Pacak et al, 2007; Chen et al, 2010). The relationship between synthesis, metabolism, and secretion of catecholamines and metanephrines may explain why there is a strong correlation between tumor size and urinary output of metanephrines, whereas the correlation between tumor size and catecholamines is weak (Eisenhofer et al, 2005a). Today, the tests with the highest sensitivity for the diagnosis of pheochromocytoma in humans are measurements of fractionated metanephrines in 24-hour urine samples and fractionated free metanephrines in plasma (Fitzgerald, 2011). There is some controversy as to which test (urine or plasma) has the higher diagnostic accuracy. Several authors have demonstrated higher sensitivity of plasma-free metanephrines compared to 24-hour urine metanephrines (Lenders et al, 2002; Kudva et al, 2003; Unger et al, 2006). Specificity has been claimed to be lower for the plasma test; however, the various studies are difficult to compare because their design differs. One recent study showed that the differences are in fact minor. Sensitivity of plasma-free metanephrines was 96% and for urinary metanephrines 95%; specificity was 89% and 86%, respectively (Grouzmann et al, 2010). The slightly superior performance of the plasma test may be explained by the fact, that the free metanephrines are direct products of the pheochromocytoma, whereas the urinary metanephrines largely reflect sulphate-conjugated metabolites, which are formed in the gastrointestinal tissue. Plasma-free normetanephrine was found to be the single best test, followed by urinary normetanephrine, whereas plasma and urinary metanephrine had lower diagnostic accuracy (Unger et al, 2006). The difference is most likely due to the fact that most pheochromocytomas produce more norepinephrine than epinephrine. So far, there are no official guidelines in humans as to which test (plasma or urine) should be used preferentially. The recommendations from the First International Symposium on Pheochromocytoma state that the initial testing for pheochromocytoma must include measurement of fractionated metanephrines in plasma, urine, or both, as available (Pacak et al, 2007). The same guidelines also address the problem of false-positive test results and advocate the use of a socalled continuous approach to test interpretation (e.g., the higher the test result, the more likely a pheochromocytoma is present). An increase of plasma or urinary normetanephrine by more than fourfold above the upper reference interval is associated with a close to 100% probability of the presence of a pheochromocytoma (Pacak et al, 2007).

Many factors may lead to false positive results, including drugs (e.g., phenoxybenzamine, β-blocker), certain foods and beverages, inadequate sampling conditions, exercise, emotional stress, and stress of other diseases. Although measurements of metanephrines are superior to measurements of catecholamines, the latter may still be of some use. Human patients with pheochromocytoma have larger increases in metanephrines than in catecholamines, whereas patients with false-positive results due to sympatho-adrenal activation usually have larger increases in catecholamines than in metanephrines (Eisenhofer et al, 2003). In patients with renal failure, total metanephrines are often severely elevated due to decreased renal elimination. Free metanephrines are less affected and therefore more suitable markers for pheochromocytoma in cases of renal failure (Eisenhofer et al, 2005b). As a reminder, total metanephrines are measured in the urinary test.

An emerging challenge in human medicine is the detection of small pheochromocytomas, which are increasingly found due to the frequent use of high-resolution imaging techniques. Biochemical confirmation, however, may be difficult, because the levels of the biochemical markers are generally lower in small than in large tumors. In a recent study, 50% of humans with small pheochromocytomas had only modestly elevated or even normal test results (Yu et al, 2012).

Other Tests

VMA is a catecholamine metabolite that is produced in the liver and excreted in the urine. VMA in 24-hour urine has previously been an established biochemical test for pheochromocytoma; however, its sensitivity has been shown to be low (64%; Lenders et al, 2005). Although the test is still offered by various laboratories, it is becoming less important.

CGA is a member of granins, which are a family of acid proteins present in secretory granules of many endocrine and non-endocrine cells. In the adrenal medulla, CGA is stored with catecholamines in storage vesicles and is also co-secreted with them. It is secreted by various tumors, including pheochromocytoma, parathyroid adenoma, medullary thyroid carcinoma (MTC), carcinoids, pancreatic islet-cell tumors, and aortic-body tumors (Bílek et al, 2008). CGA is elevated in most patients with pheochromocytomas, and the levels correlate with the tumor mass. The parameter, however, may also be elevated in other neuroendocrine and various nonendocrine diseases, as well as in renal failure, because of its excretion by the kidney (Bílek et al, 2008; Fitzgerald, 2011).

The clonidine suppression test is used as an aid to distinguish between true and false positive measurement of metanephrines. Clonidine is a centrally-acting α_2 adrenergic receptor agonist that suppresses the release of norepinephrine from sympathetic neurons but not its release from a pheochromocytoma. The test is performed by measuring plasma normetanephrine (and possibly plasma norepinephrine) before and 3 hours after the oral application of 0.3 mg clonidine. A positive response is defined as a decrease in normetanephrine of less than 40%, or a decrease in norepinephrine of less than 50%. The test has a high diagnostic accuracy, although false positive and false negative results may occur (Eisenhofer et al, 2003). Clonidine may cause marked hypotension, and the test should only be performed under close supervision (Mackenzie and Brown, 2011).

In order to identify the rare dopamine-secreting tumors, it has been recommended to include the measurement of methoxytyramine (metabolite of dopamine) in the fractionated metanephrine assay (Barron, 2010).

Dogs and Cats

Catecholamines and Metanephrines. Until recently, biochemical testing for pheochromocytoma had only infrequently been performed in dogs due to low medical awareness of pheochromocytoma, limited availability of techniques, lack of reference ranges, and problems with 24-hour urine collection with regard to the urine test. During the last few years, a small number of studies has investigated urinary and/or plasma catecholamines and metanephrines (Kook et al, 2007; 2010; Cameron et al, 2010; Quante et al, 2010; Salesov et al, 2012; Gostelow et al, 2013). Our own studies initially focused on the measurement of the parameters in urine; more recently we started to compare the diagnostic performance of the urine test with the plasma test. Due to the fact that 24-hour urine collection is hardly feasible in client-owned dogs, the urine test was established by measuring the parameters in single-voided samples, and their concentrations were expressed as ratios to the creatinine concentrations in the same urine samples (Kook et al, 2007). The objective of the first study was to evaluate if veterinary care and the stress of a hospital stay would lead to an increase of catecholamines and metanephrines, which then would require urine sampling at home. Such an increase is known for the urinary corticoid-to-creatinine ratio (van Vonderen et al, 1998). Interestingly, in staff-owned healthy dogs (who were familiar with the environment), no differences were found between urine samples taken in the hospital or at home. In contrast, in healthy client-owned dogs (who were unfamiliar with the hospital) epinephrine, norepinephrine, and metanephrine-to-creatinine ratios were significantly higher in samples taken in the hospital compared to those taken 7 days after discharge. Urinary normetanephrine ratios, however, did not differ between those two time points (Kook et al, 2007; Fig. 13-10).

The question of when to take the urine samples is of importance mainly because of two reasons. First, urine has to be acidified to a pH less than or equal to 2 after sampling and chilled until analysis; those requirements may be difficult to fulfill for some owners. Second, in dogs with a high suspicion of pheochromocytoma, an immediate start of treatment with phenoxybenzamine (an α adrenergic antagonist) may be desirable. However, it is known

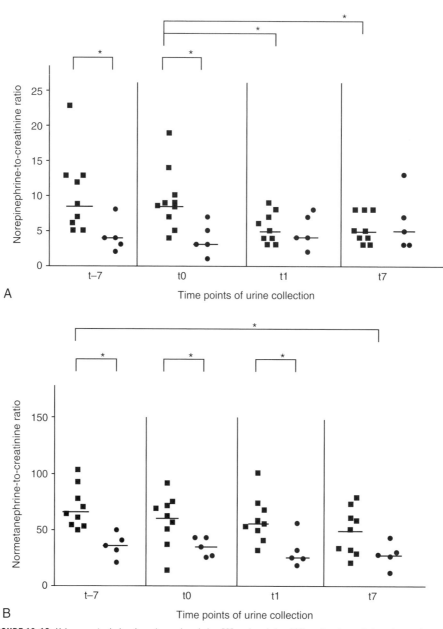

FIGURE 13-10 Urinary catecholamines (norepinephrine [A], epinephrine [C]) and metanephrines (normetanephrine [B], metanephrine [D]) to creatinine ratios in healthy client-owned dogs *(squares)* and staff-owned dogs *(circles)*. Client-owned dogs had never been to the hospital before, whereas the staff-owned dogs were familiar with the environment. Urine was sampled at various time points: *t–7* (7 days before hospital visit), *t0* (hospital visit), *t1* and *t7* (1 and 7 days after hospital visit). (Adopted and amended from Kook PH, et al.: Urinary catecholamines and metanephrines to creatinine ratios in healthy dogs at home and in a hospital environment and in 2 dogs with pheochromocytoma, *J Vet Intern Med* 21:388, 2007, with permission.) *, Significant difference; *horizontal line,* median values.

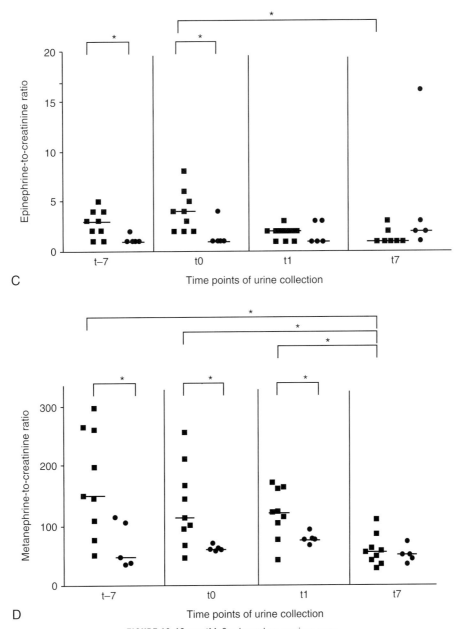

FIGURE 13-10, cont'd. See legend on previous page.

from humans that phenoxybenzamine may lead to false positive tests results, and it should be given only after samples for biochemical testing have been taken. Sending a dog home for a few days before sampling would delay this treatment. The issue of time of urine sampling was therefore explored once more in a group of dogs with hyperadrenocorticism (one of the most important differential diagnosis for pheochromocytoma). No difference was found in any of the parameters between samples taken in the hospital and samples taken at home 1 week after discharge (Quante et al, 2010). On the basis of this study and the fact that the differences in the previous study were relatively small, we concluded that urine samples may be taken in the hospital, which became the standard procedure in our institution. Most of the urine samples in the following studies were taken in the hospital. It was then shown that dogs with pheochromocytoma had significantly higher urinary norepinephrine, epinephrine, and normetanephrine ratios compared to healthy dogs. Urinary normetanephrine ratio discriminated best with no overlap between healthy dogs and dogs

with pheochromocytoma. Interestingly, urinary normetanephrine ratios were the highest in two dogs with bilateral pheochromocytomas (Kook et al, 2010). The superior performance of urinary normetanephrine over urinary catecholamines and urinary metanephrine was also demonstrated in further studies (Quante et al, 2010; Salesov et al, 2012). As discussed earlier, this finding is similar to the situation in humans. It is very likely, that canine pheochromocytomas (as human pheochromocytomas) produce predominantly norepinephrine, which is then metabolized into normetanephrine. The superior performance of the metabolite over the parent catecholamine has been extensively shown in humans (see the earlier paragraph about humans and Fig. 13-9).

Hyperadrenocorticism is one of the most important differential diagnoses for pheochromocytoma. Both diseases may present with similar clinical signs, such as weakness, tachypnea, panting, polyuria/polydipsia, and adrenal abnormalities detected by ultrasonography. It is therefore important that biochemical tests established for the diagnosis of pheochromocytoma enable differentiation

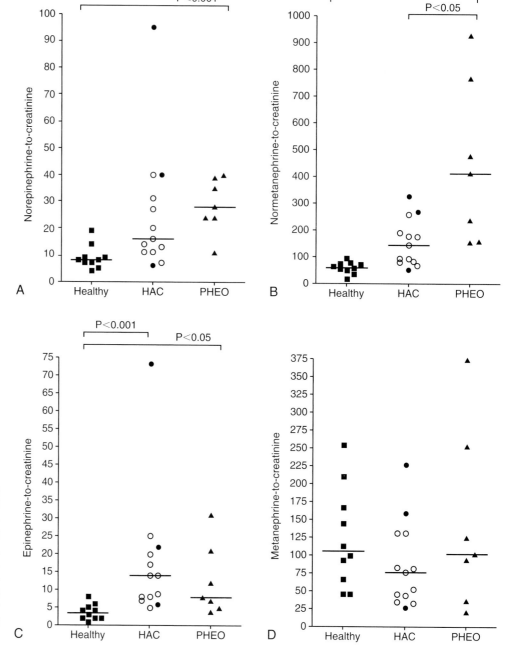

FIGURE 13-11 Urinary catecholamines (norepinephrine **[A]**, epinephrine **[C]**) and metanephrines (normetanephrine **[B]**, metanephrine **[D]**) to creatinine ratios in healthy dogs, dogs with hyperadrenocorticism (HAC), and dogs with pheochromocytoma (PHEO). (Modified from Quante S, et al.: Urinary catecholamine and metanephrine to creatinine ratios in dogs with hyperadrenocorticism or pheochromocytoma, and in healthy dogs, *J Vet Intern Med* 24:1093, 2010, with permission.)

between the two diseases. It was shown, however, that hyperadrenocorticism might be associated with increased catecholamine production. Approximately 50% of dogs with hyperadrenocorticism had urinary norepinephrine, epinephrine, and normetanephrine ratios above those of healthy dogs, and the difference was significant. Although urinary norepinephrine and epinephrine did not differ between dogs with hyperadrenocorticism and dogs with pheochromocytoma, urinary normetanephrine ratio was the single parameter that was significantly higher in dogs with pheochromocytoma compared to dogs with hyperadrenocorticism (Quante et al, 2010). As shown in Fig. 13-11, there was some overlap between the two groups. The problem that test results of individuals with pheochromocytoma overlap to some extent with those of individuals with other diseases also exists in human medicine. There, it has led to the recommendation to use cut-off values

of two to four times the upper limit of normal. By working with a cut-off value of four times the upper limit of normal, the probability of a pheochromocytoma is nearly 100% in humans (Pacak et al, 2007). The same seems to apply for dogs: A cut-off urinary normetanephrine ratio of four times the highest level measured in healthy dogs discriminates with no overlap between dogs with hyperadrenocorticism and dogs with pheochromocytoma. However, the diagnosis of a pheochromocytoma would have been missed in three of seven dogs with pheochromocytoma. The use of lower cut-offs, such as two or three times normal, would increase sensitivity at the expense of specificity, which is a well-known phenomenon. So far, we have seen urinary normetanephrine ratios above four times normal only in dogs with pheochromocytoma. Cameron, et al., (2010) found higher levels in a group of critically ill dogs. The difference from our own results may be in part

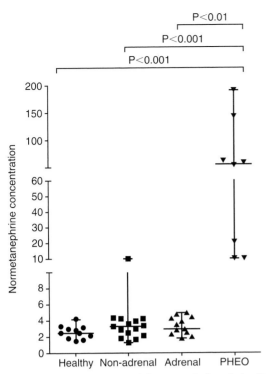

FIGURE 13-12 Plasma-free normetanephrine concentrations in healthy dogs, dogs with non-adrenal diseases, dogs with adrenocortical tumors, and dogs with pheochromocytoma *(PHEO)*. The *horizontal lines* represent the median values. (Adopted from Gostelow R, et al.: Plasma-free metanephrine and free normetanephrine measurement for the diagnosis of pheochromocytoma in dogs, *J Vet Intern Med* 27:83, 2013, with permission.)

due to methodological differences; another explanation would be that the severity of illness in the dogs studied by Cameron, et al., (2010) was higher than in our studies. In our hospital, we first stabilize patients as much as possible before taking samples for the biochemical tests.

The plasma test (i.e., plasma-free normetanephrine and plasma-free metanephrine) was recently investigated by Gostelow, et al. (2013). The two parameters were measured in healthy dogs, dogs with non-adrenal disease, dogs with adrenocortical tumors, and dogs with pheochromocytoma. Plasma-free normetanephrine was superior to plasma-free metanephrine, and it was significantly higher in dogs with pheochromocytoma compared to all other groups with nearly no overlap (Fig. 13-12). Another finding was that dogs have much higher free metanephrine and free normetanephrine concentrations than humans. It is therefore important to use species-specific reference ranges (Gostelow et al, 2013). The same, of course, is true for the urinary parameters. With regard to the latter, the laboratories usually provide human reference ranges for parameters measured in 24-hour urine samples, which have to be ignored.

In human medicine, the question of which of the tests, urine or plasma, performs best is controversial. We recently compared the two tests in healthy dogs and dogs with pheochromocytoma, hyperadrenocorticism, and non-adrenal diseases.

As expected from the previous studies, catecholamines (norepinephrine and epinephrine) overlapped to a large degree between the groups and were of little diagnostic usefulness. This was true for the urine as well as for the plasma test. The two metabolites, normetanephrine and metanephrine, were significantly higher in dogs with pheochromocytoma than in the other three groups in both urine and plasma. Again, the discrimination

between groups was clearly superior for normetanephrine compared to metanephrine. There was some difference between the urine and the plasma test. Unlike in the study of Gostelow, et al., (2013), plasma-free normetanephrine levels overlapped to some degree between dogs with pheochromocytoma and dogs with hyperadrenocorticism or non-adrenal disease. In contrast, no overlap was found with regard to the urinary normetanephrine ratio (Fig. 13-13). The absence of overlap in the urine test is, however, considered just to be a matter of coincidence, because we have found overlap in previous series of dogs. Much larger numbers of dogs with pheochromocytoma have to be evaluated before a more definitive statement about the performance of the urine and plasma test can be made. It is likely, however, that the differences will be small, as in human medicine. At the moment, the veterinarian should choose between urine and plasma test according to availability of techniques and availability of species-specific reference ranges. Some laboratories still only measure the parent catecholamines, which are of minor importance for the diagnosis of canine pheochromocytoma. Diagnosis should be based on metanephrines, the metabolites of catecholamines, and it is highly recommended that normetanephrine and metanephrine are measured as separate parameters (in urine or plasma). Sampling conditions are critical, and the user of any of the tests should discuss those with the laboratory beforehand. The protocols for urine sampling usually include acidification of urine until pH is less than or equal to 2 and storage should be at − 20° C; the protocols for plasma sampling include sampling into chilled tubes, immediate centrifugation, and storage at − 80° C. The shipping of both urine and plasma samples has to be on dry ice.

So far, only one study investigated metanephrines in cats. Plasma-free normetanephrine was found to be markedly higher in the one cat with suspected pheochromocytoma compared to healthy cats and cats with non-adrenal diseases. Plasma-free metanephrine was not different (Wimpole et al, 2010).

Other Tests

VMA, CGA and the clonidine test (see Other Tests earlier) have not been evaluated in dogs. Dopamine and its metabolite, methoxytyramine, have been measured so far in a small number of dogs with pheochromocytoma in our hospital; however, isolated increases were not found. It is therefore not known whether dopamine-secreting pheochromocytomas exist in dogs.

Measurement of serum inhibin concentration has recently been described as a valuable parameter to differentiate pheochromocytomas from adrenocortical tumors in neutered dogs. Inhibin is a glycoprotein that is mainly synthesized in the gonads; however, it may also derive from the adrenal glands. In healthy neutered dogs and in neutered dogs with pheochromocytoma, serum inhibin concentrations were shown to be very low (i.e., below the detection limit of the assay). Dogs with adrenocortical tumors had significantly higher inhibin concentrations. Therefore, an undetectable inhibin concentration in a neutered dog with an adrenal tumor is highly supportive of a pheochromocytoma (Brömel et al, 2013).

Establishing a Diagnosis

The diagnosis of a pheochromocytoma is challenging, and a high index of suspicion is required. Most pheochromocytomas are overlooked due to low medical awareness. Dogs with pheochromocytoma may present with a large variety of clinical signs. The most frequent are weakness, lethargy, tachypnea or panting, and acute or episodic collapse. Hypertension may or may

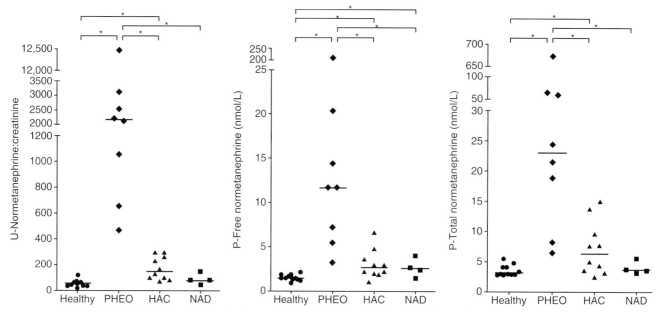

FIGURE 13-13 Comparison of urinary normetanephrine-to-creatinine ratio, plasma-free and plasma-total normetanephrine concentrations in healthy dogs, dogs with pheochromocytoma *(PHEO)*, hyperadrenocorticism *(HAC)*, and non-adrenal diseases *(NAD)*. Urinary normetanephrine-to-creatinine ratio showed less overlap than plasma-free or plasma-total normetanephrine in dogs with pheochromocytoma compared to the other groups. Plasma-total normetanephrine, which was measured for the first time in this study, performed in a similar way to plasma-free normetanephrine and has therefore no advantage (Parts of the data are from Salesov E, et al.: Urinary and plasma catecholamine and metanephrine in dogs with pheochromocytoma, hyperadrenocorticism and in healthy dogs, *J Vet Intern Med* 26:1524 (abstract), 2012.) *, Significant difference; *horizontal line*, median value; *P-Free*, plasma-free, *P-Total*, plasma-total; *U*, urinary.

not be present at the time of investigation. It is, however, not pathognomonic for pheochromocytoma and is often also seen in dogs with hyperadrenocorticism. The higher the systolic blood pressure, the more likely a pheochromocytoma is present (e.g., systolic blood pressures > 300 mm Hg so far have only been seen in dogs with pheochromocytoma). CBC, chemistry profile, and urinalysis are not helpful due to the lack of consistent abnormalities. It is important to remember that in some dogs with pheochromocytoma, laboratory findings may be similar to those in dogs with hyperadrenocorticism (e.g., increased ALP, ALT, and cholesterol and urine specific gravity in the hyposthenuric or isosthenuric range). Often, a pheochromocytoma is only considered after detection of an adrenal mass on abdominal ultrasonography. Unfortunately, no pattern of echogenicity or architecture is specific for a pheochromocytoma, and therefore, all differential diagnosis for an adrenal mass have to be considered (see sections Abdominal Ultrasonography and Incidental Discovered Adrenal Mass). Ultrasonography is helpful to determine the size and invasiveness of the mass. If the degree of the latter cannot be determined by ultrasonography (e.g., extent of vascular invasion), evaluation of the mass by CT or MRI is helpful. However, both modalities require anesthesia, which may be associated with hypertensive crisis and/or arrhythmias in dogs with pheochromocytoma. Preferentially, CT/MRI should be delayed either until a pheochromocytoma has been ruled out or until a dog with confirmed pheochromocytoma has been pretreated with phenoxybenzamine and/or an experienced anesthetist is available.

Cortisol-producing adrenocortical tumors are much more common than pheochromocytomas. Therefore, in questionable cases (i.e., all findings could be explained by hyperadrenocorticism or

pheochromocytoma), hyperadrenocorticism should be ruled first by the appropriate screening tests. There are two points to consider that demonstrate how difficult a correct approach may be. First, screening tests for hyperadrenocorticism may be false-positive in dogs with other diseases, and we have seen false-positive results in several of our dogs with pheochromocytoma. Of note, both diseases may be present in the same dog, which then poses an even bigger diagnostic challenge. The second point has so far only been described in humans with pheochromocytoma, namely that dexamethasone and ACTH may induce a hypertensive crisis (Rosas et al, 2008, Yi et al, 2010; see Box 13-1). So far, we have not seen problems after the low-dose dexamethasone test or the ACTH stimulation test in dogs with pheochromocytoma. However, close monitoring of the patients for approximately 12 hours after the tests may be a valuable consideration.

In dogs in which hyperadrenocorticism has been ruled out or in which results of the screening tests are equivocal, biochemical testing for pheochromocytoma is the next logical step. Some laboratories still offer the sole measurement of the parent catecholamines (norepinephrine and epinephrine); however, their diagnostic accuracy is poor. It is important that the testing includes measurement of the catecholamine metabolites, normetanephrine, and metanephrine. Discrimination between dogs with pheochromocytoma and dogs with other diseases is better for normetanephrine than for metanephrine. Measurement can be performed in urine (as ratio to urinary creatinine) or in plasma. The probability of a pheochromocytoma is very high if the urinary normetanephrine ratio or the plasma-free normetanephrine concentration is greater than or equal to four times the upper limit of normal. In these patients, the diagnosis is straightforward. The major remaining problems are dogs with smaller increases (e.g., two to three times normal). In those dogs, a pheochromocytoma may or may not be present. Further steps will depend on the clinical situation and owner compliance. Usually, it is a decision between the search for another disease explaining the clinical signs, reevaluation of pheochromocytoma by biochemical testing after a few weeks, or surgical removal of the adrenal tumor after a period of treatment with phenoxybenzamine.

Surgical Treatment

Pheochromocytomas should be considered malignant tumors in dogs. Tumor growth is unpredictable, and the risk of invasion into vessels (most often into the vena cava) and into surrounding tissues is high. Adrenalectomy is the treatment of choice and should be performed as soon as possible after diagnosis. The exceptions are very old and debilitated dogs, dogs in which the tumor is considered to be unresectable due to massive local invasion, and dogs with serious concurrent diseases. It is currently not known if adrenalectomy will prolong survival in dogs that have already developed metastasis. In the rare case of bilateral pheochromocytoma, the owner has to be aware that lifelong mineralocorticoid and glucocorticoid replacement will be required after bilateral adrenalectomy. Adrenal cortex–sparing surgery may in principle be possible, however, has so far only been described in humans.

Identification of a tumor thrombus in the vena cava is not an absolute contraindication for surgery. Removal of tumor thrombi by adrenalectomy and thrombectomy without increased perioperative morbidity and mortality is possible. It requires, however, a surgeon experienced in appropriate techniques (Kyles et al, 2003).

Preoperative Medical Management

In human medicine, careful consideration is given to the preoperative stabilization of the patient. The main goal is to keep catecholamine-induced complications during surgery to a minimum. Complications may be life-threatening and include hypertensive crisis, arrhythmias, pulmonary edema, and cardiac ischemia (Lenders et al, 2005). The traditional preoperative approach is to block the effects of catecholamines for at least 10 to 14 days prior to surgery in all patients with pheochromocytoma and paraganglioma, including those with apparent normal catecholamine levels (Chen et al, 2010). The most commonly used drug is phenoxybenzamine, an oral, non-competitive, α-adrenoreceptor blocker (Pacak, 2007; Fitzgerald, 2011). It is a non-selective blocker (acting on α_1 and α_2 receptors) that has irreversible and long lasting effects until de novo α-receptor synthesis. Phenoxybenzamine does not block the synthesis of catecholamines (in fact synthesis increases) but blocks α-adrenergic response to circulating norepinephrine and epinephrine. It decreases blood pressure, supports expansion of contracted blood volume, and decreases the frequency of ventricular arrhythmias. In humans, the dose is usually increased every 2 to 3 days; a dose titration is necessary to reduce side effects, such as postural hypotension, dizziness, syncope, nasal congestion, and others (Pacak, 2007). In some human centers α_1-adrenoreceptor blockers (e.g., doxazosin, prazosin, terazosin, and urapidil) are preferred over phenoxybenzamine. They are competitive and short-acting antagonists that may have fewer side effects than phenoxybenzamine; however, there is no consensus as to which drug is best.

In human patients with catecholamine- or α-blocker induced tachyarrhythmias, β-adrenoreceptor blockers are often added to the preoperative treatment regimen. They should, however, never be initiated before α-adrenoreceptor blockers have been

given for at least 2 days. Hypertension may become more severe with β-blockade alone, because α_1 mediated vasoconstriction is unopposed (Lenders et al, 2005; Pacak, 2007). Selective β_1 blockers (e.g., atenolol) are generally preferred over non-selective β-blockers (e.g., propranolol); however, at higher doses β_1 blockers also block β_2 receptors (Fitzgerald, 2011).

Another option for preoperative preparation of humans with pheochromocytoma are calcium-channel blockers. They are better tolerated than α-blockers, but they may be less effective (Pacak, 2007).

The preoperative targets for humans differ slightly between centers. Blood pressure should decrease to approximately 120 to 130/80 mm Hg, and heart rate should decrease to approximately 60 to 70 mm Hg.

In dogs, the effect of preoperative treatment on anesthetic complications, surgical outcome, and survival has so far only been investigated in a single study (Herrera et al, 2008). Twenty-three of 48 dogs (48%) were treated with phenoxybenzamine for a median of 20 days prior to adrenalectomy. The dose ranged between 0.1 to 2.5 mg/kg b.i.d. (twice a day; median 0.6 mg/kg b.i.d.). Interestingly, there were no differences in anesthesia time, surgical time, intraoperative and postoperative hypertensive and hypotensive episodes, and intraoperative arrhythmia between treated and untreated dogs. However, all six untreated dogs with intraoperative arrhythmias died, whereas only one of seven treated dogs with intraoperative arrhythmias died. The mortality rate was significantly lower in the treated group than in the untreated group (13% versus 48%). Dogs pretreated with phenoxybenzamine were six times more likely to survive adrenalectomy. The results of the study strongly support the preoperative treatment with phenoxybenzamine. It should be realized, however, that so far neither the dose nor the duration of preoperative treatment required to achieve the best effect have been defined.

We are currently using phenoxybenzamine as a standard preparation for adrenalectomy in dogs with pheochromocytoma. Treatment is performed in dogs with documented hypertension as well as in dogs that are normotensive at the time of examination. In order to reduce side effects, dose is titrated similar to what is done in human medicine. Our starting dose is 0.25 mg/kg b.i.d., which is increased stepwise every 2 to 3 days until a final dose of approximately 1 mg/kg b.i.d. is reached. Surgery is scheduled approximately 2 weeks after the start of treatment. The last dose of phenoxybenzamine is given in the evening prior to surgery. Ideally, blood pressure, heart rate, and heart rhythm are monitored regularly during the preparation phase, which would allow an individualized dose titration. Often, however, dose adjustment is done on the basis of owner feedback. If the dog shows signs of hypotension (e.g., lethargy, weakness, syncope) or other adverse effects (e.g., tachycardia, vomiting), the dose should be reduced. It is possible that by adding a calcium channel blocker (e.g., amlodipine), a lower dose of phenoxybenzamine would be sufficient, which would then improve tolerability. This has not yet been investigated.

In case tachycardia or tachyarrhythmia may occur during the preoperative period, a β-blocker may be added to the treatment regimen. A selective β_1 antagonist (e.g., atenolol 0.2 to 1.0 mg/kg by mouth every 12 to 24 hours) is preferred over a non-selective β-blocker. As mentioned earlier, β-blockade should never be used before the dog has received phenoxybenzamine for several days. Otherwise, severe hypertension may result.

Despite medical management, complications may still occur during the preoperative period, and the owner should be advised to closely monitor the dog (Feldman and Nelson, 2004a).

Anesthesia and Management of Intraoperative Complications

Surgical removal of a pheochromocytoma is a high-risk procedure and should only be performed by an experienced surgeon-anesthesiologist team. Close communication between the two before and during the procedure is mandatory. During the preoperative period, blood pressure and heart rate should have been stabilized as much as possible, and the dog should be well-hydrated. Admission to the hospital at least 1 day prior to surgery and administration of intravenous fluids (e.g., 0.9% NaCl) at maintenance rates is recommended. The latter is also done in humans to further expand the intravascular volume and reduce the risk of intraoperative and postoperative hypotension (Pacak, 2007). The patient needs continuous monitoring throughout the procedure and for approximately 24 to 48 hours thereafter. Monitoring should include electrocardiogram (ECG) and blood pressure (preferentially direct arterial pressure); a central venous pressure line is helpful to optimize fluid therapy. Despite preoperative preparation, life-threatening complications may still occur—in particular during induction of anesthesia, intubation, surgical incision, and manipulation of the tumor (Fig. 13-14). The most worrisome complications are severe hypertension, severe tachycardia, cardiac arrhythmias, hypotension, and hemorrhage. Systolic blood pressure may reach levels above 300 mm Hg, and heart rate may increase above 250 bpm. Cardiac arrhythmias most often are tachyarrhythmias, such as supraventricular and ventricular tachycardia as well as atrial and ventricular premature contractions; bradyarrhythmias are rare. Hypotension with systolic blood pressure less than 80 mm Hg may occur after tumor removal due to sudden decrease of catecholamine levels, hypovolemia, residual effect of preoperative α-blockers and desensitization of α-receptors (Kinney et al, 2002; Fitzgerald, 2011). The anesthesiologist should be prepared to deal with those complications immediately and should have all drugs ready to be administered.

Many anesthetic drugs have been successfully used, and there is no widely accepted protocol for dogs with pheochromocytoma. In humans it is believed that depth of anesthesia is generally more important than the particular drug (Kinney et al, 2002).

Premedication is advisable to reduce stress before and during the induction of anesthesia, an opioid that is not considered to cause histamine release (e.g., methadone or hydromorphone) may be a suitable option. Induction of anesthesia with propofol, thiopental, or etomidate has shown to be safe in humans with pheochromocytoma (Kinney et al, 2002) and also seems to be safe in dogs. Propofol combined with fentanyl, sufentanil, alfentanil, or remifentanil may be used for total intravenous anesthesia. If anesthesia is maintained by inhalant anesthetics, isoflurane and sevoflurane are suitable agents. In humans with pheochromocytoma vecuronium is the safest agent to achieve muscle relaxation (Manelli et al, 2012b). Various drugs are considered to increase the risk of complications, such as atropine, ketamine, acepromazine, chlorpromazine, morphine, meperidine, droperidol, halothane, desflurane, succinylcholine, and atracurium. Although no studies have been performed, it may be advisable to avoid them in dogs with pheochromocytoma.

Intraoperative hypertension may often be successfully managed by deepening the anesthesia. The most commonly used drug to combat hypertension during pheochromocytoma surgery is phentolamine, a short-acting α-adrenergic antagonist. An intravenous bolus dose of 0.02 to 0.1 mg/kg is followed by constant rate infusion to effect (Ware, 2009). In dogs with persistence of tachycardia and tachyarrhythmia esmolol, an ultra-short-acting β_1 antagonist, can be given. The initial intravenous bolus of 50 to 500 μg/kg is followed by constant rate infusion of 50 to 200 μg/kg/min (Gordon, 2010). As mentioned earlier, a β-blocker should not be given before α-blockade. If α_1-receptors are unopposed, severe hypertension may result. In cases of serious ventricular arrhythmias, lidocaine is an appropriate choice. An initial bolus of 2 mg/kg is followed by constant rate infusion of 20 to 80 μg/kg/min (Ettinger, 2010). In cases of intraoperative hypotension, the dose of phentolamine (or other blood pressure reducing agents) should be decreased or its application discontinued; the next step is the expansion of the intravascular volume, preferentially with crystalloid. If those means remain ineffective, agents such as dobutamine (to increase contractility) or phenylephrine, norepinephrine, vasopressin (to increase vascular tone) need to be considered.

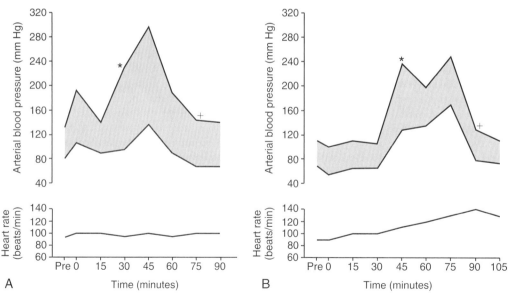

FIGURE 13-14 Direct arterial systolic and diastolic blood pressure measurements and heart rates prior to anesthesia *(Pre)*, during anesthetic induction *(0)*, and during removal of a pheochromocytoma in a Border Collie **(A)** and a West Highland White Terrier **(B)**. Hypertension developed during anesthetic induction in the Border Collie and during manual manipulation of the pheochromocytoma in both dogs. Hypertension ceased after tumor removal. *, Onset of tumor manipulation by surgeon; +, completion of tumor excision.

Surgical and Postoperative Management

The surgical techniques are described in detail in veterinary surgical textbooks. Pheochromocytomas may be resected by an open laparotomy (e.g., median celiotomy or flank laparotomy) or by a laparoscopic approach. Selection of the technique is based on tumor size and invasiveness and the surgeon's preference and experience. In humans, laparoscopic adrenalectomy has become the procedure of choice for non-invasive, solitary pheochromocytomas that are less than 6 to 8 cm in diameter (Fitzgerald, 2011; Young, 2011). In veterinary medicine, no official guidelines have yet been established, and complication rates and survival rates between the two approaches have not been compared. Open laparotomy should definitely be performed in dogs with large tumors and tumors in which preoperative imaging techniques suggest invasion into the vena cava (or other large vessels) and/or adhesion to surrounding tissue. The preoperative detection of tumor thrombi into the vena cava is by itself not a contraindication for surgery. Successful adrenalectomy and thrombectomy has been reported several times (Kyles et al, 2003; Louvet et al, 2005; Lang et al, 2011). During surgery, close communication between the surgeon and the anesthesiologist is critical, because any manipulation of the tumor may lead to a catecholamine surge followed by hypertension, tachycardia, and arrhythmias. Therefore, the area of the tumor and the tumor itself should only be touched after the anesthesiologist has been informed. The tumor has to be handled with extreme care. Because pheochromocytomas are considered potentially malignant tumors, a thorough evaluation of all surrounding tissues and abdominal organs should be performed. Careful inspection may also help to detect additional tumors, which are relatively common in dogs with pheochromocytoma. The length of surgical time has a major influence on survival (i.e., the longer the procedure lasts, the poorer the survival). According to a study, the odds of 10-day survival decreased by 75% for every hour increase in surgery time (Herrera et al, 2008). Removal of a pheochromocytoma is a demanding procedure and should only be performed by an experienced surgeon.

Postoperatively, the patient should be monitored closely for at least 48 hours, preferentially in an intensive care unit (ICU) setting. Monitoring should at least include evaluation of clinical parameters, continuous blood pressure measurement, continuous ECG, and measurement of the most important laboratory parameters (packed cell volume [PCV], total protein, glucose, and electrolytes). Postoperative complications such as hypotension, hypertension, and cardiac arrhythmias are common. Hypotension may be due to the sudden decrease of catecholamine levels or residual effect of preoperative α-blockers; however, the possibility of massive bleeding from the surgical site also needs to be considered. In theory, hypertension should no longer occur after tumor removal, and it may therefore raise concern for remnant tumor tissue and functional metastasis. In humans, however, hypertension is commonly seen in the postoperative phase. Among other reasons, it is attributed to elevated catecholamine stores in adrenergic nerve endings, resetting of baroreceptors, and structural changes of vessels (Kinney et al, 2002; Young, 2011). Management of postoperative complications follows the same principles as described earlier for intraoperative complications.

In some dogs, it may not be clear prior to surgery if the adrenal mass is a pheochromocytoma or a cortisol-producing adrenocortical tumor. Clinical signs often are alike, and results of the various tests (low-dose dexamethasone suppression test [LDDST], urinary, or plasma metanephrines) may be equivocal. It should also be remembered that both tumor types may occur together in the same dog. In questionable cases, we therefore administer dexamethasone during the surgical procedure and perform an ACTH stimulation test soon thereafter. Glucocorticoids are given until the test results show normal function of the adrenal cortex (see Chapter 10 for further details). In dogs in which bilateral adrenalectomy is performed due to bilateral pheochromocytomas, lifelong supplementation of mineralocorticoids and glucocorticoids is needed (see Chapter 12).

Histopathology

The definitive diagnosis of a pheochromocytoma is established by histopathology and immunohistochemistry. Histologically, pheochromocytoma cells are arranged in short cords, nests, or lobules separated by a fine fibrovascular stroma. The cells are round to polyhedral with lightly eosinophilic to basophilic cytoplasm. Nuclei are round to oval with coarsely granular chromatin. Mitotic activity is variable. Compression of the adrenal cortex or disruption of its zonal architecture, disruption of the adrenal capsule, as well as hemorrhage and necrosis may be seen. Invasion of small vessels and tumor thrombi may be present. Metastasis have the same histological characteristics as the primary tumor (Wilson et al, 1986; Bouayad et al, 1987; Cuervo et al, 1994; Barthez et al, 1997; Sako et al, 2001; Santamarina et al, 2003; Boes et al, 2009; Guillaumot et al, 2012).

It may be difficult to differentiate a pheochromocytoma from an adrenocortical tumor by its microscopic appearance, in particular if the tumor is large and cells have a more atypical appearance (Barthez et al, 1997; Herrera and Nelson, 2010). At times, differentiation from other tumor types may also be challenging.

In the pre-immunohistochemical era, so-called silver stains (e.g., Grimelius stain) were used as an aid to characterize the tumor as pheochromocytoma (Grimelius, 2004). Today, the use of immunohistochemical markers has widely replaced those traditional argyrophil methods. In humans, pheochromocytomas are positive for broad-spectrum neuroendocrine markers, such as CGA, synaptophysin, neuron-specific enolase (NSE), and protein gene product 9.5 (PGP 9.5). However, adrenal cortical tumors may also show immunopositivity for synaptophysin as well as for PGP 9.5, and NSE generally lacks specificity. In contrast, CGA is negative in adrenocortical tissue, rendering it a very useful marker to differentiate between tumors of the adrenal medulla and tumors of the adrenal cortex (Erickson and Lloyd, 2004). The same seems to be true in dogs, although no comprehensive studies comparing sensitivity and specificity of the various immunohistochemical markers have been performed so far. CGA is present in the adrenal medulla and absent in the adrenal cortex of dogs and therefore suitable to confirm the presence of a pheochromocytoma (Doss et al, 1998). In most published cases of canine pheochromocytoma using CGA, positive staining was demonstrated. Because staining relies on a sufficient number of secretory granules, absence of CGA does not exclude a pheochromocytoma (Doss et al, 1998). It may be difficult to distinguish between benign and malignant pheochromocytomas by means of histology. Canine pheochromocytoma often invades surrounding vessels and tissue and metastasizes to distant sites. In veterinary medicine, usually both invasion and metastasis are regarded as sign of malignancy. This is different to humans, where the traditional position of the WHO is to base the diagnosis of malignancy on the presence of metastasis and not on local invasion (Tischler et al, 2006; Carlsen et al, 2009).

Medical Treatment

After the diagnosis of pheochromocytoma has been made, medical treatment should be started to prepare the dog for surgery. We are currently using phenoxybenzamine, an oral, non-competitive, non-selective α-adrenoreceptor blocker in dogs with hypertension as well as in dogs with normal blood pressure. Phenoxybenzamine does not block the synthesis of catecholamines but blocks α-adrenergic response to circulating norepinephrine and epinephrine. A recent study showed that perioperative mortality is significantly lower in pretreated than in untreated dogs (Herrera et al, 2008). Surgery may not be an option in dogs with large and invasive tumors, metastasis, serious concurrent disease, or in cases of financial or other constraints of the owner. In those dogs, we suggest medical treatment according to the protocol used for preoperative preparation. To limit side effects, the dose of phenoxybenzamine should be increased stepwise. Our starting dose is 0.25 mg/kg b.i.d., which is increased every few days until clinical signs are controlled or until a final dose of approximately 1 mg/kg b.i.d. is reached. If the dog shows signs of hypotension (e.g., lethargy, weakness, and/or syncope) or other adverse effects (e.g., tachycardia, and/or vomiting), the dose should be reduced. In the case of tachycardia or tachyarrhythmia, a β-blocker may be added to the treatment regimen. A selective $β_1$ antagonist (e.g., atenolol 0.2 to 1.0 mg/kg by mouth every 12 to 24 hours) is preferred over a non-selective β-blocker. As mentioned earlier, β-blockade should never be used before the dog has received the α-adrenoreceptor blocker for several days. There are no studies investigating the effect of medical treatment on survival. However, several of our phenoxybenzamine treated dogs lived for more than 1 year after diagnosis.

Metyrosine (Demser) is an inhibitor of tyrosine hydroxylase, the enzyme that catalyzes the rate-limiting step in the catecholamine biosynthesis. It significantly reduces catecholamine stores and excretion. In some human centers, it is used as preoperative treatment in conjunction with α- and β-blocker or in case of metastatic disease. It has no effect on tumor progression. Serious side effects are common and include sedation, depression, anxiety, extrapyramidal signs, galactorrhea, diarrhea, crystalluria, and urolithiasis, and it has to be administered with caution in patients with hepatic and renal impairment (Pacak, 2007; Fitzgerald, 2011). In humans with advanced metastatic pheochromocytoma, chemotherapy with a combination of cyclophosphamide, vincristine, and dacarbazine has been used; however, treatment success is limited. Complete tumor response was seen in 11% and partial response in 44% of patients; median duration of response was 20 months (Huang et al, 2008).

Sunitinib (Sutent), an antiangiogenic drug, has also been used so far with limited success. There are no studies on the use of metyrosine, chemotherapy, or sunitinib in dogs with pheochromocytoma.

In humans with advanced disease, radioisotope therapy with ^{131}I-MIBG or somatostatin analog is used with some success; however, complete remission is rare. Recently, radioisotope therapy with ^{131}I-MIBG has been reported in one dog with a large, invasive pheochromocytoma. The dog improved and had clinically stable disease for 4 months. Tumor progression led to a second treatment after 5 months; however, the dog died 3 weeks thereafter (Bommarito et al, 2011).

Prognosis

The prognosis depends on various factors such as size, malignant potential, and endocrine activity of the tumor. Dogs with small tumors (maximum diameter less than 2 to 3 cm) without invasion and metastasis and low endocrine activity have better prognosis than dogs with large, invasive tumors; tumor metastasis; and with tumors secreting high amounts of catecholamines. Additional prognostic factors are age and general condition of the dog as well as presence and severity of concurrent diseases.

Adrenalectomy is the treatment of choice; it is, however, a demanding and high risk procedure. To decrease the risk of intraoperative and postoperative complications, it should only be performed by an experienced surgeon-anesthesiologist team. Perioperative mortality has been shown to be significantly lower in dogs pretreated with phenoxybenzamine compared to untreated dogs (18% versus 48%; Herrera et al, 2008). Dogs that survive the immediate perioperative period and do not suffer from metastasis or serious concurrent disease can live for several years. Tumor thrombus in the vena cava is by itself no contraindication for adrenalectomy. Dogs with and without tumor thrombus have similar perioperative morbidity and mortality, provided that the surgeon is familiar with appropriate techniques (Kyles et al, 2003). Survival times of 20, 36, and 49 months have been reported after caval venectomy or en bloc resection of the tumor and the invaded vena cava (Kyles et al, 2003; Louvet et al, 2005; Guillaumot et al, 2012).

Dogs treated medically with phenoxybenzamine without subsequent adrenalectomy can live for more than a year after diagnosis. Most dogs die because of complications caused by catecholamine excess, tumor thrombosis, tumor invasion into surrounding tissue, tumor rupture, or metastasis.

Paraganglioma

The WHO classification of endocrine tumors defines paragangliomas as tumors of the extra-adrenal sympathetic and parasympathetic paraganglia. The term *pheochromocytoma* is reserved for tumors arising from catecholamine-producing chromaffin cells in the adrenal medulla (Pacak et al, 2007). Paragangliomas are a diverse group of neuroendocrine tumors (NETs) that may develop at many body sites, such as the head, neck, thorax, and abdomen. They originate from paraganglia, which in turn derive from primitive cells of the neural crest, and are associated with autonomic ganglia throughout the body. At a microscopic and cellular level, both types (sympathetic and parasympathetic) paraganglia are similar, and both contain catecholamines, however, there are quantitative differences. In humans, clinical signs due to catecholamine secretion are usually only seen in tumors of sympathetic paraganglia (Tischler, 2007). Sympathetic paraganglioma (also called *non-head-neck paragangliomas*) account for about 10% of all pheochromocytomas/paragangliomas in adult humans. About 75% of them are intra-abdominal, and 25% are found in the thorax (Fitzgerald, 2011). Typical locations are the Zuckerkandl body (a sympathetic ganglion at the root of the caudal mesenteric artery), the sympathetic plexus of the urinary bladder, the kidneys, and the heart, as well as the sympathetic ganglia or the aortopulmonary body in the mediastinum (Timmers et al, 2012). Up to 60% are hormonally active and secrete norepinephrine and normetanephrine. They do not secrete epinephrine and metanephrine. They can be locally invasive with destruction of vertebrae and compression of nerve roots and spinal cord; metastasis occurs in 30% to 50% of human patients (Fitzgerald, 2011). Paragangliomas arising from parasympathetic paraganglia are also called *glomus tumors* or *head-and-neck paraganglia*. Most of them do not secrete relevant amounts of catecholamines (Lenders et al, 2005; Fitzgerald, 2011; Timmers et al, 2012). A substantial percentage of humans have a genetic basis for the development of paraganglia (e.g., familial paraganglioma/pheochromocytoma syndromes due to succinate dehydrogenase gene mutations; Fishbein and Nathanson, 2012).

In dogs and cats, paragangliomas are very rare NETs. Parasympathetic paragangliomas are the most common type in dogs and usually arise from the aortic or carotic body. They are also known as *glomus tumors, chemoreceptor tumors,* or *chemodectomas.* They are considered nonfunctional, and clinical signs result from space-occupying effects, local invasion, and metastasis (Capen, 2007). Other paragangliomas that may have originated from sympathetic paraganglia have only been described in a few dogs and cats. They were associated with posterior mediastinal, abdominal, or pelvic masses (Patnaik et al, 1990; Mascort and Pumarola, 1995; Davis et al, 1997). So far, endocrine activity (i.e., catecholamine secretion) has not been demonstrated, and therefore it is currently unclear if sympathetic paragangliomas secrete relevant amounts of catecholamines. Due to the fact that the mass-related signs predominate, endocrine work-up in dogs and cats with paraganglioma is usually not considered.

Incidental Discovered Adrenal Mass (Incidentaloma)

The NIH State-of-the-Science Statement (National Institutes of Health, 2002) defines the term incidentaloma for human medicine as follows:

> Incidentalomas are clinically inapparent adrenal masses that are discovered inadvertently in the course of diagnostic testing for other clinical conditions that are not related to suspicion of adrenal disease. The definition of incidentaloma excludes patients who undergo imaging procedures as part of staging and work-up for cancer.

To be regarded as incidentaloma, the mass should have a diameter of 1 cm or more (Young, 2007). The topic has become a challenging clinical problem due to the increased discovery of masses by the widespread use of diagnostic imaging techniques. In radiological studies, prevalence of incidentalomas in middle-aged people is found to be approximately 2% to 4% and increases with increasing age (Arnaldi and Boscaro, 2012). Most adrenal incidentalomas in humans are benign adenomas, which are nonfunctional. However, in 20% to 30%, the tumors are hormonally active; because the hormone excess is often only mild, the disease is either subclinical or associated with very subtle symptoms. Cortisol-producing tumors are the most frequent, followed by pheochromocytoma and aldosteronoma. Larger tumors (> 6 cm) are more likely to be malignant than smaller ones (Terzolo et al, 2011; Aron et al, 2012). The big challenge is to identify those adrenal incidentaloma that pose the patient at risk, either because of their hormonal activity or because of their malignant potential, while leaving the others alone. A pheochromocytoma has to be excluded before fine-needle aspiration (Aron et al, 2012). There is agreement that human patients with an adrenal incidentaloma should be screened for hypercortisolism, pheochromocytoma, and if hypertension is present, also for hyperaldosteronism. Routine screening for excess androgens or estrogens is not indicated, unless the patient has obvious clinical signs (Young, 2007; Zeiger et al, 2009). Adrenal biopsy is considered to be of low discriminant value and should not be done unless it is part of staging of a known malignant disease (Aron et al, 2012). Surgery is usually recommended for all functional masses, although there is some controversy as to which removal of small tumors is useful in human patients with subclinical hypercortisolism. Adrenalectomy is recommended in all nonfunctional masses more than 4 to 6 cm in diameter, due to the likelihood of malignancy (Young, 2007; Zeiger et al, 2009; Terzolo et al, 2011; Arnaldi and Boscaro, 2012; Aron et al, 2012).

In dogs and cats, the situation with regard to incidentally discovered adrenal masses shows many similarities to humans. Due to the routine use of abdominal ultrasonography in sick animals, the frequency of detection of adrenal lesions has increased tremendously. It is very common to identify an adrenal nodule or mass during work-up of a problem that is not considered to be endocrine-related. The important questions thereafter are:

- Is the nodule/mass hormonally active or inactive?
- Is the nodule/mass benign or malignant or is it a metastasis?

Unfortunately, ultrasonography is not helpful to differentiate between the different types of nodules/masses.

So far, no data are available with regard to the prevalence of the different adrenal lesions (see Box 13-5). In dogs, cortisol-producing adrenal tumors are by far the most common, followed by pheochromocytoma; aldosterone and sex-hormone producing lesions are rare. In cats, the prevalence of adrenal tumors is generally much lower than in dogs. Cortisol-producing and aldosterone-producing lesions are the most common among the functional adrenal tumors, followed by sex-hormone producing tumors; pheochromocytomas are extremely rare in cats.

Due to the similarities, it seems reasonable to use the guidelines for humans with some amendments in the management of canine and feline adrenal incidentaloma. The work-up should be done according to the following considerations:

1. Rule out adrenal metastasis by searching for a primary tumor: Adrenal involvement in case of metastatic disease is common and was found in 21% of dogs and 14.8% of cats (Labelle and De Cock, 2005).
2. Rule out hormonally active tumors: Careful review of the history, physical examination, and laboratory findings as well as blood pressure measurements should be performed. If potentially endocrine-related abnormalities are detected, hormonal evaluations are the next logical steps. See Chapters 10 and 11 for details on the different diseases and the various tests. The latter include low-dose dexamethasone test, urinary corticoid-to-creatinine ratio, and measurement of endogenous ACTH to investigate for cortisol-producing adrenal lesions, urinary, or plasma metanephrines for pheochromocytoma and plasma renin and aldosterone for primary hyperaldosteronism.

   The sequence of testing depends on clinical findings and likelihood. For instance, if clinical findings are equivocal in a dog, we usually rule out hyperadrenocorticism before performing tests for pheochromocytoma. In a cat in which hypertension is the predominant sign, we first test for primary hyperaldosteronism. Sex-hormone producing adrenal tumors usually are associated with obvious clinical signs, such as aggressive male-type or estrus-like behavior or signs similar to those of hypercortisolism. Strictly speaking, adrenal masses in patients with obvious signs of an endocrinopathy should not be considered to be an incidentaloma.
3. If the presence of a hormonally active tumor is confirmed, medical and surgical treatment options should be discussed with the owner. In most situations, adrenalectomy is the modality of choice. Knowledge of functional status prior to surgery is essential for appropriate perioperative care (e.g., pretreatment with phenoxybenzamine in the case of pheochromocytoma, or intraoperative and postoperative steroid replacement in the case of a cortisol-producing tumor).
4. In large nonfunctional masses, adrenalectomy should be considered. The likelihood that a mass is malignant increases with size, and masses larger than 4 cm in diameters are almost always malignant (Besso et al, 1997).
5. Small nodules/masses (less than 2 to 3 cm) that are thought to be nonfunctional should be monitored by ultrasonography for growth. Initially, intervals should be quite short (e.g., every

2 to 3 months). If the disease is stable, intervals may be increased to every 4 to 6 months. If size increases, adrenalectomy should be performed. It is possible that a mass initially considered to be nonfunctional will become hormonally active with time. Therefore, it may be necessary to perform or repeat hormonal evaluation later in the course of the disease.

 MULTIPLE ENDOCRINE NEOPLASIA

Multiple Endocrine Neoplasia in Human Medicine

The first published case consistent with MEN can be attributed to Jakob Erdheim, a pathologist working in Vienna, Austria, little more than 100 years ago (Erdheim, 1903). The syndrome was later classified into the two major forms, MEN-1 and MEN-2. Each form is characterized by the development of tumors within specific endocrine organs. The tumors may be functional or nonfunctional, and each form may also be associated with neoplasias in non-endocrine tissue (Gardner, 2011; Marx and Wells, 2011; Thakker et al, 2012).

Usually, MEN-1 and MEN-2 occur as distinct clinical syndromes; some patients, however, have some kind of overlapping syndrome and develop tumors of both forms (Thakker, 2011). All forms of MEN may be either inherited as autosomal dominant disease or may occur sporadically without a family history. The distinction between hereditary and sporadic disease may, however, be difficult in some cases due to death of family members before manifestation of symptoms or due to lack of symptoms in others (Thakker et al, 2012). The main genes, whose mutations are responsible for the MEN syndromes, have been identified. MEN-1 is caused by inactivation mutations of a growth suppressor gene, and MEN-2 is caused by activating mutations of a growth promoter gene (Marx and Wells, 2011). In humans and their families at risk, screening programs are available, including tumor screening by a combination of clinical, biochemical, and diagnostic imaging procedures as well as germline mutation testing (Brandi et al 2001; Marini et al, 2006a; 2006b; Thakker et al, 2012).

Multiple Endocrine Neoplasia Type 1

MEN-1, which is also known as *Wermer syndrome,* has an estimated prevalence of 2 to 20 per 100,000 in the general human population (Gardner, 2011). MEN-1 occurs as early as 5 years of age, and due to the high degree of penetrance, 80% of individuals display clinical manifestations by the fifth decade (Thakker et al, 2012). It is an autosomal dominant disease, which is due to mutations in the tumor suppressor gene MEN-1 that encodes a 610-amino acid protein named *menin.* Menin is primarily a nuclear protein and is involved in the regulation of transcription, genome stability, cell division, and proliferation. So far, more than 1300 mutations have been described, and most of them are predicted to lead to a truncated form of menin (Lemos and Thakker, 2008). Inheritance of a germline MEN-1 mutation predisposes to tumor development after a somatic mutation, which may be a deletion leading to loss of heterozygosity (Thakker et al, 2012). Additionally to the autosomal dominant disease, a nonfamilial, sporadic form may occur and genetic studies revealed de novo mutations of the MEN-1 gene in approximately 10% of patients (Thakker, 2010; 2011).

The three major components of MEN-1 are parathyroid, pancreatic, and pituitary tumors. Some patients have additional tumors, such as adrenocortical tumors, lipomas, carcinoids, facial angiofibromas, collagenomas, and others (Table 13-6). A diagnosis of MEN-1 is made if the patient has at least two of the three

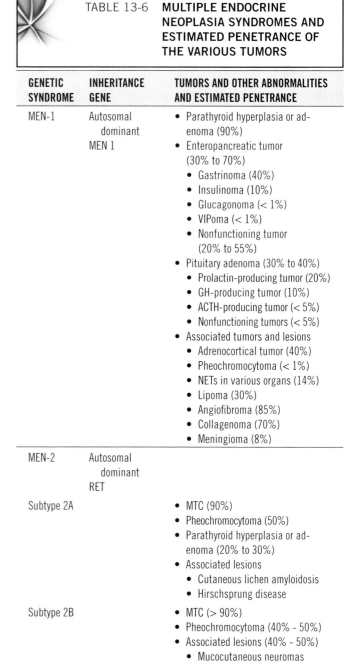

TABLE 13-6   MULTIPLE ENDOCRINE NEOPLASIA SYNDROMES AND ESTIMATED PENETRANCE OF THE VARIOUS TUMORS

GENETIC SYNDROME	INHERITANCE GENE	TUMORS AND OTHER ABNORMALITIES AND ESTIMATED PENETRANCE

MEN-1	Autosomal dominant MEN 1	• Parathyroid hyperplasia or adenoma (90%)
		• Enteropancreatic tumor (30% to 70%)
		  • Gastrinoma (40%)
		  • Insulinoma (10%)
		  • Glucagonoma (< 1%)
		  • VIPoma (< 1%)
		  • Nonfunctioning tumor (20% to 55%)
		• Pituitary adenoma (30% to 40%)
		  • Prolactin-producing tumor (20%)
		  • GH-producing tumor (10%)
		  • ACTH-producing tumor (< 5%)
		  • Nonfunctioning tumors (< 5%)
		• Associated tumors and lesions
		  • Adrenocortical tumor (40%)
		  • Pheochromocytoma (< 1%)
		  • NETs in various organs (14%)
		  • Lipoma (30%)
		  • Angiofibroma (85%)
		  • Collagenoma (70%)
		  • Meningioma (8%)

MEN-2	Autosomal dominant RET	

Subtype 2A		• MTC (90%)
		• Pheochromocytoma (50%)
		• Parathyroid hyperplasia or adenoma (20% to 30%)
		• Associated lesions
		  • Cutaneous lichen amyloidosis
		  • Hirschsprung disease

Subtype 2B		• MTC (> 90%)
		• Pheochromocytoma (40% - 50%)
		• Associated lesions (40% - 50%)
		  • Mucocutaneous neuromas
		  • Skeletal deformities, joint laxity
		  • Marfanoid habitus
		  • Myelinated corneal nerves
		  • Intestinal ganglioneuromas

FMTC	Autosomal dominant RET	• MTC (100%)

Modified from Thakker RV, et al.: Clinical practice guidelines for multiple endocrine neoplasia type 1 (MEN 1), *J Clin Endocrinol Metab* 97:2990, 2012.
ACTH, Adrenocorticotropic hormone; *FMTC,* familial medullary thyroid carcinoma; *GH,* growth hormone; *MEN-1,* multiple endocrine neoplasia type 1; *MEN-2,* multiple endocrine neoplasia type 2; *MTC,* medullary thyroid carcinoma; *NET,* neuroendocrine tumor; *VIP,* vasoactive intestinal peptide.

main MEN-1–associated tumors (parathyroid, pancreas, and/or pituitary). Familial MEN-1 is present if such a patient has at least one first degree relative with at least one of the three tumors (Brandi et al, 2001).

Primary hyperparathyroidism is the most common endocrine tumor in MEN-1 and occurs in approximately 90% of patients. It is also typically the first clinical manifestation of MEN-1. Usually three or all four parathyroid glands are enlarged due to either hyperplasia or multiple adenomas; carcinomas are rare. The increase in size is highly asymmetric. Clinical signs vary, depending on the degree of hypercalcemia. Patients may be asymptomatic or display the multiple problems associated with hypercalcemia, such as lethargy, confusion, polyuria/polydipsia, nephrocalcinosis, increased bone resorption, anorexia, constipation, and others (Marini et al, 2006a; Thakker et al, 2012). Pancreatic islet tumors, also called *pancreatic NETs,* are the second most common manifestation of MEN-1 and are present in 30% to 70% of patients. They comprise gastrinomas, insulinomas, glucagonomas, VIP-secreting tumors, and nonfunctional tumors. Because gastrinomas are often located in the duodenal mucosa, this group of tumors is also called *pancreatico-duodenal NETs.* Gastrinomas are the major cause of morbidity and mortality in MEN-1 patients. They are often malignant and metastasize, and they may manifest as Zollinger-Ellison syndrome. The latter is due to hypersecretion of gastrin and is associated with upper abdominal pain, oesophageale reflux, diarrhea, and ulcers that may perforate (Marini et al, 2006a; Gardner, 2011; Marx and Wells, 2011). Patients with insulinoma may display hypoglycemic symptoms: those with glucagonomas skin rash, weight loss, anemia, and stomatitis; those with VIPomas watery diarrhea, hypocalcemia, and achlorhydria. Pituitary tumors occur in 30% to 40% of MEN-1 patients. Compared to non–MEN-1 tumors, they tend to be larger, show more invasive behavior to surrounding pituitary tissue, and respond less to therapy. The clinical manifestations are associated with either the mass effect, such as vision field defects or headaches, and/or with the excessive secretion of hormones. Most pituitary tumors are prolactin-secreting tumors inducing galactorrhea, amenorrhea, and infertility in woman and hypogonadism, sexual dysfunction, and gynecomastia in man. The next common pituitary tumors secrete growth hormone (GH) and cause acromegaly; ACTH-producing tumors causing Cushing's syndrome are the least common (Marini et al 2006a; Thakker et al, 2012).

Multiple Endocrine Neoplasia Type 2

MEN-2 has an estimated prevalence of 1 to 10 per 100,000 in the general human population. In individuals with the defective gene, penetrance of MEN-2 is greater than 80% (Gardner, 2011). MEN-2 occurs in three clinical variants, named MEN-2A, MEN-2B, and familial medullary thyroid carcinoma (FMTC). MEN-2A accounts for 75%, FMTC for 20%, and MEN-2B for 5% of all MEN-2 cases (Martin et al, 2011). Sporadic and familial forms occur, and the latter are more common. MEN-2 is defined as the presence of at least two of the main MEN-2-related endocrine tumors. Familial MEN-2 is defined as a MEN-2 case plus a first degree relative with at least one MEN-2-related endocrine tumor (Marini et al, 2006b). MEN-2 is an autosomal dominant disease, and 98% of MEN-2 patients have activating germline point mutations of the RET protooncogene. Different from MEN-1, a strong genotype-phenotype correlation exists, and a specific RET mutation may be responsible for a more or less aggressive clinical course (Marini et al, 2006b; Romei et al, 2012). MEN-2A (Sipple syndrome) is characterized by MTC (in approximately 90% of cases), unilateral or bilateral pheochromocytoma (50% of cases),

and primary hyperparathyroidism (20% to 30% of cases). Some patients may develop additional problems, such as cutaneous lichen amyloidosis and Hirschsprung disease (congenital megacolon). The subtype MEN-2B is more aggressive than the subtype MEN-2A and FMTC. It is characterized by MTC (more than 90% of cases) and pheochromocytoma (40% to 50% of cases). In 40% to 50% of cases, additional abnormalities such as mucosal neuromas, ganglioneuromas of the gastrointestinal tract, skeletal deformities, joint laxity, marfanoid habitus, and myelinated corneal nerves are present (Marini et al, 2006b; Thakker et al, 2012; see Table 13-6). MTC is the most common manifestation of MEN-2. It is the main cause of morbidity and mortality, and it often is also the abnormality occurring first. It originates from multifocal C-cell hyperplasia as a precursor lesion and progresses to carcinoma. The progression from initial hyperplasia to benign or malignant tumors is a phenomenon also seen in other MEN-associated tumors. MTC metastasizes locally and to distant sites, such as lung, liver, and bone. Clinical manifestations are neck mass, neck pain, and diarrhea associated with excessive secretion of calcitonin (Brandi et al, 2001; Marini et al, 2006b).

Familial Medullary Thyroid Carcinoma

FMTC is defined by the isolated occurrence of MTC without other manifestations of MEN in at least four members of the same family. The clinical course is more benign than in MEN-2A and MEN-2B (Marini et al, 2006b).

Tumors of Multiple Endocrine Organs in Dogs and Cats

In dogs and cats, it is well known that tumors in several endocrine organs may be present in the same patient. Oftentimes, the tumors are diagnosed simultaneously or within a short time period; however, it is possible that a second or third endocrine tumor arises months to several years after the diagnosis of the first or second ones. The tumors may be hormonally active or inactive. In the case of hormonally active tumors, each tumor may express its own clinical picture and biochemical abnormalities. As seen in humans, it is possible that one tumor and its secretory product predominates the clinical manifestation. Tumors may also be hormonally silent and incidentally found by ultrasonography or at necropsy. A family of Alaskan Malamute-mixed breed dogs with MTC has been described. The father, as well as three female offspring, was presented at 8 to 9 years of age with neck masses and clinical signs consistent with hypothyroidism. The pattern was suggesting a dominant inheritance of autosomal or X-linked type and resembled FMTC in humans. RET mutational screening was performed; however, no mutation could be demonstrated. The authors hypothesized that there may be RET mutations outside the human hotspots or mutations in other genes (Lee et al, 2006). All other studies published so far describe single, sporadic cases. However, different from human medicine where family members are screened after the diagnosis of a MEN disorder in an individual, "family histories" of our canine and feline patients are usually unknown or are not investigated. A further limitation in veterinary medicine is that work-up oftentimes is incomplete. For instance, pituitary-dependent hyperadrenocorticism is often diagnosed by endocrine testing without the verification of the presence of a pituitary mass by diagnostic imaging, or a thyroid mass is not investigated by immunohistochemistry to define if it is a MTC. Table 13-7 provides an overview of the published canine cases harboring several endocrine tumors. In addition to the aforementioned family with a FMTC-like disease, only two dogs revealed similarity with the human MEN syndromes.

TABLE 13-7   CASE REPORTS AND CASE SERIES OF DOGS WITH MULTIPLE ENDOCRINE TUMORS

DOGS	PREDOMINANT CLINICAL SIGNS	PITUITARY TUMOR OR PITUITARY DEPENDENT HYPER-ADRENOCORTICISM	PARATHYROID HYPERPLASIA/ TUMOR	THYROID TUMOR	PHEOCHRO-MOCYTOMA	ADRENO-CORTICAL TUMOR	PANCREATIC TUMOR	TESTICULAR TUMOR	COMMENT	STUDY*
Fox Terrier, male, 15 years old	PU/PD, weakness	+	+	+ (MTC)	+			+ (ICT)	compares to MEN-2A	Peterson et al, 1982
Yorkshire Terrier, spayed, female, 13 years old	PU/PD, weakness, disorientation		+		+					Wright et al, 1995
Six dogs (four different breeds, two mixed), four males (two castrated males), two spayed females, 7- to 16 years old	Clinical signs consistent with HAC	++++			++++					Von Dehn et al, 1995
					++	++				
Australian Cattle dog, spayed female, 11 years old	PU/PD	+			+					Bennet and Norman, 1998
Standard Schnauzer, spayed female, 10 years old	Clinical signs consistent with HAC	+			+	+				Thuróczy et al, 1998
Mixed breed, male, 12 years old	PU/PD, polyphagia	+	+						compares to MEN-1	Walker et al, 2000
Mixed breed, spayed female, 12 years old	PU/PD, anorexia, weight loss, vomiting, diarrhea				(+) (Paragan-glioma)		+ (Ins)			Kiupel et al, 2000
Mixed breed, male, 15 years old	Mass in perianal region		+	+				+ (Sem)		Unterer et al, 2002
Portuguese Water dog, spayed female, 10 years old	Weight loss						++ (Somatostati-noma and gastrinoma†)			Hoenerhoff and Kiupel, 2004
Family of Alaskan Malamute-mixed breed	Clinical signs consistent with hypothyroidism, neck mass			+++ (MTC)					compares to FMTC	Lee et al, 2006
Mixed breed, male, 14 years old	PU/PD, polyphagia, abdominal enlargement			+		+		+ (ICT)		Proverbio et al, 2012

FMTC, Familial medullary thyroid carcinoma; HAC, hyperadrenocorticism; ICT, interstitial cell tumor; Ins, insulinoma; MEN-1, multiple endocrine neoplasia type 1; MEN-2A, multiple endocrine neoplasia subtype 2A; MTC, medullary thyroid carcinoma; PU/PD, polyuria and polydipsia; Sem, seminoma.

*The table only contains the major abnormalities; see the publications for details.
†Gastrinoma was found in mesenteric lymph nodes and liver.
‡Presence of tumor in individual dog

Peterson, et al., (1982) described a 15-year-old Fox Terrier with MTC, parathyroid hyperplasia, and pheochromocytoma, resembling MEN-2A in humans. Walker, et al., (2000) found a simultaneous presence of parathyroid adenoma and pituitary-dependent hyperadrenocorticism, resembling MEN-1. Additional cases have been described in textbooks and epidemiological studies. Feldman and Nelson (2004b) mention seven dogs with MTC, parathyroid tumor, and pheochromocytoma, which is similar to the case of Peterson, et al. (1982). In another four dogs, MTC was combined with pituitary tumor and pheochromocytoma. Thyroid adenoma or thyroid carcinoma (follicular or compact-follicular) in combination with various other endocrine tumors was seen in an additional 52 dogs. Many different breeds were affected, rendering familial syndromes unlikely in these cases. Hayes and Fraumeni (1975) investigated 144 dogs with thyroid tumors and found four dogs with concurrent adrenal adenoma.

In cats, tumors in multiple endocrine organs have only rarely been described. In a 13-year-old, Domestic Long-Hair cat with lethargy, exercise intolerance, and cervical ventriflexion, an aldosterone-secreting adrenal tumor, an insulinoma, and a functional parathyroid adenoma were diagnosed simultaneously (Reimer et al, 2005). Roccabianca, et al. (2006) described two male Domestic Short-Hair cats aged 12 and 13 years with a combination of tumors resembling human MEN-1. Both cats had pituitary dependent hyperadrenocorticism due to a pituitary corticotroph adenoma, thyroid C-cell and parathyroid hyperplasia, and pancreatic β-cell carcinoma.

So far, it is unknown if hereditary syndromes comparable to MEN in humans exist in dogs and cats. It may well be that the combination of endocrine tumors is different in dogs from in humans and that a different classification scheme has to be established.

However, it is important to realize that multiple endocrine tumors can occur in the same animal, underscoring the importance of a thorough evaluation in a patient in which an endocrine tumor is diagnosed.

REFERENCES

Agarwal A, et al.: Size of the tumor and pheochromocytoma of the adrenal gland scaled score (PASS): can they predict malignancy? *World J Surg* 34:3022, 2010.

Armbrust LJ, et al.: Comparison of three-view thoracic radiography and computed tomography for detection of pulmonary nodules in dogs with neoplasia, *J Am Vet Med Assoc* 240:1088, 2012.

Arnaldi G, Boscaro M: Adrenal incidentaloma, *Best Pract Res Clin Endocrinol Metab* 26:405, 2012.

Aron D, et al.: Adrenal incidentalomas, *Best Pract Res Clin Endocrinol Metab* 26:69, 2012.

Baid SK, et al.: Brief communication: radiographic contrast infusion and catecholamine release in patients with pheochromocytoma, *Ann Intern Med* 150:27, 2009.

Bailey DB, Page RL: Tumors of the endocrine system. In Withrow SJ, Vail DM, editors: *Withrow & MacEwen's small animal clinical oncology*, ed 4, St Louis, 2007, Saunders/Elsevier.

Barron J: Phaeochromocytoma: diagnostic challenges for biochemical screening and diagnosis, *J Clin Pathol* 63:669, 2010.

Barthez PY, et al.: Pheochromocytoma in dogs: 61 cases (1984-1995), *J Vet Intern Med* 11:272, 1997.

Beard CM, et al.: Occurrence of pheochromocytoma in Rochester, Minnesota, 1950 through 1979, *Mayo Clin Proc* 58:802, 1983.

Bennett PF, Norman EJ: Mitotane (o'p'-DDD) resistance in a dog with pituitary-dependent hyperadrenocorticism and phaeochromocytoma, *Aust Vet* 76:101, 1998.

Berl T, et al.: Mechanism of suppression of vasopressin during alpha-adrenergic stimulation with norepinephrine, *J Clin Invest* 53:219, 1974.

Berry CR, et al.: Use of [123]iodine metaiodobenzylguanidine scintigraphy for the diagnosis of a pheochromocytoma in a dog, *Vet Radiol Ultrasound* 34:52, 1993.

Berry CR, et al.: Imaging of pheochromocytoma in 2 dogs using p-[^{18}F] fluorobenzylguanidine, *Vet Radiol Ultrasound* 43:183, 2002.

Berzon JL: A metastatic pheochromocytoma causing progressive paraparesis in a dog, *Vet Med Small Anim Clin* 76:675, 1981.

Besso JG, et al.: Retrospective ultrasonographic evaluation of adrenal lesions in 26 dogs, *Vet Radiol Ultrasound* 38:448, 1997.

Bílek R, et al.: Chromogranin A, a member of neuroendocrine secretory proteins as a selective marker for laboratory diagnosis of pheochromocytoma, *Physiol Res* 57(Suppl 1):171, 2008. Epub.

Black HR: The paradigm has shifted to systolic blood pressure, *J Hum Hypertens* 18(Suppl 2):3, 2004.

Blake MA, et al.: Adrenal imaging, *Am J Roentgenol* 194:1450, 2010.

Boes K, et al.: What is your diagnosis? Shoulder mass in a dog with lameness, *Vet Clin Pathol* 38:511, 2009.

Bommarito DA, et al.: Treatment of a malignant pheochromocytoma in a dog using ^{131}I metaiodobenzylguanidine, *J Am Anim Hosp Assoc* 47:188, 2011.

Bouayad H, et al.: Pheochromocytoma in dogs: 13 cases (1980-1985), *J Am Vet Med Assoc* 191:1610, 1987.

Brandi ML, et al.: Consensus. Guidelines for diagnosis and therapy of MEN type 1 and type 2, *J Clin Endocrinol Metab* 86:5658, 2001.

Brömel C, et al.: Serum inhibin concentration in dogs with adrenal gland disease and in healthy dogs, *J Vet Intern Med* 27:76, 2013.

Brown AJ, et al.: Malignant pheochromocytoma presenting as a bradyarrhythmia in a dog, *J Vet Emerg Crit Care* 17:164, 2007a.

Brown S, et al.: Guidelines for the identification, evaluation, and management of systemic hypertension in dogs and cats, *J Vet Intern Med* 21:542, 2007b.

Calsyn JDR, et al.: Adrenal pheochromocytoma with contralateral adrenocortical adenoma in a cat, *J Am Anim Hosp Assoc* 46:36, 2010.

Cameron KN, et al.: The effects of illness on urinary catecholamines and their metabolites in dogs, *J Vet Intern Med* 24:1329, 2010.

Capen CC: Endocrine glands. In ed 5, Maxie MG, editor: *Jubb, Kennedy, and Palmer's pathology of domestic animals*, vol. 3. Philadelphia, 2007, Elsevier.

Carlsen E, et al.: Pheochromocytomas, PASS, and immunohistochemistry, *Horm Metab Res* 41:715, 2009.

Chen H, et al.: The NANETS Consensus Guideline for the diagnosis and management of neuroendocrine tumors: pheochromocytoma, paraganglioma & medullary thyroid cancer, *Pancreas* 39:775, 2010.

Chew SL: Diagnosis: imaging of pheochromocytomas and paragangliomas, *Nat Rev Endocrinol* 6:193, 2010.

Chobanian AV, et al.: The seventh report of the joint national committee on prevention, detection, evaluation, and treatment of high blood pressure: the JNC 7 report, *J Am Med Assoc* 289:2560, 2003.

Chun R, et al.: Apocrine gland adenocarcinoma and pheochromocytoma in a cat, *J Am Anim Hosp Assoc* 33:33, 1997.

Classics in oncology: a case of bilateral completely latent adrenal tumor and concurrent nephritis with changes in the circulatory system and retinitis: Felix Fränkel, 1886, *CA Cancer J Clin* 34:93, 1984.

Cotecchia S: The α1-adrenergic receptors: diversity of signaling networks and regulation, *J Recept Signal Transduct Res* 30:410, 2010.

Cryer PE: Diseases of the sympathochromaffin system. In Felig P, Frohman LA, editors: *Endocrinology and metabolism*, ed 4, New York, 2001, McGraw-Hill.

Cuervo L, et al.: Immunoreactivity to chromogranin and to vasoactive intestinal peptide in a canine phaeochromocytoma, *J Comp Path* 111:327, 1994.

Davis WP, et al.: Malignant cauda equina paraganglioma in a cat, *Vet Pathol* 34:243, 1997.

de Wailly P, et al.: Malignant pheochromocytoma: new malignancy criteria, *Langenbecks Arch Surg* 397:239, 2012.

Doss JC, et al.: Immunohistochemical localization of chromogranin A in endocrine tissues and endocrine tumors of dogs, *Vet Pathol Online* 35:312, 1998.

Eisenhofer G: Free or total metanephrines for diagnosis of pheochromocytoma: what is the difference? *Clin Chem* 47:988, 2001.

Eisenhofer G, et al.: Understanding catecholamine metabolism as a guide to the biochemical diagnosis of pheochromocytoma, *Rev Endocr Metab Disord* 2:297, 2001.

Eisenhofer G, et al.: Biochemical diagnosis of pheochromocytoma: how to distinguish true- from false-positive test results, *J Clin Endocrinol* 88:2656, 2003.

Eisenhofer G, et al.: Catecholamine metabolism: a contemporary view with implications for physiology and medicine, *Pharmacol Rev* 56:331, 2004a.

Eisenhofer G, et al.: Distinct gene expression profiles in norepinephrine- and epinephrine-producing hereditary and sporadic pheochromocytomas: activation of hypoxia-driven angiogenic pathways in von Hippel-Lindau syndrome, *Endocr Relat Cancer* 11:897, 2004b.

Eisenhofer G, et al.: Pheochromocytoma catecholamine phenotypes and prediction of tumor size and location by use of plasma free metanephrines, *Clin Chem* 51:735, 2005a.

Eisenhofer G, et al.: Plasma metanephrines in renal failure, *Kidney Int* 67:668, 2005b.

Eisenhofer G, et al.: Adverse drug reactions in patients with phaeochromocytoma: incidence, prevention and management, *Drug Saf* 30:1031, 2007.

Eisenhofer G, et al.: Differential expression of the regulated catecholamine secretory pathway in different hereditary forms of pheochromocytoma, *Am J Physiol Endocrinol Metab* 295:1223, 2008a.

Eisenhofer G, et al.: Current progress and future challenges in the biochemical diagnosis and treatment of pheochromocytomas and paragangliomas, *Horm Metab Res* 40:329, 2008b.

Eisenhofer G, et al.: Catecholamine metabolomic and secretory phenotypes in phaeochromocytoma, *Endocr Relat Cancer* 18:97, 2011.

Eisenhofer G, et al.: Diagnostic tests and biomarkers for pheochromocytoma and extra-adrenal paraganglioma: from routine laboratory methods to disease stratification, *Endocr Pathol* 23:4, 2012.

Elias S, et al.: Chromogranin as a crucial factor in the sorting of peptide hormones to secretory granules, *Cell Mol Neurobiol* 30:1189, 2010.

Erdheim J: Zur normalen und pathologischen Histologie der Glandula thyreoidea, *Parathyreoidea und Hypophysis, Beitr Pathol Anat 33,158*, 1903.

Erickson LA, Lloyd RV: Practical markers used in the diagnosis of endocrine tumors, *Adv Anat Pathol* 11:175, 2004.

Ettinger SJ: Therapy of arrhythmias. In ed 7, Ettinger SJ, Feldman EC, editors: *Textbook of veterinary internal medicine*, vol. 2. St Louis, 2010, Saunders/Elsevier.

Feldman JM, et al.: Deficiency of dopamine-beta-hydroxylase: a new mechanism for normotensive pheochromocytomas, *Am J Clin Pathol* 72:175, 1979.

Feldman EC, Nelson RW: Pheochromocytoma and multiple endocrine neoplasia. In Feldman EC, Nelson RW, editors: *Canine and feline endocrinology and reproduction*, ed 3, St Louis, 2004a, Saunders/Elsevier.

Feldman EC, Nelson RW: Canine thyroid tumors and hyperthyroidism. In Feldman EC, Nelson RW, editors: *Canine and feline endocrinology and reproduction*, ed 3, St Louis, 2004b, Saunders/Elsevier.

Fishbein L, Nathanson KL: Pheochromocytoma and paraganglioma: understanding the complexities of the genetic background, *Cancer Genet* 205:1, 2012.

Fitzgerald PA, Goldfien A: Adrenal medulla. In Greenspan FS, Gardner DG, editors: *Basic and clinical endocrinology*, ed 7, New York, 2004, Lang Medical Books/McGraw-Hill.

Fitzgerald PA: Adrenal medulla and paraganglia. In Gardner DA, Shoback D, editors: *Greenspan's basic and clinical endocrinology*, ed 9, New York, 2011, McGraw-Hill.

Fränkel F: Ein Fall von doppelseitigem, völlig latent verlaufenen Nebennierentumor und gleichzeitiger Nephritis mit Veränderungen am Circulationsapparat und Retinitis, *Arch Pathol Anat Physiol Klin Med* 103:244, 1886.

Fukuda I, et al.: Clinical features of insulin-like growth factor-II producing non-islet-cell tumor hypoglycemia, *Growth Horm IGF Res* 16:211, 2006.

Galac S, et al.: Adrenals. In Rijnberk A, Kooistra HS, editors: *Clinical endocrinology of dogs and cats*, ed 2, Hannover, 2010, Schlütersche Verlagsgesellschaft.

Galetta F, et al.: Cardiovascular complications in patients with pheochromocytoma: a mini-review, *Biomed Pharmacother* 64:505, 2010.

García-Sáinz JA, et al.: Mechanisms involved in α1B-adrenoceptor desensitization, *IUBMB Life* 63:811, 2011.

Gardner DG: Multiple endocrine neoplasia. In Gardner DG, Shoback D, editors: *Greenspan's basic and clinical endocrinology*, ed 9, New York, 2011, McGraw-Hill.

Gavin PR, Holmes SP: Magnetic resonance imaging of abdominal disease. In Gavin PR, Bagley RS, editors: *Practical small animal MRI*, Iowa, 2009, Wiley-Blackwell.

Gilson SD, et al.: Pheochromocytoma in 50 dogs, *J Vet Intern Med* 8:228, 1994.

Goldfarb DA, et al.: Magnetic resonance imaging for assessment of vena caval tumor thrombi: a comparative study with vena-cavography and computerized tomography scanning, *J Urol* 144:1100, 1990.

Gordon SG: Beta blocking agents. In ed 7, Ettinger SJ, Feldman EC, editors: *Textbook of veterinary internal medicine*, vol. 2. St Louis, 2010, Saunders/Elsevier.

Gostelow R, et al.: Plasma-free metanephrine and free normetanephrine measurement for the diagnosis of pheochromocytoma in dogs, *J Vet Intern Med* 27:83, 2013.

Grimelius L: Silver stains demonstrating neuroendocrine cells, *Biotech Histochem* 79:37, 2004.

Grouzmann E, et al.: Diagnostic accuracy of free and total metanephrines in plasma and fractionated metanephrines in urine of patients with pheochromocytoma, *Eur J Endocrinol* 162:951, 2010.

Guillaumot PJ, et al.: 49-month survival following caval venectomy without nephrectomy in a dog with a pheochromocytoma, *J Am Anim Hosp Assoc* 48:352, 2012.

Hayes HM, Fraumeni JF: Canine thyroid neoplasms: epidemiologic features (abstract), *J Natl Cancer Inst* 55:931, 1975.

Head LL, Daniel GB: Scintigraphic diagnosis—an unusual presentation of metastatic pheochromocytoma in a dog, *Vet Radiol Ultrasound* 45:574, 2004.

Henry CJ, et al.: Clinical vignette: adrenal pheochromocytoma, *J Vet Intern Med* 7:199, 1993.

Herrera MA, et al.: Predictive factors and the effect of phenoxybenzamine on outcome in dogs undergoing adrenalectomy for pheochromocytoma, *J Vet Intern Med* 22:1333, 2008.

Herrera M, Nelson RW: Pheochromocytoma. In ed 7, Ettinger SJ, Feldman EC, editors: *Textbook of veterinary internal medicine*, vol. 2. St Louis, 2010, Saunders/Elsevier.

Hoenerhoff M, Kiupel M: Concurrent gastrinoma and somatostatinoma in a 10-year-old Portuguese water dog, *J Comp Path* 130:313, 2004.

Hoerauf A, Reusch C: Ultrasonographic characteristics of both adrenal glands in 15 dogs with functional adrenocortical tumors, *J Am Anim Hosp Assoc* 35:193, 1999.

Howard EB, Nielsen SW: Pheochromocytomas associated with hypertensive lesions in dogs, *J Am Vet Med Assoc* 147:245, 1965.

Huang H, et al.: Treatment of malignant pheochromocytoma/paraganglioma with cyclophosphamide, vincristine, and dacarbazine: recommendation from a 22-year follow-up of 18 patients, *Cancer* 113:2020, 2008.

Kang JM, et al.: Systemic inflammatory syndrome and hepatic inflammatory cell infiltration caused by an interleukin-6 producing pheochromocytoma, *Endocr J* 52:193, 2005.

Kinney MA, et al.: Perioperative management of pheochromocytoma, *J Cardiothorac Vasc Anesth* 16:359, 2002.

Kitamura K, et al.: Adrenomedullin: a novel hypotensive peptide isolated from human pheochromocytoma, *Biochem Biophys Res Commun* 425:548, 2012.

Kiupel M, et al.: Multiple endocrine neoplasia in a dog, *J Comp Path* 123:210, 2000.

Kook PH, et al.: Urinary catecholamine and metanephrine to creatinine ratios in healthy dogs at home and in a hospital environment and in 2 dogs with pheochromocytoma, *J Vet Intern Med* 21:388, 2007.

Kook PH, et al.: Urinary catecholamine and metadrenaline to creatinine ratios in dogs with a phaeochromocytoma, *Vet Rec* 166:169, 2010.

Kudva YC, et al.: The laboratory diagnosis of adrenal pheochromocytoma: the Mayo Clinic experience, *J Clin Endocrinol Metab* 88:4533, 2003.

Kyles AE, et al.: Surgical management of adrenal gland tumors with and without associated tumor thrombi in dogs: 40 cases (1994-2001), *J Am Vet Med Assoc* 223:654, 2003.

Labelle P, De Cock HE: Metastatic tumors to the adrenal glands in domestic animals, *Vet Pathol* 42:52, 2005.

Lang, et al.: Elective and emergency surgical management of adrenal gland tumors: 60 cases (1999-2006), *J Am Anim Hosp Assoc* 47(6):428, 2011.

Lee JJ, et al.: A dog pedigree with familial medullary thyroid cancer, *Int J Oncol* 29:1173, 2006.

Lemos MC, Thakker RV: Multiple endocrine neoplasia type 1 (MEN1): analysis of 1336 mutations reported in the first decade following identification of the gene, *Hum Mutat* 29:22, 2008.

Lenders JWM, et al.: Biochemical diagnosis of pheochromocytoma, *J Am Med Assoc* 287:1427, 2002.

Lenders JWM, et al.: Phaeochromocytoma, *Lancet* 366:665, 2005.

Leung K, et al.: Pheochromocytoma: the range of appearances on ultrasound, CT, MRI, and functional imaging, *AJR Am J Roentgenol* 200:370, 2013.

Loh YP, et al.: Secretory granule biogenesis and neuropeptide sorting to the regulated secretory pathway in neuroendocrine cells, *J Mol Neurosci* 22:63, 2004.

Louvet A, et al.: Phaeochromocytoma treated by en bloc resection including the suprarenal caudal vena cava in a dog, *J Small Anim Pract* 46:591, 2005.

Mackenzie IS, Brown MJ: Phaeochromocytomas, paragangliomas and neuroblastomas. In Wass JA, Stewart PM, Amiel SA, Davies MJ, editors: *Oxford textbook of endocrinology and diabetes*, ed 2, Oxford, 2011, Oxford University Press.

Maher ER, et al.: von Hippel-Lindau disease: a clinical and scientific review, *Eur J Hum Genet* 19:617, 2011.

Manger WM: An overview of pheochromocytoma: history, current concepts, vagaries, and diagnostic challenges, *Ann N Y Acad Sci* 1073:1, 2006.

Mannelli M, et al.: Subclinical phaeochromocytoma, *Best Pract Res Clin Endocrinol Metab* 26:507, 2012a.

Mannelli M, et al.: Perioperative management of pheochromocytoma/paraganglioma: is there a state of the art? *Horm Metab Res* 44:373, 2012b.

Marini F, et al.: Multiple endocrine neoplasia type 2, *Orphanet J Rare Dis* 1:45, 2006a.

Marini F, et al.: Multiple endocrine neoplasia type I, *Orphanet J Rare Dis* 1:38, 2006b.

Martin NM, et al.: Multiple endocrine neoplasia type 2. In Wass JAH, Stwart PM, Amiel SA, Davies MJ, editors: *Oxford textbook of endocrinology and diabetes*, ed 2, Oxford, 2011, Oxford University Press.

Marx SJ, Wells SA: Multiple endocrine neoplasia. In Melmed S, Polonsky KS, Larsen PR, Kronenberg HM, editors: *Williams textbook of endocrinology*, ed 12, Philadelphia, 2011, Elsevier/Saunders.

Mascort J, Pumarola M: Posterior mediastinal paraganglioma involving the spinal cord of a dog, *J Small Anim Pract* 36:274, 1995.

McNeil AR, et al.: Phaeochromocytomas discovered during coronial autopsies in Sydney, Melbourne and Auckland, *Aust N Z J Med* 30:648, 2000.

Morandi F: Adrenal glands. In Schwarz T, Saunders J, editors: *Veterinary computed tomography*, Iowa, Wiley-Blackwell, 2011.

Mueller B, et al.: Innersekretorisch wirksame Nebennierenmarksgeschwulst (Phäochromocytom) bei einem Hund, *Zentralblatt für Veterinärmedizin* 2:289, 1955.

National Institutes of Health: NIH state-of-the-science statement on management of the clinically inapparent adrenal mass ("incidentaloma"), *NIH Consens State Sci Statements* 19(2):1, 2002.

Neumann HP, et al.: Evidence of MEN-2 in the original description of classic pheochromocytoma, *N Engl J Med* 357:1311, 2007.

Pacak K: Approach to the patient: preoperative management of the pheochromocytoma patient, *J Clin Endocrinol Metab* 92:4069, 2007.

Pacak K: Pheochromocytoma: a catecholamine and oxidative stress disorder, *Endocr Regul* 45:65, 2011.

Pacak, et al.: Pheochromocytoma: recommendations for clinical practice from the First International Symposium, *Nat Clin Pract Endocrinol Metab* 3:92, 2007.

Patnaik AK, et al.: Extra-adrenal pheochromocytoma (paraganglioma) in a cat, *J Am Vet Med Assoc* 197:104, 1990.

Peterson ME, et al.: Multiple endocrine neoplasia in a dog, *J Am Vet Med Assoc* 180:1476, 1982.

Platt SR, et al.: Pheochromocytoma in the vertebral canal of two dogs, *J Am Anim Hosp Assoc* 34:365, 1998.

Prejbisz A, et al.: Cardiovascular manifestations of phaeochromocytoma, *J Hypertens* 29:2049, 2011.

Proverbio D, et al.: Potential variant of multiple endocrine neoplasia in a dog, *J Am Anim Hosp Assoc* 48:132, 2012.

Quante S, et al.: Urinary catecholamine and metanephrine to creatinine ratios in dogs with hyperadrenocorticism or pheochromocytoma, and in healthy dogs, *J Vet Intern Med* 24:1093, 2010.

Reimer SB, et al.: Multiple endocrine neoplasia type I in a cat, *J Am Vet Med Assoc* 227:101, 2005.

Reusch CE, et al.: Endocrine hypertension in small animals, *Vet Clin North Am Small Anim Pract* 40:335, 2010.

Roccabianca P, et al.: Multiple endocrine neoplasia type-I-like syndrome in two cats, *Vet Pathol* 43:345, 2006.

Romei C, et al.: Genetic and clinical features of multiple endocrine neoplasia types 1 and 2 (abstract), *J Oncol*, 2012. Epub.

Rosas AL, et al.: Pheochromocytoma crisis induced by glucocorticoids: a report of four cases and review of the literature, *Eur J Endocrinol* 158:423, 2008.

Rosenstein DS: Diagnostic imaging in canine pheochromocytoma, *Vet Radiol Ultrasound* 41:499, 2000.

Sako T, et al.: Immunohistochemical evaluation of a malignant pheochromocytoma in a wolfdog, *Vet Pathol* 38:447, 2001.

Salesov E, et al.: Urinary and plasma catecholamine and metanephrine in dogs with pheochromocytoma, hyperadrenocorticism and in healthy dogs (abstract), *J Vet Intern Med* 26:1524, 2012.

Santamarina G, et al.: Aortic thromboembolism and retroperitoneal hemorrhage associated with a pheochromocytoma in a dog, *J Vet Intern Med* 17:917, 2003.

Schultz RM, et al.: Contrast-enhanced computed tomography as a preoperative indicator of vascular invasion from adrenal masses in dogs, *Vet Radiol Ultrasound* 50:625, 2009.

Sjaastad ØV, et al.: The endocrine system. In Sjaastad ØV, Hove K, Sand O, editors: *Physiology of domestic animals*, Norway, 2010, Scandinavian Veterinary Press.

Spall B, et al.: Imaging diagnosis—metastatic adrenal pheochromocytoma in a dog, *Vet Radiol Ultrasound* 52:534, 2011.

Stenström G, Svårdsudd K: Pheochromocytoma in Sweden 1958-1981: an analysis of the national cancer registry data, *Acta Med Scand* 220:225, 1986.

Stowater JL: Pheochromocytoma metastatic to bone in a dog, *Vet Med Small Anim Clin* 74:343, 1979.

Tamaschke C: Adrenal tumors of the dog, *Virchows Arch* 327:480, 1955.

Terzolo M, et al.: AME position statement on adrenal incidentaloma, *Eur J Endocrinol* 164:851, 2011.

Thakker RV: Multiple endocrine neoplasia type 1 (MEN1), *Best Pract Res Clin Endocrinol Metab* 24:355, 2010.

Thakker RV: Multiple endocrine neoplasia type 1. In Wass JA, Stewart PM, Amiel SA, Davies MJ, editors: *Oxford textbook of endocrinology and diabetes*, ed 2, Oxford, 2011, Oxford University Press.

Thakker RV, et al.: Clinical practice guidelines for multiple endocrine neoplasia type 1 (MEN1), *J Clin Endocrinol Metab* 97:2990, 2012.

Thouennon E, et al.: Expression of trophic peptides and their receptors in chromaffin cells and pheochromocytoma, *Cell Mol Neurobiol* 30:1383, 2010.

Thuróczy J, et al.: Multiple endocrine neoplasias in a dog: corticotrophic tumour, bilateral adrenocortical tumours, and pheochromocytoma, *Vet Quart* 20:56, 1998.

Timmers HJ, et al.: Current and future anatomical and functional imaging approaches to pheochromocytoma and paraganglioma, *Horm Metab Res* 44:367, 2012.

Tischler AS: Paraganglia. In Mills SE, editor: *Histology for pathologists*, ed 3, Philadelphia, 2007, Lippincott Williams & Wilkins.

Tischler AS, et al.: Pathology of pheochromocytoma and extra-adrenal paraganglioma, *Ann N Y Acad Sci* 1073:557, 2006.

Tokuda H, et al.: Overexpression of protein kinase C-delta plays a crucial role in interleukin-6-producing pheochromocytoma presenting with acute inflammatory syndrome: a case report, *Horm Metab Res* 41:333, 2009.

Tsujimoto G, et al.: Desensitization of beta-adrenergic receptors by pheochromocytoma, *Endocrinology* 114:1272, 1984.

Unger N, et al.: Diagnostic value of various biochemical parameters for the diagnosis of pheochromocytoma in patients with adrenal mass, *Eur J Endocrinol* 154:409, 2006.

Unterer S, et al.: Ein Fallbericht über einen Hund mit multiplen endokrinen Neoplasien (MEN): Nebenschilddrüsenadenom, Schilddrüsenkarzinom, Seminom und perianale Adenome, *Kleintierpraxis* 10:615, 2002.

Vanderveen KA, et al.: Biopsy of pheochromocytomas and paragangliomas: potential for disaster, *Surgery* 146:1158, 2009.

van Vonderen IK, et al.: Influence of veterinary care on the urinary corticoid:creatinine ratio in dogs, *J Vet Intern Med* 12:431, 1998.

Vasudevan NT, et al.: Regulation of β-adrenergic receptor function: an emphasis on receptor resensitization, *Cell Cycle* 10:3684, 2011.

Von Dehn BJ, et al.: Pheochromocytoma and hyperadrenocorticism in dogs: six cases (1982-1992), *J Am Vet Med Assoc* 207:322, 1995.

Walker MC, et al.: Multiple endocrine neoplasia type 1 in a crossbred dog, *J Small Anim Pract* 41:67, 2000.

Ware WA: Systemic arterial hypertension. In Nelson RW, Couto CG, editors: *Small animal internal medicine*, ed 4, St Louis, 2009, Mosby/Elsevier.

White RAS, Cheyne IA: Bone metastases from a phaeochromocytoma in the dog, *J Small Anim Pract* 18:579, 1977.

Whittemore JC, et al.: Nontraumatic rupture of an adrenal gland tumor causing intra-abdominal or retroperitoneal hemorrhage in four dogs, *J Am Vet Med Assoc* 219:329, 2001.

Williams JE, Hackner SG: Pheochromocytoma presenting as acute retroperitoneal hemorrhage in a dog, *J Vet Emerg Crit Care* 11:221, 2001.

Wilson RB, et al.: Leu-enkephalin and somatostatin immunoreactivities in canine and equine pheochromocytomas, *Vet Pathol* 23:96, 1986.

Wimpole JA, et al.: Plasma free metanephrines in healthy cats, cats with non-adrenal disease and a cat with suspected phaeochromocytoma, *J Feline Med Surg* 12:435, 2010.

Wright KN, et al.: Diagnostic and therapeutic considerations in a hypercalcemic dog with multiple endocrine neoplasia, *J Am Anim Hosp Assoc* 31:156, 1995.

Yi DW, et al.: Pheochromocytoma crisis after a dexamethasone suppression test for adrenal incidentaloma, *Endocr* 37:213, 2010.

Young WF: The incidentally discovered adrenal mass, *N Engl J Med* 356:601, 2007.

Young WF: Endocrine hypertension. In Melmed S, Polonsky KS, Larsen PR, Kronenberg HM, editors: *Williams textbook of endocrinology*, ed 12, St Louis, 2011, Saunders/Elsevier.

Yu Run, et al.: Small pheochromocytomas: significance, diagnosis, and outcome, *J Clin Hypertens* 14:307, 2012.

Zeiger MA, et al.: The American Association of Clinical Endocrinologists and American Association of Endocrine Surgeons medical guidelines for the management of adrenal incidentalomas, *Endocr Pract* 15(Suppl 1):1, 2009.

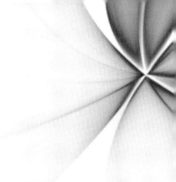

CHAPTER 14 | **Glucocorticoid Therapy**

Claudia E. Reusch

In 1949, Hench and colleagues reported on the first therapeutic use of a glucocorticoid in nine patients with rheumatoid arthritis. The substance had been known under the term "compound E" and was then named "cortisone." Later it was found that the true hormone is in fact cortisol, which is reversibly converted to its inactive metabolite cortisone. In 1950, Edward Kendall, a biochemist at the Graduate School of the Mayo Foundation, the Swiss chemist, Tadeus Reichstein, and a Mayo Clinic physician, Philip Hench, were awarded the Nobel Prize for their work on the adrenal gland hormones. The Noble Lecture held by Kendall on December 11, 1950, was titled, "The Development of Cortisone as a Therapeutic Agent" (Kendall, 1950). The finding of Hench and colleagues (1949) introduced the world to a new type of therapy and there was a saying, "Therapy was now dated BC (before cortisone) or after (AC)" (Goulding and Flower, 2000a).

The initial discovery was followed by the development of synthetic steroids mainly for use in inflammatory and immune-mediated diseases. However, it soon became obvious that their efficacy is not without costs in terms of potentially serious adverse effects (Goulding and Flower, 2000b).

Currently, glucocorticoids are among the most frequently used (and misused) drugs in veterinary medicine. Despite the widespread use of glucocorticoids, scientifically based information on optimal dose, dose interval, and physiological and pharmacological effects in dogs and cats is scarce. Therefore, treatment protocols are often extrapolated from human medicine or rodent studies or are the result of clinical experience (Ferguson et al, 2009; Boothe and Mealey, 2012). Knowledge on effects, different potencies of synthetic glucocorticoids, adverse effects, and contraindications will help the veterinarian to make informed decisions and to avoid serious complications as much as possible.

CHEMISTRY OF GLUCOCORTICOIDS AND STRUCTURE-ACTIVITY RELATIONSHIP

All hormones of the adrenal cortex are derivatives of cholesterol and contain the cyclopentanoperhydrophenanthrene nucleus (Fig. 14-1). The main products of the adrenal cortex are C_{21} and C_{19} steroids. The C_{19} steroids have a keto or hydroxyl group at position 17 and display androgenic activity. The C_{21} steroids have a two-carbon side chain at position 17 and are classified as mineralocorticoids and glucocorticoids. Those C_{21} steroids that have an additional hydroxyl group at position 17 are often called *17-hydroxycorticoids* or *17-hydroxycorticosteroids* (Barrett et al, 2012).

Cortisol (hydrocortisone) has glucocorticoid as well as mineralocorticoid properties due to its ability to stimulate both glucocorticoid and mineralocorticoid receptors (Parente, 2000). Certain structures and groups on the steroid base, as well as the orientation of the groups in the ring system, are essential for the biological activity. The groups lying below the plane of the steroid ring are indicated by α and a dashed line (···· OH), the groups lying above the ring are indicated by β and a solid line (– OH) (Parente, 2000; Barrett et al, 2012). The important features for biological activity are: a ketone group at C-3 and C-20, a double bond between C-4 and C-5, a hydroxyl group in β-orientation at C-11, a two-carbon chain in β-orientation, a hydroxyl group in α-orientation at C-17, and a methyl group in β-orientation at C-18 and C-19 (Parente, 2000) (Fig. 14-2).

Chemical modifications of the cortisol molecule have generated compounds with higher glucocorticoid activity and less mineralocorticoid activity (Fig. 14-3). Modifications of the molecular structure also alter the protein binding and hepatic metabolism thereby prolonging duration of action. High anti-inflammatory properties are unfortunately also associated with higher glucocorticoid activity

555

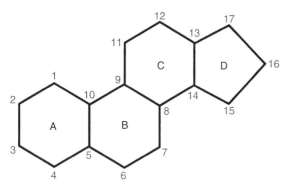

FIGURE 14-1 Basic chemical structure of the glucocorticoids (steroid nucleus).

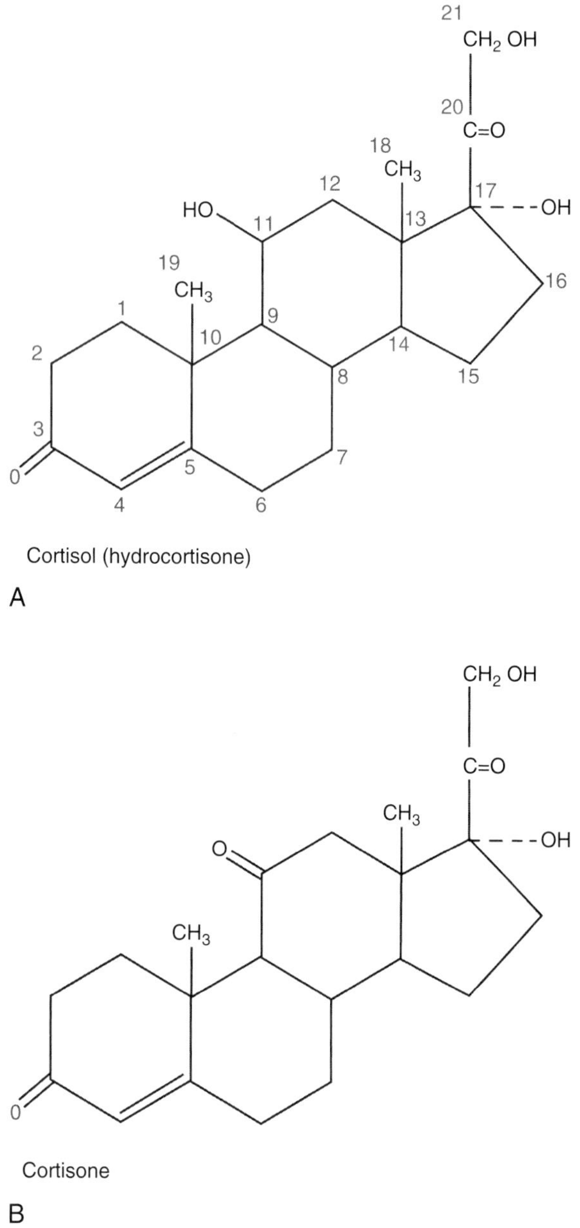

Cortisol (hydrocortisone)

A

Cortisone

B

FIGURE 14-2 Structure of **(A)** cortisol (hydrocortisone) and its inactive metabolite cortisone **(B)**.

(i.e., effects on carbohydrate and protein metabolism) (Boothe and Mealey, 2012). Introduction of a double bond between C-1 and C-2 resulted in prednisone and prednisolone, revealing increased anti-inflammatory and reduced mineralocorticoid activity compared with cortisone and cortisol. Of note, cortisone and prednisone are inactive compounds (or prodrugs) until the 11-keto group is converted into a hydroxyl group in the liver by the enzyme 11-β hydroxysteroid dehydrogenase (11β-HSD) type 1 (Parente, 2000; Ferguson et al, 2009). The addition of a methyl group in position C-6α resulted in methylprednisolone, which has slightly higher anti-inflammatory and less mineralocorticoid effect than prednisolone. The insertion of a 16α-hydroxy group decreases mineralocorticoid activity and leads to the synthesis of triamcinolone (which also has a 9α-fluoro group). The most potent anti-inflammatory glucocorticoids, dexamethasone and betamethasone, were designed by adding a fluorine atom at C-9α, which increases glucocorticoid activity, and a methyl group at C-16, reducing mineralocorticoid effects (adding was in α-orientation for dexamethasone and β-orientation for betamethasone) (Parente, 2000). The effects of glucocorticoids are dose dependent, and they are classified according to their potency in relation to the potency of cortisol (Table 14-1). There is an ongoing search to identify compounds or mechanism by which adverse effects can be minimized (McMaster and Ray, 2007; Vandevyver et al, 2013). One mechanism is the topical administration of drugs, which are rapidly metabolized if absorbed into the systemic circulation. This goal is mainly reached by manipulation of chemical groups of the D ring of the steroid base (Ferguson et al, 2009). Examples of those so-called "soft" glucocorticoids include beclomethasone, budesonide, fluticasone propionate, ciclesonide, and loteprednol etabonate (Ferguson et al, 2009; Boothe and Mealey, 2012). In particular the use of budesonide as an oral drug for the treatment of inflammatory bowel disease and budesonide and fluticasone propionate as inhaled medications for chronic inflammatory airway disease has recently gained popularity in dogs and cats (Bexfield et al, 2006; Padrid, 2006; Dye et al, 2013; Galler et al, 2013; Pietra et al, 2013).

MOLECULAR MECHANISM OF ACTION

Genomic Effects

Glucocorticoid activities can roughly be divided into genomic and nongenomic effects. The classical genomic effect is mediated by a cytoplasmic glucocorticoid receptor (GR) that belongs to the nuclear receptor superfamily, which includes all of the steroid receptors. GRs are widely distributed throughout the body: every cell appears to have GRs (Boothe and Mealey, 2012). The GRs consist of three domains with different functions: a poorly conserved N-terminal domain, a highly conserved DNA-binding domain, and a well-conserved C-terminal glucocorticoid-binding domain. Several splice variants of the GR exist, of which GRα is the most widely expressed and is the variant exerting most of the glucocorticoid actions. The variant GRβ is unable to bind glucocorticoids, but it may act as an inhibitor of GRα. The β variant may play a role in glucocorticoid resistance and possibly in autoimmune and inflammatory disorders (Ferguson et al, 2009; Nixon et al, 2013). In the resting (ligand-free) state, GR is located in the cytoplasm, where it exists as a multiprotein complex containing several heat-shock proteins (Hsp90, Hsp70, Hsp56, Hsp40); there is also interaction with other molecules, such as immunophilins and several additional factors (Stahn et al, 2007; Vandevyver et al, 2013). The GR is inactive until bound to a glucocorticoid ligand.

Glucocorticoids enter the cell by passive diffusion through the cell membrane, although there may also be an active transport mechanism. After binding of the glucocorticoid, the heat shock proteins dissociate from the GR, resulting in conformational changes that unmask nuclear localization sequences. Thereafter, the GR/glucocorticoid complex is translocated into the nucleus, where it activates or represses target gene transcription (Nixon et al, 2013). Although the main actions of glucocorticoids are mediated through the GR, some effects are also mediated through another nuclear receptor, the mineralocorticoid receptor (MR). The MR has a high affinity for endogenous glucocorticoids, which are generally present in much higher concentrations than mineralocorticoids. One of the major mechanism by which the body limits the access of endogenous glucocorticoids to the MR is through the activity of the enzyme 11β-HSD type 2 that converts cortisol to inactive cortisone. Therefore, when the MR is co-expressed with 11β-HSD type 2, its activation results in mineralocorticoid activity; in the absence of 11β-HSD type 2, the MR is

a high-affinity GR (Nixon et al, 2013). The best characterized mechanism of transcriptional activation is the binding of the GR/glucocorticoid complex to specific DNA binding-sites (glucocorticoid response elements [GREs]) in the promoter regions of target genes after entering the nucleus (Vandevyver et al, 2013). Binding to positive GRE induces synthesis of anti-inflammatory proteins as well as regulator proteins that are important for metabolism (e.g., enzymes involved in gluconeogenesis). The process mediated through positive GRE is also called *transactivation* and is considered to be responsible for numerous side effects of glucocorticoids. Binding to negative GRE leads to inhibition of gene transcription (transrepression) of the pro-opiomelanocortin (the precursor of adrenocorticotropic hormone—ACTH), α-fetoprotein, and prolactin gene, as well as suppression of inflammatory genes, such as interleukin-1β (IL-1β) and interleukin-2 (IL-2) Löwenberg et al, 2007; Stahn et al, 2007). Besides binding to GRE, other mechanisms for the upregulation and downregulation of genes exist. For instance, suppressed target gene

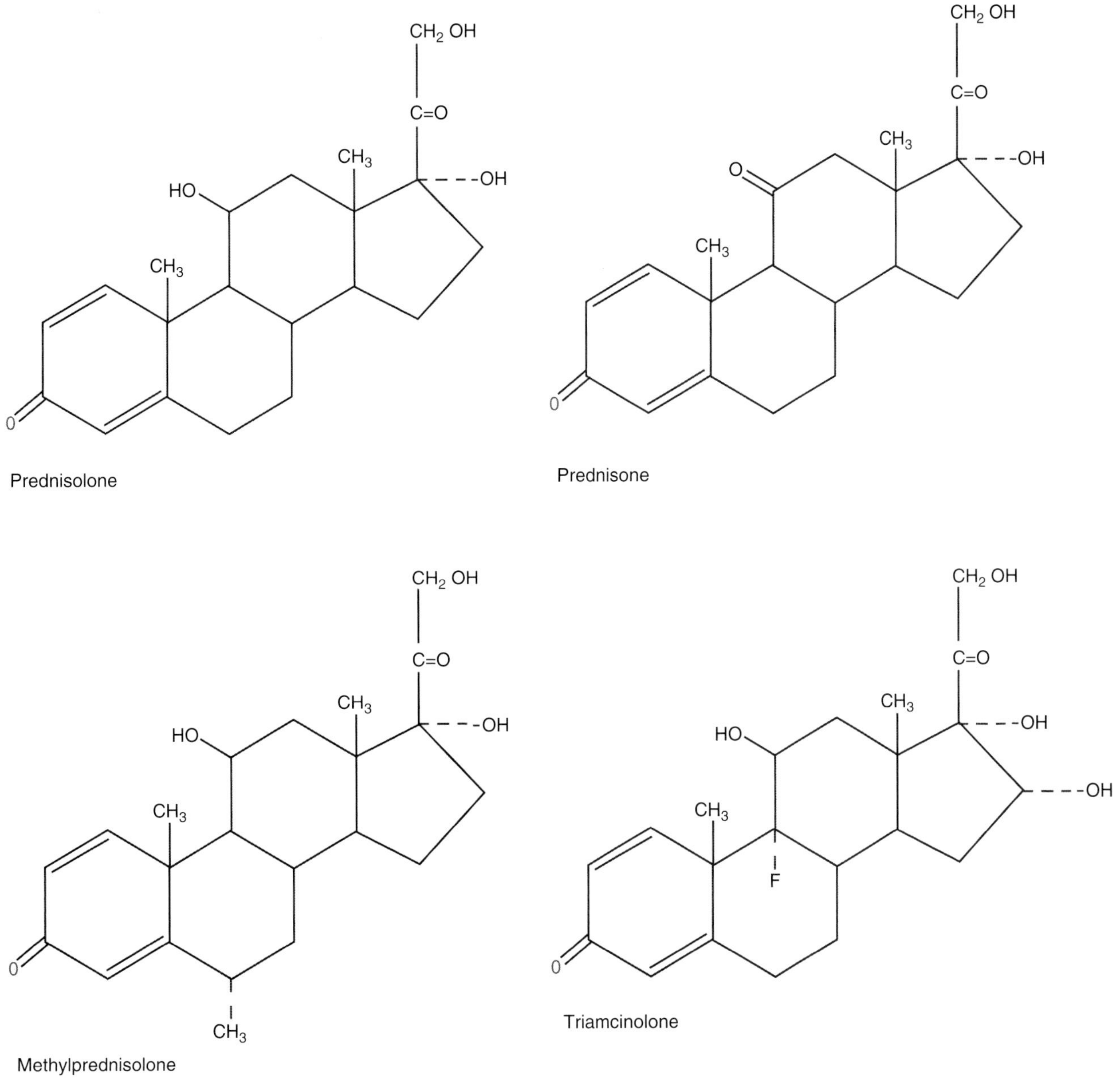

FIGURE 14-3 Structure of selected synthetic glucocorticoids.

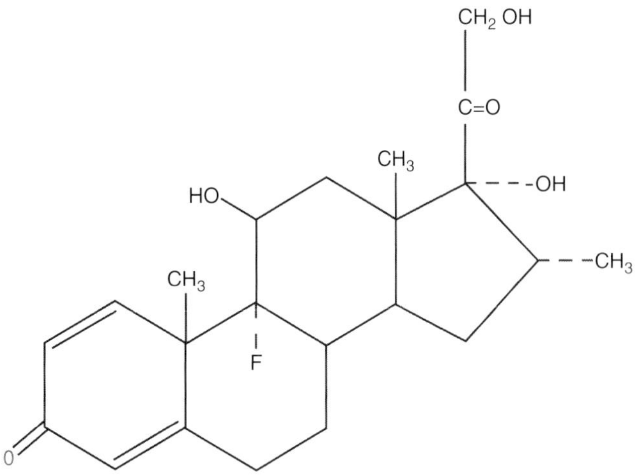

Dexamethasone

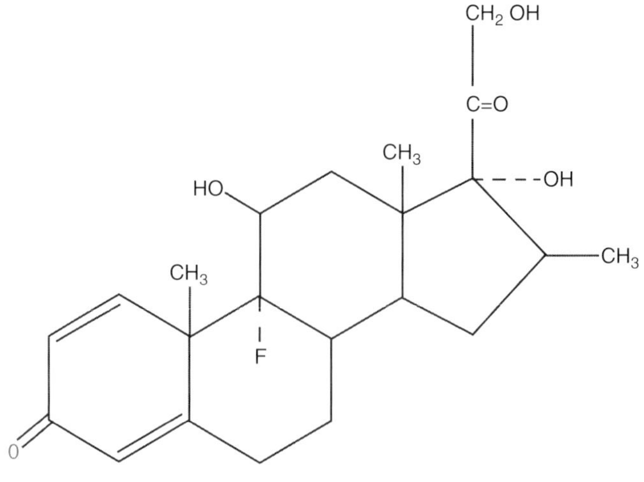

Betamethasone

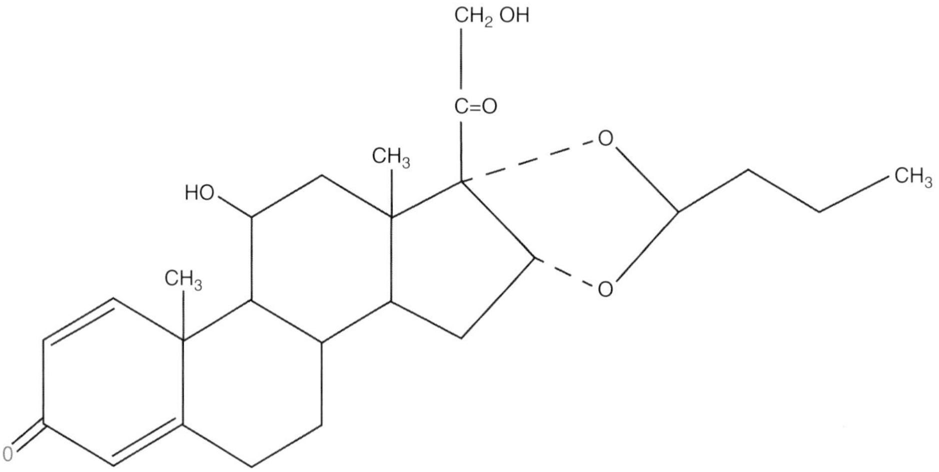

Budenoside

FIGURE 14-3, cont'd

expression can be achieved through direct protein-protein interaction with pro-inflammatory transcription factors, such as activator protein-1 (AP-1), nuclear factor kappa-light-chain-enhancer of activated B cells (NF-κB), nuclear factor of activated T-cells (NFAT), or signal transducers and activator of transcription (STAT; Löwenberg et al, 2007). It takes approximately 30 minutes for the activation of the GR, nuclear transportation of the GR/glucocorticoid complex, binding to promoter regions, and initiation of transcription and translation. Hours to days are required until changes on cellular, tissue or organism level become obvious (Stahn et al, 2007). For many years, it was thought that the undesirable side effects of glucocorticoid therapy are due to dimer-mediated transactivation, whereas its beneficial anti-inflammatory activity is mainly caused by monomer-mediated transrepressive effects. Research was therefore focused on the development of dissociated compounds that only exhibit those actions of glucocorticoids that are monomer-dependent. The dimer/monomer dogma has recently been challenged, because it was demonstrated that the GR dimer-dependent transactivation is

essential for the anti-inflammatory actions (Nixon et al, 2013; Vandevyver et al, 2013).

Nongenomic Effects

In addition to the classic genomic mode of action, glucocorticoids may exert effects through nongenomic mechanisms. It has been recognized that some of the immunosuppressive, anti-inflammatory, anti-allergic effects, and effects when used during shock occur too fast to be regulated via transcription. Rapid clinical effects may be seen when glucocorticoids are administered intravenously or intra-articularly at high doses. Various underlying mechanisms for the nongenomic effects have been described, such as nonspecific interactions of glucocorticoids with cellular membranes, nongenomic effects that are mediated by the cytosolic GR, and specific interactions with a membrane-bound GR (Löwenberg et al, 2007; Stahn et al, 2007).

It has been shown that glucocorticoids at high concentrations intercalate into membranes, thereby changing their physiological properties and the activities of membrane-associated proteins. For

TABLE 14-1 COMPARISON OF THE CHARACTERISTICS OF THE MAJOR GLUCOCORTICOID PREPARATIONS

DRUG	GLUCOCORTICOID/ANTI-INFLAMMATORY POTENCY	MINERALOCORTICOID POTENCY	EQUIVALENT ORAL DOSE (mg)	BIOLOGIC HALF-LIFE (h)
Short-Acting				
Cortisol (hydrocortisone)	1	1	20	8-12
Cortisone	0.8	0.8	25	8-12
Intermediate-Acting				
Prednisolone/Prednisone	4	0.8	5	12-36
Methylprednisolone	5	0.5	4	12-36
Triamcinolone	5	0	4	12-36
Long-Acting				
Betamethasone	25-30	0	0.7-0.8	36-72
Dexamethasone	25-30	0	0.7-0.8	36-72
Mineralocorticoids				
Aldosterone	0	200-1000		
Fludrocortisone	10	125-200		

Data from Parente L: The development of synthetic glucocorticoids. In Goulding NJ, Flower RJ, editors: *Glucocorticoids,* Basel, 2000, Springer Basel AG; and Boothe DM, Mealey KA: Glucocorticoids and mineralocorticoids. In Boothe DM, editor: *Small animal clinical pharmacology and therapeutics,* ed 2, St Louis, 2012, Saunders/Elsevier.

instance, this results in reduced calcium and sodium cycling across the cell membrane of immune cells, which contributes to rapid immunosuppression and reduction of the inflammatory process. Binding of glucocorticoids to the cytosolic GR leads to dissociation of signaling molecules, which mediate rapid responses; the cytosolic GR is also involved in inhibition of the release of arachidonic acid, an essential mediator for cell growth and various metabolic/inflammatory reactions. Binding of glucocorticoids to a membrane-bound GR, which may be a variant of the cytosolic GR, seems to be involved in apoptosis and T cell receptor–mediated signal transduction (Stahn et al, 2007). The physiological significance of the nongenomic effects is not totally clear. It is assumed that they play an important role during stress when the concentration of endogenous glucocorticoids is high (Jiang et al, 2014). Fig. 14-4 summarizes genomic and nongenomic mechanisms of glucocorticoids.

BIOLOGIC EFFECTS OF GLUCOCORTICOIDS

The name *glucocorticoid* is derived from the words *glucose* and *cortex,* and it relates to the role of glucocorticoids in glucose metabolism and their origin from the adrenal cortex. Glucocorticoids, however, have a much broader spectrum of function, they influence most cells in the body, and without them an individual will not survive a stressful event.

Effects on Carbohydrate, Protein, and Lipid Metabolism

The physiological effects of glucocorticoids in the fed state are small; however, during fasting, they contribute to the maintenance of blood glucose levels by increasing hepatic gluconeogenesis and decreasing uptake of glucose in peripheral tissues (muscle, fat). These effects protect glucose-dependent organs (e.g., brain and heart) from starvation. Glucocorticoids stimulate glycogen deposition and inhibit glycogen-mobilizing enzymes. This allows other hormones (e.g., glucagon and epinephrine) to mobilize glucose when needed (e.g., between meals). Glucocorticoids exert catabolic effects on muscle (i.e., decreased glucose uptake and

metabolism), decreased protein synthesis, and increased release of amino acids, providing precursors for gluconeogenesis in the liver. In adipose tissue, glucocorticoids stimulate lipolysis, which generates free fatty acids and glycerol, thereby providing energy and substrate for gluconeogenesis (Carroll et al, 2011; Hall, 2011).

In healthy individuals, the increase in blood glucose is counterbalanced by an increase in insulin secretion. High levels of glucocorticoids (endogenous or exogenous) reduce the sensibility of many tissues, in particular muscle and fat, to the stimulatory effects of insulin on glucose uptake and utilization (i.e., lead to insulin resistance). In this way, glucocorticoids may induce glucose intolerance and diabetes mellitus or worsen glycemic control in an individual with pre-existing diabetes. Glucocorticoid excess also leads to increased breakdown of protein, clinically seen as muscle wasting, thinning of the skin, and delayed wound healing (Boothe and Mealey, 2012). Although glucocorticoids stimulate lipolysis, increased fat deposition is a common clinical sign. The paradox has been explained by steroid-induced stimulation of appetite and the lipogenic effect of hyperinsulinemia. The reason for the abnormal fat distribution is unknown (Carroll et al, 2011).

Effects on Other Tissues

Growth and Development

Glucocorticoids play an important role in normal fetal development. They stimulate lung maturation through synthesis of surfactant proteins in the near-term fetus, allowing adaption to air breathing. In physiological concentrations, glucocorticoids stimulate gene transcription of growth hormone (GH); glucocorticoid excess, however, inhibits skeletal growth by catabolic effects on bone, muscle, and connective tissue and inhibition of insulin-like growth factor-1 (IGF-1) effects (Ferguson et al, 2009).

Bone, Cartilage, and Calcium

The effects of glucocorticoids on bone are complex and include direct and indirect effects. Under physiological circumstances, bone formation and bone resorption are tightly coupled; in cases of

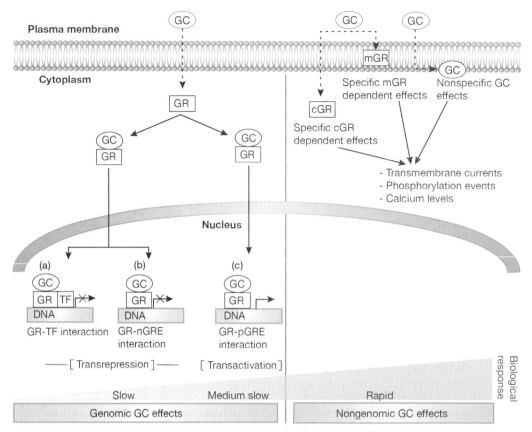

FIGURE 14-4 Genomic and nongenomic immunoregulation by glucocorticoids (GCs). GCs passively diffuse into cells and bind to the cytoplasmic glucocorticoid receptor (GR), after which the GC-GR complex translocates into the nucleus for gene regulation. *Left:* Ligated GR directly inhibits pro-inflammatory transcription factors (i.e., activator protein-1 [AP-1], nuclear factor of activated T-cells [NFAT], nuclear factor kappa-light-chain-enhancer of activated B cells [NF-κB], and signal transducers and activator of transcription [STAT]) *(a)* or actively suppresses transcription (transrepression) of inflammatory genes (i.e., interleukin-1β [IL-1β] and IL-2) through binding to negative glucocorticoid response elements (nGRE) *(b)*. Activated GR induces transcription (transactivation) of immunosuppressive genes (i.e., IκB, annexin-1, IL-10, mitogen-activated protein kinase [MAPK] phosphatase-1, lipocortin-1, and annexin-1) via positive GREs (pGRE) *(c)*. GC-induced biological responses, which are based on transrepression, are slow because some time is required before RNA and protein levels of target genes are fully degraded *(a,b)*. GC-dependent transactivation of genes that encode regulator proteins is less slow ("medium slow") compared with transrepression *(c)*. *Right:* GCs induce rapid effects (occurring within minutes) on transmembrane currents, signal transduction (e.g., T-cell receptor [TCR] and MAPK signaling pathways), second-messenger cascades or intracellular Ca2+ mobilization. It is currently assumed that nongenomic GC effects are mediated by cytosolic or membrane-bound GRs, or via nonspecific interactions with cell membranes. In this simplified scheme, no GR-chaperones are depicted. (Reproduced with permission from Loewenberg M, Verhaar AP, van den Brink GR, et al.: Glucocorticoid signaling: a nongenomic mechanism for T-cell immunosuppression, *Trends Mol Med* 13:158, 2007.) *cGR,* Cytosolic glucocorticoid receptor; *mGR,* membrane-bound glucocorticoid receptor; *TF,* transcription factor.

glucocorticoid excess, those processes are uncoupled (van Brussel et al, 2009). Glucocorticoid excess decreases number and function of osteoblasts, induces apoptosis of osteocytes, and increases the formation of osteoclasts. Indirect effects include disturbed calcium metabolism, muscle weakening, and decrease of GH and gonadotropin secretion (Canalis et al, 2007; van Brussel et al, 2009). In humans, glucocorticoid-induced osteoporosis belongs to the most devastating side effects of long-term glucocorticoid therapy (van Brussel et al, 2009). In dogs and cats, effects of glucocorticoids are rarely described. Recently, the effect of glucocorticoids on mineral density of the vertebral spine was investigated. Application of 2 mg/kg prednisone over 30 days led to a significant loss of bone mass (Costa et al, 2010). Pathological fractures were not seen in

the study by Costa and colleagues (2010) and also do not occur in dogs with long-standing glucocorticoid excess (e.g., in dogs with endogenous hyperadrenocorticism).

At physiological concentrations, glucocorticoids stimulate collagen; glucocorticoid excess results in inhibition of collagen synthesis, depression of chondrocyte metabolism, and decrease of the proteoglycan content of cartilage (Boothe and Mealey, 2012).

Glucocorticoids inhibit calcium absorption from the intestinal tract by antagonizing the effect of active vitamin D_3 and by decreasing the expression of specific calcium channels in the duodenum. The inhibition is not due to decreased levels of vitamin D_3, as those are normal, or even increased in the presence of glucocorticoid excess. Glucocorticoids also increase renal calcium excretion as well as the excretion of phosphorous. Serum phosphate concentrations are reduced, whereas calcium concentrations are usually maintained normal (Canalis et al, 2007; Carroll et al, 2011). Theoretically, the reduced absorption and increased secretion of calcium would promote secondary hyperparathyroidism. In humans on glucocorticoid therapy, however, increased parathyroid hormone (PTH) levels have not been consistently demonstrated. Glucocorticoids may alter the secretory dynamics of PTH with a decrease in its tonic release and an increase in pulsatile bursts. Additionally, they may enhance sensitivity of skeletal cells to PTH by increasing the number and affinity of PTH receptors (Canalis et al, 2007). So far, no detailed studies on calcium balance in dogs and cats with endogenous or exogenous glucocorticoid excess have been performed. In dogs, the administration of approximately 1 mg/kg prednisolone every other day for 6 weeks did not result in significant changes in concentrations of total and ionized calcium, phosphate, vitamin D metabolites (25(OH)D and 1,25(OH)$_2$D$_3$), and PTH in blood and urinary fractional excretion of calcium and phosphate (Kovalik et al, 2012). The results contrast in part those of Ramsey, et al., (2005) who assessed parameters of calcium metabolism in dogs with endogenous hyperadrenocorticism. Total and ionized calcium concentrations were not different to a matched control group. Different from humans and the study of Kovalik, et al, (2012), phosphate and PTH concentrations were significantly higher. Approximately one third of the dogs had PTH concentrations greater than three times the reference range. No explanation for the increased phosphate concentrations could be given; it was assumed to play a role in the increase in PTH concentrations (Ramsey et al, 2005).

Renal Function

Glucocorticoids increase the glomerular filtration rate, sodium transport in the proximal tubule, and free water clearance. They have an inhibitory effect on antidiuretic hormone (ADH) and may decrease permeability of the distal tubules to water through a direct effect (Boothe and Mealey, 2012). Cortisol and several synthetic glucocorticoids have mineralocorticoid activity. Depending on the concentration or dose and the activity of the 11β-HSD type 2, they act on the MR and cause sodium retention and potassium loss. The polyuria and polydipsia commonly seen in dogs (infrequently in non-diabetic cats treated with glucocorticoids) is considered to be mainly due to inhibition of ADH release and action.

Cardiovascular and Respiratory Functions

Glucocorticoids have positive inotrope and positive chronotropic actions on the heart. Because glucocorticoids are necessary for maximal catecholamine sensitivity, they contribute to the maintenance of normal vascular tone. They decrease capillary permeability through inhibition of the activity of kinins and bacterial endotoxins and by decreasing the amount of histamine released by basophils (Ferguson et al, 2009). Refractory shock may occur when individuals deficient in glucocorticoids are exposed to stress (Carroll et al, 2011).

Glucocorticoid excess may lead to hypertension through various mechanisms, such as their intrinsic mineralocorticoid activity, activation of the renin-angiotensin-aldosterone system; enhancement of cardiovascular inotropic and pressor activity of vasoactive substances, including catecholamines, vasopressin and angiotensin II; and suppression of the vasodilatory system, including the nitric oxide (NO) synthase, prostacyclin and kinin-kallikrein systems. The exact mechanisms in dogs and cats have not been elucidated (Reusch et al, 2010). The studies on the potential role of

aldosterone revealed conflicting results (Goy-Thollot et al, 2002; Javadi et al, 2003; Wenger et al, 2004). Martinez and colleagues (2005) demonstrated increased vascular reactivity to increasing doses of norepinephrine in dogs with experimentally induced hypercortisolism.

Glucocorticoids increase the number and affinity of β$_2$ receptors, thus promoting bronchodilatation (Boothe and Mealey, 2012).

Gastrointestinal Tract

Glucocorticoids are involved in normal function and integrity of the gastrointestinal tract. Glucocorticoid excess is associated with reduced gastric mucosal cell growth and renewal and decreased mucus production, resulting in impairment of the protective barrier of the gastric mucosa (Boothe and Mealey, 2012). Glucocorticoid therapy in dogs with neurological disease may result in gastrointestinal hemorrhage, ulcers, and colonic perforations. Gastric hemorrhage has also been described in healthy dogs given high doses of methylprednisolone sodium succinate (Rohrer et al, 1999a).

Central Nervous System Function

Glucocorticoids are involved in maintaining adequate blood glucose concentrations for cerebral functions, maintaining cerebral blood flow, and influencing electrolyte balance in the central nervous system (CNS). They also decrease formation of cerebrospinal fluid, appear to regulate neuronal excitation, and appear to have neuroprotective effects (Boothe and Mealey, 2012). In humans, glucocorticoid excess initially causes euphoria, and prolonged exposure may result in various psychologic abnormalities, including irritability, emotional lability, and depression; impairment in cognitive functions is also common (Carroll et al, 2011). In dogs treated with glucocorticoids, euphoric effects are also commonly seen.

Blood Cells

Glucocorticoids have only little effects on erythrocytes, although mild polycythemia may be seen. The underlying mechanism may be glucocorticoid-induced enhancement of erythroid progenitor proliferation (von Lindern et al, 1999).

Endogenous or exogenous glucocorticoid excess may induce leukocytosis in dogs and cats. The leukogram ("stress leukogram") is characterized by mature neutrophilia, lymphopenia, and eosinopenia. In dogs, monocytosis may be an additional finding, which is usually not present in cats. The mature neutrophilia is due to several factors, such as increased release of neutrophils from bone marrow, shift of marginated neutrophils in the circulating neutrophil pool, and decreased movement of neutrophils from blood into tissue. Lymphopenia is the result of a redistribution of circulating lymphocytes; lysis of lymphocytes may occur with high doses of glucocorticoids. Eosinopenia is caused by inhibition of eosinophil release from the bone marrow and sequestration of eosinophils within tissues (Schultze, 2010; Valenciano et al, 2010). In dogs, glucocorticoid excess may provoke thrombocytosis (Neel et al, 2012); knowledge on potential glucocorticoid-induced thrombocytosis in cats is scarce.

Hypothalamic Pituitary Adrenal Axis

Glucocorticoids inhibit synthesis and secretion of ACTH from the corticotropic cells in the anterior pituitary and of corticotropin-releasing hormone (CRH) and ADH from neurons in the hypothalamus in a negative feedback fashion. Exogenous glucocorticoids have profound effects on the hypothalamic pituitary adrenal

(HPA) axis. Even "physiological" doses of glucocorticoids (0.22 mg/kg prednisolone once daily) may result in suppression of the HPA axis, which is reflected by reduced increase of cortisol after ACTH stimulation and lead to a reduction of the zona fasciculate and reticularis to the zona glomerulosa in the adrenal gland (Ferguson et al, 2009). Generally, the degree and duration of suppression of the HPA axis depends on dose, potency, half-life, and duration of administration of the glucocorticoid preparation. HPA axis suppression can occur with any form of glucocorticoid. Glucocorticoids possessing anti-inflammatory effects but no suppressive effects on the HPA axis have not yet been identified (Ferguson et al, 2009). For more details on HPA axis suppression, see the Adverse Effects section.

Thyroid Function

Glucocorticoids have a major impact on the hypothalamic pituitary thyroid axis and also influence peripheral metabolism of thyroid hormones. Main proposed mechanisms include inhibition of synthesis and release of thyroid-stimulating hormone (also known as thyrotropin; TSH), decrease in thyroxine (T_4) binding proteins, and impairment of peripheral 5′-deiodination. Studies in dogs do not point as clearly to a suppressive effect on TSH secretion in dogs as compared to humans. In dogs with hyperadrenocorticism, reduced T_4 and triiodothyronine (T_3) concentrations were found in more than 50% of cases. The concentrations of both hormones normalized during treatment of the hyperadrenocorticism. The T_4 response after TSH administration was also reduced (Peterson et al, 1984). TSH concentrations in dogs with hyperadrenocorticism were not different from that of control dogs in another study (Meij et al, 1997). The effect of exogenous glucocorticoids on thyroid hormones has been evaluated in various studies. The duration and extent of thyroid hormone suppression varies with type, dose, and route of administration, and duration of therapy and is certainly also influenced by individual sensitivity. In dogs, the application of immunosuppressive doses of prednisone/prednisolone (1.1 to 2.0 mg/kg twice a day) for 3 weeks significantly decreased T_4; it also decreased free T_4, albeit to a lesser extent. The effect on T_4 was seen as early as 1 day after start of therapy. Endogenous TSH concentrations were not affected (Torres et al, 1991; Daminet et al, 1999; Daminet and Ferguson, 2003). See Chapter 3 for more details.

Growth Hormone and Gonadotropins

Glucocorticoids decrease GH secretion, most likely by increasing somatostatin release. Dogs with hyperadrenocorticism have decreased response of GH after stimulation with xylazine, clonidine, and growth hormone-releasing hormone (GHRH) (Frank, 2005). Exogenous glucocorticoid excess presumably has the same effect.

Hyperadrenocorticism is also frequently associated with reproductive disturbances, such as testicular atrophy, reduced libido, and persistent anestrus. Similarly, exogenous glucocorticoid (prednisone) leads to a decrease in circulating testosterone concentrations in male dogs. Prednisone treatment also resulted in a reduction of basal luteinizing hormone (LH) concentration, which suggested that glucocorticoids inhibit the gonadal axis at the hypothalamic or pituitary level (Kemppainen et al, 1983; Kemppainen, 1984). Interestingly, however, basal LH concentrations in dogs with hyperadrenocorticism were not different from controls. It was hypothesized that glucocorticoids have a direct inhibitory effect on gonads and/or on transport and metabolism of their secretory products and influence the sensitivity of the feedback control at the hypothalamic/pituitary level (Meij et al, 1997). Glucocorticoid administration to pregnant dogs may lead to abortion.

Anti-Inflammatory and Immunosuppressive Effects

Glucocorticoids suppress inflammatory and immune-mediated responses of the body, and this fact has been the stimulus for the development of potent glucocorticoid preparations. The anti-inflammatory and immunosuppressive effects only occur when supraphysiological doses (i.e., pharmacological doses) are given. Both effects are closely related, and which of the two predominates in a clinical situation is a question of the dose given. Many hundreds of glucocorticoid response genes have been identified. Additional to the genomic effects, rapid actions of glucocorticoids on inflammation are mediated by nongenomic mechanisms (Rhen and Cidlowski, 2005). It is important to remember that the encompassing properties render glucocorticoid therapy dangerous, because it can mask severity and progression of the disease and serious side effects may occur. Glucocorticoids limit early and late manifestations of inflammation, including edema formation, fibrin deposition, leukocyte migration, phagocytic activity, collagen deposition, and capillary and fibroblast proliferation. Many of these processes involve lymphokines, and other soluble mediators of inflammation and glucocorticoids exert their anti-inflammatory effects through those mediators (Boothe and Mealey, 2012).

Generally, due to the fact that GR expression is ubiquitous, glucocorticoids can affect nearly all cells of the immune system. Glucocorticoids inhibit proliferation, growth and differentiation, adhesion, migration, and chemotaxis of monocytes/macrophages, neutrophils, and T cells (Box 14-1). Antigen processing by monocytes/macrophages is suppressed, and antibody production by B cells may be impaired; apoptosis of monocytes/macrophages, T cells, and B cells is increased (Vollmar and Dingermann, 2005). Of note, B

BOX 14-1   Selected Effects of Glucocorticoids on the Immune System

Neutrophils
Neutrophilia
Depressed chemotaxis
Depressed margination
Depressed phagocytosis
Depressed antibody-dependent cellular cytotoxicity
Depressed bactericidal activity
Stabilization of membranes
Inhibition of phospholipase $A_2\alpha$

Macrophages
Depressed chemotaxis
Depressed phagocytosis
Depressed bactericidal activity
Depressed IL-1 and IL-6 production
Depressed antigen processing

Lymphocytes
Depressed proliferation
Depressed T-cell responses
Impaired T-cell mediated cytotoxicity
Depressed IL-2 production
Depressed lymphokine production

Immunoglobulins
Decreased antibody synthesis only after high dose, long-term therapy
Interference with antibody function

Modified from Tizard IR, *Veterinary immunology*, ed 9, St Louis, 2013, Elsevier.
IL, Interleukin.

cells are thought to have greater resistance to the effects of glucocorticoids, although the inhibition of T-cell help will have indirect consequences for B-cell activation. Glucocorticoids may inhibit the action of complement molecules and interfere with the function of immunoglobulins by down-regulation of Fc receptor expression (Day, 2011). Usually, high doses of glucocorticoid are required to suppress antibody production, and therapeutic doses do not significantly decrease the antibody response to an antigenic challenge (e.g., vaccinations; Boothe and Mealey, 2012; Tizard, 2013).

Inflammatory and immunologic reactions are mediated by various signaling pathways. The pathways that are associated with the activation of NF-κB are of particular importance (Fig. 14-5). In its inactive state, NF-κB is sequestered in the cytoplasm by the inhibitory factor IκB-α. Tumor necrosis factor alpha (TNFα), interleukin-1 (IL-1), microbial pathogens, viral infections, and other inflammatory signals trigger signaling cascades that activate IκB-α kinases, resulting in liberation and translocation of NF-κB into the nucleus. NF-κB stimulates the transcription of cytokines (e.g., IL-1, IL-2, IL-6, and TNFα), chemokines (e.g., IL-8, monocyte chemotactic protein-1 [MCP-1]), cell-adhesion molecules, complement factors, and receptors for these molecules. After binding to its receptor, glucocorticoids inhibit NF-κB by direct protein-protein interaction; glucocorticoids also induce the synthesis of IκB-α, thereby inhibiting translocation of NF-κB into the nucleus (Rhen and Cidlowksi, 2005; Steinfelder and Oetjen, 2009; see also http://www.bu.edu/nf-kb/gene-resources/target-genes/).

Similar to NF-κB, the transcription factor AP-1 is one of the key mediators of the inflammatory response; AP-1 is inhibited by glucocorticoids as well (Busillo and Cidlowski, 2013). NF-κB also induces the transcription of cyclooxygenase 2 (COX2), an enzyme that is essential for prostaglandin production; glucocorticoids inhibit COX2 through inhibition of NF-κB. Other mechanisms by which glucocorticoids inhibit prostaglandin synthesis are mediated through induction and activation of annexin I (also called *lipocortin-1*) and through induction of mitogen-activated protein kinase (MAPK) phosphatase 1. Annexin I is an anti-inflammatory protein that inhibits phospholipase $A_2\alpha$, thereby blocking the release of arachidonic acid and its subsequent conversion to eicosanoids. Phospholipase $A_2\alpha$ is also inhibited by MAPK phosphatase 1. MAPKs are pivotal in the regulation of immune responses; they are involved in the production of inflammatory mediators (e.g., TNFα, IL-1, IL-6, prostaglandin, NO, and inducible nitric-oxide synthase) and in T-cell development and function. Removal of the phosphatases (which is induced by glucocorticoids) renders MAPK inactive (Rhen and Cidlowski, 2005; Liu et al, 2007). Glucocorticoids reduce local inflammation by preventing the actions of histamine and plasminogen activators (Stewart and Krone, 2011). In summary, the anti-inflammatory and immunosuppressive effects of glucocorticoids are attributed to partial or complete suppression of an extremely complex interplay of cells and cell mediators. The potent effects of glucocorticoids on leukocytes are responsible for most of the anti-inflammatory activity. These effects are also immunosuppressive, which explains their efficacy in immune-mediated disease. It should be remembered, however, that glucocorticoids can lead to an increased susceptibility to infection (Papich and Davis, 1989).

PHARMACOKINETICS AND CLINICAL PHARMACOLOGY

Duration of Action

A distinction has to be made between plasma half-life and biological half-life of glucocorticoids. Plasma half-life is the amount of time required for 50% of a drug's concentration to disappear from plasma, whereas the biological half-life refers to the duration of effect. The biologic half-life of glucocorticoids is disparate, because many of the biological effects are due to alterations in genetic regulation of protein production; biological effects are delayed and prolonged compared to the drug concentration in plasma (Cohn, 2010). It is the biological half-life that needs to be considered when a treatment protocol is established. Glucocorticoids are usually divided into three groups according to the duration of HPA axis suppression. Cortisol (hydrocortisone) and cortisone are considered short-acting (biologic half-life < 12 hours); prednisolone, prednisone, methylprednisolone, and triamcinolone are intermediate-acting (biologic half-life 12 to 36 hours); and dexamethasone and betamethasone are long-acting drugs (biologic half-life 36 to 72 hours) (see Table 14-1). Duration of action is influenced by factors such as route of administration, the preparation used (e.g., soluble or insoluble steroid ester), and other variables, such as health of the patient and concurrent use of other drugs.

Route of Administration

Glucocorticoids of varying potency are available in oral, parenteral, and topical formulations.

Oral

Cortisol (hydrocortisone) and synthetic glucocorticoids are orally effective, and oral administration is the preferred route for systemic application (except in emergency situations). It is the safest, most convenient, and most economical route. The main disadvantages and limitations of the oral route include vomiting as a result of irritation of the gastric mucosa, variable absorption due to many factors (gastrointestinal disease, local blood flow, and/or presence of food or other drugs), and the need for cooperation of the pet. The oral bioavailability differs between glucocorticoids; it is generally highest for cortisol, prednisolone, and methylprednisolone and lower for dexamethasone. Triamcinolone and budesonide have a very low oral bioavailability; in the case of budesonide, the low bioavailability is a desired effect because it is designed for local application (e.g., for treatment of inflammatory bowel disease [IBD]).

Previously, it had been thought that prednisolone and the prodrug prednisone are equivalent in terms of dosing when used as oral drugs. However, this belief does not seem to be correct. It was shown in cats that only 21% of orally-administered prednisone appeared in the blood as active prednisolone. It is not clear if the differences are due to decreased gastrointestinal absorption or to decreased hepatic conversion of prednisone to prednisolone (Graham-Mize and Rosser, 2004). According to these data, the dose of prednisone must be three- to fivefold higher than that of prednisolone to achieve equivalent activity (Boothe and Mealey, 2012). Because prednisone is commonly used in cats, its poor absorption (or poor conversion) may contribute to the perceived glucocorticoid resistance in cats (Lowe et al, 2008a). Also in dogs, oral administration of prednisone may not result in systemic prednisolone concentrations, which are achieved with oral prednisolone. The relative bioavailability of prednisolone was only 65% when prednisone was administered compared to the administration of prednisolone (Boothe and Mealey, 2012). These data suggest that prednisolone should be preferred over prednisone.

Parenteral

Most glucocorticoids for parenteral use are synthesized as glucocorticoid esters, which either improves solubility or increases

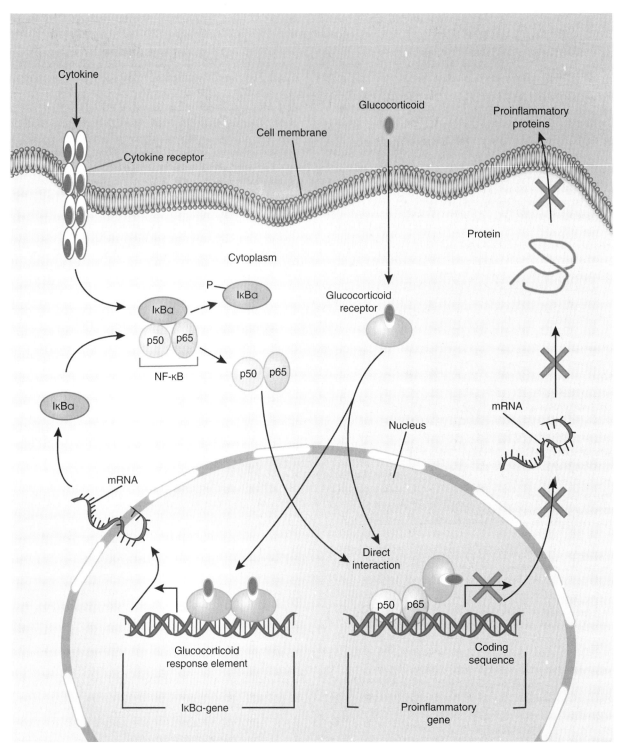

FIGURE 14-5 Inhibition of the transcription factor nuclear factor kappa-light-chain-enhancer of activated B cells (NF-κB) by glucocorticoids. NF-κB is a dimer and consists of two subunits (p50, p65). In its inactive state, it is sequestered in the cytoplasm by the inhibitory factor IκB-α. Upon stimulation by, for example, cytokines NF-κB is released and translocates into the nucleus. After binding to specific DNA sites, NF-κB increases the transcription of target genes, which include genes of cytokines, chemokines, growth factors, cell adhesion molecules, complement factors, immunoreceptors, and cyclooxygenase 2 (COX2). Glucocorticoids inhibit NF-κB after their binding to the glucocorticoid receptor (GR) through direct protein-protein interaction between the GR and the p65 subunit. Glucocorticoids can also stimulate the transcription of the IκB-α gen, thereby augmenting the inhibition of NF-κB. Inhibition of NF-κB is one of the major mechanisms of the anti-inflammatory and immunosuppressive effect of glucocorticoids. (Redrawn from Steinfelder HJ, Oetjen E: Nebennierenrindenhormone. In Aktories K, Foerstermann U, Hofmann F, Starke K, editors: *Allgemeine und Spezielle Pharmakologie und Toxikologie,* ed 10, 2009, Elsevier Urban & Fischer.) *mRNA,* Messenger ribonucleic acid.

TABLE 14-2 SOME CHARACTERISTICS OF COMMON ROUTES OF DRUG ADMINISTRATION

ROUTE	ABSORPTION PATTERN	SPECIAL UTILITY	LIMITATIONS AND PRECAUTIONS
Intravenous (IV)	Absorption circumvented Potentially immediate effects	Valuable for emergency use Permits titration of dosage Suitable for large volumes and for irritating substances when diluted	Increased risk of adverse effects Must inject solutions slowly as a rule Not suitable for oily solutions or insoluble substances
Subcutaneous (SC)	Prompt, from aqueous solution Slow and sustained, from repository preparations	Suitable for some insoluble suspensions and for implantation of solid pellets	Not suitable for large volumes Possible pain or necrosis from irritating substances
Intramuscular (IM)	Prompt, from aqueous solution Slow and sustained, from repository preparations	Suitable for moderate volumes, oily vehicles, and some irritating substances	Precluded during anticoagulant medication May interfere with interpretation of certain diagnostic tests (e.g., creatine phosphokinase)
Oral ingestion	Variable, depends upon many factors (see text)	Most convenient and economical; usually safer than other routes	Requires patient cooperation Absorption potentially erratic and incomplete for drugs that are poorly soluble, slowly absorbed, or unstable

duration of action. Water-soluble esters of cortisol and synthetic glucocorticoids can be given intravenously to achieve high concentrations rapidly. Prolonged effects are obtained by intramuscular (IM) injection of water-insoluble esters (suspensions) of cortisol and its synthetic derivatives (see later). Injection of drugs has certain advantages over oral administration. Absorption is usually more predictable than oral application, and therefore, the effective dose can be accurately selected. In particular, intravenous (IV) administration circumvents absorption issues and permits titration of dose. It also allows the administration of large volumes. Disadvantages include the need for asepsis, possible pain and necrosis, and costs. See Table 14-2 for some characteristics of the major routes of glucocorticoids.

Topical

Topical steroids for dermatological indications are available in ointments, creams, gels, solutions, shampoos, and rinses. Glucocorticoids for ophthalmological indications come as eye drops (aqueous solutions and suspensions) and ointments; intra-articular application is usually in form of crystal suspensions. Glucocorticoids are also used as inhalants in patients with lung disease. Topical therapy can provide high concentrations of a potent glucocorticoid at a specific site while reducing systemic side effects. However, topical glucocorticoids can be absorbed to a certain extent, exerting the same adverse reaction as systemically administered steroids. The extent of percutaneous absorption depends on various factors, including the preparation vehicle, ester form of the steroid (greater lipid solubility enhances percutaneous absorption), integrity of epidermal barriers (e.g., absorption is increased in case of inflammation), size of treated area, and duration of treatment. Absorption is enhanced by use of occlusive wraps and possibly by clipping the skin (Behrend and Kemppainen, 1997; Boothe and Mealey, 2012). Systemic effects (e.g., suppression of the HPA axis) may also occur with inhaled glucocorticoids and in conjunction with intra-articular, intra-lesional, or ocular application.

Distribution, Metabolism, and Excretion

After absorption, cortisol and synthetic glucocorticoids are bound to corticosteroid binding protein (CBP, also called *transcortin*) and albumin. Only the unbound, free fraction of glucocorticoids is active and can enter cells. CBP is α-globulin secreted by the liver, which has a high affinity for glucocorticoids but a relatively low binding capacity. Albumin, on the other hand, has a low affinity but large binding capacity. Glucocorticoids compete with one another for binding sites and will displace one another at high concentrations (Boothe and Mealey, 2012). Compared to cortisol, binding to CBP is less for synthetic glucocorticoids; they are mainly bound to albumin or circulate as free hormones, thereby diffusing more readily into tissues. Glucocorticoids distribute widely in all tissues of the body, and they pass the blood brain and placental barrier. Glucocorticoids are metabolized in the liver and to a lesser extent in the kidney; synthetic drugs are metabolized slower than cortisol. Metabolism is by oxidation or reduction followed by glucuronidation or sulfation, and excretion of the metabolites is mainly via the kidney. Only small amounts of glucocorticoids are excreted in the unmodified form. Biliary and fecal elimination do not appear to be significant; enterohepatic cycling takes place to a small extent (Ungemach, 2010; Boothe and Mealey, 2012).

Synthetic steroids with an 11-ketogroup, such as cortisone and prednisolone, must be enzymatically reduced to the 11-β-hydroxy derivative before they become biologically active. The enzyme 11β-HSD type 1, which catalyzes this reaction, is expressed mainly in the liver but also in other tissues, including adipose tissue, immune system cells, and brain tissue. Similarly, also in natural situations, this enzyme generates active (endogenous) cortisol from inactive (endogenous) cortisone. The isoform 11β-HSD type 2 is predominantly expressed in classic mineralocorticoid targets, such as distal nephron, salivary glands, colon, and placenta. It inactivates cortisol by mediating the conversion to inactive cortisone and thereby ensures that only aldosterone binds to the MR (Chapman et al, 2013; Fig. 14-6).

Dose Equivalents of Glucocorticoids

The glucocorticoid activity is closely related to the anti-inflammatory activity, and the effective anti-inflammatory time usually equals the time of HPA axis suppression (Ferguson et al, 2009). The anti-inflammatory and mineralocorticoid activities of cortisol (hydrocortisone) are used as a baseline for comparison with the synthetic glucocorticoids and are arbitrarily assigned as being 1. Chemical modifications have generated glucocorticoids with greater glucocorticoid/anti-inflammatory activity and less mineralocorticoid activity. Some derivatives (e.g., triamcinolone, dexamethasone) have no or negligible mineralocorticoid effects even at high doses. Increased anti-inflammatory potency is also associated with longer duration of action. The latter can be prolonged

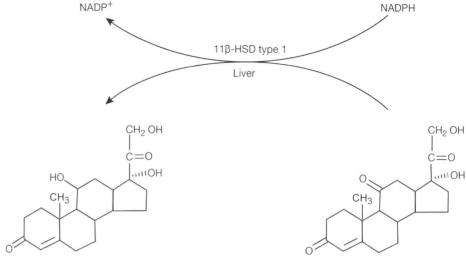

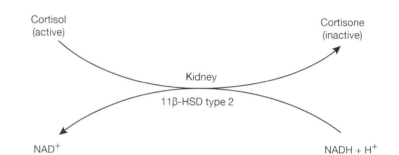

FIGURE 14-6 Interconversion of cortisol and cortisone by 11β-hydroxysteroid dehydrogenase (11β-HSD) type 1 and 2. Similar to the conversion of cortisone to cortisol, prednisone has to be converted to prednisolone to be able to bind to the glucocorticoid receptor (GR). *NAD+,* Nicotinamide adenine dinucleotide; *NADH,* nicotinamide adenine dinucleotide plus hydrogen; *NADP+,* nicotinamide adenine dinucleotide phosphate; *NADPH,* nicotinamide adenine dinucleotide phosphate plus hydrogen.

substantially by esterification. See the Chemistry of Glucocorticoids and Structure-Activity Relationship section and Box 14-1 for more details; the effects of esterification are discussed later.

There is a general belief that there are no relevant qualitative differences between the various glucocorticoid preparations because they all bind to the GR. Equipotent amounts of any glucocorticoid exert similar effects, meaning that a higher dose of a less potent glucocorticoid can achieve the same effect as a lower dose of a more potent preparation (Cohn, 2010). When choosing a treatment protocol, the veterinarian has to be aware of the equivalent doses of glucocorticoids. Failure to make dose adjustments for different glucocorticoids will result in the administration of inadequate or excessive doses, leading to either inefficacy or dangerous overdose. For instance, a dose of 1 mg/kg prednisolone in a dog is a reasonable anti-inflammatory dose; the equivalent dose of dexamethasone is only approximately 0.14 mg/kg (Calvert and Cornelius, 1990a). Generally, the anti-inflammatory dose is considered to be approximately 10 times the physiological dose, and immunosuppressive doses are roughly twice the anti-inflammatory dose. In contrast to the aforementioned belief of equal effects, it is possible that there are indeed some qualitative differences between the various synthetic steroids. In an in vitro model, it was shown that dexamethasone was more effective than prednisone and cortisol in inhibiting the clearance of immunoglobulin G (IgG)-coated cells by its effect on Fc receptors of splenic macrophages (Ruiz et al, 1991). In healthy cats, dexamethasone showed a greater diabetogenic effect than equipotent doses of prednisolone (Lowe et al, 2009).

Galenic Formulations and Steroid Esters

Water solubility of glucocorticoids is generally low and can be altered by pharmaceutical manipulations. Esterification and the

kind of ester at C-21 of the glucocorticoid base determine to a large extent the lipid/water solubility ratio and the duration of action (Ferguson et al, 2009). The ester moiety also determines if the drug can be given intravenously, intramuscularly, or topically (Fig. 14-7; Table 14-3). Glucocorticoid preparations for oral use are either free alcohols or they are esterified; however, in this case, esterification does not impair bioavailability.

For parenteral application, three galenic formulations are available.

Water-Soluble Ester (Aqueous Solutions)

The most commonly used esters are succinate, hemisuccinate, and phosphate; common formulations are hydrocortisone sodium succinate, prednisolone sodium succinate, prednisolone sodium phosphate, methylprednisolone sodium phosphate, and dexamethasone sodium phosphate. Those esters are hydrolyzed within minutes, resulting in immediate availability of the glucocorticoid. They can be administered intravenously, as well as intramuscularly and subcutaneously. These characteristics render them ideal for emergency situations. The duration of action of these esterified glucocorticoids is equivalent to that of the unmodified glucocorticoid (Cohn, 2010).

Free Alcohol Solutions

These preparations are unique to veterinary medicine as dexamethasone solutions. Dexamethasone is poorly soluble in water, but it is available as an injectable preparation in solution with polyethylene glycol. The glucocorticoid is released within minutes to a few hours. Free alcohol solutions can be administered intramuscularly as well as intravenously. IV application, however, may be associated with CNS side effects. If IV application of larger doses is required, water soluble esters should be used.

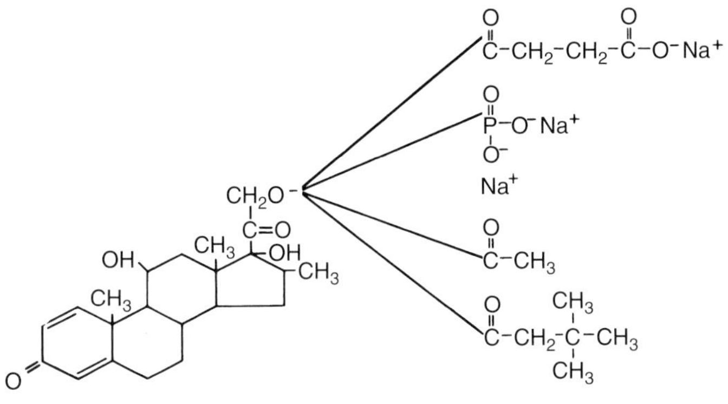

Sodium succinate

Sodium phosphate

Acetate

Acetonide

FIGURE 14-7 Esters of glucocorticoids. Glucocorticoid structure illustrating various esters that may bind to C-21.

	TABLE 14-3	**DURATION OF ACTION OF VARIOUS STEROID ESTERS AFTER INTRAMUSCULAR ADMINISTRATION**	

STEROID ESTER	ABSORPTION FOLLOWING INTRAMUSCULAR APPLICATION	DURATION OF ACTION	MOST COMMONLY USED GLUCOCORTICOID BASES
Sodium succinate	Minutes to hours	Hours	Hydrocortisone, prednisolone, prednisone, methylprednisolone, dexamethasone, betamethasone
Sodium phosphate			
Acetate	Days to weeks	Days to weeks	Methylprednisolone, triamcinolone, betamethasone
Diacetate			
Acetonide	Weeks	Weeks	Triamcinolone
Dipropionate			
Pivalate			

Insoluble Steroid Ester (Suspensions)

Suspensions can be administered intramuscularly, intra-articularly, and intralesionally. They are not to be given intravenously. They are used as depot preparation because of their slow release of the active glucocorticoid from the site of administration. They provide long-term, low level therapy and are not indicated in situations in which a quick effect and high blood levels are needed (Feldman and Nelson, 2004). The duration of action depends on the extent of water-solubility. Water solubility of acetate and diacetate esters is moderate and duration of action ranges from days to weeks. Pivalate, dipropionate, and acetonide esters are the least water soluble and have duration of actions of several weeks. It is of utmost importance to realize that glucocorticoid preparations esterified with those esters do not compare with the native base with regard to duration of effect. For instance, the duration of effect of methylprednisolone is 12 to 36 hours; the duration of methylprednisolone acetate, however, is 3 to 6 weeks (Cohn et al, 2010). The major advantage of the suspensions is convenience of administration. However, they have major disadvantages, such as unpredictability of blood concentrations, long-term suppression of the HPA axis (may be up to several months after a single dose), possible induction of glucocorticoid resistance, and the fact that the drug cannot be withdrawn in case adverse reactions occur (Boothe and Mealey, 2012). Steroid suspensions should be handled with care, and the guidelines of the manufacturer with regard to storage temperature and shelf life should be followed. The steroid suspensions represent some of the most abused and overused drugs in veterinary medicine. Other than for intralesional and intra-articular therapy, those long-acting preparations are hardly ever needed. The exceptions are fractious cats and cats that live outdoors and are only seen occasionally by their owners. The same anti-inflammatory effects can be achieved with much shorter acting oral preparations. Use of short-acting drugs allows the dose to be altered as needed and helps to minimize HPA axis suppression and other adverse effects (Feldman and Nelson, 2004).

Combination Products

Combination products between glucocorticoids and other pharmaceutical products (e.g., antibiotics) are available. However, their use is associated with various problems, such as dose discrepancies and variable duration of effects of the constituent drugs. Dose discrepancy means that administrations based on recommended dose for one of the drugs may result in underdosing or overdosing of the other drug in the product. The use of those drugs is discouraged.

THERAPEUTIC APPLICATION AND CLASSES OF GLUCOCORTICOID USAGE

Goals and General Guidelines

Except in case of physiological replacement, therapy with glucocorticoids is not directed at the inciting agent. Glucocorticoids are used to reduce the processes that are activated in response to a disease (Boothe and Mealey, 2012). Oftentimes, glucocorticoids are applied, although there is no indication or even a clear contraindication in higher than recommended doses and/or as depot preparations that lead to long-term suppression of the HPA axis. The goal is to bring the disease process under control with the lowest dose necessary. In serious conditions, initial IV application may be required. For this purpose, water-soluble ester preparations should be used. Thereafter, treatment should be continued with oral glucocorticoids (e.g., prednisolone). Parenteral use of depot preparations (insoluble steroid esters) should only be used in exceptional cases (i.e., if application of shorter acting steroids is not possible [fractious cats]). After achieving disease remission, the latter should be maintained with the lowest possible dose; alternate-day regimens using oral prednisolone should be used whenever indicated. Cats have fewer GRs than dogs and require higher doses. For the discussion on the preferred use of prednisolone over prednisone, see the Route of Administration section.

Generally, given dose ranges should be regarded as approximate guidelines, because glucocorticoid sensitivity differs between individuals. Frequent reevaluations of patients treated with glucocorticoids are of utmost importance. It is the predominant opinion that cats require higher doses of glucocorticoids than dogs. This belief is supported by a study demonstrating that cats have approximately half the density of GRs in skin and liver as compared to dogs, and the receptors have lower binding affinity (van den Broek and Stafford, 1992; Lowe et al, 2008a). Physiological effects of glucocorticoids occur at much lower doses than do anti-inflammatory and immunosuppressive doses (see Dose Equivalents of Glucocorticoids). Before initiating glucocorticoid therapy, the clinician should identify the goal (e.g., physiological replacement, suppression of inflammation, suppression of the immune system, or other actions like in neurological or neoplastic disorders) (Cohn, 2010). Other questions that should be answered prior to glucocorticoid therapy are (Ferguson et al, 2009):

- Has an exact diagnosis been made and specific treatment been initiated?
- Have other types of treatment been explored to minimize glucocorticoid dose and side effects?
- Are there contraindications or known risk factors?
- How serious is the disease?
- What is the anticipated length of glucocorticoid therapy?

Physiological Replacement Therapy

Animals with primary or secondary adrenocortical insufficiency require replacement of glucocorticoids. In case of primary disease (Addison's disease), the majority of patients also need mineralocorticoid replacement. Replacement means to provide glucocorticoids in amounts similar to those of the naturally produced glucocorticoids (mainly cortisol). Ideal replacement mimics the hormonal output of the adrenal gland under basal conditions, which is roughly 1 mg/kg cortisol per day in dogs and cats. Dose increase is needed in times of stress (Ferguson et al, 2009). A perfect replacement is difficult to reach because of the dynamic function of the adrenal gland with minute-to-minute adaption of cortisol secretion according to the actual requirement. Prednisolone is the glucocorticoid preparation most commonly used for replacement therapy in a dose of 0.1 to 0.25 mg/kg once daily. Glucocorticoid sensitivity varies widely between individuals, and therefore, replacement doses have to be curtailed to the patient's need. In some dogs in which the mineralocorticoid deficiency is replaced by fludrocortisone (which also has glucocorticoid activity), additional prednisolone may not be required under normal conditions. During times of stress, the need for glucocorticoid activity increases. As a rough guideline, the replacement dose should be

increased two to five times in case of moderate stress, and five to twenty times in case of severe stress (e.g., surgery) (Ferguson et al, 2009). See Chapter 12 for more details.

Anti-Inflammatory Therapy

Inflammatory and allergic disorders are the most common reasons for the use of glucocorticoids. If no specific treatment can be initiated or is insufficient, glucocorticoids can help to combat the clinical signs. However, there is a great potential for misuse in this category. If an infectious disease goes unnoticed, the use of glucocorticoids may have deleterious effects because the disease can progress and the outcome can potentially be fatal. Due to the general effects of glucocorticoids (e.g., reduction of fever, stimulation of appetite, feeling of euphoria, and suppression of the clinical signs of inflammation), the clinician may have the impression of improvement, while in fact the disease is worsening (Cohn, 2010). Calvert and Cornelius (1990b) described this as, "When glucocorticoids are misused, the patient may walk all the way to the necropsy laboratory." There are a few exceptions, as in some infectious diseases (e.g., bacterial or Malassezia-induced otitis externa or severe ehrlichiosis), the concurrent administration of glucocorticoids may have beneficial effects. It is understood that in the latter disease the application should be limited to a few days (2 to 7 days) (Cohn, 2003; Rougier et al, 2005; Bensignor and Grandemange, 2006). Generally, before using glucocorticoids for their anti-inflammatory effects, information regarding specific conditions should be reviewed.

Except in emergency cases (e.g., acute bronchial disease) in which IV administration of sodium succinate or sodium phosphate esters of prednisolone or methylprednisolone is indicated, oral prednisolone is usually the treatment of choice. In dogs, the anti-inflammatory dose of prednisolone is 0.5 to 1.0 mg/kg per day. In cats, it is usually recommended to give twice the dose of dogs (e.g., 1.0 to 2.0 mg/kg) (Lowe et al, 2008a; Cohn, 2010). As soon as clinical signs of inflammation are under control, the dose should be reduced to the lowest necessary concentration. The induction period usually ranges between 5 and 7 days (Behrend and Kemppainen, 1997). Prednisolone (or methylprednisolone) enables accurate dose titration and the possibility of withdrawal in case of adverse effect. It is also the glucocorticoid that can be most appropriately used every other day after remission is achieved, thereby allowing the HPA axis to recover to a certain extent (Boothe and Mealey, 2012). There is some controversy as to whether the daily dose of prednisolone should be given at once or divided twice daily. As studies supporting either frequency are lacking, once-daily dosing seems reasonable—in particular in animals that are difficult to medicate (Lowe et al, 2008a).

Topical instead of systemic glucocorticoids may be useful in inflammatory conditions of the eye, skin, respiratory tract, gastrointestinal tract, and joints. Topical steroids reduce inflammation by their local activity while minimizing systemic effects. Newer generation glucocorticoids (also called "soft glucocorticoids") were designed specifically for topical use in humans, and some of them have also been investigated in small animals. Inhalant glucocorticoids are used in nebulizers or metered dose inhaler (MDI) in patients with chronic inflammatory airway inflammation. They have relatively low systemic bioavailability because of their poor absorption and extensive first-pass metabolism in the liver into inactive metabolites. Examples are fluticasone and budesonide; their local potencies are extremely high. In the case of budesonide, the potency compared to cortisol is 60, that of fluticasone is 540 (Viviano, 2013). Both have been successfully used as inhaled glucocorticoids in dogs and cats (Bexfield et al, 2006; Padrid, 2006; Cohn et al, 2010; Galler et al, 2013). Budesonide is also available as an oral drug and exerts its inflammatory action locally in the intestinal tract. It is mainly used to treat IBD in dogs (Dye et al, 2013; Pietra et al, 2013). Mometasone is a potent topical glucocorticoid with low systemic effects designed for use in dermatological diseases; it is 25 times more potent than cortisol (Mendelsohn, 2009).

Immunosuppressive Therapy

Glucocorticoids are considered the initial first-line therapy in various immune-mediated diseases, including immune-mediated hemolytic anemia, immune-mediated thrombocytopenia, immune-mediated polyarthritis, systemic lupus erythematosus, and pemphigus complex. They are also used to prevent organ rejection after transplantation and to reduce immunological reactions associated with some infectious diseases, such as feline infectious peritonitis (FIP) and ehrlichiosis (Cohn, 2003; Gregory et al, 2006; Case et al, 2007; Addie et al, 2009; Hopper et al, 2012). It should be noted, however, that treatment protocols for small animals are mostly empirical and adapted from human medicine. Rigorous evaluations by randomized double-blinded placebo-controlled trials have not been performed (Whitley and Day, 2011).

The goal of immune-suppressive therapy is to achieve disease remission quickly, which usually requires high doses; thereafter, the dose is tapered slowly to the lowest level that will maintain remission. Oral application of prednisolone is the preferred modality. In acute or emergency situations, IV application of water-soluble esters of prednisolone or methylprednisolone may be indicated. Depot preparations do not allow dose adjustments and should not be used. The initial oral dose of prednisolone typically is 2 to 4 mg/kg in dogs and 2 to 8 mg/kg in cats per day (Cohn, 1997; 2010; Lowe et al, 2008a). The dose is usually divided twice daily, based on the belief that this division will decrease gastrointestinal side effects. Generally, larger dogs should be treated with the lower end of the dose range (Cohn, 2010). In the opinion of the author, the high-end dose in cats should be used with great caution. The recommendation may in part be based on the frequent use of prednisone instead of prednisolone. As mentioned earlier, it is now known that only a small part of oral prednisone appears as prednisolone in the systemic circulation in cats (Graham-Mize and Rosser, 2004). Some clinicians prefer to use dexamethasone for the first few doses and thereafter switch to oral prednisolone. There are no controlled clinical studies to confirm any advantage of this approach. In one experimental study, dexamethasone was more effective than prednisone and cortisol in inhibiting the clearance of IgG-coated cells (Ruiz et al, 1991) (see Dose Equivalents of Glucocorticoids).

If dexamethasone is used, equipotent doses have to be calculated (e.g., 2 mg/kg prednisolone equals approximately 0.3 mg/kg dexamethasone). High doses of prednisolone are continued for several days after remission is achieved; usually, high doses are needed for 1 to 4 weeks.

Thereafter, the dose should be tapered slowly over many weeks to months (see Glucocorticoid Reduction Protocol). Adverse effects are commonly seen with immunosuppressive doses, and the owner has to be warned about them. The addition of other immunosuppressive agents may have steroid-sparing effects and may allow disease control at lower glucocorticoid doses and faster tapering of the dose (Cohn, 2010).

Antineoplastic Therapy

Prednisolone is often included in combination chemotherapy protocols for their cytotoxic activity. Additional desired effects of prednisolone are reduction of edema and inflammation, appetite-stimulations, and decrease of nausea and vomiting. Oral prednisolone is also used for alleviation of chronic cancer pain; the recommended dose in dogs is 0.25 to 1.0 mg/kg, and for cats it is 0.5 to 1.0 mg/kg (Mealey et al, 2003; Lascelles, 2013). Interestingly, in dogs with multicentric lymphoma using a multidrug protocol, the benefit of prednisolone with regard to outcome was recently questioned (Zandvliet et al, 2013). In case of financial or other restrictions, prednisone/prednisolone (initial dose, 2 mg/kg) is sometimes used as a single agent in lymphoma cases with a possible tumor control of 1 to 2 months. Besides the short remission period, other disadvantages include serious side effects and the potential induction of multidrug resistance. The latter would limit the success of more aggressive drug therapy in case the owner changes his or her mind (Chun, 2009; Vail et al, 2013). Besides the potential risk of decreased response to later chemotherapy, glucocorticoids induce apoptosis of neoplastic lymphocytes and may interfere with the diagnosis; they should therefore only be used after the diagnosis has been made.

Glucocorticoids may also be used in patients with hypercalcemia of malignancy (see Chapter 15) and to increase blood glucose concentrations in cases with insulinoma (see Chapter 9).

Shock

The use of high-dose glucocorticoid therapy for shock has fallen repeatedly in and out of favor (Cohn, 2010). Different from the past, high-dose glucocorticoids are nowadays mentioned only in the treatment protocols of anaphylactic shock. In humans, epinephrine is the first line treatment with a rapid onset of action; and although glucocorticoids are often used, their onset of action is considered quite slow (Lieberman, 2014). A systemic review of databases failed to identify adequately designed studies, and no relevant evidence for the use of glucocorticoids was found. The authors were therefore unable to make any recommendations for the use of glucocorticoids in the treatment of anaphylaxis in humans (Choo et al, 2013). Similarly, in dogs and cats, epinephrine is the drug of choice for treatment of anaphylaxis (Shmuel and Cortes, 2013). Glucocorticoids continue to be frequently used in small animals with anaphylaxis; however, as in humans, no studies support their benefit. Of note, glucocorticoids themselves may cause allergic reaction and even anaphylaxis. The application of methylprednisolone sodium succinate 30 mg/kg intravenously is commonly mentioned for cases with anaphylactic shock (Dowling, 2009).

In humans with septic shock, relative adrenal insufficiency may be present and low-dose glucocorticoid therapy for a few days appeared to be safe and may have some benefit for shock reversal and short-term survival (Annane et al, 2009; Sligl et al, 2009). Although relative adrenal insufficiency may also exist in dogs and cats, no clinical studies have investigated the use of low-dose glucocorticoid therapy in cases with septic shock. The results of one experimental study using low-dose corticosteroids showed beneficial effects in dogs with severe sepsis; however, results also pointed to reduced bacterial clearance even with short term treatment (Hicks et al, 2012). Therefore, no recommendation can be made for the application of glucocorticoids in septic shock. They should only be used at low doses, if at all, under close monitoring of the patient.

Neurological Diseases

Previously, glucocorticoids were advocated for the treatment of traumatic brain injury on the basis that they decreased brain edema. However, in humans, high-dose methylprednisolone was associated with an increase in mortality. Their use in humans as well as in small animals with brain injury is no longer recommended (DiFazio and Fletcher, 2013). In acute spinal cord injury, methylprednisolone is considered to reveal free radical-scavenging effects, which other glucocorticoids are lacking. It is suggested that methylprednisolone has a positive effect if administered within 8 hours of the time of insult. Suggested initial dose of methylprednisolone sodium succinate is 30 mg/kg followed by repeated boluses of 15 mg/kg at 2 and 6 hours, then every 8 hours up to 48 hours after the trauma (Park et al, 2012). However, these doses are enormous and have the potential of serious side effects (e.g., gastrointestinal ulceration, immunosuppression, and impaired wound healing). Sound data to support the use of this protocol is lacking in small animals, and its use in acute spinal cord injury is currently controversial (Park et al, 2012).

ADVERSE EFFECTS

Adverse effects are common with glucocorticoid therapy, in particular if the protocol includes high doses and/or long-term application. Severely reduced quality of life and even fatal outcomes are possible. On the other hand, glucocorticoids may be life-saving and have major therapeutic benefits when used adequately. As with any therapy, benefits must be weighed against potential adverse effects. Glucocorticoids can also alter the effectiveness or toxicity of other drugs. One of the most important examples is the substantially increased risk of gastric ulceration when glucocorticoids are co-administered with non-steroidal anti-inflammatory agents (Table 14-4). Numerous adverse effects may occur; the most important ones are discussed in the following section.

Iatrogenic Hyperadrenocorticism

In a significant percentage of dogs with hyperadrenocorticism, the disease is in fact caused by exogenous glucocorticoids. Clinical signs and laboratory abnormalities of iatrogenic hyperadrenocorticism are identical to those of the endogenous form of the disease. Polyuria, polydipsia, polyphagia, and panting usually manifest within the first 1 to 2 weeks of therapy in dogs (e.g., with oral prednisolone in anti-inflammatory or immunosuppressive doses). These signs may even occur within hours after the first dose. They dissipate as the dose is tapered or discontinued (Feldman and Nelson, 2004). More severe signs such as cutaneous lesions (thin hair coat, alopecia, hyperpigmentation, pyoderma, calcinosis cutis, and thin skin), poor wound healing, muscle weakness and atrophy, hepatomegaly due to steroid hepatopathy, pendulous abdomen, urinary tract infection, and myotonia usually require a longer time and develop within weeks to months (Behrend and Kemppainen, 1997; Huang et al, 1999; Feldman and Nelson, 2004). Lethargy may

TABLE 14-4	POTENTIAL DRUG INTERACTIONS OF GLUCOCORTICOIDS
DRUG	**POTENTIAL INTERACTION**
Antacids	Reduced oral glucocorticoid absorption
Anticholinesterase agents	Muscle weakness
Aspirin (salicylates)	Reduced salicylate blood levels
Cyclophosphamide	Inhibition of hepatic metabolism of cyclophosphamide
Cyclosporine	Increase blood levels of each, by inhibiting hepatic metabolism of each other
Digoxin	Secondary to hypokalemia, increased risk for arrhythmias
Diuretics (furosemide, thiazides)	Increased risk of hypokalemia
Ephedrine	Increased metabolism of glucocorticoids
Estrogens	Potentiation of glucocorticoid effect
Insulin	Decreased insulin effect
Ketoconazole	Decreased metabolism of glucocorticoids
Macrolide antibiotics (erythromycin, clarithromycin)	Decreased metabolism of glucocorticoids
Nonsteroidal anti-inflammatory drugs (NSAIDs)	Increased risk of gastric ulceration
Phenobarbital	Increased metabolism of glucocorticoids
Phenytoin	Increased metabolism of glucocorticoids
Rifampin	Increased metabolism of glucocorticoids
Vaccines	Immunosuppressive doses of glucocorticoids may augment virus replication, avoid live-attenuated vaccines

Modified from Plumb DC, editor: *Plumb's veterinary drug handbook*, ed 7, Ames, IA, 2011, Wiley-Blackwell.

be seen either as a short- or long-term effect. Resolution of those signs takes considerably longer than cessation of polyuria, polydipsia, polyphagia, and panting. Improvement may be seen within a few weeks; however, depending on severity, resolution may take up to 6 months or longer. Resolution may not always be complete; for instance, persistence of calcinosis cutis and of pulmonary mineralization has been reported, and there may be color change in new hair growth (Huang et al, 1999; Blois et al, 2009). Exogenous glucocorticoids lead to atrophy of the adrenal glands, which may be seen ultrasonographically as reduction in length and height of the cranial and caudal pole. The decrease in size is progressive during therapy and percentage change varies between dogs (Pey et al, 2012). Generally, there is a large individual variation with regard to glucocorticoid sensitivity. The same dose may be tolerated well in one dog, whereas substantial side effects are seen in another dog. Even low doses (e.g., suggested for physiological replacement) may induce side effects in sensitive dogs. In particular, large breed dogs may develop profound weakness and paraparesis when treated with high doses of glucocorticoids.

Cats are considered to be more resistant than dogs toward the development of iatrogenic hyperadrenocorticism. Associated signs occur most often after repeated injections of long-acting glucocorticoid preparations; however, occurrence of signs (e.g., polyphagia and weight gain) have also been reported after a single injection of methylprednisolone acetate (Ferasin, 2001). It is often assumed that polyuria and polydipsia do not occur in cats until diabetes mellitus is induced by exogenous glucocorticoids. Although this may be true for the majority of cases, polyuria and polydipsia have also been reported in cats without diabetes (Lien et al, 2006; Lowe et al, 2008a). Other signs of iatrogenic hyperadrenocorticism are similar to those seen in dogs. Unique to the cat is the development of spontaneous tearing and sloughing of the skin and, in rare cases, medial curling of the pinnae (Scott et al, 1982; Lowe et al, 2008a; 2008b). Steroid hepatopathy does occur in cats, but is considered to be less common than in dogs (Schaer and Ginn, 1999). Of note, signs of iatrogenic hyperadrenocorticism may not only occur with oral or parenteral application but also with topical treatment. Exceptions are the newer generations of topical glucocorticoids (budesonide, fluticasone), which seem to have minimal side effects. There is no treatment for iatrogenic hyperadrenocorticism. The only measure consists in cessation of glucocorticoid therapy. Because the HPA axis is usually suppressed, adrenocortical insufficiency may develop if therapy is abruptly stopped (see later and Glucocorticoid Reduction Protocol section).

Alteration of the Hypothalamic Pituitary Adrenal Axis

Closely related to the development of clinical signs of glucocorticoid excess is the suppression of the HPA axis. Of note, however, suppression of the HPA axis may be present without the animal displaying clinical signs of hyperadrenocorticism. All synthetic glucocorticoids suppress CRH and ACTH secretion, but their effects are not equivalent. Generally, the greater the anti-inflammatory potency, the greater is the capacity to suppress the HPA axis. Over time, the glucocorticoid-producing cells of the two inner zones of the adrenal cortex atrophy and the responsiveness of the HPA axis decrease progressively (Behrend and Kemppainen, 1997). Animals with suppression of the HPA lack the ability to secrete cortisol sufficiently in response to stress and may develop signs of acute adrenocortical insufficiency. The zona glomerulosa and its function are preserved, and therefore, electrolyte abnormalities associated with mineralocorticoid deficiency are not seen. Suppression of the HPA axis may occur quite soon after the onset of glucocorticoid therapy.

Oral, parenteral, and topical administration all lead to HPA axis suppression, which is most serious and prolonged after repeated injection of long-acting preparations (water-insoluble esters). In experimental dogs, a single dose of methylprednisolone acetate (2.5 mg/kg IM) suppressed the HPA axis, as demonstrated by reduced response of cortisol after ACTH, for at least 5 weeks (Kemppainen et al, 1981). A dog that was treated for pruritus with a similar single dose of methylprednisolone acetate experienced HPA axis suppression for 7 weeks (Meyer, 1982). A single dose of triamcinolone acetonide (0.22 mg/kg IM) suppressed the HPA axis for 2 to 4 weeks (Kemppainen et al, 1982). Single IV doses of 0.01 mg/kg and 0.1 mg/kg dexamethasone (as free alcohol) resulted in reduced cortisol response after ACTH for 16 to 24 hours and 32 hours, respectively. Dexamethasone sodium phosphate was associated with a somewhat shorter suppression compared with the free alcohol with the 0.01 mg/kg dose (Kemppainen and Sartin, 1984). A single

dose of prednisone (2.2 mg/kg IM) did not result in adrenocortical suppression (Kemppainen et al, 1982). However, even prednisone/prednisolone given at physiological doses can suppress the HPA axis when given for some time. Oral application of 0.22 mg/kg (physiological dose) or 0.55 mg/kg per day led to a significantly depressed cortisol after ACTH stimulation after 1 week. Administration of 1 mg/kg prednisone daily resulted in HPA axis suppression within 2 weeks; administration of 1 mg/kg prednisolone every other day was associated with HPA axis suppression after 3 weeks (Chastain and Graham, 1979; Moore and Hoenig, 1992). Cats are more resistant to the development of clinical signs of iatrogenic hyperadrenocorticism; however, they experience HPA suppression similar to dogs (Behrend and Kemppainen, 1997). The application of a single dose of methylprednisolone acetate (20 mg IM) to healthy cats led to a reduced cortisol response after ACTH within 1 week (Scott et al, 1979). In a cat treated with subcutaneous (SC) methylprednisolone acetate (20 mg) weekly for 4 weeks, complete suppression of the HPA axis was still seen 1 month after the last injection (Ferasin, 2001). Daily oral administration of prednisolone (2 mg/kg) resulted in HPA axis suppression after 1 week and was more pronounced after 2 weeks of daily therapy (Middleton et al, 1987). Similarly, daily oral methylprednisolone (4 mg/kg) was associated with HPA axis suppression within 1 week (Crager et al, 1994).

Any topically applied glucocorticoid can suppress the HPA axis. Application of triamcinolone, fluocinonide, and betamethasone valerate on the skin of healthy dogs (once daily for 5 days) resulted in decreased cortisol after stimulation with ACTH within 5 days. The HPA axis remained suppressed for 3 to 4 weeks after the last treatment (Zenoble and Kemppainen, 1987). Ophthalmic instillation of 1% prednisolone acetate or 0.1% dexamethasone four times daily in both eyes resulted in HPA axis suppression within 2 weeks, intensifying throughout the treatment period (Roberts et al, 1984; Glaze et al, 1988). Ototopical administration of therapeutic doses of dexamethasone-containing ointment daily to healthy dogs resulted in HPA axis suppression within 11 days (Abraham et al, 2005). The new generation of topical steroids cause minimal signs of iatrogenic hyperadrenocorticism but are associated with HPA axis suppression. Oral budesonide in dogs with IBD resulted in significantly lower post-ACTH cortisol concentrations after 30 days of therapy (Tumulty et al, 2004). Inhalant budesonide in cats with chronic bronchial disease resulted in HPA axis suppression in three of 15 cases (Galler et al, 2013). Inhaled fluticasone in healthy dogs and inhaled flunisolide in healthy cats suppressed the HPA axis within 2 to 3 weeks (Reinero et al, 2006; Cohn et al, 2008).

Diagnosis of HPA axis suppression is made by performing an ACTH stimulation test. Depending on the severity, post-ACTH cortisol concentrations can be below the detection limit of the cortisol assay, low (e.g., 2 to 5 µg/dL, 55 to 138 nmol/L) or low-normal. Animals with undetectable or low concentrations are at risk for signs of adrenal insufficiency, in particular when encountering a stressful situation. Potentially lethal situations may arise. If clinical signs (e.g., lethargy, anorexia, or vomiting) develop after cessation of steroids, prednisolone administrations should be instituted. The dose is somewhat arbitrary and depends on the clinical situation. If severity of signs and extent of stress are moderate, prednisolone doses between 0.5 to 1 mg/kg/day may be sufficient; doses up to 2 to 4 mg/kg/day may be needed temporarily in life-threatening situations. The prednisolone dose should then be tapered slowly. Generally, glucocorticoids should be reduced slowly after a longer period of glucocorticoid administration (e.g., > 2 weeks). Suppression of the HPA axis is usually reversible. The length of time required for full axis recovery depends on duration, dose, preparation, and frequency of application of the steroid. Single doses of triamcinolone acetonide or methylprednisolone acetate can suppress adrenal responsiveness for up to 5 weeks (see earlier). Multiple injections of long-acting preparations will aggravate the suppressive effect, and HPA axis malfunction may persist for months. Oral administration of shorter-acting or less-potent preparations may result in quicker normalization (Behrend and Kemppainen, 1997).

Abrupt cessation of glucocorticoids may result in a so-called glucocorticoid withdrawal syndrome (Greco and Behrend, 1995). Several subgroups are known in humans; one of them is attributed to the sudden lack of the high concentration of steroids. In this situation, the body perceives the glucocorticoid withdrawal as a relative deficiency. The signs are vague and can easily be mistaken with those of true adrenal insufficiency. The syndrome has been poorly characterized in dogs and cats. In questionable cases, an ACTH stimulation test should be performed to differentiate between absolute or relative adrenal insufficiency. Prednisolone administration may be needed in either situation.

Diabetes Mellitus

Glucocorticoids may exert diabetogenic properties thereby inducing hyperglycemia in previously normoglycemic patients, as well as worsening glycemic control in patients already known to have diabetes mellitus. Glucocorticoids increase insulin resistance in peripheral tissues (muscle, fat) and increase hepatic glucose production, and they may also inhibit insulin release from the β cells. In humans, overt diabetes or impaired glucose tolerance is seen in 14% to 28% of individuals receiving long-term glucocorticoids. Prevalence of diabetes induced by exogenous glucocorticoids has not been systematically studied in dogs and cats. It is well known that cats are more susceptible to the diabetogenic effects of glucocorticoids than dogs. Approximately 80% of cats with endogenous hyperadrenocorticism are diabetic, whereas in dogs, the prevalence is only about 10%. Steroid diabetes can occur after oral or parenteral, as well as after topical administration of any of the traditional glucocorticoids, but it has not been reported with the newer class of topical drugs (budesonide, fluticasone). Glucocorticoid sensitivity varies between individuals and therefore dose, duration, and frequency of application that will ultimately lead to hyperglycemia cannot be predicted. Experimental studies have shown that abnormalities may already become apparent after short-term therapy. Administration of 2 mg/kg prednisolone once daily for 8 days resulted in reduced glucose tolerance after an IV glucose load in all six cats, and three of the six cats developed hyperglycemia (Middleton and Watson, 1985). Weekly injections of 20 mg methylprednisolone subcutaneously lead to hyperglycemia within 4 weeks in the two cats studied (Scott et al, 1982). Within 1 month of daily administration of immunosuppressive doses of prednisolone or dexamethasone, 29% and 71% of cats developed glucosuria (Lowe et al, 2009). The later study points to a greater diabetogenic effect of dexamethasone than equipotent doses of prednisolone. Steroid-induced diabetes is also seen in dogs but with much lower frequency than in cats (Campbell and Latimer, 1984; Jeffers et al, 1991). Administration of antiinflammatory/immunosuppressive doses of prednisone (1.1 mg/kg/day) or prednisolone (1 to 2 mg/kg/day) for 28 days to normal dogs has not produced hyperglycemia, glucose intolerance, or insulin resistance (Wolfsheimer et al, 1986; Moore and Hoenig, 1993).

Diagnosis of steroid-induced diabetes should result in cessation of glucocorticoid therapy whenever possible; depending on the disease, alternative drugs (e.g., cyclosporine) or topical use of the new generation of glucocorticoids should be considered. In cats, steroid-induced diabetes often goes into remission, provided that the glucocorticoid application is ceased immediately and insulin treatment is initiated. In dogs, diabetic remission has been seen; however, too few data have been published to make a general statement. In a dog or cat with known diabetes, glycemic control usually worsens when glucocorticoids are administered. Diabetes mellitus should not be regarded as an absolute contraindication for glucocorticoids, because in some diseases they may be life-saving. The glucocorticoid dose should be as low as possible to control the disease. In short-term glucocorticoid therapy (1 to 2 weeks), the insulin dose may be maintained while awaiting the withdrawal of the drug. If long-term glucocorticoid therapy is needed, an increase in the daily insulin doses is usually necessary to maintain control over the diabetic state. The amount of increase is variable and should follow the guidelines discussed in Chapters 6 and 7. Careful monitoring of blood glucose levels is important. After the effect of the glucocorticoid on insulin sensitivity wears off, the insulin requirement decreases, resulting in the need to also decrease the insulin dose. Remission may fail to appear if treatment is inadequate or if the cat has substantial islet pathology. If glucocorticoid therapy cannot be terminated and no alternative drug can be used, the insulin dose has to be adjusted based on the severity of the insulin resistance. In those cases, glycemic control oftentimes remains difficult.

Gastrointestinal Hemorrhage and Ulceration

In the physiological state, glucocorticoids exert protective effects for the gastrointestinal integrity by various mechanisms. The administration of glucocorticoids in pharmacological doses may alter mucosal defense mechanisms in many ways (e.g., by decreasing mucus production, altering the biochemical structure of mucus, decreasing mucosal cell turnover, increasing acid output, and impairing mucosal blood flow). Other mechanisms are decreased healing rate and promotion of bacterial colonization of ulcers (Hanson et al, 1997; Rohrer et al, 1999a; Feldman and Nelson, 2004). In most situations, it is unlikely that glucocorticoids are the sole factor for gastrointestinal problems. The exception may be when extremely high doses of steroids are used. The application of methylprednisolone sodium succinate (30 mg/kg initially, and then 15 mg/kg 2 and 6 hours later and every 6 hours thereafter for 48 hours) was associated with gastric hemorrhage in all of the 10 dogs and was severe in nine of them (Rohrer et al, 1999a). Similarly, the application of extremely high doses of dexamethasone (4.4 mg/kg/day for 8 days) or prednisone (8.8 mg/kg/day for 7 days) to experimental dogs did result in endoscopic evidence of hemorrhage but not in ulcers (Sorjonen et al, 1983; Behrend and Kemppainen, 1997).

In clinical patients, the most striking gastrointestinal side effects have been reported in dogs with neurological disease. However, because a neurological problem can result in gastrointestinal lesions itself, it is difficult to say how much glucocorticoids contributed to the development of the problems. In one study, 23 of 155 dogs with intervertebral disk herniation had gastrointestinal problems, and 10 of them had not received glucocorticoids (Moore and Withrow, 1982). More than 75% of dogs with acute intervertebral disc disease treated with glucocorticoids had gastric mucosal lesions as detected by endoscopy. In 8% of dogs, gastric ulcers developed during the treatment period. Only 24% of the dogs had clinical signs such as vomiting or melena (Neiger et al, 2000). The most catastrophic of the gastrointestinal complications is colon perforation. Colonic perforation in 13 dogs treated with glucocorticoids was uniformly fatal (Toombs et al, 1986). Ten of the 13 dogs were neurosurgical patients, one was treated for head-trauma and non-ambulatory paresis, and two others had undergone major surgery for other reasons. Dexamethasone was the most frequently used steroid and was given in a mean cumulative dose of 6.4 mg/kg/day over a period of 5 days. The most common clinical signs were depression, anorexia, and vomiting. Signs became evident 3 to 8 days after surgery and preceded death by an average of 22 hours (Toombs et al, 1986).

Because of the potential association between glucocorticoids and gastrointestinal side effects, certain precautions should be taken, in particular in patients with neurological disease. Non-ambulatory patients certainly have an increased risk (Behrend and Kemppainen, 1997). The following recommendations have been made: to use prednisolone or methylprednisolone instead of the more potent dexamethasone, limit treatment to the lowest possible dose and duration, avoid concurrent or successive use of other drugs with known ulcerogenic potential (in particular nonsteroidal anti-inflammatory drugs), avoid urinary retention by closed urine drainage, and correct fecal retention problems prior to surgery (Toombs et al, 1986).

Misoprostol, cimetidine, or sucralfate were evaluated for their potential preventative role for gastrointestinal hemorrhage but did not show any effect (Hanson et al, 1997; Rohrer et al, 1999b).

Laboratory Abnormalities

The most common biochemical abnormalities in dogs receiving exogenous glucocorticoids are elevation of liver enzymes. Any glucocorticoid and any form of application (oral, parenteral, or topical) can lead to an increase of alkaline phosphatase (ALP), alanine aminotransferase (ALT), and gamma glutamyl transferase (GGT). However, there is a tremendous amount of variation between individual dogs; in some, the elevation may reach several-fold of normal, whereas others only have minor increase or even no change. In part, the changes may be dose-related. The administration of 1.1 mg/kg/day prednisone by mouth for 35 days did not result in a significant increase of ALP and the glucocorticoid-induced ALP isoenzyme. Only five of the 18 healthy dogs had ALP activities above the reference range (Moore et al, 1992). A prednisone dose of 4.4 mg/kg/day IM for 14 days was associated with a significant increase in ALP activity within 2 days, in ALT activity within 3 days, and in GGT activity within 6 days. Six weeks after the end of the study, the enzyme activities were still slightly to moderately increased (Badylak and Van Vleet, 1981).

The application of other glucocorticoids, such as dexamethasone, methylprednisolone (acetate), and triamcinolone, has similar effects. The contributory role of the glucocorticoid induced isoenzyme of ALP to the increase of total ALP activity seems to be inconsistent. In the study of Moore and colleagues (1992), it contributed only to a small extent to the total ALP activity. In a study by Solter and colleagues (1994), the initial increase of ALP was mainly due to the liver ALP isoenzyme, followed by the glucocorticoid and bone isoenzyme 7 and 10 days after initiating treatment with prednisone. Serum bile acids may also increase during glucocorticoid therapy, whereas ammonia tolerance test does not seem to be affected (Meyer, 1982; DeNovo and Prasse, 1983; Solter et al, 1994). For effects on blood glucose and lipase activity, see the Diabetes Mellitus section and the Pancreatitis section. Otic medications containing triamcinolone or dexamethasone were also associated with an increase in ALP, ALT, and GGT (Meyer et al, 1990; Abraham et al, 2005). Increase in liver enzyme activities

may also be seen with the new generation of glucocorticoids. A short term (30 days) oral application of budesonide was associated with an increase in ALP activity in dogs, but the difference to pretreatment levels was not significant (Tumulty et al, 2004). Cats are generally considered more resistant to the effects of glucocorticoids and do not have a glucocorticoid induced isoenzyme. Increases in liver enzyme activities after administration of glucocorticoids do occur, and the most consistent increase is seen in ALT activity. The ALP activity may also increase; however, it often still remains within the normal range (Scott et al, 1982; Sharkey et al, 2007; Lowe et al, 2008b). As in dogs, glucocorticoid administration in cats may result in steroid (vacuolar) hepatopathy, although the frequency is lower (Schaer and Ginn, 1999). Increase in serum lipids (cholesterol, triglycerides) may be seen in both species.

Glucocorticoids also affect hematological parameters. In dogs with iatrogenic hyperadrenocorticism, eosinopenia was seen in 18 out of 28 dogs and was the most frequent finding. Other constituents of the "stress leukogram" were also found, but to a lesser extent (Huang et al, 1999). In 14 cats treated with glucocorticoids (4.4 mg/kg prednisolone or 0.55 mg/kg dexamethasone for 56 days), neutrophils were significantly higher, and lymphocytes and eosinophils were significantly lower after treatment (Lowe et al, 2008b). In this study, monocytes were also increased, which is usually considered not a typical finding in steroid-treated cats.

Pancreatitis

More than 500 drugs have been reported to the World Health Organization (WHO) because they were suspected to induce pancreatitis in humans. In many of them, evidence of causality is weak, and for only 31 of those drugs a definitive causality has been established. Among them are steroids, but they do not belong to the group of high risk drugs (Nitsche et al, 2010). Previously, glucocorticoids were also assumed to cause pancreatitis in small animals. Much of the evidence regarding this association, however, is related to an increased viscosity of pancreatic secretion shown in rabbits. In dogs, increased viscosity of pancreatic secretions has been shown only when isolated pancreases were perfused with a huge dose of methylprednisolone (400 mg); a lower dose (200 mg) did not change the viscosity (Kimura et al, 1979; Behrend and Kemppainen, 1997). Pancreatitis has also been seen in dogs treated with glucocorticoids. However, these were sporadic cases, and the dogs suffered from intervertebral disc disease, which may alone be a risk factor (Behrend and Kemppainen, 1997). The administration of dexamethasone to healthy dogs in various doses for up to 3 weeks did not cause pancreatitis. However, it increased lipase activity without any histological damage to the pancreas (Parent, 1982). In a more recent study, evaluating the canine pancreatic lipase immunoreactivity (cPLI), immunosuppressive doses of prednisone (2.2 mg/kg once daily) given for 6 weeks did not result in an increase in cPLI (Steiner et al, 2009).

In dogs and cats, the early concerns that glucocorticoids could cause pancreatitis have now largely been dismissed. Steroids are no longer included in the list of drugs suspected of being associated with pancreatitis (Armstrong and Williams, 2012; Mansfield, 2012). It is possible, however, that glucocorticoids are a contributing factor in sick animals or that only a subset of patients is susceptible for steroid-induced pancreatitis.

Miscellaneous

Glucocorticoids may have numerous other adverse effects, including growth retardation in young animals, induction or worsening of hypertension, disposing the animal to infections due to immunosuppression (e.g., urinary tract infection), interference with fertility, induction of abortion, and behavior changes.

GLUCOCORTICOID REDUCTION PROTOCOL

There are various ways to taper an animal from glucocorticoids, and there are no studies demonstrating that one way is better than the other. Several principles, however, are widely accepted. Tapering of the glucocorticoid dose should always be done if therapy was longer than or equal to 2 weeks, or if high doses have been used (> 1 mg/kg prednisolone/day or its equivalent) (Ferguson et al, 2009). In the latter case (i.e., short duration of high dose), tapering can be done quickly over a few days. Tapering of the steroid dose should be started after the disease being addressed is in remission (e.g., normalized hematocrit in immune-mediated anemia, and/or absence of gastrointestinal signs in IBD). Inflammatory diseases usually require 5 to 7 days of induction therapy, whereas immunosuppressive diseases may need 10 to 28 days (Behrend and Kemppainen, 1997). Worsening of the disease soon after the start of tapering suggests that the tapering was done too fast. If an immune-mediated disease recrudesces, a second remission is more difficult to obtain than previously. If recrudescence occurs, the glucocorticoid dose should be increased immediately to a dose equivalent even higher than the initial dose. If remission is lost in an inflammatory disease, the dose should be increased to the last dose that kept the animal disease free (Behrend and Kemppainen, 1997). In general, the longer the induction phase and/or the greater the induction dose, the more stepwise and longer the period between dose reductions has to be. Glucocorticoids used for life-threatening diseases should be tapered more slowly than glucocorticoids used for other diseases (Cohn, 2010). Tapering for immune-mediated disease can take several months; some cases may even need life-long therapy.

The initial dose reduction step may be done by consolidating the dose, thereby achieving longer dosing intervals; this might spare the HPA axis suppression while the desired effects are maintained. For instance, if prednisolone is administered twice daily, the daily dose is given at once (e.g., 10 mg prednisolone once daily instead of 5 mg prednisolone twice daily). The daily dose is then reduced incrementally (Cohn, 2010). Usually, when the daily prednisolone dose has been reduced to 0.25 to 0.5 mg/kg/day, the dose interval is switched to alternate-day therapy. The latter should allow the HPA axis to recover on the "off-days" and is assumed to provide greater safety than if therapy is suddenly discontinued. Successful alternate-day therapy depends upon the therapeutic effects lasting longer than the suppressive effects on the HPA axis (Ferguson et al, 2009). Alternate-day therapy should not be applied during the initial phase of glucocorticoid therapy because it will not be effective to bring the disease under control. Prednisolone is the preferred glucocorticoid for alternate-day therapy; the action of cortisol (hydrocortisone) is too short and that of dexamethasone is too long for this approach. When changing to alternate-dose therapy, the same daily dose of prednisolone can be given every other day (e.g., change from 5 mg every day to 5 mg every other day), which results in a 50% reduction of dose. Alternatively, the same dose can be maintained by doubling the dose on the "on-days" (e.g., change from 5 mg every day to 10 mg every other day) (Behrend and Kemppainen, 1997). In case of serious immune-mediated diseases, this latter approach for moving from daily to alternate-day therapy is preferred. If alternate-dose therapy is successful to maintain the disease in remission, further reduction to every third day can be attempted (Behrend and Kemppainen, 1997).

Tapering of oral prednisolone used for immune-mediated disease in dogs could be done as follows (Behrend and Kemppainen, 1997):

Induction:	2.0 mg/kg divided b.i.d. for 10 to 28 days
Tapering:	1.5 mg/kg divided b.i.d. or once daily for 10 to 28 days
	1.0 mg/kg divided b.i.d. or once daily for 10 to 28 days
	0.5 mg/kg divided b.i.d. or once daily for 10 to 28 days
	0.25 mg/kg once daily for 10 to 28 days
	0.25 mg/kg every other day, for 21 days or more

It should be understood that the animal should be reevaluated before every reduction step to ensure that the disease is still in remission. The glucocorticoid dose used for induction in inflammatory diseases is substantially lower (0.5 to 1.0 mg/kg/day in dogs) and the induction period is shorter (5 to 7 days). Tapering, therefore, can be done faster, usually within 10 to 14 days. Tapering of the higher anti-inflammatory and immune-suppressive doses in cats should be done accordingly.

REFERENCES

Abraham G, et al.: Evidence for ototopical glucocorticoid-induced decrease in hypothalamic-pituitary-adrenal axis response and liver function, *Endocrinol* 146:3163, 2005.

Addie D, et al.: Feline infectious peritonitis: ABCD guidelines on prevention and management, *J Feline Med Surg* 11:594, 2009.

Annane D, et al.: Corticosteroids in the treatment of severe sepsis and septic shock in adults: a systematic review, *J Am Med Assoc* 301:2362, 2009.

Armstrong PJ, Williams DA: Pancreatitis in cats, *Top Companion Anim Med* 27:140, 2012.

Badylak SF, Van Vleet JF: Sequential morphologic and clinicopathologic alterations in dogs with experimentally induced glucocorticoid hepatopathy, *Am J Vet Res* 42:1310, 1981.

Barrett KE, et al.: The adrenal medulla and adrenal cortex. In Barrett KE, Barman SM, Boitano S, Brooks HL, editors: *Ganong's review of medical physiology*, ed 24, New York, 2012, McGraw-Hill Lange.

Behrend EN, Kemppainen RJ: Glucocorticoid therapy: pharmacology, indications, and complications, *Vet Clin North Am Small Anim Pract* 27:187, 1997.

Bensignor E, Grandemange E: Comparison of an antifungal agent with a mixture of antifungal, antibiotic and corticosteroid agents for the treatment of Malassezia species otitis in dogs, *Vet Rec* 158:193, 2006.

Bexfield NH, et al.: Management of 13 cases of canine respiratory disease using inhaled corticosteroids, *J Small Anim Pract* 47:377, 2006.

Blois SL, et al.: Diagnosis and outcome of a dog with iatrogenic hyperadrenocorticism and secondary pulmonary mineralization, *Can Vet* 50:397, 2009.

Boothe DM, Mealey KA: Glucocorticoids and mineralocorticoids. In Boothe DM, editor: *Small animal clinical pharmacology and therapeutics*, ed 2, St Louis, 2012, Saunders/Elsevier.

Busillo JM, Cidlowski JA: The five Rs of glucocorticoid action during inflammation: ready, reinforce, repress, resolve, and restore, *Trends Endocrinol Metab* 24:109, 2013.

Calvert CA, Cornelius LM: The pharmacodynamic differences among glucocorticoid preparations, *Vet Med* 85:860, 1990a.

Calvert CA, Cornelius LM: Corticosteroid hormones: endogenous regulation and the effects of exogenous administration, *Vet Med* 85:810, 1990b.

Campbell KL, Latimer KS: Transient diabetes mellitus associated with prednisone therapy in a dog, *J Am Vet Med Assoc* 185:299, 1984.

Canalis E, et al.: Glucocorticoid-induced osteoporosis: pathophysiology and therapy, *Osteoporos Int* 18:1319, 2007.

Carroll TB, et al.: Glucocorticoids and adrenal androgens. In Gardner DG, Shoback D, editors: *Greenspan's basic and clinical endocrinology*, ed 9, New York, 2011, McGraw-Hill.

Case JB, et al.: Incidence of and risk factors for diabetes mellitus in cats that have undergone renal transplantation: 187 cases (1986-2005), *J Am Vet Med Assoc* 230:880, 2007.

Chapman K, et al.: 11β-hydroxysteroid dehydrogenases: intracellular gate-keepers of tissue glucocorticoid action, *Physiol Rev* 93:1139, 2013.

Chastain CB, Graham CL: Adrenocortical suppression in dogs on daily and alternate-day prednisone administration, *Am J Vet Res* 40:936, 1979.

Choo KJ, et al.: Glucocorticoids for the treatment of anaphylaxis, *Cochrane Database Syst Rev* 18:1276, 2013.

Chun R: Lymphoma: Which chemotherapy protocol and why? *Top Companion Anim Med* 24:157, 2009.

Cohn LA: Glucocorticosteroids as immunosuppressive agents, *Semin Vet Med Surg (Small Anim)* 12:150, 1997.

Cohn LA: Ehrlichiosis and related infections, *Vet Clin Small Anim* 33:863, 2003.

Cohn LA: Glucocorticoid therapy. In Ettinger SJ, Feldman EC, editors: *Textbook of veterinary internal medicine*, ed 7, St Louis, 2010, Saunders/Elsevier.

Cohn LA, et al.: Endocrine and immunologic effects of inhaled fluticasone propionate in healthy dogs, *J Vet Intern Med* 22:37, 2008.

Cohn LA, et al.: Effects of fluticasone propionate dosage in an experimental model of feline asthma, *J Feline Med Surg* 12:91, 2010.

Costa LAVS, et al.: Bone demineralization in the lumbar spine of dogs submitted to prednisone therapy, *J Vet Pharmacol Therap* 33:583, 2010.

Crager CS, et al.: Adrenocorticotropic hormone and cortisol concentrations after corticotropin-releasing hormone stimulation testing in cats administered methylprednisolone, *Am J Vet Res* 55:704, 1994.

Daminet S, Ferguson DC: Influence of drugs on thyroid function in dogs, *J Vet Intern Med* 17:463, 2003.

Daminet S, et al.: Short-term influence of prednisone and phenobarbital on thyroid function in euthyroid dogs, *Can Vet J* 40:411, 1999.

Day MJ: Immunotherapy. In Day MJ, Schultz RD, editors: *Veterinary immunology, principles and practice*, London, 2011, Manson Publishing Ltd.

DeNovo RC, Prasse KW: Comparison of serum biochemical and hepatic functional alterations in dogs treated with corticosteroids and hepatic duct ligation, *Am J Vet Res* 44:1703, 1983.

DiFazio J, Fletcher DJ: Update in the management of the small animal patient with neurologic trauma, *Vet Clin Small Anim* 43:915, 2013.

Dowling PM: Anaphylaxis. In Silverstein DC, Hopper K, editors: *Small animal critical care medicine*, St Louis, 2009, Saunders/Elsevier.

Dye TL, et al.: Randomized, controlled trial of budesonide and prednisone for the treatment of idiopathic inflammatory bowel disease in dogs, *J Vet Intern Med* 27:1385, 2013.

Feldman EC, Nelson RW: Glucocorticoid therapy. In Feldman EC, Nelson RW, editors: *Canine and feline endocrinology and reproduction*, ed 3, St Louis, 2004, Saunders/Elsevier.

Ferasin L: Iatrogenic hyperadrenocorticism in a cat following a short therapeutic course of methylprednisolone acetate, *J Feline Med Surg* 3:87, 2001.

Ferguson DC, et al.: Glucocorticoids, mineralocorticoids and adrenolytic drugs. In Riviere JE, Papich MG, editors: *Veterinary pharmacology and therapeutics*, ed 9, Ames, IA, 2009, Wiley-Blackwell.

Frank LA: Growth hormone-responsive alopecia in dogs, *J Am Vet Med Assoc* 226:1494, 2005.

Galler A, et al.: Inhaled budesonide therapy in cats with naturally occurring chronic bronchial disease (feline asthma and chronic bronchitis), *J Small Anim Pract* 54:531, 2013.

Glaze MB, et al.: Ophthalmic corticosteroid therapy: systemic effects in the dog, *J Am Vet Med Assoc* 192:73, 1988.

Goulding NJ, Flower RJ: Preface. In Goulding NJ, Flower RJ, editors: *Glucocorticoids*, Basel, 2000a, Springer Basel AG.

Goulding NJ, Flower RJ: Glucocorticoid biology—a molecular maze and clinical challenge. In Goulding NJ, Flower RJ, editors: *Glucocorticoids*, Basel, 2000b, Springer Basel AG.

Goy-Thollot I, et al.: Investigation of the role of aldosterone in hypertension associated with spontaneous pituitary-dependent hyperadrenocorticism in dogs, *J Small Anim Pract* 43:489, 2002.

Graham-Mize CA, Rosser EJ: Bioavailability and activity of prednisone and prednisolone in the feline patient, Plenary Session Abstracts, *Vet Dermatol* 15(Suppl. 1):9, 2004.

Greco CS, Behrend EN: Corticosteroid withdrawal syndrome. In Bonagura JD, editor: *Kirk's current veterinary therapy XII*, Philadelphia, 1995, Saunders/Elsevier.

Gregory CR: Results of clinical renal transplantation in 15 dogs using triple drug immunosuppressive therapy, *Vet Surg* 35:105, 2006.

Hall JE: Adrenocortical hormones. In Hall JE, editor: *Guyton and Hall textbook of medical physiology*, ed 12, Philadelphia, 2011, Saunders/Elsevier.

Hanson SM, et al.: Clinical evaluation of cimetidine, sucralfate, and misoprostol for prevention of gastrointestinal tract bleeding in dogs undergoing spinal surgery, *Am J Vet Res* 58:1320, 1997.

Hench P, et al.: The effects of a hormone of the adrenal cortex (17-hydroxy-11-dehydrocorticosterone; compound E) and of pituitary adrenocorticotropic hormone on rheumatoid arthritis, *Proc Staff Meet Mayo Clin* 24:181, 1949.

Hicks CW, et al.: Beneficial effects of stress-dose corticosteroid therapy in canines depend on the severity of staphylococcal pneumonia, *Intensive Care Med* 38:2063, 2012.

Hopper K, et al.: Outcome after renal transplantation in 26 dogs, *Vet Surg* 41:316, 2012.

Huang HP, et al.: Iatrogenic hyperadrenocorticism in 28 dogs, *J Am Anim Hosp Assoc* 35:200, 1999.

Javadi S, et al.: Plasma aldosterone concentrations and plasma renin activity in healthy dogs and dogs with hyperadrenocorticism, *Vet Rec* 153:521, 2003.

Jeffers JG, et al.: Diabetes mellitus induced in a dog after administration of corticosteroids and methylprednisolone pulse therapy, *J Am Vet Med Assoc* 199:77, 1991.

Jiang CL, et al.: Why do we need nongenomic glucocorticoid mechanisms? *Front Neuroendocrinol* 35:72, 2014.

Kemppainen RJ: Effects of glucocorticoids on endocrine function in the dog, *Vet Clin North Am Small Anim Pract* 14:721, 1984.

Kemppainen RJ, Sartin JL: Effects of single intravenous doses of dexamethasone on baseline plasma cortisol concentrations and responses to synthetic ACTH in healthy dogs, *Am J Vet Res* 45:742, 1984.

Kemppainen RJ, et al.: Adrenocortical suppression in the dog after a single dose of methylprednisolone acetate, *Am J Vet Res* 42:822, 1981.

Kemppainen RJ, et al.: Adrenocortical suppression in the dog given a single intramuscular dose of prednisone or triamcinolone acetonide, *Am J Vet Res* 42:204, 1982.

Kemppainen RJ, et al.: Effects of prednisone on thyroid and gonadal endocrine function in dogs, *J Endocrinol* 96:293, 1983.

Kendall EC: The development of cortisone as a therapeutic agent, *Nobel Lecture*, December 11, 1950. Nobelprize.org: (PDF online): http://www.nobelprize.org/nobel_prizes/medicine/laureates/1950/kendall-lecture.pdf. Accessed June 19, 2014.

Kimura T, et al.: Steroid administration and acute pancreatitis: studies with an isolated, perfused canine pancreas, *Surgery* 85:520, 1979.

Kovalik M, et al.: Short-term prednisolone therapy has minimal impact on calcium metabolism in dogs with atopic dermatitis, *Vet J* 193:439, 2012.

Lascelles BDX: Supportive care for the cancer patient. In Withrow SJ, Vail DM, Page RL, editors: *Withrow & MacEwen's small animal clinical oncology*, ed 5, St Louis, 2013, Elsevier/Saunders.

Lieberman PL: Recognition and first-line treatment of anaphylaxis, *Am J Med* 127:S6, 2014.

Lien YH, et al.: Iatrogenic hyperadrenocorticism in 12 cats, *J Am Anim Hosp Assoc* 42:414, 2006.

Liu Y, et al.: MAPK phosphatases—regulating the immune response, *Nat Rev Immunol* 7:202, 2007.

Lowe AD, et al.: Glucocorticoids in the cat, *Vet Dermatol* 19:340, 2008a.

Lowe AD, et al.: Clinical, clinicopathological and histological changes observed in 14 cats treated with glucocorticoids, *Vet Rec* 162:777, 2008b.

Lowe AD, et al.: A pilot study comparing the diabetogenic effects of dexamethasone and prednisolone in cats, *J Am Anim Hosp Assoc* 45:215, 2009.

Löwenberg M, et al.: Glucocorticoid signaling: a nongenomic mechanism for T-cell immunosuppression, *Trends Mol Med* 13:158, 2007.

Mansfield C: Acute pancreatitis in dogs: advances in understanding, diagnostics, and treatment, *Top Companion Anim Med* 27:123, 2012.

Martinez NI, et al.: Evaluation of pressor sensitivity to norepinephrine infusion in dogs with iatrogenic hyperadrenocorticism. Pressor sensitivity in dogs with hyperadrenocorticism, *Res Vet Sci* 78:25, 2005.

McMaster A, Ray DW: Modelling the glucocorticoid receptor and producing therapeutic agents with anti-inflammatory effects but reduced side-effects, *Exp Physiol* 92:299, 2007.

Mealey KL, et al.: Dexamethasone treatment of a canine, but not human, tumour cell line increases chemoresistance independent of P-glycoprotein and multidrug resistance-related protein expression, *Vet Comp Oncol* 1:67, 2003.

Meij BP, et al.: Alterations in anterior pituitary function of dogs with pituitary-dependent hyperadrenocorticism, *J Endocrinol* 154:505, 1997.

Mendelsohn C: Topical therapy for otitis externa. In Bonagura JD, Twedt DC, editors: *Kirk's current veterinary therapy*, ed 14, St Louis, 2009, Saunders/Elsevier.

Meyer DJ: Prolonged liver test abnormalities and adrenocortical suppression in a dog following a single intramuscular glucocorticoid dose, *J Am Anim Hosp Assoc* 18:725, 1982.

Meyer DJ, et al.: Effect of otic medications containing glucocorticoids on liver function test results in healthy dogs, *J Am Vet Med Assoc* 196:743, 1990.

Middleton DJ, Watson AD: Glucose intolerance in cats given short-term therapies of prednisolone and megestrol acetate, *Am J Vet Res* 46:2623, 1985.

Middleton DJ, et al.: Suppression of cortisol responses to exogenous adrenocorticotrophic hormone, and the occurrence of side effects attributable to glucocorticoid excess, in cats during therapy with megestrol acetate and prednisolone, *Can J Vet Res* 51:60, 1987.

Moore GE, Hoenig M: Duration of pituitary and adrenocortical suppression after long-term administration of anti-inflammatory doses of prednisone in dogs, *Am J Vet Res* 53:716, 1992.

Moore GE, Hoenig M: Effects of orally administered prednisone on glucose tolerance and insulin secretion in clinically normal dogs, *Am J Vet Res* 54:126, 1993.

Moore GE, et al.: Hematologic and serum biochemical effects of long-term administration of anti-inflammatory doses of prednisone in dogs, *Am J Vet Res* 53:1033, 1992.

Moore GE, et al.: Effects of oral administration of anti-inflammatory doses of prednisone on thyroid hormone response to thyrotropin-releasing hormone and thyrotropin in clinically normal dogs, *Am J Vet Res* 54:130, 1993.

Moore RW, Withrow SJ: Gastrointestinal hemorrhage and pancreatitis associated with intervertebral disk disease in the dog, *J Am Vet Med Assoc* 180:1443, 1982.

Neel JA, et al.: Thrombocytosis: a retrospective study of 165 dogs, *Vet Clin Pathol* 41:216, 2012.

Neiger R, et al.: Gastric mucosal lesions in dogs with acute intervertebral disc disease: characterization and effects of omeprazole or misoprostol, *J Vet Intern Med* 14:33, 2000.

Nitsche CJ, et al.: Drug induced pancreatitis, *Best Pract Res Clin Gastroenterol* 24:143, 2010.

Nixon M, et al.: It takes two to tango: dimerisation of glucocorticoid receptor and its anti-inflammatory functions, *Steroids* 78:59, 2013.

Padrid P: Use of inhaled medications to treat respiratory diseases in dogs and cats, *J Am Anim Hosp Assoc* 42:165, 2006.

Papich MG, Davis LE: Glucocorticoid therapy. In Kirk RW, editor: *Current veterinary therapy X: small animal practice*, Philadelphia, 1989, Saunders/Elsevier.

Parent J: Effects of dexamethasone on pancreatic tissue and on serum amylase and lipase activities in dogs, *J Am Vet Med Assoc* 180:743, 1982.

Parente L: The development of synthetic glucocorticoids. In Goulding NJ, Flower RJ, editors: *Glucocorticoids*, Basel, 2000, Springer Basel AG.

Park EH, et al.: Mechanisms of injury and emergency care of acute spinal cord injury in dogs and cats, *J Vet Emerg Crit Care* 22:160, 2012.

Peterson ME, et al.: Effects of spontaneous hyperadrenocorticism on serum thyroid hormone concentrations in the dog, *Am J Vet Res* 45:2034, 1984.

Pey P, et al.: Effect of glucocorticoid administration on adrenal gland size and sonographic appearance in beagle dogs, *Vet Radiol Ultrasound* 53:204, 2012.

Pietra M, et al.: Plasma concentrations and therapeutic effects of budesonide in dogs with inflammatory bowel disease, *Am J Vet Res* 74:78, 2013.

Plumb DC, editor: *Plumb's veterinary drug handbook*, ed 7, Ames, IA, 2011, Wiley-Blackwell.

Ramsey IK, et al.: Hyperparathyroidism in dogs with hyperadrenocorticism, *J Small Anim Pract* 46:531, 2005.

Reinero CR, et al.: Inhaled flunisolide suppresses the hypothalamic-pituitary-adrenocortical axis, but has minimal systemic immune effects in healthy cats, *J Vet Intern Med* 20:57, 2006.

Reusch CE, et al.: Endocrine hypertension in small animals, *Vet Clin North Am Small Anim Pract* 40:335, 2010.

Rhen T, Cidlowski JA: Antiinflammatory action of glucocorticoids—new mechanisms for old drugs, *N Engl J Med* 353:1711, 2005.

Roberts SM, et al.: Effect of ophthalmic prednisolone acetate on the canine adrenal gland and hepatic function, *Am J Vet Res* 45:1711, 1984.

Rohrer CR, et al.: Gastric hemorrhage in dogs given high doses of methylprednisolone sodium succinate, *Am J Vet Res* 60:977, 1999a.

Rohrer CR, et al.: Efficacy of misoprostol in prevention of gastric hemorrhage in dogs treated with high doses of methylprednisolone sodium succinate, *Am J Vet Res* 60:982, 1999b.

Rougier S, et al.: A comparative study of two antimicrobial/anti-inflammatory formulations in the treatment of canine otitis externa, *Vet Dermatol* 16:299, 2005.

Ruiz P, et al.: In vivo glucocorticoid modulation of guinea pig splenic macrophage Fc gamma receptors, *J Clin Invest* 88:149, 1991.

Schaer M, Ginn PE: Iatrogenic Cushing's syndrome and steroid hepatopathy in a cat, *J Am Anim Hosp Assoc* 35:48, 1999.

Schultze AE: Interpretation of canine leukocyte responses. Interpretation of feline leukocyte response. In Weiss DJ, Wardrop KJ, editors: *Schalm's veterinary hematology*, ed 6, Ames, IA, 2010, Wiley-Blackwell.

Scott DW: Some effects of short-term methylprednisolone therapy in normal cats, *Cornell Vet* 69:104, 1979.

Scott DW, et al.: Iatrogenic Cushing's syndrome in the cat, *Feline Pract* 12:30, 1982.

Sharkey LC, et al.: Effects of a single injection of methylprednisolone acetate on serum biochemical parameters in 11 cats, *Vet Clin Pathol* 36:184, 2007.

Shmuel DL, Cortes Y: Anaphylaxis in dogs and cats, *J Vet Emerg Crit Care* 23:377, 2013.

Sligl WI, et al.: Safety and efficacy of corticosteroids for the treatment of septic shock: a systematic review and meta-analysis, *Clin Infect Dis* 49:93, 2009.

Solter PF, et al.: Hepatic total 3α-hydroxy bile acids concentration and enzyme activities in prednisone-treated dogs, *Am J Vet Res* 55:1086, 1994.

Sorjonen DC, et al.: Effects of dexamethasone and surgical hypotension on the stomach of dogs: clinical, endoscopic, and pathologic evaluations, *Am J Vet Res* 44:1233, 1983.

Stahn C, et al.: Molecular mechanisms of glucocorticoid action and selective glucocorticoid receptor agonists, *Mol Cell Endocrinol* 275:71, 2007.

Steiner JM, et al.: Stability of canine pancreatic lipase immunoreactivity concentration in serum samples and effects of long-term administration of prednisone to dogs on serum canine pancreatic lipase immunoreactivity concentrations, *Am J Vet Res* 70:1001, 2009.

Steinfelder HJ, Oetjen E: Nebennierenrindenhormone. In Aktories K, Foerstermann U, Hofmann F, Starke K, editors: *Allgemeine und spezielle Pharmakologie und Toxikologie*, ed 10, 2009, Elsevier Urban & Fischer.

Stewart PM, Krone NP: The adrenal cortex. In Melmed S, Polonsky K, Larsen PR, Kronenberger HM, editors: *Williams textbook of endocrinology*, ed 12, Philadelphia, 2011, Elsevier/Saunders.

Tizard IR: Drugs and other agents that affect the immune system. In Tizard IR, editor: *Veterinary immunology*, ed 9, St Louis, 2013, Elsevier/Saunders.

Toombs JP, et al.: Colonic perforation in corticosteroid-treated dogs, *J Am Vet Med Assoc* 188:145, 1986.

Torres SM, et al.: Effect of oral administration of prednisolone on thyroid function in dogs, *Am J Vet Res* 52:416, 1991.

Tumulty JW, et al.: Clinical effects of short-term oral budesonide on the hypothalamic-pituitary-adrenal axis in dogs with inflammatory bowel disease, *J Am Anim Hosp Assoc* 40:120, 2004.

Ungemach FR: Pharmaka zur Beeinflussung von Entzündungen. In Loescher W, Ungemach FR, Kroker R, editors: *Pharmakotherapie bei Haus- und Nutztieren*, ed 8, Stuttgart, 2010, Enke Verlag.

Vail DM, et al.: Hematopoietic tumors. In Withrow SJ, Vail DM, Page RL, editors: *Withrow & MacEwen's small animal clinical oncology*, ed 5, St Louis, 2013, Elsevier/Saunders.

Valenciano AC, et al.: Interpretation of feline leukocyte response. In Weiss DJ, Wardrop KJ, editors: *Schalm's veterinary hematology*, ed 6, Ames, IA, 2010, Wiley-Blackwell.

van Brussel MS, et al.: Prevention of glucocorticoid-induced osteoporosis, *Expert Opin Pharmacother* 10:997, 2009.

van den Broek AH, Stafford WL: Epidermal and hepatic glucocorticoid receptors in cats and dogs, *Res Vet Sci* 52:312, 1992.

Vandevyver S, et al.: New insights into the anti-inflammatory mechanisms of glucocorticoids: an emerging role for glucocorticoid-receptor-mediated transactivation, *Endocrinol* 154:993, 2013.

Viviano KR: Update on immunosuppressive therapies for dogs and cats, *Vet Clin Small Anim* 43:1149, 2013.

Vollmar A, Dingermann T: Immunosuppressiva. In Vollmar A, Dingermann T, editors: *Immunologie, Grundlagen und Wirkstoffe*, Stuttgart, 2005, Wissenschaftliche Verlagsgesellschaft.

von Lindern M, et al.: The glucocorticoid receptor cooperates with the erythropoietin receptor and c-Kit to enhance and sustain proliferation of erythroid progenitors in vitro, *Blood* 94:550, 1999.

Wenger M, et al.: Effect of trilostane on serum concentrations of aldosterone, cortisol, and potassium in dogs with pituitary-dependent hyperadrenocorticism, *Am J Vet Res* 65:1245, 2004.

Whitley NT, Day MJ: Immunomodulatory drugs and their application to the management of canine immune-mediated disease, *J Small Anim Pract* 52:670, 2011.

Wolfsheimer KJ, et al.: Effects of prednisolone on glucose tolerance and insulin secretion in the dog, *Am J Vet Res* 47:1011, 1986.

Zandvliet M, et al.: Prednisolone inclusion in a first-line multidrug cytostatic protocol for the treatment of canine lymphoma does not affect therapy results, *Vet J* 197:656, 2013.

Zenoble RD, Kemppainen RJ: Adrenocortical suppression by topically applied corticosteroids in healthy dogs, *J Am Vet Med Assoc* 191:685, 1987.

CHAPTER CONTENTS

CALCIUM REGULATION AND HYPERCALCEMIA

 ## CALCIUM FUNCTION AND CONTROL

Overview

Calcium serves two principal physiologic functions. First, insoluble calcium salts (primarily hydroxyapatite) provide the structural characteristics that allow bones to protect internal organs and bear weight. Second, soluble calcium ions in the extracellular fluid (ECF) and cytosol are critically important for a myriad of biochemical intracellular and extracellular functions. For example, calcium is necessary for various enzymatic reactions, transport of substances across membranes and membrane stability, blood coagulation, nerve conduction, neuromuscular transmission, muscle contraction, smooth muscle tone, hormone secretion, bone formation, hepatic glycogen metabolism, cell growth, and cell division (Rasmussen, 1989; Brown et al, 1995; Rosol et al, 2000; Wysolmerski and Insogna, 2012). Approximately 1% of total body calcium is contained within the ECF and soft tissue, 99% is found in bone. The skeleton, therefore, is a reservoir of available calcium when ECF concentrations decline, and it acts as a storehouse for excess calcium. About 50% of circulating calcium (0.5% of total body calcium) is bound to serum proteins, primarily albumin, and to a

lesser extent, complexed with anions, such as citrate or sulfate. The remaining 50% is in the ionized biologically active form (Fig. 15-1).

The concentration of serum ionized calcium (iCa) and the calcium content of skeleton is maintained within narrow limits by a complicated homeostatic system involving multiple organs and several hormones. The organs involved in the regulation of calcium metabolism are the parathyroid glands, kidneys, skeleton, and gut (Fig. 15-2). The hormones include parathyroid hormone (PTH), vitamin D, and PTH-related protein (PTHrP). The actions of PTH on bone resorption, renal calcium excretion, and metabolism of vitamin D are responsible for maintaining homeostasis (Fig. 15-3; Table 15-1). Abnormalities in any of these organs, hormones, or receptors may cause disturbances in calcium metabolism that can lead to hypercalcemia or hypocalcemia.

Parathyroid Hormone

PTH is an 84–amino acid, single-chain polypeptide, synthesized, stored, and secreted by chief cells in the four parathyroid glands (Fig. 15-4). PTH is synthesized initially as a single-chain, preproparathyroid peptide. The 25 residue presequence is cleaved twice to generate the biologically active full-length protein (PTH 1-84). PTH has a half-life of minutes in circulation and is degraded in the liver and kidneys. The degradative process releases carboxyterminal (C-terminal) fragments of PTH into the circulation. In

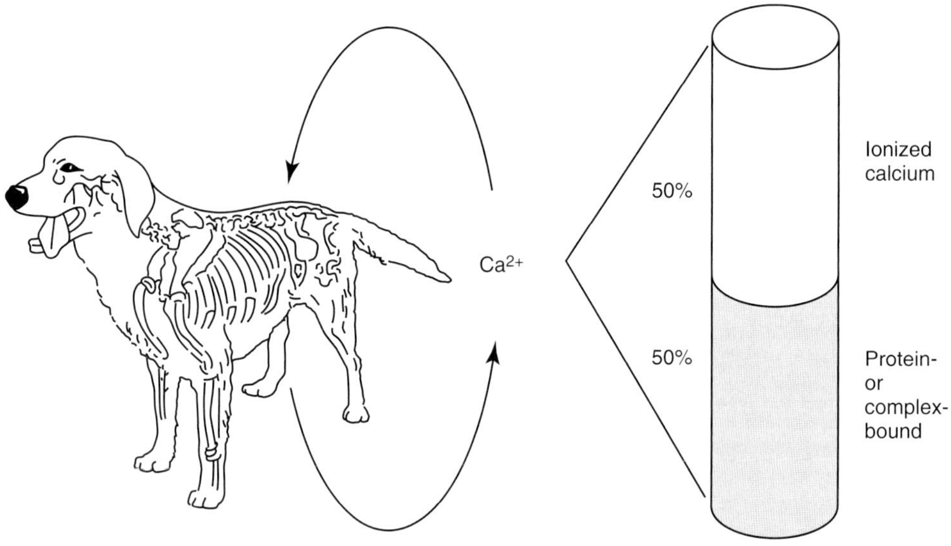

FIGURE 15-1 Skeletal calcium acts as a reservoir so that calcium can be stored or mobilized, depending on need. (From Skelly BJ: Hyperparathyroidism. In Mooney CT, Peterson ME, editors: *BSAVA manual of canine and feline endocrinology,* ed 4, Gloucester, England, 2012, British Small Animal Veterinary Association; used with permission.)

Ca²⁺

Ionized calcium

50%

50%

Protein- or complex-bound

response to subtle hypercalcemia, proteases found within parathyroid secretory granules digest the amino-terminal portions of PTH, leaving the inactive C-terminal fragments to be secreted. Thus, biologically inactive C-terminal fragments, known to accumulate in the circulation of patients with chronic kidney disease (CKD), are a product of both parathyroid secretion and peripheral metabolism of full-length PTH (Wysolmerski and Insogna, 2012).

PTH secretion is regulated by the extracellular iCa concentration. A steep inverse sigmoidal relationship exists between PTH secretion and calcium concentration. The steep portion of this curve encompasses the normal physiologic range for extracellular calcium, over which small changes in serum concentrations of iCa elicit large changes in the rate of PTH secretion. Increased serum calcium concentrations inhibit secretion of PTH and decreased concentrations stimulate PTH synthesis and secretion (Aurbach et al, 1985; Brown et al, 1999; see Fig. 15-3). For parathyroid cells to regulate PTH secretion, they must sense changes in extracellular calcium concentration. This is accomplished through a G protein-coupled receptor (GPCR) known as the *calcium-sensing receptor (CaR)*. Calcium

binding to the CaR activates downstream signaling pathways, primarily induction of phospholipases, and intracellular calcium transients (Stewart, 2004). This, in turn, suppresses PTH secretion. In addition to parathyroid cells, the CaR is prominently expressed in kidneys, where they regulate the calcium handling by renal tubules. Subtle hypercalcemia activates the CaR, suppressing renal calcium reabsorption. In this manner, hypercalcemia directly promotes calcium excretion in urine, and hypocalcemia directly enhances its reabsorption (Wysolmerski and Insogna, 2012; see Fig. 15-2).

The actions of PTH are mediated by the type 1 PTH/PTHrP receptor (PTH1R). The calcium-regulating effects of the receptor appear to be primarily the result of activating adenylyl cyclase. During usual conditions, this receptor is activated equally well by the amino-terminal portions of PTH and PTHrP (see later). The PTH1P is most abundant in bone and kidney, where it mediates the systemic functions of PTH. However, PTH1P is also expressed in cells throughout the body, where it serves as a PTHrP receptor. In this capacity, PTH1P has important functions during bone development, and it mediates many of PTHrP's effects on

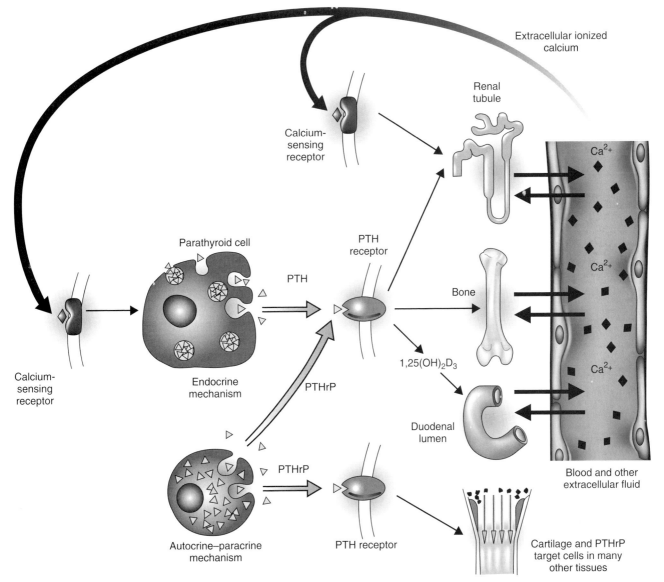

FIGURE 15-2 The parathyroid axis. The synthesis of parathyroid hormone *(PTH)* and parathyroid hormone–related protein *(PTHrP)* is shown on the left and the target sites on the right. Both act by means of the same receptor (also called the *type 1 receptor*). Negative feedback of 1,25-dihydroxyvitamin D_3—*1,25(OH)$_2$D$_3$*—is not shown. (Modified from Marx SJ: Hyperparathyroid and hypoparathyroid disorders, *N Engl J Med* 343:1863, 2000.)

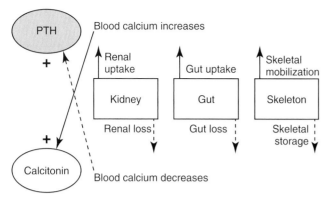

FIGURE 15-3 Calcium homeostasis. The release of parathyroid hormone *(PTH)* causes increased uptake of calcium in the kidney and gut and mobilization from the skeleton. (From Skelly BJ: Hyperparathyroidism. In Mooney CT, Peterson ME, editors: *BSAVA manual of canine and feline endocrinology,* ed 4, Gloucester, England, 2012, British Small Animal Veterinary Association; used with permission.)

TABLE 15-1	**APPROXIMATE REFERENCE INTERVALS FOR SERUM CONCENTRATIONS OF TOTAL CALCIUM, IONIZED CALCIUM, PARATHYROID HORMONE, PARATHYROID HORMONE–RELATED PROTEIN, AND CALCITRIOL**

	DOG	**CAT**
Total calcium (TCa)		
(mg/dL)	9.0-11.7	8.0-10.5
(mmol/L)	2.2-2.9	2.0-2.6
Ionized calcium (iCa)		
(mg/dL)	4.6-5.6	4.5-5.5
(mmol/L)	1.1-1.4	1.1-1.4
Parathyroid hormone (PTH) (variability among laboratories)		
(pmol/L)	0.5-5.8	0-4
(pg/mL)		6-16*
Parathyroid hormone–related protein (PTHrP)		
(pmol/L)	< 2	< 2
1,25-Dihydroxyvitamin D_3 (calcitriol) (pg/mL)		
Adults	20-50[†]	20-40[†]
10 to 12 weeks old (pg/mL)	60-120[†]	20-80[†]

*From Pineda et al.: Feline parathyroid hormone: validation of hormonal assays and dynamics of secretion, *Domest Anim Endocrinol* 42:256, 2012.
[†]From Rosol et al.: Disorders of calcium. In DiBartola SP, editor: *Fluid therapy in small animal practice,* ed 2, Philadelphia, 2000, WB Saunders, pp. 108-162.

cellular proliferation, apoptosis, and differentiation (Wysolmerski and Insogna, 2012).

The amino acid sequence of PTH is known for humans, dogs, cows, pigs, rats, chickens, and cats. Based on immunologic reactivities, most mammals appear to have similar amino-terminal portions of the molecule (Toribio et al, 2002). It is recognized that the amino terminal of PTH binds to CaR, whereas the carboxyl

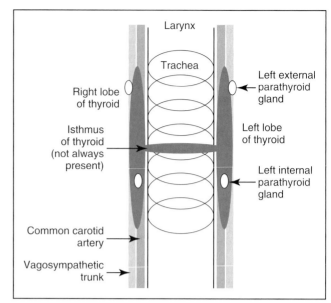

FIGURE 15-4 Schematic representation of the anatomical position of the parathyroid glands. (From Skelly BJ: Hyperparathyroidism. In Mooney CT, Peterson ME, editors: *BSAVA manual of canine and feline endocrinology,* ed 4, Gloucester, England, 2012, British Small Animal Veterinary Association; used with permission.)

terminus is thought to serve only as a guide for PTH through the cellular secretory pathway (Orloff and Stewart, 1995). A synthetic 1-34 amino-terminal fragment is biologically active, but relatively minor modifications, especially at the first two residues, can completely abolish this effect (Marx, 2000).

Parathyroid Hormone–Related Protein

PTHrP was discovered in the course of exploring the pathogenesis of humoral hypercalcemia of malignancy (HHM). PTH and PTHrP share structural features suggesting that they arose from a common ancestor: in people eight of the first 13 amino-terminal amino acids are identical. This amino-terminal homology allows both PTH and PTHrP to bind to the receptor PTH1P with equal affinity, thereby activating the same pathways. PTH is made only in parathyroid glands and is secreted into the circulation. PTHrP is synthesized in many cells, is secreted locally, and acts in a paracrine or autocrine fashion to activate PTH1P on neighboring cells. In veterinary medicine, PTHrP is best recognized as having a central role in the pathogenesis of HHM and is used as a "tumor marker" in both dogs and cats (Williams et al, 2003; Henry, 2010). Since its discovery in the early 1980s, assay of PTHrP has been used in the evaluation of hypercalcemic patients in whom cancer is a possibility (Philbrick et al, 1996).

Vitamin D

Inactive vitamin D is produced in skin and is available in some foods. It appears that dogs are less able to synthesize vitamin D in the skin than are other mammals (Gross et al, 2000; Mellanby et al, 2005). Thus, dogs have a greater requirement for dietary vitamin D. PTH stimulates activity of renal enzymes responsible for synthesizing biologically-active 1,25-dihydroxyvitamin D_3 $(1,25[OH]_2D_3)$, also known as calcitriol. The main function of vitamin D is to support circulating calcium concentrations. Vitamin D stimulates calcium (and phosphorus) absorption from the gut lumen by enterocytes, and it stimulates bone resorption via osteoblastic release of cytokines (see Figs. 15-2 and 15-3).

PATHOPHYSIOLOGY OF PRIMARY HYPERPARATHYROIDISM

Introduction: Extensive Effects of Excess PTH

Hypercalcemia in primary hyperparathyroidism (PHPTH) is the result of PTH inducing osteoclast-mediated bone resorption, stimulating intestinal absorption of calcium, and stimulating renal tubular resorption of calcium (Mundy, 1988; Hruska and Teitelbaum, 1995).

Kidney

In the setting of accelerated bone resorption, the kidneys become the principal defense against hypercalcemia (Bilezikian, 1992a; Hruska and Teitelbaum, 1995). In the kidney, PTH has three principal effects. First, PTH acts on proximal tubules to inhibit reabsorption of phosphate. Second, it stimulates the activity of renal 1α-hydroxylase in proximal tubular cells leading to formation of biologically active $1,25(OH)_2D_3$ from its circulating precursor 25-hydroxyvitamin D (25[OH]D) (also known as calcidiol) while inhibiting synthesis of inactive vitamin D forms. Third, PTH increases kidney calcium reabsorption. Most calcium is reclaimed from glomerular filtrate in the proximal tubules via a PTH-independent process. The primary target of PTH's action to promote calcium reabsorption is in distal tubules, where it stimulates directional, transcellular calcium transport from the tubule lumen, across the cell, and into the ECF. Early in the course of PHPTH, when hypercalcemia is mild, urinary calcium excretion is relatively low. PTH action, at the renal level, enhances tubular resorption of calcium. When serum calcium concentrations are greater than 12 to 14 mg/dL, the renal tubular mechanism for reabsorbing calcium becomes overwhelmed. Here, the kidney's adaptive mechanism for correcting hypercalcemia becomes operative despite excessive concentrations of PTH. This hypercalciuria, however, is not sufficient to correct the hypercalcemia but can lead to nephrocalcinosis. Nephrocalcinosis may be mild and reversible or severe and progressive, leading to continued renal damage and uremia. Most dogs with PHPTH have normal blood urea nitrogen (BUN) and serum creatinine concentrations. As has been described in people with PHPTH untreated for as many as 10 years, virtually no changes in serum renal or other biochemical profiles (aside from increasing calcium and decreasing phosphate concentrations) are noted (Silverberg et al, 1999).

Bone

In the skeleton, PTH activates bone turnover and liberates stored calcium. The immediate action of PTH is to stimulate the transport of calcium across bone lining cells from an easily mobilized pool of calcium at the bone surface (Attie, 1989). The activity of these cells, caused by PTH or PTHrP, is the foundation for virtually all cases of marked hypercalcemia. Associated with accelerated osteocytic and osteoclastic bone resorption, mineral is removed and replaced by immature fibrous connective tissue. The bone lesion of fibrous osteodystrophy in afflicted dogs is reported to be generalized throughout the skeleton but accentuated in certain areas, such as the cancellous bone of the skull (Capen and Martin, 1983). Iliac crest bone biopsies from virtually all humans with PHPTH reveal histomorphometric evidence of the effects of excess PTH (Arnaud and Kolb, 1991; Hruska and Teitelbaum, 1995). These findings may include increased bone resorption surfaces, increased numbers of osteoclasts, osteocytic osteolysis, and marrow fibrosis. Bone histomorphometric findings in dogs with PHPTH were similar to those reported in humans (i.e., parallel increases in osteoblastic and osteoclastic activity) (Meuten et al, 1983a; Weir et al, 1986). Excessive absorption of calcium from the gastrointestinal tract is not usually an important cause of hypercalcemia, although it is a contributor to the hypercalcemia resulting from vitamin D toxicosis.

Uroliths and Urinary Tract Infections

Hypercalciuria resulting from PHPTH is a cause of the urolithiasis and urinary tract infections that are "common" with this disorder. The incidence of urinary tract infection is about 20% to 30% of afflicted dogs and about 25% to 40% have urinary calculi (Berger and Feldman, 1987; Klausner et al, 1987). Hypercalciuria from increased glomerular filtration of calcium predisposes individuals to urolithiasis. Additional factors may play a role in urolith formation or urinary solute saturation, including pH, ionic strength, and crystal aggregation inhibitors. Calcium phosphate, for example, is markedly less soluble in alkaline urine than in acidic urine. Other hypercalcemic conditions are not usually associated with urolithiasis. This discrepancy may be explained, perhaps, by the chronic nature of the hypercalcemia in dogs with PHPTH as opposed to the short-term nature of hypercalcemia in dogs with neoplasia, toxin exposure, and other such conditions. In these other conditions, dogs tend to develop their clinical signs quickly, which either resolve or worsen in the short-term.

In PHPTH, hypercalcemia is aggravated by increased production of vitamin D and decreased amount of serum phosphate available to form complexes with serum iCa. The result is decreased tubular resorption of phosphate, hyperphosphaturia, and hypophosphatemia. These actions are responsible for the development of the biochemical triad classic for PHPTH: hypercalcemia, hypophosphatemia, and hyperphosphaturia. Vitamin D deficiency, after chronic PTH-stimulated use of vitamin D stores, is a possible natural adaptive mechanism to PHPTH in people. People with vitamin D deficiency caused by PHPTH may develop osteomalacia, a problem considered uncommon or not clinically relevant in animals (Meuten et al, 1983a; Weir et al, 1986).

Calcitonin

Calcitonin, a 32–amino acid polypeptide hormone produced by parafollicular or "C cells" located in the thyroid, is secreted in response to increases in serum calcium (Mol et al, 1991). This hormone has the primary responsibility of limiting postprandial hypercalcemia in normal mammals. Calcitonin decreases bone resorption by reducing the size of osteoclast brush borders, the number of osteoclasts, and osteoclast motility. Calcitonin does not affect the kidney or intestine. It may, however, influence the satiety center, decreasing appetite. The role of calcitonin in dogs with PHPTH is not known. Increased calcitonin secretion in response to hypercalcemia seems a reasonable physiologic response. Parafollicular cells are markedly hyperplastic and appear as small white foci in the thyroid gland of dogs with PHPTH (Capen and Martin, 1983). Hyperplastic parafollicular cells may displace colloid-containing follicles lined by thyroid follicular cells, implying the presence of an adaptive response by the parafollicular cells. Studies in humans suggest that this adaptive mechanism is inconsistent (Arnaud and Kolb, 1991).

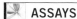 **ASSAYS**

Total Calcium

Serum or heparinized plasma samples are suitable for routine analysis of total calcium (TCa). Fasted blood samples may reduce problems with lipemia. Mean serum TCa concentrations in healthy mature dogs is about 10.5 mg/dL (reference interval of about 9.6 to 11.6 mg/dL; 2.4 to 2.9 mmol/L). Results from healthy cats are usually slightly lower. Dogs younger than 3 months of age have slightly higher results than dogs older than 1 year (Schenck and Chew, 2012). Oxalate, citrate, and ethylenediaminetetraacetic acid (EDTA) anticoagulants should not be used because they bind calcium. Calcium status of dogs and cats is often initially based on the *total* concentration because this is the result provided in most general biochemistry "profiles." Estimation of iCa based on the TCa is not a perfect science. For example, when estimating the iCa based on the TCa in dogs, there is a tendency to overestimate the number of normocalcemic patients and underestimate those with hypocalcemia. In cats, using the TCa to estimate the iCa tends to underestimate normocalcemia and hypercalcemia, overestimating hypocalcemia (Schenck and Chew, 2005a; 2005b). Adjustment formulas previously used to predict the iCa are not recommended (Schenck and Chew, 2012). Because iCa is available to most veterinary clinicians, it is wise to assess the iCa directly whenever there is suspicion of a calcium imbalance.

Ionized Calcium

Typically, serum is analyzed for iCa measurement, but heparinized plasma or whole blood can be used. Results from heparinized whole blood samples tend to be lower than results using serum (Schenck and Chew, 2008). The analysis of serum eliminates potential interference by heparin and allows longer storage periods. Silicone separator tubes should not be used. Analysis utilizing an ion-selective electrode allows easy and accurate measurement. Serum iCa concentration in healthy adult dogs and cats is about 1.1 to 1.4 mmol/L. Young dogs and cats have slightly higher values. Accurate determination of iCa requires that samples be collected and processed correctly. Therefore, adhering to laboratory protocol is imperative.

Parathyroid Hormone

The development of an assay for serum PTH in 1963 by Berson and colleagues was a major breakthrough in the diagnosis of human parathyroid disorders. It is now appreciated that complete (84–amino acid) molecules of PTH and numerous incomplete "pieces" of PTH are found in the circulation of all animals. Primary bioactivity resides in the intact molecule, the major secretory product of parathyroid glands (see Fig. 15-4). Excellent valid assays are available for PTH in dogs and cats. It is imperative for clinicians to follow their laboratories' protocols regarding sample collection and processing, usually including shipping samples on ice (Torrance and Nachreiner, 1989a; 1989b). Development of the "two-site" PTH assay system used by many laboratories depended on production of two different polyclonal antibodies. The two-site immunoradiometric assay (IRMA) system for intact human PTH was demonstrated to be valid for measurement of dog and cat PTH (Torrance and Nachreiner, 1989a; Flanders and Reimers, 1991; Barber et al, 1993). One antibody binds only the midregion and C-terminal 39-84 amino acids of human PTH. The other antibody binds only the N-terminal amino acids of human PTH. Samples being assayed are incubated simultaneously with

both antibodies, with a "sandwich" comprised of the N-terminal antibody plus the patient's intact hormone plus the 39-84 antibody. Only these "sandwiches" are detected by the assay system, eliminating interference by midregion or C-terminal fragments, even if present in large concentrations. These assays usually require several days to receive results.

Two-site immunochemiluminometric assays for intact PTH in humans use similar antibodies and a similar range of applicability to animal sera (Michelangeli et al, 1997; Estepa et al, 2003). One chemiluminescent PTH assay system required only about 20 minutes to perform, making this method potentially of use during surgery (Bilezikian et al, 2001; Ham et al, 2009; Cortadellas et al, 2010). As can be appreciated, assay systems often become unavailable for various reasons. A whole intact molecule PTH assay system is now being used that has lower reference values, but good correlation with previously-used systems (Refsal and Nachreiner, 2012). Currently, enzyme-linked immunosorbent assay (ELISA) is the most common assay used to measure PTH in the Great Britain and Europe. A canine-specific intact ELISA, which is also validated for cats, is available (Skelly, 2012). Reference intervals and units used in reporting results vary among laboratories, necessitating good communication to avoid confusion. Assay of 1-84 amino acid PTH is now considered to be most reliable (Gao et al, 2001).

Determination of the serum PTH concentration is a useful diagnostic aid in the evaluation of dogs and cats suspected of having parathyroid disease. As with most hormone assays, evaluation of the serum hormone concentration "out of context" is not as consistently informative as evaluation in the proper context is. With this in mind, the serum PTH concentration must be evaluated relative to the total and, ideally, ionized serum calcium concentrations. Decreases in the serum calcium concentration are normally associated with increases in the serum PTH concentration. Increases in the serum calcium concentration are normally associated with decreases in the PTH concentration (Fig. 15-5). As with any laboratory value, a single PTH result may not be the "expected" value. Therefore practitioners are encouraged to complete a thorough evaluation of hypercalcemic dogs or cats. If any test result does not seem logical, it may need to be repeated. Serum hormone concentrations may fluctuate significantly.

Vitamin D

Measurement of vitamin D metabolites, although not commonly used in veterinary medicine, would occasionally be helpful in the diagnosis of calcium disorders. 25(OH)D (calcidiol) and $1,25(OH)_2D_3$ (calcitriol) are the metabolites of greatest clinical interest for detection of hypovitaminosis or hypervitaminosis D syndromes and in CKD (Carothers et al, 1994). These metabolites are stable during refrigeration and freezing, but samples should not be exposed to light for any length of time. Both metabolites are chemically identical among species, therefore receptor-binding assays or radioimmunoassays (RIAs) used for people may be satisfactory for dogs and cats (Hollis et al, 1996). Young growing individuals have higher calcitriol concentrations than adults.

Calcitriol assays have demonstrated genetic errors of vitamin D metabolism and normal-to-increased concentrations in PHPTH, whereas patients with hypercalcemia of malignancy have levels that may be low, normal, or high. Dogs and cats with possible exposure to rat and mouse poisons containing vitamin D may present challenging diagnostic problems. Serum concentrations of vitamin D have been increased in these animals (Dougherty et al, 1990).

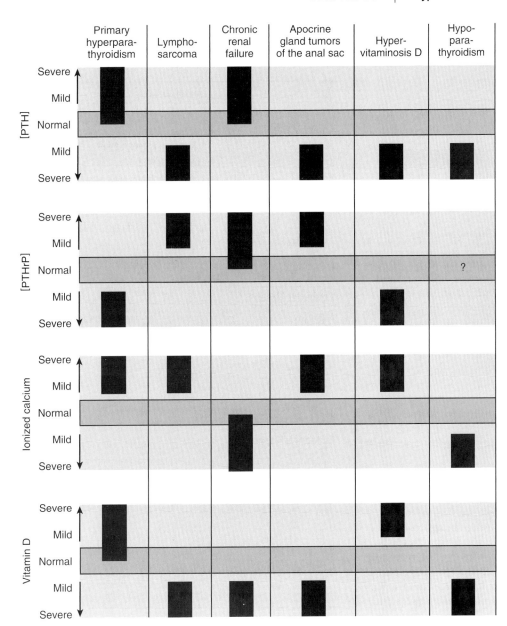

FIGURE 15-5 Graph showing the serum parathyroid hormone *(PTH)*, parathyroid hormone–related protein *(PTHrP)*, ionized calcium (iCa), and vitamin D concentrations in the most common causes for hypercalcemia of dogs.

Parathyroid Hormone–Related Protein

PTHrP resembles PTH not only in terms of its genetic sequence but also in terms of structure (Fig. 15-6); thus, PTHrP is a second member of the PTH family of hormones (Broadus and Stewart, 1994). In marked contrast to PTH, found only in parathyroid glands, PTHrP is found in many tissues (Table 15-2; Fig. 15-7) (Strewler, 2000). Two-site IRMA and N-terminal RIAs are available for the measurement of human PTHrP, and these same assay systems have been validated for the dog (Brown et al, 1987; Burtis, 1992). Because PTHrP is susceptible to degradation by serum proteases, assays should use fresh or frozen plasma using EDTA as anticoagulant. The EDTA complexes with plasma calcium, limiting the action of most proteases. The addition of protease inhibitors, such as aprotinin, may provide further protection. Use of serum is not recommended (Budayr et al, 1989; Henderson et al, 1990; Rosol et al, 2000). Valid assays for dog and cat PTHrP can be used to screen for certain cancers. Simultaneously assaying PTH and PTHrP in hypercalcemic dogs and cats has the potential to be a quick,

reliable, noninvasive, and inexpensive aide in distinguishing HHM from nonmalignant hypercalcemia. Animals with renal insufficiency may also have increased concentrations of PTHrP (see Fig. 15-5).

DIFFERENTIAL DIAGNOSIS OF HYPERCALCEMIA

See Box 15-1.

Primary Hyperparathyroidism

See the next section.

Hypercalcemia of Malignancy

General Overview

Malignancies are the most common causes of hypercalcemia in dogs and cats (Messinger et al, 2009). Neoplasms can cause hypercalcemia by several recognized physiologic processes (Fig. 15-8): HHM is caused by secretion of PTHrP, while some lymphomas

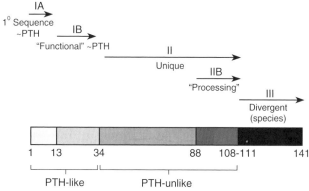

FIGURE 15-6 Structural and functional domains of parathyroid hormone–related protein (PTHrP). The 1 to 13 region of PTHrP is 70% homologous with the corresponding region of parathyroid hormone *(PTH)* and is believed to be involved in activation of adenylate cyclase and other second-messenger systems in target tissues. The 14 to 34 region shares no homology with the 14 to 34 region of PTH but has been shown to bind effectively to the PTH receptor. The 35 to 108 region of PTHrP is unique, sharing no homology with any other known peptide. This region is extraordinarily highly conserved among species, which suggests that it has a crucial but as yet unknown function or functions. The 88 to 108 region of the peptide is rich in potential proteolytic cleavage sites and contains several amidation signals and is therefore presumed to be the site of posttranslational processing, at least in some tissues. The 112 to 141 region of the peptide is poorly conserved among species. Preliminary evidence suggests that at least in some situations, C-terminal fragments derived from this region enter the circulation. The functional consequences of this are unknown. (From Broadus AE, et al.: Humoral hypercalcemia of cancer: identification of a novel parathyroid hormone-like peptide, *N Engl J Med* 319:556, 1988.)

synthesize vitamin D in addition to PTHrP. Hypercalcemia is then induced by marked increase in osteoclastic bone resorption in areas surrounding the malignant cells within the marrow (Rosol et al, 2000; Stewart, 2005). Ectopic PTH synthesis and secretion is a rare cause of hypercalcemia in people (Stewart, 2005). Some dogs with lymphosarcoma, apocrine gland carcinomas of the anal sac, or multiple myeloma are hypercalcemic. Some tumors that metastasize to bone can cause hypercalcemia through the induction of local bone resorption. These include malignancies of mammary tissue, prostate, liver, and lung. Primary bone tumors do not typically cause hypercalcemia. Hypercalcemia has been associated with nasal adenocarcinomas, thyroid carcinoma, thymoma, squamous cell carcinoma of the gastrointestinal system or vagina, and melanoma (Pressler et al, 2002; Schenck and Chew, 2012).

Humoral Hypercalcemia of Malignancy

Humoral Factors, Including Parathyroid Hormone–Related Protein. Tumor tissue at a site distant from bone may synthesize and secrete PTHrP, stimulating bone resorption, leading to hypercalcemia. Excessive secretion of biologically active PTHrP plays a central role in the pathogenesis of hypercalcemia in most forms of HHM. Cytokines, such as interleukin-1 (IL-1), tumor necrosis factor alpha (TNFα), transforming growth factor-a (TGF-a), transforming growth factor-b (TGF-b), or calcitriol, can have synergistic or cooperative actions with PTHrP (Fig. 15-9) (Rosol et al, 2000). PTHrP binds to the PTH1R, as described earlier. PTHrP, via interaction with PTH1R, stimulates osteoclastic bone resorption, increases renal tubular calcium resorption, and decreases renal tubular phosphate resorption. IL-1 and the transforming growth factors (TGFs) also have the potential to stimulate bone resorption (McCauley et al, 1991; Rosol et al,

TABLE 15-2	SITES AND PROPOSED ACTIONS OF PARATHYROID HORMONE–RELATED PROTEIN (PTHrP)
SITE	**PROPOSED ACTIONS**
Mesenchymal Tissues	
Cartilage	Promotes proliferation of chondrocytes; inhibits terminal differentiation and apoptosis of chondrocytes
Bone	Stimulates or inhibits bone resorption
Smooth muscle	Released in response to stretching; relaxes smooth muscle in the vascular system, myometrium, and urinary bladder
Cardiac muscle	Positive chronotropic stimulus; indirect positive inotropic stimulus
Skeletal muscle	Unknown
Epithelial Tissues	
Mammary	Induces branching morphogenesis; secreted in milk; possible roles in lactation
Epidermis	Unknown
Hair follicle	Inhibits anagen
Intestine	Unknown
Tooth enamel	Induces osteoclastic resorption of overlying bone
Endocrine Tissues	
Parathyroid glands	Stimulates placental transport of calcium (?)
Pancreatic islets	Stimulates insulin secretion and somatic growth
Pituitary	Unknown
Placenta	Calcium transport (?)
Central Nervous System (CNS)	Released from cerebellar granular neurons in response to activation of L-type calcium channels; receptors in cerebellum, hippocampus, hypothalamus

From Strewler GL: The physiology of parathyroid hormone–related protein, *N Engl J Med* 342:177, 2000.

2000). Identification of PTHrP provides an explanation of why some tumors (those that do not synthesize PTHrP) are not associated with hypercalcemia. PTHrP concentrations are abnormal usually only in individuals with malignancies and renal failure (see Fig. 15-5). Serum PTH concentrations in dogs with malignancy-associated hypercalcemia are typically low or undetectable. This should be seen as a normal response by the parathyroid glands to hypercalcemia. Assay of PTH and PTHrP concentrations should not be viewed as a replacement for a complete physical examination, thoracic radiography, abdominal ultrasonography, or any other key parameter used to identify neoplasia. These assay results are as integral as other components of an evaluation.

Hematopoietic Neoplasia. T cell lymphoma is the most common cause of hypercalcemia in dogs, accounting for almost 60% of dogs with hypercalcemia and almost 80% of dogs with hypercalcemia due to cancer (Messinger et al, 2009). Lymphoma afflicts dogs of any age and either sex. Approximately 20% to 40% of

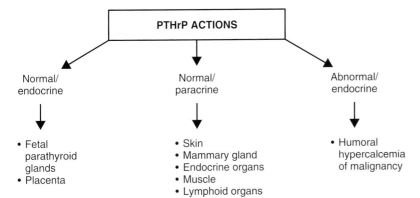

FIGURE 15-7 Actions of parathyroid hormone–related protein *(PTHrP).* (From Rosol TJ, et al.: Disorders of calcium. In DiBartola SP, editor: *Fluid therapy in small animal practice,* ed 2, Philadelphia, 2000, WB Saunders, pp. 108-162.)

BOX 15-1 Differential Diagnoses for Hypercalcemia

Non-Pathologic
Spurious, laboratory error
Young growing animal

Common
Lymphosarcoma
Hypoadrenocorticism
Primary hyperparathyroidism (PHPTH)
Chronic kidney disease (CKD)
Idiopathic hypercalcemia of cats (IHC)

Less Common
Apocrine gland carcinoma of the anal sac
Multiple myeloma
Vitamin D toxicosis
   Overzealous dietary supplementation
   Plants (calcitriol glycosides)
   Rodenticides (cholecalciferol)
   Anti-psoriasis creams (calcipotriol or calcipotriene)

Uncommon to Rare
Hemoconcentration, hyperproteinemia
Carcinomas
   Lung
   Mammary
   Nasal
   Pancreas
   Testicular
   Thymus
   Thyroid
   Vaginal
   Adrenal medullary
Melanoma
Acute kidney injury (AKI)
Hyperthyroidism
Nutritional secondary hyperparathyroidism
   (Serum calcium concentrations usually within reference intervals)
Granulomatous disease
   Blastomycosis
   Histoplasmosis
   Schistosomiasis
Hypervitaminosis A
Raisin/grape toxicity

Cancer-Associated Hypercalcemia

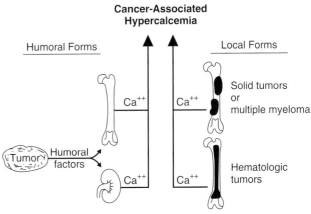

FIGURE 15-8 Pathogenesis of cancer-associated hypercalcemia. Humoral and local forms of cancer-associated hypercalcemia increase circulating concentrations of calcium by stimulating osteoclastic bone resorption and increased renal tubular resorption of calcium. (From Rosol TJ, et al.: Disorders of calcium. In DiBartola SP, editor: *Fluid therapy in small animal practice,* ed 2, Philadelphia, 2000, WB Saunders, pp. 108-162.)

dogs with lymphosarcoma are hypercalcemic (Weller et al, 1982; Matus et al, 1986; Rosol et al, 2000). Clinical signs may be subtle, moderate, or severe. About one-third of cats with lymphoma are hypercalcemic (Savary et al, 2000). Studies on affected dogs have demonstrated parameters consistent with influence by PTHrP, including increased fractional excretion of phosphorus, increased nephrogenous cyclic adenosine monophosphate (cAMP), and increased osteoclastic bone resorption. PTHrP appears to differ from natural PTH in its inability to stimulate renal formation of $1,25(OH)_2D_3$ and its lack of cross-reactivity with specific, two-site, intact PTH assays. A significant percentage of these dogs have increased serum concentrations of PTHrP (Fig. 15-10) (Weir et al, 1988a; 1988b; 1988c). Studies in cats have revealed similar findings (i.e., some cats with cancer have hypercalcemia secondary to tumor-synthesis and secretion of PTHrP). In seven cats with HHM and increases in serum or plasma PTHrP, one had lymphoma, four had lung carcinomas, one had a thyroid carcinoma, and one had an undifferentiated carcinoma. These authors demonstrated that IRMA assays for human 1-84 PTHrP can be used to measure PTHrP in cats and that malignancies in cats, particularly carcinomas, may secrete PTHrP and induce HHM in cats (Bollinger et al, 2002).

Humoral Factor and HHM

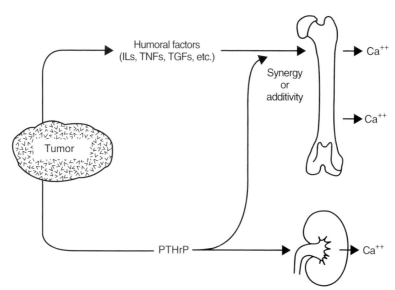

FIGURE 15-9 Humoral factors, such as parathyroid hormone–related protein *(PTHrP)*, interleukin-1 (IL-1), tumor necrosis factors *(TNFs)*, and transforming growth factors *(TGFs)* produced by tumors induce humoral hypercalcemia of malignancy *(HHM)* by acting as systemic hormones and stimulating osteoclastic bone resorption or by increasing tubular resorption of calcium. (From Rosol TJ, et al.: Disorders of calcium. In DiBartola SP, editor: *Fluid therapy in small animal practice,* ed 2, Philadelphia, 2000, WB Saunders, pp. 108-162.)

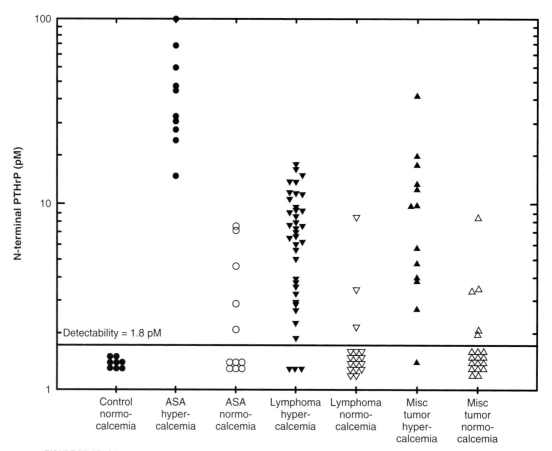

FIGURE 15-10 Circulating N-terminal parathyroid hormone–related protein *(PTHrP)* concentrations in normal dogs (control); dogs with hypercalcemia (>12 mg/dL) and anal sac adenocarcinoma *(ASA),* lymphoma, or miscellaneous tumors *(misc tumor);* and dogs with normocalcemia (< 12 mg/dL) and anal sac adenocarcinoma, lymphoma, or miscellaneous tumors. (From Rosol TJ, et al.: Disorders of calcium. In DiBartola SP, editor: *Fluid therapy in small animal practice,* ed 2, Philadelphia, 2000, WB Saunders, pp. 108-162.)

Lymphomas can synthesize vitamin D in addition to PTHrP, in which case afflicted patients would not only have the expected increases in serum PTHrP but also would have increased vitamin D concentrations (Seymour and Gagel, 1993). Some lymphocytes contain the 1α-hydroxylase (similar to that found in renal tubules) that converts 25(OH)D to the active metabolite, 1,25(OH)$_2$D$_3$ (Rosol et al, 2000). Therefore lymphomas that retain this capability may synthesize excessive amounts of calcitriol, which would increase calcium absorption from the intestinal tract and exacerbate the hypercalcemia resulting from PTHrP synthesis and secretion (see Figs. 15-1 and 15-5).

Although the clinical signs associated with lymphoma are variable, a dog with lymphoma and HHM is typically far more ill than dogs with PHPTH. Lymphoma must remain a possible explanation for hypercalcemia in any dog or cat until a different cause has been confirmed. Lymphosarcoma may or may not be apparent to the veterinarian during the physical examination. At least 40% of dogs with both lymphoma and HHM do not have peripheral lymph node, liver, spleen, or renal enlargement. Most of these dogs have a mediastinal mass, usually obvious on thoracic radiographs. The finding of a mediastinal mass in a dog with hypercalcemia should suggest a diagnosis of lymphoma, although other forms of neoplasia (e.g., thymoma) may account for both the mass and the hypercalcemia (Foley et al, 2000). In addition to lymphoma and thymoma, hypercalcemia due to HHM can be caused by melanoma, myeloma, or by carcinomas of the lung, pancreas, thyroid, skin, mammary gland, nasal cavity, or adrenal medulla. Concentrations of PTHrP are highest in dogs with apocrine gland carcinomas of the anal sac (Pressler et al, 2002; Williams et al, 2003; Schenck and Chew, 2012).

Apocrine Gland Adenocarcinoma of the Anal Sac. Adenocarcinomas of the anal sac represent a classic example of cancer associated hypercalcemia. Like lymphosarcoma, this neoplasm is known to synthesize PTHrP (Matus and Weir, 1989; Williams et al, 2003). This is a well-defined but relatively uncommon tumor of older dogs; their mean age at presentation is 10 to 11 years (range, 3 to 17 years) (Bennett et al, 2002). Slightly more than half of the dogs with this cancer were female. Dogs of almost any breed and mixed breed dogs can develop this condition (Ross et al, 1991; Goldschmidt and Shofer, 1992; Bennett et al, 2002; Williams et al, 2003). In one study, the serum calcium concentrations (upper reference value of 12.6 mg/dL) at the time of diagnosis ranged from 12.7 to 21.7 mg/dL (Bennett et al, 2002). Clinical signs associated with this condition include (among many owner observations) recognition of a mass near the rectum, tenesmus, poor appetite or anorexia, polyuria/polydipsia, and lethargy. HHM is reported in about 25% of dogs with apocrine gland carcinoma of the anal sac (Ross et al, 1991; Williams et al, 2003).

Local reappearance of the cancer or metastasis causes recurrence of hypercalcemia if surgery resulted in transient resolution. Dogs afflicted with this form of cancer have increases in urinary cAMP and fractional phosphorus excretion. Serum PTH concentrations are suppressed, PTHrP concentrations are excessive, bone histomorphometry reveals increased bone resorption, and there is no compensatory increase in formation. These changes are consistent with excesses in PTH or PTHrP (Meuten et al, 1983b). Apocrine gland adenocarcinoma cell lines established in mice have also demonstrated potential factors responsible for HHM, although only PTHrP is increased in the serum (Grone et al, 1998). This form of malignancy carries a guarded prognosis (Rosol et al, 1992a; 1992b; Williams et al, 2003).

With recognition of hypercalcemia in any dog, a rectal examination and careful palpation of the anal sac areas should be routine.

In affected dogs, rectal examination usually demonstrates a space-occupying mass that may be invasive and occasionally ulcerated. Careful digital rectal palpation is necessary to identify the presence of sublumbar lymph node enlargement. Although radiography may also be used to evaluate the sublumbar area, abdominal ultrasonography has been a sensitive diagnostic aid. Radiography of the thorax and abdomen can be used in searching for pulmonary metastases and/or bony metastases (lytic areas).

Other Nonneoplastic and Solid Tumors That May Synthesize Parathyroid Hormone–Related Protein. Thymoma, melanoma, carcinomas of the lung, pancreas, thyroid, skin, mammary gland, nasal cavity, adrenal medulla, and interstitial cell tumors of the testicle are less commonly encountered solid tumors that cause hypercalcemia without bone metastasis (Grain and Walder, 1982; Meuten et al, 1983a; Pressler et al, 2002; Williams et al, 2003). Dogs or cats with any of these neoplastic conditions are not usually hypercalcemic, but when present, the value of a randomly collected serum or plasma sample for PTHrP measurement can be quite informative. In people, a small percentage of bronchogenic non–small-cell carcinomas, breast cancers, squamous cell carcinomas of the esophagus, renal-cell carcinomas, and hepatomas have synthesized and secreted PTHrP (Harris et al, 2002). PTHrP has also been associated with hypercalcemia in nonneoplastic diseases, such as schistosomiasis (Fradkin et al, 2001).

Hematologic Malignancies of the Bone Marrow: Osteolytic Hypercalcemia

Background. Some types of hematologic malignances present in bone (e.g., lymphoma and multiple myeloma) produce hypercalcemia by inducing bone resorption locally (Rosol et al, 2000). In humans, metastatic breast cancer is another example, although this association is not common in dogs or cats. A number of paracrine factors may be responsible for the stimulation of local bone resorption in dogs or cats with such tumors, such as the previously discussed cytokines and PTHrP (see Humoral Hypercalcemia of Malignancy; Black and Mundy, 1994). Production of small amounts of PTHrP by a tumor in bone may stimulate local bone resorption without inducing a systemic response. Prostaglandins (especially prostaglandin E$_2$) may also contribute to local stimulation of bone resorption (Rosol et al, 2000). Together, these cytokines and prostaglandins comprise the osteoclast-activating factors.

Multiple Myeloma. Multiple myeloma is a tumor of B-lymphocytes or plasma cell lines that may be associated with the development of osteolytic bone lesions and, occasionally, hypercalcemia. The hypercalcemia develops secondary to production of the previously described interleukin-1β (IL-1β; previously described as "osteoclast-activating factor"), plus transforming growth factor-β (TGF-β), and the receptor activator of nuclear factor k-B ligand (RAN kL). The latter is a membrane-associated protein that stimulates osteoclast activity by binding to surface receptors (Henry, 2010). There is correlation between extent of bone destruction, tumor cell burden, and the amount of IL-1β produced by myeloma cell cultures (Durie et al, 1981; Wysolmerski and Insogna, 2012). Approximately 17% of dogs afflicted with this cancer are hypercalcemic and 50% of dogs with multiple myeloma have radiographic evidence of bone lysis (Matus et al, 1986; Henry, 2010).

Bone pain may be associated with the lytic areas. The initial database from afflicted dogs often reveals abnormal increases in the total serum globulin concentration as a result of a monoclonal spike. A "monoclonal gammopathy" can be demonstrated via serum protein electrophoresis. Bone marrow aspiration may aid in confirming the diagnosis. Analysis of urine for light chains of myeloma protein (Bence Jones protein) has not been of value (Matus et al, 1986; Henry, 2010).

Hypercalcemia Induced by Metastases of Solid Tumors to Bone

Certain malignant neoplasms with osseous metastasis may cause hypercalcemia and hypercalciuria. Primary bone tumors, by contrast, do not typically induce hypercalcemia. For example, hypercalcemia would be rare in a dog with osteosarcoma, whereas malignant mammary adenocarcinoma or squamous cell carcinoma are (albeit infrequently) associated with both bone metastasis and hypercalcemia. Several different types of cells may be involved in the actual destruction of bone at sites of metastasis, including osteoclasts, tumor cells, lymphocytes, and monocytes. Lymphocytes and monocytes may accumulate as part of the cell-mediated immune response to a tumor (Mundy et al, 1984). Osteolysis is a result of the physical disruption of bone by proliferating neoplastic cells, but it also can be caused by secretion of cytokines or prostaglandins that stimulate local bone resorption (Garrett, 1993; Henry, 2010).

Epithelial tumors, especially squamous cell carcinomas, are the most likely neoplasms to metastasize to bone in dogs and cats (Quigley and Leedale, 1983). Common metastatic bone sites in the dog include the humerus, femur, and vertebrae, whereas in the cat, local invasion of bone rather than distant metastasis is more common. Although reported, these tumors are not commonly associated with hypercalcemia (Grain and Walder, 1982).

Hypervitaminosis D

Background

Vitamin D can be cumulative in its toxic action if a dog or cat consumes excess quantities in food, for example, and may require weeks before effects on mineral metabolism become clinically obvious. However, acute toxicity after massive ingestion of cholecalciferol appears to be the more commonly reported cause of vitamin D toxicosis in dogs. Hypercalcemia and hyperphosphatemia are the anticipated electrolyte abnormalities in vitamin D toxicity, although normophosphatemia and transient periods of normocalcemia have been reported (Harrington and Page, 1983; Mellanby et al, 2005; Figs. 15-11 and 15-12). Hypercalcemia begins as soon as 12 to 18 hours after massive ingestion, and peak concentrations are usually demonstrated by 48 to 72 hours, coinciding with increases in BUN and creatinine (Rumbeiha, 2000). Increased resorption from bone, coupled with increased gastrointestinal absorption of calcium and phosphorus, are responsible for these abnormalities. Skeletal disease is usually not detectable radiographically, probably because of the acute nature of the toxicosis. The osteoclastic phase of bone resorption occurs early and is followed by osteoid deposition and hyperosteoidosis (Boyce and Weisbrode, 1983). Extensive soft tissue mineralization of the endocardium, blood vessels, tendons, kidney, and lung is frequently associated with vitamin D toxicity (Meuten, 1984).

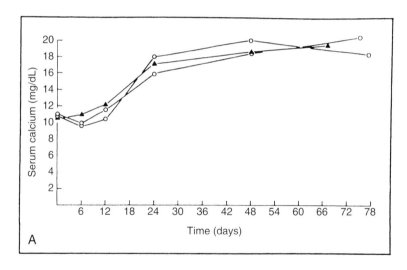

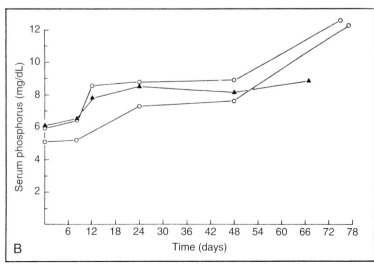

FIGURE 15-11 Serum calcium **(A)** and phosphorus **(B)** concentrations of dogs given vitamin D₃ at a dosage of 10 mg/kg *(circles)* and 20 mg/kg *(triangles)*. (From Gunther R, et al.: Toxicity of a vitamin D₃ rodenticide to dogs, *J Am Vet Med Assoc* 193:211, 1988.)

Rodenticide Toxicosis

Hypercalcemia that develops secondary to cholecalciferol rodenticide toxicosis in dogs and cats is a recognized concern (Gunther et al, 1988; Moore et al, 1988; Bahri, 1990; Dougherty et al, 1990; Fooshee and Forrester, 1990; Rumbeiha et al, 1999; Murphy, 2002). A variety of rat bait products contain cholecalciferol (Nicholson, 2000; Rumbeiha, 2000; Morrow, 2001). Dogs studied after being given this type of poison became weak, lethargic, and anorexic within 48 hours. Within 60 to 70 hours of consumption, all dogs became recumbent, exhibited hematemesis, and progressed into shock before dying or being euthanized (Gunther et al, 1988). Although the median lethal dose of cholecalciferol in dogs is widely reported to be 43 to 88 mg/kg, studies have shown that as little as 10 mg/kg given once orally can be lethal. Dogs that ingest as little as 4 to 6 mg/kg, once, can become ill. Clinically healthy dogs that ingest single doses of 2 mg/kg may develop hypercalcemia (Rumbeiha, 2000).

Most dogs and cats exposed to these toxins have had rapid increases in the serum calcium and phosphate concentrations (see Fig. 15-11). Diffuse gastrointestinal hemorrhage was obvious. Histologic lesions consisting of hemorrhage or mineralization or both were identified in the gastrointestinal tract, kidneys, myocardium, and in the blood vessels of many organs (Gunther et al, 1988). The incidence of acute and/or severe renal failure was variable. Three exposed cats survived (Moore et al, 1988).

Other Causes of Vitamin D Toxicosis (Creams, Plants, and Dietary Supplements)

Since 1997, perhaps the most common accidental cause of vitamin D toxicosis in pets has been ingestion of human psoriasis medications containing the vitamin D analogs calcipotriol or calcipotriene. Excess dietary supplementation and overzealous administration of vitamin D by veterinarians to dogs or cats with hypoparathyroidism have been reported (Mellanby et al, 2005). Vitamin D given after removal of a parathyroid tumor when hypocalcemia is recognized or anticipated can be overdosed.

Lilies and *Cestrum diurnum* (day-blooming jessamine) are popular houseplants that should be considered sources of vitamin D toxicity in pets because they contain active metabolite of vitamin D. Jasmine, an indoor climbing plant without active vitamin D metabolites, should not be confused with day-blooming jessamine. Other plants containing glycosides of vitamin D include *Solanum malacoxylon and Trisetum flavescens.*

Diagnosis

The diagnosis of vitamin D toxicosis is based on a history of exposure. In acute cases, one may see dark or bloody feces, azotemia, oliguria or polyuria, proteinuria, and sometimes glucosuria. An additional clue in diagnosing chronic hypervitaminosis D, such as with a dietary excess, would be hyperphosphatemia in a hypercalcemic dog or cat. Most other causes of hypercalcemia are associated with hypophosphatemia or normal serum phosphate concentrations. The history and signs of vitamin D toxicosis can be strikingly similar to those seen in dogs with hypoadrenocorticism, acute kidney injury (AKI), and CKD. Various assays are available as diagnostic aides. Calcidiol (25[OH]D) concentration is a good indicator of vitamin D ingestion and can be used to help identify hypervitaminosis D, because vitamin D metabolites resulting from rodenticides will be measured. The vitamin D analog found in skin creams is not measured with this assay but should be detectable with a calcitriol assay (Peterson, 2012).

Hypoadrenocorticism

Hypoadrenocorticism (Addison's disease) is one of the more common causes of hypercalcemia in dogs, accounting for approximately 10% to 50% of cases (Uehlinger et al, 1998; Rosol et al, 2000). Serum calcium concentrations have been reported to be increased in as many as 33% of dogs with adrenocortical insufficiency (hypoadrenocorticism) (Peterson and Feinman, 1982; Peterson et al, 1996; Scott-Moncrieff, 2010) as well as in a smaller percentage of hypoadrenal cats (Johnessee et al, 1982; Peterson et al, 1989). A correlation has been noted between

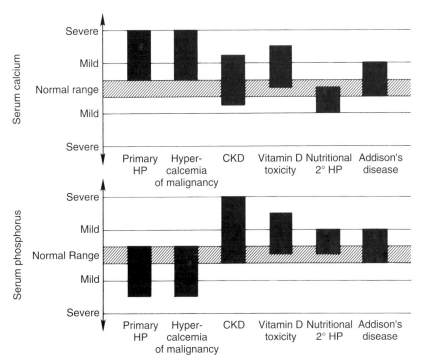

FIGURE 15-12 The range in serum calcium and phosphorus concentrations for the more common causes of hypercalcemia and/or hyperparathyroidism in the dog. *CKD,* Chronic kidney disease; *HP,* hyperparathyroidism; *2° HP,* secondary hyperparathyroidism.

the degree of hyperkalemia and the level of hypercalcemia (see Chapter 12). If the serum potassium concentration exceeds 6.0 to 6.5 mEq/L, a large percentage of these animals have serum calcium concentrations of 12 to 13.5 mg/dL. Hypercalcemia is not restricted to the extremely ill hypoadrenal dog. It is not common, however, for the serum calcium concentration to exceed 13.5 mg/dL, and it rarely exceeds 15 to 16 mg/dL. Despite the increased serum TCa concentrations, serum iCa concentrations usually remain in the reference range. Serum phosphate concentrations also correlate with serum calcium concentrations, with the hyperphosphatemic animal more likely to exhibit hypercalcemia (see Fig. 15-12).

Clinical signs and laboratory abnormalities associated with hypoaldosteronism (a primary component of Addison's disease) are often striking and overshadow concerns related to hypercalcemia (see Chapter 12). Most dogs and cats with hypoadrenocorticism have hyperkalemia, hyponatremia, azotemia, hyperphosphatemia, and may be severely ill. The only differential diagnoses for this combination of clinical and serum abnormalities are hypoadrenocorticism, significant (acute?) kidney injury, and vitamin D (rodenticide) toxicosis. Hypercalcemia rapidly resolves after saline fluid therapy for adrenal insufficiency, but does not respond as quickly or at all in dogs with vitamin D toxicosis or primary renal disease.

The pathogenesis of the hypercalcemia associated with hypoadrenocorticism is probably multifactorial. Any combination of the following may be involved: volume contraction, decreased glomerular filtration rate (GFR), increased intestinal absorption of calcium, hyperproteinemia resulting from dehydration and hemoconcentration, increased plasma protein binding affinity for calcium, increased concentrations of calcium-citrate complexes, and increased renal tubular resorption of calcium (Peterson and Feinman, 1982; Scott-Moncrieff, 2010).

Chronic Kidney Disease (CKD)

A majority of dogs and cats with CKD have normal serum TCa concentrations, a small minority have hypocalcemia, and a larger minority (14% of dogs and 38% of cats) have increases in TCa, making CKD the second or third most common cause of hypercalcemia (Schenck and Chew, 2012). The prevalence of hypercalcemia increases with CKD severity. The finding of hypercalcemia and renal azotemia presents a diagnostic dilemma because hypercalcemia can lead to renal failure or develop as a consequence of it. Deleterious effects of hypercalcemia only follow increases in serum iCa concentrations, making assessment of this parameter of particular importance. About 10% of dogs and almost 30% of cats with CKD have increases in serum iCa concentrations. The pathogenesis of hypercalcemia associated with CKD usually involves diffuse hyperplasia of the parathyroid glands (Fig. 15-13). The actual presence or incidence of a syndrome involving "autonomously functioning" parathyroid glands that are the result of chronic stimulation due to CKD (i.e., tertiary hyperparathyroidism) is not known. *Tertiary hyperparathyroidism* is the name given to the syndrome of chronic renal secondary hyperparathyroidism, in which one or more of the parathyroid glands begin to autonomously secrete PTH ("tertiary" disease). Dogs or cats with no or minimal clinical signs, persistent hypercalcemia of a magnitude greater than 13.0 mg/dL, and a serum phosphate that is normal or low usually do not have CKD. Those with serum calcium concentrations less than 12.5 mg/dL and hyperphosphatemia are more likely to have CKD. The dog or cat for which the diagnosis remains vague despite these guidelines may need further

evaluation. Measurement of serum iCa concentrations should help distinguish primary kidney disease (normal or low) from a primary parathyroid problem (increased) (see Fig. 15-5). Cervical ultrasonography may aid in distinguishing enlargement of more than one gland (consistent with renal secondary hyperparathyroidism) versus identifying one parathyroid nodule (consistent with PHPTH). If the underlying disease process is still uncertain, the results of PTH and PTHrP assays may be helpful (Schenck and Chew, 2012).

Acute Kidney Injury (AKI)

Dogs with acute and severe hyperphosphatemia as a component of AKI usually have normal or low serum calcium concentrations. Mild hypercalcemia is occasionally seen. As with hypercalcemia associated with CKD, the pathogenesis of hypercalcemia induced by AKI is multifactorial. In the oliguric phase of acute failure, deposition of calcium and phosphorus in soft tissues may occur. During the polyuric phase, as kidney function improves, this mineral may be mobilized, and hypercalcemia and hyperphosphatemia may develop (Llach et al, 1981). Alternatively, rapid improvement in both renal function and serum phosphate concentrations may lead to transient hypercalcemia as a result of changing mass law interactions.

Raisin/Grape Toxicity

Of 132 dogs reported to have had raisin or grape ingestion, 33 had no adverse effects, 14 became ill but did not have azotemia, and 43 had clinical signs and AKI. More than 90% of dogs with grape or raisin ingestion associated AKI have had increases in both serum TCa and phosphate concentrations. Ingestion of even small quantities can lead to acute life threatening kidney failure. Any dog suspected of ingesting raisins or grapes should be induced to vomit while gastric lavage and administration of activated charcoal are considered. Intravenous (IV) fluid therapy is recommended for at least 48 hours. Pathogenesis of the kidney injury and of the hypercalcemia is multifactorial (Gwaltney-Brant et al, 2001; Morrow et al, 2001; Eubig et al, 2005; Schenck and Chew, 2012). As many as 50% of these dogs do not survive, whereas many of those who have survived required days or even weeks of fluid therapy or dialysis. Higher serum TCa and TCa x phosphate products are associated with poorer prognosis.

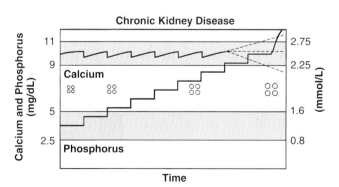

FIGURE 15-13 Diagrammatic illustration of progressive renal failure with time. Note the progressive loss in the ability to excrete phosphate, the small fluctuations in the serum calcium concentration until late in the disease, and the progressive enlargement of all four parathyroids secondary to the progressive renal failure. *Open circles,* Parathyroid gland size over time, illustrating renal secondary hyperparathyroidism.

Nutritional Secondary Hyperparathyroidism

Increased secretion of PTH associated with nutritional secondary hyperparathyroidism represents a normal compensatory response to nutritionally induced hypocalcemia. Dietary mineral imbalances capable of inducing this syndrome include diets low in calcium or vitamin D or diets containing excessive amounts of phosphorus with normal or low calcium levels (Crager and Nachreiner, 1993). Nutritional secondary hyperparathyroidism most commonly develops after the exclusive ingestion of all-meat diets, classically diets consisting solely of liver or beef heart (Capen and Martin, 1983).

Subtle and chronic decreases in the serum calcium concentration (usually not below normal reference concentrations) develop in animals fed these diets. Subtle decreases in serum iCa concentration stimulate the parathyroid glands to secrete PTH. With prolonged stimulation, chief cell hyperplasia and secondary hyperparathyroidism develop. Depletion of skeletal calcium leads to clinical signs in these animals. Pathologic bone fractures are common. Acute lameness is the most common owner observation. Because renal function is normal, hyperparathyroidism diminishes renal tubular resorption of phosphate (hyperphosphaturia) and increases resorption of calcium. These dogs and cats usually have a low-normal serum calcium concentration and a normal serum phosphorus concentration (Schenck and Chew, 2012).

Septic Bone Disease, Sepsis, Schistosomiasis, and Systemic Mycoses

Bacterial or fungal osteomyelitis and primary or secondary tumors of bone are rare causes of hypercalcemia. Neonatal septicemia in puppies with septic emboli and lysis of bone is also rare. Hypercalcemia has been associated with blastomycosis, histoplasmosis, schistosomiasis, aspergillosis, and coccidioidomycosis in dogs without apparent bone involvement (Legendre et al, 1981; Dow et al, 1986; Troy et al, 1987; Meuten and Armstrong, 1989; Rohrer et al, 2000, Fradkin et al, 2001; Parker, 2001). In one of these reports, increases in PTHrP concentration were believed to cause hypercalcemia in two dogs with schistosomiasis (Fradkin et al, 2001). The pathogenesis for sepsis-induced hypercalcemia is not certain, but inflammation associated with sepsis may cause sufficient bone destruction and mobilization of calcium to cause hypercalcemia (Meuten, 1984). The production of bone-resorbing factors such as prostaglandins and cytokines comprise the osteoclast-activating factors produced by monocytes and lymphocytes that may be involved in the pathogenesis (Mundy et al, 1984). Viable macrophages have osteolytic capabilities that may be enhanced by endotoxin (McArthur et al, 1980). Abnormal metabolism of vitamin D may also be involved in the hypercalcemia associated with granulomatous disease (Lemann and Gray, 1984).

Disuse Osteoporosis/Tumors Metastasizing to Bone

Disuse osteoporosis is a rare cause of hypercalcemia seen in animals immobilized because of extensive musculoskeletal or neurologic injury. This form of hypercalcemia is mild and is associated with bone resorption and urinary hydroxyproline excretion, decreased bone production, hypercalciuria, and osteopenia (Chew and Meuten, 1982). While metastasis of cancers to bone is relatively common in dogs and cats, hypercalcemia is not common.

Hemoconcentration, Sodium Bicarbonate Infusion, and Plasma Transfusion

Hypercalcemia occasionally may develop in severely dehydrated animals. Hypercalcemia is usually mild, perhaps resulting from volume contraction and secondary hyperproteinemia. Hypercalcemia should resolve with fluid therapy. Sodium bicarbonate infusions have been demonstrated to decrease the TCa and iCa concentrations (Chew et al, 1989). Increases in the serum TCa concentration and decreases in the iCa concentration can transiently follow plasma transfusion, presumably secondary to excesses in citrate–calcium ion complexes (Mischke et al, 1996).

Hypothermia, Fetal Retention, and Endometritis

A dog and a cat have been described with severe, environmentally induced hypothermia and hypercalcemia (Ross and Goldstein, 1981). Hypercalcemia rapidly resolved after rewarming and fluid therapy. The pathogenesis is not known. Similarly, one dog with a retained fetus and concurrent endometritis had hypercalcemia (Hirt et al, 2000). It remains to be demonstrated whether or not these conditions warrant being included in differential diagnosis lists for hypercalcemia.

Age

See Serum Total Calcium Concentration.

Laboratory Error

See Serum Total Calcium Concentration.

PRIMARY HYPERPARATHYROIDISM IN DOGS

SIGNALMENT

Age, Gender, and Weight

PHPTH is typically diagnosed in older dogs and appears to be much less common, or at least less frequently diagnosed, in cats. The mean age of dogs with PHPTH is about 11 years with a range of about 4 to 17 years (Fig. 15-14). More than 95% of dogs with this condition are 7 years of age or older. There is no apparent gender predilection.

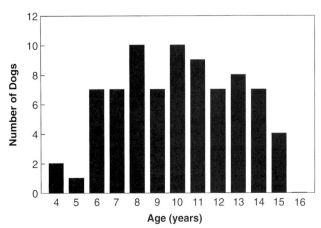

FIGURE 15-14 Age distribution of 78 dogs with primary hyperparathyroidism (PHPTH). Their mean age at the time of diagnosis was 10½ years.

TABLE 15-3	BREED DISTRIBUTION OF 210 DOGS WITH PRIMARY HYPERPARATHYROIDISM

BREED	PERCENTAGE
Keeshond	20
Mixed Breed	14
Labrador Retriever	9
German Shepherd dog	6
Golden Retriever	6
Springer Spaniel	5
Poodle	4
Shih Tzu	4
Australian Shepherd	3
Cocker Spaniel	3
Doberman Pinscher	2
Rhodesian Ridgeback	2
Breeds represented once	22

Data from Feldman EC et al.: Pretreatment clinical and laboratory findings in dogs with primary hyperparathyroidism: 210 cases (1987-2004), *J Am Vet Med Assoc* 227:756, 2005.

The mean body weight (22 kg) in one study of dogs with PHPTH included a range of 2.6 to 60 kg (Feldman et al, 2005).

Breed

PHPTH has been diagnosed in dogs from almost every breed and mixed breed. The etiology of the condition in most is unknown. PHPTH has been demonstrated to be an autosomal dominant, genetically transmitted disease in Keeshonden with possible age-dependent penetrance (Skelly and Franklin, 2006; Goldstein et al, 2007). The breeds most commonly encountered, in addition to the Keeshond are dogs of mixed breeding, Labrador Retrievers, German Shepherd dogs, Golden Retrievers, Poodles, Shih Tzu, or Springer Spaniels (Table 15-3). Hereditary neonatal PHPTH (an extremely rare condition) with a possible autosomal recessive mode of inheritance was reported in two German Shepherd dogs (Thompson et al, 1984).

ANAMNESIS: CLINICAL SIGNS

Overview

Between 20% and 50% of owners do not observe clinical signs in their dog with PHPTH, even after being told of the signs to expect. Early, mild, or even more dramatic hypercalcemia due to PHPTH may not be associated with owner observed signs. In these dogs, hypercalcemia was identified serendipitously only after a standard biochemical panel had been obtained for unrelated reasons. This serendipitous finding of hypercalcemia is also true in a majority of people with PHPTH, in whom "occult PHPTH" is more prevalent than the symptomatic form (Heath, 1989; Potts, 1990; Consensus Development Conference Panel, 1991; Silverberg et al, 1999; Wysolmerski and Insogna, 2012). When present, initial clinical signs in dogs tend to be mild, insidious, and nonspecific. Many owners can only estimate duration of signs (Table 15-4). In some cases, it is not until the pet has been treated for PHPTH that owners realize in retrospect that their dog had signs. This concept

TABLE 15-4	APPROXIMATE DURATION OF CLINICAL SIGNS IN 210 DOGS WITH NATURALLY OCCURRING PRIMARY HYPERPARATHYROIDISM

DURATION (MONTHS)	PERCENTAGE OF DOGS
< 1	20
1–3	20
3–6	20
6–12	25
> 12	15

Data from Feldman EC et al.: Pretreatment clinical and laboratory findings in dogs with primary hyperparathyroidism: 210 cases (1987-2004), *J Am Vet Med Assoc* 227:756, 2005.

TABLE 15-5	FREQUENCY OF CLINICAL SIGNS REPORTED PROSPECTIVELY OR RETROSPECTIVELY IN 210 DOGS WITH PRIMARY HYPERPARATHYROIDISM*

SIGN	PERCENTAGE OF DOGS

Urinary tract signs
   Straining (stranguria)
   Frequency (pollakiuria)
   Blood (hematuria)
	50

Polyuria/polydipsia	48
Weakness	46
Exercise intolerance	46
Listlessness	43
"Incontinence" (polyuria?)	39
Inappetence	37
Weight loss	18
Muscle wasting	18
Vomiting	13
Shivering	10
Constipation	6
Stiff gait	5

Data from Feldman EC et al.: Pretreatment clinical and laboratory findings in dogs with primary hyperparathyroidism: 210 cases (1987-2004), *J Am Vet Med Assoc* 227:756, 2005.
*Sixty-nine out of 210 owners reported no abnormalities.

promoted the suggestion that people with PHPTH be treated regardless of perceived symptoms (Utiger, 1999).

As many as half of dogs with PHPTH have had or have signs at the time of a diagnosis related to stones or a urinary tract infection (pollakiuria, stranguria, and/or hematuria). Additional common owner observations include polyuria/polydipsia "incontinence", decreased activity, lethargy, and muscle weakness; decreased appetite; weight loss; and muscle atrophy (Feldman et al, 2005; Gear et al, 2005; Ham et al, 2009; Sawyer et al, 2011; Arbaugh et al, 2012; Milovancev and Schmiedt, 2013). Less commonly, owners have noted shivering/trembling, vomiting, constipation, diarrhea, and stiff or painful gait. Although quite uncommon, some PHPTH dogs were extremely ill when first examined due to renal failure. Central nervous system (CNS) signs include mental dullness and, far less commonly, signs of obtundation, seizures, collapse, or coma

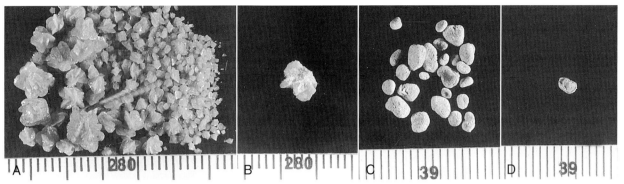

FIGURE 15-15 Calcium-containing cystic calculi from two dogs with primary hyperparathyroidism (PHPTH) **(A** and **C)** and individual cracked calculi from each dog **(B** and **D).**

(Table 15-5). In general, the more worrisome the clinical signs in a hypercalcemic dog, the greater the likelihood that the increase in calcium is not due to PHPTH. Extremely serious signs are usually the result of the underlying cause for the hypercalcemia (e.g., cancer, renal failure, hypoadrenocorticism, and/or toxin). However, in one report, about one third of 29 dogs with PHPTH were described as having renal failure (Gear et al, 2005).

Polydipsia and/or Polyuria

The most common clinical signs in dogs with PHPTH are polyuria, polydipsia, and/or urinary "incontinence." Polyuria develops as a result of impaired renal tubular response to antidiuretic hormone (ADH). In the normal state, ADH binds to V2 receptors located in the basolateral membrane of principal cells in the renal collecting tubules. Binding causes increased expression of aquaporin-2 water channels within apical cell membranes, increasing permeability to water and promoting water reabsorption (Shiel, 2012). Hypercalcemia interferes with ADH binding to V2 receptors. This acquired and reversible nephrogenic diabetes insipidus causes production of relatively dilute, solute-free urine (polyuria) and compensatory polydipsia.

Urinary Tract Calculi and Infections

Nephrocalcinosis, the diffuse deposition of calcium phosphate complexes in the renal parenchyma, and ureteroliths have not been commonly reported in dogs with PHPTH. Cystic calculi are common in dogs with PHPTH with the most common stone being calcium oxalate or mixed calcium oxalate and calcium phosphate (Fig. 15-15). The risk factors for stone formation in patients with PHPTH are hypercalciuria and a tendency to have renal losses of bicarbonate and phosphate. The loss of bicarbonate leads to relatively alkaline urine, favoring the precipitation of calcium phosphate. The incidence of urinary tract infection is increased with the presence of uroliths. Further, it is possible that the relatively dilute urine and, perhaps, some degree of decreased bladder tone following chronic excess urine production may also contribute to their incidence of infection. Both of these latter factors can lead to urine retention because of an inability to completely void.

Chronic Kidney Disease or Acute Kidney Injury

It is unclear in people whether PHPTH impairs renal function. In the majority of untreated human PHPTH patients followed over time, some for longer than a decade, renal function remains both normal and stable (Silverberg et al, 1999; Wysolmerski and Insogna, 2012). Why PHPTH seems to adversely affect kidney function in a few dogs and not the majority is not understood. Hydronephrosis

and loss of function secondary to obstruction caused by nephroliths or ureteroliths is logical, but some dogs with severe kidney failure and PHPTH have not been described as having had obstructive disease. Dogs with PHPTH typically have decreases in serum phosphate concentrations and their calcium x phosphate products, usually similar or less than values in healthy dogs, have been considered a predictor of stable kidney function. In more than 300 dogs with PHPTH, renal failure was extremely uncommon (Feldman et al, 2005; Ham et al, 2009; Sawyer et al, 2011; Arbaugh et al, 2012; Milovancev and Schmiedt, 2013). However, in one report of 29 dogs with PHPTH, 13 had mild to severe kidney failure (Gear et al, 2005).

Lethargy, Weakness, Shivering, and Muscle Atrophy

Listlessness, decreases in activity and/or weakness are observed in one third to one half of dogs with PHPTH, whereas the signs of shivering, trembling, or stiff gait are less common (Feldman et al, 2005; Gear et al, 2005; Ham et al, 2009; Sawyer et al, 2011; Arbaugh et al, 2012; Milovancev and Schmiedt, 2013). Increased serum calcium concentrations tend to hyperpolarize membranes. This may cause a range of muscular, neuromuscular, and/or neurologic abnormalities in people with PHPTH—some of whom have been described as developing fatigue, weakness, and myopathies. Some, but not all affected individuals, comment on their weakness, fatigue, listlessness, and difficulty concentrating. However, the specificity and origin of these symptoms are debated (Wysolmerski and Insogna, 2012). Analogous abnormalities in dogs may explain the common observation of listlessness and/or "depression" associated with this disorder. Shivering and muscle twitching have uncommonly been observed in hypercalcemic dogs, as has the extremely unusual problems of circling or ataxia (Chew and Capen, 1980). Seizure activity has been reported in several dogs with PHPTH (Ihle et al, 1988; Gear et al, 2005; Arbaugh et al, 2012). The mechanism for these problems is not well understood but in rare cases may progress to stupor or coma. "Collapse" was described in two of 29 dogs in one report (Gear et al, 2005).

Inappetence, Weight Loss, and Abdominal or Nonspecific Pain

Hypercalcemia impairs gastrointestinal motility via decreases in excitability of smooth muscle. This may contribute to the signs of reduced appetite and subsequent weight loss observed in one-third to one half of PHPTH people (Wysolmerski and Insogna, 2012) and dogs. Abdominal pain, vomiting, and diarrhea are recognized but seem uncommon. Constipation, described in some people with PHPTH, is quite uncommon in dogs. The development of gastric or duodenal ulcers secondary to increases in gastrin

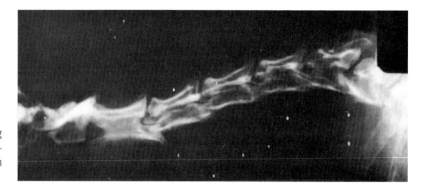

FIGURE 15-16 Lateral radiograph of the cervical spine from a dog with multiple myeloma and hypercalcemia. Note the severe osteolysis involving several vertebrae. These findings are consistent with a diagnosis of the hypercalcemia of malignancy syndrome.

secretion has been documented in hypercalcemic people but has not yet been reported in dogs (Aurbach et al, 1985a). Weight loss and decreases in appetite are far more common. Nonspecific arthralgias are complications recognized in humans with PHPTH (Arnaud and Kolb, 1991) and may account for the pain or stiff gait occasionally observed in dogs.

Stiff Gait, Fractures, and Skeletal Pain

Stiff gait and fractures are both uncommon but have been associated with PHPTH (see Table 15-5). Excessive subperiosteal bone resorption and osteoporosis induced by PHPTH can result in replacement of bone matrix with fibrous tissue (Fig. 15-16). This thinning and weakening is more likely in cortical bone, leading to fracture predisposition (Wysolmerski and Insogna, 2012). Lameness may be associated with pain as skeletal changes progress.

 ## PHYSICAL EXAMINATION

General Observations

The physical examination was unremarkable in about 66% to 75% of dogs with PHPTH (Feldman et al, 2005). When abnormalities are found, they typically are related to the presence of uroliths, some concurrent and unrelated condition, or they are subtle and nonspecific. This concept is important, because the differential diagnoses for dogs with a serendipitous finding of hypercalcemia include lymphosarcoma, CKD, apocrine gland carcinoma of the anal sac, hypoadrenocorticism, multiple myeloma, vitamin D toxicosis, and granulomatous diseases. Dogs with any of these other conditions are usually ill or quite ill. In other words, a relatively stable or apparently healthy older dog with hypercalcemia is more likely to have PHPTH than one of the serious conditions that cause secondary hypercalcemia.

Common Abnormalities

Potential physical examination findings in dogs with PHPTH, other than those caused by uroliths, include thin body composition, generalized muscle atrophy, and/or weakness. Severity of these abnormalities is variable, but they are usually mild. Bone deformities involving the mandible or maxilla and fractures of long bones have been reported (Capen and Martin, 1983; Gear et al, 2005) but are extremely rare.

Ophthalmologic Changes

Infrequent ocular abnormalities in humans with PHPTH include "band keratopathy" and subconjunctival deposits of calcium

(Aurbach et al, 1985a). Band keratopathy results from the deposition of calcium phosphate in the cornea. The condition is recognized as opaque material appearing as parallel lines in the limbus of the eye, best visualized on slit lamp examination.

Palpable Parathyroid Masses

It is extremely unusual to palpate an enlarged parathyroid gland in dogs. A palpable parathyroid mass has been reported in only one of more than 300 dogs with PHPTH (Feldman et al, 2005; Ham et al, 2009; Sawyer et al, 2011; Arbaugh et al, 2012; Milovancev and Schmiedt, 2013). Even with confirmed PHPTH, a nodule felt in the neck is much more likely to involve the thyroid or some other structure than a parathyroid. About 10% to 20% of dogs with PHPTH had an incidentally discovered thyroid mass on cervical ultrasonography in one study (Pollard et al, in press). Parathyroid masses are not palpable because they are located dorsolateral to the trachea, are usually 4 to 8 mm in diameter, and they are covered by several muscle layers. Although an enlarged parathyroid gland was not palpable in any of our dogs, palpable tumors have been identified in cats with PHPTH.

Importance of a Thorough Physical Examination

A thorough physical examination is imperative in any animal with documented hypercalcemia. Physical examination results are usually normal in dogs with PHPTH. Because the more common causes of hypercalcemia in dogs include malignant cancers, hypoadrenocorticism, toxicosis, CKD, and other worrisome conditions, the diagnostic approach to the dog with confirmed hypercalcemia is to rule out these differential diagnoses as completely as possible. Careful palpation of peripheral lymph nodes, mammary glands, perineal region, as well as digital rectal and vaginal examinations should be included. Lymphosarcoma, for example, can be extremely easy or extremely difficult to diagnose, and it is a condition not removed from a list of differential diagnoses until an alternative diagnosis has been confirmed. In addition to hypercalcemia of malignancy, other causes of hypercalcemia may be suspected after a thorough physical examination. Dogs with CKD or AKI may have palpably abnormal kidneys. Dogs with hypoadrenocorticism may have bradycardia, weak femoral pulses, melena, or a bloody rectal discharge.

 ## CLINICAL PATHOLOGY

Hemogram

The hemogram is usually unremarkable in dogs, whereas people with PHPTH may have a nonregenerative anemia and elevation in erythrocyte sedimentation rates. In dogs with PHPTH,

TABLE 15-6   **SERUM BLOOD UREA NITROGEN, CREATININE AND INORGANIC PHOSPHORUS (PHOSPHATE) CONCENTRATIONS, AND URINE SPECIFIC GRAVITIES AT TIME OF DIAGNOSIS OF PRIMARY HYPERPARATHYROIDISM IN 210 DOGS**

	BLOOD UREA NITROGEN (mg/dL)	SERUM CREATININE (mg/dL)	SERUM PHOSPHATE (mg/dL)	URINE SPECIFIC GRAVITY
Reference range	18-28	0.5-1.6	3.0-6.2	—
Mean	16.9	0.8	2.8	1.012
Median	15	0.8	2.7	1.010
Ranges	5-92	0.4-4.1	1.3-6.1	1.008-1.037
Number / % ↑ reference range	9/4%	7/3%	0	—
Number / % ↓ reference range	132/63%	9/4%	136/65%	—

Data from Feldman EC et al.: Pretreatment clinical and laboratory findings in dogs with primary hyperparathyroidism: 210 cases (1987-2004), *J Am Vet Med Assoc* 227:756, 2005.

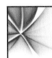

TABLE 15-7   **DOGS WITH PRIMARY HYPERPARATHYROIDISM: SERUM TOTAL AND IONIZED CALCIUM CONCENTRACTIONS (210 DOGS), SERUM PARATHYROID HORMONE CONCENTRATIONS (185 DOGS), AND ULTRASONOGRAPHICALLY IDENTIFIED PARATHYROID MASSES (117 DOGS, EACH WITH A SOLITARY NODULE, AND 13 DOGS, EACH WITH TWO NODULES)**

	TOTAL CALCIUM (mg/dL)	IONIZED CALCIUM (mmol/L)	PARATHYROID HORMONE (pmol/L)	ULTRASOUND MASS SIZE (mm)
Reference range	9.9-11.7	1.12-1.41	2-13	< 4
Mean	14.5	1.71	11.3	6
Median	14.3	1.77	11.3	5
Range	12.1-23.4	1.22-2.41	2.3-121	3-23
Number / % ↓ reference range	0	0	0	—
Number / % ↑ reference range	210/100%	191/91%	50/27%	—

Data from Feldman EC et al.: Pretreatment clinical and laboratory findings in dogs with primary hyperparathyroidism: 210 cases (1987-2004), *J Am Vet Med Assoc* 227:756, 2005.

no specific changes in bone marrow aspirates or peripheral blood smears are seen.

Biochemical Profile

Serum Total Calcium Concentration

Various factors can alter the reported serum TCa concentration and the differential diagnoses for hypercalcemia includes a number of possibilities. This increases the importance of many serum biochemistry parameters. Specifically, the serum calcium concentration should be assessed relative to serum albumin, phosphorus, BUN, and creatinine concentrations (Table 15-6).

Hypercalcemia is the hallmark abnormality of PHPTH (see Figs. 15-5 and 15-12). The mean serum calcium concentrations from four reports were 13.9, 14.3, 13.6, and 13.6 mg/dL, respectively, with an approximate range of 12.1 to 23.4 mg/dL (Feldman et al, 2005; Gear et al, 2005; Ham et al, 2009; Milovancev and Schmiedt, 2013; Table 15-7). These mean values could be slightly inflated because evaluation of hypercalcemia is often limited to animals with a serum TCa concentration greater than 12.0 mg/dL (the upper reference range limit is often about 11.5 to 11.8 mg/dL). After initial recognition of hypercalcemia and referral, 52% of dogs with PHPTH had an initial TCa concentration more than 12 but less than 14 mg/dL; about 30% had concentrations between 14 and 16 mg/dL, 12% had results of 16 to 18 mg/dL, and 6% had values in excess of 18 mg/dL (Feldman et al, 2005). One of eight dogs with serum TCa

concentration more than 18 mg/dL in that study had a mildly increased BUN concentration; the other seven had results within or below the reference range.

It seems logical that untreated PHPTH would result in progressively increasing serum calcium concentrations over time. This, however, has not been the experience in people. A group of 60 people with untreated PHPTH were evaluated periodically for 10 years. The mean total serum calcium concentration at the time of diagnosis was 10.5 mg/dL (reference range, 8.4 to 10.2 mg/dL); after 5 years it was 10.6 mg/dL and after a total of 10 years, it was 10.3 mg/dL (Silverberg et al, 1999). However, eight individuals developed uroliths during the decade, leaving 52 who remained asymptomatic. Two of 52 individuals (3.8%) developed "marked hypercalcemia" (defined as a serum calcium concentration greater than 12 mg/dL) during the study period, eight had significant hypercalciuria, and six had decreasing bone density. All 52, however, remained relatively asymptomatic. Dogs with PHPTH have persistent hypercalcemia and our subjective experience suggests that their hypercalcemia slowly increases with time.

Factors Affecting the Serum Calcium Concentration

Sample Error and Other Non-Pathologic Conditions. Marked lipemia can falsely increase serum TCa concentrations determined by some automated analyzers. Hemoconcentration (dehydration) and hyperproteinemia can produce mild increases in TCa. Hemolysis can also falsely increase the serum

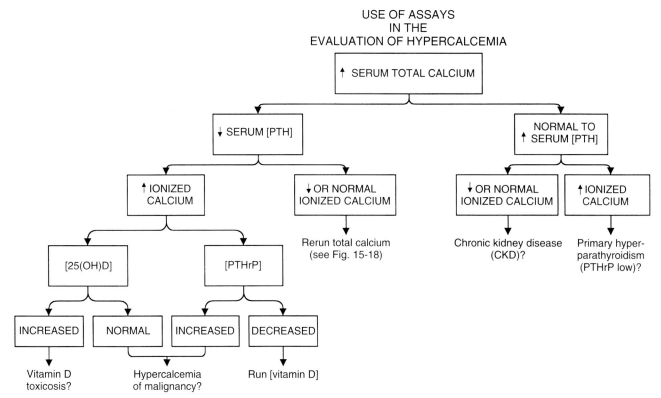

FIGURE 15-17 Algorithm showing the potential value and use of various assays in the evaluation of hypercalcemic dogs. *25(OH)D*, 25-hydroxyvitamin D; *PTH*, parathyroid hormone; *PTHrP*, parathyroid hormone–related protein.

TCa concentration measured with some automated analyzers. Young growing animals may have mild increases in serum calcium concentration, and postprandial samples may, rarely, yield false increases. Excess use of oral phosphate binders may cause the serum calcium concentration to increase. Collection and storage of samples in glassware or plastic containers that have been washed with detergents may falsely increase or decrease calcium values. Simple prolonged storage may yield artifactual decreases in the calcium concentration, and contamination (chalk writing boards in the laboratory) may yield false increases. Confirmation of hypercalcemia with a fresh blood sample would help rule out any of these concerns (Schenck and Chew, 2012).

Acid-Base Status. Acidosis decreases plasma protein–binding affinity for calcium, increasing iCa concentrations and creating mild physiologic hypercalcemia. Alkalosis has the opposite effect, creating a physiologic hypocalcemia. The total serum calcium concentration appears to change with the acid-base status in a manner roughly parallel to the change in iCa concentration (Meuten, 1984).

Age. Age should be considered when serum concentrations of calcium, phosphorus, and alkaline phosphatase are evaluated. Young dogs have higher concentrations than adults (Meuten, 1984; Schenck and Chew, 2012). Reference values for TCa concentrations in young dogs were approximately 11.1 ± 0.4 mg/dL (10.5 to 11.5 mg/dL), higher than those observed in adults (8.8 to 11.0 mg/dL) (Meuten et al, 1982).

Serum Ionized Calcium Concentration

The iCa fraction of total circulating calcium concentrations is biologically active. Valid assays for iCa can be an integral component of determining the cause for a hypercalcemic condition (Figs. 15-17 and 15-18). The mean iCa concentration from more than 135 dogs with PHPTH reported in five studies was consistently above the reference range (Gear et al, 2005; Ham et al, 2009; Sawyer et al, 2011; Arbaugh et al, 2012; Milovancev and Schmiedt, 2013). In one study, 19 (9%) of 210 dogs with PHPTH had a serum iCa concentration within the reference range. These reference range results may have been affected by external factors (aerobic collection, pH) affecting the ionized result without altering serum TCa concentrations. In that latter study, about 25% had mildly increased serum iCa concentrations (1.42 to 1.65 mg/dL), about 50% had results of 1.66 to 1.90 mg/dL, and less than 20% had iCa concentrations more than1.9 mg/dL (Feldman et al, 2005).

Serum Phosphorus Concentration

Low or low-normal serum phosphorus concentrations (< 4.0 mg/dL) are typical of PHPTH (see Fig. 15-12). Hypophosphatemia develops after PTH-induced inhibition of renal tubular phosphorus resorption, resulting in excessive urinary losses. In three reports on more than 300 dogs with PHPTH, the mean serum PO₄ concentration was 2.9, 2.8, and 2.86 mg/dL (Feldman et al, 2005; Gear et al, 2005; Milovancev and Schmiedt, 2013). Reference ranges were similar in these reports (about 3.0 to 6.2 mg/dL). In one report, dogs with PHPTH had results that ranged from 1.3 to 6.1 mg/dL, with none above the reference range, and in another report, only two of 29 dogs had values above their reference range despite 13 of 29 dogs having increases in BUN and evidence of CKD and/or AKI (Feldman et al, 2005; Gear et al, 2005).

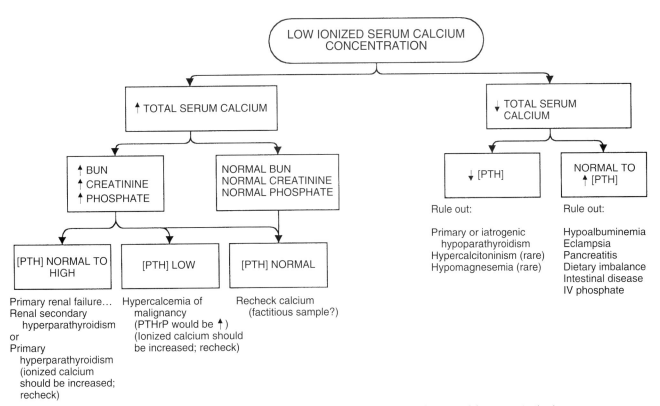

FIGURE 15-18 Algorithm for determining the cause of decreases in the ionized serum calcium concentration in dogs. *BUN,* Blood urea nitrogen; *IV,* intravenous; *PTH,* parathyroid hormone; *PTHrP,* parathyroid hormone–related protein.

The serum phosphorus concentration should always be evaluated relative to the serum calcium concentration and renal parameters. Hypophosphatemia, when dietary phosphate is adequate and oral phosphate-binding agents are not being given, is consistent with either PHPTH or hypercalcemia of malignancy (see Fig. 15-12). Other causes of hypophosphatemia are less common (Box 15-2). Hyperphosphatemia in the absence of azotemia suggests a non-parathyroid cause of hypercalcemia. When both hyperphosphatemia and azotemia are present, the clinician must rely on the history, physical examination, and other parameters to determine the primary disorder. Differentiation remains a diagnostic dilemma. Dogs with CKD and an increased TCa concentration usually have iCa concentrations that are normal or mildly low, in contrast to dogs with PHPTH, in which both total and the ionized fractions are increased.

Age should also be considered when evaluating the serum phosphorus concentration. Young dogs (< 1 year old) tend to have a higher serum phosphorus concentrations than adults. Puppies may have similar serum phosphorus and calcium concentrations (i.e., both approximately 10 to 12 mg/dL). However, the serum phosphorus concentration gradually declines during puppyhood, reaching normal adult concentrations by 4 to 12 months of age.

Blood Urea Nitrogen and Serum Creatinine

Blood Urea Nitrogen. Almost all dogs with PHPTH have normal renal parameters (BUN, creatinine; see Table 15-6). Among about 320 dogs with PHPTH, the incidence of abnormally increased renal parameters was 4% or less. In one study of 210 dogs with PHPTH, their mean BUN of 16.9 mg/dL was below the reference

---

BOX 15-2   Potential Causes of Hypophosphatemia

Decreased Intestinal Absorption
Decreased dietary intake
Malabsorption/steatorrhea
Vomiting/diarrhea
Phosphate-binding antacids
Vitamin D deficiency

Increased Urinary Excretion
Primary hyperparathyroidism (PHPTH)
Diabetes mellitus ± ketoacidosis
Hyperadrenocorticism (naturally occurring/iatrogenic)
Fanconi syndrome (renal tubular defects)
Diuretic or bicarbonate administration
Hypothermia recovery
Hyperaldosteronism
Aggressive parenteral fluid administration
Hypercalcemia of malignancy (early stages)

Transcellular Shifts
Insulin administration
Parenteral glucose administration
Hyperalimentation
Respiratory alkalosis

range of 18 to 30 mg/dL. Three percent had a BUN less than 10, and 60% had concentrations of 10 to 17. Thus, almost two thirds of dogs with PHPTH had BUN concentrations less than the lower limit of the reference range. About 25% had results in the lower half of the reference range, and 10% had results in the upper half of the reference range. Nine of the 210 dogs had abnormally increased BUN concentrations, ranging from 31 to 92 mg/dL. The serum TCa concentrations from these nine dogs were not significantly different from the dogs whose BUN concentrations were within or below the reference range (Feldman et al, 2005). One report on 29 dogs with PHPTH, however, included 13 dogs with increases in BUN, 10 of which were "marked" (Gear et al, 2005). By contrast, renal failure was not mentioned or rare in the reports on about 110 dogs with PHPTH (Ham et al, 2009; Sawyer et al, 2011; Arbaugh et al, 2012; Milovancev and Schmiedt, 2013).

Creatinine. Mean serum creatinine concentrations for 210 dogs with PHPTH were 0.8 mg/dL. Sixty percent of the dogs had results less than 1.0, and 37% had values of 1.0 to 1.5 mg/dL. Thus, 97% had results within the reference range. Three percent (seven dogs) had results above 1.5 mg/dL. The highest serum creatinine concentration in any dog was 4.1 mg/dL, and six of the seven dogs had increases in both BUN and creatinine concentrations. Four dogs with increases in both BUN and creatinine concentrations had been diagnosed with CKD 3 to 24 months before becoming hypercalcemic.

Renal Values in Dogs Who Do Not Have Primary Hyperparathyroidism. In the study on 210 dogs with PHPTH, 200 control dogs that did not have PHPTH had significantly higher mean BUN and creatinine concentrations. It would appear that dogs with PHPTH are less likely to have abnormal renal parameters than dogs that do not have PHPTH. Whether this is the result of the low calcium x phosphate product or some other factor is not known. In one study, the TCa x phosphate product was not predictive of renal failure (Gear et al, 2005) and that study had far more dogs with renal failure than was seen in five studies on 320 dogs with PHPTH (Feldman et al, 2005; Ham et al, 2009; Sawyer et al, 2011; Arbaugh et al, 2012; Milovancev and Schmiedt, 2013).

The uncommonly encountered combination of azotemia, hypercalcemia, hyperphosphatemia, and increases in serum PTH concentrations represents a diagnostic challenge. Such changes could lead to renal failure or develop as a consequence of renal failure. Increases in serum TCa concentration have been documented in as many as 10% to 15% of dogs with CKD, with hypercalcemia worsening severity of azotemia. However, the deleterious effects of hypercalcemia may only be associated with abnormally increased serum iCa concentrations. Fewer than 10% of all dogs with CKD have increases in iCa, most have normal or low concentrations. As discussed, the serum iCa is usually normal or low in CKD and almost always increased with PHPTH. Rarely, tertiary hyperparathyroidism occurs in dogs with CKD as an extremely unusual progression of renal secondary hyperparathyroidism. It is most likely due to an alteration in the set point for circulating iCa (Schenck and Chew, 2012). Use of both serum iCa and PTH concentrations are useful in determining cause (see Figs. 15-17 and 15-18). It is possible for PHPTH to predispose a small percentage of dogs to kidney injury, that some dogs with PHPTH may also have CKD, or that some dogs with CKD develop tertiary hyperparathyroidism, accounting for what might be autonomous secretion of PTH.

Serum Alkaline Phosphatase

In humans, an increase in serum alkaline phosphatase (SAP) is more common in hypercalcemia of malignancy than in PHPTH (Arnaud and Kolb, 1991). Increases in SAP activity are nonspecific

in veterinary medicine; about 40% of dogs with PHPTH had an increased result. When present, increases were generally mild (twofold to sixfold) with a mean of 240 IU/L (range, 12 to more than 4,000 IU/L; reference range, 5 to 92 IU/L). The increased activity of this enzyme, when present, is thought to result from a compensatory increase in osteoblastic activity in bone trabeculae as a response to mechanical stress in bone weakened by excessive resorption (Capen and Martin, 1983).

Serum Alanine Aminotransferase

Serum alanine aminotransferase (ALT) concentrations are usually normal in dogs with PHPTH. Mild increases are nonspecific and not usually worrisome. The suggestion that mild increases may reflect hepatic ischemia due to systemic dehydration seems unlikely. Moderate to marked increases in ALT should raise concern that a separate and concurrent liver condition exists.

Serum Chloride Concentration

In people, excess PTH secretion decreases the proximal renal tubular resorption of bicarbonate, leading to increased resorption of chloride and the production of mild hyperchloremic renal tubular acidosis. Increased serum chloride concentrations in people with PHPTH often are associated with serum chloride-to-phosphate ratios greater than 33 (Arnaud and Kolb, 1991). With the availability of reliable PTH and PTHrP assays, the increases in the serum chloride concentration are less critical as a diagnostic tool but may aggravate existing hypercalcemia by impairing binding of calcium to albumin and by increasing the dissolution of bone mineral.

Urinalysis

Urine Specific Gravity

Many dogs with PHPTH have relatively dilute urine on randomly collected home-caught or in-hospital obtained samples. In 210 dogs with PHPTH, their mean urine specific gravity (USG) was 1.012. Fifty dogs (24%) had a USG less than 1.008 on randomly collected urine; 75 (36%) had a result of 1.008 to 1.012; 70 (33%) had a results ranging from 1.013 to 1.020; eight (4%) had a USG of 1.021 to 1.030; and seven had a result greater than 1.030 (see Table 15-6). These results reflect the effect of hypercalcemia interfering with the action of ADH action at the renal tubular level causing a reversible form of nephrogenic diabetes insipidus. Randomly obtained USG from 140 age-matched control dogs that did not have PHPTH had a significantly higher mean of 1.025 (Feldman et al, 2005).

Isosthenuria (or hyposthenuria) is a common consequence of hypercalcemia, regardless of its etiology. The combination of hypercalcemia and dilute urine is considered a cause and effect phenomenon, but it is not specific for any condition. Confusion regarding cause may arise because CKD is a differential diagnosis for isosthenuria. A thorough review of the serum chemistry profile and other parameters may be necessary to determine cause of isosthenuria or hyposthenuria.

Urine Sediment

Hematuria, pyuria, bacteriuria, and/or crystalluria are often identified in the urine sediment of dogs with PHPTH. Hypercalciuria, proximal renal tubular acidosis with impaired bicarbonate resorption, and the production of alkaline urine may predispose dogs to the development of bacterial cystitis and urolith formation. Urinary tract infection, at the time of PHPTH diagnosis, was identified in almost 30% of 210 dogs. One third of those dogs had concurrent cystic calculi. Cystic calculi had been surgically removed from 42 of 210 dogs (20%) in the 6 month period preceding diagnosis of PHPTH. Fifty dogs (24%) had cystic calculi when seen at our hospital, but 27 of those 50 were among the 42 who had already had surgery, indicating recurrence. Thus, a total of 65 dogs (31%) with PHPTH had cystic calculi. All analyzed calculi were calcium oxalate, calcium phosphate, or both (Feldman et al, 2005; see Fig. 15-15).

Electrocardiography

Experimentally induced hypercalcemia may increase myocardial contractility, shorten mechanical ventricular systole, and decrease myocardial automaticity. Potential electrocardiographic changes caused by hypercalcemia include a prolongation of the P-R interval and a shortening of the QT interval as a result of a shortened ST segment (Feldman, 1989). Theoretically, the decrease in myocardial conduction velocity and the shortened refractory period could predispose to arrhythmias. Cardiac abnormalities are rare in dogs with PHPTH.

IMAGING

Radiography

General

Conventional radiography plays an integral role in the diagnostic evaluation of hypercalcemic dogs or cats. Thoracic radiographs should be obtained in order to screen for neoplasia. Abdominal ultrasonography may be preferred over radiographs, although these imaging modalities are complementary. Lack of thoracic or abdominal radiographic or ultrasonographic abnormalities in a dog with hypercalcemia is consistent with PHPTH.

Thoracic Radiographs

The anterior mediastinum, perihilar, and sternal lymph nodes should be evaluated for mass effect or lymphadenopathy. The classic finding in hypercalcemic dogs with lymphosarcoma is an anterior mediastinal mass (Fig. 15-19). The ribs, vertebrae, and any long bones included in the study should be evaluated for osteolytic areas arising from myeloma or other metastatic tumors. The lung fields should be carefully assessed for nodules that might represent primary or metastatic lesions.

Abdomen and Skeleton

Other than urinary tract calculi, radiographic alterations associated with PHPTH are rare. As previously discussed, cystic calculi are common and urethral calculi are always a concern, especially in male dogs. Uroliths have quite uncommonly been identified in the kidneys and ureters. The sublumbar area and mesenteric lymph nodes can be evaluated for any mass effect that might be indicative of metastatic apocrine gland carcinoma of the anal sac, lymphoma, or other neoplastic process (Fig. 15-20). The liver and spleen should be similarly evaluated for enlargement or irregularities associated with neoplasia.

Osteitis fibrosa cystica, the classic bony abnormality of primary and secondary hyperparathyroidism in humans, is rarely seen in dogs. It is manifested radiographically as generalized osteopenia due to increased bone resorption, especially at the subperiosteal surfaces, and the formation of cysts or cystlike areas in bone. In humans the phalanges and skull are usually involved. In severe cases, the long bones, patella, and ribs may become involved. The clinical manifestations of osteitis fibrosa cystica are bone pain, pathologic fractures, bone cysts, and localized swelling of bone (Hruska and Teitelbaum, 1995). Radiographic changes rarely associated with PHPTH in dogs include loss of the lamina dura, fractures of the long bones and vertebrae, and soft tissue calcification. Fractures have been described in only one of more than 340 dogs with PHPTH (Feldman et al, 2005; Gear et al, 2005; Ham et al, 2009; Arbaugh et al, 2012; Milovancev and Schmiedt, 2013).

Ultrasonography

Neck

Background. Parathyroid ultrasonography has been used extensively in people as part of the diagnostic evaluation for hypercalcemia. Applications have included differentiation of primary and secondary hyperparathyroidism; confirmation of suspect lesions by ultrasound-guided, fine-needle aspiration biopsy; and presurgical localization of parathyroid adenomas (Attie et al, 1988; Krubsack et al, 1989; Lloyd et al, 1990). Reported sensitivity of ultrasonography in identifying one or more abnormal parathyroid glands in people is well over 90% (Wysolmerski and Insogna, 2012). In dogs, parathyroid glands as small as 1 to 2 mm

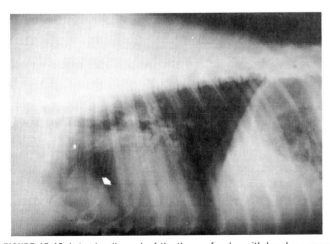

FIGURE 15-19 Lateral radiograph of the thorax of a dog with lymphosarcoma and hypercalcemia. Note the sternal lymphadenopathy *(arrow)*.

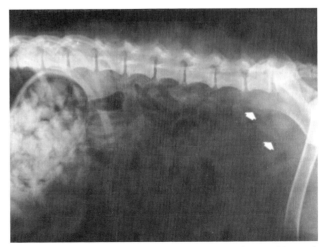

FIGURE 15-20 Lateral radiograph of the caudal abdomen of a dog with apocrine gland adenocarcinoma of the anal sac and hypercalcemia. Note the multiple masses in the sublumbar region and pelvic canal *(arrows)*, which are suggestive of sublumbar lymph nodes that have been invaded by the neoplasia.

in diameter can be visualized. Accuracy of ultrasonographic evaluation is determined by facilities as well as the skill and experience of the ultrasonographer.

An "ectopic" location for parathyroid tumors is possible. Although reported in humans, ectopic parathyroid tumors have not been reported in dogs or cats. Localization of ectopic abnormal parathyroid tissue can be difficult. In humans, noninvasive procedures that can be used include esophagoscopy, computed tomography (CT), and radionuclide scans. Invasive procedures include thyroid arteriography, selective venous catheterization of the neck and mediastinal veins, and surgical exploration of the anterior mediastinum (Arnaud and Kolb, 1991). Although ectopic parathyroid tissue or tumor is rare, this condition may be considered in any dog whose testing is indicative of PHPTH but whose cervical ultrasonographic examination is negative. Visualization of "normal" parathyroid glands without seeing a "nodule" is not consistent with PHPTH. If the parathyroid glands seem small or not visualized, one may suspect an ectopic location. This would also be a concern should a surgeon be unable to see any abnormal thyroid-parathyroid tissue.

Dogs. The parathyroid glands in healthy dogs can be routinely visualized (Wisner et al, 1991; Reusch et al, 2000; Pollard et al, in press). Parathyroid masses are usually solitary, round or oval, well marginated, and hypoechoic to anechoic compared with surrounding thyroid gland parenchyma (Fig. 15-21). Occasionally two enlarged parathyroid glands may be identified in dogs with PHPTH. Seeing three or four enlarged glands is not typical. Not every nodule in the parathyroid anatomic region is obvious. Some masses have not been seen, whereas the cell type of others is sometimes questioned. The most common concern was whether an identified mass was thyroid or parathyroid (see Incidentally Discovered Thyroid Masses).

Parathyroid masses (usually adenomas) from dogs with PHPTH have been as small as 2 mm to as large as 23 mm in diameter. Most adenomas are 4 to 10 mm in diameter and easily visualized (Wisner et al, 1993; Wisner and Nyland, 1994). A statistically significant size difference was reported for solitary hyperplastic parathyroid glands (2 to 6 mm, mean 2.9 mm) as compared with solitary parathyroid adenomas or adenocarcinomas (4 to 20 mm, mean 7.5 mm) (Wisner et al, 1997).

Similar to reports in people, ultrasonography correctly identified parathyroid mass size and location (as determined by surgery) in 63% to 100% of dogs with PHPTH (Feldman et al, 2005; Gear et al, 2005; Ham et al, 2009; Sawyer et al, 2011; Arbaugh et al, 2012; Milovancev and Schmiedt, 2013). Although a reference range for parathyroid gland size on ultrasonographic examination has not been established for dogs, it has been suggested that most healthy dogs have glands 1 to 3 mm in greatest diameter. For the 142 masses correctly identified in one study, the mean abnormal parathyroid gland was 6 mm (range, 3 to 23 mm) in greatest diameter. Sixty percent of the nodules were 3 to 6 mm in greatest diameter, 24% were 7 to 10 mm, 10% were 11 to 15 mm, and 6% were greater than 15 mm in greatest diameter. In this study, 116 dogs had a solitary parathyroid mass and 13 dogs (10%) had 2 distinct masses. No dog had more than two masses identified (Feldman et al, 2005; see Table 15-7). In another study, 76% of the ultrasonographic assessments were correct as determined by the tissue identified and removed. However, in 19% of the dogs, ultrasonography results did not agree with surgical findings regarding laterality of the parathyroid mass location (Milovancev and Schmiedt, 2013). In another study, 12 ultrasonographic-identified parathyroid masses were confirmed at surgery, but five enlarged masses seen at surgery had not been identified via ultrasonography and two masses identified with ultrasonography were not seen at surgery (Ham et al, 2009). By contrast, all 17 parathyroid carcinomas in another study were correctly identified via ultrasonography (Sawyer et al, 2011).

Because results of cervical ultrasonography are often of use in establishing a diagnosis of PHPTH, we include and recommend cervical ultrasonography as a diagnostic aid for any hypercalcemic dog. Failure to identify a parathyroid mass in a dog suspected as having PHPTH is cause for reconsidering the differential diagnosis for hypercalcemia. Experience of the operator and equipment quality (including use of the correct transducer) must be considered (Wisner et al, 1993; Wisner and Nyland, 1994).

Abdomen

Ultrasonographic scanning of the abdomen, when possible, should be a component of the diagnostic evaluation of hypercalcemic dogs and cats. If the liver, spleen, mesenteric lymph nodes, or other abdominal structures appear abnormal, percutaneous fine needle aspiration or biopsy should be considered. Ultrasonography has proven to be an excellent tool for identifying uroliths as well. Most uroliths are found in the bladder, but renal, ureter, and urethral stones also have been identified.

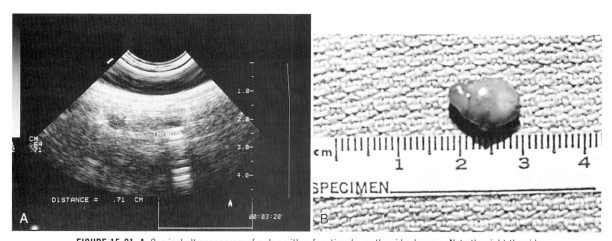

FIGURE 15-21 A, Cervical ultrasonogram of a dog with a functional parathyroid adenoma. Note the right thyroid lobe, in which a well-marginated, hypoechoic mass *(arrows)* is visible at the cranial pole of the thyroid. **B,** Solitary parathyroid adenoma removed from a dog with primary hyperparathyroidism (PHPTH; see Fig. 15-26, *C*). (**A,** Courtesy of Dr. Tom Nyland and Dr. Erik Wisner.)

Incidentally Discovered Thyroid Masses

One study has assessed the prevalence of subclinical thyroid nodules in dogs undergoing cervical ultrasonography as a component of evaluating hypercalcemia. No dog had a palpable mass, and in no dog was the thyroid believed responsible for hypercalcemia. At least one "incidentally discovered" thyroid nodule was identified in 14 of 91 PHPTH dogs. The thyroid gland masses had a mean length, width, and height of 1.5, 1.0, and 0.75 cm, respectively. Histologic diagnoses included thyroid cysts, adenomas, adenocarcinomas, and one dog with nodular hyperplasia. These results suggest that subclinical thyroid nodules are present in some hypercalcemic dogs that do not have a palpable neck mass (Pollard et al, in press). The clinical significance and management of incidentally identified thyroid nodules in dogs remains to be elucidated.

USE OF PARATHYROID HORMONE AND PARATHYROID HORMONE–RELATED PROTEIN ASSAYS

In dogs with PHPTH, serum PTH concentrations are typically mid/normal to increased (Figs. 15-5 and 15-22), serum PTHrP concentrations should be undetectable, and serum calcitriol

concentrations would be expected to be normal to increased. Serum PTH concentration must always be evaluated relative to the serum calcium concentration. In normal animals, as the serum calcium concentration increases, the serum PTH concentration decreases. Therefore, a serum PTH concentration in the reference range from a hypercalcemic dog is not ***normal.*** Relative to their hypercalcemia (using TCa or iCa) dogs with PHPTH have excessive concentrations of serum PTH even though the result may be within the reference range. These results are consistent with a condition associated with autonomous secretion of PTH (Fig. 15-23).

The challenge for laboratories that offer serum PTH assays is that companies either go out of business or discontinue products. Therefore, assays utilized by laboratories invariably must change. Regarding PTH assays, quality of the results using newer products has either been similar or more reliable as compared with older products (see Fig. 15-5). Comparison of PTH assay results from different studies performed at various times and locations is difficult. Currently, the PTH assay that provides excellent correlation in dogs and cats is an intact-molecule assay, which has numerically lower test values as compared with previously reported results. The N-terminal antibody in previously utilized "intact sandwich" assay systems cross reacted with a biologically inactive PTH 7-83 amino acid fragment. The new intact-molecule PTH assay antibody requires the first four amino acids of the N-terminal be present for binding (Refsal, 2014). One study compared the "intact sandwich" PTH assay system that requires several days to complete with a rapid, 20-minute chemiluminescent assay. Within-run and day-to-day precisions were comparable, and there was a high correlation in results. Numerical results from the rapid chemiluminescent assay system were usually lower than the intact assay (Ham et al, 2009).

In one study, serum PTH concentrations were determined using an immunoradiometric "intact sandwich" assay for PTH in randomly obtained serum samples from 185 dogs with PHPTH. The mean serum PTH concentration of 11.3 pmol/L was within the reference range (2 to 13 pmol/L). Almost 75% of these dogs had a serum PTH concentration within the reference range, about 45% in the lower half and almost 30% in the upper half of the reference range. About 10% of the 185 dogs had "mildly increased" serum PTH concentration, and about 15% had moderate or extreme increases (see Table 15-7; Feldman et al, 2005). Other studies have reported similar results: a mean serum PTH concentration in dogs with PHPTH of 13.6 pmol/L

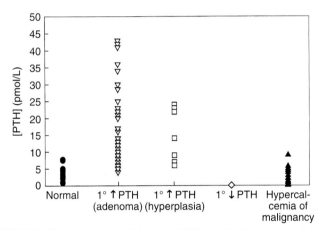

FIGURE 15-22 Serum parathyroid hormone *(PTH)* concentrations for normal dogs and those with various disorders of calcium homeostasis. Note that some overlap exists in test results and that the results shown in Fig. 15-23 are easier to interpret. *1° ↑ PTH,* primary hyperparathyroidism; *1° ↓ PTH,* primary hypoparathyroidism.

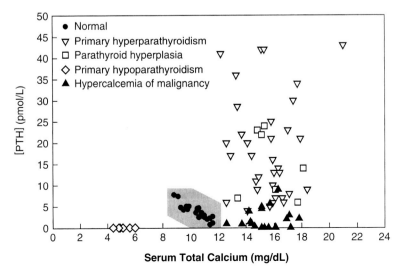

FIGURE 15-23 Serum parathyroid hormone *(PTH)* concentrations plotted against simultaneous serum calcium concentrations from normal dogs and those with abnormalities in calcium homeostasis. Note that the various groups are more distinguishable than would be the case if only the serum calcium or only the serum PTH concentrations were evaluated. The shaded area represents the approximate reference range.

BOX 15-3   Differential Diagnosis for Humoral Hypercalcemia of Malignancy

Hematologic Cancers
Lymphosarcoma
Lymphocytic leukemia
Myeloproliferative disease
Myeloma

Solid Tumors with Bone Metastasis
Mammary adenocarcinoma
Nasal adenocarcinoma
Epithelial-derived tumors
Pancreatic adenocarcinoma
Lung carcinoma

Solid Tumors without Bone Metastasis
Apocrine gland adenocarcinoma of the anal sac
Interstitial cell tumor
Squamous cell carcinoma
Thyroid adenocarcinoma
Lung carcinoma
Pancreatic adenocarcinoma
Fibrosarcoma

(reference range, 2 to 13 pmol/L) (Arbaugh et al, 2012); 8 out of 12 dogs (75%) with PHPTH had serum PTH concentrations within the reference range, and 4 out of 12 were increased (Ham et al, 2009); and a mean of 17.7 pmol/L in 19 dogs with PHPTH with a range of 4.7 to 156 pmol/L (reference range, 3 to 17 pmol/L) (Sawyer et al, 2011).

 DIAGNOSTIC APPROACH TO THE HYPERCALCEMIC PATIENT

General Comments

The list of differential diagnoses for hypercalcemia is relatively short (see Boxes 15-1 and 15-3), allowing a logical approach to identification of its cause. At the same time, serum inorganic phosphorus should be assessed, and if low, that differential diagnosis can be considered as well (Box 15-2). The most common cause of hypercalcemia and hypophosphatemia in the dog is malignancy-associated hypercalcemia. In an attempt to be practical, logical, and cost-effective, the veterinarian should design the diagnostic approach to first identify or rule out an underlying malignancy. Diagnostic testing can proceed to assess each patient for PHPTH simultaneously as the testing is interwoven.

Review of the History and Physical Examination

First Steps

The diagnostic approach to the hypercalcemic patient is usually relatively straightforward (see Box 15-1; Fig. 15-24). One may wish to submit a second blood sample to recheck the calcium and phosphorus results, although the second sample is rarely different. Next, submit appropriate samples for a serum iCa concentration to confirm the presence of hypercalcemia. If the iCa concentration is within or below the reference range in a dog with confirmed increases in serum TCa concentration, CKD should be among the conditions considered (see Fig. 15-18). Rechecking an "illogical" iCa result is always wise.

Signalment

Review of breed is emphasized because of the genetic predisposition for developing PHPTH in the Keeshond. PHPTH typically occurs in dogs 7 years of age or older. CKD can occur at any age. Dogs of any age are at risk for malignancy (lymphosarcoma), toxin exposure, granulomatous disease, or hypoadrenocorticism, whereas apocrine gland carcinoma of the anal sac and some other malignancies occur in older dogs.

History

The owner should be asked about their pet's diet, travel history, vitamin-mineral supplementation, and exposure to rat or mouse poisons or houseplants that contain vitamin D analogs. An attempt can be made to determine whether the pet is in pain (lytic bone lesions). Response to questions about the presence of polydipsia, polyuria, appetite, activity, change in body weight, ability to exercise, vomiting, diarrhea, and any other pertinent information, may be important. Generally, as the pet appears more ill, PHPTH becomes less likely.

Physical Examination

After assessment of the dog's hydration status and severity of illness, the physical examination should include careful palpation of peripheral lymph nodes and the mammary glands (lymphoma and mammary cancer). A thorough rectal and perirectal examination is imperative to help rule in or out apocrine gland carcinoma of the anal sac. Anal sac tumors may be covered by haired skin and may not be identified unless rectal and perirectal examinations are performed. A digital vaginal examination should also be performed (vaginal tumor). The veterinarian should gently palpate as much of the skeleton as possible, searching for any area of focal bone pain, which then could be examined further with radiographs (multiple myeloma). The kidneys should be palpated in an attempt to assess size or irregularities.

Initial Database

Blood and Urine

The initial database should include a hemogram (complete blood count [CBC]), serum biochemical profile, serum iCa, urinalysis, and thoracic radiographs. The abdomen should be evaluated with ultrasonography, radiography, or both. If the serum phosphorus concentration is normal or low, CKD and rodenticide toxicosis are less likely (see Fig. 15-24). Dogs with hypoadrenocorticism usually have hyperphosphatemia in addition to their hyperkalemia and hyponatremia. Serum creatinine and BUN concentrations are also critically important. Evaluation of the sodium-to-potassium ratio should help identify hypoadrenocorticism. A sodium-to-potassium ratio less than 27:1 is consistent with but not necessarily diagnostic of adrenal insufficiency. An ACTH stimulation test should be performed if Addison's disease is considered likely, whereas a basal serum cortisol can be assessed if Addison's disease is considered a possibility. If the serum phosphorus concentration is increased and renal function is normal, bone osteolysis secondary to metastatic disease should be considered. Low, low-normal, or normal serum phosphate concentrations are consistent with PHPTH and malignancy-associated hypercalcemia (see Fig. 15-12). A striking increase in the total protein concentration, specifically due to a monoclonal spike, is classic for multiple myeloma.

Primary Parathyroid Disease Versus Primary Renal Disease

A diagnostic dilemma exists when hyperphosphatemia and hypercalcemia coexist with azotemia. The clinician must determine

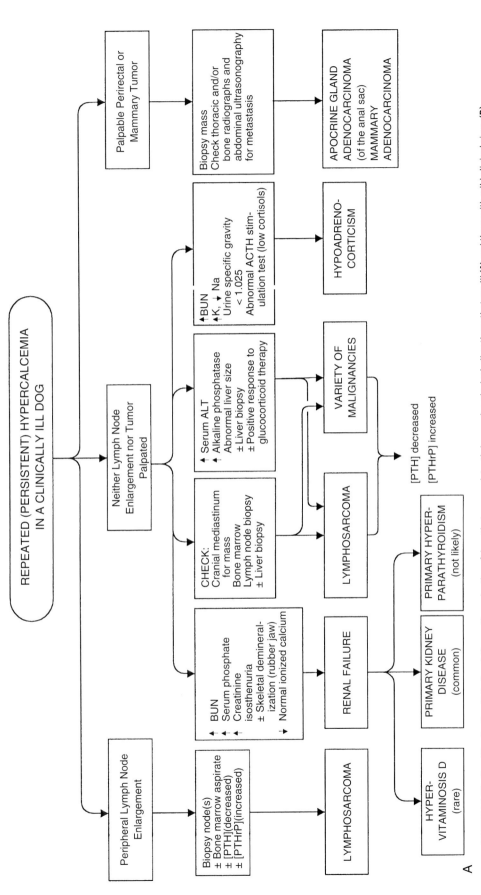

FIGURE 15-24 Algorithm for the clinical and diagnostic evaluation of dogs that are persistently hypercalcemic, including those that are ill (**A**) and those with mild clinical signs (**B**).

Continued

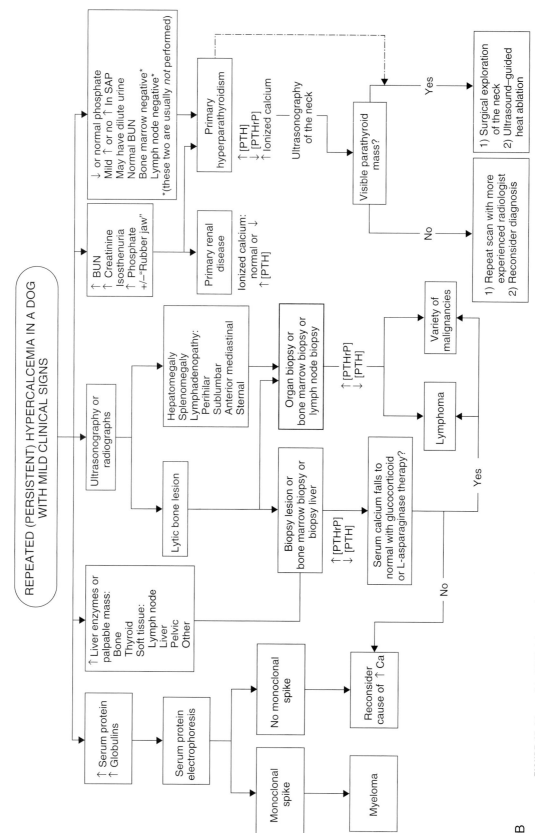

FIGURE 15-24, cont'd *ACTH,* Adrenocorticotropic hormone; *ALT,* alanine aminotransferase; *BUN,* blood urea nitrogen; *PTH,* parathyroid hormone; *PTHrP,* parathyroid hormone–related protein; *SAP,* serum alkaline phosphatase.

whether the hypercalcemia is the cause or the consequence of renal disease. Other abnormalities in the initial database supportive of CKD as the primary problem include mild to marked increase in the serum phosphorus concentration, a normal to low serum iCa concentration, nonregenerative anemia, proteinuria, and/or palpably or radiographically small and irregular kidneys. The serum iCa fraction in dogs with PHPTH is increased. If hypercalcemia dissipates with aggressive fluid therapy and diuresis, PHPTH is less likely. Furthermore, dogs with renal failure usually have a TCa concentration less than 12.5 mg/dL. Dogs with PHPTH and secondary renal disease typically have a total serum calcium concentration greater than 13 mg/dL (see Figs. 15-5, 15-17, 15-18, and 15-24).

Radiography and Ultrasonography

Radiographs of the thorax and ultrasonographic examination of the abdomen should be evaluated for soft tissue masses, soft tissue calcification, evidence of fungal disease, organomegaly, osteolysis, and/or osteoporosis. The goal is to identify an abnormal area that could be biopsied in the hope of providing a definitive explanation for hypercalcemia. An anterior mediastinal mass is demonstrable radiographically in as many as 40% of hypercalcemic dogs with lymphosarcoma (see Fig. 15-19; Greenlee et al, 1990). If hepatomegaly or splenomegaly is identified, histologic evaluation of a fine needle aspirate or of a biopsy could be considered.

Adenocarcinomas derived from the apocrine glands of the anal sac may appear radiographically as a mass in the pelvic canal. Sublumbar lymphadenopathy caused by tumor metastasis is also common (see Fig. 15-20; Meuten et al, 1983b; Meuten, 1984). Soft tissue calcification is most frequently observed with hypervitaminosis D or CKD, although mineralization can be seen with any hypercalcemic disorder in association with hyperphosphatemia and a calcium x phosphorus product greater than 60 to 80.

Discrete lytic lesions in the vertebrae or long bones are suggestive of either myeloma or malignancy-associated hypercalcemia with bone metastasis (see Fig. 15-16). Radionuclide bone scans (Fig. 15-25) may identify or exclude focal bone lesions not detected with plain radiography (Chew et al, 1991). One dog with PHPTH had the uncommon finding of fractures at the time of presentation (Gear et al, 2005). Concurrent hyperproteinemia is supportive of myeloma. Solid tumors with metastasis to bone are more likely if lytic bone lesions and normoproteinemia (especially a normal serum globulin concentration) are present. A core biopsy of a lytic lesion may be necessary to establish a definitive diagnosis of neoplasia. Mild generalized osteoporosis is difficult to diagnose with plain survey radiographs. If present, however, it is suggestive of PHPTH or hypercalcemia of malignancy.

Ultrasonography of the cervical region has been reviewed. This tool is noninvasive and can be quite valuable (see Fig. 15-21).

Identification of a solitary mass in or near one thyroid lobe supports the presence of an autonomously functioning parathyroid mass if the dog does not have CKD (Reusch et al, 2000).

Lymph Node and Bone Marrow Evaluations

If the initial database has not established a diagnosis, the clinician may consider histologic evaluation of lymph nodes, bone marrow, or both. Lymphosarcoma is the most common cancer associated with hypercalcemia in the dog and cat. Involvement of the peripheral lymph nodes in lymphosarcoma can be present without enlargement of those nodes, although such a finding would be unusual. Ideally, the largest lymph node (not the submandibular node) should be assessed for histologic evaluation. Needle aspirates for cytology are often diagnostic, but biopsy samples may be requested. These steps may be omitted in dogs that are relatively healthy according to their owners and veterinarians, who have unremarkable CBCs, and no abnormalities seen on thoracic radiographs.

A bone marrow aspirate may be considered in the hypercalcemic pet because the lymphosarcoma may invade the marrow (Meuten et al, 1983b). As with the peripheral lymph node evaluation, the presence of a normal bone marrow aspirate does not definitively rule out lymphosarcoma. As with the lymph node aspirate or biopsy, we usually omit this diagnostic tool when a dog is clinically well and when a CBC is unremarkable.

Specific Assays: Parathyroid Hormone, Parathyroid Hormone–Related Protein, and Calcitriol

See previous discussions.

Trial Therapy—Why This Approach Is *Strongly* Discouraged

If the diagnostic evaluation described fails to identify a cause for hypercalcemia, the clinician is faced with a diagnostic decision:
* Wait and retest?
* Trial medical therapy?
* Exploratory surgery of the neck?

If a hypercalcemic dog is stable, eating, and not significantly ill, we recommend rechecking any vague test result after a few days or weeks. The clinician should also consider referring the client and patient to a colleague more familiar with hypercalcemia and/or capable of performing high quality cervical ultrasonography, fine needle aspiration under ultrasonographic guidance, or some other diagnostic aid. Ill hypercalcemic dogs may also benefit from referral and a new opinion.

Most of the disorders that cause hypercalcemia are not "occult," but a diagnosis may occasionally be difficult. Diagnosis of PHPTH or malignancy-associated hypercalcemia (usually lymphosarcoma) can be straightforward (common) or problematic (uncommon). The veterinarian is reminded to complete a thorough history, bearing in mind the importance of diet, supplements, and potential exposure to toxins (Mellanby et al, 2005). The ability to utilize the combination of cervical and abdominal ultrasonography together with assessment of PTH and PTHrP assays usually leads to a correct diagnosis. Occasionally, the results of these tests are nebulous, and the clinician may consider one of two options: (1) surgical exploration of the neck to look for a parathyroid tumor, or (2) trial therapy with a chemotherapeutic drug effective against lymphosarcoma to see if the hypercalcemia can be alleviated.

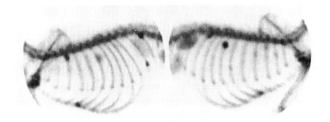

FIGURE 15-25 Bone scan from a dog with hypercalcemia caused by multiple myeloma. Note that the focal "black" areas are those of increased bone activity, as is typical for a metastatic lesion. (Courtesy of Dr. William Hornof, Davis, CA.)

Nonspecific Medical Treatment for Hypercalcemia

If hypercalcemia is caused by a lymphosarcoma (or other hematopoietic tumor), a rapid decline in the serum calcium concentration is common within 48 hours of glucocorticoid administration (Chew et al, 1991). The actions of glucocorticoids in inhibiting the growth of neoplastic lymphoid tissue and lymphocytolysis account for their rapid beneficial effect in most dogs with hematologic cancers, such as lymphoma or multiple myeloma (Goodwin et al, 1986). Glucocorticoids also counteract the effects of vitamin D, which accounts for their value, while limited, in animals with vitamin D toxicosis or granulomatous diseases (Sandler et al, 1984). In general, glucocorticoid therapy is ineffective in PHPTH or nonhematologic cancers (Bilezikian, 1992b). If the serum calcium concentration fails to decline after glucocorticoid administration, PHPTH may be considered as a possible explanation, but this represents a dangerous and inappropriate protocol for diagnosis. Unfortunately, glucocorticoids have nonspecific effects on calcium homeostasis and may cause transient declines in TCa or iCa. If the serum calcium concentration decreases into the reference range after administration of a chemotherapeutic agent, lymphosarcoma and other malignancies should be suspected and further diagnostic tests implemented to confirm this diagnosis. However, confirmation of lymphosarcoma in dogs who have received glucocorticoids may be challenging, and their response to adjunct therapy may be adversely affected.

Exploratory Surgery—No Longer Necessary?

Surgical exploration of the neck is an alternative approach for attempting to manage a dog with hypercalcemia of undetermined origin. The use of PTH, PTHrP, and iCa assays together with cervical and abdominal ultrasonography should negate the need for a true "exploratory" procedure. In other words, PHPTH can be confirmed in almost all dogs with PHPTH prior to surgery. Thus, surgery becomes a therapeutic regimen rather than a diagnostic tool. We again emphasize, *confidence in a diagnosis prior to surgery or medical therapy is preferred over "exploratory" or "trial" therapies.*

Spontaneous Resolution of Primary Hyperparathyroidism

Acute hypocalcemia has been described in two dogs with histories of chronic hypercalcemia. The acute hypocalcemia may have been the result of parathyroid gland tumor infarction and necrosis. Hypocalcemia may have resulted because the remaining parathyroid glands were atrophied and transiently unable to compensate for acute loss of PTH (Rosol et al, 1988).

ACUTE MEDICAL THERAPY FOR HYPERCALCEMIA (*NOT* PRIMARY HYPERPARATHYROIDISM)

Primary Hyperparathyroidism Versus Other Disorders

Dogs with Primary Hyperparathyroidism Do Not Require Immediate Therapy for Hypercalcemia

Treatment of dogs and cats with PHPTH involves ablation or surgical excision of abnormal tissue. Their hypercalcemia would rarely be "acute," and the calcium x phosphate product is usually normal or low. Although hypercalcemia can be theoretically cause mineralization of nephrons, this not a concern among most dogs with PHPTH. We have not employed any "acute" or other long-term medical therapy in dogs that we suspect as having PHPTH, other than strongly advising owners to provide their dog with ready access to water at all times. The following discussion on medical therapies is directed at ill or extremely ill dogs whose hypercalcemia is not caused by PHPTH. If a dog with PHPTH is ill, there should be concern of a concurrent problem. Despite a dramatic increase in the serum calcium concentration (mean serum TCa concentration > 14 mg/dL), dogs and cats with PHPTH are typically stable and not in need of emergency therapy (Table 15-8).

Therapy for Renal Failure or Vitamin D Toxicosis

Severity of clinical signs and degree of kidney injury depends, in part, on both serum calcium and phosphorus concentrations. Renal damage induced by metastatic mineralization is thought to correlate with the serum TCa x phosphate product. Products greater than 60 to 80 may be associated with nephrotoxicity. Thus hypercalcemia associated with PHPTH (low-normal or low serum phosphate concentrations) is less worrisome and dangerous than the hypercalcemia associated conditions like renal failure or hypervitaminosis D (high-normal to increased concentrations; see Table 15-8).

Indications and Alternatives for Acute Therapy in Hypercalcemia

Dogs with hypercalcemia of malignancy, vitamin D toxicosis, or other non-PHPTH causes of hypercalcemia often exhibit extremely worrisome clinical signs that are caused by their underlying malignancy as well as their hypercalcemia. Treatment for cancer may indirectly decrease serum calcium concentrations. Dogs that have mild hypercalcemia and CKD also have worrisome clinical signs, moderate to severe hyperphosphatemia, and are at risk for tissue mineralization. They may benefit from treatment directed at maintaining fluid homeostasis while decreasing the calcium x phosphorus product.

| | | TABLE 15-8 | **"CLASSIC" SERUM TOTAL CALCIUM AND INORGANIC PHOSPHORUS (PHOSPHATE) CONCENTRATIONS FOR VARIOUS CONDITIONS TO DEMONSTRATE THEIR TYPICAL NUMERICAL PRODUCTS** |

	TYPICAL SERUM CALCIUM (mg/dL)	TYPICAL SERUM PHOSPHATE (mg/dL)	TYPICAL CALCIUM × PHOSPHATE PRODUCT
Normal dog	10	4.5	45
Primary hyperparathyroidism (PHPTH)	15	3.0	45
Lymphosarcoma	15	3.0	45
Apocrine cell carcinoma of the anal sac	15	3.0	45
Chronic kidney disease (CKD)	11.5	10	115
Vitamin D toxicosis	11.5	10	115

Note that therapy is likely indicated if the product of these two electrolytes exceeds 60 to 80.

There is no single treatment protocol consistently effective for all causes of hypercalcemia. Removal of the underlying cause is definitive, but this is not always possible. The goals of supportive treatment are to enhance renal excretion of calcium and to prevent calcium reabsorption from bone. Hemoconcentration contributes to increases in serum iCa concentration. Parenteral fluid therapy (saline is often the fluid of choice) is the single most important and potentially effective therapy. IV fluids should correct dehydration and, once fluid volume and blood pressure have been restored, induce diuresis. Renal calcium excretion is enhanced by sodium, thus the recommendation of saline. In the hydrated or rehydrated dog, furosemide should be the next therapy considered to further enhance renal calcium excretion.

Thiazide diuretics should be avoided as they may promote renal reabsorption of calcium (Schenck and Chew, 2008; 2012). Glucocorticoids are an effective therapy by inducing cytolysis (lymphosarcoma), as well as reducing bone resorption, decreasing intestinal absorption, and increasing renal excretion of calcium. Glucocorticoids have had demonstrable effect in dogs with hypercalcemia secondary to lymphosarcoma, multiple myeloma, hypoadrenocorticism, hypervitaminosis D, or granulomatous diseases, but have minimal effect on other causes.

Glucocorticoid therapy should be withheld if a definitive diagnosis has not been established. A bisphosphonate may be utilized for chronic control of hypercalcemia. Bisphosphonates lower calcium by reducing the number and action of osteoclasts. Several bisphosphonates have been employed in dogs (Box 15-4 and Table 15-9; Schenck and Chew, 2012; Skelly, 2012). Oral administration is not typically effective because of poor intestinal absorption. IV pamidronate, which is about 100 times more potent than etidronate, has been more reliable, is relatively well tolerated, lasts as long as 3 weeks, and repeat dosing can be considered if necessary (Hostutler et al, 2005).

BOX 15-4   General Treatment of Hypercalcemia

Definitive
Remove underlying cause

Supportive
Initial considerations
    Fluid (0.9% sodium chloride)
    Furosemide
    Sodium bicarbonate
    Glucocorticosteroids
Secondary considerations
    Bisphosphonates
    Calcitonin
Tertiary considerations
    Mithramycin
    Ethylenediaminetetraacetic acid (EDTA)
    Peritoneal dialysis
    Hemodialysis
Future considerations
    Calcium channel blockers
    Somatostatin congeners
    Calcium receptor agonists
    Non-hypercalcemic calcitriol analogues

SURGICAL THERAPY FOR PRIMARY HYPERPARATHYROIDISM

Introduction

Surgical techniques for the thyroid-parathyroid complex have been adequately described. Usually the surgery is not difficult; it is often described to owners as "easier than a spay and less time consuming than a dental prophylaxis." Recognition and surgical excision of autonomously functioning abnormal parathyroid tissue is the most commonly employed treatment for dogs with PHPTH (see Fig. 15-21, *B;* Fig. 15-26). The cure rate has been estimated at about 95% (Rasor et al, 2007; Ham et al, 2009). Failure to cure can be due to the presence of multiglandular disease known to occur in about 10% of dogs with PHPTH, incorrect intraoperative decisions that result in incomplete excision of all autonomously functioning tissue, ectopic autonomously functioning parathyroid tissue (extremely unlikely), or the presence of malignant disease with functioning distant metastases (extremely unlikely; Bilezikian et al, 2001; Ham et al, 2009). Correctly identifying all abnormal tissue can, uncommonly, be problematic because visible changes may be subtle or inapparent. Alternatively, after removing an abnormal nodule, another nodule may be present but not seen (Ham et al, 2009). An attempt must be made to ensure that at least one parathyroid gland remains intact to maintain calcium homeostasis and prevent permanent hypoparathyroidism. If none of the parathyroid glands appears abnormal, if all appear small, or if all are enlarged, the diagnosis of PHPTH must be questioned. The reader is reminded that 5% to 15% of dogs with PHPTH due to an abnormal parathyroid gland(s) may also have an incidentally identified thyroid mass.

Surgical Observations

In three studies describing 53 dogs with PHPTH, each had a solitary nodule successfully identified and removed (Gear et al, 2005; Sawyer et al, 2011; Arbaugh et al, 2012). In another study, seven of 12 dogs (58%) had a solitary nodule and five (42%) had two (Ham et al, 2009). One study included the only four dogs with three nodules excised (6% of 62 dogs). In that report, each of 16 dogs (26%) had two nodules and 42 dogs (68%) had a solitary nodule (Milovancev and Schmiedt, 2013). In our series, about 90% of dogs with PHPTH have had a solitary mass, and about 10% have had two. It is rare to diagnose PHPTH associated with more than two abnormal and autonomously secreting glands.

Cervical Imaging

Ultrasonography

The potential for excellence in sensitivity and specificity of cervical ultrasonography has been previously discussed. In three reports, ultrasonography results correctly identified the abnormal parathyroid tissue in 58 of 61 dogs (95%) (Gear et al, 2005; Sawyer et al, 2011; Arbaugh et al, 2012). However, in another study, ultrasonography correctly identified all abnormal tissue in only 44 of 55 dogs (80%) with PHPTH (Milovancev and Schmiedt, 2013). In a study of 12 dogs with PHPTH, ultrasonography correctly identified 12 abnormal nodules but also identified two nodules that were not seen at surgery and failed to identify five masses that were seen at surgery (Ham et al, 2009).

Cervical ultrasonography should be an integral component of evaluating hypercalcemic dogs and cats. We are reluctant to recommend surgery in any dog suspected to have PHPTH but that

TABLE 15-9   TREATMENT OPTIONS FOR HYPERCALCEMIA NOT CAUSED BY PRIMARY HYPERPARATHYROIDISM

TREATMENT	DOSE	INDICATIONS	COMMENTS
Volume Expansion			
SC saline (0.9%)	Small volumes		Rarely indicated or beneficial
IV saline (0.9%)*	100 to 125 mL/kg/day or "as needed"	Moderate to severe hypercalcemia	Careful in patients with congestive heart failure or hypertension (rarely indicated in dogs with PHPTH)
Diuretics			
Furosemide	2 to 4 mg/kg every 8 to 12 hours, IV, SC, or by mouth	Moderate to severe hypercalcemia	Volume expansion is necessary before use of this drug
Alkalinizing Agent			
Sodium bicarbonate	1 mEq/kg IV slow bolus; may continue at 0.3 × base deficit × weight in kg/day	Severe hypercalcemia	Requires close monitoring
Glucocorticoids			
Prednisone	1 to 2.2 mg/kg every 12 hours by mouth, SC, or IV	Moderate to severe hypercalcemia	Use of these drugs before identification of etiology may make definitive diagnosis difficult
Dexamethasone	0.1 to 0.22 mg/kg every 12 hours, IV or SC	Same	Same
Bone Resorption Inhibitors			
Calcitonin	4 to 6 IU/kg as IV infusion and then SC every 8 or 12 hours	Hypervitaminosis D	Response may be short-lived; vomiting and anorexia may occur
Bisphosphonates			
Etidronate	5 to 15 mg/kg every 12 to 24 hours	Moderate to severe hypercalcemia	Expensive and use in dogs is limited
Clodronate	20 to 25 mg/kg in a 4-hour IV infusion	Same	Same
Pamidronate	1.3 mg/kg in 150 mL 0.9% saline in a 2-hour IV infusion; can repeat in 1 week	Same	Same
Alendronate	5 to 20 mg orally every 7 days	Same	Must ensure complete passage of medication into stomach to avoid esophagitis
Miscellaneous			
Sodium EDTA	25 to 75 mg/kg/h	Severe hypercalcemia	Nephrotoxicity
Peritoneal dialysis	Low calcium dialysate	Severe hypercalcemia	Short duration of response; use in hypercalcemia not reported

EDTA, Ethylenediaminetetraacetic acid; *IHC*, idiopathic hypercalcemia of cats; *IV*, intravenous; *PHPTH*, primary hyperparathyroidism; *SC*, subcutaneous.
*Potassium supplementation may be necessary.

fails to demonstrate at least one abnormal parathyroid nodule on cervical ultrasonography. If a relatively inexperienced individual is performing the examination in which no abnormal nodules are seen or if more than one is seen, we recommend that the examination be repeated when one of our more experienced radiologists is available. Disagreement between ultrasonography and surgical observations are not common. Incidentally identified thyroid masses are encountered.

Radionuclide Scans

Radionuclide procedures have been used for the detection and localization of parathyroid adenomas in humans (Fine, 1987). The most commonly used radionuclide imaging technique is a dual radioisotope procedure combining thallous chloride (^{201}Tl) with either pertechnetate (^{99m}Tc) or radioactive iodine (^{123}I) (Picard et al, 1987). Various problems with this methodology led to the use of one radionuclide: technetium-99m-sestamibi (^{99m}Tc-sestamibi) (O'Dougherty et al, 1992; Taillefer et al, 1992). The procedure and hospitalization time for radionuclide scans using ^{99m}Tc-sestamibi in humans are similar to those for ^{99m}Tc scans in dogs. ^{99m}Tc-sestamibi

radionuclide scans provide excellent results for localizing parathyroid adenomas in people (O'Dougherty et al, 1992; Taillefer et al, 1992).

Two reports suggested that this procedure might be helpful in localizing parathyroid adenomas in dogs with PHPTH (Wright et al, 1995; Matwichuk et al, 1996). In a subsequent study, double-phase parathyroid scintigraphy was evaluated in a group of PHPTH dogs with one of 10 having a scan that correlated with surgery. The poor sensitivity and specificity of parathyroid gland scintigraphy led the authors to conclude that use of this tool could not be recommended (Matwichuk et al, 2000).

Selective Venous Sampling

An attempt was made to determine the side on which an autonomously functioning parathyroid nodule was located by taking blood from both jugular veins and measuring PTH concentrations in each. The hypothesis was that the vein draining the side of the autonomously functioning tissue would have greater amounts of PTH than the opposite side. PTH concentrations were compared from the samples obtained from each jugular vein prior to surgery. Each dog had PHPTH caused by a solitary functioning adenoma.

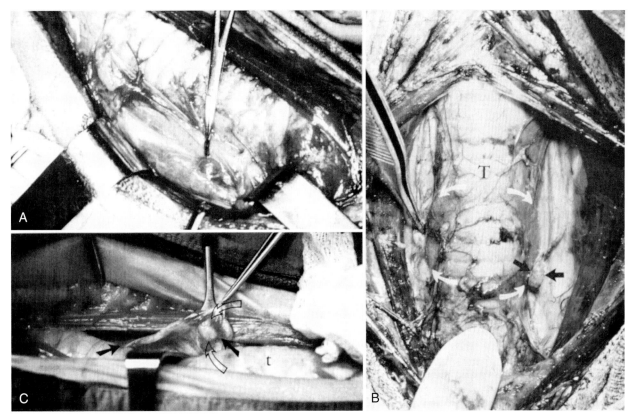

FIGURE 15-26 A, Surgical site during removal of a solitary parathyroid adenoma (tip of forceps). **B,** Surgical site during removal of a solitary parathyroid adenoma (*T,* trachea). *White arrows* delineate the cranial and caudal poles of the thyroid glands; *black arrows* point out the parathyroid adenoma. **C,** Surgical site during removal of an "internal" parathyroid adenoma (*t,* trachea). *Solid arrows* delineate the cranial and caudal poles of the thyroid, which is being retracted from the trachea to reveal the parathyroid adenoma *(open arrows)* on the dorsal surface of the thyroid.

Unfortunately, a gradient between samples was identified in only one of 11 dogs and this is not recommended (Feldman et al, 1997).

A rapid chemiluminescent PTH assay was employed on blood samples obtained during surgery from local veins to help identify laterality (left or right side) of autonomously functioning parathyroid tumors. In addition, plasma PTH concentrations were obtained from local veins to determine if all abnormal tissue had likely been removed. Systemic and local PTH concentrations decreased more than 50% from presurgical values in all dogs after complete excision of abnormal tissue. Mean preoperative systemic plasma PTH concentrations were significantly higher than mean postoperative concentrations. The mean local pre-excision PTH concentration from the affected side was significantly higher than mean pre-excision concentration taken from the unaffected side. Unfortunately, local PTH concentrations from the affected side were greatly increased in comparison to the opposite side in a minority of the dogs. Thus, the side on which an autonomously nodule was located and removed was not consistently detected with intraoperative PTH sampling. Results of this elegant study did not support intraoperative blood sampling for PTH to locate the side on which an autonomously functioning gland resided (Ham et al, 2009).

New Methylene Blue Infusions

IV infusion of new methylene blue (3 mg/kg) has been described as a means of improving the surgeon's ability to recognize abnormal glands. Three dogs with PHPTH were evaluated, and in each

a tumor was identified after the infusion. However, two of three dogs developed Heinz body anemia and red blood cell "blistering" after the procedure (Fingeroth and Smeak, 1988).

Solitary Adenoma, Hyperplastic Nodule, or Carcinoma?

In surgery, a large majority of dogs with PHPTH have had a solitary nodule identified and removed. One cannot predict the histologic classification from gross appearance. About 50% of nodules are identified on the ventral surface of the thyroid glands. If the mass is not seen on the ventral surface, careful inspection of the dorsal surface of each thyroid lobe should be conducted. "External" parathyroid nodules are usually removed easily and without damage to surrounding tissue (see Figs. 15-4 and 15-26). In some dogs with an "internal" parathyroid adenoma, surgeons may choose to remove the entire thyroid-parathyroid complex from the affected side. In a small number of dogs, tissue removed was based on cervical ultrasonography identifying an intrathyroidal nodule.

Enlargement of Multiple Parathyroid Glands

Approximately 10% of dogs with PHPTH have enlargement of more than one gland in our experience. Others have identified more than one gland enlarged in more than 20% of dogs with PHPTH (Gear et al, 2005). Histologic classification of removed tissue may or may be similar. A dog may have more than one adenoma, carcinoma, or hyperplastic gland or have any combination (DeVries et al, 1993). When more than one enlarged gland is identified, the concern is primary versus secondary hyperparathyroidism. The presurgical evaluation, as reviewed, should discriminate dogs with PHPTH from non-surgical causes of hypercalcemia. If the clinician is convinced that primary disease is present, the decision to remove two glands is straightforward. However, if three or four glands are involved, the decision regarding removal should be based on one's confidence in the presurgical diagnosis and, potentially, the owner's ability to treat permanent hypoparathyroidism.

Recurrence of Primary Hyperparathyroidism

About 8% to 10% of dogs with treated PHPTH have complete resolution of their condition for 6 months to longer than 5 years and then have had a recurrence (Ham et al, 2009). In each, their second diagnosis of PHPTH was caused by a solitary, autonomously functioning parathyroid nodule, in a gland not previously affected. Nodules surgically removed after recurrence have had the same range of histologic diagnoses; adenoma is the most common, whereas "carcinoma" or "hyperplasia" is each diagnosed in about 5% to 10% of the cases. Because recurrence of PHPTH has been documented, periodic rechecks are warranted.

Absence of a Parathyroid Mass at Surgery

If an abnormal parathyroid nodule is not seen at surgery (or with ultrasonography), one must first consider the confidence with which the diagnosis of PHPTH was established. If convinced of the condition, the most likely diagnoses include hypercalcemia due to PTH production by a parathyroid tumor in an aberrant location or the presence of a non-parathyroid tumor producing PTH (i.e., ectopic hyperparathyroidism). Either would be extremely rare. The ventral neck should be carefully explored and any suspicious mass excised. New methylene blue infusion, as previously described, can also be considered (Fingeroth and Smeak, 1988).

 ## PERCUTANEOUS THERAPIES FOR PRIMARY HYPERPARATHYROIDISM IN DOGS

Percutaneous Ultrasound-Guided Ethanol Ablation

Based on experience using cervical ultrasonography as a diagnostic aid for dogs and on the use of chemical ablation for small nodules in people (Bennedbaek et al, 1997), the efficacy of ethanol ablation as a treatment for dogs with PHPTH was evaluated (Long et al, 1999). Ethanol causes coagulation necrosis and vascular thrombosis. PHPTH was diagnosed in twelve dogs whose clinical and biochemical evaluation was typical for the condition. Each dog had a solitary, hypoechoic, round or oval mass near a thyroid lobe on cervical ultrasonography. Parathyroid nodules were identified on the right side in eight and left side in four dogs. The nodules ranged from 4 to 10 mm in greatest diameter; they were located at the cranial aspect of a thyroid lobe in six, within the caudal pole of a thyroid lobe in three, and in the midbody of a thyroid lobe in three dogs. The calculated volume of the nodules ranged from 0.06 to 0.16 cm³.

Each dog was placed under general anesthesia, and the ventral cervical region was clipped and aseptically prepared. The parathyroid nodule was identified and continuously monitored throughout the procedure via ultrasonography, using an appropriate transducer. The tip of a 27-gauge needle, with arterial tubing attached to a syringe containing about 50% more ethanol than

the estimated nodular volume, was inserted into the nodule (Fig. 15-27). That volume was slowly injected, with a goal of having the entire parenchyma exposed to ethanol. Because parathyroid nodules are small, considerable experience with ultrasonographic-guided needle placement is necessary. Parathyroid nodules may also be in close proximity to the carotid artery and vagosympathetic trunk; therefore absolute certainty about needle placement is required prior to and during injection.

Because ethanol is hyperechoic, it is easily visualized with ultrasonography (see Fig. 15-27). The parathyroid nodules received different calculated volumes, as dictated by the monitored diffusion. The injected volumes ranged from 50% to 150% of the calculated nodular volume. No dog was under anesthesia for more than an hour, and the mean duration of anesthesia was 38 minutes. A single injection was administered to 11 of the 12 dogs. One dog was injected a second time 48 hours after the first dose failed to reduce the serum calcium concentration into the reference range. In all 12 dogs, the serum TCa concentrations decreased into the reference range. In 11 dogs this decrease was documented within 48 hours of injection (10 after the first injection and one after the second injection). One dog remained hypercalcemic for 4 days, but the serum calcium concentration decreased into the reference range 5 days after treatment (Fig. 15-28). One dog had a recurrence of hypercalcemia 30 days after injection and was treated surgically. Each of the other 11 dogs remained normocalcemic for more than 12 months. The only adverse side effect was a transient change in the bark of two dogs, both of whom were believed, retrospectively, to have suffered transient, unilateral laryngeal paralysis.

Ethanol ablation was an efficacious mode of therapy for PHPTH in dogs (Long et al, 1999). The cost of the procedure was considerably less than for surgery. Chemical ablation of parathyroid masses may be more effective in dogs than in humans because canine parathyroid nodules are considerably smaller, thus requiring a smaller volume of ethanol for complete ablation. One group treated five dogs utilizing this approach without success (Gear et al, 2005). A subsequent study concluded that ethanol ablation was an effective mode of therapy but not as effective as surgery or heat ablation. Control of hypercalcemia for a median of 540 days was achieved in 13 of 18 dogs (72%) (Rasor et al, 2007).

Percutaneous Ultrasound-Guided Radio Frequency Heat Ablation

Based on experience with cervical ultrasonography both as a diagnostic aid and for ethanol ablation, the efficacy of treatment with percutaneous ultrasonographic-guided radio frequency heat ablation was evaluated. Radio frequency waves are converted to heat at the needle tip causing thermal necrosis at the needle tip (Pollard et al, 2001). This treatment modality has several advantages over ethanol ablation. Radio frequency damages a discrete amount of tissue surrounding the uninsulated portion of the needle. (There is no potential for "leakage," as there is with ethanol.) Radio frequency offers the additional advantage of not damaging regional vasculature. Vascular blood flow disperses heat. In humans, this treatment modality has a higher success rate than ethanol for mass ablation and fewer retreatments required to achieve remission. Radio frequency heat ablation has been used in the treatment of multifocal hepatic, breast and nasal masses, as well as for prostatic hypertrophy (Jiao et al, 1999; Livraghi et al, 1999). One disadvantage of the radio frequency technique is equipment cost.

In the first report using this treatment modality for dogs with PHPTH, 27 dogs were treated, 22 with a solitary parathyroid nodule and five dogs each had two nodules. In three of the five

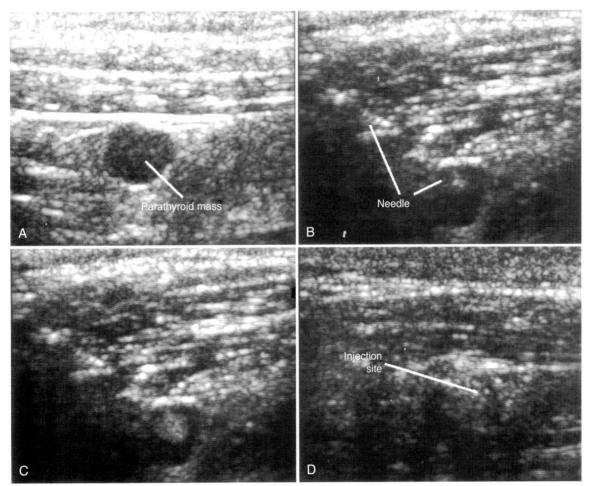

FIGURE 15-27 Ultrasonographic appearance of chemical ablation of a parathyroid mass in a dog. **A,** Sagittal view of the parathyroid mass prior to treatment. **B,** A 27-gauge needle is inserted into the mass. **C,** A test injection of 96% ethanol is used to confirm placement of the needle inside the mass. Note that the ethanol is hyperechoic in relation to the parenchyma of the mass. **D,** After injection of the target dose of ethanol, the entire mass has an echogenic appearance. (From Long CD, et al.: Percutaneous ultrasound–guided chemical parathyroid ablation for treatment of primary hyperparathyroidism in dogs, *J Am Vet Med Assoc* 215:217, 1999.)

dogs with two nodules, both were on the left side of the neck, and two dogs had one nodule on each side. Ultrasonographic appearance of each nodule was similar: spherical to ovoid and hypoechoic to the surrounding thyroid parenchyma. Length of the masses ranged from 3 to 15 mm. Each dog with a solitary parathyroid mass was treated once. When two parathyroid nodules were present and located on the same side, as in the three dogs, both were ablated during the first anesthesia. In the two dogs with one nodule on either side of the neck, each nodule was treated separately, 30 days apart. Preparation was the same as utilized for ethanol ablation. The parathyroid nodule was identified and continuously monitored with ultrasonography, including guiding the tip of a 20-gauge, over-the-needle (insulated) catheter into the mass. The needle hub was removed, allowing for an insulated wire to connect the needle to the radio frequency unit (Radiotherapeutics Inc., Redwood City, CA). Initially, 10 watts of energy were applied to the tissue for 10 to 20 seconds. If echogenic bubbles were not seen via ultrasonography at the needle tip, the wattage was increased by 2 watts every 5 to 10 seconds until echogenic foci became apparent (Fig. 15-29). Also, if a "popping sound" could be heard, the maximum heat application was assumed to have been reached and no additional increases in wattage were made. The needle tip was arbitrarily redirected multiple times, as necessary, in an attempt

to expose all the parenchyma to heat. Mean anesthesia time was 41 minutes, but with experience it now averages about 15 minutes.

The procedure was successful in 26 of the 27 dogs with a dramatic reduction in the serum PTH concentration and normalization of both the TCa and iCa concentrations within 24 hours (Fig. 15-30). Serum calcium concentrations remained within the reference range for more than a year in each dog. One dog improved for only 1 month and was treated surgically after hypercalcemia recurred. Immediately after heat ablation, one dog with a unilateral parathyroid nodule developed a transient voice change, which resolved within 5 days. It is unclear whether this voice change occurred secondary to intubation or to the ablation procedure. Signs of pain, swelling, or respiratory distress were not detected in any dog. Eleven of the 26 successfully treated dogs required vitamin D therapy for postablation hypocalcemia (see next section). In a retrospective evaluation of ultrasonographic-guided heat ablation in dogs with PHPTH, success rates were comparable to those achieved with surgery. Forty-four of 49 dogs with PHPTH (90%) experienced rapid resolution (hours to days) of their condition following heat ablation, resulting in normal calcium concentrations for a median of 580 days (Rasor et al, 2007). Inclusion criteria for heat ablation include having a readily seen abnormal parathyroid nodule more than 2 mm but less than 16 mm in greatest diameter, not too close to the carotid or

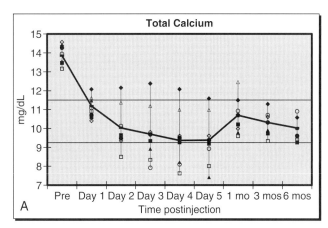
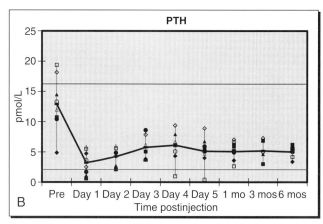

FIGURE 15-28 A, Serum total calcium (TCa) concentration in eight dogs before *(Pre)* and after chemical ablation of a parathyroid mass. The *horizontal black lines* indicate the reference range. Dog 6 developed clinical signs of hypocalcemia 4 days after the ablation procedure. Dog 8 received two injections of ethanol (the data given represent values obtained after the second injection). Dog 7 underwent surgical removal of a parathyroid mass after the 1-month reevaluation. Dog 5 died of unrelated causes after the 3-month reevaluation. **B,** Serum parathyroid hormone *(PTH)* concentrations in eight dogs before *(Pre)* and after chemical ablation of a parathyroid mass. The *horizontal black lines* indicate the reference range. (From Long CD, et al.: Percutaneous ultrasound–guided chemical parathyroid ablation for treatment of primary hyperparathyroidism in dogs, *J Am Vet Med Assoc* 215:217, 1999.)

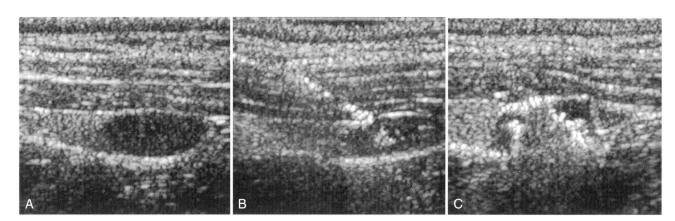

FIGURE 15-29 Left lateral sonographic images of an oval hypoechoic parathyroid nodule in a dog prior to heat ablation **(A),** with the insulated needle passing through the superficial soft tissues into the cranial aspect of the mass **(B),** and after heat ablation **(C).** Note the hyperechoic foci in the parenchyma of the gland in **C.** (From Pollard RE, et al.: Percutaneous ultrasonographically guided radio frequency heat ablation for treatment of primary hyperparathyroidism in dogs, *J Am Vet Med Assoc* 218:1106, 2001.)

any other vital structure, and no cystic calculi documented. It is recommended that dogs with PHPTH and cystic calculi have parathyroid and abdominal surgery performed during the same anesthesia.

 POSTTREATMENT MANAGEMENT OF POTENTIAL HYPOCALCEMIA

A full discussion of vitamin D and calcium supplementation is presented in Chapter 16.

Background

Physiologically, the long-term response to autonomous secretion of PTH by an abnormal parathyroid nodule is atrophy of normal glands. Duration of hypercalcemia is apparent for some dogs but is unknown for most. Thus, the use of pretreatment serum calcium

concentrations has been used in an attempt to predict dogs most likely to become seriously hypocalcemic after therapy. Surgical removal or percutaneous ablation of an autonomous source of PTH results in rapid disappearance of circulating PTH (see Fig. 15-30; Fig. 15-31) and decreases in serum calcium concentrations. Potential for serious decreases in serum calcium concentration (see Figs. 15-28 and 15-30; Fig. 15-32) exist for any dog treated successfully for PHPTH. After resolution of PHPTH, decreases in serum calcium concentrations usually continue for a period of 1 to 7 days but rarely longer. Our hypothesis and experience has been that posttreatment hypocalcemia correlates with severity of hypercalcemia prior to surgery. We compared 50 dogs with PHPTH who did not become seriously hypocalcemic (TCa < 7mg/dL; iCa < 0.8mmol/L) with 50 who did following treatment. The mean pretreatment serum TCa and iCa concentrations of those who did not become seriously hypoglycemic (13.88 mg/dL, 1.61 mmol/L,

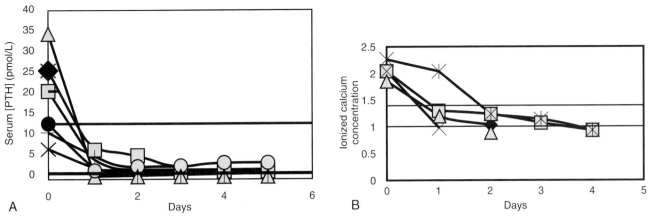

FIGURE 15-30 A, Serum parathyroid hormone *(PTH)* concentration (pmol/L: individual data points) of eight dogs that were successfully treated for primary hyperparathyroidism (PHPTH). The reference range is 2 to 13 pmol/L. **B,** Serum ionized calcium (iCa) concentrations (mmol/L; individual data points) in five dogs that were successfully treated for PHPTH on day 0 and eventually required vitamin D supplementation 1 to 4 days after treatment. The reference range is 1.1 to 1.4 (From Pollard RE, et al.: Percutaneous ultrasonographically guided radio frequency heat ablation for treatment of primary hyperparathyroidism in dogs, *J Am Vet Med Assoc* 218:1106, 2001.)

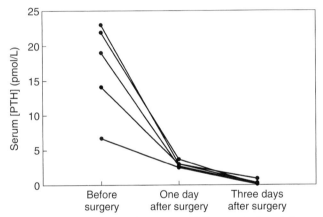

FIGURE 15-31 Serum parathyroid hormone *(PTH)* concentrations before and after surgery in eight dogs in which a solitary functional parathyroid adenoma was removed.

respectively) were significantly lower than results from those who did (16.12 mg/dL, 1.87 mmol/L). These unpublished data are comparable to those reported by another group: Mean pretreatment TCa concentration of those who did not develop posttreatment hypocalcemia (13.6 mg/dL) was significantly lower than the TCa pretreatment of those who did become seriously hypocalcemic (16.8 mg/dL) (Gear et al, 2005).

Although we and Gear and colleagues (2005) have noted correlation between presurgical TCa or iCa concentrations and development of posttreatment hypocalcemia, this has not been appreciated in other studies (Arbaugh et al, 2012; Milovancev and Schmiedt, 2013). Size of unaffected parathyroid tissue is another consideration with dogs that have undetectable atrophied parathyroid glands being at greater risk for posttreatment hypocalcemia than dogs with small but visible parathyroid glands.

Some veterinarians have suggested that it is imperative to document a decline in the serum calcium concentration after surgery to subnormal levels before considering supportive therapy. Although such a protocol allows further confirmation that PHPTH existed and was corrected, it places a dog at risk

for discomfort as well as life-threatening hypocalcemia. The next sections review dogs for which no therapy or immediate therapy (posttreatment) is suggested. Beginning therapy before or soon after surgery or ablation but before documented decreases in the serum calcium concentration has not prevented the serum calcium concentration to decline into or below the reference range, but it has prevented serious hypocalcemia and tetany.

Protocol Based on the Pretreatment Total Calcium Concentration

Pretreatment Total Calcium Less Than 14 mg/dL

If the serum calcium concentration prior to surgery is less than 14 mg/dL, the risk of postsurgical hypocalcemia is relatively small, *but we now recommend that all dogs with PHPTH receive prophylactic treatment to prevent posttreatment hypocalcemia.* If prophylactic treatment is withheld, the dog should be hospitalized for 3 to 5 days after treatment to monitor the TCa and/or iCa concentrations once or twice daily. Hospitalization also reduces activity levels of most dogs. Dogs sent home are likely to be more active and, if hypocalcemic, at much greater risk of clinical tetany than one kept quiet. If the serum TCa concentration remains above about 8.5 mg/dL (assuming a lower reference limit of about 9.5 mg/dL) and/or the serum iCa concentration remains above about 0.95 mmol/L (assuming a lower reference limit of 1.10 mmol/L), vitamin D treatment can be withheld. It should be noted, however, that these are general guidelines and prophylactic treatment of all PHPTH dogs to prevent hypocalcemia may be warranted (Box 15-5). Chapter 16 presents a complete discussion of the acute and chronic management of hypocalcemia in dogs and cats.

Chronicity of Primary Hyperparathyroidism

Experience indicates an association between posttreatment hypocalcemia and chronicity of PHPTH in dogs. Often, duration of hypercalcemia secondary to PHPTH is unknown. Occasionally, however, PHPTH has been documented for extended time periods. Dogs with protracted histories of confirmed disease often have not been treated because owners have not observed worrisome signs and they are monitoring the condition. Another cause

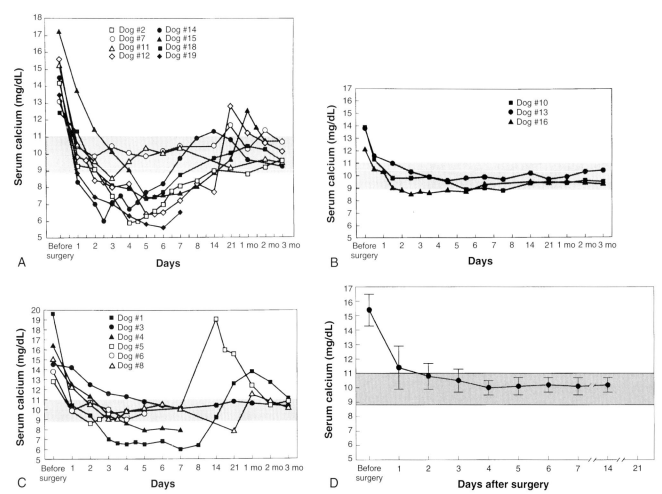

FIGURE 15-32 Serial calcium concentrations before and after removal of a parathyroid tumor from dogs with primary hyperparathyroidism (PHPTH). **A,** These eight dogs were placed on vitamin D_2 and calcium supplementation after hypocalcemia was identified. **B,** These three dogs had mild hypercalcemia prior to surgery, and they were not treated with vitamin D or calcium after surgery. **C,** These six dogs began receiving vitamin D_2 and calcium immediately after recovery from anesthesia. **D,** Serum calcium concentrations from 34 dogs that began receiving dihydrotachysterol immediately after recovery from anesthesia.

BOX 15-5	**Clinical Signs Associated with the Acute Onset of Hypocalcemia**

Panting
Nervousness
Anxiety
Muscle trembling, twitching
Leg cramping, pain (may be seen as "weakness")
Ataxia
Atypical aggressive behavior
Stiff gait
Facial rubbing
Biting at feet
Vocalizing
Hypersensitivity
Seizures: focal or generalized

for longer histories is the client/veterinarian team who choose a more deliberate approach. We now recommend prophylactic treatment with vitamin D in an attempt to prevent hypocalcemia or, at least, to reduce its severity clinically and biochemically.

Pretreatment Serum Calcium Concentration (More Than 15 mg/dL; Ionized Calcium More Than 1.75 mmol/L)

We assume that dogs with a serum TCa or iCa persistently greater than 15 mg/dL or 1.75 mmol/L, respectively, due to PHPTH have been hypercalcemic "chronically" or their level of negative feedback and resultant atrophy of normal glands greater. The recommendation is to prophylactically attempt to avoid hypocalcemia after PHPTH therapy by beginning vitamin D (calcitriol, 20 to 30 ng/kg/day, divided b.i.d. [twice a day]) that morning (see Chapter 16). In some cases we have begun calcitriol therapy 24 to 36 hours before surgery, but this may not be necessary. Initiation of calcitriol has not prevented decreases in the serum calcium concentration to or below reference ranges after surgery, but it has prevented or decreased the severity of clinical and biochemical hypocalcemia. Each dog should be kept quiet in a cage or run for at least 3 to 5 days after treatment.

Timing of Posttreatment Hypocalcemia and Recommendations Regarding Vitamin D

Postsurgical hypocalcemia has been observed as early as 12 hours to as late as 20 days after curative therapy. Most dogs that become hypocalcemic, usually do so between the second and sixth days posttreatment.

Tetany, when it has occurred, has usually been seen 4 to 7 days after treatment. The serum calcium concentration should be monitored once or twice daily. The goal of vitamin D therapy is to maintain serum calcium concentrations in the low to low-normal range (i.e., TCa, 8 to 9.5 mg/dL; iCa, 0.9 to 1.2 mmol/L). Such serum calcium concentrations are well above those associated with clinical signs, are not likely to be a cause of iatrogenic vitamin D toxicosis, and are low enough to stimulate functional recovery in atrophied parathyroid glands. Mid- to high-normal or greater serum calcium concentrations in dogs being given vitamin D should be avoided. Such concentrations may be associated with worrisome increases in serum phosphate concentration, and they predispose the dog to AKI.

The Tapering Process

In order to stimulate the remaining parathyroid glands to regain control of calcium homeostasis, vitamin D supplements must be gradually withdrawn. This process of returning parathyroid function in remaining glands is not completely predictable. Once serum calcium concentrations have stabilized and the dog has been returned to the owner, tapering vitamin D (calcitriol) begins. It is usually withdrawn by gradually extending the time between administration (e.g., twice daily to once daily for 2 weeks; to once every other day for 2 weeks; then once every third day for 2 weeks; then once every fourth day for 2 weeks; and finally, once weekly for 2 to 4 weeks). The serum calcium concentration should be checked prior to each adjustment in the dosing interval to prevent the development of occult hypo- or hypercalcemia. If the serum calcium concentration drops below 8 mg/dL, reduction of the vitamin D supplementation should be delayed or the dose increased. The serum calcium concentration should remain above 8 mg/dL to minimize the risk of tetany. However, if the serum calcium concentrations are high-normal or increased, vitamin D should be discontinued (permanently or transiently, as determined by the patient). Once the vitamin D supplementation has been reduced to once weekly for 2 to 4 weeks, it may be discontinued. Also, if serum calcium concentrations remain in reference ranges after the dose has been reduced to once weekly, any calcium supplements should then be withdrawn. Specific calcium supplementation should not be needed if the dog is being fed quality food. If calcium content of the diet is questionable, supplemental calcium can be given (see Chapter 16). Using this protocol, the withdrawal process for vitamin D and calcium usually takes 3 to 4 months. It is important to remember that there is considerable individual variation in response to therapy, and it is difficult, therefore, to check the serum calcium concentration too frequently.

Prophylactic Vitamin D (Calcitriol) Therapy in All Dogs Treated for Primary Hyperparathyroidism

Background

Prediction of posttreatment hypocalcemia in dogs with PHPTH has proven difficult and may depend on multiple factors, including but not limited to signalment, history, physical examination findings, clinicopathologic results, and imaging results (Arbaugh et al, 2012; Milovancev and Schmiedt, 2013). Prophylactic vitamin D treatment strategies have been employed based on pretreatment factors used to identify dogs most likely to suffer serious hypocalcemia after being treated for PHPTH. Many dogs with PHPTH develop posttreatment subclinical hypocalcemia (Arbaugh et al, 2012). Further, some dogs with PHPTH develop posttreatment clinical tetany, and a few have had serious life-threatening hypocalcemia persist (Sawyer et al, 2011; Arbaugh et al, 2012; Milovancev and Schmiedt, 2013).

Current Recommended Protocol

We have embarked on a new, more aggressive protocol to avoid posttreatment hypocalcemia in dogs being treated for PHPTH. Results have been encouraging to date, and time will tell if this protocol is satisfactory. All dogs being treated for PHPTH should be given calcitriol the morning of the planned treatment at a dose of 20 to 30 ng/kg. That posttreatment night, the dog should be given 10 to 15 ng/kg, and that dose should be continued (20 to 30 ng/kg/day divided b.i.d.) for the first 2 days following treatment. The third day after therapy, and every 4 days thereafter, the dose of calcitriol should then be reduced by 10%, continuing for about 45 to 60 days. Twice daily monitoring of serum TCa and iCa concentrations are strongly recommended while in the hospital. Both parameters should be checked prior to every planned dose reduction. As described in the previous section, monitoring serum calcium concentrations are required in an attempt to avoid under or over dosage. If calcium concentrations are less than 8.5 mg/dL (TCa) or 0.95 mmol/L (iCa) at any time, the dose of vitamin D should be at least transiently increased to a previously used and safe dose. Monitoring of serum calcium concentrations is also required in an attempt to avoid iatrogenic vitamin D toxicosis. If calcium concentrations are within the upper portion of the reference range, the dose of calcitriol should be decreased by 50%. If the serum calcium concentrations are above reference ranges, the calcitriol should be stopped for 48 hours and the values again rechecked. If hypercalcemia and hyperphosphatemia are documented, IV saline therapy for 24 hours or longer should be considered.

Vitamin D Resistance/Time Until an Effect Is Documented

It is not common for calcitriol to begin to have an immediate effect. Rather, vitamin D gradually takes effect during the first several days of therapy and almost always within 4 to 7 days. Individual variation is typical.

 PATHOLOGY

Subjectivity of Histologic Interpretation

Abnormal, autonomously functioning parathyroid glands from people, dogs, and cats have been characterized histologically as adenoma, carcinoma, and hyperplasia. Controlled studies reviewing histologic interpretations by pathologists have shown that classifying a parathyroid nodule as adenoma, hyperplasia, or carcinoma is not straightforward (Aurbach et al, 1985a; DeVries et al, 1993; Ham et al, 2009). Histologic classification of parathyroid tissue may be influenced to some degree by gross features observed during surgery. The surgeon determines the number, size, and appearance of normal and abnormal glands. The pathologist then determines whether removed tissue is parathyroid and further classifies the tissue, when possible, as benign or malignant.

As previously discussed, single-gland involvement (adenoma, carcinoma, or hyperplasia) occurs in about 80% to 90% of people and dogs with PHPTH. Multiple-gland involvement has been documented in 10% to 20% (Arnaud and Kolb, 1991; Gear et al, 2005; Ham et al, 2009; Sawyer et al, 2011; Arbaugh et al, 2012; Milovancev and Schmiedt, 2013). The diagnosis of carcinoma is based on gross appearance, histologic features, and ultimately the biologic behavior of the lesion. Fewer than 2% of autonomously secreting parathyroid nodules in people are malignant. Five percent to 10% of parathyroid tissue removed from dogs with PHPTH has been assigned the diagnosis of carcinoma, but we are aware of only one dog being described as having "multicentric disease" not amenable to surgical extirpation (Ham et al, 2009).

Solitary Parathyroid Mass

Background

In people, dogs, and cats, the most common cause of PHPTH is a solitary functioning chief cell adenoma, resulting in the secretion of excessive amounts of PTH. Adenomas are usually solitary (developing in an existing parathyroid gland), light brown-red in color, and located in close proximity to that thyroid lobe (see Figs. 15-21 and 15-26). Because of the difficulty involved in histologically classifying an enlarged parathyroid gland as an adenoma, carcinoma, or adenomatous hyperplasia, a "nodule" is tentatively diagnosed during surgery when a solitary abnormal parathyroid gland is identified and the remaining glands are normal, atrophied, or not seen. The term *adenoma* may also be arbitrary as applied to such tissue.

Adenoma

"Adenoma" is diagnosed when a single nodule is easily seen, well demarcated, and histologically compresses a rim of atrophied but otherwise normal parathyroid tissue (Capen and Martin, 1983; DeVries et al, 1993). Adenomas are generally composed of a diffuse pattern of parathyroid chief cells. About 75% to 85% of dogs with PHPTH have a solitary parathyroid adenoma identified and removed during surgical exploration of the neck. Multiple adenomas have been reported in people (Aurbach et al, 1985a) and are found in 3% to 5% of dogs with PHPTH (Pollard et al, 2001).

About 5% to 10% of dogs with PHPTH experience complete resolution of their condition after removal or ablation of a solitary parathyroid nodule but have a recurrence of the condition 6 months or more afterward. Each of those dogs then had this second nodule ablated or removed. In most cases the second mass was also an adenoma, but carcinoma and hyperplasia have been diagnosed. In none of these dogs were two masses present initially, demonstrated in part by resolution of hypercalcemia for an extended period. Thorough exploration of the neck, initially, also failed to demonstrate two masses.

Carcinoma

Chief cell carcinomas are identified in fewer than 3% to 4% of people with PHPTH (Shane and Bilezikian, 1982). In as many as 50% of these people, the malignant lesion may be palpable in the neck, and at surgery the mass is often firm and densely adherent to local structures (Aurbach et al, 1985a). Capsular and vascular invasion are characteristic histologic findings. Parathyroid carcinomas in people tend to be locally invasive with the potential to spread to regional lymph nodes, lung, liver, and bone. Parathyroid gland carcinomas in dogs behave as an adenoma (Berger and Feldman, 1987; DeVries et al, 1993: Sawyer et al, 2011). In one study, each of 19 dogs with PHPTH caused by a parathyroid carcinoma had a solitary nodule identified at surgery. Each nodule was described as having a benign gross appearance. Hypercalcemia resolved in 18 of 19 after surgery, and no dog was confirmed to develop recurrent or metastatic PHPTH (Sawyer et al, 2011).

Primary Hyperplasia

Hyperplasia implies an abnormality involving all parathyroid tissue and is frequently diagnosed when more than one parathyroid gland is grossly and microscopically abnormal. Gross enlargement of all four glands is not a prerequisite for a diagnosis of hyperplasia because microscopic alterations may be present in a normal-sized gland (Aurbach et al, 1985a). An accurate histologic diagnosis requires clear criteria for distinguishing adenoma from hyperplasia and for distinguishing either of these from normal. A tentative differentiation often is based on the number of glands involved (i.e., one gland supports a diagnosis of adenoma and multiple glands a diagnosis of hyperplasia) (Verdonk and Edis, 1981).

We reported a group of six dogs with PHPTH (8% of the 72 in our series at the time) that had hyperplasia as determined by board certified pathologists (DeVries et al, 1993). That percentage approximates the experience in the literature since. The terms *nodular hyperplasia* and *adenomatous hyperplasia* may be applied to parathyroids that contain multiple nodules less than 5 mm in diameter as opposed to adenomas, which are often defined as parathyroid tumors consisting of a solitary nodule greater than 5 mm in diameter.

Differentiation of hyperplasia and adenoma has important implications regarding surgery, medical therapy, and long-term prognosis. A dog or cat with PHPTH may be cured after complete surgical removal of a solitary adenoma with three normal parathyroid glands (albeit atrophied in the immediate postsurgical period) remaining to prevent permanent hypoparathyroidism. In contrast, parathyroid hyperplasia implies that if all abnormal parathyroid tissue is not removed, the chance for persistent or recurrent hyperparathyroidism is high. However, this has not consistently been observed in dogs with PHPTH. Most PHPTH dogs diagnosed as having a solitary hyperplastic parathyroid nodule removed at surgery have complete resolution of the condition. Their PHPTH seems no different than for dogs diagnosed as having a parathyroid adenoma or carcinoma (DeVries et al, 1993).

Summary

In our series of dogs with PHPTH that have had surgery and that had a solitary mass, about 87% had a solitary parathyroid adenoma, about 8% had a diagnosis of solitary primary parathyroid hyperplasia, and 5% had a diagnosis of carcinoma. In general, long-term response to therapy was similar regardless of histologic classification. Recurrences occur regardless of the initial histologic diagnosis. When recurrences occur (approximately 10% of our dogs), the histologic diagnosis of tissue removed at second surgery is just as likely to be different from the initial diagnosis as it is to be similar. Distant metastasis from a parathyroid carcinoma and/or local invasion has been described, but is extremely uncommon (Ham et al, 2009). It is also worth repeating that about 10% of dogs with PHPTH have two parathyroid nodules at the time of initial diagnosis. Again, the histologic classification of these masses is as likely to be different (e.g., one adenoma and one carcinoma or one hyperplasia and one adenoma) as they are to be the same. The recurrence rate in dogs with two masses at the time of diagnosis is less than the recurrence rate of dogs with a single solitary mass.

Mediastinal Parathyroid Tissue

Parathyroid tissue, displaced into the anterior mediastinum during the embryologic expansion of the thymus and often referred to as "ectopic" because its location is not associated with the thyroid, may become autonomously functioning. In humans, this is an uncommon but recognized location for a solitary adenoma (Heath, 1989). Mediastinal parathyroid tissue that results in PHPTH has been reported in a dog, and a mediastinal parathyroid cyst was diagnosed in a normocalcemic cat (Swainson et al, 2000; Ham et al, 2009).

Multiple Endocrine Neoplasia and Adrenal Secondary Hyperparathyroidism

Multiple Endocrine Neoplasia

Multiple endocrine neoplasia (MEN) refers to a group of syndromes in humans (often familial) consisting of hyperplasia or neoplasia in two or more endocrine glands. Two patterns of MEN involve the parathyroid gland: (1) MEN type I, parathyroid hyperplasia with pancreatic islet cell adenoma/carcinoma or adenoma/hyperplasia of the anterior pituitary; and (2) MEN type IIa, medullary carcinoma of the thyroid with pheochromocytoma and/or parathyroid hyperplasia (see Chapter 5). In both conditions, hyperplasia, not neoplasia, is the most common parathyroid abnormality. Although the clinical expression of the MEN components is variable, hyperparathyroidism usually predominates in MEN type I, whereas medullary thyroid carcinoma predominates in MEN type IIa (Leshin, 1985). Sporadic cases of dogs and cats with multiple endocrine disorders are occasionally reported. Our experience of multiple endocrine conditions involving PHPTH would include the common combination with Cushing's syndrome. It remains elucidated if dogs with these concurrent conditions have pituitary dependent Cushing's and parathyroid hyperplasia. Further, as we recognize more thyroid tumors incidentally on cervical ultrasonography, this may add to the combinations seen (Pollard et al, in press).

Adrenal Secondary Hyperparathyroidism

Hypercortisolism is associated with dysregulation of calcium homeostasis as illustrated by dogs with calcinosis cutis and/or bronchial tree calcification. A majority of dogs with hypercortisolism were demonstrated to have increases in circulating PTH concentrations, although not associated with changes in TCa or iCa (Ramsey et al, 2005). With successful treatment of hypercortisolism, serum PTH concentrations returned to reference range concentrations (Tebb et al, 2005).

Hereditary Neonatal Primary Hyperparathyroidism

A rare form of hereditary neonatal PHPTH has been described in humans, which is associated with diffuse hyperplasia of the parathyroid chief cells. Primary parathyroid hyperplasia has also been reported in two German Shepherd pups from a litter of four females (Thompson et al, 1984). Clinical signs were apparent in these dogs by 2 weeks of age, including stunted growth, muscular weakness, and polyuria/polydipsia. An autosomal recessive mode of inheritance for the PHPTH was suggested, and an analogous condition is recognized in children.

 PROGNOSIS: DOGS WITH PRIMARY HYPERPARATHYROIDISM

The prognosis for most dogs with PHPTH is excellent. Hypocalcemia may occur after therapy, but clinical hypocalcemia should not be common with use of posttreatment calcitriol. Care must be taken not to overdose vitamin D.

HYPERCALCEMIA IN CATS

 BACKGROUND

In general, the same differential diagnoses for hypercalcemia in dogs can be used in cats. In a study of 71 hypercalcemic cats, their mean age was about 9 years and their mean serum TCa concentration was 12.2 mg/dL. Anorexia and lethargy were their most common clinical signs (70%). Vomiting, diarrhea, and/or constipation were observed in 27%, polyuria and/or polydipsia were observed in 24%, urinary signs were seen in 23%, and neurologic signs were observed in 14% (Savary et al, 2000). Hypercalcemia secondary to malignancy was diagnosed in 30% of these cats. The most common cancers diagnosed included lymphoma and squamous cell carcinoma. Less common neoplasms included leukemia, osteosarcoma, fibrosarcoma, undifferentiated sarcoma, and bronchogenic carcinoma (Anderson et al, 2000; Bollinger et al, 2002; Geddes, 2013). CKD was diagnosed in 25% of the cats, and half of those had urolithiasis. In a separate study, CKD in cats was usually associated with a serum TCa concentration in the reference range and a low-normal to low serum iCa concentration (Barber and Elliott, 1998). Of cats with hypercalcemia, several had urolithiasis without renal injury. Four cats (6%) had PHPTH. One cat had hypoadrenocorticism. Several cats had hyperthyroidism or diabetes mellitus, but it would not seem likely that either of these endocrine conditions would contribute to hypercalcemia. However, four cats (6%) had infectious or granulomatous disease (e.g., feline infectious peritonitis [FIP], toxoplasmosis, actinomycosis, or cryptococcosis). Thus the differential diagnosis for hypercalcemia in cats is not dramatically different from that in dogs (Mealey et al, 1999; Savary et al, 2000; Pineda et al, 2012).

 IDIOPATHIC HYPERCALCEMIA OF CATS

Idiopathic hypercalcemia of cats (IHC) may be their most common cause of hypercalcemia. In contrast to hypercalcemic dogs, in which a diagnosis can usually be made, this condition remains frustrating to understand and treat. IHC has been recognized in North America and in other areas (Schenck and Chew, 2012). There is no age or gender predisposition. Long-haired cats may be over represented (Barsanti, 1997; Refsal et al, 1998; Midkiff et al, 2000; Rosol et al, 2000; Schenck and Chew, 2005a). About 50% of cats with IHC have no apparent clinical signs. When present, signs include any combination of weight loss, weakness, diarrhea, constipation, vomiting, and decreases in appetite. Calcium containing uroliths have been documented in about 10% to 15% of cats with IHC. Increases in their serum iCa concentrations are similar to or higher than expected from the increases noted in TCa. Serum PTH concentrations have been within or below reference intervals, and PTHrP is not increased. Serum magnesium and 25(OH)D concentrations have usually been within reference intervals, and concentrations of $1,25(OH)_2D_3$ are decreased (Schenck and Chew, 2012). Some cats with IHC have developed CKD.

The pathogenesis of IHC is not understood, making therapies nonspecific. Increasing dietary fiber has been advocated to decrease intestinal absorption of calcium. Increasing dietary fiber has not been uniformly helpful, probably related to the many forms of fiber used. Use of diets formulated for cats with CKD have also been helpful in some but not all IHC cats. These diets are usually low in calcium and phosphorus and may have an alkalinizing effect. A positive dietary response with normalization of serum calcium concentrations, however, does not usually persist.

Prednisolone has been beneficial in some cats with IHC. Doses of 5 to 20 mg/cat/day often reduce serum calcium concentrations and in some cats contribute to long-term control. Prednisolone has also improved appetite and body weight in some cats. When diet and prednisolone fail to resolve IHC, the use of a bisphosphonate has been recommended. IV administration is not recommended because of the chronic nature of IHC. Rather, oral alendronate is recommended, 10 mg weekly after a 12 hour fast, with special note made of the medication causing esophagitis if not completely passed into the stomach. To

TABLE 15-10   CLINICAL, LABORATORY, AND HISTOLOGIC FINDINGS IN 10 CATS WITH PRIMARY, NATURALLY OCCURRING, HYPERPARATHYROIDISM IN THE UC DAVIS SERIES

SIGNALMENT	CLINICAL SIGNS	SERUM Ca (mg/dL)	SERUM PO$_4$ (mg/dL)	BLOOD UREA NITROGEN (mg/dL)	SERUM CREATININE (mg/dL)	URINE SPECIFIC GRAVITY	PARATHYROID HISTOLOGY
15 y.o. M/N, DLH	Anorexia, vomiting	14.6	3.4	35	1.8	1.011	Solitary adenoma
14 y.o. F/S, Siamese	Anorexia, vomiting, muscle fasciculation	22.8	6.6	70	3.2	1.013	Solitary adenoma
15 y.o. M/N, Siamese	None	13.5	3.3	21	2.2	1.031	Solitary adenoma
15 y.o. F/S, Siamese	Polydipsia, polyuria	13.3	2.2	31	2.7	1.010	Solitary adenoma
8 y.o. F/S, DSH	Anorexia, weight loss	13.8	1.8	15	1.0	1.015	Solitary adenoma
14 y.o. F/S, DSH	Polydipsia, polyuria, lethargy	15.4	2.5	30	1.2	1.010	Solitary adenoma
9 y.o. F/S, Siamese	Anorexia	17.1	6.2	63	2.6	1.026	Bilateral cystadenoma
9 y.o. M/N, DSH	Anorexia, vomiting, lethargy, dysuria	15.2	2.6	59	3.6	1.015	Solitary carcinoma
14 y.o. M/N, DSH	Constipation	13.4	3.7	41	2.2	1.022	Solitary adenoma
12 y.o. M/N, DSH	Weight loss, lethargy, constipation	14.1	3.2	27	1.4	1.018	Bilateral carcinomas
Reference values		8.8-11.4	2.4-6.1	10-30	0.8-2.0	—	—

DLH, Domestic Long-Haired; *DSH,* Domestic Short-Haired; *F,* female; *M,* male; *N,* neutered; *S,* spay/ovariohysterectomy; serum Ca, serum total calcium; serum PO$_4$, serum phosphate concentration; *y.o.,* years old.

avoid esophageal irritation and to enhance passage into the stomach, water should be given (Schenck and Chew, 2012).

 PRIMARY HYPERPARATHYROIDISM IN CATS

A relatively small number of cats with PHPTH have been reported (Kallet et al, 1991; Marquez et al, 1995; den Hertog et al, 1997; Savary et al, 2000; Sueda and Stefanacci, 2000). Their mean age was approximately 13 years (range, 8 to 20 years) and various breeds were represented. The most common clinical signs were anorexia, lethargy, and vomiting. Owners also observed constipation, polyuria, polydipsia, and weight loss. Other signs were uncommon. A parathyroid mass was palpable in 11 of the 19 cats. The presence of a palpable mass and the owners' observations contrast with our experience in dogs with PHPTH. A palpable parathyroid mass in dogs with PHPTH is quite uncommon (Sawyer et al, 2011).

The only consistent abnormality on CBC and serum biochemical profiles is hypercalcemia (Table 15-10). Afflicted cats have persistent increases in both the serum TCa and iCa concentrations. Several cats had cystic calculi and a large percentage had abnormalities in their BUN and serum creatinine concentrations, in

contrast to dogs. Cervical ultrasonography was described as normal in several cats, but others had visible masses that would be considered huge in a dog. On cervical ultrasonography, two cats each had a single parathyroid mass, one mass measuring 4.5 × 2 × 1 cm and the other measuring 1.7 × 1.1 × 1 cm (Sueda and Stefanacci, 2000). Serum PTH concentrations, when measured, ranged from within the reference range (0 to 4 pmol/L) to increased. In one cat, seven separate serum PTH samples were assayed; five results were in the reference range and two were increased.

Most of the 19 cats had surgical nodule removal followed by resolution of their PHPTH. Tetany has not been described in any cat treated with surgery, although several cats became subclinically hypocalcemic and were treated with vitamin D and calcium. Of the nine cats we followed after surgery, all lived well beyond 1 year, although at 1½ years, one had recurrence of hypercalcemia and at necropsy was demonstrated to have had both a parathyroid adenoma and a parathyroid carcinoma. Histologic evaluation of tissue removed showed that 13 cats had had a parathyroid adenoma, three had had parathyroid carcinomas, two had had parathyroid hyperplasia (involving all four glands), and one had had bilateral cystadenomas.

REFERENCES

Anderson TE, et al.: Probable hypercalcemia of malignancy in a cat with bronchogenic adenocarcinoma, *J Am Anim Hosp Assoc* 36:52, 2000.

Arbaugh M, et al.: Evaluation of preoperative serum concentrations of ionized calcium and parathyroid hormone as predictors of hypocalcemia following parathyroidectomy in dogs with primary hyperparathyroidism: 17 cases (2001-2009), *J Am Vet Med Assoc* 241:233, 2012.

Arnaud CD, Kolb FO: The calciotropic hormones and metabolic bone disease. In Greenspan FS, editor: *Basic and clinical endocrinology*, Los Altos, CA, 1991, Lange Medical Publications, p 247.

Attie JN, et al.: Preoperative localization of parathyroid adenomas, *Am J Surg* 156:323, 1988.

Attie MF: Treatment of hypercalcemia, *Endocrinol Metab Clin North Am* 18:807, 1989.

Aurbach GD, et al.: Parathyroid hormone, calcitonin, and the calciferols. In Wilson JD, Foster DW, editors: *Williams textbook of endocrinology*, ed 7, Philadelphia, 1985a, WB Saunders, p 1137.

Bahri LE: Poisoning in dogs by vitamin D3 containing rodenticides, *Compend Continu Ed Pract Vet* 12:1414, 1990.

Barber PJ, Elliott J: Feline chronic renal failure: calcium homeostasis in 80 cases diagnosed between 1992 and 1995, *J Small Anim Pract* 39:108, 1998.

Barber PJ, et al.: Measurement of feline intact parathyroid hormone: assay validation and sample handling studies, *J Small Anim Pract* 34:614, 1993.

Barsanti JA: Hypercalcemia and urolithiasis in cats, *Proc Am Coll Vet Intern Med Ann Forum* 15:327, 1997.

Bennedbaek FN, et al.: Percutaneous ethanol injection therapy in the treatment of thyroid and parathyroid diseases, *Eur J Endocrinol* 136:240, 1997.

Bennett PF, et al.: Canine anal sac adenocarcinomas: clinical presentation and response to therapy, *J Vet Intern Med* 16:100, 2002.

Berger B, Feldman EC: Primary hyperparathyroidism in dogs, *J Vet Med Assoc* 191:350, 1987.

Bilezikian JP: Hypercalcemic states. In Coe FL, et al.: editors: *Disorders of bone and mineral metabolism*, New York, 1992a, Raven Press, p 493.

Bilezikian JP: Management of acute hypercalcemia, *N Engl J Med* 326:1196, 1992b.

Bilezikian JP, et al.: *The parathyroids: basic and clinical concepts*, ed 2, San Diego, CA, 2001, Academic Press.

Black KS, Mundy GR: Other causes of hypercalcemia: local and ectopic secretion syndromes. In Bilezikian JP, et al.: editors: *The parathyroids*, New York, 1994, Raven Press, p 341.

Bollinger AP, et al.: Detection of parathyroid hormone-related protein in cats with humoral hypercalcemia of malignancy, *Vet Clin Pathol* 31:3, 2002.

Boyce RA, Weisbrode SE: Effect of dietary calcium on the response of bone to 1,25(OH)2D3, *Lab Invest* 48:683, 1983.

Broadus AE, Stewart AF: Parathyroid hormone–related protein: structure, processing, and physiologic actions. In Bilezikian JP, editor: *The parathyroids: basic and clinical concepts*, New York, 1994, Raven Press, pp 259–294.

Brown EM, et al.: Calcium ion–sensing cell surface receptors, *N Engl J Med* 333:234, 1995.

Brown EM, et al.: G-protein–coupled, extracellular Ca^{2+}–sensing receptor: a versatile regulator of diverse cellular functions, *Vitam Horm* 55:1, 1999.

Brown RC, et al.: Circulating intact parathyroid hormone measured by a two-site immunochemiluminometric assay, *J Clin Endocrinol Metab* 65:407, 1987.

Budayr AA, et al.: Increased serum levels of parathyroid hormone–like protein in malignancy-associated hypercalcemia, *Ann Intern Med* 111:807, 1989.

Burtis WJ: Parathyroid hormone-related protein: structure, function, and measurement, *Clin Chem* 38:2171, 1992.

Capen CC, Martin SL: Calcium-regulating hormones and diseases of the parathyroid glands. In Ettinger SJ, editor: *Textbook of veterinary internal medicine*, ed 2, Philadelphia, 1983, WB Saunders, p 1550.

Carothers MA, et al.: 25-OH-cholecalciferol intoxication in dogs, *Proc Am Coll Vet Intern Med Forum* 12:822, 1994.

Chew DJ, Capen CC: Hypercalcemic nephropathy and associated disorders. In Kirk RW, editor: *Current veterinary therapy VII*, Philadelphia, 1980, WB Saunders, p 1067.

Chew DJ, Meuten DJ: Disorders of calcium and phosphorus metabolism, *Vet Clin North Am* 12:411, 1982.

Chew DJ, et al.: Effect of sodium bicarbonate infusions on ionized calcium and total calcium concentrations in serum of clinically normal cats, *Am J Vet Res* 50:145, 1989.

Chew DJ, et al.: Hypercalcemia in dogs and cats: overview of etiology, diagnostic approach, and therapy, *Proceedings of the Waltham/OSU Symposium* 1991, p 35.

Consensus Development Conference Panel: NIH conference; diagnosis and management of asymptomatic primary hyperparathyroidism: consensus development conference statement, *Ann Intern Med* 114:593, 1991.

Cortadellas O, et al.: Calcium and phosphorus homeostasis in dogs with spontaneous chronic kidney disease at different stages of severity, *J Vet Intern Med* 24:73, 2010.

Crager CS, Nachreiner RF: Increased parathyroid hormone concentration in a Siamese kitten with nutritional secondary hyperparathyroidism, *J Am Anim Hosp Assoc* 29:331, 1993.

den Hertog E, et al.: Primary hyperparathyroidism in two cats, *Vet Q* 19:81, 1997.

DeVries SE, et al.: Primary parathyroid gland hyperplasia in dogs: six cases (1982-1991), *J Am Vet Med Assoc* 202:1132, 1993.

Dougherty SA, et al.: Salmon calcitonin as adjunct treatment for vitamin D toxicosis in a dog, *J Am Vet Med Assoc* 196:1269, 1990.

Dow SW, et al.: Hypercalcemia associated with blastomycosis in dogs, *J Am Vet Med Assoc* 188:706, 1986.

Durie BG, et al.: Relation of osteoclast activating factor production to the extent of bone disease in multiple myeloma, *Br J Haematol* 47:21, 1981.

Estepa JC, et al.: Dynamics of secretion and metabolism of PTH during hypo- and hypercalcemia in the dog as determined by the "intact" and "whole" PTH assays, *Nephrology Dialysis Transplantation* 18:1101, 2003.

Eubig PA, et al.: Acute renal failure in dogs after the ingestion of grapes or raisins: a retrospective evaluation of 43 dogs (1992-2002), *J Vet Intern Med* 19:663, 2005.

Feldman EC: Canine primary hyperparathyroidism. In Kirk RW, Bonagura JD, editors: *Current veterinary therapy X*, Philadelphia, 1989, WB Saunders, p 985.

Feldman EC, et al.: Comparison of results of hormonal analysis of samples obtained from selected venous sites versus cervical ultrasonography for localizing parathyroid masses in dogs, *J Am Vet Med Assoc* 211:54, 1997.

Feldman EC, et al.: Pretreatment clinical and laboratory findings in dogs with primary hyperparathyroidism: 210 cases (1987-2004), *J Am Vet Med Assoc* 227:756, 2005.

Fine EJ: Parathyroid imaging: its current status and future role, *Semin Nucl Med* 17:350, 1987.

Fingeroth JM, Smeak DD: Intravenous methylene blue infusion for intraoperative identification of parathyroid gland tumors in dogs: III. clinical trials and results in three dogs, *J Am Anim Hosp Assoc* 24:673, 1988.

Flanders JA, Reimers TJ: Radioimmunoassay of parathyroid hormone in cats, *Am J Vet Res* 52:422, 1991.

Foley P, et al.: Serum parathyroid hormone–related protein concentration in a dog with a thymoma and persistent hypercalcemia, *Can Vet J* 41:867, 2000.

Fooshee SK, Forrester SD: Hypercalcemia secondary to cholecalciferol rodenticide toxicosis in two dogs, *J Am Vet Med Assoc* 196:1265, 1990.

Fradkin JM, et al.: Elevated parathyroid hormone–related protein and hypercalcemia in two dogs with schistosomiasis, *J Am Anim Hosp Assoc* 37:349, 2001.

Gao P, et al.: Development of a novel immunoradiometric assay exclusively for biologically active whole parathyroid hormone 1-84: implications for improvement of accurate assessment of parathyroid function, *J Bone and Mineral Research* 16:605, 2001.

Garrett IR: Bone destruction in cancer, *Semin Oncol* 20:4, 1993.

Gear RN, et al.: Primary hyperparathyroidism in 29 dogs: diagnosis, treatment, outcome and associated renal failure, *J Small Animal Prac* 46:10, 2005.

Geddes, et al.: Eight novel polymorphisms identified in the feline calcium sensing receptor in cats with varying plasma ionized calcium concentrations, *J Am Vet Med Assoc* 687, 2013.

Goldschmidt MH, Shofer FS: *Skin tumors of the dog and cat*, Oxford, England, 1992, Pergamon Press, pp 103–108.

Goldstein RE, et al.: Inheritance, mode of inheritance and candidate genes for primary hyperparathyroidism in Keeshonden, *J Vet Intern Med* 21:199, 2007.

Goodwin JS, et al.: Mechanism of action of glucocorticoids: inhibition of T cell proliferation and interleukin-2 production by hydrocortisone is reversed by leukotriene B_4, *J Clin Invest* 77:1244, 1986.

Grain E, Walder EJ: Hypercalcemia associated with squamous cell carcinoma in a dog, *J Am Vet Med Assoc* 181:165, 1982.

Greenlee PG, et al.: Lymphomas in dogs: a morphologic, immunologic and clinical study, *Cancer* 66:480, 1990.

Grone A, et al.: Dependence of humoral hypercalcemia of malignancy on parathyroid hormone–related protein expression in the canine anal sac apocrine gland adenocarcinoma (CAC-8) nude mouse model, *Vet Pathol* 35:344, 1998.

Gross KL, et al.: Nutrients. In Hand MS, et al.: editors: *Small animal clinical nutrition*, ed 4, Kansas, 2000, Mark Morris Institute, p 84.

Gunther R, et al.: Toxicity of a vitamin D_3 rodenticide to dogs, *J Am Vet Med Assoc* 193:211, 1988.

Gwaltney-Brant S, et al.: Renal failure associated with ingestion of grapes or raisins in dogs, *J Am Vet Med Assoc* 218:1555, 2001.

Ham K, et al.: Validation of rapid parathyroid hormone assay and intraoperative measurement of parathyroid hormone in dogs with benign naturally occurring primary hyperparathyroidism, *Vet Surg* 38:122, 2009.

Harrington DD, Page EH: Acute vitamin D_2 (ergocalciferol) toxicosis in horses: case report and experimental studies, *J Am Vet Med Assoc* 182:1358, 1983.

Harris NL, et al.: Case records of the Massachusetts General Hospital, *N Engl J Med* 347:1952, 2002.

Heath DA: Primary hyperparathyroidism: clinical presentation and factors influencing clinical management, *Endocrinol Metab Clin North Am* 18:631, 1989.

Henderson JE, et al.: Circulating concentrations of parathyroid hormone–like peptide in malignancy and in hyperparathyroidism, *J Bone Miner Res* 5:105, 1990.

Henry CJ: Paraneoplastic syndromes. In Ettinger SJ, Feldman EC, editors: *Textbook of veterinary internal medicine: diseases of the dog and cat*, St Louis, 2010, Elsevier, p 2213.

Hirt RA, et al.: Severe hypercalcemia in a dog with a retained fetus and endometritis, *J Am Vet Med Assoc* 216:1423, 2000.

Hollis BW, et al.: Quantification of circulating 1,25-dihydroxyvitamin D by radioimmunoassay with an ^{125}I-labeled tracer, *Clin Chem* 42:586, 1996.

Hostutler RA, et al.: Uses and effectiveness of pamidronate disodium for treatment of dogs and cats with hypercalcemia, *J Vet Intern Med* 19:29, 2005.

Hruska KA, Teitelbaum SL: Renal osteodystrophy, *N Engl J Med* 333:166, 1995.

Ihle SL, et al.: Seizures as a manifestation of primary hyperparathyroidism in a dog, *J Am Vet Med Assoc* 192:71, 1988.

Jiao LR, et al.: Clinical short-term results of radio frequency ablation in primary and secondary liver tumors, *Am J Surg* 177:303, 1999.

Johnessee JS, et al.: Primary hypoadrenocorticism in a cat, *J Am Vet Med Assoc* 183:881, 1982.

Kallet AJ, et al.: Primary hyperparathyroidism in cats: seven cases (1984-1989), *J Am Vet Med Assoc* 199:1767, 1991.

Klausner JS, et al.: Calcium urolithiasis in two dogs with parathyroid adenomas, *J Am Vet Med Assoc* 191:1423, 1987.

Krubsack AJ, et al.: Prospective comparison of radionuclide, computed tomography, and sonographic and magnetic resonance localization of parathyroid tumors, *Surgery* 106:639, 1989.

Legendre AM, et al.: Canine blastomycosis: a review of 47 clinical cases, *J Am Vet Med Assoc* 178:1163, 1981.

Lemann J, Gray RW: Calcitriol, calcium, and granulomatous disease, *N Engl J Med* 311:1115, 1984.

Leshin M: Multiple endocrine neoplasia. In Wilson JC, Foster DW, editors: *Williams textbook of endocrinology*, ed 7, Philadelphia, 1985, WB Saunders, p 1274.

Livraghi T, et al.: Small hepatocellular carcinoma: treatment with radio frequency ablation versus ethanol ablation, *Radiology* 210:655, 1999.

Llach F, et al.: The pathophysiology of altered calcium metabolism in rhabdomyolysis-induced acute renal failure, *N Engl J Med* 305:117, 1981.

Lloyd MN, et al.: Preoperative localization in primary hyperparathyroidism, *Clin Radiol* 41:239, 1990.

Long CD, et al.: Percutaneous ultrasound–guided chemical parathyroid ablation for treatment of primary hyperparathyroidism in dogs, *J Am Vet Med Assoc* 215:217, 1999.

Marquez GA, et al.: Calcium oxalate urolithiasis in a cat with a functional parathyroid adenocarcinoma, *J Am Vet Med Assoc* 206:817, 1995.

Marx SJ: Hyperparathyroid and hypoparathyroid disorders, *N Engl J Med* 343:1863, 2000.

Matus RE, Weir EC: Hypercalcemia of malignancy. In Kirk RW, Bonagura JD, editors: *Current veterinary therapy X*, Philadelphia, 1989, WB Saunders, p 988.

Matus RE, et al.: Prognostic factors for multiple myeloma in the dog, *J Am Vet Med Assoc* 188:1288, 1986.

Matwichuk C, et al.: Use of ^{99m}Tc-sestamibi for detection of a parathyroid adenoma in a dog with primary hyperparathyroidism, *J Am Vet Med Assoc* 209:1733, 1996.

Matwichuk C, et al.: Double-phase parathyroid scintigraphy in dogs using ^{99m}Tc-sestamibi, *Vet Radiol Ultrasound* 41:461, 2000.

McArthur W, et al.: Bone solubilization by mononuclear cells, *Lab Invest* 42:452, 1980.

McCauley LK, et al.: In vivo and in vitro effects of interleukin-1a and cyclosporin A on bone and lymphoid tissues in mice, *Toxicol Pathol* 19:1, 1991.

Mealey KL, et al.: Hypercalcemia associated with granulomatous disease in a cat, *J Am Vet Med Assoc* 215:959, 1999.

Mellanby RJ, et al.: Hypercalcaemia in two dogs caused by excessive dietary supplementation of vitamin D, *J Small Animal Prac* 46:334, 2005.

Messinger JS, et al.: Ionized hypercalcemia in dogs: a retrospective study of 109 cases (1998-2003), *J Vet Intern med* 23:514, 2009.

Meuten DJ: Hypercalcemia, *Vet Clin North Am (Small Anim Pract)* 14:891, 1984.

Meuten DJ, Armstrong PJ: Parathyroid disease and calcium metabolism. In Ettinger SJ, editor: *Textbook of veterinary internal medicine: diseases of the dog and cat*, ed 3, Philadelphia, 1989, WB Saunders, p 1610.

Meuten DJ, et al.: Relationship of calcium to albumin and total proteins in dogs, *J Am Vet Med Assoc* 180:63, 1982.

Meuten DJ, et al.: Hypercalcemia in dogs with lymphosarcoma: biochemical, ultrastructural, and histomorphometric investigation, *Lab Invest* 49:553, 1983a.

Meuten DJ, et al.: Hypercalcemia in dogs with adenocarcinoma derived from apocrine glands of the anal sacs: biochemical and histomorphometric investigations, *Lab Invest* 48:428, 1983b.

Michelangeli VP, et al.: Evaluation of a new, rapid, and automated immunochemiluminometric assay for the measurement of serum intact parathyroid hormone, *Ann Clin Biochem* 34:97, 1997.

Midkiff AM, et al.: Idiopathic hypercalcemia in cats, *J Vet Intern Med* 14:619, 2000.

Milovancev M, Schmiedt CW: Preoperative factors associated with postoperative hypocalcemia in dogs that underwent parathyroidectomy: 62 cases (2004-2009), *J Am Vet Med Assoc* 242:507, 2013.

Mischke R, et al.: The effect of the albumin concentration on the relation between the concentration of ionized calcium and total calcium in the blood of dogs, *Dtsch Tierarztl Wochenschr* 103:199, 1996.

Mol JA, et al.: Elucidation of the sequence of canine (pro)-calcitonin: a molecular biological and protein chemical approach, *Regul Pept* 35:189, 1991.

Moore FM, et al.: Hypercalcemia associated with rodenticide poisoning in three cats, *J Am Vet Med Assoc* 193:1099, 1988.

Morrow C: Cholecalciferol poisoning, *Vet Med* 2001, p 905.

Mundy GR: Hypercalcemia of malignancy revisited, *J Clin Invest* 82:1, 1988.

Mundy GR, et al.: The hypercalcemia of cancer: clinical implications and pathogenic mechanisms,, *N Engl J Med* 310:1718, 1984.

Murphy MJ: Rodenticides, *Vet Clinics N Amer: Small Anim Pract* 32:469, 2002.

Nicholson SS: Toxicology. In Ettinger SJ, Feldman EC, editors: *Textbook of veterinary internal medicine: diseases of the cat and dog*, ed 5, Philadelphia, 2000, WB Saunders, p 357.

O'Dougherty MJ, et al.: Parathyroid imaging with technetium-^{99m}-sestamibi: preoperative localization and tissue uptake studies, *J Nucl Med* 33:313, 1992.

Orloff JJ, Stewart AF: The carboxy-terminus of parathyroid hormone: inert or invaluable, *Endocrinology* 136:4729, 1995.

Parker M: *Personal communication*, 2001.

Peterson ME: *Hypercalcemia in dogs and cats: differential diagnosis and treatment*, Proceedings: 84th Annual Western Veterinary Conference, Las Vegas, NV, 2012.

Peterson ME, Feinman JM: Hypercalcemia associated with hypoadrenocorticism in sixteen dogs, *J Am Vet Med Assoc* 181:804, 1982.

Peterson ME, et al.: Primary hypoadrenocorticism in ten cats, *J Vet Intern Med* 3:55, 1989.

Peterson ME, et al.: Pretreatment clinical and laboratory findings in dogs with hypoadrenocorticism: 225 cases (1979-1993), *J Am Vet Med Assoc* 208:85, 1996.

Philbrick WM, et al.: Defining the roles of parathyroid hormone–related protein in normal physiology, *Physiol Rev* 76:127, 1996.

Picard D, et al.: Localization of abnormal parathyroid glands using ^{201}thallium/^{123}iodine subtraction scintigraphy in patients with primary hyperparathyroidism, *Clin Nucl Med* 12:61, 1987.

Pineda C, et al.: Feline parathyroid hormone: validation of hormonal assays and dynamics of secretion, *Domest Anim Endocrinol* 42:256, 2012.

Pollard RE, et al.: Percutaneous ultrasonographically guided radio frequency heat ablation for treatment of primary hyperparathyroidism in dogs, *J Am Vet Med Assoc* 218:1106, 2001.

Pollard RE, et al.: Prevalence of subclinical thyroid nodules in dogs with hypercalcemia, *J Vet Radiol Ultrasonography, (2008–2013)* in press

Potts JT Jr: Management of asymptomatic hyperparathyroidism, *J Clin Endocrinol Metab* 70:1489, 1990.

Pressler BM, et al.: Hypercalcemia and high parathyroid hormone–related protein concentration associated with malignant melanoma in a dog, *J Am Vet Med Assoc* 221:263, 2002.

Quigley PJ, Leedale AH: Tumors involving bone in domestic cats: a review of fifty-eight cases, *Vet Pathol* 20:670, 1983.

Ramsey I, et al.: Hyperparathyroidism in dogs with hyperadrenocorticism, *J Small Animal Prac* 46:531, 2005.

Rasmussen H: The cycling of calcium as an intracellular messenger, *Sci Am* 261:66, 1989.

Rasor L, et al.: Retrospective evaluation of three treatment methods for primary hyperparathyroidism in dogs, *J Am Anim Hosp Assoc* 43:70, 2007.

Refsal KR: *Personal communication*, 2014.

Refsal KR, Nachreiner RF: Hormone assays and collection of samples. In Mooney CT, Peterson ME, editors: *BSAVA manual of canine and feline endocrinology*, ed 4, British Small Animal Assoc, 2012, p 1.

Refsal KR, et al.: Laboratory assessment of hypercalcemia, *Proc Am Coll Vet Intern Med Forum* 16:646, 1998.

Reusch CE, et al.: Ultrasonography of the parathyroid glands as an aid in differentiation of acute and chronic renal failure in dogs, *J Am Vet Med Assoc* 217:1849, 2000.

Rohrer CR, et al.: Hypercalcemia in a dog: a challenging case, *J Am Anim Hosp Assoc* 36:20, 2000.

Rosol TJ, et al.: Acute hypocalcemia associated with infarction of parathyroid gland adenomas in two dogs, *J Am Vet Med Assoc* 192:212, 1988.

Rosol TJ, et al.: Parathyroid hormone (PTH)–related protein, PTH, and 1,25-dihydroxyvitamin D in dogs with cancer-associated hypercalcemia, *Endocrinology* 131:1157, 1992a.

Rosol TJ, et al.: Effects of mithramycin on calcium metabolism and bone in dogs, *Vet Pathol* 29:223, 1992b.

Rosol TJ, et al.: Disorders of calcium. In DiBartola SP, editor: *Fluid therapy in small animal practice*, ed 2, Philadelphia, 2000, WB Saunders, pp 108–162.

Ross JT, et al.: Adenocarcinoma of the apocrine glands of the anal sac in dogs: a review of 32 cases, *J Am Anim Hosp Assoc* 27:349, 1991.

Ross LA, Goldstein M: *Biochemical abnormalities associated with accidental hypothermia in a dog and in a cat*, Proceedings of the Annual American College of Veterinary Internal Medicine Meeting, St Louis, 1981, p 66.

Rumbeiha WK: Nephrotoxins. In Bonagura JD, editor: *Kirk's current veterinary therapy XIII*, Philadelphia, 2000, WB Saunders, pp 212–214.

Rumbeiha WK, et al.: Use of pamidronate to reverse vitamin D_3–induced toxicosis in dogs, *Am J Vet Res* 60:1092, 1999.

Sandler LM, et al.: Studies of the hypercalcemia of sarcoidosis: effect of steroids and exogenous vitamin D_3 on the circulating concentration of 1,25-dihydroxy vitamin D_3, *O J Med* 53:165, 1984.

Savary KC, et al.: Hypercalcemia in cats: a retrospective study of 71 cases (1991-1997), *J Vet Intern Med* 14:184, 2000.

Sawyer ES, et al.: Outcome of 19 dogs with parathyroid carcinoma after surgical excision, *Vet Comp Oncol* 10:57, 2011.

Schenck PA, Chew DJ: Idiopathic hypercalcemia in cats, *Waltham Focus* 15:20, 2005a.

Schenck PA, Chew DJ: Prediction of serum ionized calcium concentration by use of serum total calcium concentration in dogs, *Am J Vet Res* 66:1330, 2005b.

Schenck PA, Chew DJ: Calcium: total or ionized? *Vet Clin North Amer: Small Anim Pract* 38:497, 2008.

Schenck PA, Chew DJ: Investigation of hypercalcaemia and hypocalcaemia. In Mooney CT, Peterson ME, editors: *BSAVA manual of canine and feline endocrinology*, ed 4, Gloucester, England, 2012, British Small Animal Veterinary Association, p 221.

Scott-Moncrieff CR: Hypoadrenocorticism. In Ettinger SJ, Feldman EC, editors: *Textbook of veterinary internal medicine: diseases of the dog and cat*, ed 7, St Louis, 2010, Elsevier, p 1847.

Seymour JF, Gagel RF: Calcitriol: the major humoral mediator of hypercalcemia in Hodgkin's and non-Hodgkin's lymphomas, *Blood* 82:1383, 1993.

Shane E, Bilezikian JP: Parathyroid carcinoma: a review of 62 patients, *Endocrinol Rev* 3:218, 1982.

Shiel RE: Disorders of vasopressin production. In Mooney CT, Peterson ME, editors: *BSAVA manual of canine and feline endocrinology*, ed 4, Gloucester, England, 2012, British Small Animal Veterinary Association, p 15.

Skelly BJ: Hyperparathyroidism. In Mooney CT, Peterson ME, editors: *BSAVA manual of canine and feline endocrinology*, ed 4, Gloucester, England, 2012, British Small Animal Veterinary Association, p 43.

Skelly BJ, Franklin RJM: Mutations in genes causing human familial isolated hyperparathyroidism do not account for hyperparathyroidism in Keeshond dogs, *Vet J* 174:652, 2006.

Silverberg SJ, et al.: A 10-year prospective study of primary hyperparathyroidism with or without parathyroid surgery, *N Engl J Med* 341:1249, 1999.

Stewart AF: Translational implications of the parathyroid calcium receptor, *N Engl J Med* 351:324, 2004.

Stewart AF: Hypercalcemia associated with cancer, *N Engl J Med* 352:373, 2005.

Strewler GL: The physiology of parathyroid hormone–related protein, *N Engl J Med* 342:177, 2000.

Sueda MT, Stefanacci JD: Ultrasound evaluation of the parathyroid glands in two hypercalcemic cats, *Vet Radiol Ultrasound* 41:448, 2000.

Swainson SW, et al.: Radiographic diagnosis: mediastinal parathyroid cyst in a cat, *Vet Radiol Ultrasound* 41:41, 2000.

Taillefer R, et al.: Detection and localization of parathyroid adenomas in patients with hyperparathyroidism using a single radionuclide imaging procedure with technetium-99m-sestamibi (double-phase study), *J Nucl Med* 33:1801, 1992.

Tebb AJ, et al.: Canine HAC effects of trilostane on parathyroid hormone, calcium and phosphate concentrations, *J Small Animal Prac* 46:537, 2005.

Thompson KG, et al.: Primary hyperparathyroidism in German Shepherd dogs: a disorder of probable genetic origin, *Vet Pathol* 21:370, 1984.

Toribio RE, et al.: Cloning and sequence analysis of the complementary DNA for feline preproparathyroid hormone, *Am J Vet Res* 63:194, 2002.

Torrance AG, Nachreiner R: Human parathormone assay for use in dogs: validation, sample handling studies, and parathyroid function testing, *Am J Vet Res* 50:1123, 1989a.

Torrance AG, Nachreiner R: Intact parathyroid hormone assay and total calcium concentration in the diagnosis of disorders of calcium metabolism in dogs, *J Vet Intern Med* 3:86, 1989b.

Troy GC, et al.: Heterobilharzia americana infection and hypercalcemia in a dog: a case report, *J Am Anim Hosp Assoc* 23:35, 1987.

Uehlinger P, et al.: Differential diagnosis of hypercalcemia: a retrospective study of 46 dogs, *Schweiz Arch Tierheilkd* 140:188, 1998.

Utiger RD: Treatment of primary hyperparathyroidism, *N Engl J Med* 341:1301, 1999.

Verdonk CA, Edis AJ: Parathyroid "double adenomas": fact or fiction? *Surgery* 90:523, 1981.

Weir EC, et al.: Primary hyperparathyroidism in a dog: biochemical, bone histomorphometric, and pathologic findings, *J Am Vet Med Assoc* 189:1471, 1986.

Weir EC, et al.: Humoral hypercalcemia of malignancy in canine lymphosarcoma, *Endocrinology* 122:602, 1988a.

Weir EC, et al.: Adenyl cyclase stimulating, bone resorbing and b-TGF–like activities in canine apocrine cell adenocarcinoma of the anal sac, *Calcif Tissue Int* 43:359, 1988b.

Weir EC, et al.: Isolation of 16,000-dalton parathyroid hormone–like proteins from two animal tumors causing humoral hypercalcemia of malignancy, *Endocrinology* 123:2744, 1988c.

Weller RE, et al.: Chemotherapeutic responses in dogs with lymphosarcoma and hypercalcemia, *J Am Vet Med Assoc* 181:891, 1982.

Williams LE, et al.: Carcinoma of the apocrine glands of the anal sac in dogs: 113 cases (1985-1995), *J Am Vet Med Assoc* 223:825, 2003.

Wisner ER, Nyland TG: Clinical vignette, *J Vet Intern Med* 8:244, 1994.

Wisner ER, et al.: Normal ultrasonographic anatomy of the canine neck, *Vet Radiol* 32:185, 1991.

Wisner ER, et al.: Ultrasonographic evaluation of the parathyroid glands in hypercalcemic dogs, *Vet Radiol Ultrasound* 34:108, 1993.

Wisner ER, et al.: High-resolution parathyroid sonography, *Vet Radiol Ultrasound* 38:462, 1997.

Wright KN, et al.: Diagnostic and therapeutic considerations in a hypercalcemic dog with multiple endocrine neoplasia, *J Am Anim Hosp Assoc* 31:156, 1995.

Wysolmerski JJ, Insogna KL: The parathyroid glands, hypercalcemia and hypocalcemia. In Goldman L, Schafer AI, editors: *Goldman's Cecil medicine*, ed 24, Philadelphia, 2012, Elsevier Saunders, p 1591.

CHAPTER 16 | Hypocalcemia and Primary Hypoparathyroidism

Edward C. Feldman

CHAPTER CONTENTS

In health, homeostatic control mechanisms maintain serum total calcium (TCa) and ionized calcium (iCa) concentrations within narrow ranges. In addition to providing skeletal support, calcium is a necessary component of numerous vital intra- and extracellular functions. Ionized calcium is required for bone formation and resorption, cell growth and division, membrane transport and stability, enzymatic reactions, nerve conduction, muscle contraction, hormone secretion, hepatic glycogen metabolism, blood coagulation, and numerous other activities. Ionized calcium in the extracellular fluid (ECF) contributes to regulation of cell function by binding to cell membrane calcium-sensing receptors (Brown et al, 1995). Intracellular calcium ions aid in cellular response to agonists by serving as messengers to transport signals received at cell surfaces to the interior (Rasmussen, 1989). Identification of abnormal serum calcium concentrations may help explain clinical signs and may aid in determining cause of illness. Ability to accurately assess concentrations of serum TCa, iCa, parathyroid hormone (PTH), parathyroid hormone–related protein (PTHrP), and vitamin D metabolites has enhanced our capacity to determine the cause of hypocalcemia in most patients.

Several historical landmarks in the understanding of parathyroid physiology and maintenance of calcium homeostasis are significant regarding current knowledge of hypocalcemia. Rickets (hypovitaminosis D) was first described in 1645. More than 200 years later (1884), an association was made between thyroidectomy in dogs and cats and the development of clinical hypocalcemia (tetany). In 1891, Gley proved that the parathyroid glands must be removed with the thyroids to produce tetany and that administration of calcium salts following parathyroidectomy successfully prevented tetany. Almost a century later, the amino acid sequence of PTH was determined (Tepperman, 1980). Soon thereafter, the amino acid sequence of a PTHrP, produced by some cancers, was described in both humans and dogs (Broadus et al, 1988; Weir et al, 1988; Yates et al, 1988).

 PHYSIOLOGY OF SYSTEMIC HYPOCALCEMIA

Maintenance of a Normal Serum Calcium Concentration

The parathyroid glands are exquisitely sensitive to small changes in the serum iCa concentration. The integrated actions of PTH on calcium resorption from bone, distal renal tubular calcium reabsorption, and 1,25-dihydroxyvitamin D_3 (1,25[OH]$_2$D$_3$) (calcitriol)–mediated intestinal calcium absorption are responsible for the fine regulation of serum iCa concentration. Precision in control is such that plasma iCa concentrations may fluctuate day-to-day by no more than 0.1 mmol/L from their "set" normal value. The "acute" phases of bone resorption and distal renal tubular calcium reabsorption are important components of minute-to-minute calcium homeostasis.

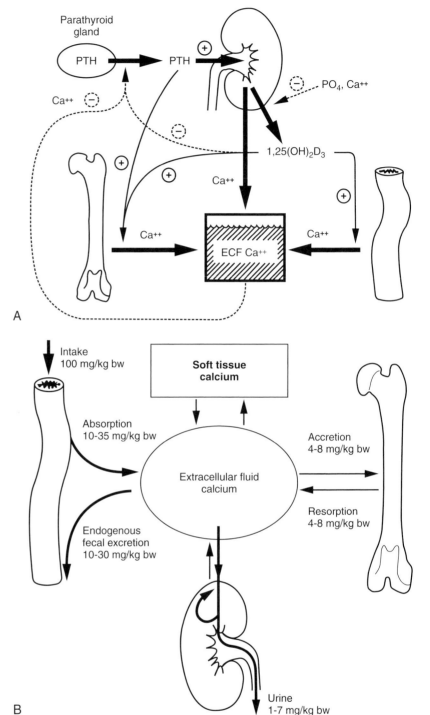

FIGURE 16-1 A, Regulation of extracellular fluid *(ECF)* calcium concentration by the effects of parathyroid hormone *(PTH)* and 1,25-dihydroxyvitamin D_3 *(1,25[OH]$_2$D$_3$;* calcitriol) on gut, kidney, bone, and parathyroid gland. The principal effect of PTH is to increase the ECF calcium concentration by mobilizing calcium from bone, increasing tubular calcium reabsorption, and, indirectly on the gut, by increasing calcitriol synthesis. The principal effect of calcitriol is to increase intestinal absorption of calcium, but it also exerts negative regulatory control of PTH synthesis and further calcitriol synthesis. **B,** Normal calcium balance showing the major organs that supply or remove calcium from ECF: bone, gut, and kidney. Total calcium (TCa) input into ECF equals TCa leaving the extracellular space. *bw,* Body weight, *Ca^{++},* ionized calcium; *PO$_4$,* phosphate. (From Rosol et al.: Disorders of calcium. In DiBartola SP, editor: *Fluid therapy in small animal practice,* ed 2, Philadelphia, 2000, WB Saunders, p 108.)

The effect of PTH on distal renal tubules is quantitatively most important. Adjustments in the rate of intestinal calcium absorption via the calcium-PTH-vitamin D axis require about 24 to 48 hours to become maximal (see full discussion in Chapter 15).

Defense Against Hypocalcemia

Physiologic responses to hypocalcemia have been characterized (Fig. 16-1). The three classic challenges to maintaining serum calcium concentrations within the narrow reference range include (1) minor transient challenges, (2) moderate challenges, and (3) severe, prolonged challenges. Hypocalcemia elicits corrective homeostatic responses that are mediated by PTH and vitamin

D. Acute effects occur in seconds to minutes, subacute or moderate effects occur over several hours and may last a few days, and chronic effects occur over days to weeks and even months (Rosol and Capen, 1997; Rosol et al, 2000).

Minor Transient Hypocalcemia Challenges

A 12- to 15-hour fast (or consumption of a diet completely deficient in calcium) in a normal mammal requires only subtle hormonal adjustments. If there are slight decreases in serum calcium concentration, slight increases in secretion of preformed PTH quickly take place. With increases in PTH secretion, renal calcium reabsorption and phosphorus excretion are enhanced within minutes, whereas bone mobilization of calcium and phosphate occurs over a period of hours (Rosol et al, 2000). Hypocalcemia also decreases the proportion of PTH that is degraded in the parathyroid chief cells, making more hormone available for secretion. By 12 hours, only minor increases in vitamin D synthesis have occurred.

Moderate Hypocalcemia Challenges

Moderate reductions in dietary calcium intake, or other causes of hypocalcemia, initiate a series of adjustments in calcium metabolism beyond those documented with minor decreases. The result is a new steady state of PTH and vitamin D (calcitriol) synthesis and secretion. Moderate increases in the secretion rate of PTH result in (1) increased calcium reabsorption from distal renal tubules, (2) increased mobilization of calcium and phosphorus from bone, and (3) increased synthesis of $1,25(OH)_2D_3$ (calcitriol). Calcitriol teams with PTH in bone resorption and increases the efficiency of calcium and phosphorus absorption from the intestine (see Fig. 16-1). The increased concentrations of circulating PTH enhance renal excretion of phosphorus, thereby compensating for the increased amounts of phosphorus mobilized from bone and absorbed from the intestine. In this new steady state, the serum calcium concentration returns to normal, the serum phosphorus concentration is unchanged or slightly reduced, and a state of mild secondary hyperparathyroidism with enhanced intestinal mineral absorption exists. Initial requirement of calcium mobilization from skeleton is largely replaced by the enhanced absorption of calcium from intestine.

Severe and Prolonged Hypocalcemia Challenges

Lactation and chronic kidney disease (CKD) with decreasing ability to excrete phosphorus represent two common examples of severe challenges to calcium homeostasis. These issues cannot be corrected by processes known to occur within minutes or hours. Assuming the four parathyroid glands are intact and functional, the previously described sequence of events resulting from "minor" and "moderate" challenges caused by hypocalcemia ensue. However, continuing losses of calcium into milk associated with lactation (for example) prevents complete compensation by the usual calcium-PTH-vitamin D absorption axis. Physiologic compensation in this setting includes (1) a maximal PTH secretion rate of approximately five times normal, (2) a maximal rate of vitamin D synthesis, and (3) initiation of maximal "rapid" and "late" phases of bone resorption in response to the combined effects of PTH and vitamin D.

Over days, weeks, or even longer periods of hypocalcemia, increases in PTH secretion (beyond those already described) are achieved largely via hyperplasia of parathyroid gland chief cells (Roth and Capen, 1974; Rosol et al, 2000). Hypocalcemia directly stimulates the growth of parathyroid cells. This effect occurs regardless of vitamin D metabolite concentrations (Li et al, 1998; Malloy et al, 1999, Marx, 2000). With hyperplasia of parathyroid chief cells, PTH secretion rates approach 10 to 50 times normal. These circulating concentrations of PTH result in recruitment of an increasing osteoclast population and the incorporation of substantial bone surfaces into the resorption process. In the final steady state, serum calcium concentrations are maintained at the expense of the skeleton, and significant bone losses ensue. Thus, the integrity of skeletal mineral homeostasis is sacrificed in an attempt to compensate for systemic mineral deficits (Broadus, 1981).

Physiology of Hypocalcemia Caused by Hypoparathyroidism

Definition

A pair of parathyroid glands is located in close proximity to each thyroid lobe in healthy individuals. Hypoparathyroidism, an

---

> **BOX 16-1** **Signs Noted by Owners of Dogs and Cats with Primary Hypoparathyroidism***
>
> **Common**
> Muscle tremors, twitching, fasciculations
>   May be focal or diffuse; often worse with activity or excitement
> Facial rubbing (possible paresthesia)
> Intense biting or licking their paws (possible paresthesia)
> Oral "chomping" (possible paresthesia)
> Generalized seizures (convulsions, "fits")
> Rear leg muscle cramping, pain, or stiff gait
>   Can occur in forelegs, but rear leg signs are more common
> Behavior changes
>   Restless, nervous, anxious
>   Aggressive, biting
>   Hypersensitive (reluctant to be petted, touched, or handled)
> Poor appetite, weight loss
> Less active, listless
>
> **Uncommon**
> Weakness
> Anorexia, vomiting, diarrhea
> Ataxia
> Pyrexia
> Prolapsed third eyelid and/or ptyalism (cats)
>
> **Rare**
> No signs observed
> Circling
> Respiratory arrest or death

*Note: Most signs are seen episodically.

---

uncommon endocrine disorder, develops as a result of an absolute or relative deficiency in synthesis and secretion of PTH, the sole product of the parathyroid glands. PTH deficiency invariably leads to hypocalcemia, usually defined as a serum TCa concentration less than about 9 mg/dL and/or an iCa less than about 1.0 mmol/L in dogs. Values defining hypocalcemia in cats are slightly lower. In dogs, the serum TCa concentration tends to underestimate the iCa. In cats, the serum TCa concentration tends to overestimate the iCa concentration (Schenck and Chew, 2005; Schenck et al, 2012). Signs of hypocalcemia are similar, regardless of cause (Box 16-1). Once hypocalcemia is identified, clinicians are encouraged to determine cause in order to formulate appropriate short- and long-term treatment strategies and a prognosis.

Initial Physiologic Alterations

The pathologic and biochemical consequences of parathyroid gland removal or loss of a critical number of parathyroid chief cells secondary to immune-mediated destruction (a less common condition) can be appreciated by referring to the "butterfly" diagram (Fig. 16-2). In this condition, the right limbs of the three feedback loops predominate with (1) decreased bone resorption; (2) decreased renal phosphate excretion, increased serum phosphate, decreased calcitriol and intestinal absorption of calcium; and (3) excess renal excretion of calcium relative to the prevailing circulating concentration. Typically, there is hypocalcemia and hyperphosphatemia if dietary phosphate intake has been normal.

All changes discussed can be explained by a PTH deficiency. The processes that are *not* taking place include (1) mobilization of calcium and phosphate from the skeleton via increased

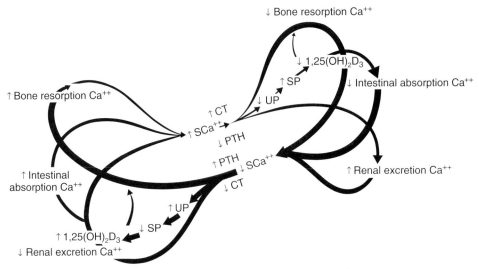

FIGURE 16-2 Regulation of calcium homeostasis. Three overlapping control loops interlock and relate to one another through the level of blood concentrations of ionic calcium, parathyroid hormone *(PTH)*, and calcitonin *(CT)*. Each loop involves a calciotropic hormone target organ (bone, intestine, or kidney). The limbs on the left depict physiologic events that increase the blood serum concentration of calcium (SCa^{++}), and the limbs on the right depict physiologic events that decrease this concentration. *1,25(OH)$_2$D$_3$,* 1,25-dihydroxyvitamin D$_3$ (calcitriol); *SP,* serum phosphorus; *UP,* urine phosphorus. (Modified and reproduced with permission from Arnaud and Kolb, 1991.)

osteoclast activity on bony surfaces, (2) retention of calcium and enhanced excretion of phosphate by kidneys as a direct effect that PTH has on the distal convoluted tubule and its indirect effects on the thin ascending loop of Henle, (3) increased absorption of calcium and phosphate from the intestine, and (4) accelerating the formation of the active metabolite of vitamin D in the kidney by both inducing synthesis and by activating 1α-hydroxylase in mitochondria of renal epithelial cells of proximal convoluted tubules (Skelly, 2012). Activation of vitamin D, under the control of PTH, increases intestinal absorption of calcium and phosphate, a process diminished without PTH (Skelly, 2012).

PTH also stimulates release of magnesium from bone, enhances magnesium uptake through the intestinal wall, and supports renal tubular magnesium resorption. An initial magnesium diuresis without significant change in plasma magnesium concentration has also been observed in hypoparathyroidism. In spite of dramatic changes in the concentrations of serum calcium and phosphate secondary to PTH deficiency, bone mineralization is normal, bone resorption rates decline, and bone formation declines only slightly. Ultimately, bones are slightly more dense than normal in humans with hypoparathyroidism and, in long-standing cases, osteosclerosis may be seen.

Peripheral Neuromuscular Observations

Although all cells are affected by deficiencies in iCa, clinical signs are typically associated with the neuromuscular system, simply because alteration in the function of these cells results in obvious visible abnormalities. Ionized calcium is involved in the release of acetylcholine during neuromuscular transmission and is essential for muscle contraction. Ionized calcium stabilizes nerve cell membranes by decreasing their permeability to sodium.

When the ECF concentration of iCa progressively declines below normal, the nervous system, in a parallel manner, becomes progressively more excitable, a result of increases in neuronal membrane permeability. This increased excitability occurs both in the central nervous system (CNS) and in peripheral nerves. With severe hypocalcemia, nerve fibers begin to discharge spontaneously, initiating nerve impulses that pass to the peripheral skeletal muscles, where they elicit tetanic contractions ("cramps" or "tetany").

Tetany is defined as a random stiffening or tightening of various muscle groups. It is reasonable to assume that nerve fibers are particularly sensitive to decreases in calcium in part because signs associated with the nervous system precede others, and because those signs are so acute, dramatic, and obvious. Dogs with tetany that had previously undergone spinal cord transection had signs above but not below the transection site, suggesting that tetany is primarily initiated in the CNS (Arnaud and Kolb, 1991). Acute hypocalcemia can be fatal secondary to respiratory muscle paralysis, decreased myocardial contractility, hypotension, or from persistent seizure activity.

Hypocalcemia, based on the serum TCa concentration, is a relatively "common" laboratory abnormality, being observed on more than 13% of serum biochemical profiles in dogs in one report (Chew and Meuten, 1982). If the diagnosis of hypocalcemia is based on the serum iCa concentration, the prevalence was 31% (Schenck and Chew, 2005). Severe hypocalcemia and/or clinical tetany are rarely observed unless the decreases in serum calcium concentration are severe. For example, tetany is likely present when the serum TCa concentration declines to or below 6 to 7 mg/dL, or the serum iCa concentration declines to less than about 0.7 mmol/L. Concentrations slightly higher than these may be worrisome but are usually clinically silent. Serum TCa concentrations below 4 mg/dL for any length of time are frequently fatal.

Although dogs with untreated hypoparathyroidism consistently have obvious decreases in serum TCa concentrations, the onset of *clinical* tetany is not entirely predictable. We tend to associate clinical signs with serum TCa concentrations below 6 to 7 mg/dL and serum iCa concentrations below about 0.7 mmol/L. It is possible for a dog to have clinical signs with serum concentrations slightly above these values, whereas others have no discernible signs despite extremely low calcium concentrations. Physical activity and/or excitement have a role in development of clinical tetany. A quiet dog is less likely than an active dog to exhibit signs. Individual variation, however, is the only consistent feature of this condition. Calcium concentrations within cerebrospinal fluid (CSF) do not decrease as rapidly as serum concentrations in parathyroidectomized dogs. Although the serum TCa concentration decreases as much as 27% (iCa, 28%) within 24 hours of surgery, decreases in CSF TCa concentration are less than 5% and in iCa less than 10% (Wysolmerski and Insogna, 2012). Rapid equilibrium does not occur between plasma and CSF iCa. Thus the concentration of calcium ions in the CSF is relatively constant despite large fluctuations in plasma. Conversely, relatively small decreases in CSF calcium concentration may result in dramatic clinical abnormalities.

When serum calcium concentrations decline to subnormal levels but not low enough to cause obvious clinical tetany, a physical state of "latent tetany" may exist. This condition is described as one in which an individual can progress from appearing clinically normal to becoming "tetanic" with minimal stimulation. Such a condition can be demonstrated to be present in people by weakly stimulating a nerve and observing an abnormal response (see Physical Examination). Another example of tetany lurking under the surface (being "latent") can be demonstrated when a human with latent tetany hyperventilates. The resulting subtle alkalinization of the body fluids can decrease the iCa concentration with increased nerve irritability, causing overt signs of tetany. It is assumed that similar situations develop in hypocalcemic dogs or cats. Some owners have described that sudden excitement, activity, or petting may unpredictably cause muscle cramping, lameness, facial rubbing, pain, irritability, or aggressive behavior. These signs usually disappear quickly, only to recur sporadically. In addition, the non-tetanic severely hypocalcemic pet is usually described by the owner as having a change in personality. Such dogs are often observed to have a poor appetite and to be irritable, non-playful, and slow-moving. Frequently, owners report that their dog "seems to be in pain." Such signs are vague, but after hypocalcemia is diagnosed, the clinical signs are most consistent with those of "latent" tetany.

The Heart

Calcium has both positive inotropic and chronotropic cardiac effects (Milnor, 1980). Hypocalcemia prolongs action potential duration in cardiac cells. This may result in decreased force of myocardial contraction (negative inotropic effect) and, in severe cases, bradycardia (negative chronotropic effect).

Miscellaneous Physiologic Effects of Hypocalcemia

Because calcium serves as a cofactor in both the intrinsic and extrinsic blood clotting systems, coagulopathies are theoretically possible in hypocalcemia. In hypocalcemic humans, disorders less common and less dramatic than tetany may be encountered, including (1) basal ganglia calcification and occasional extrapyramidal neurologic syndromes; (2) papilledema and increased intracranial pressure; (3) psychiatric disorders; (4) skin, hair, and fingernail abnormalities; (5) candidal infections; (6) inhibition of normal dental development; (7) lenticular cataracts; (8) intestinal malabsorption; and (9) increased serum concentrations of creatine phosphokinase and lactic dehydrogenase (Arnaud and Kolb, 1991; Wysolmerski and Insogna, 2012).

 ## CLINICAL FEATURES: NATURALLY OCCURRING HYPOPARATHYROIDISM IN DOGS

Signalment

The records from 57 dogs seen at University of California, Davis (UC Davis) with naturally occurring primary hypoparathyroidism (includes Bruyette and Feldman, 1988) and from an additional

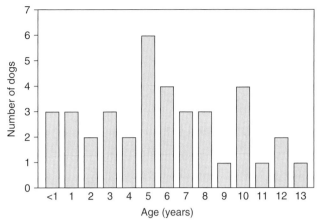

FIGURE 16-3 The ages of 38 dogs at the time of primary hypoparathyroidism diagnosis. These include 25 dogs in our series, as well as 4 dogs from Kornegay and colleagues (1980), 1 dog from Crawford and Dunstan (1985), 6 dogs from Sherding and colleagues (1980), 1 dog from Meyer and Tyrrell (1976), and 1 dog from Burk and Schaubhut (1975).

TABLE 16-1	BREEDS IDENTIFIED AS HAVING NATURALLY OCCURRING PRIMARY HYPOPARATHYROIDISM
BREED	**NUMBER OF DOGS (TOTAL = 87)***
Toy Poodle	13
German Shepherd dog	9
Labrador Retriever	8
Miniature Schnauzer	8
Terrier breeds	8
St. Bernard	4
Beagle	4
Dachshund	4
Golden Retriever	3
Chihuahua	2
Boxer	2
Breeds represented once each	12
Mixed breed	10

*Includes 57 dogs from our UC Davis series, 17 dogs from Russell and colleagues (2006), 6 dogs from Sherding and colleagues (1980), 4 dogs from Kornegay and colleagues (1980), 1 dog each from Burk and Schaubhut (1975), Meyer and Tyrrell (1976), and Crawford and Dunstan (1985).

30 dogs with hypoparathyroidism in the veterinary literature were reviewed. Hypoparathyroidism can be recognized in dogs of any age; the youngest dog being 6 weeks and the oldest being 14 years (Fig. 16-3). The average age was 5.4 years. Of 57 dogs in the ongoing UC Davis series, about half were female; and in a published series of 735 hypoparathyroid dogs, 62% were female (Refsal et al, 2001; Skelly, 2012). The breeds most frequently identified as having primary hypoparathyroidism were Toy Poodles, Labrador Retrievers, Miniature Schnauzers, German Shepherd dogs, various terrier breeds, and mixed breed dogs (Table 16-1). In a report on 17 dogs from Australia with naturally occurring hypoparathyroidism, St. Bernards, Chihuahuas, Jack Russell Terriers, and West Highland White Terriers were each represented more than

once (Russell et al, 2006). As anticipated from the various breeds described, body weights vary greatly.

History

Duration of Illness

As described by their owners, the 57 dogs in the UC Davis series commonly developed an abrupt onset of intermittent neurologic or neuromuscular disturbances (see Box 16-1). About half of the owners noted that signs were initiated or worsened by excitement, exercise, or petting. The hypocalcemia-related signs had been observed for periods of only about 24 hours in some dogs to as long as 12 months in others. Only a minority of the 57 dogs had signs for longer than 14 days before veterinary care was sought. Some dogs with prolonged histories had been symptomatic for 1 to 12 months, but some of these had been diagnosed and treated for nonspecific seizure disorders. The dogs with signs for more than several days invariably had neuromuscular disturbances that became progressively more frequent and violent despite administration of anticonvulsant medication.

Early Signs

Clinical signs observed by owners that resulted in their seeking veterinary care varied (see Box 16-1). The most common reason for seeking veterinary care was apparent grand mal convulsions (discussed in the next section). Owners also sought veterinary care after seeing apparent muscle cramping, tonic spasm of leg muscles, or pain. Focal muscle twitching, tremors, fasciculations, or trembling were commonly seen as were stiff, hunched, or rigid gait. One of the first owner observations (retrospectively) was that their pet appeared abnormally "nervous" or "anxious." Owners also commonly described their pets as having poor appetites or as being "slow," "less playful," or "not as friendly." A few were noted to have had episodes of vomiting or diarrhea. Aggressive behavior was seen in a majority of affected dogs and is assumed to be caused by pain associated with muscle cramping. The muscle cramping could be elicited by petting, possibly explaining why dogs that previously suffered acute pain from such a mild stimulus are reluctant to be handled. This likely also explains the observations of dogs appearing to be less friendly or for their change in behavior or personality. Also retrospectively, owners noted that their dogs would intensely use their paws or the ground to rub their muzzles (discussed later) or they would intensely lick or chew their paws. Although common, such signs were usually not mentioned by owners until specifically questioned or were noted as having disappeared after treatment had been instituted. In one study, "mandibular champing," possibly a reflection of masticatory muscle cramping or facial paresthesias, was observed by almost half the owners (Russell et al, 2006).

Seizures

Grand mal convulsions were observed by owners of 49 out of 57 dogs with naturally occurring primary hypoparathyroidism. As previously reported, most of these dogs had typical-appearing grand mal convulsions. However, some dogs had atypical seizures in that the dogs either did not appear to lose consciousness or were neither urinary nor fecal incontinent during the episode. Of interest was the incidence of seizure activity seen by veterinarians. Of the 57 dogs in our series, 45 were observed by a veterinarian to have seizures. This frequency of observing seizure-like episodes represents a much higher incidence of veterinarian-witnessed neuromuscular disorders than expected with idiopathic epilepsy. Also, as noted by other investigators (Sherding et al, 1980; Russell et al, 2006; Skelly, 2012), muscle tremors during some episodes began in one limb and gradually became generalized and more violent, finally culminating in a generalized seizure. In some dogs, seizure episodes were as brief as 30 to 90 seconds; in others, they lasted for more than 30 minutes. Most, but not all, of the generalized seizures lasted less than 3 minutes and spontaneously abated.

Miscellaneous Signs

As can be seen in Box 16-1, many owners observed overlapping neurologic and neuromuscular signs. Retrospectively, each dog suffered bouts of significant hypocalcemic tetany as a part of their initial signs. Some vague signs included panting, ataxia, circling, episodic weakness, complete anorexia, vomiting, diarrhea, and weight loss. Veterinarians occasionally noted an increase in body temperature. All owners observed some clinical signs. Although hypocalcemia was almost always considered a serendipitous finding on laboratory testing, it remains an abnormality that "made sense" after being demonstrated. Death remains a potential sequela of untreated hypocalcemia.

Facial Rubbing

Thirty-five out of 57 dogs in our series were observed to paw their muzzles, eyes, and ears and/or to rub their muzzles on the ground. Additionally, most owners noted their dogs intensely licking or chewing at their paws. These signs of pain are thought to be associated with masseter and temporal muscle cramping caused by hypocalcemia, or they could result from a "tingling" sensation around the mouth or at the distal extremities. Classic signs of hypocalcemia in humans include "paresthesias," which are defined as numbness and tingling that often occur around the mouth, fingers, and/or toes (Arnaud and Kolb, 1991).

Hyperventilation

Because of the acute anxiety or pain associated with tetany, hypoparathyroid humans (and presumably dogs) may episodically hyperventilate and secrete increased amounts of epinephrine. Hyperventilation may lead to hypocapnia and alkalosis, either of which can worsen hypocalcemia by causing increased binding of ionic calcium to plasma proteins. Hyperventilation in healthy people can decrease serum iCa concentration (Arnaud and Kolb, 1991).

Episodic Nature of the Illness

All neurologic and neuromuscular signs in hypocalcemic dogs tend to be episodic, often followed by asymptomatic periods. The periods of clinical well-being lasts minutes to days or even weeks. Tetany was rather unpredictable, although retrospectively, these signs were more frequent or inducible with exercise (even slow or short "leash" walks), excitement, petting (possible latent tetany), or stress (being taken to the veterinarian).

All of the dogs were persistently hypocalcemic but displayed tetany only episodically. This illustrates some adaptation in each to hypocalcemia, suggesting that minor alterations in calcium concentration could result in profound clinical signs. One dog in our series had been diagnosed as having primary hypoparathyroidism but remained untreated for almost a year. This dog was persistently hypocalcemic but had only one or two clinically obvious hypocalcemic episodes monthly. In spite of this tragic history, the dog was relatively well, suffering primarily from a poor appetite and weight loss.

Physical Examination

General Observations

Other than signs related to hypocalcemia, dogs with primary hypoparathyroidism usually do not have additional physical examination abnormalities. Physical examination findings on hypoparathyroid dogs varied (Table 16-2). Retrospectively, most

TABLE 16-2	INITIAL PHYSICAL EXAMINATION FINDINGS IN 57 DOGS WITH NATURALLY OCCURRING PRIMARY HYPOPARATHYROIDISM		
SIGN		**NUMBER OF DOGS**	**%**
Seizure or "in tetany"			
Initial examination		23	40
Total: First 4 days of hospitalization		41	72
Intense rubbing or pawing at face		35	61
Intense biting or licking at paws		34	60
Fever		31	54
Tense, splinted abdomen		30	53
Stiff gait		29	51
Thin		25	44
Generalized muscle fasciculations		24	42
Growling		23	40
Cardiac abnormalities			
Tachyarrhythmia		14	25
Muffled heart sounds/weak pulse		4	7
Neurologic examination difficult to complete and/or interpret		37	65
Cataracts		14	25
No abnormality		6	10

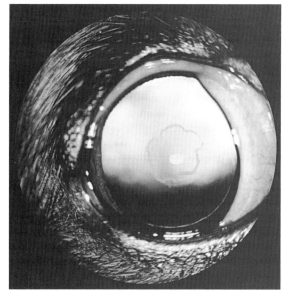

FIGURE 16-4 Lenticular cataract in the lens of a hypoparathyroid dog.

dogs were "in tetany" on presentation, an observation made after review of serum biochemical results. Forty-eight of the 57 dogs were referred for evaluation of hypocalcemia. Thus, the veterinarian examining such a dog was "primed" to observe tetany. Observations (almost all of which are noted in Table 16-2), although impressive to the uninitiated, may not have been made if the history not alerted the clinician to the underlying condition.

A minority of dogs appeared healthy, despite their previous history of neurologic or neuromuscular disorders. A number of dogs were thin and/or growled when examined. It is accepted that the growling dogs were in pain or were anticipating that handling would cause them pain, because almost all of them became friendly after resolution of their hypocalcemia. Cardiac abnormalities were suspected in 18 dogs on initial examination. These abnormalities consisted of paroxysmal tachyarrhythmias suspected in 14 dogs and muffled heart sounds with weak pulses suspected in four dogs.

Spontaneous Neurologic and Neuromuscular Signs

On initial examination, 51 of the 57 dogs with primary hypoparathyroidism had at least one abnormality that could be attributed to hypocalcemia. Most of these dogs had a convulsion or were considered to be "in tetany." Others growled, were extremely tense or "rigid," or had "splinted" abdomens, stiff gaits, and/or muscle fasciculations. Virtually every time that a dog growled, the owner would comment that this "new behavior" had been noticed at home as well. Fever was noted in 31 of the 57 dogs.

Twenty-three dogs were observed to have a convulsion during their initial examination, and an additional 18 had at least one convulsion observed within the first 96 hours of hospitalization. Complete neurologic examinations were attempted on 37 dogs revealing a variety of problems—the most common of which was that "the dog was too tense and nervous to complete a thorough evaluation." Retrospectively, these dogs were recognized to have been in tetany. Other findings included brisk reflexes, absent reflexes, clonus, and/or pain. Because these dogs were in latent or active tetany, their neurologic examinations were difficult to interpret until hypocalcemia was identified.

Induced Neurologic or Neuromuscular Signs

Two physical tests are used in humans as aids in diagnosing latent tetany (hypocalcemia). *Chvostek's sign* is elicited by tapping the facial nerve just anterior to the ear lobe. A positive sign is one of extensive facial muscle twitching or muscle contraction. *Trousseau's sign* is induced with a blood pressure cuff inflated above systolic blood pressure for at least 2 minutes. A positive response consists of carpal spasm, at least 5 to 10 seconds in duration, after release of the cuff or while the cuff is inflated (Arnaud and Kolb, 1991; Meininger and Kendler, 2000). Although such tests are not described for dogs suspected of being hypocalcemic, episodes of intense muscle spasm have been stimulated when testing reflexes.

Cataracts

Posterior lenticular cataract formation is the most common permanent sequela of hypoparathyroidism in humans (Arnaud and Kolb, 1991). Such cataracts are thought to require 5 to 10 years before visual impairment occurs. Successful treatment of hypocalcemia generally halts their progression (Arnaud and Kolb, 1991). Cataracts were first described in two hypoparathyroid dogs (Kornegay et al, 1980) and have been seen in 14 of the 57 dogs in our series. No dog was blind. Opacities are randomly distributed along the lens fibers and are separated from the capsule by an intervening zone of normal thin cortex (Fig. 16-4). Other ocular signs not yet reported in dogs include papilledema, optic neuritis, conjunctivitis, keratitis, blepharospasm, loss of lashes, strabismus, nystagmus, and anisocoria.

CLINICAL FEATURES: NATURALLY OCCURRING HYPOPARATHYROIDISM IN CATS

Hypocalcemia in cats, like dogs, is seen with hypoalbuminemia, although iCa concentrations are typically within reference limits. Hypocalcemia in cats has also been associated with renal failure, intestinal malabsorption, acute pancreatitis, lactation, and ethylene glycol toxicity. The most common iatrogenic cause of hypocalcemia is removal of all parathyroid glands as a complication of cervical surgery, such as bilateral thyroidectomy for hyperthyroidism. Surgical techniques have improved, and this complication is now uncommon. However, parathyroid damage or removal is a risk with any cervical surgery involving both sides of the trachea. Less frequently, hypocalcemia may occur after administration of phosphate containing enemas.

Naturally occurring primary hypoparathyroidism in cats is encountered less often than in dogs. Nine cats with naturally occurring primary hypoparathyroidism have been reported in the veterinary literature, and an additional seven have been seen at UC Davis. These 16 cats, 6 months to 11 years of age and of various breeds, include 11 males. The clinical course of each cat was characterized by an abrupt or gradual onset of intermittent neurologic or neuromuscular disturbances, which included focal or generalized muscle tremors, seizures, ataxia, stilted gait, disorientation, and weakness. Other concerns included lethargy, anorexia, panting, and raised nictitating membranes. Less commonly, dysphagia, pruritus, and ptyalism were observed. Physical examination findings included depression, weakness, fever, hypothermia, bradycardia, and mild to severe dehydration. Lenticular cataracts were detected in several of these cats (Forbes et al, 1990; Parker, 1991; Peterson et al, 1991; Bassett, 1998; Ruopp, 2001; Gunn-Moore, 2005; Skelly, 2012).

DIAGNOSTIC EVALUATION: ROUTINE STUDIES

Calcium

Hypocalcemia was a serendipitous finding in each of our 57 dogs with primary, naturally occurring, hypoparathyroidism. All had a history consistent with a behavioral, neurologic, muscular, or neuromuscular disorder. A complete blood count, urinalysis, and serum chemistry profile were considered necessary aids in attempting to determine the cause of abnormalities noted by owners and the veterinarian. Severe hypocalcemia was suspected in few but noted in all (Table 16-3). Because severe hypocalcemia (serum calcium concentration < 7.0 mg/dL) is an unusual finding in our clinic population, this parameter was invariably rechecked with a separate blood sample. Actually, each dog had its serum calcium concentration monitored three to five times during the first 72 hours of hospitalization as therapy was begun. Persistent hypocalcemia was

uniform. No dog had a serum calcium concentration greater than 6.1 mg/dL on any assessment until therapy began to have an effect. After serum iCa concentrations became routinely available, each of these results was also profoundly low (see Table 16-3).

"Corrected" Serum Calcium Values

Calcium in plasma or serum exists in three fractions: ionized (free calcium), complexed or chelated (bound to phosphate, bicarbonate, sulfate, citrate, and lactate), and protein-bound (Fig. 16-5). In general, between 50% and 60% of TCa is in the "ionized" form in normal animals. In clinically normal dogs, protein-bound, complexed, and iCa account for approximately 34%, 10%, and 56% of the serum TCa, respectively (Schenck et al, 1996). Laboratories generally measure these components together and report them as

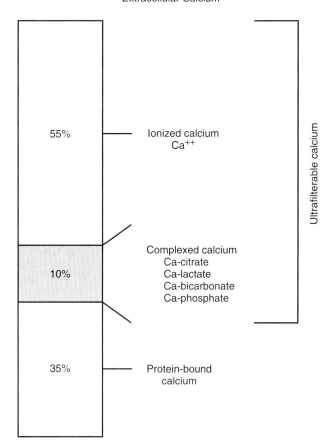

FIGURE 16-5 Serum total calcium (TCa) concentration consists of ionized (free), complexed, and protein-bound fractions. *Ca,* Calcium; *Ca⁺⁺,* ionized calcium.

TABLE 16-3	PERTINENT FINDINGS IN 57 DOGS (30 FEMALE, 27 MALE) WITH PRIMARY HYPOPARATHYROIDISM							
	AGE (YEARS)	DURATION OF SIGNS (DAYS)	TOTAL CALCIUM (mg/dL)	IONIZED CALCIUM (mm/L)	SERUM PHOSPHATE (mg/dL)	PLASMA MAGNESIUM (mg/dL)	BLOOD UREA NITROGEN (mg/dL)	PARATHYROID HORMONE (pmol/L)
Result ranges	0.5-14	1-360	3.4-6.1	0.2-0.6	4.9-10.2	1.2-2.3	8-51	0.05-3.4
Mean values	5.4	26	4.6	0.3	7.7	1.9	15	0.5
Median values	4.0	3	4.3	0.3	7.9	1.8	17	0.6
Reference ranges	—	—	8.9-11.4	1.1-1.4	3.0-4.7	1.8-2.4	12-28	2-13

a TCa value. Ionized calcium is the biologically active component, and protein-bound calcium serves as a "reservoir" or storage pool for the ionized fraction. However, changes in serum concentration of albumin and globulins may alter the measured serum TCa concentration without altering iCa levels. Despite an alteration in the total amount of serum calcium resulting from hyperproteinemia or hypoproteinemia, the biologically active iCa concentration remains stable because of homeostatic mechanisms. Any dog or cat with hypocalcemia should also have its serum albumin assessed (Chew and Meuten, 1982).

Two formulas were developed for use in dogs to account for changes in the reported serum calcium value attributed to changes in serum protein values (Meuten et al, 1982). The formulas were thought to be of significant value prior to routine availability of iCa assays. These formulas are:

corrected TCa (mg/dL) = measured TCa (mg/dL) - albumin (g/dL) + 3.5

or

corrected TCa (mg/dL) = measured TCa (mg/dL) − [0.4 × total protein (g/dL)] + 3.3

Hypoalbuminemia is a common explanation for apparent hypocalcemia. However, it is the least important, causes no hypocalcemia-related clinical signs, and is associated with only mild changes from reference ranges. Although correction to normal limits implies that the ionized fraction is "normal," the ionized fraction may yet be low. These formulas, developed more than three decades ago, were derived from serum albumin concentrations obtained with analytical methods no longer employed by modern automated analyzers. The reference range for serum albumin concentration reported then (Meuten et al, 1982) was considerably lower than those reported now. At the time, a positive correlation was noted, but only 33% of the variability in serum TCa concentration could be attributed to serum albumin concentration, and only 17% of the variability could be attributed to serum total protein. There was no association in cats between serum total protein and serum calcium concentrations, and only 18% of the variability in TCa concentration could be attributed to albumin concentration (Flanders et al, 1989). In another study, only 17% and 29% of the variability in serum TCa concentration in dogs and cats, respectively, could be attributed to serum albumin concentration (Bienzle et al, 1993). For these reasons, plus the availability of serum iCa results via commercial laboratories, these correction formulas are no longer used (Rosol et al, 2000).

Serum Phosphorus

The most consistent laboratory findings among the dogs with primary hypoparathyroidism in our series were the presence of both hypocalcemia and hyperphosphatemia. Most dogs with primary hypoparathyroidism have a serum phosphorus concentration higher than the TCa concentration on the same sample. All had had blood urea nitrogen (BUN), total protein, and serum albumin concentrations within the reference range. The absence of an absolute hyperphosphatemia in some of the dogs can be explained in part by the wide variation in what is considered "normal" by veterinary laboratories. Such reference ranges may include results of all ages, and readers are reminded that immature pets typically have a relative hyperphosphatemia. Their serum phosphorus concentrations gradually decline until puberty, at which time the levels remain relatively constant. Inappetent hypoparathyroid dogs were noted to have higher mean phosphate concentrations than those with adequate food intake (Russell et al, 2006).

Remainder of the Serum Chemistry Profile

The diagnosis of primary hypoparathyroidism in the dog is usually made "by exclusion." In other words, clinicians develop a complete differential diagnosis for hypocalcemia and then attempt to rule each condition in or out. In this context, a complete database is invaluable when assessing any nonlactating hypocalcemic animal. It has been suggested that hypoparathyroidism is the only possible diagnosis when one encounters a combination of low serum calcium concentration, increased serum phosphorous concentration, normal renal function, and a decreased (relative or absolute) serum PTH concentration (Rosol et al, 2000).

There are three potential causes of hypoparathyroidism: suppressed secretion of PTH without parathyroid gland destruction (Dhupa and Proulx, 1998); sudden correction of chronic hypercalcemia in which the remaining parathyroid glands are severely atrophied; and absence or destruction of the parathyroid glands. In reviewing the additional routine laboratory tests performed on hypoparathyroid dogs, abnormalities were not seen. Therefore the only significant alterations were hypocalcemia in all patients and hyperphosphatemia in most.

Laboratory Testing of Cats with Primary Hypoparathyroidism

Laboratory testing in 16 cats (nine reported cases and seven in our series) with naturally occurring primary hypoparathyroidism demonstrated severe hypocalcemia in each cat (range, 2.5 to 4.4 mg/dL). Serum phosphate concentrations were inappropriately increased in each cat (range, 5.2 to 19 mg/dL). Serum protein, albumin, urea nitrogen, creatinine, and magnesium concentrations were within reference limits in each cat tested (Forbes et al, 1990; Parker, 1991; Peterson et al, 1991; Bassett, 1998; Ruopp, 2001; Gunn-Moore, 2005).

Electrocardiogram

A good correlation exists between severity of hypocalcemia and duration of the electrocardiogram (ECG)-demonstrated S-T segment. Most hypoparathyroid dogs in our series had no clinical evidence of cardiovascular disease and were not assessed with an ECG. When an ECG was taken, changes observed that were consistent with hypocalcemia included (1) deep and wide T waves, (2) prolonged Q-T or S-T intervals (also noted in four out of four dogs in a separate study [Russell et al, 2006]), and (3) bradycardia (Kornegay et al, 1980; Sherding et al, 1980; Russell, et al, 2006). When the ECGs obtained during hypocalcemia were compared with those taken following restoration of normal calcium concentrations, the R waves appeared taller during hypocalcemia (Fig. 16-6). No obvious ECG explanation could be found for the arrhythmias, weak pulses, or muffled heart sounds that were suspected on several physical examinations.

Magnesium

Magnesium is an important cofactor for PTH secretion because it is required for release of stored hormone from secretory granules. In conditions of severe magnesium deficiency, suppressed parathyroid secretion with concurrent hypocalcemia and hyperphosphatemia has been documented. Another contributor to the hypocalcemia seen with hypomagnesemia is a reversible resistance

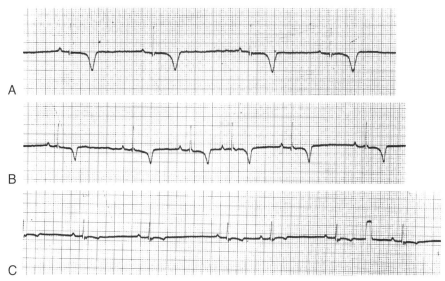

FIGURE 16-6 Electrocardiogram (ECG) illustrating various stages in the treatment of a dog with hypocalcemia secondary to primary hypoparathyroidism. **A,** The serum calcium level was 4.0 mg/dL. On this ECG, prolonged S-T and Q-T segments are obvious. The T wave itself is prolonged and deep. At this time the serum potassium (4.3 mEq/L), sodium (147 mEq/L), and chloride (103 mEq/L) levels were normal. The inorganic phosphorus level was 4.9 mg/dL. **B,** ECG taken when the serum calcium level was 6.2 mg/dL. The S-T, Q-T, and T wave durations are diminished, as is the T wave amplitude. **C,** ECG taken of a dog with a normal serum calcium level of 9.7 mg/dL. The S-T, Q-T, and T waves are normal. The three ECGs also suggest a diminishing R wave amplitude as the serum calcium level rises to normal.

BOX 16-2   Causes of Hypomagnesemia and Magnesium Depletion in Humans

Decreased Intake and/or Absorption
Protein-calorie malnutrition
Magnesium-free fluid therapy
Magnesium-free total parenteral nutrition

Gastrointestinal Disorders
Prolonged nasogastric suction
Chronic diarrhea
Malabsorption syndromes
Extensive bowel resection, intestinal fistulas

Renal Losses
Chronic parenteral fluid therapy without magnesium
Nonazotemic renal tubular dysfunction (see text)
Loop and osmotic diuretics
Hypercalcemia
Hypokalemia
Alcohol

Metabolic
Hypercalcemia
Hypophosphatemia

Endocrine
Diabetes mellitus, insulin therapy
Hyperthyroidism
Primary hyperparathyroidism
Primary and secondary hyperaldosteronism
Hyperadrenocorticism
Syndrome of inappropriate secretion of antidiuretic hormone

Redistribution
Pancreatitis
Hyperadrenergic states
Massive blood transfusion
Hypothermia
Acute respiratory alkalosis
Sepsis

Other
Burns
Excessive lactation
Excessive sweating

---

to the actions of PTH at the level of both bone and kidney (Wysolmerski and Insogna, 2012).

In humans, there are a variety causes for severe (serum concentration < 1.2 mg/dL) magnesium deficiency (Box 16-2; Yu, 2012). People with various intestinal disorders associated with small bowel malabsorption and/or steatorrhea are at risk for magnesium depletion. Responsible mechanisms include formation of magnesium soaps with unabsorbed fatty acids in addition to simple loss of magnesium into intestinal contents. Decreased renal tubular magnesium reabsorption and hypomagnesemia has been reported in people during the diuretic phase of acute renal tubular necrosis, renal tubular acidosis, pyelonephritis, and hydronephrosis. Impaired magnesium reabsorption and hypomagnesemia has been documented with gentamicin nephrotoxicity and is recognized as a potential adverse reaction to cisplatin chemotherapy. Virtually all diuretics increase magnesium excretion and symptomatic hypomagnesemia has been documented with primary and secondary states of hyperaldosteronism (Yu, 2012). The osmotic diuresis associated with diabetic ketoacidosis (DKA) can be associated with significant urinary losses of magnesium. The time course for the development of hypomagnesemia in response to treatment of ketoacidosis is similar to that for decreasing serum potassium and phosphorus concentrations. Normal pretreatment magnesium concentrations may decrease to less than 1 mg/dL during the first 24 hours of intensive therapy for DKA unless anticipated and treated. Hyperthyroidism is sometimes associated with negative magnesium balance and hypomagnesemia due to bone resorption and altered distribution of magnesium into soft tissues (Yu, 2012). Primary infantile hypomagnesemia is a rare autosomal recessive disorder in people that appears to be caused by a specific abnormality in intestinal magnesium absorption (Wysolmerski and Insogna, 2012).

Hypoparathyroidism secondary to hypomagnesemia in dogs with protein-losing enteropathies and in dogs with eclampsia have been reported (Aroch et al, 1999; Kimmel et al, 2000; Bush et al, 2001). Serum magnesium concentrations were determined in 38 of the 57 hypoparathyroid dogs included in Table 16-3. Eight of these dogs were hypomagnesemic. Hypocalcemia in people with concurrent hypomagnesemia is often refractory to calcium therapy unless magnesium is administered first (Hansen, 2000). In humans, symptoms of hypomagnesemia do not usually occur at serum levels of magnesium above 1.5 mg/dL, and obvious signs are not always seen, even at serum magnesium levels below 1.0 mg/dL (Wysolmerski and Insogna, 2012).

Poor quantitative relationships between testing and clinical relevance are limitations created by having only 0.3% of total body magnesium in plasma or serum (Elin, 1994). Serum magnesium concentrations may be normal or high in the presence of intracellular depletion. Although serum testing is the least expensive and most convenient, most authorities recognize inaccuracies associated with such assessments. Furthermore, interest in measuring serum ionized magnesium concentration has involved expensive equipment or facilities not widely available (Wysolmerski and Insogna, 2012).

It is unclear whether mild/asymptomatic hypomagnesemia needs to be treated. In humans, magnesium repletion is recommended if a patient is symptomatic, has concurrent severe hypocalcemia, hypokalemia, or an underlying cardiac arrhythmia or seizure disorder. Intravenous (IV) magnesium sulfate can be used for repletion, and its redistribution from extracellular to intracellular space is relatively slow. Normalization of serum concentrations usually precedes achievement of total magnesium replacement needs. It is recommended, therefore, that humans receiving IV supplementation continue to be treated for 24 to 48 hours beyond the time that serum concentrations normalize. In people with normal renal function, excess supplementation should be excreted. Symptoms of hypermagnesemia in people include hypotension and flaccid paralysis (Yu, 2012).

DIAGNOSTIC EVALUATION: PARATHYROID HORMONE CONCENTRATIONS

Clinical Usefulness in Humans

Measurement of serum PTH concentration is an important aid to the diagnosis of parathyroid gland disorders in people (Arnaud and Kolb, 1991; Wysolmerski and Insogna, 2012). Decreases in serum PTH concentration are consistent with primary parathyroid gland failure in hypocalcemic individuals. Increases in serum PTH concentration (an appropriate physiologic response to hypocalcemia) rules out hypoparathyroidism in individuals whose hypocalcemia is unexplained, suggesting end-organ resistance to PTH (pseudohypoparathyroidism or vitamin D deficiency) or secondary hyperparathyroidism due

to conditions such as dietary calcium deficiency or intestinal malabsorption.

Clinical Usefulness in Dogs and Cats

Undetectable serum PTH concentration in a severely hypocalcemic animal confirms the diagnosis of primary hypoparathyroidism. Reliable and validated PTH assays are commercially available for cats and dogs. Serum PTH concentrations may be detectable or "low-normal" in pets with hypoparathyroidism. A serum PTH concentration within the reference range is not a healthy response to hypocalcemia (see Figs. 15-5, 15-22, and 15-23). Low-normal to extremely low serum PTH concentrations were obtained from each of 44 dogs with primary hypoparathyroidism we tested (see Table 16-3 and Figs. 15-22 and 15-23).

Response to therapy, coupled with ruling out each differential diagnosis for hypocalcemia, has served as a relatively reliable and logical method for supporting a diagnosis of primary hypoparathyroidism. This approach allows assessment of serum PTH concentration to serve in a "confirmatory" role. Because naturally occurring primary hypoparathyroidism is a permanent condition requiring lifelong therapy, assaying serum PTH concentrations is warranted and serves to aid both veterinarian and client (Torrance, 1998). Despite inevitable changes in methodologies over the years, PTH assays for both dogs and cats have provided excellent and reliable information (Feldman and Krutzik, 1981; Torrance and Nachreiner, 1989; Flanders and Reimers, 1991; Flanders et al, 1991; Barber et al, 1993; Chew et al, 1995; see Chapter 15). The most important differential diagnoses for hypocalcemia are laboratory error, hypoalbuminemia, surgical removal of the parathyroids, use of phosphate enemas, acute or chronic kidney failure, eclampsia, malabsorption, and severe pancreatitis (Schenck and Chew, 2012).

DIFFERENTIAL DIAGNOSIS OF EPISODIC WEAKNESS

Because the clinical signs of hypocalcemia occur episodically, clinicians may consider a variety of potential causes for "episodic weakness" or paroxysmal neurologic and/or neuromuscular disorders. The differential diagnosis for episodic weakness presented in Chapter 9 is worth reviewing because those clinical signs are somewhat similar to those of hypocalcemia. Several of the dogs in this series were initially believed to have idiopathic epilepsy. Toxins were also commonly suspected (e.g., strychnine, metaldehyde, and/or lead). Other tentative diagnoses after initial examination of hypocalcemic dogs included tetanus, trauma, cardiac disease, myasthenia gravis, hepatic disease, and hypoglycemia.

DIFFERENTIAL DIAGNOSIS FOR HYPOCALCEMIA

The differential diagnosis for hypocalcemia is listed in Box 16-3 and the diagnostic algorithm is in Fig. 16-7.

Parathyroid-Related Hypocalcemia

Naturally Occurring Primary Hypoparathyroidism in Dogs and Cats

Naturally occurring hypoparathyroidism is an uncommon condition in dogs and cats. The onset of signs typically seem abrupt to owners and may be severe (e.g., tetany and/or seizures). Although the onset of signs almost always seems sudden, the condition is likely insidious with mild subclinical hypocalcemia present for some period. Surprisingly, some dogs and cats with naturally occurring disease have had signs for months at

---

BOX 16-3   Differential Diagnosis of Hypocalcemia

Parathyroid-related hypocalcemia
    Naturally occurring primary hypoparathyroidism
    Rare disorders in people
    Iatrogenic (surgically removed or damaged glands)
    Acute resolution of chronic hypercalcemia
    Pseudohypoparathyroidism
Pseudopseudohypoparathyroidism
Hypomagnesemia
Chronic Kidney Disease (CKD)
Hypoalbuminemia
Acute pancreatitis
Critically ill patients
Diabetes mellitus
Puerperal tetany (eclampsia)
Malabsorption syndromes

Nutritional secondary hyperparathyroidism
Acute kidney injury (AKI) and ethylene glycol toxicity
Urinary tract obstruction
Phosphate-containing enemas
Miscellaneous causes of hypocalcemia
    Laboratory error
    Anticonvulsant therapy
    Hyperthyroidism
    Vitamin D deficiency
    Transfusion using citrated blood
    Use of EDTA-coagulated blood
    Trauma to the neck area
    Medullary carcinoma of the thyroid
    Primary and metastatic bone cancer
    Side-effect to some cancer chemotherapies

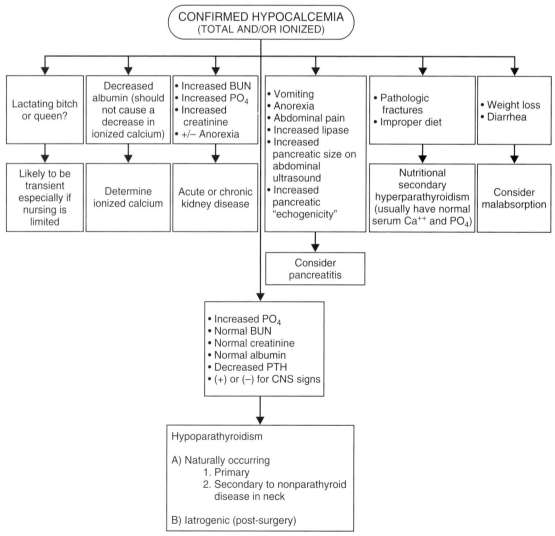

FIGURE 16-7 Algorithm for diagnosing the various causes of hypocalcemia. *BUN,* Blood urea nitrogen; *Ca,* calcium; *Ca++,* ionized calcium; *CNS,* central nervous system; *PO4,* phosphorus; *PTH,* parathyroid hormone.

the time of diagnosis (one, in our series, for about a year) and survive without appropriate treatment. Signs are not usually recognized until there has been a decline in the TCa concentration below some critical level (approximately 6 to 7 mg/dL). At such serum calcium concentrations, relatively small decreases in calcium concentration may result in obvious clinical problems. For example, a serum TCa decline of 0.3 mg/dL in a dog or cat with a serum concentration of 10.5 mg/dL has no effect and remains "normal," but the same decrease when the serum calcium concentration is 5.7 mg/dL could result in convulsions.

Diffuse lymphocytic "parathyroiditis" was described in seven dogs with hypoparathyroidism (Kornegay, 1982). Our series includes an additional 19 dogs with similar histologic findings, and a few others had their parathyroid tissue replaced by fibrous tissue. It is possible that fibrous tissue is an "end result" following lymphocytic/plasmacytic inflammation. Therefore the finding of either inflammatory infiltrates or scar tissue is most likely dependent on when tissue is obtained relative to the time course of the condition. Interestingly, two dogs with primary hypoparathyroidism from Australia had no histologic abnormalities (Russell et al, 2006). Detection of antibodies against parathyroid tissue in people with idiopathic hypoparathyroidism has confirmed presence of an autoimmune disease. An immune-mediated mechanism may explain the condition in some dogs and cats.

Rare Disorders in Humans Causing Hypoparathyroidism

The DiGeorge syndrome in humans consists of parathyroid gland absence and thymic aplasia (Rasmussen, 1981; Marx, 2000; Yu, 2012). This disorder presumably results from abnormal development of the third pharyngeal pouch during embryogenesis. Parathyroid agenesis has also been reported in dogs (Meuten and Armstrong, 1989). Another form of idiopathic hypoparathyroidism in humans is a familial immune-mediated endocrine syndrome that includes hypofunction of the adrenal cortex, ovarian failure, pernicious anemia, thyroiditis, diabetes mellitus, candidiasis, and occasionally malabsorption. Those patients who manifest disease before 6 months of age conform to an X-linked recessive inheritance pattern, and older individuals likely have an autosomal recessive inherited condition (Arnaud and Kolb, 1991; Wysolmerski and Insogna, 2012). Calcium-sensing receptor mutations have also been identified (Pearce et al, 1996).

Surgically Induced Hypoparathyroidism

An uncommon cause for primary hypoparathyroidism in dogs and cats, but relatively common in people, is surgical removal, damage, or interruption of blood supply to the glands (Marx, 2000). Hypoparathyroidism is a risk of thyroid, parathyroid, or other neck surgeries. Because the incidence of hyperthyroidism in cats is high and because canine thyroid tumors are often malignant, thyroid surgery is common in both species. One group estimated that as many as 10% of hyperthyroid cats undergoing surgery suffer from transient or permanent hypoparathyroidism (Peterson, 1986). Of 41 hyperthyroid cats that had bilateral thyroidectomy, postoperative hypocalcemia (not always associated with clinical signs) developed in 82% undergoing an extracapsular surgical technique, 36% with an intracapsular technique, and 11% with two separate thyroidectomies performed 3 to 4 weeks apart (Flanders et al, 1987). Of 106 cats studied in a subsequent report, postoperative hypocalcemia developed in 22% to 33% of cats, depending on the surgical technique (Welches et al, 1989). Clinical signs were observed only in severely hypocalcemic cats (TCa < 7.0 mg/dL). The incidence of surgically-related hypoparathyroidism is now much lower, because surgeons are more

aware of this complication and because techniques have improved (Henderson et al, 1991; Flanders, 1994; Graves, 1995; Klein et al, 1995). Because this complication is recognized as possible, autotransplantation of removed parathyroid tissue has been successfully employed in humans and has excellent veterinary potential (Padgett et al, 1998).

The transient nature of hypoparathyroidism following thyroid surgery in many cats is not well understood. The physiology of this complication may be related to the hyperphosphatemia and secondary hyperparathyroidism documented in 18% and 77%, respectively, of untreated hyperthyroid cats (Barber and Elliott, 1996). It has been postulated that this may be the result of thyroxine (T_4)-mediated alterations in bone metabolism and increased phosphate absorption (Barber and Elliott, 1996). One group of cats had significantly reduced serum PTH concentrations after thyroparathyroidectomy. During the 12 weeks following surgery, serum PTH concentrations did not recover, but the serum calcium concentration did slowly increase. The increases in serum calcium concentration in these thyroparathyroidectomized cats, it was theorized, were an "accommodation" of existing calcium-regulating systems that operate at suboptimal levels in the absence of PTH. One example of such an "accommodation" might involve changes in vitamin D metabolism, allowing continued calcium absorption from the intestine despite the PTH deficiency (Flanders et al, 1991). The onset of biochemical or clinical signs suggestive of parathyroid failure after neck surgery in dogs and cats can begin within days or take as long as several weeks. Other potential but rare destructive disorders of the parathyroids include neck injury, neoplastic conditions within the neck, irradiation, and aminoglycoside intoxication. We have not observed iodine[131]-induced parathyroid damage in any so-treated hyperthyroid cat.

Pseudohypoparathyroidism

Pseudohypoparathyroidism is a rare familial disorder in humans characterized by target tissue resistance to PTH. These individuals have hypocalcemia, increased serum concentrations of PTH, and a variety of congenital developmental growth and skeletal defects. Increases in serum PTH concentration represent an appropriate physiologic response to hypocalcemia. If the serum calcium concentration is transiently normalized by an infusion of calcium, the concentration of circulating PTH decreases. Therefore diagnosis of end-organ unresponsiveness involves (1) the inability of PTH to increase cyclic adenosine 3′,5′-monophosphate (cAMP) excretion and (2) elevated circulating PTH concentrations. The hormone secreted by patients with pseudohypoparathyroidism is presumably normal in structure. Some of these patients have no developmental abnormalities (Wysolmerski and Insogna, 2012). A deficiency in renal PTH-sensitive cAMP results in renal tubular resistance to PTH and diminished phosphaturia. Deficits in active vitamin D and/or bone cAMP have also been claimed to be the inciting factor leading to pseudohypoparathyroidism. One dog with apparent hypoparathyroidism had an increased serum PTH concentration, urine cAMP, and plasma cAMP (Kornegay et al, 1980). Another dog with hypoparathyroidism had Fanconi syndrome, which was thought to occur secondary to a 1,25–vitamin D deficiency (Freeman et al, 1994).

Pseudopseudohypoparathyroidism

Humans with this disorder have typical developmental defects (growth and skeletal abnormalities) associated with pseudohypoparathyroidism, but they are not hypocalcemic or hyperphosphatemic, nor do they have abnormalities in serum PTH concentration (Marx, 2000).

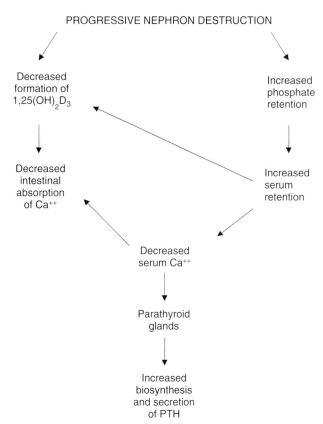

FIGURE 16-8 Pathogenesis of parathyroid hyperplasia during progressive destruction of nephrons. *1,25(OH)₂D₃,* 1,25-dihydroxyvitamin D₃ (calcitriol); *Ca,* calcium; *Ca⁺⁺,* ionized calcium; *PTH,* parathyroid hormone.

Hypomagnesemia

Magnesium deficiency can result in hypocalcemia (see earlier Magnesium section).

Chronic Kidney Disease (CKD)

Dogs and cats with CKD usually have (in addition to abnormal BUN and serum creatinine concentrations) increased serum phosphate and normal serum calcium concentrations. Despite hypocalcemia being uncommon in dogs and cats with CKD, the prevalence of CKD makes this condition one of the more frequent causes of low calcium. Low serum TCa was detected in about 10% of dogs with CKD, and the iCa concentration was low in about 30% (Schenck and Chew, 2012). In cats, as CKD progresses, the incidence of hypocalcemia increases. About 15% of cats with "moderate CKD" had low iCa, and the percentage rises to 50% if the condition is "advanced" (Schenck and Chew, 2010). In CKD patients, hypocalcemia is a biochemical problem and rarely clinically significant.

When present in CKD, hypocalcemia is the result of decreased vitamin D synthesis by diseased kidneys and mass law interactions of calcium with the sometimes markedly increased phosphate. Early stages of progressive CKD are associated with a decreased capacity to excrete phosphate. Even mild hyperphosphatemia induces subclinical ionized hypocalcemia which, in turn, stimulates PTH synthesis and secretion. This ionized hypocalcemia is the classically described genesis of renal secondary hyperparathyroidism (Fig. 16-8). In dogs with nonazotemic kidney disease (IRIS stage I; International Renal Interest Society; www.iris-kidney.com), 36% had secondary hyperparathyroidism. The hyperparathyroidism

should augment phosphate excretion, but with time, secondary hyperparathyroidism can no longer compensate for the alterations of CKD; hyperphosphatemia develops and it becomes progressively worse (Chew and Nagode, 1990). Because progressive renal disease leads to reduced capacity to form active vitamin D, intestinal absorption of calcium is limited, enhancing the potential for hypocalcemia. Also, increased urinary calcium excretion may contribute to the hypocalcemia sometimes seen in CKD.

Hypoalbuminemia

Reductions in total serum protein and/or albumin concentrations are encountered in a variety of disorders. Hypoalbuminemia is the most common and clinically least important cause of hypocalcemia. As previously described, reductions in circulating albumin concentration cause a decrease in the protein-bound fraction of circulating calcium. However, since iCa concentrations remain normal, these animals rarely have clinical signs of hypocalcemia.

Acute Pancreatitis

Hypocalcemia, when it occurs in dogs with acute pancreatitis, is usually mild and subclinical. Coexisting acidosis, which is commonly present, increases the ionized fraction of TCa and further reduces the likelihood of clinical signs related to hypocalcemia (Hess et al, 1998). The incidence of hypocalcemia may be higher in cats with pancreatitis than in dogs. Results of one study suggest that low TCa and iCa concentrations are common in cats with acute pancreatitis (41% and 61%, respectively). Furthermore, cats with ionized hypocalcemia, even though none had clinical signs related to this complication, had a poorer prognosis than those with normal concentrations. A grave prognosis and aggressive medical therapy was recommended for cats with both acute pancreatitis and a plasma iCa concentration less than 1.00 mmol/L (Kimmel et al, 2001).

The traditional theory for development of hypocalcemia in pancreatitis is that calcium precipitates into insoluble soaps via saponification of peripancreatic fatty acids formed subsequent to release of pancreatic lipase. Despite general agreement that this occurs, it is not clear whether it is sufficient to account for hypocalcemia in view of the large quantity of calcium that potentially can be mobilized from skeletal reserves. Other contributors to hypocalcemia may include hypomagnesemia, decreased secretion of or resistance to PTH secondary to magnesium deficiency, hypoproteinemia, and glucagon-stimulated calcitonin secretion (Ryzen and Rude, 1990; Dhupa and Proulx, 1998; Schenck and Chew, 2012).

Critically Ill Patients

Hypocalcemia due to decreases in TCa and/or iCa concentrations is common among critically ill people, dogs, and cats, especially those with sepsis. Magnitude of the decreases appears to correlate with severity of illness. In addition to sepsis, causes of hypocalcemia include systemic inflammatory response syndrome, hypomagnesemia, blood transfusions, and acute kidney disease (Zivin et al, 2001; Schenck and Chew, 2012).

Diabetes Mellitus

Almost 50% of diabetic dogs have ionized hypocalcemia. Because pancreatitis was diagnosed in less than 15% of these dogs, it is unlikely for pancreatitis to be the sole explanation for the hypocalcemia (Hess et al, 2000). In a study on more than 100 dogs in DKA, slightly more than 50% had ionized hypocalcemia, the severity of which correlated with mortality (Schenck and Chew, 2012).

Puerperal Tetany (Eclampsia)

Eclampsia is an acute life-threatening condition that develops secondary to extreme hypocalcemia in lactating bitches and queens (Fascetti and Hickman, 1999; Drobatz and Casey, 2000). Dogs and cats with clinical signs of eclampsia are usually severely hypocalcemic (< 6 to 7 mg/dL). Eclampsia is most common in small dogs and less common in cats and large dogs. Signs seen by veterinarians usually depend on how quickly the owner recognizes the problem and seeks professional care. Most bitches and queens are affected during the first 21 days of nursing, although eclampsia has been diagnosed as early as during the last 2 weeks of gestation and as late as 45 days after whelping. Diagnosis of eclampsia is usually based on the presence of neuromuscular signs (tetany) in a lactating bitch or queen. In most situations, the diagnosis is so obvious that the serum calcium concentration is never assessed. However, three cats with preparturient eclampsia had hypothermia rather than the expected hyperthermia, and four cats had clinical signs that included flaccid paralysis, rather than the more typical tonic-clonic muscle fasciculations noted in dogs (Fascetti and Hickman, 1999).

Hypocalcemia typically arises as a consequence of lactation and its attendant calcium loss into milk. Other possible contributors include poor use of dietary calcium and loss of calcium to fetal skeletal development. Sometimes the stress of nursing reduces a bitch's (or queen's) appetite or interferes with her ability to eat. Another predisposing factor is the parathyroid gland atrophy that can be caused by improper diet or dietary supplements. In one study, 44% of bitches with eclampsia had hypomagnesemia. Decreased magnesium-to-calcium ratios at the neuromuscular junctions can promote tetany. Magnesium therapy may be beneficial for treatment of eclampsia (Aroch et al, 1999).

Malabsorption Syndromes

Many patients with protein losing enteropathies have hypoalbuminemia and typical decreases in serum TCa concentrations but serum iCa concentrations that are within reference intervals. True enteropathy-associated vitamin D deficiency leading to hypocalcemia is uncommon but possible. Malabsorption conditions, such as inflammatory bowel disease (IBD) or intestinal lymphoma, in dogs, cats, and people are frequently associated with derangements in fat soluble vitamin metabolism (Gow et al, 2011; Wysolmerski and Insogna, 2012; Lalor et al, 2014). Various explanations have been proposed for enteropathy-associated hypocalcemia, including decreased intestinal absorption or increased intestinal loss of both albumin and vitamin D bound to vitamin D-binding protein (Lalor et al, 2014). Decreased appetite in patients with significant enteropathies may contribute to vitamin D deficiency. Serum vitamin D concentrations were significantly lower in dogs with IBD and moderate to severe decreases in appetite as compared with dogs that had similar bowel disease but normal appetites (Gow et al, 2011). A majority of 10 IBD cats and six with intestinal small cell lymphoma had low vitamin D concentrations, but only two were hypocalcemic (Lalor et al, 2014). There is also evidence from experimental models suggesting that IBD may be due to hypovitaminosis D rather than caused by it (Mora et al, 2008).

Hypocalcemia may be caused by or worsened by excess fecal calcium excretion due to decreased resorption of calcium in disorders such as lymphangiectasia. The degree of calcium malabsorption and the poor absorption of vitamin D appear to correlate with the extent of small bowel disease (Mellanby et al, 2005). Hypomagnesemia may also play a role in the physiology resulting in hypocalcemia. In two studies, it was suggested that hypomagnesemia and hypocalcemia may have a related pathogenesis involving intestinal loss, malabsorption, and abnormalities of vitamin D and PTH metabolism. Magnesium supplementation was demonstrated to normalize serum magnesium and PTH concentrations, improve plasma iCa concentrations, and alleviate clinical signs of paresis (Kimmel et al, 2000; Bush et al, 2001).

Nutritional Secondary Hyperparathyroidism

It would be rare for a pet being fed commercially available nutritionally complete and balanced diet to ever develop this condition. However, dogs or cats exclusively fed diets containing a low calcium-to-phosphorus ratio (the classical examples are beef heart and liver) can develop severe mineral deficiencies. BARF ("biologically appropriate raw food" or "bones and raw food") diets have also been implicated (DeLay and Laing, 2002). Severe gastrointestinal disease may also result in this condition by directly impairing calcium absorption or, indirectly, by interfering with vitamin D absorption (Mellanby et al, 2005; Skelly, 2012). If either a dietary deficiency or an inability to absorb calcium from intestinal content results in decreased circulating calcium concentration, a cascade of events begins. Those events include increased PTH secretion, reduction in bone mass as calcium is removed from bone to replace that not available in the diet, diffuse skeletal osteopenia, and, if persistent, "nutritional secondary hyperparathyroidism." Although renal secondary hyperparathyroidism seems to target bones of the face (fibrous osteodystrophy), nutritional hyperparathyroidism appears to target long bones and vertebrae. This process can cause bone pain and pathologic fractures. Because the skeletal disturbances are the result of physiologic processes placing the serum calcium concentrations as highest priority, affected dogs and cats usually have normal serum concentrations of TCa, iCa, and phosphorus. A minority of affected dogs and cats have had mild to severe hypocalcemia (Tomsa et al, 1999). Treatment involves providing balanced diets and restricting activity until skeletal remodeling is complete. Diagnosis is based on recognizing skeletal disorders in a dog or cat receiving an improper diet.

Acute Kidney Injury (AKI) and Ethylene Glycol Toxicity

Acute kidney injury (such as that which occurs with ethylene glycol poisoning) and postrenal failure (such as that which occurs with urinary tract obstruction) may result in abrupt and severe increases in serum phosphate concentration. Mass law effects cause a secondary reduction in serum calcium concentrations. Hypocalcemia may be exaggerated in acute failure because rapid onset of these disturbances blunts compensatory mechanisms. Dogs with acute intrinsic renal failure had a mean serum TCa concentration of 9.8 mg/dL (Vaden et al, 1997). Ethylene glycol intoxication can cause severe renal failure, acidosis, hypocalcemia, tetany, and death.

Urinary Tract Obstruction

Male cats with long-standing (more than 12 to 24 hours) urethral obstruction and severe hyperphosphatemia often have associated hypocalcemia, hyperkalemia, azotemia, and sometimes experience seizures (Chew and Meuten, 1982). Hypocalcemia was diagnosed in 26% of male cats with urethral obstruction at initial presentation, based on serum TCa assessment. On the basis of iCa concentrations, however, 75% were hypocalcemic. The hypocalcemia was defined as mild in 37.5%, moderate in 25%, and severe in 12.5% of affected cats. These abnormalities may contribute to cardiac dysfunction in severely affected cats. Although effects of IV administration of calcium were not evaluated, results in this study support their use in cats with urethral obstruction (Drobatz and Hughes, 1997).

Phosphate-Containing Enemas

Phosphate-containing enemas may result in acute and severe hyperphosphatemia following colonic absorption, especially when administered to dehydrated cats with colonic atony and mucosal disruption. Colonic absorption of sodium and phosphate from the enema solution as well as transfer of intravascular water to the colonic lumen (because of hypertonicity of the enema solution) can cause hypernatremia and hyperphosphatemia. Acute increases in serum phosphate may cause reciprocal significant declines in serum calcium concentration (Atkins et al, 1985; Jorgensen et al, 1985). Therefore use of phosphate-containing enemas is not recommended in animals predisposed to hyperphosphatemia, such as with severe obstipation, marginal renal function, or abnormal serum calcium-to-phosphorus ratios. Clinical signs of phosphate enema toxicosis (shock and neuromuscular irritability) result from hypocalcemia and hypernatremia. Treatment may require plasma volume expansion and calcium. Diagnosis is based on the history (Peterson, 1992).

Miscellaneous Causes

Laboratory Error

An uncommon cause of reported hypocalcemia is laboratory error. Incorrect reporting of the serum calcium concentration can reflect a simple mistake or artifact due to samples submitted in tubes containing ethylenediaminetetraacetic acid (EDTA) as an anticoagulant, because EDTA chelates calcium. Mixing of serum with air can significantly decrease iCa concentrations. Freshly obtained plasma for iCa determination should be transported to reference laboratories with a cold pack. If a delay in processing lasting days seems likely, plasma should be sent frozen (Schenck et al, 1995). Caution should be exercised in the interpretation of iCa measured with portable analyzers, because results for dogs and cats are lower than those obtained with standard methodology. The use of dry heparin syringes for sample collection may negate this difference (Grosenbaugh et al, 1998). Whenever the reported serum calcium concentration is unexpectedly high or low, it should be rechecked.

Anticonvulsant Therapy

Surveys of humans receiving long-term anticonvulsant therapy (principally phenobarbital and phenytoin) have shown a tendency to develop hypocalcemia, hypophosphatemia, and abnormal serum alkaline phosphatase activities. Studies of these subjects reveal a state similar to vitamin D deficiency. Bone biopsies and radiographs suggest osteomalacia without evidence of malabsorption or renal disease. Serum PTH concentrations are increased but remain normally suppressible with calcium infusions. Severity of the altered calcium metabolism is directly related to dosage (Arnaud and Kolb, 1991).

Although this problem has not been recognized in the dog, it is described here to remind practitioners that a variety of drugs have the potential to cause unexpected endocrine problems. Furthermore, several of our hypoparathyroid dogs were referred because of failure to respond to anticonvulsant therapy. The finding of hypocalcemia in dogs on relatively high doses of anticonvulsants may be mistakenly interpreted as iatrogenic.

Hyperthyroid Cats

Cats with untreated hyperthyroidism have significantly lower iCa concentrations than do control cats, although none had decreases in TCa concentration, and only 4 of 15 had iCa concentrations below the reference range. Hyperthyroid cats also had significantly increased serum PTH concentrations. These changes are likely associated with the hyperphosphatemia often noted in hyperthyroid cats. The importance of these findings is not known (Barber and Elliott, 1996).

Vitamin D Deficiency

Vitamin D deficiency is an unlikely clinical cause of hypocalcemia (Henik et al, 1999). Dogs and cats with a significant and diffuse intestinal malabsorption syndrome may lose the ability to absorb vitamin D.

Use of Citrated Blood

Blood for transfusion that contains citrates as anticoagulant may induce hypocalcemia, particularly if the volume of donor blood is small compared with the volume of anticoagulant.

Trauma

Trauma, especially soft tissue trauma, has been reported as a cause of hypocalcemia (Chew and Meuten, 1982), but this is rare.

Medullary Carcinoma of the Thyroid

Medullary carcinoma of the thyroid has been reported to cause severe hypocalcemia and tetany in one dog and represents an unusual cause of hypocalcemia in humans.

Primary and Metastatic Bone Cancer

Primary and metastatic bone tumors are common in small animal practice. Humans, dogs, and cats with tumors that have metastasized to bone usually have normal serum calcium concentrations. Hypercalcemia is occasionally associated with primary bone neoplasia and with metastasis of certain cancers to bone. However, hypocalcemia and hypophosphatemia rarely occur in humans. When osteoblastic metastases are present in humans, the incorporation of calcium into those lesions may be sufficient to result in measurable hypocalcemia and even clinical signs. This has not been reported in dogs or cats.

Chemotherapy and the "Tumor Lysis Syndrome"

The tumor lysis syndrome can follow acute release of intracellular potassium and phosphate during chemotherapy for highly sensitive neoplasms, such as lymphoid or bone marrow tumors (Persons et al, 1998). Among the multiple metabolic abnormalities that can occur in this setting is hypocalcemia due to mass law interactions induced by acute and severe hyperphosphatemia (Calia et al, 1996; Piek and Teske, 1996). Further, calcium salts can be deposited into soft tissues. Acute kidney injury may also result (Schenck and Chew, 2012). In addition to hypocalcemia, transient PTH deficiency may occur (Horn and Irwin, 2000). One salicylate-intoxicated cat developed hypocalcemia associated with sodium bicarbonate therapy (Abrams, 1987).

![hand icon] **THERAPY FOR HYPOCALCEMIA AND HYPOPARATHYROIDISM**

General Approach

Primary hypoparathyroidism can be permanent, requiring acute and then lifelong management to alleviate and prevent clinical signs. Hypoparathyroidism following surgical removal or ablation of a parathyroid adenoma that caused hyperparathyroidism may require short-term therapy but, as remaining normal-but-atrophied parathyroid cells return to function, one should be able to taper and discontinue medications. Similarly, eclampsia (puerperal tetany) is a classic condition due to hypocalcemia in which specific and acute correction of the calcium deficiency is necessary but chronic treatment is not. In contrast to these examples, no treatment is indicated for animals with hypocalcemia attributable entirely to hypoalbuminemia, assuming the iCa fraction is normal.

Treatment of hypocalcemia virtually always requires that a protocol be tailored to the individual needs of a dog or cat. Management will be effected by the magnitude of the hypocalcemia and the rate of decline in calcium concentration. The trend in serum concentrations (fluctuating, remaining stable, or quickly falling) will influence decision processes. Aggressive approaches are needed for dogs and cats with obvious clinical signs, for those with significant decreases in TCa or iCa concentrations, or when severe hypocalcemia can be anticipated (e.g., with therapy for primary hyperparathyroid dogs who have endured chronically increased serum TCa concentrations; see Chapter 15). Veterinarians should not delay treatment for hypocalcemia until clinical signs are obvious. Such an approach, at best, exposes the pet to an extremely painful condition. At worst, it places the pet at risk for developing a life-threatening event.

The goal of therapy, one that may be difficult to achieve, is to increase serum calcium concentrations smoothly above the threshold responsible for clinical signs. That threshold is usually a TCa concentration of about 6.0 mg/dL, or above a plasma iCa concentration of about 0.6 to 0.7 mmol/L. Individual differences can be significant, however. Clinical signs typically improve with slight increases in measurable calcium. Veterinarians should raise measured calcium concentrations conservatively, because values that increase into reference ranges increase risk for hypercalcemia, associated hyperphosphatemia, tissue mineralization, and stone formation. For anticipated or known postsurgical hypocalcemia that will be transient, as in pets being treated for primary hyperparathyroidism, it is physiologically ideal to maintain calcium concentrations above the threshold for tetany but below established reference ranges, because "below normal" values should enhance functional recovery of atrophied parathyroid glands.

Emergency Therapy for Tetany—Diagnosis Not Apparent

In the event that a practitioner is treating a seizing animal without a specific diagnosis, anti-convulsants are usually utilized. This approach is usually beneficial, even in hypocalcemic pets. However, if treatment fails or if a diagnosis is still not obvious, blood should be drawn for glucose, calcium, and any other parameter that may lead to a diagnosis. In the meantime, IV glucose and/or calcium can be administered.

Hypocalcemic Tetany: Intravenous Calcium

When possible, hypocalcemic tetany should immediately be treated with calcium salts. Ten percent calcium gluconate, readily available and not as caustic as calcium chloride, is recommended and should be slowly administered intravenously, usually over a 10 to 30 minute period, or to effect. ECG monitoring is advisable and, if not possible, one should listen to the heart and have a finger on the pulse during the calcium infusion. If bradycardia, pulse deficits, arrhythmias, S-T segment elevation, shortened Q-T intervals, and/or premature complexes are recognized, the IV infusion should be slowed or temporarily discontinued (Peterson, 1992). This emergency therapy is usually successful and cessation of seizures, for example, is typically noted within a minute or minutes of initiating the infusion. The total dose needed to control tetany is not predictable. Furthermore, some clinical signs may be slower to respond. Nervousness, panting, and behavioral changes may persist for as long as 30 to 60 minutes after return of eucalcemia, perhaps reflecting a lag in equilibrium between CSF and circulating calcium.

Calcium Dose and Salt Choices

The calcium content of different salts varies considerably. For example, both calcium gluconate and calcium chloride supplements are available as 10% solutions in 10-mL ampules, and each ampule provides 1 g of the parent compound. However, calcium chloride provides approximately 27 mg/mL of elemental calcium, and calcium gluconate provides approximately 9 mg/mL. The 200 mg/mL calcium borogluconate solution contains the equivalent of about 15 mg/mL of elemental calcium. Calcium borogluconate is 1.6 times more concentrated and calcium chloride is 3 times more concentrated than the 10% calcium gluconate solution. Thus, guideline doses for calcium gluconate (0.5 to 1.5 mL/kg), calcium borogluconate (0.3 to 0.9 mL/kg), and calcium chloride (0.15 to 0.5 mL/kg) reflect these different concentrations (Table 16-4). It may be easiest to achieve a slow infusion by first calculating the estimated required dose and then diluting that amount in a larger volume of 0.9% saline. Recommended doses should be used as guidelines, and patient response should be the definitive factor in determining the volume administered (Skelly, 2012). Remember that extravasation of calcium chloride outside

TABLE 16-4	SOME AVAILABLE PARENTERAL CALCIUM PREPARATIONS		
PREPARATIONS	**APPROXIMATE CALCIUM CONTENT**	**DOSE**	**COMMENT**
10% Calcium gluconate *(IV)*	9.3 mg Ca/mL	0.5-1.5 mL/kg	Administer slowly "to effect" Stop if bradycardia or shortened Q-T interval
		2.5-3.75 mg/kg/hr	Infusion to maintain safe serum Ca level
10% Calcium gluconate *(SC)*	9.3 mg Ca/mL	Dilute 2, 3, 4:1	SC to support serum calcium without IV (see text)
10% Calcium borogluconate *(IV)*	15.0 mg Ca/mL	0.3-0.9 mL/kg	Same as for Ca gluconate
10% Calcium chloride *(IV)*	27.2 mg Ca/mL	Do *not* use	Do *not* use

Ca, Calcium; *IV,* intravenous; *Q-T,* interval on an electrocardiogram (ECG); *SC,* subcutaneous.

a vein is caustic, potentially causing large areas of tissue death and sloughing. Extravasation may also cause calcinosis cutis (Schick et al, 1987). In our opinion, calcium chloride should never be stocked by small animal practitioners, thus eliminating any possibility of its use.

Hyperphosphatemia

Infusion of calcium-rich fluids should be performed with caution in any hyperphosphatemic dog or cat. Hyperphosphatemia, however, is common among hypocalcemic animals due to mass law effects. Therefore, although a concern, as calcium increases with treatment, the phosphate concentrations should decrease. However, in conditions like CKD, the combination of calcium administration and hyperphosphatemia could cause soft tissue mineralization and further renal damage to the kidneys (Chew and Meuten, 1982).

Fever

Fever, sometimes greater than 105° F, commonly accompanies tetany. Veterinarians may be tempted to treat both hypocalcemia and fever (using ice or alcohol baths and/or parenteral drugs). However, with administration of calcium, fever should be monitored but not treated. Fever usually dissipates rapidly with control of tetany. Additional measures to lower body temperature may result in hypothermia and the development of shock. Further, three of four cats reported to have had preparturient eclampsia were hypothermic (Fascetti and Hickman, 1999).

Subacute Management of Hypocalcemia: Post-Tetany Maintenance Therapy

The Issue. Once signs of hypocalcemic tetany are controlled with an IV calcium infusion, its effects usually only last minutes to an hour or so. On the other hand, long-term maintenance therapy with oral vitamin D and oral calcium supplementation usually requires 24 to 96 hours before effect is achieved. Therefore, parenteral calcium support during the initial post-tetany period is necessary.

The Alternatives. **Repeated Intravenous Boluses.** One method for managing hypocalcemia in the immediate post-tetany period is repeated IV calcium boluses. This procedure is not recommended except in emergencies, because wide fluctuations in circulating calcium concentrations result.

Continuous Intravenous Infusion. Continuous IV infusion of calcium can be utilized at doses of 60 to 90 mg/kg/day elemental calcium (2.5 to 3.75 mg/kg/hr) until oral medications provide control of serum calcium concentration. Initial doses in the high end of this protocol are recommended for dogs and cats with severe hypocalcemia. The dose should be decreased according to the serum calcium concentration achieved and as oral calcium and vitamin D become effective.

Using 10% calcium gluconate solutions, 10 mL provides 93 mg of elemental calcium. A convenient protocol for infusing calcium assumes that the IV fluids are being administered at a typical maintenance rate of about 60 mL/kg/day (2.5 mL/kg/hr). Approximately 1, 2, or 3 mg/kg/hr of elemental calcium is provided by adding 40, 80, or 120 mL of 10% calcium gluconate, respectively, to each liter of fluid solution, equivalent to 6.5 to 10 mL/kg/day. Calcium salts may precipitate if added to solutions containing lactate, acetate, bicarbonate, or phosphates. Additionally, IV solutions containing sodium bicarbonate should be avoided because systemic alkalinization can decrease circulating iCa concentrations, precipitating clinical signs in dogs or cats with borderline hypocalcemia (Rosol et al, 2000).

Subcutaneous Calcium. Once tetany has been controlled with IV calcium gluconate, administration of subcutaneous (SC) calcium has been effective, simple, and inexpensive. Continuous IV administration of fluids is expensive and requires hospitalization. However, one can utilize the dose of calcium gluconate required to control tetany initially and administer that dose SC every 6 to 8 hours. Alternatively, a calcium dose of 60 to 90 mg/kg/day, divided, can be given. The calcium gluconate should be diluted as one part of calcium to two, three, or four parts of saline. This protocol has effectively supported serum calcium concentrations and has not caused inflammation or sloughing of skin. This is true even in dogs treated subcutaneously for months. The SC regimen is an efficacious method of supporting circulating calcium while waiting for atrophied parathyroid glands to regain function, or while waiting for oral vitamin D and calcium to have effect. The procedure is easily taught to owners, further decreasing expense.

Remember, calcium chloride should never be administered subcutaneously, but calcium gluconate is usually safe. Several cases of calcinosis cutis following SC administration of calcium gluconate have been reported (Ruopp, 2001; Schaer et al, 2001; Skelly, 2012). However, our experience with repeated SC injections of diluted 10% calcium gluconate, without problems, suggests that such terrible side effects are quite uncommon.

After normal or near-normal serum calcium concentrations have been maintained for 48 hours, the frequency of SC injections should be decreased from every 6 to every 8 hours. If serum calcium concentrations remain stable for the ensuing 48 to 72 hours, the calcium can be tapered to twice daily. This protocol is continued until parenteral calcium has been completely discontinued. Obviously, the tapering process in each patient may not be this smooth, because response to oral therapy is variable. Ideally, the serum TCa concentration should be maintained above 8 mg/dL. Concentrations below 8 mg/dL indicate a need to increase the dose or frequency of parenteral calcium. Serum calcium concentrations of 8 to 9 mg/dL suggest maintaining the current parenteral dose. Concentrations greater than 9 mg/dL may indicate need for reducing the dose. The frequency and/or dosage of parenteral calcium are often increased before the therapy can be safely decreased and then discontinued. This is true regardless of the calcium supplementation protocol used.

Maintenance (Chronic) Therapy for Hypoparathyroidism

General

The most appropriate therapy for hypoparathyroidism would be some form of PTH given to maintain normal physiologic concentrations, likely determined on an individual basis. However, no long-acting commercially available PTH preparation is available at the time of writing this comment, although such a product is currently being evaluated. Parenteral PTH is available on a limited basis but lasts only hours. Thus, oral administration of both a vitamin D product and a calcium product, especially in the early phases of therapy, remains the most successful means of treating hypoparathyroidism. It is emphasized that oral calcium should be a component of any early treatment plan, especially if the animal is not eating. Active intestinal calcium uptake transport mechanisms are under control of vitamin D when calcium intake is low, but vitamin D-independent passive intestinal absorption of calcium occurs when intake is high. One can take advantage of this passive-but-enhanced calcium absorption process while administered vitamin D has time to become effective (Chew et al, 2009).

Because most commercially available pet food contains adequate calcium for daily needs, once a dog is home and stable, we typically slowly taper oral calcium therapy over a period of 12 to 16 weeks. Recurrent hypocalcemia and worrisome hypercalcemia represent potential complications of treatment if adequate calcium and phosphorus monitoring is neglected. On the other hand, we have successfully helped monitor and manage a number of primary hypoparathyroid dogs for years and encourage clients to treat their pet.

Vitamin D

General. Maintenance therapy for hypoparathyroidism consists of oral vitamin D and calcium supplementation. The need for vitamin D therapy is usually permanent in dogs and cats with primary, naturally occurring, parathyroid gland failure. Calcium supplementation, however, can often be tapered and even stopped after several months of administration, because dietary calcium is sufficient for maintaining the needs of the animal. Conservative doses of supplemental calcium given chronically, however, ensure that vitamin D, which raises serum calcium by promoting its intestinal absorption, has substrate upon which to function. Iatrogenic hypoparathyroidism in dogs and cats treated for primary hyperparathyroidism is often transient and lifelong therapy is not always needed.

In contrast to tetany, for which the immediate goal of treatment is to avoid recurrence of neuromuscular signs, the aim of long-term therapy is to maintain serum TCa concentrations at mildly low to low-normal concentrations (8.0 to 9.5 mg/dL). Such calcium concentrations are well above the risk threshold for clinical hypocalcemia and well below concentrations (even with day-to-day fluctuations) that might be associated with hypercalcemia and hyperphosphatemia, which would place the patient at risk for renal damage due to nephrocalcinosis. Maintaining the serum calcium concentration at the low end or just below the reference range also reduces risk of hypercalciuria and associated calculi formation. Mild hypocalcemia should also serve to promote return to function of atrophied parathyroid glands

Vitamin D₂ (Ergocalciferol). Vitamin D_2 is a widely available and relatively inexpensive drug (40,000 USP U/mg; Table 16-5).

Initially, large doses are required to induce normocalcemia. Dogs and cats often require 4000 to 6000 U/kg daily doses to offset the decreased biologic potency of this product in hypoparathyroid patients. Additionally, large doses are required to saturate fat depots, which is important because vitamin D is a fat-soluble vitamin. Effect of the medication is usually obvious 5 to 14 days after beginning therapy. Parenteral calcium can usually be discontinued 1 to 5 days after starting oral vitamin D treatment. The serum calcium concentrations should be below the level that might be associated with hypercalciuria (risk for calculi formation) or severe hypercalcemia and hyperphosphatemia (risk for nephrocalcinosis and renal failure).

Dogs and cats receiving vitamin D_2 should remain hospitalized until the serum TCa concentration remains between 8 and 10 mg/dL without parenteral support and the pet is eating and drinking on its own. Once these goals are achieved, the pet can be returned to the owner, and the vitamin D_2 is usually given every other day. Serum calcium concentrations should be monitored weekly, with vitamin D_2 doses adjusted to maintain a serum calcium concentration of 8 to 9.5 mg/dL. The aim of therapy is to avoid hypocalcemic tetany on one hand, while also limiting hypercalcemia.

Even after a pet appears stable, monthly rechecks are strongly advised for 6 months and should be followed by rechecks every 2 to 3 months indefinitely. These animals cannot be rechecked too often. Underdose can place the pet at risk for tetany. Vitamin D-induced hypercalcemia can result in renal damage and failure, a problem minimized through proper monitoring. Vitamin D_2 has been used in cats and dogs with success and is relatively inexpensive. Some of our dogs and cats receive medication as infrequently as twice monthly, whereas others require daily supplementation.

The drawbacks of vitamin D_2 include the length of time to achieve maximal effect and the length of time it takes to reduce effects if an overdose is documented. If hypocalcemia is documented, it may take days to weeks before an increase in dose is reflected in the serum calcium concentration. Hypercalcemia, if it occurs, is not easily resolved because fat-soluble vitamin D may need to be discontinued for as long as 1 to 4 weeks before serum concentrations decline significantly. Hypercalcemia should be aggressively treated with IV fluids, especially if the product of

DRUG	DOSE*	TIME TO MAXIMUM EFFECT	TIME FOR TOXCITIY TO RESOLVE
1,25-dihydroxyvitamin D_3 (1,25[OH]$_2$D$_3$; calcitriol)	*Initial:* 20 to 30 ng/kg/day, divided b.i.d. *Maintenance:* 5 to 15 ng/kg/day	1 to 4 days	2 to 14 days
Vitamin D_2 (ergocalciferol)	*Initial:* 4000 to 6000 U/kg/day Maintenance: 1000 to 2000 U/kg/7 days	5 to 21 days	7 to 28 days
Alfacalcidol	*Initial:* 0.01 to 0.03 µg/kg/day *Maintenance:* May need to be increased or decreased	1 to 4 days	2 to 14 days
Dihydrotachysterol (DHT)	*Initial:* 0.02 to 0.03 mg/kg/day *Maintenance:* 0.01 to 0.02 mg/kg/24 to 48 hours	1 to 7 days	2 to 14 days

TABLE 16-5 SOME VITAMIN D PREPARATIONS

*Note: Doses are listed as mg, µg, ng, and Units/kg of body weight.

the serum calcium multiplied by the serum phosphate is greater than 60 to 80. These factors make ergocalciferol the least attractive agent for long-term treatment of hypocalcemia. We restrict use of ergocalciferol to dogs whose owners have financial limitations that prevent use of calcitriol.

Calcidiol and Alfacalcidol. Alfacalcidol has about twice the potency of ergocalciferol in binding capacity to natural calcitriol receptors. It is, however, 500 times less potent than calcitriol in this regard. It is a reasonable alternative to calcitriol. This form of vitamin D must undergo 25-hydroxylation by the liver before it is metabolically active. The process occurs rapidly and is unregulated; therefore the time required for effect is similar to that of calcitriol (Skelly, 2012). The drug is available in some countries as 0.25, 0.5, and 1 µg capsules and in a liquid formulation of 2 µg/mL. As available, the drug can be used in cats and small dogs. The recommended dose is 0.01 to 0.03 µg/kg, once daily. The dose should be tailored to the needs of the individual (Skelly, 2012).

Oral 1,25-Dihydroxyvitamin D₃; Calcitriol. Calcitriol is the most potent form of vitamin D in stimulating intestinal calcium transport and osteoblastic activity in the skeleton. It also has the most rapid onset of maximal action and the shortest biologic half-life (Chew and Nagode, 2000; Rosol et al, 2000). Oral calcitriol has a direct effect on intestinal receptors, stimulating intestinal calcium absorption to a greater degree than other forms of vitamin D, including parenteral administration (Coburn, 1990). Because calcitriol only programs undifferentiated cells in intestinal crypts and turnover of these cells takes place every 24 hours, calcitriol is given twice daily to ensure continuous effect (Chew et al, 2009).

The dose of calcitriol can be adjusted and changes take effect quickly because of its rapid onset of action and brief biologic effect. If hypercalcemia occurs, the effects of this drug abate quickly after stopping therapy or with dose reduction. The peak serum concentration of calcitriol is reached after 4 hours, the half-life is 4 to 6 hours, and the biologic half-life is 2 to 4 days. A loading dose of 20 to 30 ng/kg/day can be administered for 2 to 4 days and then decreased to a maintenance dose of 5 to 15 ng/kg/day, divided and given twice a day. (Note: This dose is in nanograms.) Calcitriol (250 and 500 ng capsules as well as 1000 ng/mL liquid formulation; Rocaltrol, Hoffman-LaRoche) is formulated for humans and may require reformulation for dogs and cats. The concerns we have regarding calcitriol only relate to expense and the need for reformulation. Although reformulation should be reliable, inconsistencies occur among pharmacies. Reformulation by specialty pharmacies of calcitriol into liquid or into capsule sizes tailored to the need of specific pets may not provide the same effectiveness to each patient.

We have had experience with one dog that did not respond to oral calcitriol at any dose. This dog was known to have liver "insufficiency" because a diagnosis of vascular anomaly had been made 10 years earlier. Although calcitriol is "active," it is interesting to note lack of response in this setting. Although this dog was not tested, it is now understood that if a patient is documented to have concurrent hypomagnesemia, supplementation with the sulfate form should be considered at a dose of 1 to 2 mEq/kg/day. In some cases, normalization of serum magnesium concentrations may lead to lower requirements of calcitriol and/or calcium.

Parenteral Calcitriol. In the event that oral medication cannot be administered or if oral calcitriol is ineffective, parenteral calcitriol can be given. Empirically, the same dose as that used for oral administration can be utilized (20 to 30 ng/kg/day). The drug is usually given IV to human dialysis patients, three times weekly, immediately after dialysis (Rolla et al, 1993; Selgas et al, 1993). The drug can also be given subcutaneously or intraperitoneally. We have used parenteral calcitriol successfully by administering it IV, t.i.d.

to effect and then progressively decreasing the dose. As with other forms of vitamin D, in-hospital monitoring is recommended until circulating calcium concentrations are stable. Owners can then administer the drug subcutaneously.

Dihydrotachysterol. DHT, although not available at the time of writing, is described here, because it may be marketed in the future. It is a synthetic vitamin D analogue. The advantages of DHT over vitamin D₂ are that it raises the serum calcium concentration more rapidly (1 to 7 days) and its effect dissipates faster when administration is discontinued. Veterinarians, therefore, have more control over therapy. DHT is more potent than vitamin D₂; 1.0 mg of DHT is equivalent to 120,000 U of vitamin D₂. The rapid onset of action and the increased effectiveness of DHT are a result of its stereochemistry; the A ring of the sterol structure is rotated 180 degrees so that the hydroxyl group in the third position serves as a pseudo-1-hydroxyl group (Fig. 16-9). Therefore, after hepatic 25-hydroxylation, DHT has biologic activity that is greater than 25-hydroxyvitamin D (25[OH]D) and less than that of 1,25 dihydroxyvitamin D₃ (1,25[OH]₂D₃) (Peterson, 1982). The polarity and lower dose requirements of DHT limit its storage in fat compared with ergocalciferol.

DHT was initially given at a dose of 0.03 mg/kg/day (divided and given twice a day) for 2 days or until effect is demonstrated, then 0.02 mg/kg/day for several days, and finally 0.01 mg/kg/day in divided dosages. As suggested with the less potent forms of vitamin D, significant individual variation in dose requirements dictate that pets remain hospitalized until the serum TCa concentration remains stable between 8 and 9.5 mg/dL (or the iCa 1.0 to 1.2 mmol/L) for several days. We have seen cats and dogs that appeared to be resistant to the tablet and capsule forms of this drug (0.125, 0.25, 0.4 mg) but respond readily to the liquid (0.25 mg/mL). We have also seen dogs and cats fail to respond to any form of DHT but respond to calcitriol. Rechecks of the serum calcium concentration on a weekly basis allow dosage adjustment while avoiding prolonged hypercalcemia or hypocalcemia. As with vitamin D₂, long-term rechecks at least every 2 to 3 months are strongly encouraged. Serum calcium concentrations higher than desired (> 10.5 to 11.0 mg/dL) should be treated by lowering or discontinuing vitamin D therapy and, depending on the severity of the clinical signs and biochemistry abnormalities, possibly initiating IV fluids (see Chapter 15). The lag period between stopping DHT and noting a fall in the serum calcium concentration has been 4 to 14 days, a longer period than is needed with calcitriol but a briefer period than with vitamin D₂.

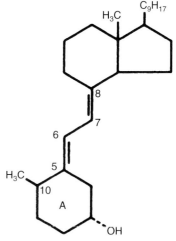

FIGURE 16-9 The chemical structure of dihydrotachysterol (DHT).

Calcium Supplementation

Initial Approach to Oral Calcium. Once tetany is controlled with bolus IV calcium, serum calcium levels should be maintained with a slow IV infusion or SC injections. When the pet is able to eat without vomiting, oral calcium and vitamin D therapy should be initiated. Within 24 hours, parenteral calcium administration can begin to be tapered, and within 72 hours it is usually discontinued. Meanwhile, oral therapy is maintained. In this manner, smooth continuous control is achieved. Calcium available within intestinal content must be adequate when treating hypoparathyroidism, because long-term success depends on the action of administered vitamin D, which increases intestinal absorption of calcium. Commercial pet food typically contains sufficient calcium to supply the needs of hypoparathyroid dogs and cats. However, because symptomatic hypocalcemia can be fatal, such catastrophic consequences of severe hypocalcemia must be avoided. For this reason, especially early in the course of therapy, we continue oral calcium at low doses indefinitely.

Calcium Supplements. Supplements can be provided by administering calcium as the gluconate, lactate, chloride, or carbonate salt. Each has disadvantages. Calcium gluconate and lactate tablets contain relatively small quantities of elemental calcium, so relatively large numbers of tablets may need to be given. Calcium chloride and carbonate tablets contain large quantities of calcium but the chloride form tends to produce gastric irritation, whereas the carbonate form could contribute to alkalosis, which has the potential to worsen hypocalcemia. Calcium carbonate is 40% calcium. One gram yields 20 mEq of calcium, and gastric acid converts the calcium carbonate to calcium chloride. Calcium lactate is 13% calcium, and 1 g yields 6.5 mEq. Calcium gluconate contains 9% calcium, and 1 g yields 4.5 mEq.

Although there are numerous calcium preparations available (Table 16-6), calcium carbonate is the preparation of choice in treating hypoparathyroid humans because of its high percentage of calcium, low cost, lack of gastric irritation, and ready availability in stores in the form of antacids (Arnaud and Kolb, 1991). No specific research to support recommendations for use of this drug is available for dogs and cats, although our success with calcium carbonate has been excellent.

Treatment Protocol. In cats, the dosage of calcium is approximately 0.5 to 1.0 g/day in divided doses. In dogs, the dosage is usually 1.0 to 4.0 g/day in divided doses. Alternatively, the dose of elemental calcium can be determined as about 25 to 50 mg/kg/day, divided into two or three daily doses. Recommendations regarding calcium are always approximate, in part because the effectiveness of administered vitamin D, the oral preparation of calcium used, and the intestinal milieu are major contributors to the stability of serum calcium concentrations. As administered vitamin D reaches a steady level, the dose of oral calcium can be gradually tapered over a period of 2 to 4 months. This method of treatment avoids unnecessary therapy, considering that dietary calcium should be sufficient to supply the needs of the pet and should decrease the demands of treatment placed on the owner. In spite of this logical approach, we tend to continue low dose calcium supplementation to our patients.

Summary of Keys to Long-Term Success

It is emphasized that the ideal serum calcium concentration in treated hypoparathyroid animals, long-term, is in the low-normal-to-slightly-low range. We attempt to achieve serum TCa concentrations of 9.0 to 10.5 mg/dL. Alternatively, one could utilize serum iCa concentrations with the goal of about 0.9 to 1.1 mmol/L. Serum TCa concentrations less than 8.0 mg/dL are a concern due to increased risk of symptomatic hypocalcemia, which can result in life-threatening convulsions or respiratory arrest. Serum TCa concentrations above 10 are unnecessarily high for avoiding tetany and increase risk of unwanted hypercalcemia, hyperphosphatemia, or a calcium-phosphorus product greater than 60 to 80. Each of these latter concerns could cause permanent renal damage and failure. Avoiding excess serum calcium concentrations also decreases calciuria (calcium in the urine) and risk of calculi within the urinary tract to which patients lacking PTH are predisposed.

It is quite valuable for the pet owner to understand as much as possible regarding hypoparathyroidism, hypocalcemia, and hypercalcemia. As owner knowledge increases, they gain a better understanding of how difficult it can be to achieve goals of therapy and

	TABLE 16-6	**SOME AVAILABLE ORAL CALCIUM PREPARATIONS***[†]	
FORMULATIONS	**PREPARATIONS AVAILABLE**	**APPROXIMATE CALCIUM CONTENT**	**COMMENT**
Calcium Carbonate	Tablets: many 500 mg 750 mg 1000 mg 1250 mg	1 mg of Ca/2.5 mg tablet 200 mg of Ca/tablet 300 mg of Ca/tablet 400 mg of Ca/tablet 500 mg of Ca/tablet	Commonly used
Calcium Gluconate	Tablets: many 325 mg 500 mg 650 mg 1000 mg	1 mg of Ca/11.2 mg tablet 30 mg of Ca/tablet 45 mg of Ca/tablet 60 mg of Ca/tablet 90 mg of Ca/tablet	Less commonly used
Calcium Lactate	Tablets: many 325 mg 650 mg	1 Ca/7.7 mg tablet 42 mg of Ca/tablet 85 mg of Ca/tablet	Less commonly used

From Schenck PA, Chew DJ: Investigation of hypercalcaemia and hypocalcaemia. In Mooney CT, Peterson ME, editors: *BSAVA manual of canine and feline endocrinology*, ed 4, British Small Animal Veterinary Association, 2012, p 221.

Ca, Calcium.

*All are dosed at 25 to 50 mg/kg/day.

[†]Usually can be tapered to low doses or stopped once vitamin D reaches effective dose.

that one of the only means of improving of long-term success is frequent monitoring of calcium, phosphorus, and renal parameters. The importance of blood monitoring is underscored by realizing that one can never predict results. Remind clients that polydipsia, polyuria, decrease in appetite, vomiting, or depression may be indicative of hypercalcemia, and veterinary attention should be sought immediately should any of these signs be observed. Most clients need little reminder regarding the clinical signs of hypocalcemia because those were the signs in their pet that first necessitated veterinary care. Regardless, if an owner observes any signs of hypocalcemia (from restlessness to convulsions), veterinary care should be sought.

Occasional calcium assessments will reveal results higher or lower than desired, but catastrophic changes are quite uncommon when frequent monitoring, changing dose as predicted from test results, and luck are linked. The need for modifying doses of vitamin D can usually be explained by changes in diet, activity, and alterations in individual health. How often should these patients be monitored? Once returned to the owner, our uncomplicated patients have been checked twice the first week or two, weekly for 3 weeks, monthly for 3 months, and then every 2 to 3 months thereafter.

If a dose of calcitriol needs to be increased or decreased, changes should be small (10% to 20%). Increasing or decreasing the vitamin D dose should be followed by adequate time to determine if it had the anticipated result. The lag period varies because a dose decrease in ergocalciferol, for example, might take several weeks before change is documented on serum testing. Use of calcitriol shortens this lag period from weeks to days (see Table 16-5). Animals that develop worrisome iatrogenic hypercalcemia secondary to excess vitamin D administration would most likely benefit from hospitalization, IV fluid therapy, and, perhaps, furosemide, steroids, bisphosphonates, or calcitonin. Until the hypercalcemia is resolved, oral calcium and vitamin D should be discontinued.

Although studies evaluating long-term response to therapy have not been published, it is fair to state that many of our patients have done well for long time periods. Success has been achieved using all forms of vitamin D, because this is something determined in part by owners. As previously discussed, it is the monitoring, owner knowledge, and luck that have significant roles in long-term success. Whenever possible, we utilize calcitriol as the source of vitamin D because its relatively quick response to increasing or decreasing doses is easier to manage than the more long acting products. It has been pointed out that hypercalciuria, nephrocalcinosis, urolithiasis, and reduced renal function have been noted in people being treated for primary hypoparathyroidism. As many as 80% of individuals treated for longer than 2 years have been reported to have decreases in creatinine clearance. All of these problems can be traced to occasional hypercalcemia due to excess vitamin D effect. Because these patients lack PTH action at the level of renal tubules, hypercalciuria occurs more readily, even if the serum calcium concentrations are within reference intervals. Therefore, as discussed, it is extremely important to maintain calcium concentrations below reference limits as much as possible while understanding that this alone may not be sufficient to avoid hypercalciuria.

PARATHYROID HISTOLOGY IN HYPOPARATHYROIDISM

Animals have been classified as having idiopathic hypoparathyroidism when there is no evidence of trauma, cervical malignancy, surgical destruction, or other obvious damage to the neck or parathyroid glands. The glands from these dogs have been difficult to locate visually or via ultrasound and are microscopically atrophied. Approximately 60% to 80% of the glands are replaced by mature lymphocytes, occasional plasma cells, extensive degeneration of chief cells, and/or fibrous connective tissue. Chief cells are randomly isolated in multiple small areas or bands at the periphery. In the early stages of an immune-mediated attack, the gland is infiltrated with lymphocytes and plasma cells with nodular regenerative hyperplasia of remaining chief cells. Later, the parathyroid gland is completely replaced by lymphocytes, fibroblasts, and neocapillaries with only an occasional viable chief cell. The final interpretation is one of lymphocytic parathyroiditis (Sherding et al, 1980; Capen and Marten, 1983).

PROGNOSIS

The prognosis in dogs and cats with primary hypoparathyroidism depends, for the most part, on the dedication of the owner, the attention of the veterinarian, and luck. With proper therapy, the prognosis is excellent. A large majority of the dogs we have treated have lived more than 5 years from the time of diagnosis and treatment. However, proper management requires close monitoring of the serum calcium concentration, ideally every 1 to 3 months once the pet is stabilized. The more frequent the rechecks, the better chance the pet has of avoiding extremes in serum calcium concentrations. The chance for a normal life expectancy is excellent with proper care.

REFERENCES

Abrams KL: Hypocalcemia associated with administration of sodium bicarbonate for salicylate intoxication in a cat, *J Am Vet Med Assoc* 191:235, 1987.

Arnaud CD, Kolb FO: The calciotropic hormones and metabolic bone disease. In Greenspan FS, Baxter JD, editors: *Basic and clinical endocrinology*, ed 5, Los Altos, CA, 1991, Lange Medical Publications, p 247.

Aroch I, et al.: Serum electrolyte concentrations in bitches with eclampsia, *Vet Rec* 145:318, 1999.

Atkins CE, et al.: Clinical, biochemical, acid-base, and electrolyte abnormalities in cats after hypertonic sodium phosphate enema administration, *Am J Vet Res* 46:980, 1985.

Barber PJ, Elliott J: Study of calcium homeostasis in feline hyperthyroidism, *J Sm Anim Pract* 37:575, 1996.

Barber PJ, et al.: Measurement of feline parathyroid hormone: assay validation and sample handling studies, *J Small Anim Pract* 34:614, 1993.

Bassett JR: Hypocalcemia and hyperphosphatemia due to primary hypoparathyroidism in a six-month-old kitten, *J Am Anim Hosp Assoc* 34:503, 1998.

Bienzle D, et al.: Relationship of serum total calcium to serum albumin in dogs, cats, horses, and cattle, *Can Vet J* 34:360, 1993.

Broadus AE: Mineral metabolism. In Felig P, et al., editor: *Endocrinology and metabolism*, New York, 1981, McGraw-Hill, p 1056.

Broadus AE, et al.: Humoral hypercalcemia of cancer: identification of a novel parathyroid hormone-like peptide, *N Engl J Med* 319:556, 1988.

Brown EM, et al.: Calcium-ion-sensing cell-surface receptors, *N Engl J Med* 333:234, 1995.

Bruyette DS, Feldman EC: Primary hypoparathyroidism in the dog: report of 15 cases and review of 13 previously reported cases, *J Vet Intern Med* 2:7, 1988.

Burk RL, Schaubhut CW: Spontaneous primary hypoparathyroidism in a dog, *J Am Anim Hosp Assoc* 11:784, 1975.

Bush WW, et al.: Secondary hypoparathyroidism attributed to hypomagnesemia in a dog with protein-losing enteropathy, *J Am Vet Med Assoc* 219:1732, 2001.

Calia CM, et al.: Acute tumor lysis syndrome in a cat with lymphoma, *J Vet Intern Med* 10:409, 1996.

Capen CC, Martin SL: Calcium-regulatory hormones and diseases of the parathyroid glands. In Ettinger SJ, editor: *Textbook of veterinary internal medicine*, Philadelphia, 1983, WB Saunders, p 1581.

Chew DJ, Meuten DJ: Disorders of calcium and phosphorus metabolism, *Vet Clin North Am Small Anim Pract* 12:411, 1982.

Chew DJ, Nagode LA: Renal secondary hyperparathyroidism, Proceedings of the 4th Annual Meeting of The Society for Comparative Endocrinology, 1990, p 17.

Chew DJ, Nagode LA: Treatment of hypoparathyroidism. In Bonagura JD, editor: *Kirk's current veterinary therapy XIII*, Philadelphia, 2000, WB Saunders, p 340.

Chew DJ, et al.: Utility of diagnostic assays in the evaluation of hypercalcemia and hypocalcemia: parathyroid hormone, vitamin D metabolites, parathyroid hormone-related peptide, and ionized calcium. In Bonagura JD, editor: *Kirk's current veterinary therapy XII*, Philadelphia, 1995, WB Saunders, p 378.

Chew DJ, et al.: Treatment of hypoparathyroidism. In Bonagura JD, Twedt DC, editors: *Kirk's current veterinary therapy XIV*, St Louis, 2009, Saunders/Elsevier, p 241.

Coburn JW: Use of oral and parenteral calcitriol in the treatment of renal osteodystrophy, *Kidney Int* 38(Suppl):S54, 1990.

Crawford MA, Dunstan RW: Hypocalcemia secondary to primary hypoparathyroidism in a dog, *Calif Vet May/June:21*, 1985.

DeLay J: Laing: Nutritional osteodystrophy in puppies fed a BARF diet, *AHL Newsletter* 6:23, 2002.

Dhupa N, Proulx J: Hypocalcemia and hypomagnesemia, *Vet Clin North Am Small Anim Pract* 28:587, 1998.

Drobatz KJ, Casey KK: Eclampsia in dogs: 31 cases (1995-1998), *J Am Vet Med Assoc* 217:216, 2000.

Drobatz KJ, Hughes D: Concentration of ionized calcium in plasma from cats with urethral obstruction, *J Am Vet Med Assoc* 211:1392, 1997.

Elin RJ: Magnesium: the fifth but forgotten electrolyte, *Clin Chem* 102:616, 1994.

Fascetti AJ, Hickman MA: Preparturient hypocalcemia in four cats, *J Am Vet Med Assoc* 215:1127, 1999.

Feldman EC, Krutzik S: Case reports of parathyroid hormone concentrations in spontaneous canine parathyroid disorders, *J Am Anim Hosp Assoc* 17:393, 1981.

Flanders JA: Surgical therapy of the thyroid, *Vet Clin N Am Small Anim Pract* 24:607, 1994.

Flanders JA, Reimers TJ: Radioimmunoassay of parathyroid hormone in cats, *Am J Vet Res* 52:422, 1991.

Flanders JA, et al.: Feline thyroidectomy: a comparison of postoperative hypocalcemia associated with three different surgical techniques, *Vet Surg* 16:362, 1987.

Flanders JA, et al.: Adjustment of total serum calcium concentration for binding to albumin and protein in cats: 291 cases (1986-1987), *J Am Vet Med Assoc* 194:1609, 1989.

Flanders JA, et al.: Functional analysis of ectopic parathyroid activity in cats, *Am J Vet Res* 52:1336, 1991.

Forbes S, et al.: Primary hypoparathyroidism in a cat, *J Am Vet Med Assoc* 196:1285, 1990.

Freeman LM, et al.: Fanconi's syndrome in a dog with primary hypoparathyroidism, *J Vet Int Med* 8:349, 1994.

Gow AG, et al.: Hypovitaminosis D in dogs with inflammatory bowel disease and hypoalbuminemia, *J Small Anim Pract* 52:411, 2011.

Graves TK: Complications of treatment and concurrent illness associated with hyperthyroidism in cats. In Bonagura JD, editor: *Kirk's current veterinary therapy XII*, Philadelphia, 1995, WB Saunders, p 369.

Grosenbaugh DA, et al.: Evaluation of a portable clinical analyzer in a veterinary hospital setting, *J Am Vet Med Assoc* 213:691, 1998.

Gunn-Moore D: Feline endocrinopathies, *Vet Clinics North Amer Small Anim Prac* 35:171, 2005.

Hansen B: Disorders of magnesium. In DiBartola SP, editor: *Fluid therapy in small animal practice*, ed 2, Philadelphia, 2000, WB Saunders, p 175.

Henderson RA, et al.: Development of hypoparathyroidism after excision of laryngeal rhabdomyosarcoma in a dog, *J Am Vet Med Assoc* 198:639, 1991.

Henik RA, et al.: Rickets caused by excessive renal phosphate loss and apparent abnormal vitamin D metabolism in a cat, *J Am Vet Med Assoc* 215:1644, 1999.

Hess RS, et al.: Clinical, clinicopathologic, radiologic, and ultrasonographic abnormalities in dogs with fatal acute pancreatitis: 70 cases (1986-1995), *J Am Vet Med Assoc* 213:665, 1998.

Hess RS, et al.: Concurrent disorders in dogs with diabetes mellitus: 221 cases (1993-1998), *J Am Vet Med Assoc* 217:1166, 2000.

Horn B, Irwin PJ: Transient hypoparathyroidism following successful treatment of hypercalcemia of malignancy in a dog, *Aust Vet J* 78:690, 2000.

Jorgensen LS, et al.: Electrolyte abnormalities induced by hypertonic phosphate enemas in two cats, *J Am Vet Med Assoc* 187:1367, 1985.

Kimmel SE, et al.: Hypomagnesemia and hypocalcemia associated with protein-losing enteropathy in Yorkshire Terriers: five cases (1992-1998), *J Am Vet Med Assoc* 217:703, 2000.

Kimmel SE, et al.: Incidence and prognostic value of low plasma ionized calcium concentration in cats with acute pancreatitis: 46 cases (1996-1998), *J Am Vet Med Assoc* 219:1105, 2001.

Klein MK, et al.: Treatment of thyroid carcinoma in dogs by surgical resection alone: 20 cases (1981-1989), *J Am Vet Med Assoc* 206:1007, 1995.

Kornegay JN: Hypocalcemia in dogs, *Comp Cont Ed Small Anim Pract* 4:103, 1982.

Kornegay JN, et al.: Idiopathic hypocalcemia in four dogs, *J Am Anim Hosp Assoc* 16:723, 1980.

Lalor AM, et al.: Cats with inflammatory bowel disease and intestinal small cell lymphoma have low serum concentrations of 25-hydroxyvitamin D, *J Vet Intern Med* 28:351, 2014.

Li YC, et al.: Normalization of mineral ion homeostasis by dietary means prevents hyperparathyroidism, rickets, and osteomalacia, but not alopecia in vitamin D-receptor ablated mice, *Endocrinol* 139:4391, 1998.

Malloy PJ, et al.: The vitamin D receptor and the syndrome of hereditary 1,25-dihydroxyvitamin D-resistant rickets, *Endocr Rev* 20:156, 1999.

Marx SJ: Hyperparathyroid and hypoparathyroid disorders, *N Engl J Med* 343:1863, 2000.

Meininger ME, Kendler JS: Trousseau's sign, *N Engl J Med* 343:1855, 2000.

Mellanby RJ, et al.: Hypocalcemia associated with low serum vitamin D metabolite concentrations in two dogs with protein-losing enteropathies, *J Small Anim Pract* 46:345, 2005.

Meuten DJ, Armstrong PJ: Parathyroid disease and calcium metabolism. In Ettinger SJ, editor: *Textbook of veterinary internal medicine*, ed 3, Philadelphia, 1989, WB Saunders, p 1610.

Meuten DJ, et al.: Relationship of serum total calcium to albumin and total protein in dogs, *J Am Vet Med Assoc* 180:63, 1982.

Meyer DJ, Tyrrell TG: Idiopathic hypoparathyroidism in a dog, *J Am Vet Med Assoc* 168:858, 1976.

Milnor WR: Properties of cardiac tissues. In Mountcastle VB, editor: *Medical physiology*, St Louis, 1980, CV Mosby Co, p 980.

Mora JR, et al.: Vitamin effects on the immune system: vitamins A and D take center stage, *Nat Rev Immunol* 8:685, 2008.

Padgett SL, et al.: Efficacy of parathyroid gland autotransplantation in maintaining serum calcium concentrations after bilateral thyroparathyroidectomy in cats, *J Am Anim Hosp Assoc* 34:219, 1998.

Parker JSL: A probable case of hypoparathyroidism in a cat, *J Small Anim Pract* 32:470, 1991.

Pearce SHS, et al.: A familial syndrome of hypocalcemia with hypercalciuria due to mutations in the calcium-sensing receptor, *N Engl J Med* 335:1115, 1996.

Persons DA, et al.: Tumor lysis syndrome and acute renal failure after treatment of non–small-cell lung carcinoma with combination irinotecan and cisplatin, *Am J Clin Oncol* 21:426, 1998.

Peterson ME: Treatment of canine and fKeline hypoparathyroidism, *J Am Vet Med Assoc* 181:1434, 1982.

Peterson ME: Hypoparathyroidism. In Kirk RW, editor: *Current veterinary therapy IX*, Philadelphia, 1986, WB Saunders, p 1039.

Peterson ME: Hypoparathyroidism and other causes of hypocalcemia in cats. In Kirk RW, Bonagura JA, editors: *Current veterinary therapy XI*, Philadelphia, 1992, WB Saunders, p 376.

Peterson ME, et al.: Idiopathic hypoparathyroidism in five cats, *J Vet Intern Med* 5:47, 1991.

Piek CJ, Teske E: Tumor lysis syndrome in a dog, *Tijdschr Diergeneeskd* 121:64, 1996.

Rasmussen H: Theoretical considerations in the treatment of osteoporosis. In De Luca HF, editor: *Osteoporosis: recent advances in pathogenesis and treatment*, Baltimore, 1981, University Park Press, p 383.

Rasmussen H: The cycling of calcium as an intracellular messenger, *Sci Am* 261:66, 1989.

Refsal KR, et al.: Update on the diagnosis and treatment of disorders of calcium regulation, *Vet Clinics N Amer Sm Anim Prac* 31:1043, 2001.

Rolla D, et al.: Effects of subcutaneous calcitriol administration on plasma calcium and parathyroid hormone concentrations in continuous ambulatory peritoneal dialysis uremic patients, *Peritoneal Dialysis Int* 13:118, 1993.

Rosol TJ, Capen CC: Calcium-regulating hormones and diseases of abnormal mineral (calcium, phosphorus, magnesium) metabolism. In Kaneko JJ, Harvey JW, Bruss ML, editors: *Clinical biochemistry of domestic animals*, San Diego, 1997, Academic Press, p 619.

Rosol TJ, et al.: Disorders of calcium. In DiBartola SP, editor: *Fluid therapy in small animal practice*, ed 2, Philadelphia, 2000, WB Saunders, p 108.

Roth SI, Capen CC: Ultrastructural and functional correlations of the parathyroid gland, *Int Rev Exp Pathol* 13:161, 1974.

Ruopp JL: Primary hypoparathyroidism in a cat complicated by suspect iatrogenic calcinosis cutis, *J Am Anim Hosp Assoc* 37:370, 2001.

Russell NJ, et al.: Primary hypoparathyroidism in dogs: a retrospective study of 17 cases, *Australian Vet J* 84:285, 2006.

Ryzen E, Rude RK: Low intracellular magnesium in patients with acute pancreatitis and hypocalcemia, *West J Med* 152:145, 1990.

Schaer M, et al.: Severe calcinosis cutis associated with treatment of hypoparathyroidism in a dog, *J Am Anim Hosp Assoc* 37:364, 2001.

Schenck PA, Chew DJ: Prediction of serum ionized calcium concentration by serum total calcium measurement in dogs, *Am J Vet Res* 66:1330, 2005.

Schenck PA, Chew DJ: Prediction of serum ionized calcium concentration by serum total calcium measurement in cats, *Can J Vet Res* 74:209, 2010.

Schenck PA, Chew DJ: Investigation of hypercalcaemia and hypocalcaemia. In Mooney CT, Peterson ME, editors: *BSAVA manual of canine and feline endocrinology*, ed 4, British Small Animal Veterinary Association, 2012, p 221.

Schenck PA, et al.: Effects of storage on normal canine serum ionized calcium and pH, *Am J Vet Res* 56:304, 1995.

Schenck PA, et al.: Effects of storage on serum ionized calcium and pH from horses with normal and abnormal ionized calcium concentrations, *Vet Clin Pathol* 25:118, 1996.

Schenck PA, et al.: Disorders of calcium: hypercalcemia and hypocalcemia. In DiBartola SP, editor: *Fluid, electrolyte, and acid-base disorders*, ed 4, St Louis, 2012, Elsevier/Saunders, p 120.

Schick MP, et al.: Calcinosis cutis secondary to percutaneous penetration of calcium chloride in dogs, *J Am Vet Med Assoc* 191:207, 1987.

Selgas R, et al.: The pharmacokinetics of a single dose of calcitriol administered subcutaneously in continuous ambulatory peritoneal dialysis patients, *Peritoneal Dialysis Int* 13:122, 1993.

Sherding RG, et al.: Primary hypoparathyroidism in the dog, *J Am Vet Med Assoc* 176:439, 1980.

Skelly BJ: Hypoparathyroidism. In Mooney CT, Peterson ME, editors: *BSAVA manual of canine and feline endocrinology*, ed 4, British Small Animal Veterinary Association, 2012, p 56.

Tepperman J: *Metabolic and endocrine physiology*, Chicago, 1980, Year Book Medical Publishers, 297.

Tomsa K, et al.: Nutritional secondary hyperparathyroidism in six cats, *J Sm Anim Pract* 40:533, 1999.

Torrance AG: Disorders of calcium metabolism. In Torrance AG, Mooney CT, editors: *Manual of small animal endocrinology*, ed 2, British Small Animal Veterinary Association, 1998, p 129.

Torrance AG, Nachreiner R: Intact parathyroid hormone assay and total calcium concentration in the diagnosis of disorders of calcium metabolism in dogs, *J Vet Intern Med* 3:86, 1989.

Vaden SL, et al.: A retrospective case-control study of acute renal failure in 99 dogs, *J Vet Intern Med* 11:58, 1997.

Weir EC, et al.: Isolation of 16,000-dalton parathyroid hormone like proteins from two animal tumors causing humoral hypercalcemia of malignancy, *Endocrinology* 123:2744, 1988.

Welches CD, et al.: Occurrence of problems after three techniques of bilateral thyroidectomy in cats, *Vet Surg* 18:392, 1989.

Wysolmerski JJ, Insogna KL: The parathyroid glands, hypercalcemia, and hypocalcemia. In Goldman L, Schafer AI, editors: *Goldman's Cecil medicine*, ed 24, Philadelphia, 2012, Elsevier/Saunders, p 1591.

Yates AJ, et al.: Effects of a synthetic peptide of a parathyroid-related protein on calcium homeostasis, renal tubular calcium reabsorption and bone metabolism in vivo and in vitro in rodents, *J Clin Invest* 81:932, 1988.

Yu ASL: Disorders of magnesium and phosphorus. In Goldman L, Schafer AI, editors: *Goldman's Cecil medicine*, ed 24, Philadelphia, 2012, Elsevier/Saunders, p 753.

Zivin JR, et al.: Hypocalcemia: a pervasive metabolic abnormality in the critically ill, *Am J Kidney Dis* 37:689, 2001.

Index

Page numbers followed by f indicate figures; t, tables; b, boxes.